COMPLETE GUIDE TO PRESCRIPTION & NON-PRESCRIPTION
DRUGS

By H. WINTER GRIFFITH, M.D.

Technical consultants:
John D. Palmer, M.D., Ph.D.
William N. Jones, B.S., M.S.

HPBooks®

Publishers: Bill and Helen Fisher
Executive Editor: Rick Bailey
Editorial Director: Randy Summerlin
Editor: Judith Wesley Allen
Editorial Assistance: Roberta Janes
Art Director: Don Burton
Typography: Cindy Coatsworth, Michelle Claridge
Cover Photo: Balfour Walker

HPBooks®
P.O. Box 5367
Tucson, AZ 85703
602-888-2150

ISBN: 0-89586-275-1
Library of Congress Catalog Card Number: 83-82397
©1983 Fisher Publishing, Inc.
Printed in U.S.A.

Contents

Drugs and You 4
Guide to Drug Charts 6
Drugs of Abuse 14
Checklist for Safer Drug Use 16
Drug Charts
(Alphabetized by
generic drug name) 18
Additional Brand Names 820
Additional Drug Interactions 832
Glossary 847
Index
(Generic names, brand
names and class names) 852
Emergency Guide
for Overdose Victims 886
Emergency Guide
for Anaphylaxis Victims 888
Emergency Telephone Numbers 888

About the Author

H. Winter Griffith has authored several medical books, including *Instructions for Patients, Drug Information for Patients, Instructions for Dental Patients, Information and Instructions for Pediatric Patients* and *Pediatrics for Parents.* Dr. Griffith received his medical degree from Emory University in 1953. After 20 years in private practice, he established a basic medical-science program at Florida State University. He then became an associate professor of family and community medicine at the University of Arizona College of Medicine.

Technical Consultants

John D. Palmer, M.D., Ph.D.
Associate professor of pharmacology, University of Arizona College of Medicine
Associate professor of medicine (clinical pharmacology), University of Arizona College of Medicine

William N. Jones, Pharmacist, B.S., M.S.
Clinical pharmacy coordinator, Veterans Administration Medical Center, Tucson, Arizona
Adjunct assistant professor, Department of Pharmacy Practice, College of Pharmacy, University of Arizona

Drugs and You

My first day of pharmacology class in medical school started with a jolt. The professor began by writing on the blackboard, "Drugs are poisons."

I thought the statement was extreme. New drug discoveries promised to solve medical problems that had baffled men for centuries. The medical community was intrigued with new possibilities for drugs.

In the 30 years since then, many drug "miracles" have lived up to those early expectations. But the years have also shown the damage drugs can cause when they are misused or not fully understood.

As a family doctor and teacher, I have developed a healthy respect for what drugs can and can't do. I now appreciate my professor's warning.

A drug cannot "cure." It aids the body's natural defenses to promote recovery.

Likewise, a manufacturer or doctor cannot guarantee a drug will be useful for everyone. The complexity of the human body, individual responses in different people and in the same person under different circumstances, past and present health, age and sex influence how well a drug works.

All effective drugs produce desirable changes in the body, but a drug can also cause undesirable adverse reactions or side effects in some people.

Despite uncertainties, the drug discoveries of the last 40 years have given us tools to save lives and reduce discomfort.

Before you decide whether to take a drug, you or your doctor must ask, "Will the benefits outweigh the risks?"

The purpose of this book is to give you enough information about the most widely used drugs so you can make a wise decision. The information will alert you to potential or preventable problems. You can learn what to do if problems arise.

The information is derived from several expert sources. Every effort has been made to ensure accuracy and completeness. When information from different sources conflicts, I have used the majority's opinion, coupled with my clinical judgment and that of my technical consultants. Drug information changes with continuing observations by clinicians and users.

Information in this book applies to generic drugs in both the United States and Canada. Generic names do not vary in these countries, but brand names do.

BE SAFE! TELL YOUR DOCTOR

Some suggestions for wise drug use apply to all drugs. Always give the following information to your physician, dentist or other health-care professional. They must have complete information to prescribe drugs safely for you. This information includes your medical history, your medical plans and progress while under medication.

MEDICAL HISTORY

Tell the important facts of your medical history dealing with drugs. Include allergic or adverse reactions you have had to any medicine in the past. Name the allergic symptoms you have, such as hay fever, asthma, eye watering and itching, throat irritation and reactions to food. People who have allergies to common substances are more likely to develop drug allergies.

List all drugs you take. Don't forget vitamin and mineral supplements, skin, rectal or vaginal medicines, antacids, antihistamines, cold and cough remedies, aspirin and aspirin combinations, motion-sickness remedies, weight-loss aids, salt and sugar substitutes, caffeine, oral contraceptives, sleeping pills or "tonics."

FUTURE MEDICAL PLANS

Discuss plans for elective surgery, pregnancy and breast-feeding.

QUESTIONS

Don't hesitate to ask questions about a drug. Your doctor, nurse or pharmacist may be able to provide more information if they are familiar with you and your medical history.

YOUR ROLE

Learn the generic names and brand names of all your medicines. Write them down to help you remember. If a drug is a mixture, learn the names of its generic ingredients.

TAKING A DRUG

Never take medicine in the dark! Recheck the label before each use. You could be taking the *wrong* drug! Tell your doctor about any unexpected new symptoms you have while taking medicine. You may need to change medicines or have a dose adjustment.

STORAGE

Keep all medicines out of children's reach. Store drugs in a cool, dry place, such as a kitchen cabinet or bedroom. Avoid medicine cabinets in bathrooms. They get too moist and warm at times.

Keep medicine in its original container, tightly closed. Don't remove the label! If directions call for refrigeration, don't freeze.

DISCARDING

Don't save leftover medicine to use later. Discard it on the expiration date shown on the container. Dispose safely to protect children and pets.

REFILLS

All refills must be ordered by your doctor or dentist, either in the first prescription or later. Only the pharmacy that originally filled the prescription can refill it. If you go elsewhere, you must get a new prescription. Pharmacies don't usually transfer prescriptions.

If you need a refill, call your pharmacist and order your refill by number and name.

Use one pharmacy for the whole family if you can. The pharmacist then has a record of all of your drugs and can communicate effectively with your doctor.

LEARN ABOUT DRUGS

Study the information in this book's charts regarding your medications. Read each chart completely. Because of space limitations, most information that fits more than one category appears only once.

Take care of yourself. You are the most important member of your health-care team.

Guide to Drug Charts

The drug information in this book is organized in condensed, easy-to-read charts. Each drug is described in a two-page format, as shown in the sample chart below and opposite. Charts are arranged alphabetically by drug generic names.

A *generic name* is the official chemical name for a drug. A *brand name* is a drug manufacturer's registered trademark for a generic drug. Brand names listed on the charts include those from the United States and Canada. A generic drug may have one or many brand names.

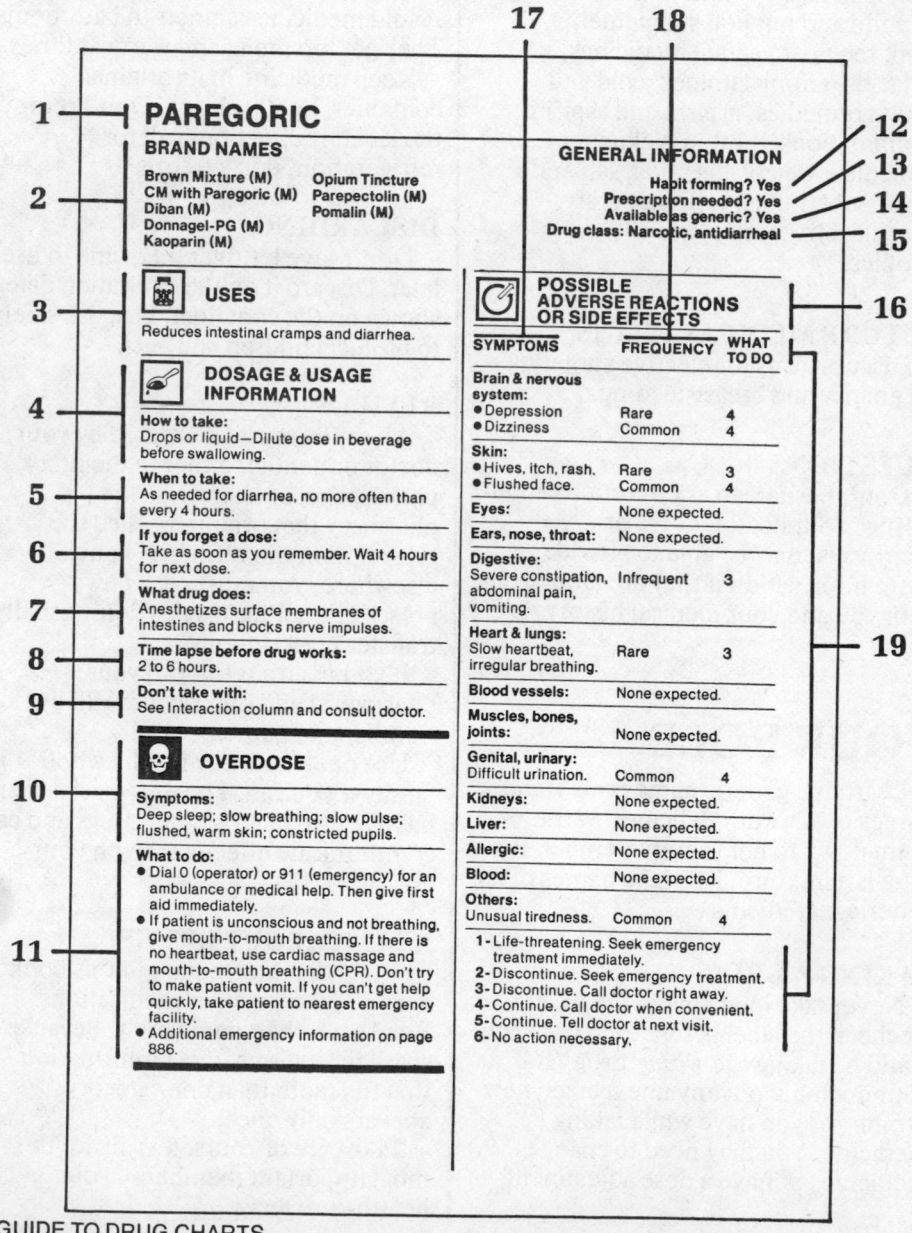

PAREGORIC

BRAND NAMES

Brown Mixture (M)
CM with Paregoric (M)
Diban (M)
Donnagel-PG (M)
Kaoparin (M)
Opium Tincture
Parepectolin (M)
Pomalin (M)

GENERAL INFORMATION

Habit forming? Yes
Prescription needed? Yes
Available as generic? Yes
Drug class: Narcotic, antidiarrheal

USES

Reduces intestinal cramps and diarrhea.

DOSAGE & USAGE INFORMATION

How to take:
Drops or liquid—Dilute dose in beverage before swallowing.

When to take:
As needed for diarrhea, no more often than every 4 hours.

If you forget a dose:
Take as soon as you remember. Wait 4 hours for next dose.

What drug does:
Anesthetizes surface membranes of intestines and blocks nerve impulses.

Time lapse before drug works:
2 to 6 hours.

Don't take with:
See Interaction column and consult doctor.

OVERDOSE

Symptoms:
Deep sleep; slow breathing; slow pulse; flushed, warm skin; constricted pupils.

What to do:
• Dial 0 (operator) or 911 (emergency) for an ambulance or medical help. Then give first aid immediately.
• If patient is unconscious and not breathing, give mouth-to-mouth breathing. If there is no heartbeat, use cardiac massage and mouth-to-mouth breathing (CPR). Don't try to make patient vomit. If you can't get help quickly, take patient to nearest emergency facility.
• Additional emergency information on page 886.

POSSIBLE ADVERSE REACTIONS OR SIDE EFFECTS

SYMPTOMS	FREQUENCY	WHAT TO DO
Brain & nervous system:		
• Depression	Rare	4
• Dizziness	Common	4
Skin:		
• Hives, itch, rash.	Rare	3
• Flushed face.	Common	4
Eyes:	None expected.	
Ears, nose, throat:	None expected.	
Digestive: Severe constipation, abdominal pain, vomiting.	Infrequent	3
Heart & lungs: Slow heartbeat, irregular breathing.	Rare	3
Blood vessels:	None expected.	
Muscles, bones, joints:	None expected.	
Genital, urinary: Difficult urination.	Common	4
Kidneys:	None expected.	
Liver:	None expected.	
Allergic:	None expected.	
Blood:	None expected.	
Others: Unusual tiredness.	Common	4

1 - Life-threatening. Seek emergency treatment immediately.
2 - Discontinue. Seek emergency treatment.
3 - Discontinue. Call doctor right away.
4 - Continue. Call doctor when convenient.
5 - Continue. Tell doctor at next visit.
6 - No action necessary.

Callout numbers: 1, 2, 3, 4, 5, 6, 7, 8, 9, 10, 11 (left side); 17, 18 (top); 12, 13, 14, 15, 16, 19 (right side)

To find information about a generic drug, look it up in the alphabetical charts. To learn about a brand name, check the index first, where brand names are followed by their generic ingredients and chart page numbers.

The chart design is the same for every drug. When you are familiar with the chart, you can quickly find information you want to know about a drug.

On the next few pages, each of the numbered chart sections below is explained. This information will guide you in reading and understanding the charts that begin on page 18.

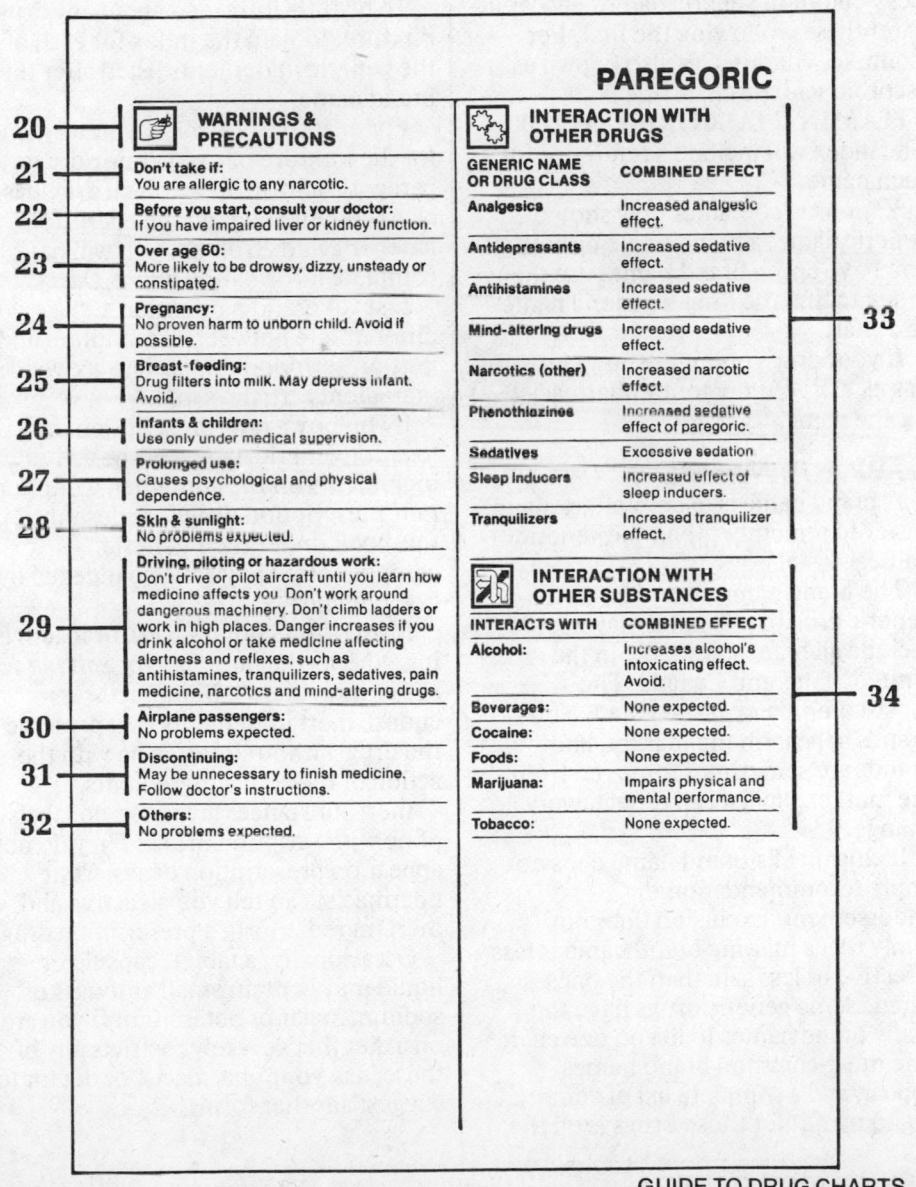

PAREGORIC

20 — WARNINGS & PRECAUTIONS

21 — Don't take if:
You are allergic to any narcotic.

22 — Before you start, consult your doctor:
If you have impaired liver or kidney function.

23 — Over age 60:
More likely to be drowsy, dizzy, unsteady or constipated.

24 — Pregnancy:
No proven harm to unborn child. Avoid if possible.

25 — Breast-feeding:
Drug filters into milk. May depress infant. Avoid.

26 — Infants & children:
Use only under medical supervision.

27 — Prolonged use:
Causes psychological and physical dependence.

28 — Skin & sunlight:
No problems expected.

29 — Driving, piloting or hazardous work:
Don't drive or pilot aircraft until you learn how medicine affects you. Don't work around dangerous machinery. Don't climb ladders or work in high places. Danger increases if you drink alcohol or take medicine affecting alertness and reflexes, such as antihistamines, tranquilizers, sedatives, pain medicine, narcotics and mind-altering drugs.

30 — Airplane passengers:
No problems expected.

31 — Discontinuing:
May be unnecessary to finish medicine. Follow doctor's instructions.

32 — Others:
No problems expected.

INTERACTION WITH OTHER DRUGS

GENERIC NAME OR DRUG CLASS	COMBINED EFFECT
Analgesics	Increased analgesic effect.
Antidepressants	Increased sedative effect.
Antihistamines	Increased sedative effect.
Mind-altering drugs	Increased sedative effect.
Narcotics (other)	Increased narcotic effect.
Phenothiazines	Increased sedative effect of paregoric.
Sedatives	Excessive sedation
Sleep inducers	Increased effect of sleep inducers.
Tranquilizers	Increased tranquilizer effect.

— 33

INTERACTION WITH OTHER SUBSTANCES

INTERACTS WITH	COMBINED EFFECT
Alcohol:	Increases alcohol's intoxicating effect. Avoid.
Beverages:	None expected.
Cocaine:	None expected.
Foods:	None expected.
Marijuana:	Impairs physical and mental performance.
Tobacco:	None expected.

— 34

GUIDE TO DRUG CHARTS

1—GENERIC NAME

Each drug chart is titled by generic name.

Sometimes a drug is known by more than one generic name. The chart is titled by the most-common one. Less-common generic names appear in parentheses following the first. For example, vitamin C is also known as ascorbic acid. Its chart title is **VITAMIN C (ASCORBIC ACID).** The index will include a reference for each name.

Your drug container may show a generic name, a brand name or both. If you have only a brand name, use the index to find the drug's generic name and chart.

If your drug container shows no name, ask your doctor or pharmacist for the name.

2—BRAND NAMES

A brand name is usually shorter and easier to remember than the generic name.

The brand names listed for each generic drug in this book may not include all brands available in the United States and Canada. The most-common ones are listed. New brands appear on the market, and brands are sometimes removed from the market. No list can reflect every change.

Inclusion of a brand name does not imply recommendation or endorsement. Exclusion does not imply that a missing brand name is less effective or less safe than the ones listed. Some generic drugs have too many brand names to list on one chart. The most-common brand names appear, and a complete list of common brand names for those drugs is on the page indicated at the bottom of the brand names list.

The letter M in parentheses (M) following some brand names indicates the brand is a mixture of two or more generic drugs.

To be fully informed about any drug mixture, look in the index for each of the generic ingredients listed after the brand name.

For example, *Diban* is a brand name for the mixture of two generic drugs, paregoric and atropine. Each drug has a chart. When you read the charts for paregoric and atropine, you will have complete information about *Diban.*

Lists of brand names don't differentiate between prescription and non-prescription drugs. The active ingredients are the same.

If you buy a non-prescription drug, look for generic names of the active ingredients on the container. Common non-prescription drugs are described in this book under their generic components. They are also indexed by brand name.

Most drugs contain *inert,* or inactive, ingredients that are *fillers* or *solvents* for active ingredients. Manufacturers choose inert ingredients that preserve the drug without interfering with the action of the active ingredients.

Inert substances are listed on labels of non-prescription drugs. They do not appear on prescription drugs. Your pharmacist can tell you all active and inert ingredients in a prescription drug.

Occasionally, a tablet, capsule or liquid may contain small amounts of sodium, sugar or potassium. If you are on a diet that severely restricts any of these, ask your pharmacist or doctor to suggest another form.

3—USES

This section lists the disease or disorder for which a drug is prescribed.

Most uses listed are approved by the U.S. Food and Drug Administration. Some uses are listed if experiments and clinical trials indicate effectiveness and safety.

Other uses are included that may not be officially sanctioned, but for which doctors commonly prescribe the drug.

The use for which your doctor prescribes the drug may not appear. You and your doctor should discuss the reason for any prescription medicine you take.

You alone will probably decide whether to take a non-prescription drug. The Uses section may help you make a decision.

4—DOSAGE & USAGE INFORMATION: HOW TO TAKE

Drugs are available in tablets, capsules, liquids, suppositories, injections, aerosol inhalers and topical forms such as drops, sprays, creams, ointments and lotions. This section gives general instructions for taking each form.

This information supplements drug-label information. If your doctor's instructions differ from the suggestions, follow your *doctor's* instructions.

Instructions are left out for how *much* to take. Dose amounts can't be generalized. They must be individualized for you by your doctor, or you must read the drug label.

5—WHEN TO TAKE

Dose schedules vary for medicines and for patients.

Drugs prescribed on a schedule should usually be taken at approximately the same times each day. Some *must* be taken at regular intervals to maintain a steady level of the drug in the body. If the schedule interferes with your sleep, consult with your doctor.

Instructions to take on an empty stomach mean the drug is absorbed best in your body this way. Many drugs must be taken with liquid or food because they irritate the stomach.

Instructions for other dose schedules are usually on the label. Variations in standard dose schedules may apply because some medicines interact with others if you take them at the same time.

6—IF YOU FORGET A DOSE

Suggestions in this section vary from drug to drug. Most tell you when to resume taking the medicine if you forget a scheduled dose.

Establish habits so you won't forget doses. Forgotten doses decrease a drug's therapeutic effect.

7—WHAT DRUG DOES

This is a simple description of the drug's action in the body. The wording is generalized and may not be a complete explanation of the complex chemical process that takes place.

8—TIME LAPSE BEFORE DRUG WORKS

The times given are approximations. Times vary a great deal from person to person, and from time to time in the same person. The figures give you some idea of when to expect improvement.

9—DON'T TAKE WITH

Some drugs create problems when

GUIDE TO DRUG CHARTS

taken in combination with other substances. Most problems are detailed in the Interaction column of each chart. This section mentions substances that don't appear in the Interaction column.

Occasionally, an interaction is singled out if the combination is particularly harmful.

10—OVERDOSE: SYMPTOMS

The symptoms listed are most likely to develop with accidental or purposeful overdose. An overdose patient may not show all symptoms listed. Sometimes symptoms are identical to ones listed as side effects. The difference is intensity and severity. You will have to judge. Consult a doctor or poison-control center if you have any doubt.

11—WHAT TO DO

If you suspect an overdose, whether symptoms are apparent or not, follow instructions in this section. Expanded instructions for emergency treatment for overdose are on page 886.

12—HABIT FORMING

A drug habit can be physical or psychological. A drug that produces physical dependence leads to addiction. It causes painful and sometimes dangerous effects when withdrawn.

Psychological dependence does not cause dangerous withdrawal effects. It may cause stress and unwanted behavior changes until the habit is broken.

13—PRESCRIPTION NEEDED?

"Yes" means a doctor must prescribe the drug for you. "No" means you can buy this drug without prescription. Sometimes low strengths of a drug are available without prescription, while high strengths require prescription.

The information about the generic drug applies whether it requires prescription or not. If the generic ingredients are the same, non-prescription drugs have the same dangers, warnings, precautions and interactions as prescribed drugs.

14—AVAILABLE AS GENERIC?

Some generic drugs have copyright restrictions that protect the manufacturer or distributor of that drug. These drugs may be purchased only by brand name.

In recent years, drug manufacturers have marketed more drugs under generic names. Drugs purchased by generic name sometimes are less expensive than brand names.

Some states allow pharmacists to fill prescriptions by brand names or generic names. This allows patients to buy the least-expensive form of a drug.

A doctor may specify a brand name because he or she trusts a known source more than an unknown manufacturer of generic drugs. You and your doctor should decide whether you should buy a medicine by generic or brand name.

Generic drugs manufactured in other countries are not subject to regulation by the U.S. Food and Drug Administration. Drugs manufactured in the United States are subject to regulation.

15—DRUG CLASS

Drugs that possess similar chemical structure and similar therapeutic effects are grouped into classes. Most drugs within a class produce similar benefits, side effects, adverse reactions and interactions with other drugs and substances. For example, there are 15 generic drugs in the narcotic drug class. All have similar effects on the body.

Some information on the charts applies to all drugs in a class. For example, a reference may be made to narcotics. The index lists the class—narcotics—and lists drugs in that class.

Drug classes are not standardized, so classes listed in other references may vary from the classes in this book.

16—POSSIBLE ADVERSE REACTIONS OR SIDE EFFECTS

Adverse reactions or side effects are symptoms that may occur when you take a drug. They are effects on the body other than the desired therapeutic effect.

The term *side effect* implies expected and usually unavoidable effects of a drug. Side effects have nothing to do with the drug's intended use.

For example, the generic drug paregoric reduces intestinal cramps and vomiting. It also often causes a flushed face. The flushing is a side effect that is harmless and does not affect the drug's therapeutic potential.

The term *adverse reaction* is more significant. For example, paregoric can cause serious adverse allergic reaction in some people. This reaction can include hives, rash and severe itch.

Some adverse reactions can be prevented, which is one reason this information is included in the book.

Most adverse reactions are minor and last only a short time. With many drugs, adverse reactions that might occur will frequently diminish in intensity as time passes.

The majority of drugs used properly for valid reasons offer benefits that outweigh potential hazards.

17—SYMPTOMS

Symptoms are grouped by various body systems. Symptoms that don't naturally apply to these body systems or which overlap systems are listed under "Others."

18—FREQUENCY

This is an estimation of how often symptoms occur in persons who take the drug. "Common" means these symptoms are expected and sometimes inevitable. "Infrequent" means the symptoms occur in approximately 1% to 10% of patients. "Rare" means symptoms occur in less than 1%.

19—WHAT TO DO

The numbers refer to the key at the bottom of the column. For example, paregoric produces the rare symptoms of slow heartbeat and irregular breathing—listed under "Heart & lungs." The chart suggests you discontinue the medicine and call your doctor right away.

20—WARNINGS AND PRECAUTIONS

Read these entries to determine special information that applies to you.

21—DON'T TAKE IF

This section lists circumstances that indicate the use of a drug may not be safe. On some drug labels and in formal medical literature, these circumstances are called *contraindications*.

22—BEFORE YOU START, CONSULT YOUR DOCTOR

This section lists conditions under which a drug should be used with caution.

GUIDE TO DRUG CHARTS

23—OVER AGE 60

As a person ages, physical changes occur that require special consideration in drug use. Liver and kidney functions decrease, metabolism slows and the prostate gland enlarges in men.

Most drugs are metabolized or excreted at a rate dependent on kidney and liver functions. Small doses or longer intervals between doses may be necessary to prevent unhealthy concentration of a drug. Toxic effects and adverse reactions occur more frequently and cause more serious problems in this age group.

24—PREGNANCY

The best rule to follow during pregnancy is to avoid all drugs, including tobacco and alcohol. Any medicine—prescription or non-prescription—requires medical advice and supervision.

This section will alert you if there is evidence that a drug harms the unborn child. Lack of evidence does not guarantee a drug's safety. If safety is undetermined, and reasonable doubt exists, "No proven problems" is indicated.

25—BREAST-FEEDING

Many drugs filter into a mother's milk. Some drugs have dangerous or unwanted effects on the nursing infant. This section suggests ways to minimize harm to the child.

26—INFANTS & CHILDREN

Many drugs carry special warnings and precautions for children because of a child's size and immaturity. In medical terminology, *newborns* are babies up to 2 weeks old, *infants* are 2 weeks to 1 year, and *children* are 1 to 12 years.

27—PROLONGED USE

Most drugs produce no ill effects during short periods of treatment. However, relatively safe drugs taken for long periods may produce unwanted effects. These are listed. Drugs should be taken in the smallest dose and for the shortest time possible. Nevertheless, some diseases and conditions require an indefinite period of treatment. Your doctor may want to change drugs occasionally or alter your treatment regimen to minimize problems.

The words "functional dependence" sometimes appear in this section. This does not mean *physical* or *psychological addiction*. Sometimes a body function ceases to work naturally because it has been replaced or interfered with by the drug. The body then becomes dependent on the drug to continue the function.

28—SKIN & SUNLIGHT

Many drugs cause *photosensitivity,* which means increased skin sensitivity to ultraviolet rays from sunlight or artificial rays from a sunlamp. This section will alert you to this potential problem.

29—DRIVING, PILOTING OR HAZARDOUS WORK

Any drug that decreases alertness, muscular coordination or reflexes may make these activities hazardous. The effects may not appear in all people, or they may disappear after a short exposure to the drug. If this section contains a warning, use caution until you determine how a new drug affects you.

30—AIRPLANE PASSENGERS

Before you fly, check this section to determine how altitude can affect you when taking a drug.

31—DISCONTINUING

Some patients stop taking a drug when symptoms begin to go away, although complete recovery may require longer treatment.

Other patients continue taking a drug when it is no longer needed. This section will tell you when you may safely discontinue a drug.

Some drugs cause symptoms days or weeks after discontinuing. This section warns you so the symptoms won't puzzle you if they occur.

32—OTHERS

Warnings and precautions appear here if they don't fit into the other categories. This section includes storage instructions, how to dispose of outdated drugs, weather influences on drug effect, changes in blood and urine tests, warnings to persons with chronic illness and other information.

33—INTERACTION WITH OTHER DRUGS

Drugs interact in your body with other drugs, whether prescription or non-prescription. Interactions affect absorption, elimination or distribution of either drug. The chart lists interactions by generic name or drug class.

If a drug class appears, the generic drug interacts with any drug in that class. Drugs in each class that are included in the book are listed in the index.

Interactions are sometimes beneficial. You may not be able to determine from the chart which interactions are good and which are bad. Don't guess! Consult your doctor if you take drugs that interact. Some combinations are fatal!

Occasionally, drugs appear in the Interaction column that are not included in this book. These drugs are listed under Interactions for your safety.

Some drugs have too many interactions to list on one chart. The additional interactions appear on the page indicated at the bottom of the list.

34—INTERACTION WITH OTHER SUBSTANCES

The substances listed here are repeated on every drug chart. All people eat food and drink beverages. Many adults consume alcohol. Many people use cocaine and smoke tobacco or marijuana. This section shows possible interactions between these substances and each drug.

Drugs of Abuse

Each of the drug charts beginning on page 18 contains a section listing the interactions of alcohol, marijuana and cocaine with the therapeutic drug in the bloodstream. These three drugs are singled out because of their widespread use and abuse. The information is factual, not judgmental.

The long-term effects of alcohol and tobacco abuse are numerous. They have been well-publicized.

Drugs of potential abuse include those that are addictive and harmful. They usually produce a temporary, false sense of well-being. The long-term effects, however, are harmful and can be devastating to the body and psyche of the addict.

Refresh your memory frequently about the potential harm from prolonged use of *any* drugs or substances you take. Avoid unwise use of habit-forming drugs.

These are the most common drugs of abuse:

MARIJUANA (CANNABIS, HASHISH)

What they do: Heighten perception, cause mood swings, relax mind and body.
Signs of use: Red eyes, lethargy, uncoordinated body movements.
Long-term effects: Decreased motivation. Possible brain, heart, lung and reproductive-system damage.

AMPHETAMINES

What they do: Speed up physical and mental processes to cause energy and excitement.
Signs of use: Dilated pupils, insomnia, trembling.
Long-term effects: Violent behavior, paranoia, possible death from overdose.

BARBITURATES

What they do: Produce drowsiness and lethargy.
Signs of use: Confused speech, lack of coordination and balance.
Long-term effects: Disrupts normal sleep pattern. Possible death from overdose, especially in combination with alcohol.

COCAINE

What it does: Stimulates the nervous system, heightens sensations and may produce hallucinations.

Signs of use: Trembling, intoxication, dilated pupils, constant sniffling.

Long-term effects: Ulceration of nasal passages where sniffed. Itching all over body, sometimes with open sores. Possible brain damage. Possible death from overdose.

OPIATES (CODEINE, HEROIN, METHADONE, MORPHINE, OPIUM)

What they do: Relieve pain, create temporary and false sense of well-being.

Signs of use: Constricted pupils, mood swings, slurred speech, sore eyes, lethargy, weight loss, sweating.

Long-term effects: Malnutrition, extreme susceptibility to infection, the need to increase drug amount to produce the same effects. Possible death from overdose.

PSYCHEDELIC DRUGS (LSD, MESCALINE)

What they do: Produce hallucinations, either pleasant or frightening.

Signs of use: Dilated pupils, sweating, trembling, fever, chills.

Long-term effects: Lack of motivation, unpredictable behavior, narcissism, recurrent hallucinations without drug use ("flashbacks"). Possible death from overdose.

VOLATILE SUBSTANCES (GLUE, SOLVENTS)

What they do: Produce hallucinations, temporary, false sense of well-being and possible unconsciousness.

Signs of use: Dilated pupils, flushed face, confusion.

Long-term effects: Permanent brain, liver, kidney damage. Possible death from overdose.

Checklist for Safer Drug Use

- Learn all you can about drugs you may take *before* you take them. Information sources are your doctor, your nurse, your pharmacist, this book and other books in your public library.

- Don't take drugs prescribed for someone else—even if your symptoms are the same.

- Keep your prescription drugs to yourself. Your drugs may be harmful to someone else.

- Tell your doctor about any symptoms you believe are caused by a drug—prescription or non-prescription—that you take.

- Take only medicines that are *necessary*. Avoid taking non-prescription drugs while taking prescription drugs for a medical problem.

- Before your doctor prescribes for you, tell him about your previous experiences with any drug—beneficial results, adverse reactions or allergies.

- Take medicine in good light after you have identified it. If you wear glasses to read, put them on to check drug labels. It is easy to take the wrong drug at the wrong time.

- Don't keep by your bedside any drugs that change mood, alertness or judgment such as sedatives, narcotics or tranquilizers. These cause many accidental overdose deaths. You may unknowingly repeat a dose when you are half asleep or confused.

- Know the names of your medicines. These include the generic name, the brand name and the generic names of all ingredients in a drug mixture. Your doctor, nurse or pharmacist can give you this information.

- Study the labels on all non-prescription drugs. If the information is incomplete or if you have questions, ask the pharmacist for more details.

- If you must deviate from your prescribed dose schedule, tell your doctor.

- Shake liquid medicines before taking.

- Store all medicines away from moisture and heat. Bathroom medicine cabinets are usually unsuitable.

- If a drug needs refrigeration, don't freeze.

- Obtain a standard measuring spoon from your pharmacy for liquid medicines. Kitchen teaspoons and tablespoons are not accurate enough.

- Follow diet instructions when you take medicines. Some work better on a full stomach, others on an empty stomach. Some drugs are more useful with special diets. For example, medicine for high blood pressure is more effective if accompanied by a sodium-restricted diet.

- Tell your doctor about any allergies you have. A previous allergy to a drug may make it dangerous to prescribe again. People with other allergies, such as eczema, hay fever, asthma, bronchitis and food allergies, are more likely to be allergic to drugs.

- Prior to surgery, tell your doctor, anesthesiologist or dentist about any drug you have taken in the past few weeks. Advise them of any cortisone drugs you have taken within two years.

- If you become pregnant while taking any medicine, including birth-control pills, tell your doctor immediately.

- Avoid *all* drugs while you are pregnant, if possible. If you must take drugs during pregnancy, record names, amounts, dates and reasons.

- If you see more than one doctor, tell each one about drugs others have prescribed.

- When you use non-prescription drugs, report it so the information is on your medical record.

- Store all drugs away from the reach of children.

- Note the expiration date on each drug label. Discard outdated ones safely.

- Pay attention to the information in the charts about safety while driving, piloting or working in dangerous places.

- Alcohol, cocaine, marijuana, other mood-altering drugs and tobacco—mixed with some drugs—can cause a life-threatening interaction, prevent your medicine from being effective or delay your return to health. Common sense dictates that you avoid them during illness.

ACETAMINOPHEN

BRAND NAMES

Arthralgen
Campain
Co-Tylenol (M)
Darvocet-N (M)

Datril
Excedrin (M)
Liquiprin
Parafon Forte (M)

Phenaphen
Robigesic
Sinarest (M)
Tylenol

See complete brand names list, page 820.

GENERAL INFORMATION

Habit forming? No
Prescription needed? No
Available as generic? Yes
Drug class: Analgesic, fever-reducer

USES

Treatment of mild to moderate pain and fever. Acetaminophen does not relieve redness, stiffness or swelling of joints or tissue inflammation. Use aspirin or other drugs for inflammation.

DOSAGE & USAGE INFORMATION

How to take:
- Tablet or capsule—Swallow with liquid.
- Effervescent granules—Dissolve granules in 4 oz. of cool water. Drink all the water.
- Suppositories—Remove wrapper and moisten suppository with water. Gently insert larger end into rectum. Push well into rectum with finger.

When to take:
As needed, no more often than every 3 hours.

If you forget a dose:
Take as soon as you remember. Wait 3 hours for next dose.

What drug does:
May affect hypothalamus—part of brain that helps regulate body heat and receives body's pain messages.

Time lapse before drug works:
15 to 30 minutes. May last 4 hours.

Don't take with:
- Other drugs with acetaminophen. Too much acetaminophen can damage liver and kidneys.
- See Interaction column and consult doctor.

OVERDOSE

Symptoms:
Stomach upset, irritability, convulsions, coma.

What to do:
- Call your doctor or poison-control center for advice if you suspect overdose, even if not sure. Symptoms may not appear until damage has occurred.
- Additional emergency information on page 886.

POSSIBLE ADVERSE REACTIONS OR SIDE EFFECTS

SYMPTOMS	FREQUENCY	WHAT TO DO
Brain & nervous system: Extreme fatigue.	Rare	3
Skin: Rash, itch, hives.	Rare	3
Eyes:	None expected.	
Ears, nose, throat: Sore throat and fever after a few days.	Rare	3
Digestive:	None expected.	
Heart & lungs:	None expected.	
Blood vessels: Unexplained bleeding or bruising.	Rare	3
Muscles, bones, joints:	None expected.	
Genital, urinary: Blood in urine, painful urination or frequent urge to urinate.	Rare	3
Kidneys: Less urine.	Rare	4
Liver: Jaundice (yellow skin and eyes).	Rare	3
Allergic:	None expected.	
Blood: Anemia	Rare	3
Others:	None expected.	

1- Life-threatening. Seek emergency treatment immediately.
2- Discontinue. Seek emergency treatment.
3- Discontinue. Call doctor right away.
4- Continue. Call doctor when convenient.
5- Continue. Tell doctor at next visit.
6- No action necessary.

ACETAMINOPHEN

 WARNINGS & PRECAUTIONS

Don't take if:
- You are allergic to acetaminophen.
- Your symptoms don't improve after 2 days use. Call your doctor.

Before you start, consult your doctor:
If you have bronchial asthma, kidney disease or liver damage.

Over age 60:
Don't exceed recommended dose. You can't eliminate drug as efficiently as younger persons.

Pregnancy:
No proven harm to unborn child. Avoid if possible.

Breast-feeding:
No proven harm to nursing infant.

Infants & children:
Use only under medical supervision.

Prolonged use:
May affect blood system and cause anemia. Limit use to 5 days for children 12 and under, and 10 days for adults.

Skin & sunlight:
No problems expected.

Driving, piloting or hazardous work:
Avoid if you feel drowsy. Otherwise, no restrictions.

Airplane passengers:
No problems expected.

Discontinuing:
Discontinue in 2 days if symptoms don't improve.

Others:
No problems expected.

 INTERACTION WITH OTHER DRUGS

GENERIC NAME OR DRUG CLASS	COMBINED EFFECT
Anticoagulants (oral)	Danger of hidden bleeding.
Phenobarbital	Quicker elimination of and decreased effect of acetaminophen.
Tetracyclines (effervescent granules or tablets)	May slow tetracycline absorption. Space doses 2 hours apart.

 INTERACTION WITH OTHER SUBSTANCES

INTERACTS WITH	COMBINED EFFECT
Alcohol:	Drowsiness
Beverages:	None expected.
Cocaine:	None expected. However, cocaine may slow body's recovery. Avoid.
Foods:	None expected.
Marijuana:	Increased pain relief. However, marijuana may slow body's recovery. Avoid.
Tobacco:	None expected.

ACETAZOLAMIDE

BRAND NAMES

Ak-Zol
Cetazol
Diamox

Habit forming? No
Prescription needed? Yes
Available as generic? No

GENERAL INFORMATION

Drug class: Diuretic (carbonic anhydrase inhibitor, sulfonamide), antiglaucoma

USES

- Treatment of glaucoma.
- Treatment of epileptic seizures.
- Treatment of body-fluid retention.
- Treatment for shortness of breath, insomnia and fatigue in high altitudes.

DOSAGE & USAGE INFORMATION

How to take:
Tablets—Swallow whole with liquid or food to lessen stomach irritation.

When to take:
- 1 dose per day—At the same time each morning.
- More than 1 dose per day—Take last dose several hours before bedtime.

If you forget a dose:
Take as soon as you remember. Continue regular schedule.

What drug does:
- Inhibits action of carbonic anhydrase, an enzyme. This lowers the internal eye pressure by decreasing fluid formation in the eye.
- Forces sodium and water excretion, reducing body fluid.

Time lapse before drug works:
2 hours.

Don't take with:
- Non-prescription drugs without consulting doctor.
- See Interaction column and consult doctor.

OVERDOSE

Symptoms:
Drowsiness, confusion, excitement, nausea, vomiting, numbness in hands and feet, coma.

What to do:
- Call your doctor or poison-control center for advice if you suspect overdose, even if not sure. Symptoms may not appear until damage has occurred.
- Additional emergency information on page 886.

POSSIBLE ADVERSE REACTIONS OR SIDE EFFECTS

SYMPTOMS	FREQUENCY	WHAT TO DO
Brain & nervous system:		
• Headache, mood changes, nervousness, clumsiness, trembling, confusion.	Rare	3
• Convulsions	Rare	1
Skin:		
Hives, itch, rash, or sores.	Rare	3
Ears, nose, throat:		
• Ringing in ears, hoarseness, dry mouth, thirst.	Rare	3
• Sore throat, fever.	Rare	3
Digestive:		
• Appetite change, nausea, vomiting.	Rare	3
• Black, tarry stool.	Rare	3
Heart & lungs:		
Breathing difficulty, irregular or weak heartbeat.	Rare	3
Blood vessels:		
Easy bleeding or bruising.	Rare	3
Muscles, bones, joints:		
Muscle cramps.	Rare	3
Genital, urinary:		
Painful or frequent urination, bloody urine.	Rare	3
Kidneys:		
Back pain.	Infrequent	3
Allergic, blood, liver, eyes:	None expected.	
Others:		
• Fatigue, weakness.	Infrequent	4
• Tingling or burning in feet or hands.	Infrequent	4

1-Life-threatening. Seek emergency treatment immediately.
2-Discontinue. Seek emergency treatment.
3-Discontinue. Call doctor right away.
4-Continue. Call doctor when convenient.

ACETAZOLAMIDE

WARNINGS & PRECAUTIONS

Don't take if:
- You are allergic to any carbonic anhydrase inhibitor.
- You have liver or kidney disease.
- You have Addison's disease (adrenal gland failure).
- You have diabetes.

Before you start, consult your doctor:
- If you have gout or lupus.
- If you are allergic to any sulfa drug.

Over age 60:
- Don't exceed recommended dose.
- If you take a digitalis preparation, eat foods high in potassium content or take a potassium supplement.

Pregnancy:
No proven harm to unborn child. Avoid if possible, especially first 3 months.

Breast-feeding:
Avoid drug or don't nurse your infant.

Infants & children:
Not recommended for children younger than 12.

Prolonged use:
May cause kidney stones, vision change, loss of taste and smell, jaundice (yellow skin and eyes) or weight loss.

Skin & sunlight:
No problems expected.

Driving, piloting or hazardous work:
Avoid if you feel drowsy or dizzy. Otherwise, no problems expected.

Airplane passengers:
No problems expected.

Discontinuing:
Don't discontinue without medical advice.

Others:
Medicine may increase sugar levels in blood and urine. Diabetics may need insulin adjustment.

INTERACTION WITH OTHER DRUGS

GENERIC NAME OR DRUG CLASS	COMBINED EFFECT
Amphetamines	Increased amphetamine effect.
Anticonvulsants	Increased loss of bone minerals.
Antidepressants (tricyclic)	Increased antidepressant effect.
Antidiabetics (oral)	Increased potassium loss.
Aspirin	Decreased aspirin effect.
Cortisone drugs	Increased potassium loss.
Digitalis preparations	Possible digitalis toxicity.
Diuretics (other)	Increased potassium loss.
Lithium	Decreased lithium effect.
Methenamine	Decreased methenamine effect.
Quinidine	Increased quinidine effect.
Sympathomimetics	Increased sympathomimetic effect.

INTERACTION WITH OTHER SUBSTANCES

INTERACTS WITH	COMBINED EFFECT
Alcohol:	None expected.
Beverages:	None expected.
Cocaine:	Decreased acetazolamide effect.
Foods: Potassium-rich foods.	Eat these to decrease potassium loss. See page 850.
Marijuana:	Increased acetazolamide effect.
Tobacco:	None expected.

ACETOHEXAMIDE

BRAND NAMES

Dymelor
Dimelor

GENERAL INFORMATION

Habit forming? No
Prescription needed? Yes
Available as generic? No
Drug class: Antidiabetic (oral), sulfonurea

 USES

Treatment for diabetes in adults who can't control blood sugar by diet, weight loss and exercise.

 DOSAGE & USAGE INFORMATION

How to take:
Tablet—Swallow with liquid or food to lessen stomach irritation. If you can't swallow whole, crumble tablet and take with liquid or food.

When to take:
At the same times each day.

If you forget a dose:
Take as soon as you remember up to 2 hours late. If more than 2 hours, wait for next scheduled dose (don't double this dose).

What drug does:
Stimulates pancreas to produce more insulin. Insulin in blood forces cells to use sugar in blood.

Time lapse before drug works:
3 to 4 hours. May require 2 weeks for maximum benefit.

Don't take with:
See Interaction column and consult doctor.

 OVERDOSE

Symptoms:
Excessive hunger, nausea, anxiety, cool skin, cold sweats, drowsiness, rapid heartbeat, weakness, unconsciousness, coma.

What to do:
- Dial 0 (operator) or 911 (emergency) for an ambulance or medical help. Then give first aid immediately.
- Additional emergency information on page 886.

POSSIBLE ADVERSE REACTIONS OR SIDE EFFECTS

SYMPTOMS	FREQUENCY	WHAT TO DO
Brain & nervous system:		
• Dizziness	Common	3
• Fatigue	Rare	3
Skin:		
Itching or rash.	Rare	3
Eyes:	None expected.	
Ears, nose, throat:		
• Sore throat, fever.	Rare	3
• Ringing in ears.	Rare	3
Digestive:		
Diarrhea, loss of appetite, nausea, stomach pain, heartburn.	Common	4
Heart & lungs, muscles, bones, joints, genital, urinary, kidneys, allergic, blood:	None expected.	
Blood vessels:		
Unusual bleeding or bruising.	Rare	3
Liver:		
Jaundice (yellow skin and eyes).	Rare	3
Others:		
Low blood sugar (ravenous hunger, nausea, anxiety, cold sweats, cool skin, chills, drowsiness, nervousness, headache, rapid heartbeat, weakness).	Infrequent	2

1- Life-threatening. Seek emergency treatment immediately.
2- Discontinue. Seek emergency treatment.
3- Discontinue. Call doctor right away.
4- Continue. Call doctor when convenient.

ACETOHEXAMIDE

 **WARNINGS &
PRECAUTIONS**

Don't take if:
- You are allergic to any sulfonurea.
- You have impaired kidney or liver function.

Before you start, consult your doctor:
- If you have a severe infection.
- If you have thyroid disease.
- If you take insulin.
- If you have heart disease.

Over age 60:
Dose usually smaller than for younger adults. Avoid "low-blood-sugar" episodes because repeated ones can damage brain permanently.

Pregnancy:
No proven harm to unborn child. Avoid if possible.

Breast-feeding:
Drug filters into milk. May lower baby's blood sugar. Avoid.

Infants & children:
Don't give to infants or children.

Prolonged use:
None expected.

Skin & sunlight:
May cause rash or intensify sunburn in areas exposed to sun or sunlamp.

Driving, piloting or hazardous work:
No problems expected unless you develop hypoglycemia (low blood sugar). If so, avoid driving or hazardous activity.

Airplane passengers:
No problems expected.

Discontinuing:
Don't discontinue without consulting doctor. Dose may require gradual reduction if you have taken drug for a long time. Doses of other drugs may also require adjustment.

Others:
- Don't exceed 1500 mg. in 1 day.
- Hypoglycemia (low blood sugar) may occur, even with proper dose schedule. You must balance medicine, diet and exercise.

 **INTERACTION WITH
OTHER DRUGS**

GENERIC NAME OR DRUG CLASS	COMBINED EFFECT
Androgens	Increased acetohexamide effect.
Anticoagulants (oral)	Unpredictable prothrombin times (see page 850).
Anticonvulsants (hydantoin)	Decreased acetohexamide effect.
Antiinflammatory drugs (non-steroidal)	Increased acetohexamide effect.
Aspirin	Increased acetohexamide effect.
Beta-adrenergic blockers	Increased acetohexamide effect.
Chloramphenicol	Increased acetohexamide effect.
Clofibrate	Increased acetohexamide effect.
Contraceptives (oral)	Decreased acetohexamide effect.
Cortisone drugs	Decreased acetohexamide effect.
Diuretics (thiazide)	Decreased acetohexamide effect.
Epinephrine	Decreased acetohexamide effect.
Estrogens	Increased acetohexamide effect.
Guanethidine	Unpredictable acetohexamide effect.

Additional Interactions on page 832.

 **INTERACTION WITH
OTHER SUBSTANCES**

INTERACTS WITH	COMBINED EFFECT
Alcohol:	Disulfiram reaction (see page 848). Avoid.
Beverages:	None expected.
Cocaine:	No proven problems.
Foods:	None expected.
Marijuana:	Decreased acetohexamide effect. Avoid.
Tobacco:	None expected.

ACETOPHENAZINE

BRAND NAMES

Tindal

GENERAL INFORMATION

Habit forming? No
Prescription needed? Yes
Available as generic? Yes
Drug class: Tranquilizer, antiemetic (phenothiazine)

USES

- Stops nausea, vomiting.
- Reduces anxiety, agitation.

DOSAGE & USAGE INFORMATION

How to take:
- Tablet or capsule—Swallow with liquid or food to lessen stomach irritation.
- Suppositories—Remove wrapper and moisten suppository with water. Gently insert into rectum, large end first.
- Drops or liquid—Dilute dose in beverage.

When to take:
- Nervous and mental disorders—Take at the same times each day.
- Nausea and vomiting—Take as needed, no more often than every 4 hours.

If you forget a dose:
- Nervous and mental disorders—Take up to 2 hours late. If more than 2 hours, wait for next scheduled dose (don't double this).
- Nausea and vomiting—Take as soon as you remember. Wait 4 hours for next dose.

What drug does:
- Suppresses brain's vomiting center.
- Suppresses brain centers that control abnormal emotions and behavior.

Time lapse before drug works:
- Nausea and vomiting—1 hour or less.
- Nervous and mental disorders—4-6 weeks.

Don't take with:
- Antacid or medicine for diarrhea.
- Non-prescription drug for cough, cold or allergy.
- See Interaction column and consult doctor.

OVERDOSE

Symptoms:
Stupor, convulsions, coma.

What to do:
- Dial 0 (operator) or 911 (emergency) for an ambulance or medical help. Then give first aid immediately.
- Additional emergency information on page 886.

POSSIBLE ADVERSE REACTIONS OR SIDE EFFECTS

SYMPTOMS	FREQUENCY	WHAT TO DO
Brain & nervous system:		
• Restlessness, tremor.	Common	3
• Fainting	Infrequent	2
• Drowsiness	Common	3
Skin:		
• Rash	Infrequent	3
• Less perspiration.	Common	4
Eyes:		
Vision changes.	Rare	3
Ears, nose, throat:		
• Sore throat, fever.	Rare	3
• Dry mouth, nasal congestion.	Common	4
Digestive:		
Constipation	Common	4
Heart & lungs, blood vessels, kidneys, allergic, blood:	None expected.	
Muscles, bones, joints:		
Muscle spasms of face and neck, unsteady gait.	Common	2
Genital, urinary:		
Urination difficulty.	Infrequent	4
Liver:		
Jaundice (yellow eyes and skin).	Rare	3
Others:		
Less interest in sex, breast swelling, change in menstrual pattern.	Infrequent	4

1 - Life-threatening. Seek emergency treatment immediately.
2 - Discontinue. Seek emergency treatment.
3 - Discontinue. Call doctor right away.
4 - Continue. Call doctor when convenient.
5 - Continue. Tell doctor at next visit.
6 - No action necessary.

ACETOPHENAZINE

WARNINGS & PRECAUTIONS

Don't take if:
- You are allergic to any phenothiazine.
- You have a blood or bone-marrow disease.

Before you start, consult your doctor:
- If you will have surgery within 2 months, including dental surgery, requiring general or spinal anesthesia.
- If you have asthma, emphysema or other lung disorder.
- If you take non-prescription ulcer medicine, asthma medicine or amphetamines.

Over age 60:
Adverse reactions and side effects may be more frequent and severe than in younger persons. More likely to develop involuntary movement of jaws, lips, tongue, chewing. Report this to your doctor immediately. Early treatment can help.

Pregnancy:
Risk to unborn child outweighs drug benefits. Don't use.

Breast-feeding:
Drug passes into milk. Avoid drug or discontinue nursing until you finish medicine. Consult doctor for advice on maintaining milk supply.

Infants & children:
Don't give to children younger than 2.

Prolonged use:
May lead to tardive dyskinesia (involuntary movement of jaws, lips, tongue, chewing).

Skin & sunlight:
May cause rash or intensify sunburn in areas exposed to sun or sunlamp. Skin may remain sensitive for 3 months after discontinuing.

Driving, piloting or hazardous work:
Don't drive or pilot aircraft until you learn how medicine affects you. Don't work around dangerous machinery. Don't climb ladders or work in high places. Danger increases if you drink alcohol or take medicine affecting alertness and reflexes.

Airplane passengers:
No problems expected.

Discontinuing:
- Nervous and mental disorders—Don't discontinue without doctor's advice until you complete prescribed dose, even though symptoms diminish or disappear.
- Nausea and vomiting—May be unnecessary to finish medicine. Follow doctor's instructions.

INTERACTION WITH OTHER DRUGS

GENERIC NAME OR DRUG CLASS	COMBINED EFFECT
Anticholinergics	Increased anticholinergic effect.
Antidepressants (tricyclic)	Increased acetophenazine effect.
Antihistamines	Increased antihistamine effect.
Appetite suppressants	Decreased suppressant effect.
Levodopa	Decreased levodopa effect.
Mind-altering drugs	Increased effect of mind-altering drugs.
Narcotics	Increased narcotic effect.
Phenytoin	Increased phenytoin effect.
Quinidine	Impaired heart function. Dangerous mixture.
Sedatives	Increased sedative effect.
Tranquilizers (other)	Increased tranquilizer effect.

INTERACTION WITH OTHER SUBSTANCES

INTERACTS WITH	COMBINED EFFECT
Alcohol:	Dangerous oversedation.
Beverages:	None expected.
Cocaine:	Decreased acetophenazine effect. Avoid.
Foods:	None expected.
Marijuana:	Drowsiness. May increase antinausea effect.
Tobacco:	None expected.

ADRENOCORTICOIDS (TOPICAL)

BRAND NAMES

Aristocort	Decadron	Medrol
Celestone	Decaspray	Neo-Cortef (M)
Cordran	Hydrocortone	Neo-Decadron (M)
Cort-Dome	Kenalog	Synalar
Cortef	Lidex	Topicort
Cortril	Locorten	Valisone

GENERAL INFORMATION

Vioform

Habit forming? No
Prescription needed? Yes
Available as generic? Yes
Drug class: Adrenocorticoid (topical)

 USES

Relieves redness, swelling, itching, skin discomfort of hemorrhoids, insect bites, poison ivy, oak, sumac, soaps, cosmetics and jewelry.

 DOSAGE & USAGE INFORMATION

How to use:
- Cream, lotion, ointment—Apply small amount and rub in gently.
- Topical aerosol—Follow directions on container. Don't breathe vapors.

When to use:
When needed or as directed. Don't use more often than directions allow.

If you forget an application:
Use as soon as you remember.

What drug does:
Reduces inflammation by affecting enzymes that produce inflammation.

Time lapse before drug works:
15 to 20 minutes.

Don't use with:
See Interaction column and consult doctor.

 OVERDOSE

Symptoms:
None expected.

What to do:
If person swallows or inhales drug, call doctor, poison-control center or hospital emergency room for instructions.

 POSSIBLE ADVERSE REACTIONS OR SIDE EFFECTS

SYMPTOMS	FREQUENCY	WHAT TO DO
Brain & nervous system:	None expected.	
Skin:		
• Infection with pain, redness, blisters, pus.	Infrequent	4
• Skin irritation with burning, itching, blistering or peeling.	Infrequent	4
• Acne-like eruptions.	Infrequent	4
Eyes:	None expected.	
Ears, nose, throat:	None expected.	
Digestive:	None expected.	
Heart & lungs:	None expected.	
Blood vessels:	None expected.	
Muscles, bones, joints:	None expected.	
Genital, urinary:	None expected.	
Kidneys:	None expected.	
Liver:	None expected.	
Allergic:	None expected.	
Blood:	None expected.	
Others:	None expected.	

1-Life-threatening. Seek emergency treatment immediately.
2-Discontinue. Seek emergency treatment.
3-Discontinue. Call doctor right away.
4-Continue. Call doctor when convenient.
5-Continue. Tell doctor at next visit.
6-No action necessary.

ADRENOCORTICOIDS (TOPICAL)

 ## WARNINGS & PRECAUTIONS

Don't take if:
You are allergic to any topical adrenocorticoid (cortisone) preparation.

Before you start, consult your doctor:
- If you plan pregnancy within medication period.
- If you have diabetes.
- If you have infection at treatment site.
- If you have stomach ulcer.
- If you have tuberculosis.

Over age 60:
Adverse reactions and side effects may be more frequent and severe than in younger persons, especially thinning of the skin.

Pregnancy:
Risk to unborn child outweighs drug benefits. Don't use.

Breast-feeding:
No problems expected.

Infants & children:
- Use only under medical supervision. Too much for too long can be absorbed into bloodstream through skin and retard growth.
- For infants in diapers, avoid plastic pants or tight diapers.

Prolonged use:
- Increases chance of absorption into bloodstream to cause side effects of oral cortisone drugs (see page 184).
- May thin skin where used.

Skin & sunlight:
No problems expected.

Driving, piloting or hazardous work:
No problems expected.

Airplane passengers:
No problems expected.

Discontinuing:
May be unnecessary to finish medicine. Follow doctor's instructions.

Others:
- Don't use a plastic dressing longer than 2 weeks.
- Aerosol spray—Store in cool place. Don't use near heat or open flame or while smoking. Don't puncture, break or burn container.

 ## INTERACTION WITH OTHER DRUGS

GENERIC NAME OR DRUG CLASS	COMBINED EFFECT
Antibiotics (topical)	Decreased antibiotic effects.
Antifungals (topical)	Decreased antifungal effect.

 ## INTERACTION WITH OTHER SUBSTANCES

INTERACTS WITH	COMBINED EFFECT
Alcohol:	None expected.
Beverages:	None expected.
Cocaine:	None expected.
Foods:	None expected.
Marijuana:	None expected.
Tobacco:	None expected.

ALLOPURINOL

BRAND NAMES

Lopurin
Purinol
Zyloprim

Habit forming? No
Prescription needed? Yes
Available as generic? Yes
Drug class: Antigout

USES

- Treatment for chronic gout.
- Prevention of kidney stones caused by uric acid.

DOSAGE & USAGE INFORMATION

How to take:
Tablet—Swallow with liquid or food to lessen stomach irritation.

When to take:
At the same times each day.

If you forget a dose:
- 1 dose per day—Take as soon as you remember up to 6 hours late. If more than 6 hours, wait for next scheduled dose (don't double this dose).
- More than 1 dose per day—Take as soon as you remember up to 3 hours late. If more than 3 hours, wait for next scheduled dose (don't double this dose).

What drug does:
Slows formation of uric acid by inhibiting enzyme (xanthine oxidase) activity.

Time lapse before drug works:
Reduces blood uric acid in 1 to 3 weeks. May require 6 months to prevent acute gout attacks.

Don't take with:
- Vitamin C.
- See Interaction column and consult doctor.

OVERDOSE

Symptoms:
None expected.

What to do:
Overdose unlikely to threaten life. If person takes much larger amount than prescribed, call doctor, poison-control center or hospital emergency room for instructions.

POSSIBLE ADVERSE REACTIONS OR SIDE EFFECTS

SYMPTOMS	FREQUENCY	WHAT TO DO
Brain & nervous system: Drowsiness	Infrequent	4
Skin: Rash, hives, itch.	Common	3
Eyes:	None expected.	
Ears, nose, throat: Sore throat, fever.	Rare	3
Digestive: Diarrhea, stomach pain, nausea, vomiting.	Infrequent	4
Heart & lungs:	None expected.	
Blood vessels: Unusual bleeding or bruising.	Rare	3
Muscles, bones, joints: Numbness, tingling, pain in hands or feet.	Rare	4
Genital, urinary:	None expected.	
Kidneys:	None expected.	
Liver: Jaundice (yellow skin and eyes).	Infrequent	3
Allergic:	None expected.	
Blood:	None expected.	
Others:	None expected.	

1-Life-threatening. Seek emergency treatment immediately.
2-Discontinue. Seek emergency treatment.
3-Discontinue. Call doctor right away.
4-Continue. Call doctor when convenient.
5-Continue. Tell doctor at next visit.
6-No action necessary.

WARNINGS & PRECAUTIONS

Don't take if:
You are allergic to allopurinol.

Before you start, consult your doctor:
If you have had liver or kidney problems.

Over age 60:
Adverse reactions and side effects may be more frequent and severe than in younger persons.

Pregnancy:
Studies inconclusive on harm to unborn child. Animal studies show fetal abnormalities. Decide with your doctor whether drug benefits justify risk to unborn child.

Breast-feeding:
Drug passes into milk. Avoid drug or discontinue nursing.

Infants & children:
Not recommended.

Prolonged use:
No problems expected.

Skin & sunlight:
No problems expected.

Driving, piloting or hazardous work:
Avoid if you feel drowsy. Use may disqualify you for piloting aircraft.

Airplane passengers:
No problems expected.

Discontinuing:
Don't discontinue without doctor's advice until you complete prescribed dose, even though symptoms diminish or disappear.

Others:
Acute gout attacks may increase during first weeks of use. If so, consult doctor about additional medicine.

INTERACTION WITH OTHER DRUGS

GENERIC NAME OR DRUG CLASS	COMBINED EFFECT
Ampicillin	Likely skin rash.
Anticoagulants (oral)	Increased anticoagulant effect.
Antidiabetics (oral)	Increased uric-acid elimination.
Azathioprine	Increased azathioprine effect.
Chlorthalidone	Decreased allopurinol effect.
Cyclophosphamide	Increased cyclophosphamide toxicity.
Diuretics (thiazide)	Decreased allopurinol effect.
Ethacrynic acid	Decreased allopurinol effect.
Furosemide	Decreased allopurinol effect.
Iron supplements	Excessive accumulation of iron in tissues.
Mercaptopurine	Increased mercaptopurine effect.

Additional interactions on page 832.

INTERACTION WITH OTHER SUBSTANCES

INTERACTS WITH	COMBINED EFFECT
Alcohol:	None expected, but may impair management of gout.
Beverages: Caffeine drinks	Decreased allopurinol effect.
Cocaine:	Decreased allopurinol effect. Avoid.
Foods:	None expected. Low-purine diet recommended (see page 851).
Marijuana:	Occasional use—None expected. Daily use—Possible increase in uric-acid level.
Tobacco:	None expected.

ALPRAZOLAM

BRAND NAMES

Xanax

GENERAL INFORMATION

Habit forming? Yes
Prescription needed? Yes
Available as generic? No
Drug class: Tranquilizer (benzodiazepine)

USES

Treatment for nervousness or tension.

DOSAGE & USAGE INFORMATION

How to take:
Tablet or capsule—Swallow with liquid. If you can't swallow whole, crumble tablet or open capsule and take with liquid or food.

When to take:
At the same time each day, according to instructions on prescription label.

If you forget a dose:
Take as soon as you remember up to 2 hours late. If more than 2 hours, wait for next scheduled dose (don't double this dose).

What drug does:
Affects limbic system of brain—part that controls emotions.

Time lapse before drug works:
2 hours. May take 6 weeks for full benefit.

Don't take with:
See Interaction column and consult doctor.

OVERDOSE

Symptoms:
Drowsiness, weakness, tremor, stupor, coma.

What to do:
- Dial 0 (operator) or 911 (emergency) for an ambulance or medical help. Then give first aid immediately.
- If patient is unconscious and not breathing, give mouth-to-mouth breathing. If there is no heartbeat, use cardiac massage and mouth-to-mouth breathing (CPR). Don't try to make patient vomit. If you can't get help quickly, take patient to nearest emergency facility.
- Additional emergency information on page 886.

POSSIBLE ADVERSE REACTIONS OR SIDE EFFECTS

SYMPTOMS	FREQUENCY	WHAT TO DO
Brain & nervous system:		
• Clumsiness, drowsiness, dizziness.	Common	4
• Hallucinations, confusion, depression, irritability.	Infrequent	3
Skin:		
Rash, itch.	Infrequent	3
Eyes:		
Vision changes.	Infrequent	3
Ears, nose, throat:		
Mouth, throat ulcers.	Rare	3
Digestive:		
Constipation or diarrhea, nausea, vomiting.	Infrequent	4
Heart & lungs:		
Slow heartbeat, breathing difficulty.	Rare	2
Blood vessels:	None expected.	
Muscles, bones, joints:	None expected.	
Genital, urinary:		
Urination difficulty.	Infrequent	4
Kidneys:	None expected.	
Liver:		
Jaundice (yellow eyes and skin).	Rare	3
Allergic:	None expected.	
Blood:	None expected.	
Others:	None expected.	

1- Life-threatening. Seek emergency treatment immediately.
2- Discontinue. Seek emergency treatment.
3- Discontinue. Call doctor right away.
4- Continue. Call doctor when convenient.
5- Continue. Tell doctor at next visit.
6- No action necessary.

ALPRAZOLAM

WARNINGS & PRECAUTIONS

Don't take if:
- You are allergic to any benzodiazepine.
- You have myasthenia gravis.
- You have glaucoma.
- You are active or recovering alcoholic.
- Patient is younger than 6 months.

Before you start, consult your doctor:
- If you have liver, kidney or lung disease.
- If you have diabetes, epilepsy or porphyria.

Over age 60:
Adverse reactions and side effects may be more frequent and severe than in younger persons. You need smaller doses for shorter periods of time. May develop agitation, rage or "hangover effect."

Pregnancy:
Risk to unborn child outweighs drug benefits. Don't use.

Breast-feeding:
Drug passes into milk. Avoid drug or discontinue nursing until you finish medicine. Consult doctor for advice on maintaining milk supply.

Infants & children:
Use only under medical supervision for children older than 6 months.

Prolonged use:
May impair liver function.

Skin & sunlight:
No problems expected.

Driving, piloting or hazardous work:
Don't drive or pilot aircraft until you learn how medicine affects you. Don't work around dangerous machinery. Don't climb ladders or work in high places. Danger increases if you drink alcohol or take medicine affecting alertness and reflexes.

Airplane passengers:
No problems expected.

Discontinuing:
Don't discontinue without consulting doctor. Dose may require gradual reduction if you have taken drug for a long time. Doses of other drugs may also require adjustment.

Others:
- Hot weather, heavy exercise and profuse sweat may reduce excretion and cause overdose.
- Blood sugar may rise in diabetics, requiring insulin adjustment.

INTERACTION WITH OTHER DRUGS

GENERIC NAME OR DRUG CLASS	COMBINED EFFECT
Anticonvulsants	Change in seizure frequency or severity.
Antidepressants	Increased sedative effect of both drugs.
Antihistamines	Increased sedative effect of both drugs.
Antihypertensives	Excessively low blood pressure.
Cimetidine	Excess sedation.
Disulfiram	Increased alprazolam effect.
MAO inhibitors	Convulsions, deep sedation, rage.
Narcotics	Increased sedative effect of both drugs.
Sedatives	Increased sedative effect of both drugs.
Sleep inducers	Increased sedative effect of both drugs.
Tranquilizers	Increased sedative effect of both drugs.

INTERACTION WITH OTHER SUBSTANCES

INTERACTS WITH	COMBINED EFFECT
Alcohol:	Heavy sedation. Avoid.
Beverages:	None expected.
Cocaine:	Decreased alprazolam effect.
Foods:	None expected.
Marijuana:	Heavy sedation. Avoid.
Tobacco:	Decreased alprazolam effect.

ALUMINUM HYDROXIDE

BRAND NAMES

Camalox (M)	Kolantyl Wafers (M)	Pepsogel
Chemgel	Maalox (M)	Robalate
Creamalin (M)	Magnatril (M)	Rolaids (M)
Delcid (M)	Maxamag (M)	Sterazolidin (M)
Di-Gel (M)	Mucotin (M)	
Ducon (M)	Mylanta (M)	

GENERAL INFORMATION

Habit forming? No
Prescription needed? No
Available as generic? Yes
Drug class: Antacid, antidiarrheal

USES

- Binds excess phosphate in intestine.
- Treatment for hyperacidity in upper gastrointestinal tract, including stomach and esophagus. Symptoms may be heartburn or acid indigestion. Diseases include peptic ulcer, gastritis, esophagitis, hiatal hernia.
- Treatment for diarrhea.

DOSAGE & USAGE INFORMATION

How to take:
- Tablet or capsule—Swallow with liquid.
- Chewable tablets or wafers—Chew well before swallowing.
- Liquid—Shake well and take undiluted.

When to take:
1 to 3 hours after meals unless directed otherwise by your doctor.

If you forget a dose:
Take as soon as you remember, but not simultaneously with any other medicine.

What drug does:
- Neutralizes some of the hydrochloric acid in the stomach.
- Reduces action of pepsin, a digestive enzyme.

Time lapse before drug works:
15 minutes.

Don't take with:
Other medicines at the same time. Decreases absorption of other drugs. Wait 2 hours between doses.

OVERDOSE

Symptoms:
Weakness, fatigue, dizziness.

What to do:
Overdose unlikely to threaten life. If person takes much larger amount than prescribed, call doctor, poison-control center or hospital emergency room for instructions.

POSSIBLE ADVERSE REACTIONS OR SIDE EFFECTS

SYMPTOMS	FREQUENCY	WHAT TO DO
Brain & nervous system: Mood changes.	Infrequent	4
Skin:	None expected.	
Eyes:	None expected.	
Ears, nose, throat:	None expected.	
Digestive:		
• Constipation, appetite loss.	Common	4
• Nausea, vomiting.	Infrequent	4
• Lower abdominal pain and swelling.	Infrequent	3
Heart & lungs:	None expected.	
Blood vessels:	None expected.	
Muscles, bones, joints: Bone pain, muscle weakness.	Infrequent	3
Genital, urinary:	None expected.	
Kidneys:	None expected.	
Liver:	None expected.	
Allergic:	None expected.	
Blood:	None expected.	
Others:		
• Swelling of wrists or ankles.	Infrequent	3
• Weight loss.	Infrequent	4

1- Life-threatening. Seek emergency treatment immediately.
2- Discontinue. Seek emergency treatment.
3- Discontinue. Call doctor right away.
4- Continue. Call doctor when convenient.
5- Continue. Tell doctor at next visit.
6- No action necessary.

ALUMINUM HYDROXIDE

WARNINGS & PRECAUTIONS

Don't take if:
You are allergic to any antacid.

Before you start, consult your doctor:
- If you have kidney disease.
- If you have chronic constipation, colitis or diarrhea.
- If you have symptoms of appendicitis.
- If you have have stomach or intestinal bleeding.

Over age 60:
Adverse reactions and side effects may be more frequent and severe than in younger persons. Diarrhea or constipation particularly likely.

Pregnancy:
Risk to unborn child outweighs drug benefits. Don't use.

Breast-feeding:
Drug passes into milk. Avoid drug or discontinue nursing until you finish medicine. Consult doctor for advice on maintaining milk supply.

Infants & children:
Use only under medical supervision.

Prolonged use:
Decreased phosphate level in blood weakens bones.

Skin & sunlight:
No problems expected.

Driving, piloting or hazardous work:
No problems expected.

Airplane passengers:
No problems expected.

Discontinuing:
May be unnecessary to finish medicine. Follow doctor's instructions.

Others:
Don't take longer than 2 weeks unless under medical supervision.

INTERACTION WITH OTHER DRUGS

GENERIC NAME OR DRUG CLASS	COMBINED EFFECT
Anticoagulants	Decreased anticoagulant effect.
Chlorpromazine	Decreased chlorpromazine effect.
Digitalis preparations	Decreased digitalis effect.
Iron supplements	Decreased iron effect.
Meperidine	Increased meperidine effect.
Nalidixic acid	Decreased effect of nalidixic acid.
Oxyphenbutazone	Decreased oxyphenbutazone effect.
Para-aminosalicylic acid (PAS)	Decreased PAS effect.
Penicillins	Decreased penicillin effect.
Pentobarbital	Decreased pentobarbital effect.
Phenylbutazone	Decreased phenylbutazone effect.
Pseudoephedrine	Increased pseudoephedrine effect.
Sulfa drugs	Decreased sulfa effect.
Tetracyclines	Decreased tetracycline effect.
Vitamins A and C	Decreased vitamin effect.

INTERACTION WITH OTHER SUBSTANCES

INTERACTS WITH	COMBINED EFFECT
Alcohol:	Decreased antacid effect.
Beverages:	No proven problems.
Cocaine:	No proven problems.
Foods:	Decreased antacid effect. Wait 1 hour after eating.
Marijuana:	No proven problems.
Tobacco:	Decreased antacid effect.

AMANTADINE

BRAND NAMES

Symmetrel

GENERAL INFORMATION

Habit forming? No
Prescription needed? Yes
Available as generic? No
Drug class: Antiviral, antiparkinsonism

USES

- Treatment for Type-A flu infections.
- Relief for symptoms of Parkinson's disease.

DOSAGE & USAGE INFORMATION

How to take:
- Tablet or capsule—Swallow with liquid or food to lessen stomach irritation.
- Syrup—Dilute dose in beverage before swallowing.

When to take:
At the same times each day. For Type-A flu it is especially important to take regular doses as prescribed.

If you forget a dose:
Take as soon as you remember. Wait 4 hours for next dose. Return to schedule.

What drug does:
- Type-A flu—May block penetration of tissue cells by infectious material from virus cells.
- Parkinson's disease—Improves muscular condition and coordination.

Time lapse before drug works:
- Type-A flu—48 hours.
- Parkinson's disease—2 days to 2 weeks.

Don't take with:
- Alcohol
- See Interaction column and consult doctor.

OVERDOSE

Symptoms:
Heart-rhythm disturbances, blood-pressure drop, convulsions, toxic psychosis.

What to do:
- Dial 0 (operator) or 911 (emergency) for an ambulance or medical help. Then give first aid immediately.
- Additional emergency information on page 886.

POSSIBLE ADVERSE REACTIONS OR SIDE EFFECTS

SYMPTOMS	FREQUENCY	WHAT TO DO
Brain & nervous system:		
● Hallucinations, confusion, mood changes.	Common	4
● Fainting, slurred speech.	Infrequent	3
● Dizziness, headache.	Common	5
Skin:		
● Purple blotches.	Common	5
● Rash	Rare	3
Eyes:		
Uncontrolled rolling of eyes, blurred vision.	Rare	3
Ears, nose, throat:		
● Dry mouth.	Common	6
● Sore throat, fever.	Rare	3
Digestive:		
● Constipation	Rare	5
● Appetite loss, nausea.	Common	5
● Vomiting	Rare	4
Heart & lungs, blood vessels, muscles, bones, joints, liver, allergic, blood:	None expected.	
Genital, urinary:		
Difficult urination.	Infrequent	4
Others:		
Faintness on standing.	Common	4

1- Life-threatening. Seek emergency treatment immediately.
2- Discontinue. Seek emergency treatment.
3- Discontinue. Call doctor right away.
4- Continue. Call doctor when convenient.
5- Continue. Tell doctor at next visit.
6- No action necessary.

WARNINGS & PRECAUTIONS

Don't take if:
You are allergic to amantadine.

Before you start, consult your doctor:
- If you have had epilepsy or other seizures.
- If you have had heart disease or heart failure.
- If you have had liver or kidney disease.
- If you have had peptic ulcers.
- If you have had eczema or skin rashes.
- If you have had emotional or mental disorders or taken drugs for them.

Over age 60:
Adverse reactions and side effects may be more frequent and severe than in younger persons.

Pregnancy:
Studies inconclusive on harm to unborn child. Animal studies show fetal abnormalities. Decide with your doctor whether benefits justify risk to unborn child.

Breast-feeding:
Drug passes into milk. Avoid drug or discontinue nursing until you finish medicine. Consult doctor for advice on maintaining milk supply.

Infants & children:
Use only under medical supervision.

Prolonged use:
Skin splotches, feet swelling, rapid weight gain, shortness of breath. Consult doctor.

Skin & sunlight:
No problems expected.

Driving, piloting or hazardous work:
Don't drive or pilot aircraft until you learn how medicine affects you. Don't work around dangerous machinery. Don't climb ladders or work in high places. Danger increases if you drink alcohol or take medicine affecting alertness and reflexes.

Airplane passengers:
No problems expected.

Discontinuing:
- Parkinson's disease—Don't discontinue without doctor's advice until you complete prescribed dose, even though symptoms diminish or disappear.
- Type-A flu—Discontinue 48 hours after symptoms disappear.

Others:
- Parkinson's disease—May lose effectiveness in 3 to 6 months. Consult doctor.
- Amantadine may increase susceptibility to German measles.

INTERACTION WITH OTHER DRUGS

GENERIC NAME OR DRUG CLASS	COMBINED EFFECT
Amphetamines	Increased amantadine effect. Possible excessive stimulation and agitation.
Anticholinergics	Increased benefit, but excessive anticholinergic dose produces mental confusion, hallucinations, delirium.
Appetite suppressants	Increased amantadine effect. Possible excessive stimulation and agitation.
Levodopa	Increased benefit of levodopa. Can cause agitation.
Sympathomimetics	Increased amantadine effect. Possible excessive stimulation and agitation.

INTERACTION WITH OTHER SUBSTANCES

INTERACTS WITH	COMBINED EFFECT
Alcohol:	Increased alcohol effect. Possible fainting.
Beverages:	None expected.
Cocaine:	Dangerous overstimulation.
Foods:	None expected.
Marijuana:	None expected.
Tobacco:	None expected.

AMBENONIUM

BRAND NAMES

Mytelase

GENERAL INFORMATION

Habit forming? No
Prescription needed? Yes
Available as generic? No
Drug class: Cholinergic (anticholinesterase)

USES

- Treatment of myasthenia gravis.
- Treatment of urinary retention and abdominal distention.

DOSAGE & USAGE INFORMATION

How to take:
Capsule—Swallow with liquid or food to lessen stomach irritation.

When to take:
As directed, usually 3 or 4 times a day.

If you forget a dose:
Take as soon as you remember up to 2 hours late. If more than 2 hours, wait for next scheduled dose (don't double this dose).

What drug does:
Inhibits the chemical activity of an enzyme (cholinesterase) so nerve impulses can cross the junction of nerves and muscles.

Time lapse before drug works:
3 hours.

Don't take with:
See Interaction column and consult doctor.

OVERDOSE

Symptoms:
Muscle weakness, cramps, twitching or clumsiness; severe diarrhea, nausea, vomiting, stomach cramps or pain; breathing difficulty; confusion, irritability, nervousness, restlessness, fear; unusually slow heartbeat; seizures.

What to do:
- Dial 0 (operator) or 911 (emergency) for an ambulance or medical help. Then give first aid immediately.
- Additional emergency information on page 886.

POSSIBLE ADVERSE REACTIONS OR SIDE EFFECTS

SYMPTOMS	FREQUENCY	WHAT TO DO
Brain & nervous system: Confusion, irritability.	Infrequent	2
Skin:	None expected.	
Eyes: Constricted pupils, watery eyes.	Infrequent	4
Ears, nose, throat: Excess saliva.	Common	4
Digestive: Mild diarrhea, nausea, vomiting, stomach cramps or pain.	Common	3
Heart & lungs: Lung congestion.	Infrequent	4
Blood vessels:	None expected.	
Muscles, bones, joints:	None expected.	
Genital, urinary: Frequent urge to urinate.	Infrequent	4
Kidneys:	None expected.	
Liver:	None expected.	
Allergic:	None expected.	
Blood:	None expected.	
Others: Unusual sweating.	Common	4

1- Life-threatening. Seek emergency treatment immediately.
2- Discontinue. Seek emergency treatment.
3- Discontinue. Call doctor right away.
4- Continue. Call doctor when convenient.
5- Continue. Tell doctor at next visit.
6- No action necessary.

WARNINGS & PRECAUTIONS

Don't take if:
- You are allergic to any cholinergic or bromide.
- You take mecamylamine.

Before you start, consult your doctor:
- If you plan to become pregnant within medication period.
- If you have bronchial asthma.
- If you have heartbeat irregularities.
- If you have urinary obstruction or urinary-tract infection.

Over age 60:
Adverse reactions and side effects may be more frequent and severe than in younger persons.

Pregnancy:
No proven harm to unborn child. Avoid if possible. May increase uterus contractions close to delivery.

Breast-feeding:
No problems expected, but consult doctor.

Infants & children:
Not recommended.

Prolonged use:
Medication may lose effectiveness. Discontinuing for a few days may restore effect.

Skin & sunlight:
No problems expected.

Driving, piloting or hazardous work:
Don't drive or pilot aircraft until you learn how medicine affects you. Don't work around dangerous machinery. Don't climb ladders or work in high places. Danger increases if you drink alcohol or take medicine affecting alertness and reflexes, such as antihistamines, tranquilizers, sedatives, pain medicine, narcotics and mind-altering drugs.

Airplane passengers:
No problems expected.

Discontinuing:
Don't discontinue without doctor's advice until you complete prescribed dose, even though symptoms diminish or disappear.

Others:
No problems expected.

INTERACTION WITH OTHER DRUGS

GENERIC NAME OR DRUG CLASS	COMBINED EFFECT
Anesthetics (local or general)	Decreased ambenonium effect.
Antiarrhythmics	Decreased ambenonium effect.
Antibiotics	Decreased ambenonium effect.
Anticholinergics	Decreased ambenonium effect. May mask severe side effects.
Cholinergics (other)	Reduced intestinal-tract function. Possible brain and nervous-system toxicity.
Mecamylamine	Decreased ambenonium effect.
Quinidine	Decreased ambenonium effect.

INTERACTION WITH OTHER SUBSTANCES

INTERACTS WITH	COMBINED EFFECT
Alcohol:	No proven problems with small doses.
Beverages:	None expected.
Cocaine:	Decreased ambenonium effect. Avoid.
Foods:	None expected.
Marijuana:	No proven problems.
Tobacco:	No proven problems.

AMILORIDE

Midamor

GENERAL INFORMATION

Habit forming? No
Prescription needed? Yes
Available as generic? No
Drug class: Diuretic

USES

Treatment for high blood pressure and congestive heart failure. Decreases fluid retention and prevents potassium loss.

DOSAGE & USAGE INFORMATION

How to take:
Tablet—Swallow with liquid.

When to take:
At the same time each day, preferably in the morning. May interfere with sleep if taken after 6 p.m.

If you forget a dose:
Take as soon as you remember up to 8 hours late. If more than 8 hours, wait for next scheduled dose (don't double this dose).

What drug does:
Blocks exchange of certain chemicals in the kidney so sodium is excreted. Conserves potassium.

Time lapse before drug works:
2 hours.

Don't take with:
See Interaction column and consult doctor.

OVERDOSE

Symptoms:
Rapid, irregular heartbeat; confusion; shortness of breath; nervousness; extreme weakness.

What to do:
- Dial 0 (operator) or 911 (emergency) for an ambulance or medical help. Then give first aid immediately.
- If patient is unconscious and not breathing, give mouth-to-mouth breathing. If there is no heartbeat, use cardiac massage and mouth-to-mouth breathing (CPR). Don't try to make patient vomit. If you can't get help quickly, take patient to nearest emergency facility.
- Additional emergency information on page 886.

POSSIBLE ADVERSE REACTIONS OR SIDE EFFECTS

SYMPTOMS	FREQUENCY	WHAT TO DO
Brain & nervous system:		
● Headache	Common	4
● Dizziness	Infrequent	4
Skin:	None expected.	
Eyes:	None expected.	
Ears, nose, throat:	None expected.	
Digestive:		
● Nausea, appetite loss, vomiting, diarrhea.	Common	4
● Constipation, pain, bloating.	Infrequent	4
Heart & lungs: Cough, shortness of breath.	Infrequent	3
Blood vessels:	None expected.	
Muscles, bones, joints: Muscle cramps.	Infrequent	4
Genital, urinary:	None expected.	
Kidneys:	None expected.	
Liver:	None expected.	
Allergic:	None expected.	
Blood:	None expected.	
Others:	None expected.	

1- Life-threatening. Seek emergency treatment immediately.
2- Discontinue. Seek emergency treatment.
3- Discontinue. Call doctor right away.
4- Continue. Call doctor when convenient.
5- Continue. Tell doctor at next visit.
6- No action necessary.

WARNINGS & PRECAUTIONS

Don't take if:
- You are allergic to amiloride.
- Your serum potassium level is high.

Before you start, consult your doctor:
- If you plan to become pregnant within medication period.
- If you have diabetes.
- If you have heart disease.
- If you have kidney or liver disease.

Over age 60:
Adverse reactions and side effects may be more frequent and severe than in younger persons. More likely to exceed safe potassium blood levels.

Pregnancy:
No proven harm to unborn child. Avoid if possible.

Breast-feeding:
No problems expected, but consult doctor.

Infants & children:
Not recommended.

Prolonged use:
No problems expected.

Skin & sunlight:
No problems expected.

Driving, piloting or hazardous work:
Don't drive or pilot aircraft until you learn how medicine affects you. Don't work around dangerous machinery. Don't climb ladders or work in high places. Danger increases if you drink alcohol or take medicine affecting alertness and reflexes, such as antihistamines, tranquilizers, sedatives, pain medicine, narcotics and mind-altering drugs.

Airplane passengers:
No problems expected.

Discontinuing:
Don't discontinue without doctor's advice until you complete prescribed dose, even though symptoms diminish or disappear.

Others:
Periodic physical checkups and potassium-level tests recommended.

 ## INTERACTION WITH OTHER DRUGS

GENERIC NAME OR DRUG CLASS	COMBINED EFFECT
Antihypertensives	Increased effect of both drugs.
Blood-bank blood	Increased potassium levels.
Diuretics (other)	Increased effect of both drugs.
Lithium	Possible lithium toxicity.
Potassium supplements	Increased potassium levels.
Sodium bicarbonate	Decreased potassium levels.

 ## INTERACTION WITH OTHER SUBSTANCES

INTERACTS WITH	COMBINED EFFECT
Alcohol:	Increased blood-pressure drop. Avoid.
Beverages: Low-salt milk	Possible excess potassium levels. Low-salt milk has extra potassium.
Cocaine:	Blood-pressure rise. Avoid.
Foods: Salt substitutes	Possible excess potassium levels.
Marijuana:	None expected.
Tobacco:	None expected.

AMINOPHYLLINE

BRAND NAMES

Aminodur   Mini-Lix
Aminophyl   Somophyllin
Amphylline
Corophyllin
Lixaminol

GENERAL INFORMATION

Habit forming? No
Prescription needed? Canada—No
U.S: High strength— Yes
Low strength— No
Available as generic? Yes
Drug class: Bronchodilator (xanthine)

 ## USES

Treatment for bronchial asthma symptoms.

 ## DOSAGE & USAGE INFORMATION

How to take:
- Tablet or capsule—Swallow with liquid.
- Extended-release tablets or capsules—Swallow each dose whole. If you take regular tablets, you may chew or crush them.
- Suppositories—Remove wrapper and moisten suppository with water. Gently insert larger end into rectum. Push well into rectum with finger.
- Syrup—Take as directed on bottle.
- Enema—Use as directed on label.

When to take:
Most effective taken on empty stomach 1 hour before or 2 hours after eating. However, may take with food to lessen stomach upset.

If you forget a dose:
Take as soon as you remember up to 2 hours late. If more than 2 hours, wait for next scheduled dose (don't double this dose).

What drug does:
Relaxes and expands bronchial tubes.

Time lapse before drug works:
15 to 30 minutes.

Don't take with:
See Interaction column and consult doctor.

 ## OVERDOSE

Symptoms:
Restlessness, irritability, confusion, delirium, convulsions, rapid pulse, coma.

What to do:
- Dial 0 (operator) or 911 (emergency) for an ambulance or medical help. Then give first aid immediately.
- Additional emergency information on page 886.

 ## POSSIBLE ADVERSE REACTIONS OR SIDE EFFECTS

SYMPTOMS	FREQUENCY	WHAT TO DO
Brain & nervous system:		
• Headache, irritability, nervousness, restlessness, insomnia.	Common	4
• Dizziness or lightheadedness.	Infrequent	4
Skin:		
• Rash or hives.	Infrequent	3
• Flushed face.	Infrequent	4
Eyes:	None expected.	
Ears, nose, throat:	None expected.	
Digestive:		
• Nausea, vomiting, stomach pain.	Common	4
• Diarrhea, appetite loss.	Infrequent	3
Heart & lungs:		
• Rapid breathing.	Infrequent	3
• Irregular heartbeat.	Infrequent	3
Blood vessels:	None expected.	
Muscles, bones, joints:	None expected.	
Genital, urinary:	None expected.	
Kidneys:	None expected.	
Liver:	None expected.	
Allergic:	None expected.	
Blood:	None expected.	
Others:	None expected.	

1- Life-threatening. Seek emergency treatment immediately.
2- Discontinue. Seek emergency treatment.
3- Discontinue. Call doctor right away.
4- Continue. Call doctor when convenient.
5- Continue. Tell doctor at next visit.
6- No action necessary.

AMINOPHYLLINE

 ## WARNINGS & PRECAUTIONS

Don't take if:
- You are allergic to any bronchodilator.
- You have an active peptic ulcer.

Before you start, consult your doctor:
- If you have had impaired kidney or liver function.
- If you have gastritis.
- If you have a peptic ulcer.
- If you have high blood pressure or heart disease.
- If you take medication for gout.

Over age 60:
Adverse reactions and side effects may be more frequent and severe than in younger persons.

Pregnancy:
Risk to unborn child outweighs drug benefits. Don't use.

Breast-feeding:
Drug passes into milk. Avoid drug or discontinue nursing until you finish medicine. Consult doctor for advice on maintaining milk supply.

Infants & children:
Use only under medical supervision.

Prolonged use:
Stomach irritation.

Skin & sunlight:
No problems expected.

Driving, piloting or hazardous work:
Avoid if lightheaded or dizzy. Otherwise, no problems expected.

Airplane passengers:
No problems expected.

Discontinuing:
May be unnecessary to finish medicine. Follow doctor's instructions.

Others:
No problems expected.

 ## INTERACTION WITH OTHER DRUGS

GENERIC NAME OR DRUG CLASS	COMBINED EFFECT
Allopurinol	Decreased allopurinol effect.
Ephedrine	Increased effect of both drugs.
Epinephrine	Increased effect of both drugs.
Erythromycin	Increased aminophylline effect.
Furosemide	Increased furosemide effect.
Lincomycins	Increased aminophylline effect.
Lithium	Decreased lithium effect.
Probenecid	Decreased effect of both drugs.
Propranolol	Decreased aminophylline effect.
Rauwolfia alkaloids	Rapid heartbeat.
Sulfinpyrazone	Decreased sulfinpyrazone effect.
Troleandomycin	Increased aminophylline effect.

 ## INTERACTION WITH OTHER SUBSTANCES

INTERACTS WITH	COMBINED EFFECT
Alcohol:	None expected.
Beverages: Caffeine drinks	Nervousness and insomnia.
Cocaine:	Excess stimulation. Avoid.
Foods:	None expected.
Marijuana:	Slightly increased antiasthmatic effect of aminophylline.
Tobacco:	Decreased aminophylline effect.

AMITRIPTYLINE

BRAND NAMES

Amitid   Endep
Amitril   Etrafon (M)
Elavil   SK-Amitriptyline

GENERAL INFORMATION

Habit forming? No
Prescription needed? Yes
Available as generic? Yes
Drug class: Antidepressant (tricyclic)

USES

- Gradually relieves, but doesn't cure, symptoms of depression.
- Decreases bed-wetting.

DOSAGE & USAGE INFORMATION

How to take:
Tablet or capsule—Swallow with liquid.

When to take:
At the same time each day, usually bedtime.

If you forget a dose:
Bedtime dose—If you forget your once-a-day bedtime dose, don't take it more than 3 hours late. If more than 3 hours, wait for next scheduled dose. Don't double this dose.

What drug does:
Probably affects part of brain that controls messages between nerve cells.

Time lapse before drug works:
Begins in 1 to 2 weeks. May require 4 to 6 weeks for maximum benefit.

Don't take with:
- Non-prescription drugs without consulting doctor.
- See Interaction column and consult doctor.

OVERDOSE

Symptoms:
Hallucinations, convulsions, coma.

What to do:
- Dial 0 (operator) or 911 (emergency) for an ambulance or medical help. Then give first aid immediately.
- If patient is unconscious and not breathing, give mouth-to-mouth breathing. If there is no heartbeat, use cardiac massage and mouth-to-mouth breathing (CPR). Don't try to make patient vomit. If you can't get help quickly, take patient to nearest emergency facility.
- Additional emergency information on page 886.

POSSIBLE ADVERSE REACTIONS OR SIDE EFFECTS

SYMPTOMS	FREQUENCY	WHAT TO DO
Brain & nervous system:		
● Hallucinations, shakiness, dizziness, fainting.	Infrequent	3
● Headache	Common	4
● Seizures	Rare	1
● Insomnia	Common	5
Skin:		
Rash, itch.	Rare	3
Eyes:		
Blurred vision, pain.	Infrequent	3
Ears, nose, throat:		
● Sore throat.	Rare	3
● Dry mouth or unpleasant taste.	Common	4
Digestive:		
● Constipation or diarrhea, nausea, indigestion.	Common	4
● Vomiting	Infrequent	3
● "Sweet tooth"	Common	5
Heart & lungs:		
Irregular heartbeat or slow pulse.	Infrequent	3
Blood vessels, muscles, bones, joints, kidneys, allergic, blood:	None expected.	
Genital, urinary:		
Difficulty urinating.	Infrequent	4
Liver:		
Jaundice (yellow skin and eyes).	Rare	3
Others:		
● Fever	Rare	3
● Fatigue, weakness.	Common	4

1 - Life-threatening. Seek emergency treatment immediately.
2 - Discontinue. Seek emergency treatment.
3 - Discontinue. Call doctor right away.
4 - Continue. Call doctor when convenient.
5 - Continue. Tell doctor at next visit.

AMITRIPTYLINE

WARNINGS & PRECAUTIONS

Don't take if:
- You are allergic to any tricyclic antidepressant.
- You drink alcohol.
- You have had a heart attack within 6 weeks.
- You have glaucoma.
- You have taken MAO inhibitors within 2 weeks.
- Patient is younger than 12.

Before you start, consult your doctor:
- If you will have surgery within 2 months, including dental surgery, requiring general or spinal anesthesia.
- If you have an enlarged prostate.
- If you have heart disease or high blood pressure.
- If you have stomach or intestinal problems.
- If you have an overactive thyroid.
- If you have asthma.
- If you have liver disease.

Over age 60:
More likely to develop urination difficulty and side effects under Brain & nervous system.

Pregnancy:
Studies inconclusive on harm to unborn child. Animal studies show fetal abnormalities. Decide with your doctor whether drug benefits justify risk to unborn child.

Breast-feeding:
Drug passes into milk. Avoid drug or discontinue nursing until you finish medicine. Consult doctor for advice on maintaining milk supply.

Infants & children:
Don't give to children younger than 12.

Prolonged use:
No problems expected.

Skin & sunlight:
May cause rash or intensify sunburn in areas exposed to sun or sunlamp.

Driving, piloting or hazardous work:
Don't drive or pilot aircraft until you learn how medicine affects you. Don't work around dangerous machinery. Don't climb ladders or work in high places. Danger increases if you drink alcohol or take medicine affecting alertness and reflexes.

Airplane passengers:
No problems expected.

Discontinuing:
Don't discontinue without consulting doctor. Dose may require gradual reduction if you have taken drug for a long time. Doses of other drugs may also require adjustment.

INTERACTION WITH OTHER DRUGS

GENERIC NAME OR DRUG CLASS	COMBINED EFFECT
Anticoagulants (oral)	Increased anticoagulant effect.
Anticholinergics	Increased sedation.
Antihistamines	Increased antihistamine effect.
Barbiturates	Decreased antidepressant effect.
Clonidine	Decreased clonidine effect.
Ethchlorvynol	Delirium
Guanethidine	Decreased guanethidine effect.
MAO inhibitors	Fever, delirium, convulsions.
Methyldopa	Decreased methyldopa effect.
Narcotics	Dangerous oversedation.
Phenytoin	Decreased phenytoin effect.
Quinidine	Irregular heartbeat.
Sedatives	Dangerous oversedation.
Sympathomimetics	Increased sympathomimetic effect.
Thiazide diuretics	Increased amitriptyline effect.
Thyroid hormones	Irregular heartbeat.

INTERACTION WITH OTHER SUBSTANCES

INTERACTS WITH	COMBINED EFFECT
Alcohol: Beverages or medicines with alcohol.	Excessive intoxication. Avoid.
Beverages:	None expected.
Cocaine:	Excessive intoxication. Avoid.
Foods:	None expected.
Marijuana:	Excessive drowsiness. Avoid.
Tobacco:	None expected.

AMOBARBITAL

BRAND NAMES

Amytal
Dexamyl
Isobec
Tuinal (M)

GENERAL INFORMATION

Habit forming? Yes
Prescription needed? Yes
Available as generic? Yes
Drug class: Sedative, hypnotic (barbiturate)

USES

- Reduces anxiety or nervous tension (low dose).
- Relieves insomnia (higher bedtime dose).

DOSAGE & USAGE INFORMATION

How to take:
Tablet, capsule or liquid—Swallow with food or liquid to lessen stomach irritation. If you can't swallow whole, crumble tablet or open capsule and take with liquid or food.

When to take:
At the same times each day.

If you forget a dose:
Take as soon as you remember up to 2 hours late. If more than 2 hours, wait for next scheduled dose (don't double this dose).

What drug does:
May partially block nerve impulses at nerve-cell connections.

Time lapse before drug works:
60 minutes.

Don't take with:
- Non-prescription drugs without consulting doctor.
- See Interaction column and consult doctor.

OVERDOSE

Symptoms:
Deep sleep, weak pulse, coma.

What to do:
- Dial 0 (operator) or 911 (emergency) for an ambulance or medical help. Then give first aid immediately.
- If patient is unconscious and not breathing, give mouth-to-mouth breathing. If there is no heartbeat use cardiac massage and mouth-to-mouth breathing (CPR). Don't try to make patient vomit. If you can't help quickly, take patient to nearest emergency facility.
- Additional emergency information on page 886.

POSSIBLE ADVERSE REACTIONS OR SIDE EFFECTS

SYMPTOMS	FREQUENCY	WHAT TO DO
Brain & nervous system:		
● Dizziness, drowsiness, "hangover effect."	Common	4
● Depression, confusion, slurred speech.	Infrequent	4
● Agitation	Rare	3
Skin:		
● Rash or hives.	Infrequent	3
● Face, lip swelling.	Infrequent	3
Eyes:		
Eyelid swelling.	Infrequent	3
Ears, nose, throat:		
Sore throat, fever.	Infrequent	3
Digestive:		
Diarrhea, nausea, vomiting.	Infrequent	4
Heart & lungs:		
● Slow heartbeat.	Rare	3
● Breathing difficulty.	Rare	3
Blood vessels:		
Unexplained bleeding or bruising.	Rare	4
Muscles, bones, joints:		
Joint or muscle pain.	Infrequent	4
Genital, urinary:	None expected.	
Kidneys:	None expected.	
Liver:		
Jaundice (yellow skin and eyes).	Rare	3
Allergic:	None expected.	
Blood:	None expected.	
Others:	None expected.	

1- Life-threatening. Seek emergency treatment immediately.
2- Discontinue. Seek emergency treatment.
3- Discontinue. Call doctor right away.
4- Continue. Call doctor when convenient.

WARNINGS & PRECAUTIONS

Don't take if:
- You are allergic to any barbiturate.
- You have porphyria.

Before you start, consult your doctor:
- If you have epilepsy.
- If you have kidney or liver damage.
- If you have asthma.
- If you have anemia.
- If you have chronic pain.
- If you will have surgery within 2 months, including dental surgery, requiring general or spinal anesthesia.

Over age 60:
Adverse reactions and side effects may be more frequent and severe than in younger persons. Use small doses.

Pregnancy:
Risk to unborn child outweighs drug benefits. Don't use.

Breast-feeding:
Drug passes into milk. Avoid drug or discontinue nursing until you finish medicine. Consult doctor for advice on maintaining milk supply.

Infants & children:
Use only under doctor's supervision.

Prolonged use:
- May cause addiction, anemia, chronic intoxication.
- May lower body temperature, making exposure to cold temperatures hazardous.

Skin & sunlight:
May cause rash or intensify sunburn in areas exposed to sun or sunlamp.

Driving, piloting or hazardous work:
Don't drive or pilot aircraft until you learn how medicine affects you. Don't work around dangerous machinery. Don't climb ladders or work in high places. Danger increases if you drink alcohol or take medicine affecting alertness and reflexes.

Airplane passengers:
No problems expected.

Discontinuing:
May be unnecessary to finish medicine. Follow doctor's instructions. If you develop withdrawal symptoms of hallucinations, agitation or sleeplessness after discontinuing, call doctor right away.

Others:
No problems expected.

INTERACTION WITH OTHER DRUGS

GENERIC NAME OR DRUG CLASS	COMBINED EFFECT
Anticoagulants (oral)	Decreased anticoagulant effect.
Anticonvulsants	Changed seizure patterns.
Antidepressants (tricyclic)	Decreased antidepressant effect.
Antidiabetics (oral)	Increased amobarbital effect.
Antihistamines	Dangerous sedation. Avoid.
Antiinflammatory drugs (non-steroidal)	Decreased antiinflammatory effect.
Aspirin	Decreased aspirin effect.
Beta-adrenergic blockers	Decreased effect of beta-adrenergic blocker.
Contraceptives (oral)	Decreased contraceptive effect.
Cortisone drugs	Decreased cortisone effect.
Digitoxin	Decreased digitoxin effect.
Doxycycline	Decreased doxycycline effect.
Griseofulvin	Decreased griseofulvin effect.

Additional interactions on page 832.

INTERACTION WITH OTHER SUBSTANCES

INTERACTS WITH	COMBINED EFFECT
Alcohol:	Possible fatal oversedation. Avoid.
Beverages:	None expected.
Cocaine:	Decreased amobarbital effect.
Foods:	None expected.
Marijuana:	Excessive sedation. Avoid.
Tobacco:	None expected.

AMOXICILLIN

BRAND NAMES

Amoxil	Robamox
Larotid	Sumox
Novamoxin	Trimox
Penamox	Utimox
Polymox	Wymox

GENERAL INFORMATION

Habit forming? N●
Prescription needed? Yes
Available as generic? Yes
Drug class: Antibiotic (penicillin)

 ## USES

Treatment of bacterial infections that are susceptible to amoxicillin.

 ## DOSAGE & USAGE INFORMATION

How to take:
- Tablet or capsule—Swallow with liquid on an empty stomach 1 hour before or 2 hours after eating.
- Liquid—Take with cold beverage. Liquid form is perishable and effective for only 7 days at room temperature. Effective for 14 days if stored in refrigerator. Don't freeze.

When to take:
Follow instructions on prescription label or side of package. Doses should be evenly spaced. For example, 4 times a day means every 6 hours.

If you forget a dose:
Take as soon as you remember. Continue regular schedule.

What drug does:
Destroys susceptible bacteria. Does not kill viruses.

Time lapse before drug works:
May be several days before medicine affects infection.

Don't take with:
See Interaction column and consult doctor.

 ## OVERDOSE

Symptoms:
Severe diarrhea, nausea or vomiting.

What to do:
Overdose unlikely to threaten life. If person takes much larger amount than prescribed, call doctor, poison-control center or hospital emergency room for instructions.

 ## POSSIBLE ADVERSE REACTIONS OR SIDE EFFECTS

SYMPTOMS	FREQUENCY	WHAT TO DO
Brain & nervous system:	None expected.	
Skin: Hives, rash, intense itch soon after a dose.	Rare	1
Eyes:	None expected.	
Ears, nose, throat: Dark or discolored tongue.	Common	5
Digestive: Mild nausea, vomiting, diarrhea.	Infrequent	4
Heart & lungs:	None expected.	
Blood vessels: Unexplained bleeding.	Rare	3
Muscles, bones, joints:	None expected.	
Genital, urinary:	None expected.	
Kidneys:	None expected.	
Liver:	None expected.	
Allergic: Life-threatening anaphylaxis may occur!	Rare	1 See Page 888.
Blood:	None expected.	
Others:	None expected.	

1 - Life-threatening. Seek emergency treatment immediately.
2 - Discontinue. Seek emergency treatment.
3 - Discontinue. Call doctor right away.
4 - Continue. Call doctor when convenient.
5 - Continue. Tell doctor at next visit.
6 - No action necessary.

WARNINGS &
PRECAUTIONS

Don't take if:
You are allergic to amoxicillin, cephalosporin antibiotics, other penicillins or penicillamine. Life-threatening reaction may occur.

Before you start, consult your doctor:
If you are allergic to any substance or drug.

Over age 60:
You may have skin reactions, particularly around genitals and anus.

Pregnancy:
Studies inconclusive on harm to unborn child. Animal studies show fetal abnormalities. Decide with your doctor whether drug benefits justify risk to unborn child.

Breast-feeding:
Drug passes into milk. Child may become sensitive to penicillins and have allergic reactions to penicillin drugs. Avoid amoxicillin or discontinue nursing until you finish medicine. Consult doctor for advice on maintaining milk supply.

Infants & children:
No problems expected.

Prolonged use:
You may become more susceptible to infections caused by germs not responsive to amoxicillin.

Skin & sunlight:
No problems expected.

Driving, piloting or hazardous work:
Usually not dangerous. Most hazardous reactions likely to occur a few minutes after taking amoxicillin.

Airplane passengers:
No problems expected.

Discontinuing:
Don't discontinue without doctor's advice until you complete prescribed dose, even though symptoms diminish or disappear.

Others:
No problems expected.

INTERACTION WITH
OTHER DRUGS

GENERIC NAME OR DRUG CLASS	COMBINED EFFECT
Chloramphenicol	Decreased effect of both drugs.
Erythromycins	Decreased effect of both drugs.
Paromomycin	Decreased effect of both drugs.
Tetracyclines	Decreased effect of both drugs.
Troleandomycin	Decreased effect of both drugs.

INTERACTION WITH
OTHER SUBSTANCES

INTERACTS WITH	COMBINED EFFECT
Alcohol:	Occasional stomach irritation.
Beverages:	None expected.
Cocaine:	No proven problems.
Foods:	None expected.
Marijuana:	No proven problems.
Tobacco:	None expected.

AMPHETAMINE

BRAND NAMES

Amphaplex 10 & 20 (M)   Declobese (M)
Benzedrine   Obetrol 10 & 20 (M)
Biphetamine (M)

GENERAL INFORMATION

Habit forming? Yes
Prescription needed? Yes
Available as generic? Yes
Drug class: Central-nervous-system
stimulant (amphetamine)

USES

- Prevents narcolepsy (attacks of uncontrollable sleepiness).
- Controls hyperactivity in children.

DOSAGE & USAGE INFORMATION

How to take:
- Tablet—Swallow with liquid.
- Extended-release capsules—Swallow each dose whole with liquid.

When to take:
- At the same times each day.
- Short-acting form—Don't take later than 6 hours before bedtime.
- Long-acting form—Take on awakening.

If you forget a dose:
- Short-acting form—Take up to 2 hours late. If more than 2 hours, wait for next dose (don't double this).
- Long-acting form—Take as soon as you remember. Wait 20 hours for next dose.

What drug does:
- Narcolepsy—Apparently affects brain centers to decrease fatigue or sleepiness and increase alertness and motor activity.
- Hyperactive children—Calms children, opposite to effect on narcoleptic adults.

Time lapse before drug works:
15 to 30 minutes.

Don't take with:
See Interaction column and consult doctor.

OVERDOSE

Symptoms:
Rapid heartbeat, hyperactivity, high fever, hallucinations, suicidal or homicidal feelings, convulsions, coma.

What to do:
- Dial 0 (operator) or 911 (emergency) for an ambulance or medical help. Then give first aid immediately.
- Additional emergency information on page 886.

POSSIBLE ADVERSE REACTIONS OR SIDE EFFECTS

SYMPTOMS	FREQUENCY	WHAT TO DO
Brain & nervous system:		
● Headache	Infrequent	4
● Dizziness, lack of alertness.	Infrequent	3
● Mood changes.	Rare	4
● Irritability, nervousness, insomnia.	Common	4
Skin:		
Rash, hives.	Rare	3
Eyes:		
Blurred vision.	Infrequent	3
Ears, nose, throat:		
Dry mouth.	Common	5
Digestive:		
Diarrhea or constipation, appetite loss, stomach pain, nausea, vomiting, weight loss.	Infrequent	5
Heart & lungs:		
● Fast, pounding heartbeat.	Infrequent	3
● Chest pain or irregular heartbeat.	Rare	3
Blood vessels, kidneys, liver, allergic, blood:	None expected.	
Muscles, bones, joints:		
Uncontrolled movements of head, neck, arms, legs.	Rare	3
Genital, urinary:		
Decreased sex drive, impotence.	Infrequent	5
Others:		
● Enlarged breasts.	Rare	4
● Unusual sweating.	Infrequent	3

1-Life-threatening. Seek emergency treatment immediately.
2-Discontinue. Seek emergency treatment.
3-Discontinue. Call doctor right away.
4-Continue. Call doctor when convenient.
5-Continue. Tell doctor at next visit.

WARNINGS & PRECAUTIONS

Don't take if:
- You are allergic to any amphetamine.
- You will have surgery within 2 months, including dental surgery, requiring general or spinal anesthesia.

Before you start, consult your doctor:
- If you plan to become pregnant within medication period.
- If you have glaucoma.
- If you have heart or blood-vessel disease, or high blood pressure.
- If you have overactive thyroid, anxiety or tension.
- If you have a severe mental illness (especially children).

Over age 60:
Adverse reactions and side effects may be more frequent and severe than in younger persons.

Pregnancy:
Risk to unborn child outweighs drug benefits. Don't use.

Breast-feeding:
Drug passes into milk. Avoid drug or discontinue nursing.

Infants & children:
Not recommended for children under 12.

Prolonged use:
Habit forming.

Skin & sunlight:
No problems expected.

Driving, piloting or hazardous work:
Don't drive or pilot aircraft until you learn how medicine affects you. Don't work around dangerous machinery. Don't climb ladders or work in high places. Danger increases if you drink alcohol or take medicine affecting alertness and reflexes.

Airplane passengers:
No problems expected.

Discontinuing:
May be unnecessary to finish medicine. Follow doctor's instructions.

Others:
- This is a dangerous drug and must be closely supervised. Don't use for appetite control or depression. Potential for damage and abuse.
- During withdrawal phase, may cause prolonged sleep of several days.

INTERACTION WITH OTHER DRUGS

GENERIC NAME OR DRUG CLASS	COMBINED EFFECT
Anesthesias (general)	Irregular heartbeat.
Antidepressants (tricyclic)	Decreased amphetamine effect.
Antihypertensives	Decreased antihypertensive effect.
Carbonic anhydrase inhibitors	Increased amphetamine effect.
Guanethidine	Decreased guanethidine effect.
Haloperidol	Decreased amphetamine effect.
MAO inhibitors	May severely increase blood pressure.
Phenothiazines	Decreased amphetamine effect.
Sodium bicarbonate	Increased amphetamine effect.

INTERACTION WITH OTHER SUBSTANCES

INTERACTS WITH	COMBINED EFFECT
Alcohol:	Decreased amphetamine effect. Avoid.
Beverages: Caffeine drinks	Overstimulation. Avoid.
Cocaine:	Dangerous stimulation of nervous system. Avoid.
Foods:	None expected.
Marijuana:	Frequent use—Severely impaired mental function.
Tobacco:	None expected.

AMPICILLIN

BRAND NAMES

Alpen	Polycillin
Amcill	Prinicipen
Ampicin	SK-Ampicillin
Omnipen	Supen
Penbritin	Totacillin

GENERAL INFORMATION

Habit forming? No
Prescription needed? Yes
Available as generic? Yes
Drug class: Antibiotic (penicillin)

USES

Treatment of bacterial infections that are susceptible to ampicillin.

DOSAGE & USAGE INFORMATION

How to take:
- Tablets or capsules—Swallow with liquid on an empty stomach 1 hour before or 2 hours after eating.
- Liquid—Take with cold beverage. Liquid form is perishable and effective for only 7 days at room temperature. Effective for 14 days if stored in refrigerator. Don't freeze.

When to take:
Follow instructions on prescription label or side of package. Doses should be evenly spaced. For example, 4 times a day means every 6 hours.

If you forget a dose:
Take as soon as you remember. Continue regular schedule.

What drug does:
Destroys susceptible bacteria. Does not kill viruses.

Time lapse before drug works:
May be several days before medicine affects infection.

Don't take with:
See Interaction column and consult doctor.

OVERDOSE

Symptoms:
Severe diarrhea, nausea or vomiting.

What to do:
Overdose unlikely to threaten life. If person takes much larger amount than prescribed, call doctor, poison-control center or hospital emergency room for instructions.

POSSIBLE ADVERSE REACTIONS OR SIDE EFFECTS

SYMPTOMS	FREQUENCY	WHAT TO DO
Brain & nervous system:	None expected.	
Skin: Hives, rash, intense itch soon after a dose.	Rare	1
Eyes:	None expected.	
Ears, nose, throat: Dark or discolored tongue.	Common	5
Digestive: Mild nausea, vomiting, diarrhea.	Infrequent	4
Heart & lungs:	None expected.	
Blood vessels: Unexplained bleeding.	Rare	3
Muscles, bones, joints:	None expected.	
Genital, urinary:	None expected.	
Kidneys:	None expected.	
Liver:	None expected.	
Allergic: Life-threatening anaphylaxis may occur!	Rare	1 See page 888.
Blood:	None expected.	
Others:	None expected.	

1- Life-threatening. Seek emergency treatment immediately.
2- Discontinue. Seek emergency treatment.
3- Discontinue. Call doctor right away.
4- Continue. Call doctor when convenient.
5- Continue. Tell doctor at next visit.
6- No action necessary.

WARNINGS & PRECAUTIONS

Don't take if:
You are allergic to ampicillin, cephalosporin antibiotics, other penicillins or penicillamine. Life-threatening reaction may occur.

Before you start, consult your doctor:
If you are allergic to any substance or drug.

Over age 60:
You may have skin reactions, particularly around genitals and anus.

Pregnancy:
Studies inconclusive on harm to unborn child. Animal studies show fetal abnormalities. Decide with your doctor whether drug benefits justify risk to unborn child.

Breast-feeding:
Drug passes into milk. Child may become sensitive to penicillins and have allergic reactions to penicillin drugs. Avoid ampicillin or discontinue nursing until you finish medicine. Consult doctor for advice on maintaining milk supply.

Infants & children:
No problems expected.

Prolonged use:
You may become more susceptible to infections caused by germs not responsive to ampicillin.

Skin & sunlight:
No problems expected.

Driving, piloting or hazardous work:
Usually not dangerous. Most hazardous reactions likely to occur a few minutes after taking ampicillin.

Airplane passengers:
No problems expected.

Discontinuing:
Don't discontinue without doctor's advice until you complete prescribed dose, even though symptoms diminish or disappear.

Others:
Urine sugar test for diabetes may show false positive result.

INTERACTION WITH OTHER DRUGS

GENERIC NAME OR DRUG CLASS	COMBINED EFFECT
Chloramphenicol	Decreased effect of both drugs.
Erythromycins	Decreased effect of both drugs.
Paromomycin	Decreased effect of both drugs.
Tetracyclines	Decreased effect of both drugs.
Troleandomycin	Decreased effect of both drugs.

INTERACTION WITH OTHER SUBSTANCES

INTERACTS WITH	COMBINED EFFECT
Alcohol:	Occasional stomach irritation.
Beverages:	None expected.
Cocaine:	No proven problems.
Foods:	None expected.
Marijuana:	No proven problems.
Tobacco:	None expected.

ANESTHETICS (TOPICAL)

BRAND NAMES

Aero Caine Aerosol	Lidocaine Ointment
Americaine Aerosol	Nupercainal Cream
Americaine Ointment	Nupercainal Ointment
Benzocaine Topical	Nupercainal Spray
Cyclaine Solution	Xylocaine Ointment

See complete brand names list, page 820.

GENERAL INFORMATION

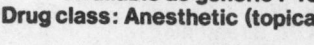

Habit forming? No
Prescription needed? High strength: Yes
Low strength: No
Available as generic? Yes
Drug class: Anesthetic (topical)

 ## USES

- Relieves pain and itch of sunburn, insect bites, scratches and other minor skin irritations.
- Relieves discomfort and itch of hemorrhoids and other disorders of anus and rectum.

 ## DOSAGE & USAGE INFORMATION

How to use:
- Suppositories—Remove wrapper and moisten suppository with water. Gently insert larger end into rectum. Push well into rectum with finger.
- All other forms—Use only enough to cover irritated area. Follow instructions on label.

When to use:
When needed for discomfort, no more often than every hour.

If you forget an application:
Use as needed.

What drug does:
Blocks pain impulses from skin to brain.

Time lapse before drug works:
3 to 15 minutes.

Don't take with:
See Interaction column and consult doctor.

 ## OVERDOSE

Symptoms:
If swallowed or inhaled—Dizziness, nervousness, trembling, seizures.

What to do:
- Dial 0 (operator) or 911 (emergency) for an ambulance or medical help. Then give first aid immediately.
- Additional emergency information on page 886.

 ## POSSIBLE ADVERSE REACTIONS OR SIDE EFFECTS

SYMPTOMS	FREQUENCY	WHAT TO DO
Brain & nervous system:		
• Dizziness	Infrequent	4
• Nervousness, trembling.	Infrequent	3
Skin: Hives, rash, itch, inflammation or tenderness not present before application.	Infrequent	3
Eyes: Blurred vision.	Infrequent	4
Ears, nose, throat:	None expected.	
Digestive:	None expected.	
Heart & lungs: Slow heartbeat.	Infrequent	3
Blood vessels:	None expected.	
Muscles, bones, joints: Swelling of feet.	Infrequent	4
Genital, urinary:		
• Bloody urine.	Rare	3
• Increased or painful urination.	Rare	4
Kidneys:	None expected.	
Liver:	None expected.	
Allergic:	None expected.	
Blood:	None expected.	
Others:	None expected.	

1- Life-threatening. Seek emergency treatment immediately.
2- Discontinue. Seek emergency treatment.
3- Discontinue. Call doctor right away.
4- Continue. Call doctor when convenient.

WARNINGS & PRECAUTIONS

Don't use if:
You are allergic to any topical anesthetic.

Before you start, consult your doctor:
- If you have skin infection at site of treatment.
- If you have had severe or extensive skin disorders such as eczema or psoriasis.
- If you have bleeding hemorrhoids.

Over age 60:
Adverse reactions and side effects may be more frequent and severe than in younger persons.

Pregnancy:
No proven harm to unborn child. Avoid if possible.

Breast-feeding:
No problems expected.

Infants & children:
Use caution. More likely to be absorbed through skin and cause adverse reactions.

Prolonged use:
Possible excess absorption. Don't use longer than 3 days for any one problem.

Skin & sunlight:
No problems expected.

Driving, piloting or hazardous work:
No problems expected.

Airplane passengers:
No problems expected.

Discontinuing:
May be unnecessary to finish medicine. Follow doctor's instructions.

Others:
No problems expected.

INTERACTION WITH OTHER DRUGS

GENERIC NAME OR DRUG CLASS	COMBINED EFFECT
Sulfa drugs	Decreased antiinfective effect of sulfa drugs.

INTERACTION WITH OTHER SUBSTANCES

INTERACTS WITH	COMBINED EFFECT
Alcohol:	None expected.
Beverages:	None expected.
Cocaine:	Possible nervous-system toxicity. Avoid.
Foods:	None expected.
Marijuana:	None expected.
Tobacco:	None expected.

ANISINDIONE

BRAND NAMES

Miradon

GENERAL INFORMATION

Habit forming? No
Prescription needed? Yes
Available as generic? Yes
Drug class: Anticoagulant

 USES

Reduces blood clots. Used for abnormal clotting inside blood vessels.

 DOSAGE & USAGE INFORMATION

How to take:
Tablet—Swallow with liquid. If you can't swallow whole, crumble tablet and take with liquid or food.

When to take:
At the same time each day.

If you forget a dose:
Take as soon as you remember up to 12 hours late. If more than 12 hours, wait for next scheduled dose (don't double this dose). Inform your doctor of any missed doses.

What drug does:
Blocks action of vitamin K necessary for blood clotting.

Time lapse before drug works:
36 to 48 hours.

Don't take with:
See Interaction column and consult doctor.

 OVERDOSE

Symptoms:
Bloody vomit and bloody or black stools, red urine.

What to do:
- Dial 0 (operator) or 911 (emergency) for an ambulance or medical help. Then give first aid immediately.
- Additional emergency information on page 886.

POSSIBLE ADVERSE REACTIONS OR SIDE EFFECTS

SYMPTOMS	FREQUENCY	WHAT TO DO
Brain & nervous system: Dizziness, headache.	Rare	3
Skin: Rash, hives, itch.	Infrequent	3
Eyes: Blurred vision.	Infrequent	3
Ears, nose, throat:		
• Sore throat.	Infrequent	3
• Mouth sores.	Rare	3
Digestive:		
• Black stools or bloody vomit.	Infrequent	2
• Diarrhea, cramps, nausea, vomiting.	Infrequent	4
• Bloating, gas.	Common	5
Heart & lungs: Coughing up blood.	Infrequent	2
Blood vessels: Easy bruising, bleeding.	Infrequent	3
Muscles, bones, joints: Swollen feet, legs.	Infrequent	4
Genital, urinary: Cloudy or red urine.	Infrequent	3
Kidneys: Back pain.	Infrequent	3
Liver: Jaundice (yellow skin and eyes).	Infrequent	3
Allergic, blood:	None expected.	
Others:		
• Fever, chills.	Infrequent	3
• Hair loss.	Infrequent	4
• Fatigue, weakness.	Infrequent	3

1- Life-threatening. Seek emergency treatment immediately.
2- Discontinue. Seek emergency treatment.
3- Discontinue. Call doctor right away.
4- Continue. Call doctor when convenient.
5- Continue. Tell doctor at next visit.

WARNINGS & PRECAUTIONS

Don't take if:
- You have been allergic to any oral anticoagulant.
- You have a bleeding disorder.
- You have an active peptic ulcer.
- You have ulcerative colitis.

Before you start, consult your doctor:
- If you take any other drugs, including non-prescription drugs.
- If you have high blood pressure.
- If you have heavy or prolonged menstrual periods.
- If you have diabetes.
- If you have a bladder catheter.
- If you have serious liver or kidney disease.
- If you will have surgery within 2 months, including dental surgery, requiring general or spinal anesthesia.

Over age 60:
Adverse reactions and side effects may be more frequent and severe than in younger persons.

Pregnancy:
Risk to unborn child outweighs drug benefits. Don't use.

Breast-feeding:
Drug filters into milk. May harm child. Avoid.

Infants & children:
Use only under doctor's supervision.

Prolonged use:
No problems expected.

Skin & sunlight:
No problems expected.

Driving, piloting or hazardous work:
- Avoid hazardous activities that could cause injury.
- Don't drive if you feel dizzy or have blurred vision.

Airplane passengers:
No problems expected.

Discontinuing:
Don't discontinue without consulting doctor. Dose may require gradual reduction if you have taken drug for a long time. Doses of other drugs may also require adjustment.

Others:
Carry identification to state you take anticoagulants.

INTERACTION WITH OTHER DRUGS

GENERIC NAME OR DRUG CLASS	COMBINED EFFECT
Acetaminophen	Increased anisindione effect.
Allopurinol	Increased anisindione effect.
Androgens	Increased anisindione effect.
Antacids (large doses)	Decreased anisindione effect.
Antibiotics	Increased anisindione effect.
Anticonvulsants (hydantoin)	Increased effect of both drugs.
Antidepressants (tricyclic)	Increased anisindione effect.
Antidiabetics (oral)	Increased anisindione effect.
Antihistamines	Unpredictable increased or decreased anticoagulant effect.
Barbiturates	Decreased anisindione effect.
Benzodiazepines	Unpredictable increased or decreased anticoagulant effect.

Additional interactions on page 832

INTERACTION WITH OTHER SUBSTANCES

INTERACTS WITH	COMBINED EFFECT
Alcohol:	Can increase or decrease effect of anticoagulant. Use with caution.
Beverages:	None expected.
Cocaine:	None expected.
Foods: High in vitamin K such as fish, liver, spinach, cabbage.	May decrease anticoagulant effect.
Marijuana:	None expected.
Tobacco:	None expected.

ASPIRIN

BRAND NAMES

Alka-Seltzer (M)   A.P.C.-   Bayer   Empirin
Anacin (M)   Demerol (M)   Bufferin   St. Joseph
See complete brand names
list on page 821.

USES

- Reduces pain, fever, inflammation.
- Relieves swelling, stiffness, joint pain of arthritis or rheumatism.

DOSAGE & USAGE INFORMATION

How to take:
- Tablet or capsule—Swallow with liquid.
- Extended-release tablets or capsules—Swallow each dose whole.
- Suppositories—Remove wrapper and moisten suppository with water. Gently insert into rectum, large end first.

When to take:
Pain, fever, inflammation—As needed, no more often than every 4 hours.

If you forget a dose:
- Pain, fever—Take as soon as you remember. Wait 4 hours for next dose.
- Arthritis—Take as soon as you remember up to 2 hours late. Return to regular schedule.

What drug does:
- Affects hypothalamus, part of brain which regulates temperature by dilating small blood vessels in skin.
- Prevents clumping of platelets (small blood cells) so blood vessels remain open.
- Decreases prostaglandin effect.
- Suppresses body's pain messages.

Time lapse before drug works:
30 minutes for pain, fever, arthritis.

Don't take with:
- Tetracyclines. Space doses 1 hour apart.
- See Interaction column and consult doctor.

OVERDOSE

Symptoms:
Ringing in ears; nausea; vomiting; dizziness; fever; deep, rapid breathing; hallucinations; convulsions; coma.

What to do:
- Dial 0 (operator) or 911 (emergency) for an ambulance or medical help. Then give first aid immediately.
- Additional emergency information on page 886.

GENERAL INFORMATION

Habit forming? No
Prescription needed? No
Available as generic? Yes
Drug class: Analgesic, antinflammatory (salicylate)

POSSIBLE ADVERSE REACTIONS OR SIDE EFFECTS

SYMPTOMS	FREQUENCY	WHAT TO DO
Brain & nervous system: Drowsiness	Rare	4
Skin: Rash, hives, itch.	Rare	3
Eyes: Diminished vision.	Rare	3
Ears, nose, throat: Ringing in ears.	Common	5
Digestive: • Nausea, vomiting, abdominal pain.	Common	2
• Black stools.	Rare	2
• Black or bloody vomit.	Rare	1
• Heartburn, indigestion.	Common	4
Heart & lungs: Shortness of breath, wheezing.	Rare	3
Blood vessels, muscles, bones, joints, kidneys, blood:	None expected.	
Genital, urinary: Blood in urine.	Rare	1
Liver: Jaundice (yellow eyes and skin).	Rare	3
Allergic: Life-threatening anaphylaxis may occur!	Rare	1 See page 888.
Others: Unexplained fever.	Rare	2

1 - Life-threatening. Seek emergency treatment immediately.
2 - Discontinue. Seek emergency treatment.
3 - Discontinue. Call doctor right away.
4 - Continue. Call doctor when convenient.
5 - Continue. Tell doctor at next visit.
6 - No action necessary.

WARNINGS & PRECAUTIONS

Don't take if:
- You need to restrict sodium in your diet. Buffered effervescent tablets and sodium salicylate are high in sodium.
- Aspirin has a strong vinegar-like odor, which means it has decomposed.
- You have a peptic ulcer of stomach or duodenum.
- You have a bleeding disorder.

Before you start, consult your doctor:
- If you have had stomach or duodenal ulcers.
- If you have had gout.
- If you have asthma or nasal polyps.

Over age 60:
More likely to cause hidden bleeding in stomach or intestines. Watch for dark stools.

Pregnancy:
Risk to unborn child outweighs drug benefits. Don't use.

Breast-feeding:
Drug passes into milk. Avoid drug or discontinue nursing until you finish medicine. Consult doctor for advice on maintaining milk supply.

Infants & children:
Overdose frequent and severe. Keep bottles out of children's reach.

Prolonged use:
Kidney damage. Periodic kidney-function test recommended.

Skin & sunlight:
Aspirin combined with sunscreen may decrease sunburn.

Driving, piloting or hazardous work:
No restrictions unless you feel drowsy.

Airplane passengers:
No problems expected.

Discontinuing:
For chronic illness—Don't discontinue without doctor's advice until you complete prescribed dose, even though symptoms diminish or disappear.

Others:
- Aspirin can complicate surgery, pregnancy, labor and delivery, and illness.
- For arthritis—Don't change dose without consulting doctor.
- Urine tests for blood sugar may be inaccurate.

 INTERACTION WITH OTHER DRUGS

GENERIC NAME OR DRUG CLASS	COMBINED EFFECT
Allopurinol	Decreased allopurinol effect.
Antacids	Decreased aspirin effect.
Anticoagulants	Increased anticoagulant effect. Abnormal bleeding.
Antidiabetics (oral)	Low blood sugar.
Antiinflammatory drugs (non-steroid)	Risk of stomach bleeding and ulcers.
Aspirin (other)	Likely aspirin toxicity.
Cortisone drugs	Increased cortisone effect. Risk of ulcers and stomach bleeding.
Furosemide	Possible aspirin toxicity.
Indomethacin	Risk of stomach bleeding and ulcers.
Methotrexate	Increased methotrexate effect.
Para-aminosalicylic acid (PAS)	Possible aspirin toxicity.
Penicillins	Increased effect of both drugs.
Phenobarbital	Decreased aspirin effect.
Phenytoin	Increased phenytoin effect.

Additional interactions on page 833.

 INTERACTION WITH OTHER SUBSTANCES

INTERACTS WITH	COMBINED EFFECT
Alcohol:	Possible stomach irritation and bleeding. Avoid.
Beverages:	None expected.
Cocaine:	None expected.
Foods:	None expected.
Marijuana:	Possible increased pain relief, but marijuana may slow body's recovery. Avoid.
Tobacco:	None expected.

ATENOLOL

BRAND NAMES

Tenormin

GENERAL INFORMATION

Habit forming? No
Prescription needed? Yes
Available as generic? No
Drug class: Beta-adrenergic blocker

USES

- Reduces angina attacks.
- Stabilizes irregular heartbeat.
- Lowers blood pressure.
- Reduces frequency of migraine headaches. (Does not relieve headache pain.)
- Other uses prescribed by your doctor.

DOSAGE & USAGE INFORMATION

How to take:
Tablet or capsule—Swallow with liquid. If you can't swallow whole, crumble tablet or open capsule and take with liquid or food.

When to take:
With meals or immediately after.

If you forget a dose:
Take as soon as you remember. Return to regular schedule, but allow 3 hours between doses.

What drug does:
- Blocks certain actions of sympathetic nervous system.
- Lowers heart's oxygen requirements.
- Slows nerve impulses through heart.
- Reduces blood vessel contraction in heart, scalp and other body parts.

Time lapse before drug works:
1 to 4 hours.

Don't take with:
Non-prescription drugs or drugs in Interaction column without consulting doctor.

OVERDOSE

Symptoms:
Weakness, slow or weak pulse, blood pressure drop, fainting, convulsions, cold and sweaty skin.

What to do:
- Dial O (operator) or 911 (emergency) for an ambulance or medical help. Then give first aid immediately.
- Additional emergency information on page 886.

POSSIBLE ADVERSE REACTIONS OR SIDE EFFECTS

SYMPTOMS	FREQUENCY	WHAT TO DO
Brain & nervous system:		
• Hallucinations, nightmares, insomnia, headache.	Infrequent	3
• Confusion, depression, reduced alertness.	Infrequent	4
• Drowsiness, numbness or tingling of fingers or toes, dizziness.	Common	4
Skin: Rash	Rare	3
Eyes:	None expected.	
Ears, nose, throat: Sore throat, fever.	Rare	3
Digestive:		
• Diarrhea, nausea.	Common	4
• Constipation	Infrequent	5
Heart & lungs:		
• Pulse slower than 50 beats per minute.	Common	3
• Breathing difficulty.	Infrequent	3
Blood vessels: Cold hands, feet.	Common	5
Muscles, bones, joints, genital, urinary, kidneys, liver, allergic:	None expected.	
Blood: Unusual bleeding and bruising.	Rare	4
Others:		
• Fatigue, weakness.	Common	4
• Dry mouth, eyes, skin.	Common	5

1-Life-threatening. Seek emergency treatment immediately.
2-Discontinue. Seek emergency treatment.
3-Discontinue. Call doctor right away.
4-Continue. Call doctor when convenient.
5-Continue. Tell doctor at next visit.

ATENOLOL

 WARNINGS & PRECAUTIONS

Don't take if:
- You are allergic to any beta-adrenergic blocker.
- You have asthma.
- You have hay fever symptoms.
- You have taken MAO inhibitors in past 2 weeks.

Before you start, consult your doctor:
- If you have heart disease or poor circulation to the extremities.
- If you have hay fever, asthma, chronic bronchitis, emphysema.
- If you have overactive thyroid function.
- If you have impaired liver or kidney function.
- If you will have surgery within 2 months, including dental surgery, requiring general or spinal anesthesia.
- If you have diabetes or hypoglycemia.

Over age 60:
Adverse reactions and side effects may be more frequent and severe than in younger persons.

Pregnancy:
Risk to unborn child outweighs drug benefits. Don't use.

Breast-feeding:
Drug passes into milk. Avoid drug or discontinue nursing until you finish medicine. Consult doctor for advice on maintaining milk supply.

Infants & children:
Not recommended.

Prolonged use:
Weakens heart muscle contractions.

Skin & sunlight:
No problems expected.

Driving, piloting or hazardous work:
Don't drive or pilot aircraft until you learn how medicine affects you. Don't work around dangerous machinery. Don't climb ladders or work in high places. Danger increases if you drink alcohol or take medicine affecting alertness and reflexes.

Airplane passengers:
No problems expected.

Discontinuing:
Don't discontinue without consulting doctor. Dose may require gradual reduction if you have taken drug for a long time. Doses of other drugs may also require adjustment.

Others:
May mask hypoglycemia.

 INTERACTION WITH OTHER DRUGS

GENERIC NAME OR DRUG CLASS	COMBINED EFFECT
Antidiabetics	Increased antidiabetic effect.
Antihistamines	Decreased antihistamine effect.
Antihypertensives	Increased antihypertensive effect.
Antiinflammatory drugs	Decreased antiinflammatory effect.
Barbiturates	Increased barbiturate effect. Dangerous sedation.
Digitalis preparations	Can either increase or decrease heart rate. Improves irregular heartbeat.
Narcotics	Increased narcotic effect. Dangerous sedation.
Phenytoin	Increased atenolol effect.
Quinidine	Slows heart excessively.
Reserpine	Increased reserpine effect. Excessive sedation and depression.

 INTERACTION WITH OTHER SUBSTANCES

INTERACTS WITH	COMBINED EFFECT
Alcohol:	Excessive blood pressure drop. Avoid.
Beverages:	None expected.
Cocaine:	Irregular heartbeat. Avoid.
Foods:	None expected.
Marijuana:	Daily use—Impaired circulation to hands and feet.
Tobacco:	Possible irregular heartbeat.

ATROPINE

BRAND NAMES

Atrobarbital (M)	Bellergal-S (M)	Donnamine (M)
Atrosed (M)	Butibel (M)	Donnatal (M)
Barbidonna (M)	Chardonna (M)	Isopto Atropine
Belladenal (M)	Contac (M)	Kinesed (M)
Bellergal (M)	Donnagel (M)	Prydon

See complete brand names list, page 822.

GENERAL INFORMATION

Habit forming? No
Prescription needed? Low strength: No
High strength: Yes
Available as generic? Yes
Drug class: Antispasmodic, anticholinergic

USES

Reduces spasms of digestive system, bladder and urethra.

DOSAGE & USAGE INFORMATION

How to take:
Tablet—Swallow with liquid or food to lessen stomach irritation.

When to take:
30 minutes before meals (unless directed otherwise by doctor).

If you forget a dose:
Take as soon as you remember up to 2 hours late. If more than 2 hours, wait for next scheduled dose (don't double this dose).

What drug does:
Blocks nerve impulses at parasympathetic nerve endings, preventing muscle contractions and gland secretions of organs involved.

Time lapse before drug works:
15 to 30 minutes.

Don't take with:
See Interaction column and consult doctor.

OVERDOSE

Symptoms:
Dilated pupils; rapid pulse and breathing; dizziness; fever; hallucinations; confusion; slurred speech; agitation; flushed face; convulsions; coma.

What to do:
- Dial 0 (operator) or 911 (emergency) for an ambulance or medical help. Then give first aid immediately.
- Additional emergency information on page 886.

POSSIBLE ADVERSE REACTIONS OR SIDE EFFECTS

SYMPTOMS	FREQUENCY	WHAT TO DO
Brain & nervous system:		
• Headache	Infrequent	4
• Confusion, delirium.	Common	3
Skin:		
Rash or hives.	Rare	3
Eyes:		
Pain, blurred vision.	Rare	3
Ears, nose, throat:		
Dryness	Common	6
Digestive:		
• Constipation	Common	5
• Nausea, vomiting.	Common	4
Heart & lungs:		
Rapid heartbeat.	Common	3
Blood vessels:	None expected.	
Muscles, bones, joints:	None expected.	
Genital, urinary:		
Difficult urination.	Infrequent	4
Kidneys:	None expected.	
Liver:	None expected.	
Allergic:	None expected.	
Blood:	None expected.	
Others:		
Less perspiration.	Common	4

1- Life-threatening. Seek emergency treatment immediately.
2- Discontinue. Seek emergency treatment.
3- Discontinue. Call doctor right away.
4- Continue. Call doctor when convenient.
5- Continue. Tell doctor at next visit.
6- No action necessary.

WARNINGS & PRECAUTIONS

Don't take if:
- You are allergic to any anticholinergic.
- You have trouble with stomach bloating.
- You have difficulty emptying your bladder completely.
- You have narrow-angle glaucoma.
- You have severe ulcerative colitis.

Before you start, consult your doctor:
- If you have open-angle glaucoma.
- If you have angina.
- If you have chronic bronchitis or asthma.
- If you have liver disease.
- If you have hiatal hernia.
- If you have enlarged prostate.
- If you have myasthenia gravis.
- If you have peptic ulcer.
- If you will have surgery within 2 months, including dental surgery, requiring general or spinal anesthesia.

Over age 60:
Adverse reactions and side effects may be more frequent and severe than in younger persons.

Pregnancy:
Studies inconclusive on harm to unborn child. Animal studies show fetal abnormalities. Decide with your doctor whether drug benefits justify risk to unborn child.

Breast-feeding:
Drug passes into milk and decreases milk flow. Avoid drug or discontinue nursing until you finish medicine. Consult doctor for advice on maintaining milk supply.

Infants & children:
Use only under medical supervision.

Prolonged use:
Chronic constipation, possible fecal impaction. Consult doctor immediately.

Skin & sunlight:
No problems expected.

Driving, piloting or hazardous work:
Use disqualifies you for piloting aircraft. Otherwise, no problems expected.

Airplane passengers:
No problems expected.

Discontinuing:
May be unnecessary to finish medicine. Follow doctor's instructions.

Others:
No problems expected.

 ## INTERACTION WITH OTHER DRUGS

GENERIC NAME OR DRUG CLASS	COMBINED EFFECT
Amantadine	Increased atropine effect.
Anticholinergics (other)	Increased atropine effect.
Antidepressants (tricyclic)	Increased atropine effect.
Antihistamines	Increased atropine effect.
Cortisone drugs	Increased internal-eye pressure.
Haloperidol	Increased internal-eye pressure.
MAO inhibitors	Increased atropine effect.
Meperidine	Increased atropine effect.
Methylphenidate	Increased atropine effect.
Orphenadrine	Increased atropine effect.
Phenothiazines	Increased atropine effect.
Pilocarpine	Loss of pilocarpine effect in glaucoma treatment.
Vitamin C	Decreased atropine effect. Avoid large doses of vitamin C.

 ## INTERACTION WITH OTHER SUBSTANCES

INTERACTS WITH	COMBINED EFFECT
Alcohol:	None expected.
Beverages:	None expected.
Cocaine:	Excessively rapid heartbeat. Avoid.
Foods:	None expected.
Marijuana:	Drowsiness and dry mouth.
Tobacco:	None expected.

AZATADINE

BRAND NAMES

Optimine

GENERAL INFORMATION

Habit forming? No
Prescription needed? Yes
Available as generic? No
Drug class: Antihistamine

 ## USES

- Reduces allergic symptoms such as hay fever, hives, rash or itching.
- Induces sleep.

 ## DOSAGE & USAGE INFORMATION

How to take:
Tablet—Swallow with liquid or food to lessen stomach irritation.

When to take:
Varies with form. Follow label directions.

If you forget a dose:
Take as soon as you remember up to 2 hours late. If more than 2 hours, wait for next scheduled dose (don't double this dose).

What drug does:
Blocks action of histamine after an allergic response triggers histamine release in sensitive cells.

Time lapse before drug works:
30 minutes.

Don't take with:
See Interaction column and consult doctor.

 ## OVERDOSE

Symptoms:
Convulsions, red face, hallucinations, coma.

What to do:
- Dial 0 (operator) or 911 (emergency) for an ambulance or medical help. Then give first aid immediately.
- If patient is unconscious and not breathing, give mouth-to-mouth breathing. If there is no heartbeat, use cardiac massage and mouth-to-mouth breathing (CPR). Don't try to make patient vomit. If you can't get help quickly, take patient to nearest emergency facility.
- Additional emergency information on page 886.

POSSIBLE ADVERSE REACTIONS OR SIDE EFFECTS

SYMPTOMS	FREQUENCY	WHAT TO DO
Brain & nervous system:		
• Nightmares, agitation, irritability.	Rare	3
• Drowsiness, dizziness.	Common	5
Skin:	None expected.	
Eyes:		
• Vision changes.	Infrequent	3
• Less tolerance for contact lenses.	Infrequent	4
Ears, nose, throat:		
• Sore throat, fever.	Rare	3
• Dry mouth, nose, throat.	Common	5
Digestive:		
• Nausea	Common	5
• Appetite loss.	Infrequent	5
Heart & lungs: Rapid heartbeat.	Rare	3
Blood vessels: Unusual bleeding or bruising.	Rare	3
Muscles, bones, joints, kidneys, liver, allergic, blood:	None expected.	
Genital, urinary: Urination difficulty.	Infrequent	4
Others: Fatigue, weakness.	Rare	3

1 - Life-threatening. Seek emergency treatment immediately.
2 - Discontinue. Seek emergency treatment.
3 - Discontinue. Call doctor right away.
4 - Continue. Call doctor when convenient.
5 - Continue. Tell doctor at next visit.
6 - No action necessary.

AZATADINE

WARNINGS & PRECAUTIONS

Don't take if:
You are allergic to any antihistamine.

Before you start, consult your doctor:
- If you have glaucoma.
- If you have enlarged prostate.
- If you have asthma.
- If you have kidney disease.
- If you have peptic ulcer.
- If you will have surgery within 2 months, including dental surgery, requiring general or spinal anesthesia.

Over age 60:
Don't exceed recommended dose. Adverse reactions and side effects may be more frequent and severe than in younger persons, especially urination difficulty, diminished alertness and other brain and nervous-system symptoms.

Pregnancy:
No proven harm to unborn child. Avoid if possible.

Breast-feeding:
Drug passes into milk. Avoid drug or discontinue nursing until you finish medicine. Consult doctor for advice on maintaining milk supply.

Infants & children:
Not recommended for premature or newborn infants. Otherwise, no problems expected.

Prolonged use:
Avoid. May damage bone-marrow and nerve cells.

Skin & sunlight:
May cause rash or intensify sunburn in areas exposed to sun or sunlamp.

Driving, piloting or hazardous work:
Don't drive or pilot aircraft until you learn how medicine affects you. Don't work around dangerous machinery. Don't climb ladders or work in high places. Danger increases if you drink alcohol or take medicine affecting alertness and reflexes, such as antihistamines, tranquilizers, sedatives, pain medicine, narcotics and mind-altering drugs.

Airplane passengers:
No problems expected.

Discontinuing:
No problems expected.

Others:
May mask symptoms of hearing damage from aspirin, other salicylates, cisplatin, paromomycin, vancomycin or anticonvulsants. Consult doctor if you use these.

INTERACTION WITH OTHER DRUGS

GENERIC NAME OR DRUG CLASS	COMBINED EFFECT
Anticholinergics	Increased anticholinergic effect.
Antidepressants	Excess sedation. Avoid.
Antihistamines (other)	Excess sedation. Avoid.
Hypnotics	Excess sedation. Avoid.
MAO inhibitors	Increased azatadine effect.
Mind-altering drugs	Excess sedation. Avoid.
Narcotics	Excess sedation. Avoid.
Sedatives	Excess sedation. Avoid.
Sleep inducers	Excess sedation. Avoid.
Tranquilizers	Excess sedation. Avoid.

INTERACTION WITH OTHER SUBSTANCES

INTERACTS WITH	COMBINED EFFECT
Alcohol:	Excess sedation. Avoid.
Beverages: Caffeine drinks	Less azatadine sedation.
Cocaine:	Decreased azatadine effect. Avoid.
Foods:	None expected.
Marijuana:	Excess sedation. Avoid.
Tobacco:	None expected.

BACAMPICILLIN

BRAND NAMES

Spectrobid

GENERAL INFORMATION

Habit forming? No
Prescription needed? Yes
Available as generic? No
Drug class: Antibiotic (penicillin)

USES

Treatment of bacterial infections that are susceptible to bacampicillin.

DOSAGE & USAGE INFORMATION

How to take:
- Tablets or capsules—Swallow with liquid on an empty stomach 1 hour before meals or 2 hours after eating.
- Liquid—Take with cold beverage. Liquid form is perishable and effective for only 7 days at room temperature. Effective for 14 days if stored in refrigerator. Don't freeze.

When to take:
Follow instructions on prescription label or side of package. Doses should be evenly spaced. For example, 4 times a day means every 6 hours.

If you forget a dose:
Take as soon as you remember. Continue regular schedule.

What drug does:
Destroys susceptible bacteria. Does not kill viruses.

Time lapse before drug works:
May be several days before medicine affects infection.

Don't take with:
See Interaction column and consult doctor.

OVERDOSE

Symptoms:
Severe diarrhea, nausea or vomiting.

What to do:
Overdose unlikely to threaten life. If person takes much larger amount than prescribed, call doctor, poison-control center or hospital emergency room for specific instructions.

POSSIBLE ADVERSE REACTIONS OR SIDE EFFECTS

SYMPTOMS	FREQUENCY	WHAT TO DO
Brain & nervous system:	None expected.	
Skin: Hives, rash, intense itch soon after a dose.	Rare	1
Eyes:	None expected.	
Ears, nose, throat: Dark or discolored tongue.	Common	5
Digestive: Mild nausea, vomiting, diarrhea.	Infrequent	4
Heart & lungs:	None expected.	
Blood vessels: Unexplained bleeding.	Rare	3
Muscles, bones, joints:	None expected.	
Genital, urinary:	None expected.	
Kidneys:	None expected.	
Liver:	None expected.	
Allergic: Life-threatening anaphylaxis may occur!	Rare	1 See Page 888.
Blood:	None expected.	

1- Life-threatening. Seek emergency treatment immediately.
2- Discontinue. Seek emergency treatment.
3- Discontinue. Call doctor right away.
4- Continue. Call doctor when convenient.
5- Continue. Tell doctor at next visit.
6- No action necessary.

WARNINGS & PRECAUTIONS

Don't take if:
You are allergic to bacampicillin, cephalosporin antibiotics, other penicillins or penicillamine. Life-threatening reaction may occur.

Before you start, consult your doctor:
If you are allergic to any substance or drug.

Over age 60:
You may have skin reactions, particularly around genitals and anus.

Pregnancy:
Studies inconclusive on harm to unborn child. Animal studies show fetal abnormalities. Decide with your doctor whether drug benefits justify risk to unborn child.

Breast-feeding:
Drug passes into milk. Child may become sensitive to this and all penicillins. Avoid bacampicillin or discontinue nursing until you finish medicine. Consult doctor for advice on maintaining milk supply.

Infants & children:
No problems expected.

Prolonged use:
You may become more susceptible to infections caused by germs not responsive to bacampicillin.

Skin & sunlight:
No problems expected.

Driving, piloting, or hazardous work:
Usually not dangerous. Most hazardous reactions likely to occur a few minutes after taking bacampicillin.

Airplane passengers:
No problems expected.

Discontinuing:
Don't discontinue without doctor's advice until you complete prescribed dose, even though symptoms diminish or disappear.

Others:
Urine sugar test for diabetes may show false positive result.

INTERACTION WITH OTHER DRUGS

GENERIC NAME OR DRUG CLASS	COMBINED EFFECT
Chloramphenicol	Decreased effect of both drugs.
Erythromycins	Decreased effect of both drugs.
Paromomycin	Decreased effect of both drugs.
Tetracyclines	Decreased effect of both drugs.
Troleandomycin	Decreased effect of both drugs.

INTERACTION WITH OTHER SUBSTANCES

INTERACTS WITH	COMBINED EFFECT
Alcohol:	Occasional stomach irritation.
Beverages:	None expected.
Cocaine:	No proven problems.
Foods:	None expected.
Marijuana:	No proven problems.
Tobacco:	None expected.

BECLOMETHASONE

BRAND NAMES

Beclovent Inhaler
Vanceril Inhaler

GENERAL INFORMATION

Habit forming? No
Prescription needed? Yes
Available as generic? No
Drug class: Cortisone drug (adrenocorticosteroid),
antiasthmatic

 ## USES

Prevents attacks of bronchial asthma and allergic hay fever. Does not stop an active asthma attack.

 ## DOSAGE & USAGE INFORMATION

How to take:
Follow package instructions. Don't inhale more than twice per dose. Rinse mouth after use to prevent hoarseness, throat irritation and mouth infection.

When to take:
Regularly at the same times each day.

If you forget a dose:
Take as soon as you remember up to 2 hours late. If more than 2 hours, wait for next scheduled dose (don't double this dose).

What drug does:
Reduces inflammation in bronchial tubes.

Time lapse before drug works:
1 to 4 weeks.

Don't take with:
See Interaction column and consult doctor.

 ## OVERDOSE

Symptoms:
Fluid retention, flushed face, nervousness, stomach irritation.

What to do:
Overdose unlikely to threaten life. If person inhales much larger amount than prescribed, call doctor, poison-control center or hospital emergency room for instructions.

 ## POSSIBLE ADVERSE REACTIONS OR SIDE EFFECTS

SYMPTOMS	FREQUENCY	WHAT TO DO
Brain & nervous system:	None expected.	
Skin: Rash	Infrequent	3
Eyes:	None expected.	
Ears, nose, throat: Fungus infection with white patches in mouth, dryness, sore throat.	Common	4
Digestive:	None expected.	
Heart & lungs: Lung inflammation, spasm of bronchial tubes.	Infrequent	4
Blood vessels:	None expected.	
Muscles, bones, joints:	None expected.	
Genital, urinary:	None expected.	
Kidneys:	None expected.	
Liver:	None expected.	
Allergic:	None expected.	
Blood:	None expected.	
Others:	None expected.	

1- Life-threatening. Seek emergency treatment immediately.
2- Discontinue. Seek emergency treatment.
3- Discontinue. Call doctor right away.
4- Continue. Call doctor when convenient.
5- Continue. Tell doctor at next visit.
6- No action necessary.

WARNINGS & PRECAUTIONS

Don't take if:
- You are allergic to beclomethasone.
- You have had tuberculosis.
- You are having an asthma attack.

Before you start, consult your doctor:
- If you take other cortisone drugs.
- If you have an infection.

Over age 60:
More likely to develop lung infections.

Pregnancy:
Risk to unborn child outweighs drug benefits. Don't use.

Breast-feeding:
Drug passes into milk. Avoid drug or discontinue nursing.

Infants & children:
Use only under medical supervision.

Prolonged use:
No problems expected.

Skin & sunlight:
No problems expected.

Driving, piloting or hazardous work:
No problems expected.

Airplane passengers:
No problems expected.

Discontinuing:
Don't discontinue without doctor's advice until you complete prescribed dose, even though symptoms diminish or disappear.

Others:
- Unrelated illness or injury may require cortisone drugs by mouth or injection. Notify your doctor.
- Consult doctor as soon as possible if your asthma returns while using beclamethasone as a preventive.
- Drug can reactivate tuberculosis.

INTERACTION WITH OTHER DRUGS

GENERIC NAME OR DRUG CLASS	COMBINED EFFECT
Antiasthmatics (other)	Increased antiasthmatic effect.
Ephedrine	Increased beclomethasone effect.
Epinephrine	Increased beclomethasone effect.
Isoetharine	Increased beclomethasone effect.
Isoproterenol	Increased beclomethasone effect.
Terbutaline	Increased beclomethasone effect.
Theophylline	Increased beclomethasone effect.

INTERACTION WITH OTHER SUBSTANCES

INTERACTS WITH	COMBINED EFFECT
Alcohol:	None expected.
Beverages:	None expected.
Cocaine:	None expected.
Foods:	None expected.
Marijuana:	Decreased beclomethasone effect.
Tobacco:	Decreased beclomethasone effect.

BELLADONNA

BRAND NAMES

Atrosed (M)   Chardonna (M)
Barbidonna (M) Spasnil (M)
Butabar Elixir   Wigraine (M)
Butibel Elixir
See complete brand names list, page 822.

See complete brand names list, page 822.

GENERAL INFORMATION

Habit forming? No
Prescription needed? Low strength: No
High strength: Yes
Available as generic? Yes
Drug class: Antispasmodic, anticholinergic

USES

Reduces spasms of digestive system, bladder and urethra.

DOSAGE & USAGE INFORMATION

How to take:
- Tablet, elixir or capsule—Swallow with liquid or food to lessen stomach irritation.
- Drops—Dilute dose in beverage before swallowing.

When to take:
30 minutes before meals (unless directed otherwise by doctor).

If you forget a dose:
Take as soon as you remember up to 2 hours late. If more than 2 hours, wait for next scheduled dose (don't double this dose).

What drug does:
Blocks nerve impulses at parasympathetic nerve endings, preventing muscle contractions and gland secretions of organs involved.

Time lapse before drug works:
15 to 30 minutes.

Don't take with:
See Interaction column and consult doctor.

OVERDOSE

Symptoms:
Dilated pupils; rapid pulse and breathing; dizziness; fever; hallucinations; confusion; slurred speech; agitation; flushed face; convulsions; coma.

What to do:
- Dial 0 (operator) or 911 (emergency) for an ambulance or medical help. Then give first aid immediately.
- Additional emergency information on page 886.

POSSIBLE ADVERSE REACTIONS OR SIDE EFFECTS

SYMPTOMS	FREQUENCY	WHAT TO DO
Brain & nervous system:		
• Headache	Infrequent	4
• Confusion, delirium.	Common	3
Skin:		
Rash or hives.	Rare	3
Eyes:		
Pain, blurred vision.	Rare	3
Ears, nose, throat:		
Dryness	Common	6
Digestive:		
• Constipation	Common	5
• Nausea, vomiting.	Common	4
Heart & lungs:		
Rapid heartbeat.	Common	3
Blood vessels:	None expected.	
Muscles, bones, joints:	None expected.	
Genital, urinary:		
Difficult urination.	Infrequent	4
Kidneys:	None expected.	
Liver:	None expected.	
Allergic:	None expected.	
Blood:	None expected.	
Others:		
Less perspiration.	Common	4

1- Life-threatening. Seek emergency treatment immediately.
2- Discontinue. Seek emergency treatment.
3- Discontinue. Call doctor right away.
4- Continue. Call doctor when convenient.
5- Continue. Tell doctor at next visit.
6- No action necessary.

WARNINGS & PRECAUTIONS

Don't take if:
- You are allergic to any anticholinergic.
- You have trouble with stomach bloating.
- You have difficulty emptying your bladder completely.
- You have narrow-angle glaucoma.
- You have severe ulcerative colitis.

Before you start, consult your doctor:
- If you have open-angle glaucoma.
- If you have angina.
- If you have chronic bronchitis or asthma.
- If you have hiatal hernia.
- If you have liver disease.
- If you have enlarged prostate.
- If you have myasthenia gravis.
- If you have peptic ulcer.
- If you will have surgery within 2 months, including dental surgery, requiring general or spinal anesthesia.

Over age 60:
Adverse reactions and side effects may be more frequent and severe than in younger persons.

Pregnancy:
Studies inconclusive on harm to unborn child. Animal studies show fetal abnormalities. Decide with your doctor whether drug benefits justify risk to unborn child.

Breast-feeding:
Drug passes into milk and decreases milk flow. Avoid drug or discontinue nursing until you finish medicine. Consult doctor for advice on maintaining milk supply.

Infants & children:
Use only under medical supervision.

Prolonged use:
Chronic constipation, possible fecal impaction. Consult doctor immediately.

Skin & sunlight:
No problems expected.

Driving, piloting or hazardous work:
Use disqualifies you for piloting aircraft. Otherwise, no problems expected.

Airplane passengers:
No problems expected.

Discontinuing:
May be unnecessary to finish medicine. Follow doctor's instructions.

Others:
No problems expected.

INTERACTION WITH OTHER DRUGS

GENERIC NAME OR DRUG CLASS	COMBINED EFFECT
Amantadine	Increased belladonna effect.
Anticholinergics (other)	Increased belladonna effect.
Antidepressants (tricyclic)	Increased belladonna effect.
Antihistamines	Increased belladonna effect.
Cortisone drugs	Increased internal-eye pressure.
Haloperidol	Increased internal-eye pressure.
MAO inhibitors	Increased belladonna effect.
Meperidine	Increased belladonna effect.
Methylphenidate	Increased belladonna effect.
Orphenadrine	Increased belladonna effect.
Phenothiazines	Increased belladonna effect.
Pilocarpine	Loss of pilocarpine effect in glaucoma treatment.
Vitamin C	Decreased belladonna effect. Avoid large doses of vitamin C.

INTERACTION WITH OTHER SUBSTANCES

INTERACTS WITH	COMBINED EFFECT
Alcohol:	None expected.
Beverages:	None expected.
Cocaine:	Excessively rapid heartbeat. Avoid.
Foods:	None expected.
Marijuana:	Drowsiness and dry mouth.
Tobacco:	None expected.

BENDROFLUMETHIAZIDE

BRAND NAMES

Naturetin

GENERAL INFORMATION

Habit forming? No
Prescription needed? Yes
Available as generic? Yes
Drug class: Antihypertensive
diuretic (thiazide)

USES

- Controls, but doesn't cure, high blood pressure.
- Reduces fluid retention (edema) caused by conditions such as heart disorders and liver disease.

DOSAGE & USAGE INFORMATION

How to take:
Tablet or capsule—Swallow with liquid. If you can't swallow whole, crumble tablet or open capsule and take with liquid or food. Don't exceed dose.

When to take:
At the same time each day.

If you forget a dose:
Take as soon as you remember up to 2 hours late. If more than 2 hours, wait for next scheduled dose (don't double this dose).

What drug does:
- Forces sodium and water excretion, reducing body fluid.
- Relaxes muscle cells of small arteries.
- Reduced body fluid and relaxed arteries lower blood pressure.

Time lapse before drug works:
4 to 6 hours. May require several weeks to lower blood pressure.

Don't take with:
- See Interaction column and consult doctor.
- Non-prescription drugs without consulting doctor.

OVERDOSE

Symptoms:
Cramps, weakness, drowsiness, weak pulse, coma.

What to do:
- Dial O (operator) or 911 (emergency) for an ambulance or medical help. Then give first aid immediately.
- Additional emergency information on page 886.

POSSIBLE ADVERSE REACTIONS OR SIDE EFFECTS

SYMPTOMS	FREQUENCY	WHAT TO DO
Brain & nervous system:		
• Dizziness	Infrequent	4
• Mood changes.	Infrequent	4
• Headaches	Infrequent	4
Skin:		
Rash or hives.	Rare	2
Eyes:		
Blurred vision.	Infrequent	3
Ears, nose, throat:		
• Sore throat, fever.	Rare	3
• Dry mouth, thirst.	Infrequent	5
Digestive:		
Severe abdominal pain, nausea, vomiting.	Infrequent	3
Heart & lungs:		
Irregular heartbeat, weak pulse.	Infrequent	3
Blood vessels:	None expected.	
Muscles, bones, joints:		
Weakness, tiredness.	Infrequent	4
Genital, urinary:	None expected.	
Kidneys:	None expected.	
Liver:		
Jaundice (yellow skin and eyes).	Rare	3
Blood:	None expected.	
Allergic:	None expected.	
Others:		
Weight changes.	Infrequent	4

1- Life-threatening. Seek emergency treatment immediately.
2- Discontinue. Seek emergency treatment.
3- Discontinue. Call doctor right away.
4- Continue. Call doctor when convenient.
5- Continue. Call doctor at next visit.
6- No action necessary.

BENDROFLUMETHIAZIDE

WARNINGS & PRECAUTIONS

Don't take if:
You are allergic to any thiazide diuretic drug.

Before you start, consult your doctor:
- If you are allergic to any sulfa drug.
- If you have gout.
- If you have liver, pancreas or kidney disorder.

Over age 60:
Adverse reactions and side effects may be more frequent and severe than in younger persons, especially dizziness and excessive potassium loss.

Pregnancy:
Risk to unborn child outweighs drug benefits. Don't use.

Breast-feeding:
Drug passes into milk. Avoid this medicine or discontinue nursing.

Infants & children:
No problems expected.

Prolonged use:
You may need medicine to treat high blood pressure for the rest of your life.

Skin & sunlight:
May cause rash or intensify sunburn in areas exposed to sun or sunlamp.

Driving, piloting or hazardous work:
Don't drive or pilot aircraft until you learn how medicine affects you. Don't work around dangerous machinery. Don't climb ladders or work in high places. Danger increases if you drink alcohol or take medicine affecting alertness and reflexes, such as antihistamines, tranquilizers, sedatives, pain medicine, narcotics and mind-altering drugs.

Airplane passengers:
No problems expected.

Discontinuing:
Don't discontinue without medical advice.

Others:
- Hot weather and fever may cause dehydration and drop in blood pressure. Dose may require temporary adjustment. Weigh daily and report any unexpected weight decreases to your doctor.
- May cause rise in uric acid, leading to gout.
- May cause blood-sugar rise in diabetics.

INTERACTION WITH OTHER DRUGS

GENERIC NAME OR DRUG CLASS	COMBINED EFFECT
Allopurinol	Decreased allopurinol effect.
Antidepressants (tricyclic)	Dangerous drop in blood pressure. Avoid combination unless under medical supervision.
Barbiturates	Increased bendroflumethiazide effect.
Cholestyramine	Decreased bendroflumethiazide effect.
Cortisone drugs	Excessive potassium loss that causes dangerous heart rhythms.
Digitalis preparations	Excessive potassium loss that causes dangerous heart rhythms.
Diuretics (thiazide)	Increased effect of other thiazide diuretics.
Lithium	Increased effect of lithium.
MAO inhibitors	Increased bendroflumethiazide effect.
Probenecid	Decreased probenecid effect.

INTERACTIONS WITH OTHER SUBSTANCES

INTERACTS WITH	COMBINED EFFECT
Alcohol:	Dangerous blood-pressure drop.
Beverages:	None expected.
Cocaine:	None expected.
Foods: Licorice	Excessive potassium loss that causes dangerous heart rhythms.
Marijuana:	May increase blood pressure.
Tobacco:	None expected.

BENZOYL PEROXIDE

BRAND NAMES

Benoxyl	Desquam-X	Panoxyl	Xerac BP
Benzac	Dry and Clean	Persadox	
Benzagel	Epi-Clear	Persa-Gel	
Clearasil BP(M)	Fostex BPO	Porox 7	
Clear By Design	Oxy-5	Teen	
Dermodex	Oxy-10	Topex	

GENERAL INFORMATION

Habit forming? No
Prescription needed? No
Available as generic? Yes
Drug class: Antiacne (topical)

USES

Treatment for acne.

DOSAGE & USAGE INFORMATION

How to use:
Cream, gel, pads, sticks or lotion—Wash affected area with plain soap and water. Dry gently with towel. Rub medicine into affected areas. Keep away from eyes, nose, mouth.

When to use:
Apply 1 or more times daily. If you have a fair complexion, start with single application at bedtime.

If you forget an application:
Use as soon as you remember.

What drug does:
Slowly releases oxygen from skin, which controls some skin bacteria. Also causes peeling and drying, helping control blackheads and whiteheads.

Time lapse before drug works:
1 to 2 weeks.

Don't use with:
See Interaction column and consult doctor.

OVERDOSE

Symptoms:
None expected.

What to do:
If person swallows drug, call doctor, poison-control center or hospital emergency room for instructions.

POSSIBLE ADVERSE REACTIONS OR SIDE EFFECTS

SYMPTOMS	FREQUENCY	WHAT TO DO
Brain & nervous system:	None expected.	
Skin:		
• Painful skin irritation.	Infrequent	4
• Rash	Infrequent	3
• Excessive dryness.	Infrequent	3
Eyes:	None expected.	
Ears, nose, throat:	None expected.	
Digestive:	None expected.	
Heart & lungs:	None expected.	
Blood vessels:	None expected.	
Muscles, bones, joints:	None expected.	
Genital, urinary:	None expected.	
Kidneys:	None expected.	
Liver:	None expected.	
Allergic:	None expected.	
Blood:	None expected.	
Others:	None expected.	

1- Life-threatening. Seek emergency treatment immediately.
2- Discontinue. Seek emergency treatment.
3- Discontinue. Call doctor right away.
4- Continue. Call doctor when convenient.
5- Continue. Tell doctor at next visit.
6- No action necessary.

WARNINGS & PRECAUTIONS

Don't take if:
You are allergic to benzoyl peroxide.

Before you start, consult your doctor:
- If you plan to become pregnant within medication period.
- If you take oral contraceptives.

Over age 60:
No problems expected.

Pregnancy:
No proven problems. Consult doctor.

Breast-feeding:
No proven problems. Consult doctor.

Infants & children:
Not recommended.

Prolonged use:
Permanent rash or scarring.

Skin & sunlight:
No problems expected.

Driving, piloting or hazardous work:
No problems expected.

Airplane passengers:
No problems expected.

Discontinuing:
- May be unnecessary to finish medicine. Discontinue when acne improves.
- If acne doesn't improve in 2 weeks, call doctor.

Others:
- Keep away from hair and clothing. May bleach.
- Store away from heat in cool, dry place.
- Avoid contact with eyes, lips, nose and sensitive areas of the neck.

INTERACTION WITH OTHER DRUGS

GENERIC NAME OR DRUG CLASS	COMBINED EFFECT
Antiacne topical preparations (other)	Excessive skin irritation.
Skin-peeling agents (salicylic acid, sulfur, resorcinol, tretinoin)	Excessive skin irritation.

INTERACTION WITH OTHER SUBSTANCES

INTERACTS WITH	COMBINED EFFECT
Alcohol:	None expected.
Beverages:	None expected.
Cocaine:	None expected.
Foods: Cinnamon, foods with benzoic acid.	Skin rash.
Marijuana:	None expected.
Tobacco:	None expected.

BENZPHETAMINE

BRAND NAMES

Didrex

GENERAL INFORMATION

Habit forming? Yes
Prescription needed? Yes
Available as generic? Yes
Drug class: Appetite suppressant

 ## USES

Suppresses appetite.

 ## DOSAGE & USAGE INFORMATION

How to take:
● Tablet—Swallow with liquid.

When to take:
1 hour before meals. Last dose no later than 4 to 6 hours before bedtime.

If you forget a dose:
Wait for next scheduled dose. Don't double this dose.

What drug does:
Apparently stimulates brain's appetite-control center.

Time lapse before drug works:
Begins in 1 hour. Lasts 4 hours.

Don't take with:
● Non-prescription drugs without consulting doctor.
● See Interaction column and consult doctor.

 ## OVERDOSE

Symptoms:
Irritability, overactivity, trembling, insomnia, mood changes, rapid heartbeat, confusion, disorientation, hallucinations, convulsions, coma.

What to do:
● Dial 0 (operator) or 911 (emergency) for an ambulance or medical help. Then give first aid immediately.
● Additional emergency information on page 886.

POSSIBLE ADVERSE REACTIONS OR SIDE EFFECTS

SYMPTOMS	FREQUENCY	WHAT TO DO
Brain & nervous system:		
● Irritability, nervousness, insomnia.	Common	4
● Mood changes.	Rare	3
Skin:		
● Hair loss.	Rare	4
● Rash or hives.	Rare	3
Eyes:		
Blurred vision.	Infrequent	4
Ears, nose, throat:		
Unpleasant taste or dry mouth.	Infrequent	4
Digestive:		
Constipation or diarrhea, nausea, vomiting, cramps.	Infrequent	4
Heart & lungs:		
● Irregular or pounding heartbeat.	Infrequent	3
● Breathing difficulty.	Rare	3
Blood vessels, muscles, bones, joints, kidneys, liver, allergic, blood:	None expected.	
Genital, urinary:		
Urinary urgency and difficulty.	Infrequent	3
Others:		
● False sense of well-being.	Common	4
● Changes in sex drive.	Infrequent	4
● Sweat increase.	Infrequent	4

1 - Life-threatening. Seek emergency treatment immediately.
2 - Discontinue. Seek emergency treatment.
3 - Discontinue. Call doctor right away.
4 - Continue. Call doctor when convenient.

BENZPHETAMINE

 WARNINGS &
PRECAUTIONS

Don't take if:
- You are allergic to any sympathomimetic or phenylpropanolamine.
- You have glaucoma.
- You have taken MAO inhibitors within 2 weeks.
- You plan to become pregnant within medication period.
- You have a history of drug abuse.

Before you start, consult your doctor:
- If you have high blood pressure or heart disease.
- If you have an overactive thyroid, nervous tension or "anxiety."
- If you have epilepsy.

Over age 60:
Adverse reactions and side effects may be more frequent and severe than in younger persons.

Pregnancy:
Safety not established. Avoid.

Breast-feeding:
No proven problems. Consult doctor.

Infants & children:
Don't give to children younger than 12.

Prolonged use:
Loses effectiveness. Avoid.

Skin & sunlight:
No problems expected.

Driving, piloting or hazardous work:
Don't drive or pilot aircraft until you learn how medicine affects you. Don't work around dangerous machinery. Don't climb ladders or work in high places. Danger increases if you drink alcohol or take medicine affecting alertness and reflexes, such as antihistamines, tranquilizers, sedatives, pain medicine, narcotics and mind-altering drugs.

Airplane passengers:
No problems expected.

Discontinuing:
Don't discontinue without consulting doctor. Dose may require gradual reduction if you have taken drug for a long time. Doses of other drugs may also require adjustment.

Others:
Don't increase dose.

 INTERACTION WITH
OTHER DRUGS

GENERIC NAME OR DRUG CLASS	COMBINED EFFECT
Appetite suppressants (other)	Dangerous overstimulation.
Caffeine	Increased stimulant effect of benzphetamine.
Guanethidine	Decreased guanethidine effect.
Hydralazine	Decreased hydralazine effect.
MAO inhibitors	Dangerous blood-pressure rise.
Methyldopa	Decreased methyldopa effect.
Phenothiazines	Decreased benzphetamine effect.
Rauwolfia alkaloids	Decreased effect of rauwolfia alkaloids.

 INTERACTION WITH
OTHER SUBSTANCES

INTERACTS WITH	COMBINED EFFECT
Alcohol: Beer, chianti wines, vermouth.	Dangerous blood-pressure rise.
Beverages: • Caffeine drinks	Excessive stimulation.
• Drinks containing tyramine (see page 851).	Blood-pressure rise
Cocaine:	Excessive stimulation.
Foods: Foods containing tyramine (see page 851).	Blood-pressure rise.
Marijuana:	Frequent use—Irregular heartbeat.
Tobacco:	None expected.

BENZTHIAZIDE

BRAND NAMES

Aquastat
Aquatag
Exna
Hydrex

GENERAL INFORMATION

Habit forming? No
Prescription needed? Yes
Available as generic? Yes
Drug class: Antihypertensive,
diuretic (thiazide)

USES

- Controls, but doesn't cure, high blood pressure.
- Reduces fluid retention (edema) caused by conditions such as heart disorders and liver disease.

DOSAGE & USAGE INFORMATION

How to take:
Tablet or capsule—Swallow with liquid. If you can't swallow whole, crumble tablet or open capsule and take with liquid or food. Don't exceed dose.

When to take:
At the same time each day.

If you forget a dose:
Take as soon as you remember up to 2 hours late. If more than 2 hours, wait for next scheduled dose (don't double this dose).

What drug does:
- Forces sodium and water excretion, reducing body fluid.
- Relaxes muscle cells of small arteries.
- Reduced body fluid and relaxed arteries lower blood pressure.

Time lapse before drug works:
4 to 6 hours. May require several weeks to lower blood pressure.

Don't take with:
- See Interaction column and consult doctor.
- Non-prescription drugs without consulting doctor.

OVERDOSE

Symptoms:
Cramps, weakness, drowsiness, weak pulse, coma.

What to do:
- Dial 0 (operator) or 911 (emergency) for an ambulance or medical help. Then give first aid immediately.
- Additional emergency information on page 886.

POSSIBLE ADVERSE REACTIONS OR SIDE EFFECTS

SYMPTOMS	FREQUENCY	WHAT TO DO
Brain & nervous system:		
• Dizziness	Infrequent	4
• Mood changes.	Infrequent	4
• Headaches	Infrequent	4
Skin:		
Rash or hives.	Rare	2
Eyes:		
Blurred vision.	Infrequent	3
Ears, nose, throat:		
• Sore throat, fever.	Rare	3
• Dry mouth, thirst.	Infrequent	5
Digestive:		
Severe abdominal pain, nausea, vomiting.	Infrequent	3
Heart & lungs:		
Irregular heartbeat, weak pulse.	Infrequent	3
Blood vessels:	None expected.	
Muscles, bones, joints:		
Weakness, tiredness.	Infrequent	4
Genital, urinary:	None expected.	
Kidneys:	None expected.	
Liver:		
Jaundice (yellow skin and eyes).	Rare	3
Allergic:	None expected.	
Blood:	None expected.	
Others:		
Weight changes.	Infrequent	4

1- Life-threatening. Seek emergency treatment immediately.
2- Discontinue. Seek emergency treatment.
3- Discontinue. Call doctor right away.
4- Continue. Call doctor when convenient.
5- Continue. Tell doctor at next visit.
6- No action necessary.

WARNINGS & PRECAUTIONS

Don't take if:
You are allergic to any thiazide diuretic drug.

Before you start, consult your doctor:
- If you are allergic to any sulfa drug.
- If you have gout.
- If you have liver, pancreas or kidney disorder.

Over age 60:
Adverse reactions and side effects may be more frequent and severe than in younger persons, especially dizziness and excessive potassium loss.

Pregnancy:
Risk to unborn child outweighs drug benefits. Don't use.

Breast-feeding:
Drug passes into milk. Avoid drug or discontinue nursing.

Infants & children:
No problems expected.

Prolonged use:
You may need medicine to treat high blood pressure for the rest of your life.

Skin & sunlight:
May cause rash or intensify sunburn in areas exposed to sun or sunlamp.

Driving, piloting or hazardous work:
Don't drive or pilot aircraft until you learn how medicine affects you. Don't work around dangerous machinery. Don't climb ladders or work in high places. Danger increases if you drink alcohol or take medicine affecting alertness and reflexes, such as antihistamines, tranquilizers, sedatives, pain medicine, narcotics and mind-altering drugs.

Airplane passengers:
No problems expected.

Discontinuing:
Don't discontinue without medical advice.

Others:
- Hot weather and fever may cause dehydration and drop in blood pressure. Dose may require temporary adjustment. Weigh daily and report any unexpected weight decreases to your doctor.
- May cause rise in uric acid, leading to gout.
- May cause blood-sugar rise in diabetics.

INTERACTION WITH OTHER DRUGS

GENERIC NAME OR DRUG CLASS	COMBINED EFFECT
Allopurinol	Decreased allopurinol effect.
Antidepressants (tricyclic)	Dangerous drop in blood pressure. Avoid combination unless under medical supervision.
Barbiturates	Increased benzthiazide effect.
Cholestyramine	Decreased benzthiazide effect.
Cortisone drugs	Excessive potassium loss that causes dangerous heart rhythms.
Digitalis preparations	Excessive potassium loss that causes dangerous heart rhythms.
Diuretics (thiazide)	Increased effect of other thiazide diuretics.
Lithium	Increased effect of lithium.
MAO inhibitors	Increased benzthiazide effect.
Probenecid	Decreased probenecid effect.

INTERACTION WITH OTHER SUBSTANCES

INTERACTS WITH	COMBINED EFFECT
Alcohol:	Dangerous blood-pressure drop.
Beverages:	None expected.
Cocaine:	None expected.
Foods: Licorice	Excessive potassium loss that causes dangerous heart rhythms.
Marijuana:	May increase blood pressure.
Tobacco:	None expected.

BENZTROPINE

BRAND NAMES

Bensylate
Cogentin

GENERAL INFORMATION

Habit forming? No
Prescription needed? Yes
Available as generic? No
Drug class: Antidyskinetic, antiparkinsonism

 ## USES

- Treatment of Parkinson's disease.
- Treatment of adverse effects of phenothiazines.

 ## DOSAGE & USAGE INFORMATION

How to take:
Tablets or capsules—Take with food to lessen stomach irritation.

When to take:
At the same times each day.

If you forget a dose:
Take as soon as you remember up to 2 hours late. If more than 2 hours, wait for next scheduled dose (don't double this dose).

What drug does:
- Balances chemical reactions necessary to send nerve impulses within base of brain.
- Improves muscle control and reduces stiffness.

Time lapse before drug works:
1 to 2 hours.

Don't take with:
- Non-prescription drugs for colds, cough or allergy.
- See Interaction column and consult doctor.

 ## OVERDOSE

Symptoms:
Agitation, dilated pupils, hallucinations, dry mouth, rapid heartbeat, sleepiness.

What to do:
- Dial 0 (operator) or 911 (emergency) for an ambulance or medical help. Then give first aid immediately.
- If patient is unconscious and not breathing, give mouth-to-mouth breathing. If there is no heartbeat, use cardiac massage and mouth-to-mouth breathing (CPR). Don't try to make patient vomit. If you can't get help quickly, take patient to nearest emergency facility.
- Additional emergency information on page 886.

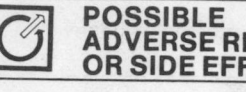 ## POSSIBLE ADVERSE REACTIONS OR SIDE EFFECTS

SYMPTOMS	FREQUENCY	WHAT TO DO
Brain & nervous system: Confusion, dizziness.	Rare	4
Skin: Rash	Rare	3
Eyes:		
• Pain	Rare	3
• Blurred vision, light sensitivity.	Common	4
Ears, nose, throat: Sore mouth or tongue.	Rare	4
Digestive:		
• Constipation	Common	4
• Nausea, vomiting.	Common	4
Heart & lungs:	None expected.	
Blood vessels:	None expected.	
Muscles, bones, joints:		
• Muscle cramps.	Rare	4
• Numbness, weakness in hands or feet.	Rare	4
Genital, urinary: Difficult or painful urination.	Common	5
Kidneys:	None expected.	
Liver:	None expected.	
Allergic:	None expected.	
Blood:	None expected.	
Others:	None expected.	

1 - Life-threatening. Seek emergency treatment immediately.
2 - Discontinue. Seek emergency treatment.
3 - Discontinue. Call doctor right away.
4 - Continue. Call doctor when convenient.
5 - Continue. Tell doctor at next visit.
6 - No action necessary.

BENZTROPINE

 **WARNINGS &
PRECAUTIONS**

Don't take if:
You are allergic to any antidyskinetic.

Before you start, consult your doctor:
- If you have had glaucoma.
- If you have had high blood pressure or heart disease.
- If you have had impaired liver function.
- If you have had kidney disease or urination difficulty.

Over age 60:
More sensitive to drug. Aggravates symptoms of enlarged prostate. Causes impaired thinking, hallucinations, nightmares. Consult doctor about any of these.

Pregnancy:
Studies inconclusive on harm to unborn child. Animal studies show fetal abnormalities. Decide with your doctor whether drug benefits justify risk to unborn child.

Breast-feeding:
No problems expected.

Infants & children:
Not recommended for children 3 and younger. Use for older children only under doctor's supervision.

Prolonged use:
Possible glaucoma.

Skin & sunlight:
No problems expected.

Driving, piloting or hazardous work:
Don't drive or pilot aircraft until you learn how medicine affects you. Don't work around dangerous machinery. Don't climb ladders or work in high places. Danger increases if you drink alcohol or take medicine affecting alertness and reflexes, such as antihistamines, tranquilizers, sedatives, pain medicine, narcotics and mind-altering drugs.

Airplane passengers:
No problems expected.

Discontinuing:
Don't discontinue without consulting doctor. Dose may require gradual reduction if you have taken drug for a long time. Doses of other drugs may also require adjustment.

Others:
- Internal eye pressure should be measured regularly.
- Avoid becoming overheated.

 **INTERACTION WITH
OTHER DRUGS**

GENERIC NAME OR DRUG CLASS	COMBINED EFFECT
Amantadine	Increased amantadine effect.
Antidepressants (tricyclic)	Increased benztropine effect. May cause glaucoma.
Antihistamines	Increased benztropine effect.
Levodopa	Increased levodopa effect. Improved results in treating Parkinson's disease.
Meperidine	Increased benztropine effect.
MAO inhibitors	Increased benztropine effect.
Orphenadrine	Increased benztropine effect.
Phenothiazines	Behavior changes.
Primidone	Excessive sedation.
Procainamide	Increased procainamide effect.
Quinidine	Increased benztropine effect.
Tranquilizers	Excessive sedation.

 **INTERACTION WITH
OTHER SUBSTANCES**

INTERACTS WITH	COMBINED EFFECT
Alcohol:	None expected.
Beverages:	None expected.
Cocaine:	Decreased benztropine effect. Avoid.
Foods:	None expected.
Marijuana:	None expected.
Tobacco:	None expected.

BETAMETHASONE

BRAND NAMES

Beconase
Betnelan
Betnesol

Celestoject
Celestone
Cel-U-Sec

Vancerace

GENERAL INFORMATION

Habit forming? No
Prescription needed? Yes
Available as generic? Yes
Drug class: Cortisone drug (adrenal corticosteroid)

USES

- Reduces inflammation caused by many different medical problems.
- Treatment for some allergic diseases, blood disorders, kidney diseases, asthma and emphysema.
- Replaces corticosteroid deficiencies.

DOSAGE & USAGE INFORMATION

How to take:
- Tablet or liquid—Swallow with liquid or food to lessen stomach irritation. If you can't swallow whole, crumble tablet and take with liquid or food.
- Inhaler—Follow label instructions.

When to take:
At the same times each day. Take once-a-day or once-every-other-day doses in mornings.

If you forget a dose:
- Several-doses-per-day prescription—Take as soon as you remember up to 2 hours late. If more than 2 hours, wait for next scheduled dose (don't double this dose).
- Once-a-day dose or less—Wait for next dose. Double this dose.

What drug does:
Decreases inflammatory responses.

Time lapse before drug works:
2 to 4 days.

Don't take with:
See Interaction column and consult doctor.

OVERDOSE

Symptoms:
Headache, convulsions, heart failure.

What to do:
- Dial 0 (operator) or 911 (emergency) for an ambulance or medical help. Then give first aid immediately.
- Additional emergency information on page 886.

POSSIBLE ADVERSE REACTIONS OR SIDE EFFECTS

SYMPTOMS	FREQUENCY	WHAT TO DO
Brain & nervous system:		
Mood changes, insomnia, restlessness.	Infrequent	4
Skin:		
• Acne	Common	4
• Rash	Rare	3
• Poor wound healing.	Common	4
Eyes:		
Blurred vision, halos around lights.	Infrequent	3
Ears, nose, throat:		
• Sore throat, fever.	Infrequent	3
• Thirst	Common	4
Digestive:		
• Indigestion, nausea, vomiting.	Common	4
• Bloody or black, tarry stool.	Infrequent	2
Heart & lungs:		
Irregular heartbeat.	Rare	2
Blood vessels, kidneys, liver, allergic, blood:	None expected.	
Muscles, bones, joints:		
Muscle cramps, swollen legs, feet.	Infrequent	3
Genital, urinary:		
Frequent urination.	Infrequent	4
Others:		
• Weight gain, round face.	Infrequent	4
• Fatigue, weakness.	Infrequent	4
• TB recurrence.	Infrequent	4
• Irregular menstrual periods.	Infrequent	4

1- Life-threatening. Seek emergency treatment immediately.
2- Discontinue. Seek emergency treatment.
3- Discontinue. Call doctor right away.
4- Continue. Call doctor when convenient.

BETAMETHASONE

 ## WARNINGS & PRECAUTIONS

Don't take if:
- You are allergic to any cortisone drug.
- You have tuberculosis or fungus infection.
- You have herpes infection of eyes, lips or genitals.

Before you start, consult your doctor:
- If you have had tuberculosis.
- If you have congestive heart failure.
- If you have diabetes.
- If you have peptic ulcer.
- If you have glaucoma.
- If you have underactive thyroid.
- If you have high blood pressure.
- If you have myasthenia gravis.
- If you have blood clots in legs or lungs.

Over age 60:
Adverse reactions and side effects may be more frequent and severe than in younger persons. Likely to aggravate edema, diabetes or ulcers. Likely to cause cataracts and osteoporosis (softening of the bones).

Pregnancy:
Risk to unborn child outweighs drug benefits. Don't use.

Breast-feeding:
Drug passes into milk. Avoid drug or discontinue nursing until you finish medicine. Consult doctor for advice on maintaining milk supply.

Infants & children:
Use only under medical supervision.

Prolonged use:
- Retards growth in children.
- Possible glaucoma, cataracts, diabetes, fragile bones and thin skin.
- Functional dependence.

Skin & sunlight:
No problems expected.

Driving, piloting or hazardous work:
No problems expected.

Airplane passengers:
No problems expected.

Discontinuing:
- Don't discontinue without doctor's advice until you complete prescribed dose, even though symptoms diminish or disappear.
- Drug affects your response to surgery, illness, injury or stress for 2 years after discontinuing. Tell about drug to anyone who takes medical care of you within 2 years.

Others:
Avoid immunizations if possible.

 ## INTERACTION WITH OTHER DRUGS

GENERIC NAME OR DRUG CLASS	COMBINED EFFECT
Amphoterecin B	Potassium depletion.
Anticholinergics	Possible glaucoma.
Anticoagulants (oral)	Decreased anticoagulant effect.
Anticonvulsants (hydantoin)	Decreased betamethasone effect.
Antidiabetics (oral)	Decreased antidiabetic effect.
Antihistamines	Decreased betamethasone effect.
Aspirin	Increased betamethasone effect.
Barbiturates	Decreased betamethasone effect. Oversedation.
Beta-adrenergic blockers	Decreased betamethasone effect.
Chloral hydrate	Decreased betamethasone effect.
Chlorthalidone	Potassium depletion.
Cholinergics	Decreased cholinergic effect.
Contraceptives (oral)	Increased betamethasone effect.
Digitalis preparations	Dangerous potassium depletion. Possible digitalis toxicity.
Diuretics (thiazide)	Potassium depletion.

Additional interactions on page 834.

 ## INTERACTION WITH OTHER SUBSTANCES

INTERACTS WITH	COMBINED EFFECT
Alcohol:	Risk of stomach ulcers.
Beverages:	No proven problems.
Cocaine:	Overstimulation. Avoid.
Foods:	No proven problems.
Marijuana:	Decreased immunity.
Tobacco:	Increased betamethasone effect. Possible toxicity.

BETHANECHOL

BRAND NAMES

Duvoid
Myotonachol
Urecholine

GENERAL INFORMATION

Habit forming? No
Prescription needed? Yes
Available as generic? Yes
Drug class: Cholinergic

USES

Helps initiate urination following surgery, or for persons with urinary infections or enlarged prostate.

DOSAGE & USAGE INFORMATION

How to take:
Tablet or capsule—Swallow with liquid, 1 hour before or 2 hours after eating.

When to take:
At the same times each day.

If you forget a dose:
Take as soon as you remember up to 2 hours late. If more than 2 hours, wait for next scheduled dose (don't double this dose).

What drug does:
Affects chemical reactions in the body that strengthen bladder muscles.

Time lapse before drug works:
30 to 90 minutes.

Don't take with:
See Interaction column and consult doctor.

OVERDOSE

Symptoms:
Shortness of breath, wheezing or chest tightness, unconsciousness, coma.

What to do:
- Dial 0 (operator) or 911 (emergency) for an ambulance or medical help. Then give first aid immediately.
- If patient is unconscious and not breathing, give mouth-to-mouth breathing. If there is no heartbeat, use cardiac massage and mouth-to-mouth breathing (CPR). Don't try to make patient vomit. If you can't get help quickly, take patient to nearest emergency facility.
- Additional emergency information on page 886.

POSSIBLE ADVERSE REACTIONS OR SIDE EFFECTS

SYMPTOMS	FREQUENCY	WHAT TO DO
Brain & nervous system: Dizziness, headache, faintness.	Infrequent	4
Skin:	None expected.	
Eyes: Blurred or changed vision.	Infrequent	4
Ears, nose, throat:	None expected.	
Digestive: Diarrhea, nausea, vomiting, stomach discomfort, belching.	Infrequent	4
Heart & lungs: Shortness of breath, wheezing, tightness in chest.	Rare	3
Blood vessels:	None expected.	
Muscles, bones, joints:	None expected.	
Genital, urinary: Excessive urge to urinate.	Infrequent	4
Kidneys:	None expected.	
Liver:	None expected.	
Allergic:	None expected.	
Blood:	None expected.	
Others:	None expected.	

1- Life-threatening. Seek emergency treatment immediately.
2- Discontinue. Seek emergency treatment.
3- Discontinue. Call doctor right away.
4- Continue. Call doctor when convenient.
5- Continue. Tell doctor at next visit.
6- No action necessary.

WARNINGS & PRECAUTIONS

Don't take if:
You are allergic to any cholinergic.

Before you start, consult your doctor:
- If you plan to become pregnant within medication period.
- If you have asthma.
- If you have epilepsy.
- If you have heart or blood-vessel disease.
- If you have high or low blood pressure.
- If you have overactive thyroid.
- If you have intestinal blockage.
- If you have Parkinson's disease.
- If you have stomach problems (including ulcer).
- If you have had bladder or intestinal surgery within 1 month.

Over age 60:
Adverse reactions and side effects may be more frequent and severe than in younger persons.

Pregnancy:
Risk to unborn child outweighs drug benefits. Don't use.

Breast-feeding:
Drug filters into milk. May harm child. Avoid.

Infants & children:
Use only under medical supervision.

Prolonged use:
No problems expected.

Skin & sunlight:
No problems expected.

Driving, piloting or hazardous work:
Don't drive or pilot aircraft until you learn how medicine affects you. Don't work around dangerous machinery. Don't climb ladders or work in high places. Danger increases if you drink alcohol or take medicine affecting alertness and reflexes, such as antihistamines, tranquilizers, sedatives, pain medicine, narcotics and mind-altering drugs.

Airplane passengers:
No problems expected.

Discontinuing:
May be unnecessary to finish medicine. Follow doctor's instructions.

Others:
- Be cautious about standing up suddenly.
- Interferes with laboratory studies of liver and pancreas function.
- Side effects more likely with injections.

INTERACTION WITH OTHER DRUGS

GENERIC NAME OR DRUG CLASS	COMBINED EFFECT
Cholinergics (other)	Increased effect of both drugs. Possible toxicity.
Procainamide	Decreased bethanechol effect.
Quinidine	Decreased bethanechol effect.

INTERACTION WITH OTHER SUBSTANCES

INTERACTS WITH	COMBINED EFFECT
Alcohol:	None expected.
Beverages:	None expected.
Cocaine:	None expected.
Foods:	None expected.
Marijuana:	None expected.
Tobacco:	None expected.

BIPERIDINE

BRAND NAMES

Akineton

GENERAL INFORMATION

Habit forming? No
Prescription needed? Yes
Available as generic? No
Drug class: Antidyskinetic, antiparkinsonism

USES

- Treatment of Parkinson's disease.
- Treatment of adverse effects of phenothiazines.

DOSAGE & USAGE INFORMATION

How to take:
Tablets or capsules—Take with food to lessen stomach irritation.

When to take:
At the same times each day.

If you forget a dose:
Take as soon as you remember up to 2 hours late. If more than 2 hours, wait for next scheduled dose (don't double this dose).

What drug does:
- Balances chemical reactions necessary to send nerve impulses within base of brain.
- Improves muscle control and reduces stiffness.

Time lapse before drug works:
1 to 2 hours.

Don't take with:
- Non-prescription drugs for colds, cough or allergy.
- See Interaction column and consult doctor.

OVERDOSE

Symptoms:
Agitation, dilated pupils, hallucinations, dry mouth, rapid heartbeat, sleepiness.

What to do:
- Dial 0 (operator) or 911 (emergency) for an ambulance or medical help. Then give first aid immediately.
- If patient is unconscious and not breathing, give mouth-to-mouth breathing. If there is no heartbeat, use cardiac massage and mouth-to-mouth breathing (CPR). Don't try to make patient vomit. If you can't get help quickly, take patient to nearest emergency facility.
- Additional emergency information on page 886.

POSSIBLE ADVERSE REACTIONS OR SIDE EFFECTS

SYMPTOMS	FREQUENCY	WHAT TO DO
Brain & nervous system: Confusion, dizziness.	Rare	4
Skin: Rash	Rare	3
Eyes:		
• Pain	Rare	3
• Blurred vision, light sensitivity.	Common	4
Ears, nose, throat: Sore mouth or tongue.	Rare	4
Digestive:		
• Constipation	Common	4
• Nausea, vomiting.	Common	4
Heart & lungs:	None expected.	
Blood vessels:	None expected.	
Muscles, bones, joints:		
• Muscle cramps.	Rare	4
• Numbness, weakness in hands or feet.	Rare	4
Genital, urinary: Difficult or painful urination.	Common	5
Kidneys:	None expected.	
Liver:	None expected.	
Allergic:	None expected.	
Blood:	None expected.	
Others:	None expected.	

1- Life-threatening. Seek emergency treatment immediately.
2- Discontinue. Seek emergency treatment.
3- Discontinue. Call doctor right away.
4- Continue. Call doctor when convenient.
5- Continue. Tell doctor at next visit.
6- No action necessary.

BIPERIDINE

WARNINGS & PRECAUTIONS

Don't take if:
You are allergic to any antidyskinetic.

Before you start, consult your doctor:
- If you have had glaucoma.
- If you have had high blood pressure or heart disease.
- If you have had impaired liver function.
- If you have had kidney disease or urination difficulty.

Over age 60:
More sensitive to drug. Aggravates symptoms of enlarged prostate. Causes impaired thinking, hallucinations, nightmares. Consult doctor about any of these.

Pregnancy:
Studies inconclusive on harm to unborn child. Animal studies show fetal abnormalities. Decide with your doctor whether drug benefits justify risk to unborn child.

Breast-feeding:
May inhibit milk secretion. Consult doctor.

Infants & children:
Not recommended for children 3 and younger. Use for older children only under doctor's supervision.

Prolonged use:
Possible glaucoma.

Skin & sunlight:
No problems expected.

Driving, piloting or hazardous work:
Don't drive or pilot aircraft until you learn how medicine affects you. Don't work around dangerous machinery. Don't climb ladders or work in high places. Danger increases if you drink alcohol or take medicine affecting alertness and reflexes, such as antihistamines, tranquilizers, sedatives, pain medicine, narcotics and mind-altering drugs.

Airplane passengers:
No problems expected.

Discontinuing:
Don't discontinue without consulting doctor. Dose may require gradual reduction if you have taken drug for a long time. Doses of other drugs may also require adjustment.

Others:
- Internal eye pressure should be measured regularly.
- Avoid becoming overheated.

INTERACTION WITH OTHER DRUGS

GENERIC NAME OR DRUG CLASS	COMBINED EFFECT
Amantadine	Increased amantadine effect.
Antidepressants (tricyclic)	Increased biperidine effect. May cause glaucoma.
Antihistamines	Increased biperidine effect.
Levodopa	Increased levodopa effect. Improved results in treating Parkinson's disease.
Meperidine	Increased biperidine effect.
MAO inhibitors	Increased biperidine effect.
Orphenadrine	Increased biperidine effect.
Phenothiazines	Behavior changes.
Primidone	Excessive sedation.
Procainamide	Increased procainamide effect.
Quinidine	Increased biperidine effect.
Tranquilizers	Excessive sedation.

INTERACTION WITH OTHER SUBSTANCES

INTERACTS WITH	COMBINED EFFECT
Alcohol:	None expected.
Beverages:	None expected.
Cocaine:	Decreased biperidine effect. Avoid.
Foods:	None expected.
Marijuana:	None expected.
Tobacco:	None expected.

BISACODYL

BRAND NAMES

Bisco-Lax	Deficol
Cenalax	Dulcolax
Clysodrast	Nulac
Codylax	Theralax

GENERAL INFORMATION

Habit forming? No
Prescription needed? No
Available as generic? Yes
Drug class: Laxative (stimulant)

 ## USES

Constipation relief.

 ## DOSAGE & USAGE INFORMATION

How to take:
- Tablet—Swallow with liquid.
- Suppository—Remove wrapper and moisten suppository with water. Gently insert larger end into rectum. Push well into rectum with finger.

When to take:
Usually at bedtime with a snack, unless directed otherwise.

If you forget a dose:
Take as soon as you remember.

What drug does:
Acts on smooth muscles of intestine wall to cause vigorous bowel movement.

Time lapse before drug works:
6 to 10 hours.

Don't take with:
- See Interaction column and consult doctor.
- Don't take within 2 hours of taking another medicine. Laxative interferes with medicine absorption.

 ## OVERDOSE

Symptoms:
Vomiting, electrolyte depletion.

What to do:

Overdose unlikely to threaten life. If person takes much larger amount than prescribed, call doctor, poison-control center or hospital emergency room for instructions.

POSSIBLE ADVERSE REACTIONS OR SIDE EFFECTS

SYMPTOMS	FREQUENCY	WHAT TO DO
Brain & nervous system: Irritability, confusion, headache.	Rare	3
Skin: Rash	Rare	3
Eyes:	None expected.	
Ears, nose, throat:	None expected.	
Digestive: Belching, cramps, nausea.	Infrequent	4
Heart & lungs: Breathing difficulty, irregular heartbeat.	Rare	3
Blood vessels:	None expected.	
Muscles, bones, joints: Muscle cramps.	Rare	3
Genital, urinary:	None expected.	
Kidneys: Burning on urination.	Rare	4
Liver:	None expected.	
Allergic:	None expected.	
Blood:	None expected.	
Others: • Rectal irritation.	Common	4
• Dangerous potassium loss.	Infrequent	3
• Unusual tiredness or weakness.	Rare	3

1- Life-threatening. Seek emergency treatment immediately.
2- Discontinue. Seek emergency treatment.
3- Discontinue. Call doctor right away.
4- Continue. Call doctor when convenient.
5- Continue. Tell doctor at next visit.
6- No action necessary.

WARNINGS & PRECAUTIONS

Don't take if:
- You have symptoms of appendicitis, inflamed bowel or intestinal blockage.
- You are allergic to a stimulant laxative.
- You have missed a bowel movement for only 1 or 2 days.

Before you start, consult your doctor:
- If you have a colostomy or ileostomy.
- If you have congestive heart disease.
- If you have diabetes.
- If you have high blood pressure.
- If you have a laxative habit.
- If you have rectal bleeding.
- If you take other laxatives.

Over age 60:
Adverse reactions and side effects may be more frequent and severe than in younger persons.

Pregnancy:
Risk to mother and unborn child outweighs drug benefits. Don't use.

Breast-feeding:
Drug passes into milk. Avoid drug or discontinue nursing until you finish medicine. Consult doctor for advice on maintaining milk supply.

Infants & children:
Use only under medical supervision.

Prolonged use:
Don't take for more than 1 week unless under doctor's supervision. May cause laxative dependence.

Skin & sunlight:
No problems expected.

Driving, piloting or hazardous work:
No problems expected.

Airplane passengers:
No problems expected.

Discontinuing:
May be unnecessary to finish medicine. Follow doctor's instructions.

Others:
Don't take to "flush out" your system or as a "tonic."

INTERACTION WITH OTHER DRUGS

GENERIC NAME OR DRUG CLASS	COMBINED EFFECT
Antacids	Tablet coating may dissolve too rapidly, irritating stomach or bowel.
Antihypertensives	May cause dangerous low potassium level.
Cimetidine	Stomach or bowel irritation.
Diuretics	May cause dangerous low potassium level.
Ranitidine	Stomach or bowel irritation.

INTERACTION WITH OTHER SUBSTANCES

INTERACTS WITH	COMBINED EFFECT
Alcohol:	None expected.
Beverages:	None expected.
Cocaine:	None expected.
Foods:	None expected.
Marijuana:	None expected.
Tobacco:	None expected.

BROMODIPHENHYDRAMINE

BRAND NAMES

Ambenyl Expectorant (M)
Ambodryl

GENERAL INFORMATION

Habit forming? No
Prescription needed? Yes
Available as generic? No
Drug class: Antihistamine

USES

- Reduces allergic symptoms such as hay fever, hives, rash or itching.
- Induces sleep.

DOSAGE & USAGE INFORMATION

How to take:
Capsule or liquid—Swallow with liquid or food to lessen stomach irritation.

When to take:
Varies with form. Follow label directions.

If you forget a dose:
Take as soon as you remember up to 2 hours late. If more than 2 hours, wait for next scheduled dose (don't double this dose).

What drug does:
Blocks action of histamine after an allergic response triggers histamine release in sensitive cells.

Time lapse before drug works:
30 minutes.

Don't take with:
See Interaction column and consult doctor.

OVERDOSE

Symptoms:
Convulsions, red face, hallucinations, coma.

What to do:
- Dial 0 (operator) or 911 (emergency) for an ambulance or medical help. Then give first aid immediately.
- If patient is unconscious and not breathing, give mouth-to-mouth breathing. If there is no heartbeat, use cardiac massage and mouth-to-mouth breathing (CPR). Don't try to make patient vomit. If you can't get help quickly, take patient to nearest emergency facility.
- Additional emergency information on page 886.

POSSIBLE ADVERSE REACTIONS OR SIDE EFFECTS

SYMPTOMS	FREQUENCY	WHAT TO DO
Brain & nervous system:		
• Nightmares, agitation, irritability.	Rare	3
• Drowsiness, dizziness.	Common	5
Skin:	None expected.	
Eyes:		
• Vision changes.	Infrequent	3
• Less tolerance for contact lenses.	Infrequent	4
Ears, nose, throat:		
• Sore throat, fever.	Rare	3
• Dry mouth, nose, throat.	Common	5
Digestive:		
• Nausea	Common	5
• Appetite loss.	Infrequent	5
Heart & lungs:		
Rapid heartbeat.	Rare	3
Blood vessels:		
Unusual bleeding or bruising.	Rare	3
Muscles, bones, joints, kidneys, liver, allergic, blood:	None expected.	
Genital, urinary:		
Urination difficulty.	Infrequent	4
Others:		
Fatigue, weakness.	Rare	3

1 - Life-threatening. Seek emergency treatment immediately.
2 - Discontinue. Seek emergency treatment.
3 - Discontinue. Call doctor right away.
4 - Continue. Call doctor when convenient.
5 - Continue. Tell doctor at next visit.
6 - No action necessary.

BROMODIPHENHYDRAMINE

 ## WARNINGS & PRECAUTIONS

Don't take if:
You are allergic to any antihistamine.

Before you start, consult your doctor:
- If you have glaucoma.
- If you have enlarged prostate.
- If you have asthma.
- If you have kidney disease.
- If you have peptic ulcer.
- If you will have surgery within 2 months, including dental surgery, requiring general or spinal anesthesia.

Over age 60:
Don't exceed recommended dose. Adverse reactions and side effects may be more frequent and severe than in younger persons, especially urination difficulty, diminished alertness and other brain and nervous-system symptoms.

Pregnancy:
No proven harm to unborn child. Avoid if possible.

Breast-feeding:
Drug passes into milk. Avoid drug or discontinue nursing until you finish medicine. Consult doctor for advice on maintaining milk supply.

Infants & children:
Not recommended for premature or newborn infants. Otherwise, no problems expected.

Prolonged use:
Avoid. May damage bone-marrow and nerve cells.

Skin & sunlight:
May cause rash or intensify sunburn in areas exposed to sun or sunlamp.

Driving, piloting or hazardous work:
Don't drive or pilot aircraft until you learn how medicine affects you. Don't work around dangerous machinery. Don't climb ladders or work in high places. Danger increases if you drink alcohol or take medicine affecting alertness and reflexes, such as antihistamines, tranquilizers, sedatives, pain medicine, narcotics and mind-altering drugs.

Airplane passengers:
No problems expected.

Discontinuing:
No problems expected.

Others:
May mask symptoms of hearing damage from aspirin, other salicylates, cisplatin, paromomycin, vancomycin or anticonvulsants. Consult doctor if you use these.

 ## INTERACTION WITH OTHER DRUGS

GENERIC NAME OR DRUG CLASS	COMBINED EFFECT
Anticholinergics	Increased anticholinergic effect.
Antidepressants	Excess sedation. Avoid.
Antihistamines (other)	Excess sedation. Avoid.
Hypnotics	Excess sedation. Avoid.
MAO inhibitors	Increased bromodiphenhydramine effect.
Mind-altering drugs	Excess sedation. Avoid.
Narcotics	Excess sedation. Avoid.
Sedatives	Excess sedation. Avoid.
Sleep inducers	Excess sedation. Avoid.
Tranquilizers	Excess sedation. Avoid.

 ## INTERACTION WITH OTHER SUBSTANCES

INTERACTS WITH	COMBINED EFFECT
Alcohol:	Excess sedation. Avoid.
Beverages: Caffeine drinks	Less bromodiphenhydramine sedation.
Cocaine:	Decreased bromodiphenhydramine effect. Avoid.
Foods:	None expected.
Marijuana:	Excess sedation. Avoid.
Tobacco:	None expected.

BROMPHENIRAMINE

BRAND NAMES

Brocon (M)	Drixoral	Rynatapp
Bromepath	Eldatapp	Symptom 3
Bromphen	Histatapp	Taltapp
Dimetane	Poly-Histine	Tapp
Dimetapp	Ralabromophen	Veltap

See complete brand names list, page 822.

GENERAL INFORMATION

Habit forming? No
Prescription needed? Yes
Available as generic? Yes
Drug class: Antihistamine

USES

- Reduces allergic symptoms such as hay fever, hives, rash or itching.
- Induces sleep.

DOSAGE & USAGE INFORMATION

How to take:
- Tablet, capsule or syrup—Swallow with liquid or food to lessen stomach irritation.
- Extended-release tablets or capsules—Swallow each dose whole.

When to take:
Varies with form. Follow label directions.

If you forget a dose:
Take as soon as you remember up to 2 hours late. If more than 2 hours, wait for next scheduled dose (don't double this dose).

What drug does:
Blocks action of histamine after an allergic response triggers histamine release in sensitive cells.

Time lapse before drug works:
30 minutes.

Don't take with:
See Interaction column and consult doctor.

OVERDOSE

Symptoms:
Convulsions, red face, hallucinations, coma.

What to do:
- Dial 0 (operator) or 911 (emergency) for an ambulance or medical help. Then give first aid immediately.
- Additional emergency information on page 886.

POSSIBLE ADVERSE REACTIONS OR SIDE EFFECTS

SYMPTOMS	FREQUENCY	WHAT TO DO
Brain & nervous system:		
• Nightmares, agitation, irritability.	Rare	3
• Drowsiness, dizziness.	Common	5
Skin:	None expected.	
Eyes:		
• Vision changes.	Infrequent	3
• Less tolerance for contact lenses.	Infrequent	4
Ears, nose, throat:		
• Sore throat, fever.	Rare	3
• Dry mouth, nose, throat.	Common	5
Digestive:		
• Nausea	Common	5
• Appetite loss.	Infrequent	5
Heart & lungs:		
Rapid heartbeat.	Rare	3
Blood vessels:		
Unusual bleeding or bruising.	Rare	3
Muscles, bones, joints, kidneys, liver, allergic, blood:	None expected.	
Genital, urinary:		
Urination difficulty.	Infrequent	4
Others:		
Fatigue, weakness.	Rare	3

1- Life-threatening. Seek emergency treatment immediately.
2- Discontinue. Seek emergency treatment.
3- Discontinue. Call doctor right away.
4- Continue. Call doctor when convenient.
5- Continue. Tell doctor at next visit.
6- No action necessary.

BROMPHENIRAMINE

WARNINGS & PRECAUTIONS

Don't take if:
You are allergic to any antihistamine.

Before you start, consult your doctor:
• If you have glaucoma.
• If you have enlarged prostate.
• If you have asthma.
• If you have kidney disease.
• If you have peptic ulcer.
• If you will have surgery within 2 months, including dental surgery, requiring general or spinal anesthesia.

Over age 60:
Don't exceed recommended dose. Adverse reactions and side effects may be more frequent and severe than in younger persons, especially urination difficulty, diminished alertness and other brain and nervous-system symptoms.

Pregnancy:
No proven harm to unborn child. Avoid if possible.

Breast-feeding:
Drug passes into milk. Avoid drug or discontinue nursing until you finish medicine. Consult doctor for advice on maintaining milk supply.

Infants & children:
Not recommended for premature or newborn infants. Otherwise, no problems expected.

Prolonged use:
Avoid. May damage bone marrow and nerve cells.

Skin & sunlight:
May cause rash or intensify sunburn in areas exposed to sun or sunlamp.

Driving, piloting or hazardous work:
Don't drive or pilot aircraft until you learn how medicine affects you. Don't work around dangerous machinery. Don't climb ladders or work in high places. Danger increases if you drink alcohol or take medicine affecting alertness and reflexes, such as antihistamines, tranquilizers, sedatives, pain medicine, narcotics and mind-altering drugs.

Airplane passengers:
No problems expected.

Discontinuing:
No problems expected.

Others:
May mask symptoms of hearing damage from aspirin, other salicylates, cisplatin, paromomycin, vancomycin or anticonvulsants. Consult doctor if you use these.

INTERACTION WITH OTHER DRUGS

GENERIC NAME OR DRUG CLASS	COMBINED EFFECT
Anticholinergics	Increased anticholinergic effect.
Antidepressants	Excess sedation. Avoid.
Antihistamines (other)	Excess sedation. Avoid.
Hypnotics	Excess sedation. Avoid.
MAO inhibitors	Increased brompheniramine effect.
Mind-altering drugs	Excess sedation. Avoid.
Narcotics	Excess sedation. Avoid.
Sedatives	Excess sedation. Avoid.
Sleep inducers	Excess sedation. Avoid.
Tranquilizers	Excess sedation. Avoid.

INTERACTION WITH OTHER SUBSTANCES

INTERACTS WITH	COMBINED EFFECT
Alcohol:	Excess sedation. Avoid.
Beverages: Caffeine drinks	Less brompheniramine sedation.
Cocaine:	Decreased brompheniramine effect. Avoid.
Foods:	None expected.
Marijuana:	Excess sedation. Avoid.
Tobacco:	None expected.

BUCLIZINE

BRAND NAMES

Bucladin-S

GENERAL INFORMATION

Habit forming? No
Prescription needed? U.S.: No
Canada: Yes
Available as generic? No
Drug class: Antihistamine, antiemetic

USES

Prevents motion sickness.

DOSAGE & USAGE INFORMATION

How to take:
Tablet—Swallow with liquid or food to lessen stomach irritation. If you can't swallow whole, crumble tablet and chew or take with liquid or food.

When to take:
30 minutes to 1 hour before traveling.

If you forget a dose:
Take as soon as you remember. Wait 4 hours for next dose.

What drug does:
Reduces sensitivity of nerve endings in inner ear, blocking messages to brain's vomiting center.

Time lapse before drug works:
30 to 60 minutes.

Don't take with:
See Interaction column and consult doctor.

OVERDOSE

Symptoms:
Drowsiness, confusion, incoordination, stupor, coma, weak pulse, shallow breathing.

What to do:
- Dial 0 (operator) or 911 (emergency) for an ambulance or medical help. Then give first aid immediately.
- Additional emergency information on page 886.

POSSIBLE ADVERSE REACTIONS OR SIDE EFFECTS

SYMPTOMS	FREQUENCY	WHAT TO DO
Brain & nervous system:		
• Drowsiness	Common	5
• Headache	Infrequent	4
• Restlessness, excitement, insomnia.	Rare	4
Skin:		
Rash or hives.	Rare	3
Eyes:		
Blurred vision.	Rare	4
Ears, nose, throat:		
Dry mouth, nose, throat.	Infrequent	5
Digestive:		
• Appetite loss, nausea.	Rare	5
• Diarrhea or constipation.	Infrequent	4
Heart & lungs:		
Fast heartbeat.	Infrequent	4
Blood vessels:	None expected.	
Muscles, bones, joints:	None expected.	
Genital, urinary:		
Urinary frequency, difficult urination.	Rare	4
Kidneys:	None expected.	
Liver:	None expected.	
Allergic:	None expected.	
Blood:	None expected.	
Others:	None expected.	

1- Life-threatening. Seek emergency treatment immediately.
2- Discontinue. Seek emergency treatment.
3- Discontinue. Call doctor right away.
4- Continue. Call doctor when convenient.
5- Continue. Tell doctor at next visit.

WARNINGS & PRECAUTIONS

Don't take if:
- You are allergic to meclizine, buclizine or cyclizine.
- You have taken MAO inhibitors in the past 2 weeks.

Before you start, consult your doctor:
- If you have glaucoma.
- If you have prostate enlargement.
- If you have reacted badly to any antihistamine.

Over age 60:
Adverse reactions and side effects may be more frequent and severe than in younger persons, especially impaired urination from enlarged prostate gland.

Pregnancy:
Studies inconclusive on harm to unborn child. Animal studies show fetal abnormalities. Decide with your doctor whether drug benefits justify risk to unborn child.

Breast-feeding:
Drug passes into milk. Avoid drug or discontinue nursing until you finish medicine. Consult doctor for advice on maintaining milk supply.

Infants & children:
No problems expected.

Prolonged use:
No problems expected.

Skin & sunlight:
No problems expected.

Driving, piloting or hazardous work:
Don't fly aircraft. Don't drive until you learn how medicine affects you. Don't work around dangerous machinery. Don't climb ladders or work in high places. Danger increases if you drink alcohol or take medicine affecting alertness and reflexes, such as antihistamines, tranquilizers, sedatives, pain medicine, narcotics and mind-altering drugs.

Airplane passengers:
Take 30 minutes before takeoff and every 4 hours while in the air.

Discontinuing:
No problems expected.

Others:
No problems expected.

 INTERACTION WITH OTHER DRUGS

GENERIC NAME OR DRUG CLASS	COMBINED EFFECT
Amphetamines	May decrease drowsiness caused by buclizine.
Anticholinergics	Increased effect of both drugs.
Antidepressants (tricyclic)	Increased effect of both drugs.
MAO inhibitors	Increased buclizine effect.
Narcotics	Increased effect of both drugs.
Pain relievers	Increased effect of both drugs.
Sedatives	Increased effect of both drugs.
Sleep inducers	Increased effect of both drugs.
Tranquilizers	Increased effect of both drugs.

 INTERACTION WITH OTHER SUBSTANCES

INTERACTS WITH	COMBINED EFFECT
Alcohol:	Increased sedation. Avoid.
Beverages: Caffeine drinks	May decrease drowsiness.
Cocaine:	None expected.
Foods:	None expected.
Marijuana:	Increased drowsiness, dry mouth.
Tobacco:	None expected.

BUTABARBITAL

BRAND NAMES

Butalan   Cytospaz SR
Butatran   Levamine
Buticaps   Quibron Plus
Butisol   Sarisol No. 2
See complete brand names list, page 823.

See complete brand names list, page 823.

GENERAL INFORMATION

Habit forming? Yes
Prescription needed? Yes
Available as generic? Yes
Drug class: Sedative, hypnotic (barbiturate)

USES

- Reduces anxiety or nervous tension (low dose).
- Relieves insomnia (higher bedtime dose).

DOSAGE & USAGE INFORMATION

How to take:
Tablet, capsule or liquid—Swallow with food or liquid to lessen stomach irritation. If you can't swallow whole, crumble tablet or open capsule and take with liquid or food.

When to take:
At the same times each day.

If you forget a dose:
Take as soon as you remember up to 2 hours late. If more than 2 hours, wait for next scheduled dose (don't double this dose).

What drug does:
May partially block nerve impulses at nerve-cell connections.

Time lapse before drug works:
60 minutes.

Don't take with:
- Non-prescription drugs without consulting doctor.
- See Interaction column and consult doctor.

OVERDOSE

Symptoms:
Deep sleep, weak pulse, coma.

What to do:
- Dial 0 (operator) or 911 (emergency) for an ambulance or medical help. Then give first aid immediately.
- Additional emergency information on page 886.

POSSIBLE ADVERSE REACTIONS OR SIDE EFFECTS

SYMPTOMS	FREQUENCY	WHAT TO DO
Brain & nervous system:		
● Dizziness, drowsiness, "hangover effect."	Common	4
● Depression, confusion, slurred speech.	Infrequent	4
● Agitation	Rare	3
Skin:		
● Rash or hives.	Infrequent	3
● Face, lip swelling.	Infrequent	3
Eyes:		
Eyelid swelling.	Infrequent	3
Ears, nose, throat:		
Sore throat, fever.	Infrequent	3
Digestive:		
Diarrhea, nausea, vomiting.	Infrequent	4
Heart & lungs:		
● Slow heartbeat.	Rare	3
● Breathing difficulty.	Rare	3
Blood vessels:		
Unexplained bleeding or bruising.	Rare	4
Muscles, bones, joints:		
Joint or muscle pain.	Infrequent	4
Genital, urinary:	None expected.	
Kidneys:	None expected.	
Liver:		
Jaundice (yellow skin and eyes).	Rare	3
Allergic:	None expected.	
Blood:	None expected.	
Others:	None expected.	

1- Life-threatening. Seek emergency treatment immediately.
2- Discontinue. Seek emergency treatment.
3- Discontinue. Call doctor right away.
4- Continue. Call doctor when convenient.

WARNINGS & PRECAUTIONS

Don't take if:
- You are allergic to any barbiturate.
- You have porphyria.

Before you start, consult your doctor:
- If you have epilepsy.
- If you have kidney or liver damage.
- If you have asthma.
- If you have anemia.
- If you have chronic pain.
- If you will have surgery within 2 months, including dental surgery, requiring general or spinal anesthesia.

Over age 60:
Adverse reactions and side effects may be more frequent and severe than in younger persons. Use small doses.

Pregnancy:
Risk to unborn child outweighs drug benefits. Don't use.

Breast-feeding:
Drug passes into milk. Avoid drug or discontinue nursing until you finish medicine. Consult doctor for advice on maintaining milk supply.

Infants & children:
Use only under doctor's supervision.

Prolonged use:
- May cause addiction, anemia, chronic intoxication.
- May lower body temperature, making exposure to cold temperatures hazardous.

Skin & sunlight:
May cause rash or intensify sunburn in areas exposed to sun or sunlamp.

Driving, piloting or hazardous work:
Don't drive or pilot aircraft until you learn how medicine affects you. Don't work around dangerous machinery. Don't climb ladders or work in high places. Danger increases if you drink alcohol or take medicine affecting alertness and reflexes.

Airplane passengers:
No problems expected.

Discontinuing:
May be unnecessary to finish medicine. Follow doctor's instructions. If you develop withdrawal symptoms of hallucinations, agitation or sleeplessness after discontinuing, call doctor right away.

Others:
No problems expected.

INTERACTION WITH OTHER DRUGS

GENERIC NAME OR DRUG CLASS	COMBINED EFFECT
Anticoagulants (oral)	Decreased anticoagulant effect.
Anticonvulsants	Changed seizure patterns.
Antidepressants (tricyclic)	Decreased antidepressant effect.
Antidiabetics (oral)	Increased butabarbital effect.
Antihistamines	Dangerous sedation. Avoid.
Antiinflammatory drugs (non-steroidal)	Decreased antiinflammatory effect.
Aspirin	Decreased aspirin effect.
Beta-adrenergic blockers	Decreased effect of beta-adrenergic blocker.
Contraceptives (oral)	Decreased contraceptive effect.
Cortisone drugs	Decreased cortisone effect.
Digitoxin	Decreased digitoxin effect.
Doxycycline	Decreased doxycycline effect.
Griseofulvin	Decreased griseofulvin effect.

Additional interactions on page 834.

INTERACTION WITH OTHER SUBSTANCES

INTERACTS WITH	COMBINED EFFECT
Alcohol:	Possible fatal oversedation. Avoid.
Beverages:	None expected.
Cocaine:	Decreased butabarbital effect.
Foods:	None expected.
Marijuana:	Excessive sedation. Avoid.
Tobacco:	None expected.

BUTAPERAZINE

BRAND NAMES

Repoise

GENERAL INFORMATION

Habit forming? No
Prescription needed? Yes
Available as generic? Yes
Drug class: Tranquilizer, antiemetic (phenothiazine)

USES

- Stops nausea, vomiting.
- Reduces anxiety, agitation.

DOSAGE & USAGE INFORMATION

How to take:
- Tablet or capsule—Swallow with liquid or food to lessen stomach irritation.
- Suppositories—Remove wrapper and moisten suppository with water. Gently insert into rectum, large end first.
- Drops or liquid—Dilute dose in beverage.

When to take:
- Nervous and mental disorders—Take at the same times each day.
- Nausea and vomiting—Take as needed, no more often than every 4 hours.

If you forget a dose:
- Nervous and mental disorders—Take up to 2 hours late. If more than 2 hours, wait for next scheduled dose (don't double this).
- Nausea and vomiting—Take as soon as you remember. Wait 4 hours for next dose.

What drug does:
- Suppresses brain's vomiting center.
- Suppresses brain centers that control abnormal emotions and behavior.

Time lapse before drug works:
- Nausea and vomiting—1 hour or less.
- Nervous and mental disorders—4-6 weeks.

Don't take with:
- Antacid or medicine for diarrhea.
- Non-prescription drug for cough, cold or allergy.
- See Interaction column and consult doctor.

OVERDOSE

Symptoms:
Stupor, convulsions, coma.

What to do:
- Dial 0 (operator) or 911 (emergency) for an ambulance or medical help. Then give first aid immediately.
- Additional emergency information on page 886.

POSSIBLE ADVERSE REACTIONS OR SIDE EFFECTS

SYMPTOMS	FREQUENCY	WHAT TO DO
Brain & nervous system:		
● Restlessness, tremor.	Common	3
● Fainting	Infrequent	2
● Drowsiness	Common	3
Skin:		
● Rash	Infrequent	3
● Less perspiration.	Common	4
Eyes:		
Vision changes.	Rare	3
Ears, nose, throat:		
● Sore throat, fever.	Rare	3
● Dry mouth, nasal congestion.	Common	4
Digestive:		
Constipation	Common	4
Heart & lungs, blood vessels, kidneys, allergic, blood:	None expected.	
Muscles, bones, joints:		
Muscle spasms of face and neck, unsteady gait.	Common	2
Genital, urinary:		
Urination difficulty.	Infrequent	4
Liver:		
Jaundice (yellow eyes and skin).	Rare	3
Others:		
Less interest in sex, breast swelling, change in menstrual pattern.	Infrequent	4

1- Life-threatening. Seek emergency treatment immediately.
2- Discontinue. Seek emergency treatment.
3- Discontinue. Call doctor right away.
4- Continue. Call doctor when convenient.
5- Continue. Tell doctor at next visit.
6- No action necessary.

WARNINGS & PRECAUTIONS

Don't take if:
- You are allergic to any phenothiazine.
- You have a blood or bone-marrow disease.

Before you start, consult your doctor:
- If you will have surgery within 2 months, including dental surgery, requiring general or spinal anesthesia.
- If you have asthma, emphysema or other lung disorder.
- If you take non-prescription ulcer medicine, asthma medicine or amphetamines.

Over age 60:
Adverse reactions and side effects may be more frequent and severe than in younger persons. More likely to develop involuntary movement of jaws, lips, tongue, chewing. Report this to your doctor immediately. Early treatment can help.

Pregnancy:
Risk to unborn child outweighs drug benefits. Don't use.

Breast-feeding:
Drug passes into milk. Avoid drug or discontinue nursing until you finish medicine. Consult doctor for advice on maintaining milk supply.

Infants & children:
Don't give to children younger than 2.

Prolonged use:
May lead to tardive dyskinesia (involuntary movement of jaws, lips, tongue, chewing).

Skin & sunlight:
May cause rash or intensify sunburn in areas exposed to sun or sunlamp. Skin may remain sensitive for 3 months after discontinuing.

Driving, piloting or hazardous work:
Don't drive or pilot aircraft until you learn how medicine affects you. Don't work around dangerous machinery. Don't climb ladders or work in high places. Danger increases if you drink alcohol or take medicine affecting alertness and reflexes.

Airplane passengers:
No problems expected.

Discontinuing:
- Nervous and mental disorders—Don't discontinue without doctor's advice until you complete prescribed dose, even though symptoms diminish or disappear.
- Nausea and vomiting—May be unnecessary to finish medicine. Follow doctor's instructions.

INTERACTION WITH OTHER DRUGS

GENERIC NAME OR DRUG CLASS	COMBINED EFFECT
Anticholinergics	Increased anticholinergic effect.
Antidepressants (tricyclic)	Increased butaperazine effect.
Antihistamines	Increased antihistamine effect.
Appetite suppressants	Decreased suppressant effect.
Levodopa	Decreased levodopa effect.
Mind-altering drugs	Increased effect of mind-altering drugs.
Narcotics	Increased narcotic effect.
Phenytoin	Increased phenytoin effect.
Quinidine	Impaired heart function. Dangerous mixture.
Sedatives	Increased sedative effect.
Tranquilizers (other)	Increased tranquilizer effect.

INTERACTION WITH OTHER SUBSTANCES

INTERACTS WITH	COMBINED EFFECT
Alcohol:	Dangerous oversedation.
Beverages:	None expected.
Cocaine:	Decreased butaperazine effect. Avoid.
Foods:	None expected.
Marijuana:	Drowsiness. May increase antinausea effect.
Tobacco:	None expected.

BUTORPHANOL

BRAND NAMES

Stadol

GENERAL INFORMATION

Habit forming? Yes
Prescription needed? Yes
Available as generic? Yes
Drug class: Narcotic

USES

Relieves pain.

DOSAGE & USAGE INFORMATION

How to take:
- Tablet or capsule—Swallow with liquid. If you can't swallow whole, crumble tablet or open capsule and take with liquid or food.
- Drops or liquid—Dilute dose in beverage before swallowing.

When to take:
When needed. No more often than every 4 hours.

If you forget a dose:
Take as soon as you remember. Wait 4 hours for next dose.

What drug does:
Blocks pain messages to brain and spinal cord.

Time lapse before drug works:
30 minutes.

Don't take with:
See Interaction column and consult doctor.

OVERDOSE

Symptoms:
Deep sleep; slow breathing; slow pulse; flushed, warm skin; constricted pupils.

What to do:
- Dial 0 (operator) or 911 (emergency) for an ambulance or medical help. Then give first aid immediately.
- If patient is unconscious and not breathing, give mouth-to-mouth breathing. If there is no heartbeat, use cardiac massage and mouth-to-mouth breathing (CPR). Don't try to make patient vomit. If you can't get help quickly, take patient to nearest emergency facility.
- Additional emergency information on page 886.

POSSIBLE ADVERSE REACTIONS OR SIDE EFFECTS

SYMPTOMS	FREQUENCY	WHAT TO DO
Brain & nervous system: Depression, confusion, hallucinations.	Infrequent	4
Skin:		
• Hives, rash, itch, face swelling.	Rare	3
• Flushed face.	Common	4
Eyes: Blurred vision.	Rare	4
Ears, nose, throat:	None expected.	
Digestive: Severe constipation, abdominal pain, vomiting.	Infrequent	3
Heart & lungs: Slow heartbeat, irregular breathing.	Rare	3
Blood vessels:	None expected.	
Muscles, bones, joints:	None expected.	
Genital, urinary: Difficult urination.	Common	4
Kidneys: Less urine.	Common	4
Liver:	None expected.	
Allergic:	None expected.	
Blood:	None expected.	
Others: Unusual tiredness.	Common	4

1 - Life-threatening. Seek emergency treatment immediately.
2 - Discontinue. Seek emergency treatment.
3 - Discontinue. Call doctor right away.
4 - Continue. Call doctor when convenient.
5 - Continue. Tell doctor at next visit.
6 - No action necessary.

BUTORPHANOL

WARNINGS & PRECAUTIONS

Don't take if:
You are allergic to any narcotic.

Before you start, consult your doctor:
If you have impaired heart, liver or kidney function.

Over age 60:
More likely to be drowsy, dizzy, unsteady or constipated. Avoid prolonged use.

Pregnancy:
Studies inconclusive on harm to unborn child. Animal studies show fetal abnormalities. Decide with your doctor whether drug benefits justify risk to unborn child. Abuse by pregnant woman will result in addicted newborn. Withdrawal can be life-threatening.

Breast-feeding:
Drug filters into milk. May harm child. Avoid.

Infants & children:
Not recommended.

Prolonged use:
Causes psychological and physical dependence.

Skin & sunlight:
No problems expected.

Driving, piloting or hazardous work:
Don't drive or pilot aircraft until you learn how medicine affects you. Don't work around dangerous machinery. Don't climb ladders or work in high places. Danger increases if you drink alcohol or take medicine affecting alertness and reflexes, such as antihistamines, tranquilizers, sedatives, pain medicine, other narcotics and mind-altering drugs.

Airplane passengers:
No proven problems.

Discontinuing:
May be unnecessary to finish medicine. Follow doctor's instructions.

Others:
No problems expected.

INTERACTION WITH OTHER DRUGS

GENERIC NAME OR DRUG CLASS	COMBINED EFFECT
Analgesics	Increased analgesic effect.
Antidepressants	Increased sedative effect.
Antihistamines	Increased sedative effect.
Mind-altering drugs	Increased sedative effect.
Narcotics (other)	Increased narcotic effect.
Phenothiazines	Increased phenothiazine effect.
Sedatives	Increased sedative effect.
Sleep inducers	Increased sedative effect.
Tranquilizers	Increased sedative effect.

INTERACTION WITH OTHER SUBSTANCES

INTERACTS WITH	COMBINED EFFECT
Alcohol:	Increases alcohol's intoxicating effect. Avoid.
Beverages:	None expected.
Cocaine:	Increased cocaine effect.
Foods:	None expected.
Marijuana:	Impairs physical and mental performance.
Tobacco:	None expected.

CAFFEINE

BRAND NAMES

A.P.C.-Demerol (M)   Cafetrate
Ban-Drow 2   Nodoz
Cafacetin (M)   Percodan (M)
Cafecon   Tirend
Cafergot (M)   Vivarin
Cafermine (M)
See complete brand names list, page 823.

GENERAL INFORMATION

Habit forming? Yes
Prescription needed? No
Available as generic? Yes
Drug class: Stimulant (xanthine), vasoconstrictor

USES

- Treatment for drowsiness and fatigue.
- Treatment for migraine and other vascular headaches in combination with ergot.

DOSAGE & USAGE INFORMATION

How to take:
- Tablet—Swallow with liquid or food to lessen stomach irritation. If you can't swallow whole, crumble tablet or open capsule and take with liquid or food.
- Extended-release capsules—Swallow whole with liquid.

When to take:
At the same times each day.

If you forget a dose:
Take as soon as you remember up to 2 hours late. If more than 2 hours, wait for next scheduled dose (don't double this dose).

What drug does:
- Constricts blood-vessel walls.
- Stimulates central nervous system.

Time lapse before drug works:
30 minutes.

Don't take with:
- Non-prescription drugs without consulting doctor.
- See Interaction column and consult doctor.

OVERDOSE

Symptoms:
Excitement, rapid heartbeat, hallucinations, convulsions, coma.

What to do:
- Dial 0 (operator) or 911 (emergency) for an ambulance or medical help. Then give first aid immediately.
- Additional emergency information on page 886.

POSSIBLE ADVERSE REACTIONS OR SIDE EFFECTS

SYMPTOMS	FREQUENCY	WHAT TO DO
Brain & nervous system:		
• Nervousness, insomnia.	Common	5
• Confusion, irritability.	Infrequent	3
Skin:	None expected.	
Eyes:	None expected.	
Ears, nose, throat:	None expected.	
Digestive: Nausea, indigestion, burning feeling in stomach.	Infrequent	4
Heart & lungs: Rapid heartbeat.	Common	4
Blood vessels:	None expected.	
Muscles, bones, joints:	None expected.	
Genital, urinary: Increased urination.	Common	6
Kidneys:	None expected.	
Liver:	None expected.	
Allergic:	None expected.	
Blood:	None expected.	
Others: Low blood sugar with tremor, irritability, weakness, sweating.	Common	4

1- Life-threatening. Seek emergency treatment immediately.
2- Discontinue. Seek emergency treatment.
3- Discontinue. Call doctor right away.
4- Continue. Call doctor when convenient.
5- Continue. Tell doctor at next visit.
6- No action necessary.

WARNINGS & PRECAUTIONS

Don't take if:
- You are allergic to any stimulant.
- You have heart disease.
- You have active peptic ulcer of stomach or duodenum.

Before you start, consult your doctor:
- If you have irregular heartbeat.
- If you have hypoglycemia (low blood sugar).
- If you have epilepsy.

Over age 60:
Adverse reactions and side effects may be more frequent and severe than in younger persons.

Pregnancy:
Risk to unborn child outweighs drug benefits. Don't use.

Breast-feeding:
Drug passes into milk. Avoid drug or discontinue nursing until you finish medicine. Consult doctor for advice on maintaining milk supply.

Infants & children:
Not recommended.

Prolonged use:
Stomach ulcers.

Skin & sunlight:
No problems expected.

Driving, piloting or hazardous work:
No problems expected.

Airplane passengers:
No problems expected.

Discontinuing:
Will cause withdrawal symptoms of headache, irritability, drowsiness. Discontinue gradually if you use caffeine for a month or more.

Others:
May produce or aggravate fibrocystic disease of the breast in women.

INTERACTION WITH OTHER DRUGS

GENERIC NAME OR DRUG CLASS	COMBINED EFFECT
Contraceptives (oral)	Increased caffeine effect.
Isoniazid	Increased caffeine effect.
MAO inhibitors	Dangerous blood-pressure rise.
Sedatives	Decreased sedative effect.
Sleep inducers	Decreased sedative effect.
Sympathomimetics	Overstimulation.
Thyroid hormones	Increased thyroid effect.
Tranquilizers	Decreased tranquilizer effect.

INTERACTION WITH OTHER SUBSTANCES

INTERACTS WITH	COMBINED EFFECT
Alcohol:	Decreased alcohol effect.
Beverages: Caffeine drinks	Increased caffeine effect.
Cocaine:	Overstimulation. Avoid.
Foods:	No proven problems.
Marijuana:	Increased effect of both drugs. May lead to dangerous, rapid heartbeat. Avoid.
Tobacco:	Increased heartbeat. Avoid.

CALCIUM CARBONATE

BRAND NAMES

Alka-2	Ducon (M)	Tums
Alkets (M)	Gustalac	
Amitone	Pepto-Bismol	
Camalox (M)	Ratio	
Chooz	Titralac	
Dicarbosil	Trialka	

GENERAL INFORMATION

Habit forming? No
Prescription needed? No
Available as generic? Yes
Drug class: Antacid

 USES

Treatment for hyperacidity in upper gastrointestinal tract, including stomach and esophagus. Symptoms may be heartburn or acid indigestion. Diseases include peptic ulcer, gastritis, esophagitis, hiatal hernia.

 DOSAGE & USAGE INFORMATION

How to take:
- Tablet—Swallow with liquid.
- Chewable tablets or wafers—Chew well before swallowing.

When to take:
1 to 3 hours after meals unless directed otherwise by your doctor.

If you forget a dose:
Take as soon as you remember.

What drug does:
- Neutralizes some of the hydrochloric acid in the stomach.
- Reduces action of pepsin, a digestive enzyme.

Time lapse before drug works:
15 minutes.

Don't take with:
Other medicines at the same time. Decreases absorption of other drugs.

 OVERDOSE

Symptoms:
Weakness, fatigue, dizziness.

What to do:
Overdose unlikely to threaten life. If person takes much larger amount than prescribed, call doctor, poison-control center or hospital emergency room for instructions.

 POSSIBLE ADVERSE REACTIONS OR SIDE EFFECTS

SYMPTOMS	FREQUENCY	WHAT TO DO
Brain & nervous system: Mood changes.	Infrequent	4
Skin:	None expected.	
Eyes:	None expected.	
Ears, nose, throat:	None expected.	
Digestive:		
• Constipation, appetite loss.	Common	4
• Nausea, vomiting.	Infrequent	4
• Lower abdominal pain and swelling.	Infrequent	3
Heart & lungs: Difficult or painful urination.	Rare	3
Blood vessels:	None expected.	
Muscles, bones, joints: Bone pain, muscle weakness.	Infrequent	3
Genital, urinary:	None expected.	
Kidneys:	None expected.	
Liver:	None expected.	
Allergic:	None expected.	
Blood:	None expected.	
Others:		
• Swelling of wrists or ankles.	Infrequent	3
• Unusual tiredness or weakness.	Rare	3
• Weight loss.	Infrequent	4

1- Life-threatening. Seek emergency treatment immediately.
2- Discontinue. Seek emergency treatment.
3- Discontinue. Call doctor right away.
4- Continue. Call doctor when convenient.
5- Continue. Tell doctor at next visit.
6- No action necessary.

CALCIUM CARBONATE

 **WARNINGS &
PRECAUTIONS**

Don't take if:
- You are allergic to any antacid.
- You have a high blood-calcium level.

Before you start, consult your doctor:
- If you have kidney disease.
- If you have chronic constipation, colitis or diarrhea.
- If you have symptoms of appendicitis.
- If you have stomach or intestinal bleeding.
- If you have irregular heartbeat.

Over age 60:
Adverse reactions and side effects may be more frequent and severe than in younger persons. Diarrhea or constipation particularly likely.

Pregnancy:
Risk to unborn child outweighs drug benefits. Don't use.

Breast-feeding:
Drug passes into milk. Avoid drug or discontinue nursing until you finish medicine. Consult doctor for advice on maintaining milk supply.

Infants & children:
Use only under medical supervision.

Prolonged use:
- High blood level of calcium which disturbs electrolyte balance.
- Kidney stones, Impaired kidney function.

Skin & sunlight:
No problems expected.

Driving, piloting or hazardous work:
No problems expected.

Airplane passengers:
No problems expected.

Discontinuing:
May be unnecessary to finish medicine. Follow doctor's instructions.

Others:
Don't take longer than 2 weeks unless under medical supervision.

 **INTERACTION WITH
OTHER DRUGS**

GENERIC NAME OR DRUG CLASS	COMBINED EFFECT
Anticoagulants	Decreased anticoagulant effect.
Calcitonin	Decreased calcitonin effect.
Chlorpromazine	Decreased chlorpromazine effect.
Digitalis preparations	Decreased digitalis effect.
Diuretics	Increased calcium in blood.
Iron supplements	Decreased iron effect.
Meperidine	Increased meperidine effect.
Nalidixic acid	Decreased effect of nalidixic acid.
Oxyphenbutazone	Decreased oxyphenbutazone effect.
Para-aminosalicylic acid (PAS)	Decreased PAS effect.
Penicillins	Decreased penicillin effect.
Pentobarbital	Decreased pentobarbital effect.
Phenylbutazone	Decreased phenylbutazone effect.
Pseudoephedrine	Increased pseudoephedrine effect.

Additional interactions on page 834.

 **INTERACTION WITH
OTHER SUBSTANCES**

INTERACTS WITH	COMBINED EFFECT
Alcohol:	Decreased antacid effect.
Beverages:	No proven problems.
Cocaine:	No proven problems.
Foods:	Decreased antacid effect if taken with food. Wait 1 hour after eating.
Marijuana:	No proven problems.
Tobacco:	Decreased antacid effect.

CAPTOPRIL

BRAND NAMES

Capoten

GENERAL INFORMATION

Habit forming? No
Prescription needed? Yes
Available as generic? No
Drug class: Antihypertensive

 USES

Treatment for high blood pressure and congestive heart failure.

 DOSAGE & USAGE INFORMATION

How to take:
Tablets—Swallow with liquid. Instructions to take on empty stomach mean 1 hour before or 2 hours after eating.

When to take:
At the same times each day, usually 3 times daily. Take first dose at bedtime and lie down immediately.

If you forget a dose:
Take as soon as you remember up to 2 hours late. If more than 2 hours, wait for next scheduled dose (don't double this dose).

What drug does:
● Reduces resistance in arteries.
● Strengthens heartbeat.

Time lapse before drug works:
60 to 90 minutes.

Don't take with:
See Interaction column and consult doctor.

 OVERDOSE

Symptoms:
Fever, chills, sore throat, fainting, convulsions, coma.

What to do:
● Dial 0 (operator) or 911 (emergency) for an ambulance or medical help. Then give first aid immediately.
● Additional emergency information on page 886.

 POSSIBLE ADVERSE REACTIONS OR SIDE EFFECTS

SYMPTOMS	FREQUENCY	WHAT TO DO
Brain & nervous system: Dizziness, fainting.	Infrequent	3
Skin: Rash	Common	3
Eyes:	None expected.	
Ears, nose, throat: ● Sore throat. ● Loss of taste.	Rare Common	3 3
Digestive: Nausea, vomiting, indigestion, abdominal pain.	Rare	4
Heart & lungs: Chest pain, fast or irregular heartbeat.	Infrequent	3
Blood vessels:	None expected.	
Muscles, bones, joints:	None expected.	
Genital, urinary: Cloudy urine.	Rare	3
Kidneys:	None expected.	
Liver:	None expected.	
Allergic: Swelling of face, hands, mouth or feet.	Infrequent	2
Blood:	None expected.	
Others: Fever, chills.	Rare	3

1- Life-threatening. Seek emergency treatment immediately.
2- Discontinue. Seek emergency treatment.
3- Discontinue. Call doctor right away.
4- Continue. Call doctor when convenient.
5- Continue. Tell doctor at next visit.
6- No action necessary.

WARNINGS & PRECAUTIONS

Don't take if:
- You are allergic to captopril.
- You have any autoimmune disease, including AIDS or lupus.
- You are receiving blood from a blood bank.
- You take drugs for cancer.
- You will have surgery within 2 months, including dental surgery, requiring general or spinal anesthesia.

Before you start, consult your doctor:
- If you have had a stroke.
- If you have angina or heart or blood-vessel disease.
- If you have high level of potassium in blood.
- If you have kidney disease.
- If you are on severe salt-restricted diet.
- If you have lupus.

Over age 60:
Adverse reactions and side effects may be more frequent and severe than in younger persons.

Pregnancy:
Risk to unborn child outweighs drug benefits. Don't use.

Breast-feeding:
Drug passes into milk. Avoid drug or discontinue nursing.

Infants & children:
Not recommended.

Prolonged use:
May decrease white cells in blood or cause protein loss in urine. Request periodic laboratory blood counts and urine tests.

Skin & sunlight:
No problems expected.

Driving, piloting or hazardous work:
Avoid if you become dizzy or faint. Otherwise, no problems expected.

Airplane passengers:
No problems expected.

Discontinuing:
Don't discontinue without consulting doctor. Dose may require gradual reduction if you have taken drug for a long time. Doses of other drugs may also require adjustment.

Others:
- Stop taking diuretics or increase salt intake 1 week before starting captopril.
- Avoid exercising in hot weather.

INTERACTION WITH OTHER DRUGS

GENERIC NAME OR DRUG CLASS	COMBINED EFFECT
Amiloride	Possible excessive potassium in blood.
Antihypertensives (other)	Possible excessive blood-pressure drop.
Chloramphenicol	Possible blood disorders.
Diuretics	Severe blood-pressure drop with first dose.
Potassium supplements	Excessive potassium in blood.
Spironolactone	Possible excessive potassium in blood.
Triamterene	Possible excessive potassium in blood.

INTERACTION WITH OTHER SUBSTANCES

INTERACTS WITH	COMBINED EFFECT
Alcohol:	Possible excessive blood-pressure drop.
Beverages: Low-salt milk	Possible excessive potassium in blood.
Cocaine:	Increased dizziness and chest pain.
Foods: Salt substitutes	Possible excessive potassium.
Marijuana:	Increased dizziness.
Tobacco:	May decrease captopril effect.

CARBAMAZEPINE

BRAND NAMES

Tegretol

Habit forming? No
Prescription needed? Yes

GENERAL INFORMATION

Available as generic? No
Drug class: Analgesic, anticonvulsant

USES

- Decreased frequency, severity and duration of attacks of tic douloureux.
- Prevents seizures.

DOSAGE & USAGE INFORMATION

How to take:
Regular or chewable tablet—Swallow with liquid or food to lessen stomach irritation.

When to take:
At the same times each day.

If you forget a dose:
Take as soon as you remember up to 2 hours late. If more than 2 hours, wait for next scheduled dose (don't double this dose).

What drug does:
- Reduces transmission of pain messages at certain nerve terminals.
- Reduces excitability of nerve fibers in brain, thus inhibiting repetitive spread of nerve impulses.

Time lapse before drug works:
- Tic douloureaux—24 to 72 hours.
- Seizures—1 to 2 weeks.

Don't take with:
See Interaction column and consult doctor.

OVERDOSE

Symptoms:
Involuntary movements, dilated pupils, flushed skin, stupor, coma.

What to do:
- Dial 0 (operator) or 911 (emergency) for an ambulance or medical help. Then give first aid immediately.
- If patient is unconscious and not breathing, give mouth-to-mouth breathing. If there is no heartbeat, use cardiac massage and mouth-to-mouth breathing (CPR). Don't try to make patient vomit. If you can't get help quickly, take patient to nearest emergency facility.
- Additional emergency information on page 886.

POSSIBLE ADVERSE REACTIONS OR SIDE EFFECTS

SYMPTOMS	FREQUENCY	WHAT TO DO
Brain & nervous system: Confusion, slurred speech, fainting, depression, headache, hallucinations.	Infrequent	3
Skin: Hives, rash.	Infrequent	3
Eyes: • Blurred vision.	Common	4
• Back-and-forth eye movements.	Rare	3
Ears, nose, throat: Sores in mouth, sore throat, fever.	Infrequent	3
Digestive: Diarrhea	Infrequent	4
Heart & lungs: Breathing difficulty; irregular, pounding or slow heartbeat; pain in chest.	Rare	3
Blood vessels: Unusual bleeding or bruising.	Infrequent	3
Muscles, bones, joints: Uncontrolled body jerks; numbness, weakness, tingling in hands and feet; tender, bluish legs or feet.	Rare	3
Genital, urinary: Frequent urination.	Rare	4
Kidneys: Less urine.	Rare	3
Liver, allergic, blood:	None expected.	
Others: • Unusual fatigue.	Infrequent	3
• Swollen lymph glands.	Rare	3

1-Life-threatening. Seek emergency treatment immediately.
2-Discontinue. Seek emergency treatment.
3-Discontinue. Call doctor right away.
4-Continue. Call doctor when convenient.

CARBAMAZEPINE

WARNINGS & PRECAUTIONS

Don't take if:
- You are allergic to carbamazepine.
- You have had liver or bone-marrow disease.
- You have taken MAO inhibitors in the past 2 weeks.

Before you start, consult your doctor:
- If you have high blood pressure, thrombophlebitis or heart disease.
- If you have glaucoma.
- If you have emotional or mental problems.
- If you have liver or kidney disease.
- If you drink more than 2 alcoholic drinks per day.

Over age 60:
Adverse reactions and side effects may be more frequent and severe than in younger persons.

Pregnancy:
Studies inconclusive on harm to unborn child. Animal studies show fetal abnormalities. Decide with your doctor whether drug benefits justify risk to unborn child.

Breast-feeding:
Drug passes into milk. Avoid drug or discontinue nursing until you finish medicine. Consult doctor for advice on maintaining milk supply.

Infants & children:
Not recommended.

Prolonged use:
- Jaundice and liver damage.
- Hair loss.
- Ringing in ears.
- Lower sex drive.

Skin & sunlight:
May cause rash or intensify sunburn in areas exposed to sun or sunlamp.

Driving, piloting or hazardous work:
Don't drive or pilot aircraft until you learn how medicine affects you. Don't work around dangerous machinery. Don't climb ladders or work in high places. Danger increases if you drink alcohol or take medicine affecting alertness and reflexes.

Airplane passengers:
No problems expected.

Discontinuing:
Don't discontinue without doctor's advice until you complete prescribed dose, even though symptoms diminish or disappear.

Others:
Use only if less-hazardous drugs are not effective. Stay under medical supervision.

INTERACTION WITH OTHER DRUGS

GENERIC NAME OR DRUG CLASS	COMBINED EFFECT
Anticoagulants (oral)	Decreased anticoagulant effect.
Anticonvulsants (hydantoin)	Decreased effect of both drugs.
Antidepressants (tricyclic)	Confusion. Possible psychosis.
Contraceptives (oral)	Reduced contraceptive protection. Use another birth-control method.
Digitalis preparations	Excess slowing of heart.
Doxycycline	Decreased doxycycline effect.
MAO inhibitors	Dangerous overstimulation. Avoid.
Tranquilizers (benzodiazepine)	Increased carbamazepine effect.

INTERACTION WITH OTHER SUBSTANCES

INTERACTS WITH	COMBINED EFFECT
Alcohol:	Increased sedative effect of alcohol. Avoid.
Beverages:	None expected.
Cocaine:	Increased adverse effect of carbamazepine. Avoid.
Foods:	None expected.
Marijuana:	Increased adverse effects of carbamazepine. Avoid.
Tobacco:	None expected.

CARBENICILLIN

BRAND NAMES

Geocillin
Geopen
Pyopen

GENERAL INFORMATION

Habit forming? No
Prescription needed? Yes
Available as generic? Yes
Drug class: Antibiotic (penicillin)

USES

Treatment of bacterial infections that are susceptible to carbenicillin.

DOSAGE & USAGE INFORMATION

How to take:
- Tablets or capsules—Swallow with liquid on an empty stomach 1 hour before or 2 hours after eating.
- Liquid—Take with cold beverage. Liquid form is perishable and effective for only 7 days at room temperature. Effective for 14 days if stored in refrigerator. Don't freeze.

When to take:
Follow instructions on prescription label or side of package. Doses should be evenly spaced. For example, 4 times a day means every 6 hours.

If you forget a dose:
Take as soon as you remember. Continue regular schedule.

What drug does:
Destroys susceptible bacteria. Does not kill viruses.

Time lapse before drug works:
May be several days before medicine affects infection.

Don't take with:
See Interaction column and consult doctor.

OVERDOSE

Symptoms:
Severe diarrhea, nausea or vomiting.

What to do:
Overdose unlikely to threaten life. If person takes much larger amount than prescribed, call doctor, poison-control center or hospital emergency room for instructions.

POSSIBLE ADVERSE REACTIONS OR SIDE EFFECTS

SYMPTOMS	FREQUENCY	WHAT TO DO
Brain & nervous system:	None expected.	
Skin: Hives, rash, intense itch soon after a dose.	Rare	1
Eyes:	None expected.	
Ears, nose, throat: Dark or discolored tongue.	Common	5
Digestive: Mild nausea, vomiting, diarrhea.	Infrequent	4
Heart & lungs:	None expected.	
Blood vessels: Unexplained bleeding.	Rare	3
Muscles, bones, joints:	None expected.	
Genital, urinary:	None expected.	
Kidneys:	None expected.	
Liver:	None expected.	
Allergic: Life-threatening anaphylaxis may occur!	Rare	1 See Page 888.
Blood:	None expected.	
Others:	None expected.	

1 - Life-threatening. Seek emergency treatment immediately.
2 - Discontinue. Seek emergency treatment.
3 - Discontinue. Call doctor right away.
4 - Continue. Call doctor when convenient.
5 - Continue. Tell doctor at next visit.
6 - No action necessary.

WARNINGS & PRECAUTIONS

Don't take if:
You are allergic to carbenicillin, cephalosporin antibiotics, other penicillins or penicillamine. Life-threatening reaction may occur.

Before you start, consult your doctor:
If you are allergic to any substance or drug.

Over age 60:
You may have skin reactions, particularly around genitals and anus.

Pregnancy:
Studies inconclusive on harm to unborn child. Animal studies show fetal abnormalities. Decide with your doctor whether drug benefits justify risk to unborn child.

Breast-feeding:
Drug passes into milk. Child may become sensitive to penicillins and have allergic reactions to penicillin drugs. Avoid carbenicillin or discontinue nursing until you finish medicine. Consult doctor for advice on maintaining milk supply.

Infants & children:
No problems expected.

Prolonged use:
You may become more susceptible to infections caused by germs not responsive to carbenicillin.

Skin & sunlight:
No problems expected.

Driving, piloting or hazardous work:
Usually not dangerous. Most hazardous reactions likely to occur a few minutes after taking carbenicillin.

Airplane passengers:
No problems expected.

Discontinuing:
Don't discontinue without doctor's advice until you complete prescribed dose, even though symptoms diminish or disappear.

Others:
Injection forms may cause fluid retention (edema) with weakness and low potassium in the blood.

INTERACTION WITH OTHER DRUGS

GENERIC NAME OR DRUG CLASS	COMBINED EFFECT
Chloramphenicol	Decreased effect of both drugs.
Erythromycins	Decreased effect of both drugs.
Paromomycin	Decreased effect of both drugs.
Tetracyclines	Decreased effect of both drugs.
Troleandomycin	Decreased effect of both drugs.

INTERACTION WITH OTHER SUBSTANCES

INTERACTS WITH	COMBINED EFFECT
Alcohol:	Occasional stomach irritation.
Beverages:	None expected.
Cocaine:	No proven problems.
Foods:	Decreased effect of oral carbenicillin.
Marijuana:	No proven problems.
Tobacco:	None expected.

CARBIDOPA & LEVODOPA

BRAND NAMES

Sinemet

GENERAL INFORMATION

Habit forming? No
Prescription needed? Yes
Available as generic? Yes
Drug class: Antiparkinsonism

 USES

Controls Parkinson's disease symptoms such as rigidity, tremor and unsteady gait.

 DOSAGE & USAGE INFORMATION

How to take:
Tablet or capsule—Swallow with liquid or food to lessen stomach irritation. If you can't swallow whole, crumble tablet or open capsule and take with liquid or food.

When to take:
At the same times each day.

If you forget a dose:
Take as soon as you remember up to 2 hours late. If more than 2 hours, wait for next scheduled dose (don't double this dose).

What drug does:
Restores chemical balance necessary for normal nerve impulses.

Time lapse before drug works:
2 to 3 weeks to improve; 6 weeks or longer for maximum benefit.

Don't take with:
See Interaction column and consult doctor.

 OVERDOSE

Symptoms:
Muscle twitch, spastic eyelid closure, nausea, vomiting, diarrhea, irregular and rapid pulse, weakness, fainting, confusion, agitation, hallucination, coma.

What to do:
- Dial 0 (operator) or 911 (emergency) for an ambulance or medical help. Then give first aid immediately.
- If patient is unconscious and not breathing, give mouth-to-mouth breathing. If there is no heartbeat, use cardiac massage and mouth-to-mouth breathing (CPR). Don't try to make patient vomit. If you can't get help quickly, take patient to nearest emergency facility.
- Additional emergency information on page 886.

 POSSIBLE ADVERSE REACTIONS OR SIDE EFFECTS

SYMPTOMS	FREQUENCY	WHAT TO DO
Brain & nervous system:		
• Fainting, severe dizziness, headache, insomnia, nightmares.	Infrequent	3
• Mood changes, uncontrolled body movements.	Common	4
Skin:		
• Flushed face.	Infrequent	4
• Rash, itch.	Infrequent	3
Eyes:		
Blurred vision.	Infrequent	4
Ears, nose, throat:		
Dry mouth.	Common	6
Digestive:		
• Duodenal ulcer.	Rare	4
• Diarrhea	Common	4
• Constipation	Infrequent	5
• Nausea, vomiting.	Infrequent	3
Heart & lungs:		
Irregular heartbeat.	Infrequent	3
Blood vessels:		
High blood pressure.	Rare	3
Muscles, bones, joints:		
Muscle twitching.	Infrequent	4
Genital, urinary:		
• Discolored or dark urine.	Infrequent	4
• Difficult urination.	Infrequent	4
Kidneys, liver, allergic:	None expected.	
Blood:		
Anemia	Rare	4
Others:		
• Tiredness	Infrequent	5
• Body odor.	Common	6

1-Life-threatening. Seek emergency treatment immediately.
2-Discontinue. Seek emergency treatment.
3-Discontinue. Call doctor right away.
4-Continue. Call doctor when convenient.
5-Continue. Tell doctor at next visit.
6-No action necessary.

CARBIDOPA & LEVODOPA

WARNINGS & PRECAUTIONS

Don't take if:
- You are allergic to levodopa or carbidopa.
- You have taken MAO inhibitors in past 2 weeks.
- You have glaucoma (narrow-angle type).

Before you start, consult your doctor:
- If you have diabetes or epilepsy.
- If you have had high blood pressure, heart or lung disease.
- If you have had liver or kidney disease.
- If you have a peptic ulcer.
- If you have malignant melanoma.
- If you will have surgery within 2 months, including dental surgery, requiring general or spinal anesthesia.

Over age 60:
Adverse reactions and side effects may be more frequent and severe than in younger persons.

Pregnancy:
Risk to unborn child outweighs drug benefits. Don't use.

Breast-feeding:
Drug filters into milk. May harm child. Avoid.

Infants & children:
Not recommended.

Prolonged use:
May lead to uncontrolled movements of head, face, mouth, tongue, arms or legs.

Skin & sunlight:
No problems expected.

Driving, piloting or hazardous work:
Don't drive or pilot aircraft until you learn how medicine affects you. Don't work around dangerous machinery. Don't climb ladders or work in high places. Danger increases if you drink alcohol or take medicine affecting alertness and reflexes, such as antihistamines, tranquilizers, sedatives, pain medicine, narcotics and mind-altering drugs.

Airplane passengers:
No problems expected.

Discontinuing:
Don't discontinue without doctor's advice until you complete prescribed dose, even though symptoms diminish or disappear.

Others:
Expect to start with small dose and increase gradually to lessen frequency and severity of adverse reactions.

INTERACTION WITH OTHER DRUGS

GENERIC NAME OR DRUG CLASS	COMBINED EFFECT
Antiparkinsonism drugs (other)	Increased effect of carbidopa and levodopa.
Haloperidol	Decreased effect of carbidopa and levodopa.
MAO inhibitors	Dangerous rise in blood pressure.
Methyldopa	Decreased effect of carbidopa and levodopa.
Papaverine	Decreased effect of carbidopa and levodopa.
Phenothiazines	Decreased effect of carbidopa and levodopa.
Pyridoxine (Vitamin B-6)	Decreased effect carbidopa and levodopa.
Rauwolfia alkaloids	Decreased effect carbidopa and levodopa.

INTERACTION WITH OTHER SUBSTANCES

INTERACTS WITH	COMBINED EFFECT
Alcohol:	None expected.
Beverages:	None expected.
Cocaine:	Decreased carbidopa and levodopa effect.
Foods:	None expected.
Marijuana:	Increased fatigue, lethargy, fainting.
Tobacco:	None expected.

CARBINOXAMINE

BRAND NAMES

Clistin

GENERAL INFORMATION

Habit forming? No
Prescription needed? Yes
Available as generic? No
Drug class: Antihistamine

 USES

Reduces allergic symptoms such as hay fever, hives, rash or itching.

 DOSAGE & USAGE INFORMATION

How to take:
- Tablet—Swallow with liquid or food to lessen stomach irritation.
- Extended-release tablets—Swallow each dose whole. If you take regular tablets, you may chew or crush them.

When to take:
Varies with form. Follow label directions.

If you forget a dose:
Take as soon as you remember up to 2 hours late. If more than 2 hours, wait for next scheduled dose (don't double this dose).

What drug does:
Blocks action of histamine after an allergic response triggers histamine release in sensitive cells.

Time lapse before drug works:
30 minutes.

Don't take with:
See Interaction column and consult doctor.

 OVERDOSE

Symptoms:
Convulsions, red face, hallucinations, coma.

What to do:
- Dial 0 (operator) or 911 (emergency) for an ambulance or medical help. Then give first aid immediately.
- If patient is unconscious and not breathing, give mouth-to-mouth breathing. If there is no heartbeat, use cardiac massage and mouth-to-mouth breathing (CPR). Don't try to make patient vomit. If you can't get help quickly, take patient to nearest emergency facility.
- Additional emergency information on page 886.

POSSIBLE ADVERSE REACTIONS OR SIDE EFFECTS

SYMPTOMS	FREQUENCY	WHAT TO DO
Brain & nervous system:		
• Nightmares, agitation, irritability.	Rare	3
• Drowsiness, dizziness.	Common	5
Skin:	None expected.	
Eyes:		
• Vision changes.	Infrequent	3
• Less tolerance for contact lenses.	Infrequent	4
Ears, nose, throat:		
• Sore throat, fever.	Rare	3
• Dry mouth, nose, throat.	Common	5
Digestive:		
• Nausea	Common	5
• Appetite loss.	Infrequent	5
Heart & lungs:		
Rapid heartbeat.	Rare	3
Blood vessels:		
Unusual bleeding or bruising.	Rare	3
Muscles, bones, joints, kidneys, liver, allergic, blood:	None expected.	
Genital, urinary:		
Urination difficulty.	Infrequent	4
Others:		
Fatigue, weakness.	Rare	3

1- Life-threatening. Seek emergency treatment immediately.
2- Discontinue. Seek emergency treatment.
3- Discontinue. Call doctor right away.
4- Continue. Call doctor when convenient.
5- Continue. Tell doctor at next visit.
6- No action necessary.

CARBINOXAMINE

WARNINGS & PRECAUTIONS

Don't take if:
You are allergic to any antihistamine.

Before you start, consult your doctor:
● If you have glaucoma.
● If you have enlarged prostate.
● If you have asthma.
● If you have kidney disease.
● If you have peptic ulcer.
● If you will have surgery within 2 months, including dental surgery, requiring general or spinal anesthesia.

Over age 60:
Don't exceed recommended dose. Adverse reactions and side effects may be more frequent and severe than in younger persons, especially urination difficulty, diminished alertness and other brain and nervous-system symptoms.

Pregnancy:
No proven harm to unborn child. Avoid if possible.

Breast-feeding:
Drug passes into milk. Avoid drug or discontinue nursing until you finish medicine. Consult doctor for advice on maintaining milk supply.

Infants & children:
Not recommended for premature or newborn infants. Otherwise, no problems expected.

Prolonged use:
Avoid. May damage bone marrow and nerve cells.

Skin & sunlight:
May cause rash or intensify sunburn in areas exposed to sun or sunlamp.

Driving, piloting or hazardous work:
Don't drive or pilot aircraft until you learn how medicine affects you. Don't work around dangerous machinery. Don't climb ladders or work in high places. Danger increases if you drink alcohol or take medicine affecting alertness and reflexes, such as antihistamines, tranquilizers, sedatives, pain medicine, narcotics and mind-altering drugs.

Airplane passengers:
No problems expected.

Discontinuing:
No problems expected.

Others:
May mask symptoms of hearing damage from aspirin, other salicylates, cisplatin, paromomycin, vancomycin or anticonvulsants. Consult doctor if you use these.

INTERACTION WITH OTHER DRUGS

GENERIC NAME OR DRUG CLASS	COMBINED EFFECT
Anticholinergics	Increased anticholinergic effect.
Antidepressants	Excess sedation. Avoid.
Antihistamines (other)	Excess sedation. Avoid.
Hypnotics	Excess sedation. Avoid.
MAO inhibitors	Increased carbinoxamine effect.
Mind-altering drugs	Excess sedation. Avoid.
Narcotics	Excess sedation. Avoid.
Sedatives	Excess sedation. Avoid.
Sleep inducers	Excess sedation. Avoid.
Tranquilizers	Excess sedation. Avoid.

INTERACTION WITH OTHER SUBSTANCES

INTERACTS WITH	COMBINED EFFECT
Alcohol:	Excess sedation. Avoid.
Beverages: Caffeine drinks	Less carbinoxamine sedation.
Cocaine:	Decreased carbinoxamine effect. Avoid.
Foods:	None expected.
Marijuana:	Excess sedation. Avoid.
Tobacco:	None expected.

CARISOPRODOL

BRAND NAMES

Rela
Soma
Soma Compound
Soprodol

Habit forming? No
Prescription needed? Yes
Available as generic? Yes
Drug class: Muscle relaxant (skeletal)

 ## USES

Treatment for sprains, strains and muscle spasms.

 ## DOSAGE & USAGE INFORMATION

How to take:
Tablet or capsule—Swallow with liquid.

When to take:
As needed, no more often than every 4 hours.

If you forget a dose:
Take as soon as you remember. Wait 4 hours for next dose.

What drug does:
Blocks body's pain messages to brain. May also sedate.

Time lapse before drug works:
60 minutes.

Don't take with:
See Interaction column and consult doctor.

 ## OVERDOSE

Symptoms:
Nausea, vomiting, diarrhea, headache. May progress to severe weakness, difficult breathing, sensation of paralysis, coma.

What to do:
- Dial 0 (operator) or 911 (emergency) for an ambulance or medical help. Then give first aid immediately.
- Additional emergency information on page 886.

POSSIBLE ADVERSE REACTIONS OR SIDE EFFECTS

SYMPTOMS	FREQUENCY	WHAT TO DO
Brain & nervous system:		
• Drowsiness, fainting, dizziness.	Common	4
• Agitation	Infrequent	3
Skin: Rash, hives or itch.	Rare	3
Eyes:	None expected.	
Ears, nose, throat: Sore throat, fever.	Rare	3
Digestive:		
• Constipation or diarrhea; nausea, cramps, vomiting.	Infrequent	3
• Bloody or tarry, black stool.	Rare	2
Heart & lungs: Wheezing, shortness of breath.	Infrequent	3
Blood vessels:	None expected.	
Muscles, bones, joints:	None expected.	
Genital, urinary: Orange or red-purple urine.	Common	6
Kidneys:	None expected.	
Liver: Jaundice (yellow eyes and skin).	Rare	3
Allergic:	None expected.	
Blood:	None expected.	
Others: Tiredness, weakness.	Rare	3

1- Life-threatening. Seek emergency treatment immediately.
2- Discontinue. Seek emergency treatment.
3- Discontinue. Call doctor right away.
4- Continue. Call doctor when convenient.
5- Continue. Tell doctor at next visit.
6- No action necessary.

CARISOPRODOL

WARNINGS & PRECAUTIONS

Don't take if:
- You are allergic to any skeletal-muscle relaxant.
- You have porphyria.

Before you start, consult your doctor:
- If you have had liver or kidney disease.
- If you plan pregnancy within medication period.

Over age 60:
Adverse reactions and side effects may be more frequent and severe than in younger persons.

Pregnancy:
No proven harm to unborn child. Avoid if possible.

Breast-feeding:
Drug passes into milk. Avoid drug or discontinue nursing until you finish medicine. Consult doctor for advice on maintaining milk supply.

Infants & children:
Not recommended.

Prolonged use:
Periodic liver-function tests recommended if you use this drug for a long time.

Skin & sunlight:
No problems expected.

Driving, piloting or hazardous work:
Don't drive or pilot aircraft until you learn how medicine affects you. Don't work around dangerous machinery. Don't climb ladders or work in high places. Danger increases if you drink alcohol or take medicine affecting alertness and reflexes, such as antihistamines, tranquilizers, sedatives, pain medicine, narcotics and mind-altering drugs.

Airplane passengers:
No problems expected.

Discontinuing:
Don't discontinue without doctor's advice until you complete prescribed dose, even though symptoms diminish or disappear.

Others:
No problems expected.

INTERACTION WITH OTHER DRUGS

GENERIC NAME OR DRUG CLASS	COMBINED EFFECT
Antidepressants	Increased sedation.
Antihistamines	Increased sedation.
Mind-altering drugs	Increased sedation.
Muscle relaxants (others)	Increased sedation.
Narcotics	Increased sedation.
Sedatives	Increased sedation.
Sleep inducers	Increased sedation.
Testosterone	Decreased carisoprodol effect.
Tranquilizers	Increased sedation.

INTERACTION WITH OTHER SUBSTANCES

INTERACTS WITH	COMBINED EFFECT
Alcohol:	Increased sedation.
Beverages:	None expected.
Cocaine:	Lack of coordination, increased sedation.
Foods:	None expected.
Marijuana:	Lack of coordination, drowsiness, fainting.
Tobacco:	None expected.

CARPHENAZINE

BRAND NAMES

Proketazine

GENERAL INFORMATION

Habit forming? No
Prescription needed? Yes
Available as generic? Yes
Drug class: Tranquilizer, antiemetic (phenothiazine)

USES

- Stops nausea, vomiting.
- Reduces anxiety, agitation.

DOSAGE & USAGE INFORMATION

How to take:
- Tablet or capsule—Swallow with liquid or food to lessen stomach irritation.
- Suppositories—Remove wrapper and moisten suppository with water. Gently insert into rectum, large end first.
- Drops or liquid—Dilute dose in beverage.

When to take:
- Nervous and mental disorders—Take at the same times each day.
- Nausea and vomiting—Take as needed, no more often than every 4 hours.

If you forget a dose:
- Nervous and mental disorders—Take up to 2 hours late. If more than 2 hours, wait for next scheduled dose (don't double this).
- Nausea and vomiting—Take as soon as you remember. Wait 4 hours for next dose.

What drug does:
- Suppresses brain's vomiting center.
- Suppresses brain centers that control abnormal emotions and behavior.

Time lapse before drug works:
- Nausea and vomiting—1 hour or less.
- Nervous and mental disorders—4-6 weeks.

Don't take with:
- Antacid or medicine for diarrhea.
- Non-prescription drug for cough, cold or allergy.
- See Interaction column and consult doctor.

OVERDOSE

Symptoms:
Stupor, convulsions, coma.

What to do:
- Dial 0 (operator) or 911 (emergency) for an ambulance or medical help. Then give first aid immediately.
- Additional emergency information on page 886.

POSSIBLE ADVERSE REACTIONS OR SIDE EFFECTS

SYMPTOMS	FREQUENCY	WHAT TO DO
Brain & nervous system:		
• Restlessness, tremor.	Common	3
• Fainting	Infrequent	2
• Drowsiness	Common	3
Skin:		
• Rash	Infrequent	3
• Less perspiration.	Common	4
Eyes:		
Vision changes.	Rare	3
Ears, nose, throat:		
• Sore throat, fever.	Rare	3
• Dry mouth, nasal congestion.	Common	4
Digestive:		
Constipation	Common	4
Heart & lungs, blood vessels, kidneys, allergic, blood:	None expected.	
Muscles, bones, joints:		
Muscle spasms of face and neck, unsteady gait.	Common	2
Genital, urinary:		
Urination difficulty.	Infrequent	4
Liver:		
Jaundice (yellow eyes and skin).	Rare	3
Others:		
Less interest in sex, breast swelling, change in menstrual pattern.	Infrequent	4

1 - Life-threatening. Seek emergency treatment immediately.
2 - Discontinue. Seek emergency treatment.
3 - Discontinue. Call doctor right away.
4 - Continue. Call doctor when convenient.
5 - Continue. Tell doctor at next visit.
6 - No action necessary.

CARPHENAZINE

WARNINGS & PRECAUTIONS

Don't take if:
- You are allergic to any phenothiazine.
- You have a blood or bone-marrow disease.

Before you start, consult your doctor:
- If you will have surgery within 2 months, including dental surgery, requiring general or spinal anesthesia.
- If you have asthma, emphysema or other lung disorder.
- If you take non-prescription ulcer medicine, asthma medicine or amphetamines.

Over age 60:
Adverse reactions and side effects may be more frequent and severe than in younger persons. More likely to develop involuntary movement of jaws, lips, tongue, chewing. Report this to your doctor immediately. Early treatment can help.

Pregnancy:
Risk to unborn child outweighs drug benefits. Don't use.

Breast-feeding:
Drug passes into milk. Avoid drug or discontinue nursing until you finish medicine. Consult doctor for advice on maintaining milk supply.

Infants & children:
Don't give to children younger than 2.

Prolonged use:
May lead to tardive dyskinesia (involuntary movement of jaws, lips, tongue, chewing).

Skin & sunlight:
May cause rash or intensify sunburn in areas exposed to sun or sunlamp. Skin may remain sensitive for 3 months after discontinuing.

Driving, piloting or hazardous work:
Don't drive or pilot aircraft until you learn how medicine affects you. Don't work around dangerous machinery. Don't climb ladders or work in high places. Danger increases if you drink alcohol or take medicine affecting alertness and reflexes.

Airplane passengers:
No problems expected.

Discontinuing:
- Nervous and mental disorders—Don't discontinue without doctor's advice until you complete prescribed dose, even though symptoms diminish or disappear.
- Nausea and vomiting—May be unnecessary to finish medicine. Follow doctor's instructions.

INTERACTION WITH OTHER DRUGS

GENERIC NAME OR DRUG CLASS	COMBINED EFFECT
Anticholinergics	Increased anticholinergic effect.
Antidepressants (tricyclic)	Increased carphenazine effect.
Antihistamines	Increased antihistamine effect.
Appetite suppressants	Decreased suppressant effect.
Levodopa	Decreased levodopa effect.
Mind-altering drugs	Increased effect of mind-altering drugs.
Narcotics	Increased narcotic effect.
Phenytoin	Increased phenytoin effect.
Quinidine	Impaired heart function. Dangerous mixture.
Sedatives	Increased sedative effect.
Tranquilizers (other)	Increased tranquilizer effect.

INTERACTION WITH OTHER SUBSTANCES

INTERACTS WITH	COMBINED EFFECT
Alcohol:	Dangerous oversedation.
Beverages:	None expected.
Cocaine:	Decreased carphenazine effect. Avoid.
Foods:	None expected.
Marijuana:	Drowsiness. May increase antinausea effect.
Tobacco:	None expected.

CASCARA

BRAND NAMES

Cascara Sagrada
Cas-Evac

GENERAL INFORMATION

Habit forming? No
Prescription needed? No
Available as generic? Yes
Drug class: Laxative (stimulant)

 USES

Constipation relief.

 DOSAGE & USAGE INFORMATION

How to take:
- Tablet—Swallow with liquid. If you can't swallow whole, chew or crumble tablet and take with liquid or food.
- Liquid—Drink 6 to 8 glasses of water each day, in addition to one taken with each dose.

When to take:
Usually at bedtime with a snack, unless directed otherwise.

If you forget a dose:
Take as soon as you remember.

What drug does:
Acts on smooth muscles of intestine wall to cause vigorous bowel movement.

Time lapse before drug works:
6 to 10 hours.

Don't take with:
- See Interaction column and consult doctor.
- Don't take within 2 hours of taking another medicine. Laxative interferes with medicine absorption.

 OVERDOSE

Symptoms:
Vomiting, electrolyte depletion.

What to do:
Overdose unlikely to threaten life. If person takes much larger amount than prescribed, call doctor, poison-control center or hospital emergency room for instructions.

 POSSIBLE ADVERSE REACTIONS OR SIDE EFFECTS

SYMPTOMS	FREQUENCY	WHAT TO DO
Brain & nervous system: Irritability, confusion, headache.	Rare	3
Skin: Rash	Rare	3
Eyes:	None expected.	
Ears, nose, throat:	None expected.	
Digestive: Belching, cramps, nausea.	Infrequent	4
Heart & lungs: Breathing difficulty, irregular heartbeat.	Rare	3
Blood vessels:	None expected.	
Muscles, bones, joints: Muscle cramps.	Rare	3
Genital, urinary:	None expected.	
Kidneys: Burning on urination.	Rare	4
Liver:	None expected.	
Allergic:	None expected.	
Blood:	None expected.	
Others: • Rectal irritation.	Common	4
• Dangerous potassium loss.	Infrequent	3
• Unusual tiredness or weakness.	Rare	3

1- Life-threatening. Seek emergency treatment immediately.
2- Discontinue. Seek emergency treatment.
3- Discontinue. Call doctor right away.
4- Continue. Call doctor when convenient.
5- Continue. Tell doctor at next visit.
6- No action necessary.

CASCARA

WARNINGS & PRECAUTIONS

Don't take if:
- You have symptoms of appendicitis, inflamed bowel or intestinal blockage.
- You are allergic to a stimulant laxative.
- You have missed a bowel movement for only 1 or 2 days.

Before you start, consult your doctor:
- If you have a colostomy or ileostomy.
- If you have congestive heart disease.
- If you have diabetes.
- If you have high blood pressure.
- If you have a laxative habit.
- If you have rectal bleeding.
- If you take other laxatives.

Over age 60:
Adverse reactions and side effects may be more frequent and severe than in younger persons.

Pregnancy:
Risk to mother and unborn child outweighs drug benefits. Don't use.

Breast-feeding:
Drug passes into milk. Avoid drug or discontinue nursing until you finish medicine. Consult doctor for advice on maintaining milk supply.

Infants & children:
Use only under medical supervision.

Prolonged use:
Don't take for more than 1 week unless under a doctor's supervision. May cause laxative dependence.

Skin & sunlight:
No problems expected.

Driving, piloting or hazardous work:
No problems expected.

Airplane passengers:
No problems expected.

Discontinuing:
May be unnecessary to finish medicine. Follow doctor's instructions.

Others:
Don't take to "flush out" your system or as a "tonic."

INTERACTION WITH OTHER DRUGS

GENERIC NAME OR DRUG CLASS	COMBINED EFFECT
Antihypertensives	May cause dangerous low potassium level.
Diuretics	May cause dangerous low potassium level.

INTERACTION WITH OTHER SUBSTANCES

INTERACTS WITH	COMBINED EFFECT
Alcohol:	None expected.
Beverages:	None expected.
Cocaine:	None expected.
Foods:	None expected.
Marijuana:	None expected.
Tobacco:	None expected.

CASTOR OIL

BRAND NAMES

Alphamul
Emulsoil
Neoloid
Purge

GENERAL INFORMATION

Habit forming? No
Prescription needed? No
Available as generic? Yes
Drug class: Laxative (stimulant)

 ## USES

Constipation relief.

 ## DOSAGE & USAGE INFORMATION

How to take:
Liquid—Drink 6 to 8 glasses of water each day, in addition to one taken with each dose.

When to take:
Usually at bedtime with a snack, unless directed otherwise.

If you forget a dose:
Take as soon as you remember.

What drug does:
Acts on smooth muscles of intestine wall to cause vigorous bowel movement.

Time lapse before drug works:
2 to 6 hours.

Don't take with:
- See Interaction column and consult doctor.
- Don't take within 2 hours of taking another medicine. Laxative interferes with medicine absorption.

 ## OVERDOSE

Symptoms:
Vomiting, electrolyte depletion.

What to do:
Overdose unlikely to threaten life. If person takes much larger amount than prescribed, call doctor, poison-control center or hospital emergency room for instructions.

POSSIBLE ADVERSE REACTIONS OR SIDE EFFECTS

SYMPTOMS	FREQUENCY	WHAT TO DO
Brain & nervous system: Irritability, confusion, headache.	Rare	3
Skin: Rash	Rare	3
Eyes:	None expected.	
Ears, nose, throat:	None expected.	
Digestive: Belching, cramps, nausea.	Infrequent	4
Heart & lungs: Breathing difficulty, irregular heartbeat.	Rare	3
Blood vessels:	None expected.	
Muscles, bones, joints: Muscle cramps.	Rare	3
Genital, urinary:	None expected.	
Kidneys: Burning on urination.	Rare	4
Liver:	None expected.	
Allergic:	None expected.	
Blood:	None expected.	
Others: • Rectal irritation.	Common	4
• Dangerous potassium loss.	Infrequent	3
• Unusual tiredness or weakness.	Rare	3

1- Life-threatening. Seek emergency treatment immediately.
2- Discontinue. Seek emergency treatment.
3- Discontinue. Call doctor right away.
4- Continue. Call doctor when convenient.
5- Continue. Tell doctor at next visit.
6- No action necessary.

WARNINGS & PRECAUTIONS

Don't take if:
- You have symptoms of appendicitis, inflamed bowel or intestinal blockage.
- You are allergic to a stimulant laxative.
- You have missed a bowel movement for only 1 or 2 days.

Before you start, consult your doctor:
- If you have a colostomy or ileostomy.
- If you have congestive heart disease.
- If you have diabetes.
- If you have high blood pressure.
- If you have a laxative habit.
- If you have rectal bleeding.
- If you take other laxatives.

Over age 60:
Adverse reactions and side effects may be more frequent and severe than in younger persons.

Pregnancy:
Risk to mother and unborn child outweighs drug benefits. Don't use.

Breast-feeding:
Drug passes into milk. Avoid drug or discontinue nursing until you finish medicine. Consult doctor for advice on maintaining milk supply.

Infants & children:
Use only under medical supervision.

Prolonged use:
Don't take for more than 1 week unless under doctor's supervision. May cause laxative dependence.

Skin & sunlight:
No problems expected.

Driving, piloting or hazardous work:
No problems expected.

Airplane passengers:
No problems expected.

Discontinuing:
May be unnecessary to finish medicine. Follow doctor's instructions.

Others:
Don't take to "flush out" your system or as a "tonic."

INTERACTION WITH OTHER DRUGS

GENERIC NAME OR DRUG CLASS	COMBINED EFFECT
Antihypertensives	May cause dangerous low potassium level.
Diuretics	May cause dangerous low potassium level.

INTERACTION WITH OTHER SUBSTANCES

INTERACTS WITH	COMBINED EFFECT
Alcohol:	None expected.
Beverages:	None expected.
Cocaine:	None expected.
Foods:	None expected.
Marijuana:	None expected.
Tobacco:	None expected.

CEFACLOR

BRAND NAMES

Ceclor

GENERAL INFORMATION

Habit forming? No
Prescription needed? Yes
Available as generic? Yes
Drug class: Antibiotic (cephalosporin)

 ## USES

Treatment of bacterial infections. Will not cure viral infections such as cold and flu.

 ## DOSAGE & USAGE INFORMATION

How to take:
- Tablet or capsule—Swallow with liquid. If you can't swallow whole, crumble tablet or open capsule and take with liquid or food.
- Liquid—Use measuring spoon.

When to take:
At same times each day, 1 hour before or 2 hours after eating.

If you forget a dose:
Take as soon as you remember or double next dose. Return to regular schedule.

What drug does:
Kills susceptible bacteria.

Time lapse before drug works:
May require several days to affect infection.

Don't take with:
See Interaction column and consult doctor.

 ## OVERDOSE

Symptoms:
Abdominal cramps, nausea, vomiting, severe diarrhea with mucus or blood in stool.

What to do:
Overdose unlikely to threaten life. If person takes much larger amount than prescribed, call doctor, poison-control center or hospital emergency room for instructions.

POSSIBLE ADVERSE REACTIONS OR SIDE EFFECTS

SYMPTOMS	FREQUENCY	WHAT TO DO
Brain & nervous system:	None expected.	
Skin:		
• Rash, redness, itching.	Common	3
• Rectal itching.	Infrequent	4
Eyes:	None expected.	
Ears, nose, throat:	None expected.	
Digestive: Mild, nausea, vomiting, cramps, severe diarrhea with mucus or blood in stool.	Rare	3
Heart & lungs:	None expected.	
Blood vessels:	None expected.	
Muscles, bones, joints:	None expected.	
Genital, urinary:	None expected.	
Kidneys:	None expected.	
Liver:	None expected.	
Allergic: Life-threatening anaphylaxis may occur!	Rare	1 See page 888.
Blood:	None expected.	
Others: Unusual weakness, tiredness, weight loss or fever.	Rare	3

1- Life-threatening. Seek emergency treatment immediately.
2- Discontinue. Seek emergency treatment.
3- Discontinue. Call doctor right away.
4- Continue. Call doctor when convenient.
5- Continue. Tell doctor at next visit.
6- No action necessary.

CEFACLOR

WARNINGS & PRECAUTIONS

Don't take if:
You are allergic to any cephalosporin antibiotic.

Before you start, consult your doctor:
- If you are allergic to any penicillin antibiotic.
- If you have a kidney disorder.
- If you have colitis or enteritis.

Over age 60:
Adverse reactions and side effects may be more frequent and severe than in younger persons. More likely to itch around rectum and genitals.

Pregnancy:
No proven harm to unborn child. Avoid if possible.

Breast-feeding:
Drug passes Into milk. Avoid drug or discontinue nursing until you finish medicine. Consult doctor for advice on maintaining milk supply.

Infants & children:
No special warnings.

Prolonged use:
Kills beneficial bacteria that protect body against other germs. Unchecked germs may cause secondary infections.

Skin & sunlight:
No problems expected.

Driving, piloting or hazardous work:
No problems expected.

Airplane passengers:
No problems expected.

Discontinuing:
Don't discontinue without doctor's advice until you complete prescribed dose, even though symptoms diminish or disappear.

Others:
No problems expected.

INTERACTION WITH OTHER DRUGS

GENERIC NAME OR DRUG CLASS	COMBINED EFFECT
Anticoagulants	Increased anticoagulant effect.
Probenecid	Increased cefaclor effect.

INTERACTION WITH OTHER SUBSTANCES

INTERACTS WITH	COMBINED EFFECT
Alcohol:	None expected.
Beverages:	None expected.
Cocaine:	None expected, but cocaine may slow body's recovery. Avoid.
Foods:	Slow absorption. Take with liquid 1 hour before or 2 hours after eating.
Marijuana:	None expected, but marijuana may slow body's recovery. Avoid.
Tobacco:	None expected.

CEFADROXIL

BRAND NAMES

Duricef
Ultracef

GENERAL INFORMATION

Habit forming? No
Prescription needed? Yes
Available as generic? Yes
Drug class: Antibiotic (cephalosporin)

 USES

Treatment of bacterial infections. Will not cure viral infections such as cold and flu.

 DOSAGE & USAGE INFORMATION

How to take:
- Tablet or capsule—Swallow with liquid. If you can't swallow whole, crumble tablet or open capsule and take with liquid or food.
- Liquid—Use measuring spoon.

When to take:
At same times each day, 1 hour before or 2 hours after eating.

If you forget a dose:
Take as soon as you remember or double next dose. Return to regular schedule.

What drug does:
Kills susceptible bacteria.

Time lapse before drug works:
May require several days to affect infection.

Don't take with:
See Interaction column and consult doctor.

 OVERDOSE

Symptoms:
Abdominal cramps, nausea, vomiting, severe diarrhea with mucus or blood in stool.

What to do:
Overdose unlikely to threaten life. If person takes much larger amount than prescribed, call doctor, poison-control center or hospital emergency room for instructions.

POSSIBLE ADVERSE REACTIONS OR SIDE EFFECTS

SYMPTOMS	FREQUENCY	WHAT TO DO
Brain & nervous system:	None expected.	
Skin:		
• Rash, redness, itching.	Common	3
• Rectal itching.	Infrequent	4
Eyes:	None expected.	
Ears, nose, throat:	None expected.	
Digestive: Mild nausea, vomiting, cramps, severe diarrhea with mucus or blood in stool.	Rare	3
Heart & lungs:	None expected.	
Blood vessels:	None expected.	
Muscles, bones, joints:	None expected.	
Genital, urinary:	None expected.	
Kidneys:	None expected.	
Liver:	None expected.	
Allergic: Life-threatening anaphylaxis may occur!	Rare	1 See page 888.
Blood:	None expected.	
Others: Unusual weakness, tiredness, weight loss or fever.	Rare	3

1- Life-threatening. Seek emergency treatment immediately.
2- Discontinue. Seek emergency treatment.
3- Discontinue. Call doctor right away.
4- Continue. Call doctor when convenient.
5- Continue. Tell doctor at next visit.
6- No action necessary.

CEFADROXIL

 WARNINGS & PRECAUTIONS

Don't take if:
You are allergic to any cephalosporin antibiotic.

Before you start, consult your doctor:
- If you are allergic to any penicillin antibiotic.
- If you have a kidney disorder.
- If you have colitis or enteritis.

Over age 60:
Adverse reactions and side effects may be more frequent and severe than in younger persons. More likely to itch around rectum and genitals.

Pregnancy:
No proven harm to unborn child. Avoid if possible.

Breast-feeding:
Drug passes into milk. Avoid drug or discontinue nursing until you finish medicine. Consult doctor for advice on maintaining milk supply.

Infants & children:
No special warnings.

Prolonged use:
Kills beneficial bacteria that protect body against other germs. Unchecked germs may cause secondary infections.

Skin & sunlight:
No problems expected.

Driving, piloting or hazardous work:
No problems expected.

Airplane passengers:
No problems expected.

Discontinuing:
Don't discontinue without doctor's advice until you complete prescribed dose, even though symptoms diminish or disappear.

Others:
No problems expected.

 INTERACTION WITH OTHER DRUGS

GENERIC NAME OR DRUG CLASS	COMBINED EFFECT
Anticoagulants	Increased anticoagulant effect.
Probenecid	Increased cefadroxil effect.

 INTERACTION WITH OTHER SUBSTANCES

INTERACTS WITH	COMBINED EFFECT
Alcohol:	None expected.
Beverages:	None expected.
Cocaine:	None expected, but cocaine may slow body's recovery. Avoid.
Foods:	Slow absorption. Take with liquid 1 hour before or 2 hours after eating.
Marijuana:	None expected, but marijuana may slow body's recovery. Avoid.
Tobacco:	None expected.

CEPHALEXIN

BRAND NAMES

Ceporex
Keflex

GENERAL INFORMATION

Habit forming? No
Prescription needed? Yes
Available as generic? Yes
Drug class: Antibiotic (cephalosporin)

USES

Treatment of bacterial infections. Will not cure viral infections such as cold and flu.

DOSAGE & USAGE INFORMATION

How to take:
- Tablet or capsule—Swallow with liquid. If you can't swallow whole, crumble tablet or open capsule and take with liquid or food.
- Liquid—Use measuring spoon.

When to take:
At same times each day, 1 hour before or 2 hours after eating.

If you forget a dose:
Take as soon as you remember or double next dose. Return to regular schedule.

What drug does:
Kills susceptible bacteria.

Time lapse before drug works:
May require several days to affect infection.

Don't take with:
See Interaction column and consult doctor.

OVERDOSE

Symptoms:
Abdominal cramps, nausea, vomiting, severe diarrhea with mucus or blood in stool.

What to do:
Overdose unlikely to threaten life. If person takes much larger amount than prescribed, call doctor, poison-control center or hospital emergency room for instructions.

POSSIBLE ADVERSE REACTIONS OR SIDE EFFECTS

SYMPTOMS	FREQUENCY	WHAT TO DO
Brain & nervous system:	None expected.	
Skin:		
• Rash, redness, itching.	Common	3
• Rectal itching.	Infrequent	4
Eyes:	None expected.	
Ears, nose, throat:	None expected.	
Digestive: Mild nausea, vomiting, cramps, severe diarrhea with mucus or blood in stool.	Rare	3
Heart & lungs:	None expected.	
Blood vessels:	None expected.	
Muscles, bones, joints:	None expected.	
Genital, urinary:	None expected.	
Kidneys:	None expected.	
Liver:	None expected.	
Allergic: Life-threatening anaphylaxis may occur!	Rare	1 See page 888.
Blood:	None expected.	
Others: Unusual weakness, tiredness, weight loss or fever.	Rare	3

1- Life-threatening. Seek emergency treatment immediately.
2- Discontinue. Seek emergency treatment.
3- Discontinue. Call doctor right away.
4- Continue. Call doctor when convenient.
5- Continue. Tell doctor at next visit.
6- No action necessary.

WARNINGS & PRECAUTIONS

Don't take if:
You are allergic to any cephalosporin antibiotic.

Before you start, consult your doctor:
- If you are allergic to any penicillin antibiotic.
- If you have a kidney disorder.
- If you have colitis or enteritis.

Over age 60:
Adverse reactions and side effects may be more frequent and severe than in younger persons. More likely to itch around rectum and genitals.

Pregnancy:
No proven harm to unborn child. Avoid if possible.

Breast-feeding:
Drug passes into milk. Avoid drug or discontinue nursing until you finish medicine. Consult doctor for advice on maintaining milk supply.

Infants & children:
No special warnings.

Prolonged use:
Kills beneficial bacteria that protect body against other germs. Unchecked germs may cause secondary infections.

Skin & sunlight:
No problems expected.

Driving, piloting or hazardous work:
No problems expected.

Airplane passengers:
No problems expected.

Discontinuing:
Don't discontinue without doctor's advice until you complete prescribed dose, even though symptoms diminish or disappear.

Others:
No problems expected.

INTERACTION WITH OTHER DRUGS

GENERIC NAME OR DRUG CLASS	COMBINED EFFECT
Anticoagulants	Increased anticoagulant effect.
Probenecid	Increased cephalexin effect.

INTERACTION WITH OTHER SUBSTANCES

INTERACTS WITH	COMBINED EFFECT
Alcohol:	None expected.
Beverages:	None expected.
Cocaine:	None expected, but cocaine may slow body's recovery. Avoid.
Foods:	Slow absorption. Take with liquid 1 hour before or 2 hours after eating.
Marijuana:	None expected, but marijuana may slow body's recovery. Avoid.
Tobacco:	None expected.

CEPHRADINE

BRAND NAMES

Anspor
Velosef

GENERAL INFORMATION

Habit forming? No
Prescription needed? Yes
Available as generic? Yes
Drug class: Antibiotic (cephalosporin)

 ## USES

Treatment of bacterial infections. Will not cure viral infections such as cold and flu.

 ## DOSAGE & USAGE INFORMATION

How to take:
- Tablet or capsule—Swallow with liquid. If you can't swallow whole, crumble tablet or open capsule and take with liquid or food.
- Liquid—Use measuring spoon.

When to take:
At same times each day, 1 hour before or 2 hours after eating.

If you forget a dose:
Take as soon as you remember or double next dose. Return to regular schedule.

What drug does:
Kills susceptible bacteria.

Time lapse before drug works:
May require several days to affect infection.

Don't take with:
See Interaction column and consult doctor.

 ## OVERDOSE

Symptoms:
Abdominal cramps, nausea, vomiting, severe diarrhea with mucus or blood in stool.

What to do:
Overdose unlikely to threaten life. If person takes much larger amount than prescribed, call doctor, poison-control center or hospital emergency room for instructions.

POSSIBLE ADVERSE REACTIONS OR SIDE EFFECTS

SYMPTOMS	FREQUENCY	WHAT TO DO
Brain & nervous system:	None expected.	
Skin:		
• Rash, redness, itching.	Common	3
• Rectal itching.	Infrequent	4
Eyes:	None expected.	
Ears, nose, throat:	None expected.	
Digestive: Mild nausea, vomiting, cramps, severe diarrhea with mucus or blood in stool.	Rare	3
Heart & lungs:	None expected.	
Blood vessels:	None expected.	
Muscles, bones, joints:	None expected.	
Genital, urinary:	None expected.	
Kidneys:	None expected.	
Liver:	None expected.	
Allergic: Life-threatening anaphylaxis may occur!	Rare	1 See page 888.
Blood:	None expected.	
Others: Unusual weakness, tiredness, weight loss or fever.	Rare	3

1-Life-threatening. Seek emergency treatment immediately.
2-Discontinue. Seek emergency treatment.
3-Discontinue. Call doctor right away.
4-Continue. Call doctor when convenient.
5-Continue. Tell doctor at next visit.
6-No action necessary.

WARNINGS & PRECAUTIONS

Don't take if:
You are allergic to any cephalosporin antibiotic.

Before you start, consult your doctor:
- If you are allergic to any penicillin antibiotic.
- If you have a kidney disorder.
- If you have colitis or enteritis.

Over age 60:
Adverse reactions and side effects may be more frequent and severe than in younger persons. More likely to itch around rectum and genitals.

Pregnancy:
No proven harm to unborn child. Avoid if possible.

Breast-feeding:
Drug passes into milk. Avoid drug or discontinue nursing until you finish medicine. Consult doctor for advice on maintaining milk supply.

Infants & children:
No special warnings.

Prolonged use:
Kills beneficial bacteria that protect body against other germs. Unchecked germs may cause secondary infections.

Skin & sunlight:
No problems expected.

Driving, piloting or hazardous work:
No problems expected.

Airplane passengers:
No problems expected.

Discontinuing:
Don't discontinue without doctor's advice until you complete prescribed dose, even though symptoms diminish or disappear.

Others:
No problems expected.

 ## INTERACTION WITH OTHER DRUGS

GENERIC NAME OR DRUG CLASS	COMBINED EFFECT
Anticoagulants	Increased anticoagulant effect.
Probenecid	Increased cephradine effect.

 ## INTERACTION WITH OTHER SUBSTANCES

INTERACTS WITH	COMBINED EFFECT
Alcohol:	None expected.
Beverages:	None expected.
Cocaine:	None expected, but cocaine may slow body's recovery. Avoid.
Foods:	Slow absorption. Take with liquid 1 hour before or 2 hours after eating.
Marijuana:	None expected, but marijuana may slow body's recovery. Avoid.
Tobacco:	None expected.

CHLORAL HYDRATE

BRAND NAMES

Aquachloral
Colidrate
Noctec
Oradrate
SK-Chloral Hydrate

GENERAL INFORMATION

Habit forming? Yes
Prescription needed? Yes
Available as generic? Yes
Drug class: Hypnotic

 ## USES

- Reduces anxiety.
- Relieves insomnia.

 ## DOSAGE & USAGE INFORMATION

How to take:
- Tablet or capsule—Swallow with milk or food to lessen stomach irritation.
- Drops—Dilute dose in beverage before swallowing.
- Suppositories—Remove wrapper and moisten suppository with water. Gently insert larger end into rectum. Push well into rectum with finger.

When to take:
At the same time each day.

If you forget a dose:
Take as soon as you remember up to 2 hours late. If more than 2 hours, wait for next scheduled dose (don't double this dose).

What drug does:
Affects brain centers that control wakefulness and alertness.

Time lapse before drug works:
30 to 60 minutes.

Don't take with:
See Interaction column and consult doctor.

 ## OVERDOSE

Symptoms:
Confusion, weakness, breathing difficulty, stagger, slow or irregular heartbeat.

What to do:
- Dial 0 (operator) or 911 (emergency) for an ambulance or medical help. Then give first aid immediately.
- If patient is unconscious and not breathing, give mouth-to-mouth breathing. If there is no heartbeat, use cardiac massage and mouth-to-mouth breathing (CPR). Don't try to make patient vomit. If you can't get help quickly, take patient to nearest emergency facility.
- Additional emergency information on page 886.

POSSIBLE ADVERSE REACTIONS OR SIDE EFFECTS

SYMPTOMS	FREQUENCY	WHAT TO DO
Brain & nervous system:		
• Hallucinations, agitation, confusion.	Rare	3
• "Hangover" effect, clumsiness or unsteadiness, drowsiness, dizziness or lightheadedness.	Infrequent	4
Skin: Hives, rash.	Rare	4
Eyes:	None expected.	
Ears, nose, throat:	None expected.	
Digestive: Nausea, stomach pain, vomiting.	Common	3
Heart & lungs:	None expected.	
Blood vessels:	None expected.	
Muscles, bones, joints:	None expected.	
Genital, urinary:	None expected.	
Kidneys:	None expected.	
Liver:	None expected.	
Allergic:	None expected.	
Blood:	None expected.	
Others:	None expected.	

1- Life-threatening. Seek emergency treatment immediately.
2- Discontinue. Seek emergency treatment.
3- Discontinue. Call doctor right away.
4- Continue. Call doctor when convenient.
5- Continue. Tell doctor at next visit.
6- No action necessary.

WARNINGS & PRECAUTIONS

Don't take if:
You are allergic to chloral hydrate.

Before you start, consult your doctor:
- If you have had liver, kidney or heart trouble.
- If you are prone to stomach upsets (if medicine is in oral form).
- If you have colitis or a rectal inflammation (if medicine is in suppository form).

Over age 60:
Adverse reactions and side effects may be more frequent and severe than in younger persons. More likely to have "hangover" effect.

Pregnancy:
Risk to unborn child outweighs drug benefits. Unborn child may become addicted to drug. Don't use.

Breast-feeding:
Drug filters into milk. May harm child. Avoid.

Infants & children:
Use only under medical supervision.

Prolonged use:
Addiction and possible kidney damage.

Skin & sunlight:
No problems expected.

Driving, piloting or hazardous work:
Don't drive or pilot aircraft until you learn how medicine affects you. Don't work around dangerous machinery. Don't climb ladders or work in high places. Danger increases if you drink alcohol or take medicine affecting alertness and reflexes, such as antihistamines, tranquilizers, sedatives, pain medicine, narcotics and mind-altering drugs.

Airplane passengers:
No problems expected.

Discontinuing:
Don't discontinue without consulting doctor. Dose may require gradual reduction if you have taken drug for a long time. Doses of other drugs may also require adjustment.

Others:
Frequent kidney-function tests recommended when drug is used for long time.

 INTERACTION WITH OTHER DRUGS

GENERIC NAME OR DRUG CLASS	COMBINED EFFECT
Anticoagulants	Possible hemorrhaging.
Antidepressants	Increased chloral hydrate effect.
Antihistamines	Increased chloral hydrate effect.
Cortisone drugs	Decreased cortisone effect.
MAO inhibitors	Increased chloral hydrate effect.
Mind-altering drugs	Increased chloral hydrate effect.
Narcotics	Increased chloral hydrate effect.
Pain relievers	Increased chloral hydrate effect.
Phenothiazines	Increased chloral hydrate effect.
Sedatives	Increased chloral hydrate effect.
Sleep inducers	Increased chloral hydrate effect.
Tranquilizers	Increased chloral hydrate effect.

 INTERACTION WITH OTHER SUBSTANCES

INTERACTS WITH	COMBINED EFFECT
Alcohol:	Increased sedative effect of both. Avoid.
Beverages:	None expected.
Cocaine:	Decreased chloral hydrate effect. Avoid.
Foods:	None expected.
Marijuana:	May severely impair mental and physical functioning. Avoid.
Tobacco:	None expected.

CHLORAMPHENICOL

BRAND NAMES

Amphicol   Econochlor
Antibiopto   Mychel
Chloromycetin   Ophthochlor
Chloroptic

GENERAL INFORMATION

Habit forming? No
Prescription needed? Yes
Available as generic? Yes
Drug class: Antibiotic

 USES

Treatment of infections susceptible to
chloramphenicol.

 **DOSAGE & USAGE
INFORMATION**

How to take:
- Tablet or capsule—Swallow with liquid.
- Eye solution or ointment, ear solution or
  cream—Follow label instructions.

When to take:
Tablet or capsule—1 hour before or 2 hours
after eating.

If you forget a dose:
Take as soon as you remember up to 2 hours
late. If more than 2 hours, wait for next
scheduled dose (don't double this dose).

What drug does:
Prevents bacteria from growing and
reproducing. Will not kill viruses.

Time lapse before drug works:
2 to 5 days, depending on type and severity
of infection.

Don't take with:
See Interaction column and consult doctor.

 OVERDOSE

Symptoms:
Nausea, vomiting, diarrhea.

What to do:
Overdose unlikely to threaten life. If person
takes much larger amount than prescribed,
call doctor, poison-control center or hospital
emergency room for instructions.

POSSIBLE ADVERSE REACTIONS OR SIDE EFFECTS

SYMPTOMS	FREQUENCY	WHAT TO DO
Brain & nervous system: Headache, confusion.	Infrequent	4
Skin: Rash, hives, swelling of face or extremities.	Infrequent	3
Eyes: Pain, blurred vision, possible vision loss.	Rare	3
Ears, nose, throat: Sore throat, fever.	Rare	3
Digestive: Diarrhea, nausea, vomiting.	Infrequent	3
Heart & lungs, blood vessels, genital, urinary, kidneys:	None expected.	
Muscles, bones, joints: Numbness, tingling, burning pain or weakness in hands and feet.	Infrequent	3
Liver: Jaundice (yellow eyes and skin).	Rare	3
Allergic: Life-threatening anaphylaxis!	Rare	1 See page 888.
Blood: Anemia	Rare	3

1- Life-threatening. Seek emergency
    treatment immediately.
2- Discontinue. Seek emergency treatment.
3- Discontinue. Call doctor right away.
4- Continue. Call doctor when convenient.

WARNINGS & PRECAUTIONS

Don't take if:
- You are allergic to chloramphenicol.
- It is prescribed for a minor disorder such as flu, cold or mild sore throat.

Before you start, consult your doctor:
- If you have had a blood disorder or bone-marrow disease.
- If you have had kidney or liver disease.
- If you have diabetes.

Over age 60:
Adverse reactions and side effects may be more frequent and severe than in younger persons, particularly skin irritation around rectum.

Pregnancy:
Risk to unborn child outweighs drug benefits. Don't use.

Breast-feeding:
Drug passes into milk. Avoid drug or discontinue nursing until you finish medicine. Consult doctor for advice on maintaining milk supply.

Infants & children:
Don't give to infants younger than 2.

Prolonged use:
You may become more susceptible to infections caused by germs not responsive to chloramphenicol.

Skin & sunlight:
No problems expected.

Driving, piloting or hazardous work:
Don't drive or pilot aircraft until you learn how medicine affects you. Don't work around dangerous machinery. Don't climb ladders or work in high places. Danger increases if you drink alcohol or take medicine affecting alertness and reflexes.

Airplane passengers:
No problems expected.

Discontinuing:
Don't discontinue without doctor's advice until you complete prescribed dose, even though symptoms diminish or disappear.

Others:
- Chloramphenicol can cause serious anemia. Frequent laboratory blood studies, liver and kidney tests recommended.
- Second medical opinion recommended before starting.

INTERACTION WITH OTHER DRUGS

GENERIC NAME OR DRUG CLASS	COMBINED EFFECT
Anticoagulants	Increased anticoagulant effect.
Antidiabetics (oral)	Increased antidiabetic effect.
Cyclophosphamide	Decreased cyclophosphamide effect.
Penicillins	Decreased penicillin effect.
Phenytoin	Increased phenytoin effect.

INTERACTION WITH OTHER SUBSTANCES

INTERACTS WITH	COMBINED EFFECT
Alcohol:	Possible liver problems. May cause disulfiram reaction (see page 848).
Beverages:	None expected.
Cocaine:	No proven problems.
Foods:	None expected.
Marijuana:	None expected.
Tobacco:	None expected.

CHLORDIAZEPOXIDE

BRAND NAMES

A-poxide	Librium	Relium	Tenax
C-Tran	Medilium	Reposans	Trilium
Chlordiazachel	Murcil	SK-Lygen	Zetran
Corax	Novopoxide	Sereen	
Libritabs	Relaxil	Solium	

GENERAL INFORMATION

Habit forming? Yes
Prescription needed? Yes
Available as generic? No
Drug class: Tranquilizer
(benzodiazepine)

USES

- Treatment for nervousness or tension.
- Treatment for muscle spasm.
- Treatment for convulsive disorders.

DOSAGE & USAGE INFORMATION

How to take:
Tablet or capsule—Swallow with liquid. If you can't swallow whole, crumble tablet or open capsule and take with liquid or food.

When to take:
At the same time each day, according to instructions on prescription label.

If you forget a dose:
Take as soon as you remember up to 2 hours late. If more than 2 hours, wait for next scheduled dose (don't double this dose).

What drug does:
Affects limbic system of brain—part that controls emotions.

Time lapse before drug works:
2 hours. May take 6 weeks for full benefit.

Don't take with:
See Interaction column and consult doctor.

OVERDOSE

Symptoms:
Drowsiness, weakness, tremor, stupor, coma.

What to do:
- Dial 0 (operator) or 911 (emergency) for an ambulance or medical help. Then give first aid immediately.
- If patient is unconscious and not breathing, give mouth-to-mouth breathing. If there is no heartbeat, use cardiac massage and mouth-to-mouth breathing (CPR). Don't try to make patient vomit. If you can't get help quickly, take patient to nearest emergency facility.
- Additional emergency information on page 886.

POSSIBLE ADVERSE REACTIONS OR SIDE EFFECTS

SYMPTOMS	FREQUENCY	WHAT TO DO
Brain & nervous system:		
• Clumsiness, drowsiness, dizziness.	Common	4
• Hallucinations, confusion, depression, irritability.	Infrequent	3
Skin: Rash, itch.	Infrequent	3
Eyes: Vision changes.	Infrequent	3
Ears, nose, throat: Mouth, throat ulcers.	Rare	3
Digestive: Constipation or diarrhea, nausea, vomiting.	Infrequent	4
Heart & lungs: Slow heartbeat, breathing difficulty.	Rare	2
Blood vessels:	None expected.	
Muscles, bones, joints:	None expected.	
Genital, urinary: Urination difficulty.	Infrequent	4
Kidneys:	None expected.	
Liver: Jaundice (yellow eyes and skin).	Rare	3
Allergic:	None expected.	
Blood:	None expected.	
Others:	None expected.	

1- Life-threatening. Seek emergency treatment immediately.
2- Discontinue. Seek emergency treatment.
3- Discontinue. Call doctor right away.
4- Continue. Call doctor when convenient.
5- Continue. Tell doctor at next visit.
6- No action necessary.

CHLORDIAZEPOXIDE

WARNINGS & PRECAUTIONS

Don't take if:
- You are allergic to any benzodiazepine.
- You have myasthenia gravis.
- You have glaucoma.
- You are active or recovering alcoholic.
- Patient is younger than 6 months.

Before you start, consult your doctor:
- If you have liver, kidney or lung disease.
- If you have diabetes, epilepsy or porphyria.

Over age 60:
Adverse reactions and side effects may be more frequent and severe than in younger persons. You need smaller doses for shorter periods of time. May develop agitation, rage or "hangover effect."

Pregnancy:
Risk to unborn child outweighs drug benefits. Don't use.

Breast-feeding:
Drug passes into milk. Avoid drug or discontinue nursing until you finish medicine. Consult doctor for advice on maintaining milk supply.

Infants & children:
Use only under medical supervision for children older than 6 months.

Prolonged use:
May impair liver function.

Skin & sunlight:
No problems expected.

Driving, piloting or hazardous work:
Don't drive or pilot aircraft until you learn how medicine affects you. Don't work around dangerous machinery. Don't climb ladders or work in high places. Danger increases if you drink alcohol or take medicine affecting alertness and reflexes.

Airplane passengers:
No problems expected.

Discontinuing:
Don't discontinue without consulting doctor. Dose may require gradual reduction if you have taken drug for a long time. Doses of other drugs may also require adjustment.

Others:
- Hot weather, heavy exercise and profuse sweat may reduce excretion and cause overdose.
- Blood sugar may rise in diabetics, requiring insulin adjustment.

INTERACTION WITH OTHER DRUGS

GENERIC NAME OR DRUG CLASS	COMBINED EFFECT
Anticonvulsants	Change in seizure frequency or severity.
Antidepressants	Increased sedative effect of both drugs.
Antihistamines	Increased sedative effect of both drugs.
Antihypertensives	Excessively low blood pressure.
Cimetidine	Excess sedation.
Disulfiram	Increased chlordiazepoxide effect.
MAO inhibitors	Convulsions, deep sedation, rage.
Narcotics	Increased sedative effect of both drugs.
Sedatives	Increased sedative effect of both drugs.
Sleep inducers	Increased sedative effect of both drugs.
Tranquilizers	Increased sedative effect of both drugs.

INTERACTION WITH OTHER SUBSTANCES

INTERACTS WITH	COMBINED EFFECT
Alcohol:	Heavy sedation. Avoid.
Beverages:	None expected.
Cocaine:	Decreased chlordiazepoxide effect.
Foods:	None expected.
Marijuana:	Heavy sedation. Avoid.
Tobacco:	Decreased chlordiazepoxide effect.

CHLOROQUINE

BRAND NAMES

Aralen

GENERAL INFORMATION

Habit forming? No
Prescription needed? Yes
Available as generic? Yes
Drug class: Antiprotozoal, antirheumatic

 USES

- Treatment for protozoal infections, such as malaria and amebiasis.
- Treatment for some forms of arthritis and lupus.

 DOSAGE & USAGE INFORMATION

How to take:
Tablet—Swallow with food or milk to lessen stomach irritation.

When to take:
- Depends on condition. Is adjusted during treatment.
- Malaria prevention—Begin taking medicine 2 weeks before entering areas with malaria.

If you forget a dose:
- 1 or more doses a day—Take as soon as you remember up to 2 hours late. If more than 2 hours, wait for next scheduled dose (don't double this dose).
- 1 dose weekly—Take as soon as possible, then return to regular dosing schedule.

What drug does:
- Inhibits parasite multiplication.
- Decreases inflammatory response in diseased joint.

Time lapse before drug works:
1 to 2 hours.

Don't take with:
See Interaction column and consult doctor.

 OVERDOSE

Symptoms:
Severe breathing difficulty, drowsiness, faintness.

What to do:
- Dial 0 (operator) or 911 (emergency) for an ambulance or medical help. Then give first aid immediately.
- Additional emergency information on page 886.

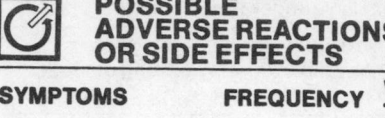 POSSIBLE ADVERSE REACTIONS OR SIDE EFFECTS

SYMPTOMS	FREQUENCY	WHAT TO DO
Brain & nervous system:		
• Mood or mental changes, seizures.	Rare	3
• Headache	Common	5
Skin:		
Rash or itch.	Infrequent	4
Eyes:		
Blurred or changed vision.	Infrequent	3
Ears, nose, throat:		
• Ringing or buzzing in ears, hearing loss.	Rare	4
• Sore throat, fever.	Rare	3
Digestive:		
Diarrhea, nausea, vomiting.	Infrequent	4
Heart & lungs:	None expected.	
Blood vessels:		
Unusual bleeding or bruising.	Rare	3
Muscles, bones, joints:		
Muscle weakness.	Rare	3
Genital, urinary:	None expected.	
Kidneys:	None expected.	
Liver:	None expected.	
Allergic:	None expected.	
Blood:	None expected.	
Others:	None expected.	

1- Life threatening. Seek emergency treatment immediately.
2- Discontinue. Seek emergency treatment.
3- Discontinue. Call doctor right away.
4- Continue. Call doctor when convenient.
5- Continue. Tell doctor at next visit.
6- No action necessary.

WARNINGS & PRECAUTIONS

Don't take if:
You are allergic to chloroquine or hydroxychloroquine.

Before you start, consult your doctor:
- If you plan to become pregnant within the medication period.
- If you have blood disease.
- If you have eye or vision problems.
- If you have a G6PD deficiency.
- If you have liver disease.
- If you have nerve or brain disease (including seizure disorders).
- If you have porphyria.
- If you have psoriasis.
- If you have stomach or intestinal disease.
- If you drink more than 3 oz. of alcohol daily.

Over age 60:
Adverse reactions and side effects may be more frequent and severe than in younger persons.

Pregnancy:
Risk to unborn child outweighs drug benefits. Don't use.

Breast-feeding:
Drug passes into milk. Avoid drug or discontinue nursing.

Infants & children:
Not recommended. Dangerous.

Prolonged use:
Permanent damage to the retina (back part of the eye) or nerve deafness.

Skin & sunlight:
May cause rash or intensify sunburn in areas exposed to sun or sunlamp.

Driving, piloting or hazardous work:
Don't drive or pilot aircraft until you learn how medicine affects you. Don't work around dangerous machinery. Don't climb ladders or work in high places. Danger increases if you drink alcohol or take medicine affecting alertness and reflexes.

Airplane passengers:
No problems expected.

Discontinuing:
Don't discontinue without doctor's advice until you complete prescribed dose, even though symptoms diminish or disappear.

Others:
- Periodic physical and blood examinations recommended.
- If you are in a malaria area for a long time, you may need to change to another preventive drug every 2 years.

INTERACTION WITH OTHER DRUGS

GENERIC NAME OR DRUG CLASS	COMBINED EFFECT
Estrogens	Possible liver toxicity.
Gold compounds	Risk of severe rash and itch.
Oxyphenbutazone	Risk of severe rash and itch.
Penicillamine	Possible blood or kidney toxicity.
Phenylbutazone	Risk of severe rash and itch.
Sulfa drugs	Possible liver toxicity.

INTERACTION WITH OTHER SUBSTANCES

INTERACTS WITH	COMBINED EFFECT
Alcohol:	Possible liver toxicity. Avoid.
Beverages:	None expected.
Cocaine:	None expected.
Foods:	None expected.
Marijuana:	None expected.
Tobacco:	None expected.

CHLOROTHIAZIDE

BRAND NAMES

Diuril
SK-Chlorothiazide

GENERAL INFORMATION

Habit forming? No
Prescription needed? Yes
Available as generic? Yes
Drug class: Antihypertensive,
diuretic (thiazide)

 USES

- Controls, but doesn't cure, high blood pressure.
- Reduces fluid retention (edema) caused by conditions such as heart disorders and liver disease.

 DOSAGE & USAGE INFORMATION

How to take:
Tablet or capsule—Swallow with liquid. If you can't swallow whole, crumble tablet or open capsule and take with liquid or food. Don't exceed dose.

When to take:
At the same time each day.

If you forget a dose:
Take as soon as you remember up to 2 hours late. If more than 2 hours, wait for next scheduled dose (don't double this dose).

What drug does:
- Forces sodium and water excretion, reducing body fluid.
- Relaxes muscle cells of small arteries.
- Reduced body fluid and relaxed arteries lower blood pressure.

Time lapse before drug works:
4 to 6 hours. May require several weeks to lower blood pressure.

Don't take with:
- See Interaction column and consult doctor.
- Non-prescription drugs without consulting doctor.

 OVERDOSE

Symptoms:
Cramps, weakness, drowsiness, weak pulse, coma.

What to do:
- Dial 0 (operator) or 911 (emergency) for an ambulance or medical help. Then give first aid immediately.
- Additional emergency information on page 886.

POSSIBLE ADVERSE REACTIONS OR SIDE EFFECTS

SYMPTOMS	FREQUENCY	WHAT TO DO
Brain & nervous system:		
• Dizziness	Infrequent	4
• Mood changes.	Infrequent	4
• Headaches	Infrequent	4
Skin:		
Rash or hives.	Rare	2
Eyes:		
Blurred vision.	Infrequent	3
Ears, nose, throat:		
• Sore throat, fever.	Rare	5
• Dry mouth, thirst.	Infrequent	5
Digestive:		
Severe abdominal pain, nausea, vomiting.	Infrequent	3
Heart & lungs:		
Irregular heartbeat, weak pulse.	Infrequent	3
Blood vessels:	None expected.	
Muscles, bones, joints:		
Weakness, tiredness.	Infrequent	4
Genital, urinary:	None expected.	
Kidneys:	None expected.	
Liver:		
Jaundice (yellow skin and eyes).	Rare	3
Allergic:	None expected.	
Blood:	None expected.	
Others:		
Weight changes.	Infrequent	4

1 - Life-threatening. Seek emergency treatment immediately.
2 - Discontinue. Seek emergency treatment.
3 - Discontinue. Call doctor right away.
4 - Continue. Call doctor when convenient.
5 - Continue. Tell doctor at next visit.
6 - No action necessary.

CHLOROTHIAZIDE

 WARNINGS & PRECAUTIONS

Don't take if:
You are allergic to any thiazide diuretic drug.

Before you start, consult your doctor:
- If you are allergic to any sulfa drug.
- If you have gout.
- If you have liver, pancreas or kidney disorder.

Over age 60:
Adverse reactions and side effects may be more frequent and severe than in younger persons, especially dizziness and excessive potassium loss.

Pregnancy:
Risk to unborn child outweighs drug benefits. Don't use.

Breast-feeding:
Drug passes into milk. Avoid drug or discontinue nursing.

Infants & children:
No problems expected.

Prolonged use:
You may need medicine to treat high blood pressure for the rest of your life.

Skin & sunlight:
May cause rash or intensify sunburn in areas exposed to sun or sunlamp.

Driving, piloting or hazardous work:
Don't drive or pilot aircraft until you learn how medicine affects you. Don't work around dangerous machinery. Don't climb ladders or work in high places. Danger increases if you drink alcohol or take medicine affecting alertness and reflexes, such as antihistamines, tranquilizers, sedatives, pain medicine, narcotics and mind-altering drugs.

Airplane passengers:
No problems expected.

Discontinuing:
Don't discontinue without medical advice.

Others:
- Hot weather and fever may cause dehydration and drop in blood pressure. Dose may require temporary adjustment. Weigh daily and report any unexpected weight decreases to your doctor.
- May cause rise in uric acid, leading to gout.
- May cause blood-sugar rise in diabetics.

 INTERACTION WITH OTHER DRUGS

GENERIC NAME OR DRUG CLASS	COMBINED EFFECT
Allopurinol	Decreased allopurinol effect.
Antidepressants (tricyclic)	Dangerous drop in blood pressure. Avoid combination unless under medical supervision.
Barbiturates	Increased chlorothiazide effect.
Cholestyramine	Decreased chlorothiazide effect.
Cortisone drugs	Excessive potassium loss that causes dangerous heart rhythms.
Digitalis preparations	Excessive potassium loss that causes dangerous heart rhythms.
Diuretics (thiazide)	Increased effect of other thiazide diuretics.
Lithium	Increased effect of lithium.
MAO inhibitors	Increased chlorothiazide effect.
Probenecid	Decreased probenecid effect.

 INTERACTION WITH OTHER SUBSTANCES

INTERACTS WITH	COMBINED EFFECT
Alcohol:	Dangerous blood-pressure drop.
Beverages:	None expected.
Cocaine:	None expected.
Foods: Licorice	Excessive potassium loss that causes dangerous heart rhythms.
Marijuana:	May increase blood pressure.
Tobacco:	None expected.

CHLOROTRIANISENE

BRAND NAMES

TACE

GENERAL INFORMATION

Habit forming? No
Prescription needed? Yes
Available as generic? Yes
Drug class: Female sex hormone (estrogen)

USES

- Treatment for symptoms of menopause and menstrual-cycle irregularity.
- Replacement for female hormone deficiency.
- Treatment for cancer of prostate.

DOSAGE & USAGE INFORMATION

How to take:
Capsule—Swallow with liquid. If you can't swallow whole, open capsule and take with liquid or food.

When to take:
At the same time each day.

If you forget a dose:
Take as soon as you remember up to 12 hours late. If more than 12 hours, wait for next scheduled dose (don't double this dose).

What drug does:
Restores normal estrogen level in tissues.

Time lapse before drug works:
10 to 20 days.

Don't take with:
See Interaction column and consult doctor.

OVERDOSE

Symptoms:
Nausea, vomiting, fluid retention, breast enlargement and discomfort, abnormal vaginal bleeding.

What to do:
Overdose unlikely to threaten life. If person takes much larger amount than prescribed, call doctor, poison-control center or hospital emergency room for instructions.

POSSIBLE ADVERSE REACTIONS OR SIDE EFFECTS

SYMPTOMS	FREQUENCY	WHAT TO DO
Brain & nervous system:		
Depression, dizziness, irritability.	Infrequent	4
Skin:		
• Rash	Infrequent	3
• Brown blotches.	Infrequent	5
• Hair loss.	Infrequent	5
Eyes, ears, nose, throat, heart & lungs, muscles, bones, joints, kidneys, allergic, blood:	None expected.	
Digestive:		
• Stomach or side pain.	Infrequent	3
• Stomach cramps.	Common	3
• Appetite loss.	Common	4
• Nausea, diarrhea.	Common	5
• Vomiting	Infrequent	4
Blood vessels:		
Swollen ankles, feet.	Common	5
Genital, urinary:		
Vaginal discharge or bleeding.	Infrequent	5
Liver:		
Jaundice (yellow skin and eyes).	Rare	3
Others:		
• Breast lumps.	Infrequent	4
• Swollen, tender breasts.	Common	5
• Changes in sex drive.	Infrequent	5

1- Life-threatening. Seek emergency treatment immediately.
2- Discontinue. Seek emergency treatment.
3- Discontinue. Call doctor right away.
4- Continue. Call doctor when convenient.
5- Continue. Tell doctor at next visit.

CHLOROTRIANISENE

WARNINGS & PRECAUTIONS

Don't take If:
- You are allergic to any estrogen-containing drugs.
- You have impaired liver function.
- You have had blood clots, stroke or heart attack.
- You have unexplained vaginal bleeding.

Before you start, consult your doctor:
- If you have had cancer of breast or reproductive organs, fibrocystic breast disease, fibroid tumors of the uterus or endometriosis.
- If you have had migraine headaches, epilepsy or porphyria.
- If you have diabetes, high blood pressure, asthma, congestive heart failure, kidney disease or gallstones.
- If you plan to become pregnant within 3 months.

Over age 60:
Controversial. You and your doctor must decide if drug risks outweigh benefits.

Pregnancy:
Risk to unborn child outweighs drug benefits. Don't use.

Breast-feeding:
Drug filters into milk. May harm child. Avoid.

Infants & children:
Not recommended.

Prolonged use:
Increased growth of fibroid tumors of uterus. Possible association with cancer of uterus.

Skin & sunlight:
May cause rash or intensify sunburn in areas exposed to sun or sunlamp.

Driving, piloting or hazardous work:
No problems expected.

Airplane passengers:
No problems expected.

Discontinuing:
You may need to discontinue chlorotrianisene periodically. Consult your doctor.

Others:
In rare instances, may cause blood clot in lung, brain or leg. Symptoms are *sudden* severe headache, coordination loss, vision change, chest pain, breathing difficulty, slurred speech, pain in legs or groin. Seek emergency treatment immediately.

INTERACTION WITH OTHER DRUGS

GENERIC NAME OR DRUG CLASS	COMBINED EFFECT
Anticoagulants (oral)	Decreased anticoagulant effect.
Anticonvulsants (hydantoin)	Increased seizures.
Antidiabetics (oral)	Unpredictable increase or decrease in blood sugar.
Clofibrate	Decreased clofibrate effect.
Carbamazepine	Increased seizures.
Meprobamate	Increased chlorotrianisene effect.
Phenobarbital	Decreased chlorotrianisene effect.
Primidone	Decreased chlorotrianisene effect.
Rifampin	Decreased chlorotrianisene effect.
Thyroid hormones	Decreased thyroid effect.

INTERACTION WITH OTHER SUBSTANCES

INTERACTS WITH	COMBINED EFFECT
Alcohol:	None expected.
Beverages:	None expected.
Cocaine:	No proven problems.
Foods:	None expected.
Marijuana:	Possible menstrual irregularities and bleeding between periods.
Tobacco:	Increased risk of blood clots leading to stroke or heart attack.

CHLORPHENIRAMINE

BRAND NAMES

Acutuss (M)	Chloramate	Naldecon (M)
Alermine	Chlor-Trimeton	Novahistine (M)
Aller-chlor	Coricidin (M)	Novopheniram
Allerest (M)	Co-Tylenol (M)	Phenetron
Allergesic (M)	Histalon	Sinarest (M)
Anamine (M)	Hycoff (M)	Teldrin

See complete brand names list, page 823.

GENERAL INFORMATION

Habit forming? No
Prescription needed? No
Available as generic? Yes
Drug class: Antihistamine

USES

- Reduces allergic symptoms such as hay fever, hives, rash or itching.
- Prevents motion sickness, nausea, vomiting.
- Induces sleep.

DOSAGE & USAGE INFORMATION

How to take:
- Tablet or syrup—Swallow with liquid or food to lessen stomach irritation.
- Extended-release tablets or capsules—Swallow each dose whole.

When to take:
Varies with form. Follow label directions.

If you forget a dose:
Take as soon as you remember up to 2 hours late. If more than 2 hours, wait for next scheduled dose (don't double this dose).

What drug does:
Blocks action of histamine after an allergic response triggers histamine release in sensitive cells.

Time lapse before drug works:
30 minutes.

Don't take with:
See Interaction column and consult doctor.

OVERDOSE

Symptoms:
Convulsions, red face, hallucinations, coma.

What to do:
- Dial 0 (operator) or 911 (emergency) for an ambulance or medical help. Then give first aid immediately.
- Additional emergency information on page 886.

POSSIBLE ADVERSE REACTIONS OR SIDE EFFECTS

SYMPTOMS	FREQUENCY	WHAT TO DO
Brain & nervous system:		•
• Nightmares, agitation, irritability.	Rare	3
• Drowsiness, dizziness.	Common	5
Skin:	None expected.	
Eyes:		
• Vision changes.	Infrequent	3
• Less tolerance for contact lenses.	Infrequent	4
Ears, nose, throat:		
• Sore throat, fever.	Rare	3
• Dry mouth, nose, throat.	Common	5
Digestive:		
• Nausea	Common	5
• Appetite loss.	Infrequent	5
Heart & lungs:		
Rapid heartbeat.	Rare	3
Blood vessels:		
Unusual bleeding or bruising.	Rare	3
Muscles, bones, joints, kidneys, liver, allergic, blood:	None expected.	
Genital, urinary:		
Urination difficulty.	Infrequent	4
Others:		
Fatigue, weakness.	Rare	3

1- Life-threatening. Seek emergency treatment immediately.
2- Discontinue. Seek emergency treatment.
3- Discontinue. Call doctor right away.
4- Continue. Call doctor when convenient.
5- Continue. Tell doctor at next visit.
6- No action necessary.

WARNINGS & PRECAUTIONS

Don't take if:
You are allergic to any antihistamine.

Before you start, consult your doctor:
- If you have glaucoma.
- If you have enlarged prostate.
- If you have asthma.
- If you have kidney disease.
- If you have peptic ulcer.
- If you will have surgery within 2 months, including dental surgery, requiring general or spinal anesthesia.

Over age 60:
Don't exceed recommended dose. Adverse reactions and side effects may be more frequent and severe than in younger persons, especially urination difficulty, diminished alertness and other brain and nervous-system symptoms.

Pregnancy:
No proven harm to unborn child. Avoid if possible.

Breast-feeding:
Drug passes into milk. Avoid drug or discontinue nursing until you finish medicine. Consult doctor for advice on maintaining milk supply.

Infants & children:
Not recommended for premature or newborn infants. Otherwise, no problems expected.

Prolonged use:
Avoid. May damage bone marrow and nerve cells.

Skin & sunlight:
May cause rash or intensify sunburn in areas exposed to sun or sunlamp.

Driving, piloting or hazardous work:
Don't drive or pilot aircraft until you learn how medicine affects you. Don't work around dangerous machinery. Don't climb ladders or work in high places. Danger increases if you drink alcohol or take medicine affecting alertness and reflexes, such as antihistamines, tranquilizers, sedatives, pain medicine, narcotics and mind-altering drugs.

Airplane passengers:
No problems expected.

Discontinuing:
No problems expected.

Others:
May mask symptoms of hearing damage from aspirin, other salicylates, cisplatin, paromomycin, vancomycin or anticonvulsants. Consult doctor if you use these.

 ## INTERACTION WITH OTHER DRUGS

GENERIC NAME OR DRUG CLASS	COMBINED EFFECT
Anticholinergics	Increased anticholinergic effect.
Antidepressants	Excess sedation. Avoid.
Antihistamines (other)	Excess sedation. Avoid.
Hypnotics	Excess sedation. Avoid.
MAO inhibitors	Increased chlorpheniramine effect.
Mind-altering drugs	Excess sedation. Avoid.
Narcotics	Excess sedation. Avoid.
Sedatives	Excess sedation. Avoid.
Sleep inducers	Excess sedation. Avoid.
Tranquilizers	Excess sedation. Avoid.

 ## INTERACTION WITH OTHER SUBSTANCES

INTERACTS WITH	COMBINED EFFECT
Alcohol:	Excess sedation. Avoid.
Beverages: Caffeine drinks	Less chlorpheniramine sedation.
Cocaine:	Decreased chlorpheniramine effect. Avoid.
Foods:	None expected.
Marijuana:	Excess sedation. Avoid.
Tobacco:	None expected.

CHLORPHENTERMINE

BRAND NAMES

Chlorophen
Pre-sate

GENERAL INFORMATION

Habit forming? Yes
Prescription needed? Yes
Available as generic? Yes
Drug class: Appetite suppressant

 USES

Suppresses appetite.

 DOSAGE & USAGE INFORMATION

How to take:
Extended-release tablets or capsules—Swallow each dose whole with liquid.

When to take:
10 to 14 hours before bedtime.

If you forget a dose:
Take as soon as you remember up to 2 hours late. If more than 2 hours, wait for next scheduled dose (don't double this dose).

What drug does:
Apparently stimulates brain's appetite-control center.

Time lapse before drug works:
Begins in 1 hour. Lasts 14 hours.

Don't take with:
- Non-prescription drugs without consulting doctor.
- See Interaction column and consult doctor.

 OVERDOSE

Symptoms:
Irritability, overactivity, trembling, insomnia, mood changes, rapid heartbeat, confusion, disorientation, hallucinations, convulsions, coma.

What to do:
- Dial 0 (operator) or 911 (emergency) for an ambulance or medical help. Then give first aid immediately.
- Additional emergency information on page 886.

 POSSIBLE ADVERSE REACTIONS OR SIDE EFFECTS

SYMPTOMS	FREQUENCY	WHAT TO DO
Brain & nervous system:		
● Irritability, nervousness, insomnia.	Common	4
● Mood changes.	Rare	3
Skin:		
● Hair loss.	Rare	4
● Rash or hives.	Rare	3
Eyes:		
Blurred vision.	Infrequent	4
Ears, nose, throat:		
Unpleasant taste or dry mouth.	Infrequent	4
Digestive:		
Constipation or diarrhea, nausea, vomiting, cramps.	Infrequent	4
Heart & lungs:		
● Irregular or pounding heartbeat.	Infrequent	3
● Breathing difficulty.	Rare	3
Blood vessels, muscles, bones, joints, kidneys, liver, allergic, blood:	None expected.	
Genital, urinary:		
Urinary urgency and difficulty.	Infrequent	3
Others:		
● False sense of well-being.	Common	4
● Changes in sex drive.	Infrequent	4
● Sweat increase.	Infrequent	4

1- Life-threatening. Seek emergency treatment immediately.
2- Discontinue. Seek emergency treatment.
3- Discontinue. Call doctor right away.
4- Continue. Call doctor when convenient.

CHLORPHENTERMINE

WARNINGS & PRECAUTIONS

Don't take if:
- You are allergic to any sympathomimetic or phenylpropanolamine.
- You have glaucoma.
- You have taken MAO inhibitors within 2 weeks.
- You plan to become pregnant within medication period.
- You have a history of drug abuse.

Before you start, consult your doctor:
- If you have high blood pressure or heart disease.
- If you have an overactive thyroid, nervous tension or "anxiety."
- If you have epilepsy.

Over age 60:
Adverse reactions and side effects may be more frequent and severe than in younger persons.

Pregnancy:
Safety not established. Avoid.

Breast-feeding:
No proven problems. Consult doctor.

Infants & children:
Don't give to children younger than 12.

Prolonged use:
Loses effectiveness. Avoid.

Skin & sunlight:
No problems expected.

Driving, piloting or hazardous work:
Don't drive or pilot aircraft until you learn how medicine affects you. Don't work around dangerous machinery. Don't climb ladders or work in high places. Danger increases if you drink alcohol or take medicine affecting alertness and reflexes, such as antihistamines, tranquilizers, sedatives, pain medicine, narcotics and mind-altering drugs.

Airplane passengers:
No problems expected.

Discontinuing:
Don't discontinue without consulting doctor. Dose may require gradual reduction if you have taken drug for a long time. Doses of other drugs may also require adjustment.

Others:
Don't increase dose.

INTERACTION WITH OTHER DRUGS

GENERIC NAME OR DRUG CLASS	COMBINED EFFECT
Appetite suppressants (other)	Dangerous overstimulation.
Caffeine	Increased stimulant effect of chlorphentermine.
Guanethidine	Decreased guanethidine effect.
Hydralazine	Decreased hydralazine effect.
MAO inhibitors	Dangerous blood-pressure rise.
Methyldopa	Decreased methyldopa effect.
Phenothiazines	Decreased chlorphentermine effect.
Rauwolfia alkaloids	Decreased effect of rauwolfia alkaloids.

INTERACTION WITH OTHER SUBSTANCES

INTERACTS WITH	COMBINED EFFECT
Alcohol: Beer, chianti wines, vermouth.	Dangerous blood-pressure rise.
Beverages: • Caffeine drinks • Drinks containing tyramine (see page 851).	Excessive stimulation. Blood-pressure rise.
Cocaine:	Excessive stimulation.
Foods: Foods containing tyramine (see page 851).	Blood-pressure rise.
Marijuana:	Frequent use—Irregular heartbeat.
Tobacco:	None expected.

CHLORPROMAZINE

BRAND NAMES

Chloramead
Chlor-Promanyl
Chlorprom
Largactil

Promapar
Promosol
Thorazine

GENERAL INFORMATION

Habit forming? No
Prescription needed? Yes
Available as generic? Yes
Drug class: Tranquilizer, antiemetic (phenothiazine)

 USES

- Stops nausea, vomiting.
- Reduces anxiety, agitation.

 DOSAGE & USAGE INFORMATION

How to take:
- Tablet or capsule—Swallow with liquid or food to lessen stomach irritation.
- Suppositories—Remove wrapper and moisten suppository with water. Gently insert into rectum, large end first.
- Drops or liquid—Dilute dose in beverage.

When to take:
- Nervous and mental disorders—Take at the same times each day.
- Nausea and vomiting—Take as needed, no more often than every 4 hours.

If you forget a dose:
- Nervous and mental disorders—Take up to 2 hours late. If more than 2 hours, wait for next scheduled dose (don't double this).
- Nausea and vomiting—Take as soon as you remember. Wait 4 hours for next dose.

What drug does:
- Suppresses brain's vomiting center.
- Suppresses brain centers that control abnormal emotions and behavior.

Time lapse before drug works:
- Nausea and vomiting—1 hour or less.
- Nervous and mental disorders—4-6 weeks.

Don't take with:
- Antacid or medicine for diarrhea.
- Non-prescription drug for cough, cold or allergy.
- See Interaction column and consult doctor.

 OVERDOSE

Symptoms:
Stupor, convulsions, coma.

What to do:
- Dial 0 (operator) or 911 (emergency) for an ambulance or medical help. Then give first aid immediately.
- Additional emergency information on page 886.

POSSIBLE ADVERSE REACTIONS OR SIDE EFFECTS

SYMPTOMS	FREQUENCY	WHAT TO DO
Brain & nervous system:		
● Restlessness, tremor.	Common	3
● Fainting	Infrequent	2
● Drowsiness	Common	3
Skin:		
● Rash	Infrequent	3
● Less perspiration.	Common	4
Eyes:		
Vision changes.	Rare	3
Ears, nose, throat:		
● Sore throat, fever.	Rare	3
● Dry mouth, nasal congestion.	Common	4
Digestive:		
Constipation	Common	4
Heart & lungs, blood vessels, kidneys, allergic, blood:	None expected.	
Muscles, bones, joints:		
Muscle spasms of face and neck, unsteady gait.	Common	2
Genital, urinary:		
Urination difficulty.	Infrequent	4
Liver:		
Jaundice (yellow eyes and skin).	Rare	3
Others:		
Less interest in sex, breast swelling, change in menstrual pattern.	Infrequent	4

1- Life-threatening. Seek emergency treatment immediately.
2- Discontinue. Seek emergency treatment.
3- Discontinue. Call doctor right away.
4- Continue. Call doctor when convenient.
5- Continue. Tell doctor at next visit.
6- No action necessary.

CHLORPROMAZINE

 WARNINGS & PRECAUTIONS

Don't take if:
- You are allergic to any phenothiazine.
- You have a blood or bone-marrow disease.

Before you start, consult your doctor:
- If you will have surgery within 2 months, including dental surgery, requiring general or spinal anesthesia.
- If you have asthma, emphysema or other lung disorder.
- If you take non-prescription ulcer medicine, asthma medicine or amphetamines.

Over age 60:
Adverse reactions and side effects may be more frequent and severe than in younger persons. More likely to develop involuntary movement of jaws, lips, tongue, chewing. Report this to your doctor immediately. Early treatment can help.

Pregnancy:
Risk to unborn child outweighs drug benefits. Don't use.

Breast-feeding:
Drug passes into milk. Avoid drug or discontinue nursing until you finish medicine. Consult doctor for advice on maintaining milk supply.

Infants & children:
Don't give to children younger than 2.

Prolonged use:
May lead to tardive dyskinesia (involuntary movement of jaws, lips, tongue, chewing).

Skin & sunlight:
May cause rash or intensify sunburn in areas exposed to sun or sunlamp. Skin may remain sensitive for 3 months after discontinuing.

Driving, piloting or hazardous work:
Don't drive or pilot aircraft until you learn how medicine affects you. Don't work around dangerous machinery. Don't climb ladders or work in high places. Danger increases if you drink alcohol or take medicine affecting alertness and reflexes.

Airplane passengers:
No problems expected.

Discontinuing:
- Nervous and mental disorders—Don't discontinue without doctor's advice until you complete prescribed dose, even though symptoms diminish or disappear.
- Nausea and vomiting—May be unnecessary to finish medicine. Follow doctor's instructions.

 INTERACTION WITH OTHER DRUGS

GENERIC NAME OR DRUG CLASS	COMBINED EFFECT
Anticholinergics	Increased anticholinergic effect.
Antidepressants (tricyclic)	Increased chlorpromazine effect.
Antihistamines	Increased antihistamine effect.
Appetite suppressants	Decreased suppressant effect.
Levodopa	Decreased levodopa effect.
Mind-altering drugs	Increased effect of mind-altering drugs.
Narcotics	Increased narcotic effect.
Phenytoin	Increased phenytoin effect.
Quinidine	Impaired heart function. Dangerous mixture.
Sedatives	Increased sedative effect.
Tranquilizers (other)	Increased tranquilizer effect.

 INTERACTION WITH OTHER SUBSTANCES

INTERACTS WITH	COMBINED EFFECT
Alcohol:	Dangerous oversedation.
Beverages:	None expected.
Cocaine:	Decreased chlorpromazine effect. Avoid.
Foods:	None expected.
Marijuana:	Drowsiness. May increase antinausea effect.
Tobacco:	None expected.

CHLORPROPAMIDE

BRAND NAMES

Chloromide
Chloronase
Diabinese

GENERAL INFORMATION

Habit forming? No
Prescription needed? Yes
Available as generic? No
Drug class: Antidiabetic (oral), sulfonurea

 ## USES

Treatment for diabetes in adults who can't control blood sugar by diet, weight loss and exercise.

 ## DOSAGE & USAGE INFORMATION

How to take:
Tablet—Swallow with liquid or food to lessen stomach irritation. If you can't swallow whole, crumble tablet and take with liquid or food.

When to take:
At the same times each day.

If you forget a dose:
Take as soon as you remember up to 2 hours late. If more than 2 hours, wait for next scheduled dose (don't double this dose).

What drug does:
Stimulates pancreas to produce more insulin. Insulin in blood forces cells to use sugar in blood.

Time lapse before drug works:
3 to 4 hours. May require 2 weeks for maximum benefit.

Don't take with:
See Interaction column and consult doctor.

 ## OVERDOSE

Symptoms:
Excessive hunger, nausea, anxiety, cool skin, cold sweats, drowsiness, rapid heartbeat, weakness, unconsciousness, coma.

What to do:
- Dial 0 (operator) or 911 (emergency) for an ambulance or medical help. Then give first aid immediately.
- Additional emergency information on page 886.

POSSIBLE ADVERSE REACTIONS OR SIDE EFFECTS

SYMPTOMS	FREQUENCY	WHAT TO DO
Brain & nervous system:		
• Dizziness	Common	3
• Fatigue	Rare	3
Skin:		
Itching or rash.	Rare	3
Eyes:	None expected.	
Ears, nose, throat:		
• Sore throat, fever.	Rare	3
• Ringing in ears.	Rare	3
Digestive:		
Diarrhea, loss of appetite, nausea, stomach pain, heartburn.	Common	4
Heart & lungs, muscles, bones, joints, genital, urinary, kidneys, allergic, blood:	None expected.	
Blood vessels:		
Unusual bleeding or bruising.	Rare	3
Liver:		
Jaundice (yellow skin, eyes).	Rare	3
Others:		
Low blood sugar (ravenous hunger, nausea, anxiety, cold sweats, cool skin, chills, drowsiness, nervousness, headache, rapid heartbeat, weakness).	Infrequent	2

1- Life-threatening. Seek emergency treatment immediately.
2- Discontinue. Seek emergency treatment.
3- Discontinue. Call doctor right away.
4- Continue. Call doctor when convenient.

CHLORPROPAMIDE

 ## WARNINGS & PRECAUTIONS

Don't take if:
- You are allergic to any sulfonurea.
- You have impaired kidney or liver function.

Before you start, consult your doctor:
- If you have a severe infection.
- If you have thyroid disease.
- If you take insulin.
- If you have heart disease.

Over age 60:
Dose usually smaller than for younger adults. Avoid "low-blood-sugar" episodes because repeated ones can damage brain permanently.

Pregnancy:
No proven harm to unborn child. Avoid if possible.

Breast-feeding:
Drug filters into milk. May lower baby's blood sugar. Avoid.

Infants & children:
Don't give to infants or children.

Prolonged use:
None expected.

Skin & sunlight:
May cause rash or intensify sunburn in areas exposed to sun or sunlamp.

Driving, piloting or hazardous work:
No problems expected unless you develop hypoglycemia (low blood sugar). If so, avoid driving or hazardous activity.

Airplane passengers:
No problems expected.

Discontinuing:
Don't discontinue without consulting doctor. Dose may require gradual reduction if you have taken drug for a long time. Doses of other drugs may also require adjustment.

Others:
- Don't exceed 1500 mg. in 1 day.
- Hypoglycemia (low blood sugar) may occur, even with proper dose schedule. You must balance medicine, diet and exercise.

 ## INTERACTION WITH OTHER DRUGS

GENERIC NAME OR DRUG CLASS	COMBINED EFFECT
Androgens	Increased chlorpropamide effect.
Anticoagulants (oral)	Unpredictable prothrombin times (see page 850).
Anticonvulsants (hydantoin)	Decreased chlorpropamide effect.
Antiinflammatory drugs (non-steroidal)	Increased chlorpropamide effect.
Aspirin	Increased chlorpropamide effect.
Beta-adrenergic blockers	Increased chlorpropamide effect.
Chloramphenicol	Increased chlorpropamide effect.
Clofibrate	Increased chlorpropamide effect.
Contraceptives (oral)	Decreased chlorpropamide effect.
Cortisone drugs	Decreased chlorpropamide effect.
Diuretics (thiazide)	Decreased chlorpropamide effect.
Epinephrine	Decreased chlorpropamide effect.
Estrogens	Increased chlorpropamide effect.
Guanethidine	Unpredictable chlorpropamide effect.

Additional interactions on page 834.

 ## INTERACTION WITH OTHER SUBSTANCES

INTERACTS WITH	COMBINED EFFECT
Alcohol:	Disulfiram reaction (see page 848). Avoid.
Beverages:	None expected.
Cocaine:	No proven problems.
Foods:	None expected.
Marijuana:	Decreased chlorpropamide effect. Avoid.
Tobacco:	None expected.

CHLORPROTHIXENE

BRAND NAMES

Taractan
Tarasan

Habit forming? No
Prescription needed? Yes
Available as generic? No

GENERAL INFORMATION

Drug class: Tranquilizer
(thioxanthine), antiemetic

USES

- Reduces anxiety, agitation, psychosis.
- Stops vomiting.

DOSAGE & USAGE INFORMATION

How to take:
- Tablet—Swallow with liquid. If you can't swallow whole, crumble tablet and take with liquid or food.
- Syrup—Dilute dose in beverage before swallowing.

When to take:
At the same time each day.

If you forget a dose:
Take as soon as you remember up to 2 hours late. If more than 2 hours, wait for next scheduled dose (don't double this dose).

What drug does:
Corrects imbalance of nerve impulses.

Time lapse before drug works:
3 weeks.

Don't take with:
See Interaction column and consult doctor.

OVERDOSE

Symptoms:
Drowsiness, dizziness, weakness, muscle rigidity, twitching, tremors, confusion, dry mouth, blurred vision, rapid pulse, shallow breathing, low blood pressure, convulsions, coma.

What to do:
- Dial 0 (operator) or 911 (emergency) for an ambulance or medical help. Then give first aid immediately.
- If patient is unconscious and not breathing, give mouth-to-mouth breathing. If there is no heartbeat, use cardiac massage and mouth-to-mouth breathing (CPR). Don't try to make patient vomit. If you can't get help quickly, take patient to nearest emergency facility.
- Additional emergency information on page 886.

POSSIBLE ADVERSE REACTIONS OR SIDE EFFECTS

SYMPTOMS	FREQUENCY	WHAT TO DO
Brain & nervous system:		
● Fainting; restlessness; jerky, involuntary movements.	Common	3
● Dizziness, drowsiness.	Common	4
Skin:		
Rash	Infrequent	3
Eyes:		
Blurred vision.	Common	3
Ears, nose, throat:		
● Sore throat, fever.	Rare	3
● Dry mouth, nasal congestion.	Common	5
Digestive:		
Constipation	Common	4
Heart & lungs:		
Rapid heartbeat.	Common	3
Blood vessels, kidneys, allergic, blood:	None expected.	
Muscles, bones, joints:		
● Muscle spasms.	Common	4
● Shuffling walk.	Common	4
Genital, urinary:		
● Less sexual ability.	Infrequent	4
● Difficult urination.	Infrequent	4
Liver:		
Jaundice (yellow skin and eyes).	Rare	3
Others:		
● Less perspiration.	Common	4
● Menstrual changes.	Infrequent	5
● Breast swelling.	Infrequent	5

1- Life-threatening. Seek emergency treatment immediately.
2- Discontinue. Seek emergency treatment.
3- Discontinue. Call doctor right away.
4- Continue. Call doctor when convenient.
5- Continue. Tell doctor at next visit.

WARNINGS & PRECAUTIONS

Don't take if:
- You are allergic to any thioxanthine or phenothiazine tranquilizer.
- You have serious blood disorder.
- You have Parkinson's disease.
- Patient is younger than 12.

Before you start, consult your doctor:
- If you have had liver or kidney disease.
- If you have epilepsy or glaucoma.
- If you have high blood pressure or heart disease (especially angina).
- If you use alcohol daily.
- If you will have surgery within 2 months, including dental surgery, requiring general or spinal anesthesia.

Over age 60:
Adverse reactions and side effects may be more frequent and severe than in younger persons.

Pregnancy:
No proven harm to unborn child. Avoid if possible.

Breast-feeding:
Studies inconclusive. Consult your doctor.

Infants & children:
Not recommended.

Prolonged use:
- Pigment deposits in lens and retina of eye.
- Involuntary movements of jaws, lips, tongue (tardive dyskinesia).

Skin & sunlight:
May cause rash or intensify sunburn in areas exposed to sun or sunlamp.

Driving, piloting or hazardous work:
Don't drive or pilot aircraft until you learn how medicine affects you. Don't work around dangerous machinery. Don't climb ladders or work in high places. Danger increases if you drink alcohol or take medicine affecting alertness and reflexes.

Airplane passengers:
No problems expected.

Discontinuing:
Don't discontinue without consulting doctor. Dose may require gradual reduction if you have taken drug for a long time. Doses of other drugs may also require adjustment.

Others:
Hot temperatures increase chance of heat stroke.

 ## INTERACTION WITH OTHER DRUGS

GENERIC NAME OR DRUG CLASS	COMBINED EFFECT
Anticholinergics	Increased anticholinergic effect.
Anticonvulsants	Change in seizure pattern.
Antidepressants (tricyclic)	Increased chlorprothixene effect. Excessive sedation.
Antihistamines	Increased chlorprothixene effect. Excessive sedation.
Antihypertensives	Excessively low blood pressure.
Barbiturates	Increased chlorprothixene effect. Excessive sedation.
Bethanechol	Decreased bethanechol effect.
Guanethidine	Decreased guanethidine effect.
Levodopa	Decreased levodopa effect.
MAO inhibitors	Excessive sedation.
Mind-altering drugs	Increased chlorprothixene effect. Excessive sedation.

Additional interactions on page 834.

 ## INTERACTION WITH OTHER SUBSTANCES

INTERACTS WITH	COMBINED EFFECT
Alcohol:	Excessive brain depression. Avoid.
Beverages:	None expected.
Cocaine:	Decreased chlorprothixene effect. Avoid.
Foods:	None expected.
Marijuana:	Daily use—Fainting likely, possible psychosis.
Tobacco:	None expected.

CHLORTHALIDONE

BRAND NAMES

Hygroton
Novothalidone
Uridon

GENERAL INFORMATION

Habit forming? No
Prescription needed? Yes
Available as generic? Yes
Drug class: Antihypertensive,
diuretic (thiazide)

 ## USES

- Controls, but doesn't cure, high blood pressure.
- Reduces fluid retention (edema) caused by conditions such as heart disorders and liver disease.

 ## DOSAGE & USAGE INFORMATION

How to take:
Tablet or capsule—Swallow with liquid. If you can't swallow whole, crumble tablet or open capsule and take with liquid or food. Don't exceed dose.

When to take:
At the same time each day.

If you forget a dose:
Take as soon as you remember up to 2 hours late. If more than 2 hours, wait for next scheduled dose (don't double this dose).

What drug does:
- Forces sodium and water excretion, reducing body fluid.
- Relaxes muscle cells of small arteries.
- Reduced body fluid and relaxed arteries lower blood pressure.

Time lapse before drug works:
4 to 6 hours. May require several weeks to lower blood pressure.

Don't take with:
- See Interaction column and consult doctor.
- Non-prescription drugs without consulting doctor.

 ## OVERDOSE

Symptoms:
Cramps, weakness, drowsiness, weak pulse, coma.

What to do:
- Dial O (operator) or 911 (emergency) for an ambulance or medical help. Then give first aid immediately.
- Additional emergency information on page 886.

POSSIBLE ADVERSE REACTIONS OR SIDE EFFECTS

SYMPTOMS	FREQUENCY	WHAT TO DO
Brain & nervous system:		
• Dizziness	Infrequent	4
• Mood changes.	Infrequent	4
• Headaches	Infrequent	4
Skin:		
Rash or hives.	Rare	2
Eyes:		
Blurred vision.	Infrequent	3
Ears, nose, throat:		
• Sore throat, fever.	Rare	3
• Dry mouth, thirst.	Infrequent	5
Digestive:		
Severe abdominal pain, nausea, vomiting.	Infrequent	3
Heart & lungs:		
Irregular heartbeat, weak pulse.	Infrequent	3
Blood vessels:	None expected.	
Muscles, bones, joints:		
Weakness, tiredness.	Infrequent	4
Genital, urinary:	None expected.	
Kidneys:	None expected.	
Liver:		
Jaundice (yellow skin and eyes).	Rare	3
Allergic:	None expected.	
Blood:	None expected.	
Others:		
Weight changes.	Infrequent	4

1- Life-threatening. Seek emergency treatment immediately.
2- Discontinue. Seek emergency treatment.
3- Discontinue. Call doctor right away.
4- Continue. Call doctor when convenient.
5- Continue. Tell doctor at next visit.
6- No action necessary.

WARNINGS & PRECAUTIONS

Don't take if:
You are allergic to any thiazide diuretic drug.

Before you start, consult your doctor:
- If you are allergic to any sulfa drug.
- If you have gout.
- If you have liver, pancreas or kidney disorder.

Over age 60:
Adverse reactions and side effects may be more frequent and severe than in younger persons, especially dizziness and excessive potassium loss.

Pregnancy:
Risk to unborn child outweighs drug benefits. Don't use.

Breast-feeding:
Drug passes into milk. Avoid this medicine or discontinue nursing.

Infants & children:
No problems expected.

Prolonged use:
You may need medicine to treat high blood pressure for the rest of your life.

Skin & sunlight:
May cause rash or intensify sunburn in areas exposed to sun or sunlamp.

Driving, piloting or hazardous work:
Don't drive or pilot aircraft until you learn how medicine affects you. Don't work around dangerous machinery. Don't climb ladders or work in high places. Danger increases if you drink alcohol or take medicine affecting alertness and reflexes, such as antihistamines, tranquilizers, sedatives, pain medicine, narcotics and mind-altering drugs.

Airplane passengers:
No problems expected.

Discontinuing:
Don't discontinue without medical advice.

Others:
- Hot weather and fever may cause dehydration and drop in blood pressure. Dose may require temporary adjustment. Weigh daily and report any unexpected weight decreases to your doctor.
- May cause rise in uric acid, leading to gout.
- May cause blood-sugar rise in diabetics.

INTERACTION WITH OTHER DRUGS

GENERIC NAME OR DRUG CLASS	COMBINED EFFECT
Allopurinol	Decreased allopurinol effect.
Antidepressants (tricyclic)	Dangerous drop in blood pressure. Avoid combination unless under medical supervision.
Barbiturates	Increased chlorthalidone effect.
Cholestyramine	Decreased chlorthalidone effect.
Cortisone drugs	Excessive potassium loss that causes dangerous heart rhythms.
Digitalis preparations	Excessive potassium loss that causes dangerous heart rhythms.
Diuretics (thiazide)	Increased effect of other thiazide diuretics.
Lithium	Increased effect of lithium.
MAO inhibitors	Increased chlorthalidone effect.
Probenecid	Decreased probenecid effect.

INTERACTION WITH OTHER SUBSTANCES

INTERACTS WITH	COMBINED EFFECT
Alcohol:	Dangerous blood-pressure drop.
Beverages:	None expected.
Cocaine:	None expected.
Foods: Licorice	Excessive potassium loss that causes dangerous heart rhythms.
Marijuana:	May increase blood pressure.
Tobacco:	None expected.

CHLORZOXAZONE

BRAND NAMES

Paraflex
Parafon Forte (M)

GENERAL INFORMATION

Habit forming? No
Prescription needed? Yes
Available as generic? No
Drug class: Muscle relaxant (skeletal)

USES

Treatment for sprains, strains and muscle spasms.

DOSAGE & USAGE INFORMATION

How to take:
Tablet or capsule—Swallow with liquid.

When to take:
As needed, no more often than every 4 hours.

If you forget a dose:
Take as soon as you remember. Wait 4 hours for next dose.

What drug does:
Blocks body's pain messages to brain. May also sedate.

Time lapse before drug works:
60 minutes.

Don't take with:
See Interaction column and consult doctor.

OVERDOSE

Symptoms:
Nausea, vomiting, diarrhea, headache, severe weakness, breathing difficulty, sensation of paralysis.

What to do:
- Overdose unlikely to threaten life. Depending on severity of symptoms and amount taken, call doctor, poison-control center or hospital emergency room for instructions.
- Additional emergency information on page 886.

POSSIBLE ADVERSE REACTIONS OR SIDE EFFECTS

SYMPTOMS	FREQUENCY	WHAT TO DO
Brain & nervous system:		
● Drowsiness, dizziness.	Common	4
● Agitation	Infrequent	3
Skin: Rash or itch.	Rare	3
Eyes:	None expected.	
Ears, nose, throat: Sore throat, fever.	Rare	3
Digestive:		
● Constipation or diarrhea, nausea, cramps, vomiting.	Infrequent	3
● Bloody or tarry, black stool.	Rare	2
Heart & lungs:	None expected.	
Blood vessels:	None expected.	
Muscles, bones, joints:	None expected.	
Genital, urinary: Orange or red-purple urine.	Common	6
Kidneys:	None expected.	
Liver: Jaundice (yellow eyes and skin).	Rare	3
Allergic:	None expected.	
Blood:	None expected.	
Others: Tiredness, weakness.	Rare	3

1- Life-threatening. Seek emergency treatment immediately.
2- Discontinue. Seek emergency treatment.
3- Discontinue. Call doctor right away.
4- Continue. Call doctor when convenient.
5- Continue. Tell doctor at next visit.
6- No action necessary.

CHLORZOXAZONE

WARNINGS & PRECAUTIONS

Don't take if:
You are allergic to any skeletal-muscle relaxant.

Before you start, consult your doctor:
- If you have had liver disease.
- If you plan pregnancy within medication period.

Over age 60:
Adverse reactions and side effects may be more frequent and severe than in younger persons.

Pregnancy:
No proven harm to unborn child. Avoid if possible.

Breast-feeding:
Drug passes into milk. Avoid drug or discontinue nursing until you finish medicine. Consult doctor for advice on maintaining milk supply.

Infants & children:
Not recommended.

Prolonged use:
No problems expected.

Skin & sunlight:
No problems expected.

Driving, piloting or hazardous work:
Don't drive or pilot aircraft until you learn how medicine affects you. Don't work around dangerous machinery. Don't climb ladders or work in high places. Danger increases if you drink alcohol or take medicine affecting alertness and reflexes, such as antihistamines, tranquilizers, sedatives, pain medicine, narcotics and mind-altering drugs.

Airplane passengers:
No problems expected.

Discontinuing:
Don't discontinue without doctor's advice until you complete prescribed dose, even though symptoms diminish or disappear.

Others:
Periodic liver-function tests recommended if you use this drug for a long time.

INTERACTION WITH OTHER DRUGS

GENERIC NAME OR DRUG CLASS	COMBINED EFFECT
Antidepressants	Increased sedation.
Antihistamines	Increased sedation.
MAO inhibitors	Increased effect of both drugs.
Mind-altering drugs	Increased sedation.
Muscle relaxants (others)	Increased sedation.
Narcotics	Increased sedation.
Sedatives	Increased sedation.
Sleep inducers	Increased sedation
Testosterone	Decreased chlorzoxazone effect.
Tranquilizers	Increased sedation.

INTERACTION WITH OTHER SUBSTANCES

INTERACTS WITH	COMBINED EFFECT
Alcohol:	Increased sedation.
Beverages:	No problems expected.
Cocaine:	Lack of coordination.
Foods:	No problems expected.
Marijuana:	Lack of coordination, drowsiness, fainting.
Tobacco:	No problems expected.

CHOLESTYRAMINE

BRAND NAMES

Questran

Habit forming? No
Prescription needed? Yes
Available as generic? No
Drug class: Antihyperlipidemic, antipruritic

USES

- Removes excess bile acids that occur with some liver problems. Reduces persistent itch caused by bile acids.
- Lowers cholesterol level.

DOSAGE & USAGE INFORMATION

How to take:
Powder, granules—Sprinkle into 8 oz. liquid. Let stand for 2 minutes, then mix with liquid before swallowing. Or mix with cereal, soup or pulpy fruit. Don't swallow dry.

When to take:
3 or 4 times a day on an empty stomach, 1 hour before or 2 hours after eating.

If you forget a dose:
Take as soon as you remember up to 2 hours late. If more than 2 hours, wait for next scheduled dose (don't double this dose).

What drug does:
Binds with bile acids to prevent their absorption.

Time lapse before drug works:
- Cholesterol reduction—1 day.
- Bile-acid reduction—3 to 4 weeks.

Don't take with:
- Any drug or vitamin simultaneously. Space doses 2 hours apart.
- See Interaction column and consult doctor.

OVERDOSE

Symptoms:
Increased side effects and adverse reactions.

What to do:
Overdose unlikely to threaten life. If person takes much larger amount than prescribed, call doctor, poison-control center or hospital emergency room for instructions.

POSSIBLE ADVERSE REACTIONS OR SIDE EFFECTS

SYMPTOMS	FREQUENCY	WHAT TO DO
Brain & nervous system:	None expected.	
Skin: Rash	Rare	3
Eyes:	None expected.	
Ears, nose, throat: Sore tongue.	Rare	4
Digestive:		
• Constipation	Common	4
• Belching, bloating, diarrhea, mild nausea, vomiting, stomach pain.	Infrequent	3
• Severe stomach pain; nausea, vomiting; black, tarry stool.	Rare	2
Heart & lungs:	None expected.	
Blood vessels:	None expected.	
Muscles, bones, joints:	None expected.	
Genital, urinary:	None expected.	
Kidneys:	None expected.	
Liver:	None expected.	
Allergic:	None expected.	
Blood:	None expected.	
Others:	None expected.	

1- Life-threatening. Seek emergency treatment immediately.
2- Discontinue. Seek emergency treatment.
3- Discontinue. Call doctor right away.
4- Continue. Call doctor when convenient.
5- Continue. Tell doctor at next visit.
6- No action necessary.

WARNINGS & PRECAUTIONS

Don't take if:
You are allergic to cholestyramine.

Before you start, consult your doctor:
- If you plan to become pregnant within medication period.
- If you have angina, heart or blood-vessel disease.
- If you have stomach problems (including ulcer).
- If you have constipation or hemorrhoids.
- If you have kidney disease.

Over age 60:
Adverse reactions and side effects may be more frequent and severe than in younger persons.

Pregnancy:
No proven harm to unborn child. Avoid if possible.

Breast-feeding:
No problems expected, but consult doctor.

Infants & children:
Not recommended.

Prolonged use:
No problems expected.

Skin & sunlight:
No problems expected.

Driving, piloting or hazardous work:
No problems expected.

Airplane passengers:
No problems expected.

Discontinuing:
Don't discontinue without doctor's advice until you complete prescribed dose, even though symptoms diminish or disappear.

Others:
No problems expected.

INTERACTION WITH OTHER DRUGS

GENERIC NAME OR DRUG CLASS	COMBINED EFFECT
Anticoagulants	Increased anticoagulant effect.
Digitalis preparations	Decreased digitalis effect.
Thyroid hormones	Decreased thyroid effect.

INTERACTION WITH OTHER SUBSTANCES

INTERACTS WITH	COMBINED EFFECT
Alcohol:	None expected.
Beverages:	None expected.
Cocaine:	None expected.
Foods:	None expected.
Marijuana:	None expected.
Tobacco:	None expected.

CIMETIDINE

BRAND NAMES

Tagamet

GENERAL INFORMATION

Habit forming? No
Prescription needed? Yes
Available as generic? No
Drug class: Histamine H-2 antagonist

USES

Treatment for duodenal ulcers and other conditions in which stomach produces excess hydrochloric acid.

DOSAGE & USAGE INFORMATION

How to take:
Tablet or capsule—Swallow with liquid.

When to take:
- 1 dose per day—Take at bedtime.
- 2 or more doses per day—Take at the same times each day.

If you forget a dose:
Take as soon as you remember up to 2 hours late. If more than 2 hours, wait for next scheduled dose (don't double this dose).

What drug does:
Blocks histamine release so stomach secretes less acid.

Time lapse before drug works:
Begins in 30 minutes. May require several days to relieve pain.

Don't take with:
See Interaction column and consult doctor.

OVERDOSE

Symptoms:
Confusion, slurred speech, breathing difficulty, rapid heartbeat, delirium.

What to do:
Overdose unlikely to threaten life. If person takes much larger amount than prescribed, call doctor, poison-control center or hospital emergency room for instructions.

POSSIBLE ADVERSE REACTIONS OR SIDE EFFECTS

SYMPTOMS	FREQUENCY	WHAT TO DO
Brain & nervous system:		
• Confusion	Rare	3
• Dizziness or headache.	Infrequent	4
Skin:		
Rash, hives.	Rare	3
Eyes, kidneys, liver, allergic, blood:	None expected.	
Ears, nose, throat:		
Sore throat, fever.	Rare	3
Digestive:		
Diarrhea	Infrequent	4
Heart & lungs:		
Slow, fast or irregular heartbeat.	Rare	3
Blood vessels:		
Unusual bleeding or bruising.	Rare	3
Muscles, bones, joints:		
Muscle cramps or pain.	Rare	3
Genital, urinary:		
Decreased sperm production.	Infrequent	4
Others:		
• Decreased sex drive, breast swelling and soreness in males; unusual milk flow in females; hair loss.	Infrequent	5
• Fatigue, weakness.	Rare	3

1- Life-threatening. Seek emergency treatment immediately.
2- Discontinue. Seek emergency treatment.
3- Discontinue. Call doctor right away.
4- Continue. Call doctor when convenient.
5- Continue. Tell doctor at next visit.

WARNINGS & PRECAUTIONS

Don't take if:
You are allergic to cimetidine.

Before you start, consult your doctor:
- If you plan to become pregnant during medication period.
- If you take aspirin. Aspirin may irritate stomach.

Over age 60:
Adverse reactions and side effects may be more frequent and severe than in younger persons.

Pregnancy:
No proven harm to unborn child. Avoid if possible.

Breast-feeding:
No problems expected.

Infants & children:
Not recommended.

Prolonged use:
Possible liver damage.

Skin & sunlight:
No problems expected.

Driving, piloting or hazardous work:
Don't drive or pilot aircraft until you learn how medicine affects you. Don't work around dangerous machinery. Don't climb ladders or work in high places. Danger increases if you drink alcohol or take medicine affecting alertness and reflexes, such as antihistamines, tranquilizers, sedatives, pain medicine, narcotics and mind-altering drugs.

Airplane passengers:
No problems expected.

Discontinuing:
Don't discontinue without consulting doctor. Dose may require gradual reduction if you have taken drug for a long time. Doses of other drugs may also require adjustment.

Others:
Patients on kidney dialysis—Take at end of dialysis treatment.

INTERACTION WITH OTHER DRUGS

GENERIC NAME OR DRUG CLASS	COMBINED EFFECT
Anticoagulants (oral)	Increased anticoagulant effect.
Anticholinergics	Decreased cimetidine effect.
Bethanechol	Increased cimetidine effect.
Carmustine (BCNU)	Severe impairment of red-blood-cell production; some interference with white-blood-cell formation.

Additional interactions on page 835.

INTERACTION WITH OTHER SUBSTANCES

INTERACTS WITH	COMBINED EFFECT
Alcohol:	No interactions expected, but alcohol may slow body's recovery. Avoid.
Beverages: Milk	Enhanced effectiveness. Small amounts useful for taking medication.
Caffeine drinks	May increase acid secretion and delay healing.
Cocaine:	Decreased cimetidine effect.
Foods:	Enhanced effectiveness. Protein-rich foods should be eaten in moderation to minimize secretion of stomach acid.
Marijuana:	Increased chance of low sperm count. Marijuana may slow body's recovery. Avoid.
Tobacco:	No interactions expected, but tobacco may slow body's recovery. Avoid.

CLEMASTINE

BRAND NAMES

Tavist

GENERAL INFORMATION

Habit forming? No
Prescription needed? No
Available as generic? No
Drug class: Antihistamine

 ## USES

Reduces allergic symptoms such as hay fever, hives, rash or itching.

 ## DOSAGE & USAGE INFORMATION

How to take:
Tablet—Swallow with liquid or food to lessen stomach irritation.

When to take:
Varies with form. Follow label directions.

If you forget a dose:
Take as soon as you remember up to 2 hours late. If more than 2 hours, wait for next scheduled dose (don't double this dose).

What drug does:
Blocks action of histamine after an allergic response triggers histamine release in sensitive cells.

Time lapse before drug works:
30 minutes.

Don't take with:
See Interaction column and consult doctor.

 ## OVERDOSE

Symptoms:
Convulsions, red face, hallucinations, coma.

What to do:
- Dial 0 (operator) or 911 (emergency) for an ambulance or medical help. Then give first aid immediately.
- If patient is unconscious and not breathing, give mouth-to-mouth breathing. If there is no heartbeat, use cardiac massage and mouth-to-mouth breathing (CPR). Don't try to make patient vomit. If you can't get help quickly, take patient to nearest emergency facility.
- Additional emergency information on page 886.

POSSIBLE ADVERSE REACTIONS OR SIDE EFFECTS

SYMPTOMS	FREQUENCY	WHAT TO DO
Brain & nervous system:		
● Nightmares, agitation, irritability.	Rare	3
● Drowsiness, dizziness.	Common	5
Skin:	None expected.	
Eyes:		
● Vision changes.	Infrequent	3
● Less tolerance for contact lenses.	Infrequent	4
Ears, nose, throat:		
● Sore throat, fever.	Rare	3
● Dry mouth, nose, throat.	Common	5
Digestive:		
● Nausea	Common	5
● Appetite loss.	Infrequent	5
Heart & lungs:		
Rapid heartbeat.	Rare	3
Blood vessels:		
Unusual bleeding or bruising.	Rare	3
Muscles, bones, joints, kidneys, liver, allergic, blood:	None expected.	
Genital, urinary:		
Urination difficulty.	Infrequent	4
Others:		
Fatigue, weakness.	Rare	3

1 - Life-threatening. Seek emergency treatment immediately.
2 - Discontinue. Seek emergency treatment.
3 - Discontinue. Call doctor right away.
4 - Continue. Call doctor when convenient.
5 - Continue. Tell doctor at next visit.
6 - No action necessary.

CLEMASTINE

WARNINGS & PRECAUTIONS

Don't take if:
You are allergic to any antihistamine.

Before you start, consult your doctor:
- If you have glaucoma.
- If you have enlarged prostate.
- If you have asthma.
- If you have kidney disease.
- If you have peptic ulcer.
- If you will have surgery within 2 months, including dental surgery, requiring general or spinal anesthesia.

Over age 60:
Don't exceed recommended dose. Adverse reactions and side effects may be more frequent and severe than in younger persons, especially urination difficulty, diminished alertness and other brain and nervous-system symptoms.

Pregnancy:
No proven harm to unborn child. Avoid if possible.

Breast-feeding:
Drug passes into milk. Avoid drug or discontinue nursing until you finish medicine. Consult doctor for advice on maintaining milk supply.

Infants & children:
Not recommended for premature or newborn infants. Otherwise, no problems expected.

Prolonged use:
Avoid. May damage bone marrow and nerve cells.

Skin & sunlight:
May cause rash or intensify sunburn in areas exposed to sun or sunlamp.

Driving, piloting or hazardous work:
Don't drive or pilot aircraft until you learn how medicine affects you. Don't work around dangerous machinery. Don't climb ladders or work in high places. Danger increases if you drink alcohol or take medicine affecting alertness and reflexes, such as antihistamines, tranquilizers, sedatives, pain medicine, narcotics and mind-altering drugs.

Airplane passengers:
No problems expected.

Discontinuing:
No problems expected.

Others:
May mask symptoms of hearing damage from aspirin, other salicylates, cisplatin, paromomycin, vancomycin or anticonvulsants. Consult doctor if you use these.

INTERACTION WITH OTHER DRUGS

GENERIC NAME OR DRUG CLASS	COMBINED EFFECT
Anticholinergics	Increased anticholinergic effect.
Antidepressants	Excess sedation. Avoid.
Antihistamines (other)	Excess sedation. Avoid.
Hypnotics	Excess sedation. Avoid.
MAO inhibitors	Increased clemastine effect.
Mind-altering drugs	Excess sedation. Avoid.
Narcotics	Excess sedation. Avoid.
Sedatives	Excess sedation. Avoid.
Sleep inducers	Excess sedation. Avoid.
Tranquilizers	Excess sedation. Avoid.

INTERACTION WITH OTHER SUBSTANCES

INTERACTS WITH	COMBINED EFFECT
Alcohol:	Excess sedation. Avoid.
Beverages: Caffeine drinks	Less clemastine sedation.
Cocaine:	Decreased clemastine effect. Avoid.
Foods:	None expected.
Marijuana:	Excess sedation. Avoid.
Tobacco:	None expected.

CLIDINIUM

BRAND NAMES

Librax (M)
Quarzan

GENERAL INFORMATION

Habit forming? No
Prescription needed? Low strength: No
High strength: Yes
Available as generic? Yes
Drug class: Antispasmodic, anticholinergic

USES

Reduces spasms of digestive system, bladder and urethra.

DOSAGE & USAGE INFORMATION

How to take:
Capsule—Swallow with liquid or food to lessen stomach irritation.

When to take:
30 minutes before meals (unless directed otherwise by doctor).

If you forget a dose:
Take as soon as you remember up to 2 hours late. If more than 2 hours, wait for next scheduled dose (don't double this dose).

What drug does:
Blocks nerve impulses at parasympathetic nerve endings, preventing muscle contractions and gland secretions of organs involved.

Time lapse before drug works:
15 to 30 minutes.

Don't take with:
See Interaction column and consult doctor.

OVERDOSE

Symptoms:
Dilated pupils; rapid pulse and breathing; dizziness; fever; hallucinations; confusion; slurred speech; agitation; flushed face; convulsions; coma.

What to do:
- Dial 0 (operator) or 911 (emergency) for an ambulance or medical help. Then give first aid immediately.
- Additional emergency information on page 886.

POSSIBLE ADVERSE REACTIONS OR SIDE EFFECTS

SYMPTOMS	FREQUENCY	WHAT TO DO
Brain & nervous system:		
• Headache	Infrequent	4
• Confusion, delirium.	Common	3
Skin:		
Rash or hives.	Rare	3
Eyes:		
Pain, blurred vision.	Rare	3
Ears, nose, throat:		
• Dryness	Common	6
• Nasal congestion, altered taste.	Infrequent	3
Digestive:		
• Constipation	Common	5
• Nausea, vomiting.	Common	4
Heart & lungs:		
Rapid heartbeat.	Common	3
Blood vessels:	None expected.	
Muscles, bones, joints:	None expected.	
Genital, urinary:		
Difficult urination.	Infrequent	4
Kidneys:	None expected.	
Liver:	None expected.	
Allergic:	None expected.	
Blood:	None expected.	
Others:		
Less perspiration.	Common	4

1- Life-threatening. Seek emergency treatment immediately.
2- Discontinue. Seek emergency treatment.
3- Discontinue. Call doctor right away.
4- Continue. Call doctor when convenient.
5- Continue. Tell doctor at next visit.
6- No action necessary.

WARNINGS & PRECAUTIONS

Don't take if:
- You are allergic to any anticholinergic.
- You have trouble with stomach bloating.
- You have difficulty emptying your bladder completely.
- You have narrow-angle glaucoma.
- You have severe ulcerative colitis.

Before you start, consult your doctor:
- If you have open-angle glaucoma.
- If you have angina.
- If you have chronic bronchitis or asthma.
- If you have hiatal hernia.
- If you have liver disease.
- If you have enlarged prostate.
- If you have myasthenia gravis.
- If you have peptic ulcer.
- If you will have surgery within 2 months, including dental surgery, requiring general or spinal anesthesia.

Over age 60:
Adverse reactions and side effects may be more frequent and severe than in younger persons.

Pregnancy:
Studies inconclusive on harm to unborn child. Animal studies show fetal abnormalities. Decide with your doctor whether drug benefits justify risk to unborn child.

Breast-feeding:
Drug passes into milk and decreases milk flow. Avoid drug or discontinue nursing until you finish medicine. Consult doctor for advice on maintaining milk supply.

Infants & children:
Use only under medical supervision.

Prolonged use:
Chronic constipation, possible fecal impaction. Consult doctor immediately.

Skin & sunlight:
No problems expected.

Driving, piloting or hazardous work:
Don't drive or pilot aircraft until you learn how medicine affects you. Don't work around dangerous machinery. Don't climb ladders or work in high places. Danger increases if you drink alcohol or take medicine affecting alertness and reflexes, such as antihistamines, tranquilizers, sedatives, pain medicine, narcotics, or mind-altering drugs.

Airplane passengers:
No problems expected.

Discontinuing:
May be unnecessary to finish medicine. Follow doctor's instructions.

INTERACTION WITH OTHER DRUGS

GENERIC NAME OR DRUG CLASS	COMBINED EFFECT
Amantadine	Increased clidinium effect.
Antacids	Decreased clidinium effect.
Anticholinergics (other)	Increased clidinium effect.
Antidepressants (tricyclic)	Increased clidinium effect.
Antihistamines	Increased clidinium effect.
Haloperidol	Increased internal-eye pressure.
MAO inhibitors	Increased clidinium effect.
Meperidine	Increased clidinium effect.
Methylphenidate	Increased clidinium effect.
Orphenadrine	Increased clidinium effect.
Phenothiazines	Increased clidinium effect.
Pilocarpine	Loss of pilocarpine effect in glaucoma treatment.
Tranquilizers	Decreased clidinium effect.
Vitamin C	Decreased clidinium effect. Avoid large doses of vitamin C.

INTERACTION WITH OTHER SUBSTANCES

INTERACTS WITH	COMBINED EFFECT
Alcohol:	None expected.
Beverages:	None expected.
Cocaine:	Excessively rapid heartbeat. Avoid.
Foods:	None expected.
Marijuana:	Drowsiness and dry mouth.
Tobacco:	None expected.

CLINDAMYCIN

BRAND NAMES

Cleocin
Cleocin-T
Dalacin C

GENERAL INFORMATION

Habit forming? No
Prescription needed? Yes
Available as generic? No
Drug class: Antibiotic (lincomycin)

 USES

Treatment of bacterial infections that are susceptible to clindamycin.

 DOSAGE & USAGE INFORMATION

How to take:
Capsule or liquid—Swallow with liquid 1 hour before or 2 hours after eating.

When to take:
At the same times each day.

If you forget a dose:
Take as soon as you remember up to 2 hours late. If more than 2 hours, wait for next scheduled dose (don't double this dose).

What drug does:
Destroys susceptible bacteria. Does not kill viruses.

Time lapse before drug works:
3 to 5 days.

Don't take with:
See Interaction column and consult doctor.

 OVERDOSE

Symptoms:
Severe nausea, vomiting, diarrhea.

What to do:
Overdose unlikely to threaten life. If person takes much larger amount than prescribed, call doctor, poison-control center or hospital emergency room for instructions.

POSSIBLE ADVERSE REACTIONS OR SIDE EFFECTS

SYMPTOMS	FREQUENCY	WHAT TO DO
Brain & nervous system:	None expected.	
Skin: Rash, itch around groin, rectum or armpits.	Infrequent	4
Eyes:	None expected.	
Ears, nose, throat:		
• Unusual thirst.	Infrequent	3
• White patches in mouth.	Infrequent	4
Digestive: Vomiting, stomach cramps, severe and watery diarrhea with blood or mucus.	Infrequent	3
Heart & lungs:	None expected.	
Blood vessels:	None expected.	
Muscles, bones, joints: Painful, swollen joints.	Infrequent	3
Genital, urinary: Vaginal discharge, itching.	Infrequent	4
Kidneys:	None expected.	
Liver: Jaundice (yellow skin and eyes).	Infrequent	3
Allergic:	None expected.	
Blood:	None expected.	
Others:		
• Fever	Infrequent	3
• Tiredness, weakness, weight loss.	Infrequent	3

1-Life-threatening. Seek emergency treatment immediately.
2-Discontinue. Seek emergency treatment.
3-Discontinue. Call doctor right away.
4-Continue. Call doctor when convenient.

CLINDAMYCIN

WARNINGS & PRECAUTIONS

Don't take if:
- You are allergic to lincomycins.
- You have had ulcerative colitis.
- Prescribed for infant under 1 month old.

Before you start, consult your doctor:
- If you have had yeast infections of mouth, skin or vagina.
- If you will have surgery within 2 months, including dental surgery, requiring general or spinal anesthesia.
- If you have kidney or liver disease.
- If you have allergies of any kind.

Over age 60:
Adverse reactions and side effects may be more frequent and severe than in younger persons.

Pregnancy:
Risk to unborn child outweighs drug benefits. Don't use.

Breast-feeding:
Drug passes into milk. Avoid drug or discontinue nursing until you finish medicine. Consult doctor for advice on maintaining milk supply.

Infants & children:
Don't give to infants younger than 1 month. Use for children only under medical supervision.

Prolonged use:
- Severe colitis with diarrhea and bleeding.
- You may become more susceptible to infections caused by germs not responsive to clindamycin.

Skin & sunlight:
No problems expected.

Driving, piloting or hazardous work:
No problems expected.

Airplane passengers:
No problems expected.

Discontinuing:
Don't discontinue without doctor's advice until you complete prescribed dose, even though symptoms diminish or disappear.

Others:
No problems expected.

INTERACTION WITH OTHER DRUGS

GENERIC NAME OR DRUG CLASS	COMBINED EFFECT
Antidiarrheal preparations	Decreased clindamycin effect.
Chloramphenicol	Decreased clindamycin effect.
Erythromycin	Decreased clindamycin effect.

INTERACTION WITH OTHER SUBSTANCES

INTERACTS WITH	COMBINED EFFECT
Alcohol:	None expected.
Beverages:	None expected.
Cocaine:	None expected.
Foods:	None expected.
Marijuana:	None expected.
Tobacco:	None expected.

CLOFIBRATE

BRAND NAMES

Atromid-S
Claripex
Liprinal

GENERAL INFORMATION

Habit forming? No
Prescription needed? Yes
Available as generic? No
Drug class: Antihyperlipidemic

 USES

Reduces fatty substances in the blood (cholesterol and triglycerides).

 DOSAGE & USAGE INFORMATION

How to take:
Capsule—Swallow with liquid or food to lessen stomach irritation.

When to take:
At the same times each day.

If you forget a dose:
Take as soon as you remember up to 2 hours late. If more than 2 hours, wait for next scheduled dose (don't double this dose).

What drug does:
Inhibits formation of fatty substances.

Time lapse before drug works:
3 months or more.

Don't take with:
See Interaction column and consult doctor.

 OVERDOSE

Symptoms:
Diarrhea, headache, muscle pain.

What to do:
Overdose unlikely to threaten life. If person takes much larger amount than prescribed, call doctor, poison-control center or hospital emergency room for instructions.

POSSIBLE ADVERSE REACTIONS OR SIDE EFFECTS

SYMPTOMS	FREQUENCY	WHAT TO DO
Brain & nervous system: Dizziness, drowsiness, headache.	Rare	4
Skin:		
• Dryness, hair loss.	Rare	4
• Rash, itch.	Rare	3
Eyes, blood vessels, allergic, blood:	None expected.	
Ears, nose, throat:		
• Sores in mouth, on lips.	Rare	3
• Sore throat.	Rare	3
Digestive: Nausea, vomiting, diarrhea, stomach pain.	Infrequent	4
Heart & lungs: Chest pain, shortness of breath, irregular heartbeat.	Infrequent	3
Muscles, bones, joints:		
• Muscle cramps.	Rare	4
• Swollen feet, legs.	Rare	3
Genital, urinary: Bloody urine, painful urination.	Rare	3
Kidneys: Backache	Rare	4
Liver: Gallstones	Infrequent	3
Others:		
• Decreased sex drive.	Rare	4
• Fever, chills.	Rare	3

1- Life-threatening. Seek emergency treatment immediately.
2- Discontinue. Seek emergency treatment.
3- Discontinue. Call doctor right away.
4- Continue. Call doctor when convenient.

WARNINGS & PRECAUTIONS

Don't take if:
You are allergic to any antihyperlipidemic.

Before you start, consult your doctor:
- If you have had liver or kidney disease.
- If you have had peptic-ulcer disease.
- If you have diabetes.

Over age 60:
Adverse reactions and side effects may be more frequent and severe than in younger persons. May develop flu-like symptoms.

Pregnancy:
Risk to unborn child outweighs drug benefits. Don't use.

Breast-feeding:
May harm child. Avoid.

Infants & children:
Not recommended.

Prolonged use:
No problems expected.

Skin & sunlight:
No problems expected.

Driving, piloting or hazardous work:
Avoid if you feel drowsy or dizzy. Otherwise, no problems expected.

Airplane passengers:
No problems expected.

Discontinuing:
Don't discontinue without doctor's advice until you complete prescribed dose, even though symptoms diminish or disappear.

Others:
- Periodic blood-cell counts and liver-function studies recommended if you take clofibrate for a long time.
- Some studies question effectiveness. Many studies warn against toxicity.

INTERACTION WITH OTHER DRUGS

GENERIC NAME OR DRUG CLASS	COMBINED EFFECT
Anticoagulants (oral)	Increased anticoagulant effect. Dose reduction of anticoagulant necessary.
Antidiabetics (oral)	Increased antidiabetic effect.
Contraceptives (oral)	Decreased clofibrate effect.
Estrogens	Decreased clofibrate effect.
Furosemide	Possible toxicity of both drugs.
Insulin	Increased insulin effect.
Thyroid hormones	Increased clofibrate effect.

INTERACTION WITH OTHER SUBSTANCES

INTERACTS WITH	COMBINED EFFECT
Alcohol:	None expected.
Beverages:	None expected.
Cocaine:	None expected.
Foods: Fatty foods	Decreased clofibrate effect.
Marijuana:	None expected.
Tobacco:	None expected.

CLOMIPHENE

BRAND NAMES

Clomid

GENERAL INFORMATION

Habit forming? No
Prescription needed? Yes
Available as generic? No
Drug class: Gonad stimulant

 USES

- Treatment for men with low sperm counts.
- Treatment for ovulatory failure in women who wish to become pregnant.

 DOSAGE & USAGE INFORMATION

How to take:
Tablet—Swallow with liquid.

When to take:
- Men—Take at the same time each day.
- Women—If you are to begin treatment on "Day 5," count your first menstrual day as "Day 1." Take a tablet each day for 5 days.

If you forget a dose:
Take as soon as you remember. If you forget a day, double next dose. If you miss 2 or more doses, consult doctor.

What drug does:
Antiestrogen effect stimulates ovulation and sperm production.

Time lapse before drug works:
Usually 3 to 6 months. Ovulation may occur 6 to 10 days after last day of treatment in any cycle.

Don't take with:
No restrictions.

 OVERDOSE

Symptoms:
Increased severity of adverse reactions and side effects.

What to do:
Overdose unlikely to threaten life. If person takes much larger amount than prescribed, call doctor, poison-control center or hospital emergency room for instructions.

 POSSIBLE ADVERSE REACTIONS OR SIDE EFFECTS

SYMPTOMS	FREQUENCY	WHAT TO DO
Brain & nervous system: Dizziness, headache, tiredness, depression, nervousness.	Rare	4
Skin: Rash, itch.	Infrequent	3
Eyes: Vision changes.	Rare	3
Ears, nose, throat:	None expected.	
Digestive:		
• Bloating, stomach pain.	Common	3
• Constipation, diarrhea, increased appetite.	Infrequent	4
Heart & lungs:	None expected.	
Blood vessels: Hot flashes.	Common	5
Muscles, bones, joints:	None expected.	
Genital, urinary:		
• Pelvic pain.	Common	3
• Heavy menstrual flow.	Infrequent	4
Kidneys: Frequent urination.	Infrequent	4
Liver: Jaundice (yellow skin and eyes).	Infrequent	3
Allergic:	None expected.	
Blood:	None expected.	
Others: Breast discomfort, weight change, hair loss.	Infrequent	4

1-Life-threatening. Seek emergency treatment immediately.
2-Discontinue. Seek emergency treatment.
3-Discontinue. Call doctor right away.
4-Continue. Call doctor when convenient.
5-Continue. Tell doctor at next visit.

WARNINGS & PRECAUTIONS

Don't take if:
You are allergic to clomiphene.

Before you start, consult your doctor:
- If you have an ovarian cyst, fibroid uterine tumors or unusual vaginal bleeding.
- If you have inflamed veins caused by blood clots.
- If you have liver disease.
- If you are depressed.

Over age 60:
Not recommended.

Pregnancy:
Stop taking at first sign of pregnancy.

Breast-feeding:
Not used.

Infants & children:
Not used.

Prolonged use:
Not recommended.

Skin & sunlight:
No problems expected.

Driving, piloting or hazardous work:
Avoid if you feel dizzy. Otherwise, no problems expected.

Airplane passengers:
No problems expected.

Discontinuing:
May be unnecessary to finish medicine. Follow doctor's instructions.

Others:
- Have a complete pelvic examination before treatment.
- If you become pregnant, twins or triplets are possible.

INTERACTION WITH OTHER DRUGS

GENERIC NAME OR DRUG CLASS	COMBINED EFFECT
None	

INTERACTION WITH OTHER SUBSTANCES

INTERACTS WITH	COMBINED EFFECT
Alcohol:	None expected.
Beverages:	None expected.
Cocaine:	None expected.
Foods:	None expected.
Marijuana:	None expected.
Tobacco:	None expected.

CLORAZEPATE

BRAND NAMES

Tranxene

GENERAL INFORMATION

Habit forming? Yes
Prescription needed? Yes
Available as generic? No
Drug class: Tranquilizer (benzodiazepine)

 USES

- Treatment for nervousness or tension.
- Treatment for convulsive disorders.

 DOSAGE & USAGE INFORMATION

How to take:
Tablet or capsule—Swallow with liquid. If you can't swallow whole, crumble tablet or open capsule and take with liquid or food.

When to take:
At the same time each day, according to instructions on prescription label.

If you forget a dose:
Take as soon as you remember up to 2 hours late. If more than 2 hours, wait for next scheduled dose (don't double this dose).

What drug does:
Affects limbic system of brain—part that controls emotions.

Time lapse before drug works:
2 hours. May take 6 weeks for full benefit.

Don't take with:
See Interaction column and consult doctor.

 OVERDOSE

Symptoms:
Drowsiness, weakness, tremor, stupor, coma.

What to do:
- Dial 0 (operator) or 911 (emergency) for an ambulance or medical help. Then give first aid immediately.
- If patient is unconscious and not breathing, give mouth-to-mouth breathing. If there is no heartbeat, use cardiac massage and mouth-to-mouth breathing (CPR). Don't try to make patient vomit. If you can't get help quickly, take patient to nearest emergency facility.
- Additional emergency information on page 886.

POSSIBLE ADVERSE REACTIONS OR SIDE EFFECTS

SYMPTOMS	FREQUENCY	WHAT TO DO
Brain & nervous system:		
• Clumsiness, drowsiness, dizziness.	Common	4
• Hallucinations, confusion, depression, irritability.	Infrequent	3
Skin:		
Rash, itch.	Infrequent	3
Eyes:		
Vision changes.	Infrequent	3
Ears, nose, throat:		
Mouth, throat ulcers.	Rare	3
Digestive:		
Constipation or diarrhea, nausea, vomiting.	Infrequent	4
Heart & lungs:		
Slow heartbeat, breathing difficulty.	Rare	2
Blood vessels:	None expected.	
Muscles, bones, joints:	None expected.	
Genital, urinary:		
Urination difficulty.	Infrequent	4
Kidneys:	None expected.	
Liver:		
Jaundice (yellow eyes and skin).	Rare	3
Allergic:	None expected.	
Blood:	None expected.	
Others:	None expected.	

1- Life-threatening. Seek emergency treatment immediately.
2- Discontinue. Seek emergency treatment.
3- Discontinue. Call doctor right away.
4- Continue. Call doctor when convenient.
5- Continue. Tell doctor at next visit.
6- No action necessary.

WARNINGS & PRECAUTIONS

Don't take if:
- You are allergic to any benzodiazepine.
- You have myasthenia gravis.
- You have glaucoma.
- You are active or recovering alcoholic.
- Patient is younger than 6 months.

Before you start, consult your doctor:
- If you have liver, kidney or lung disease.
- If you have diabetes, epilepsy or porphyria.

Over age 60:
Adverse reactions and side effects may be more frequent and severe than in younger persons. You need smaller doses for shorter periods of time. May develop agitation, rage or "hangover effect."

Pregnancy:
Risk to unborn child outweighs drug benefits. Don't use.

Breast-feeding:
Drug passes into milk. Avoid drug or discontinue nursing until you finish medicine. Consult doctor for advice on maintaining milk supply.

Infants & children:
Use only under medical supervision for children older than 6 months.

Prolonged use:
May impair liver function.

Skin & sunlight:
No problems expected.

Driving, piloting or hazardous work:
Don't drive or pilot aircraft until you learn how medicine affects you. Don't work around dangerous machinery. Don't climb ladders or work in high places. Danger increases if you drink alcohol or take medicine affecting alertness and reflexes.

Airplane passengers:
No problems expected.

Discontinuing:
Don't discontinue without consulting doctor. Dose may require gradual reduction if you have taken drug for a long time. Doses of other drugs may also require adjustment.

Others:
- Hot weather, heavy exercise and profuse sweat may reduce excretion and cause overdose.
- Blood sugar may rise in diabetics, requiring insulin adjustment.

INTERACTION WITH OTHER DRUGS

GENERIC NAME OR DRUG CLASS	COMBINED EFFECT
Anticonvulsants	Change in seizure frequency or severity.
Antidepressants	Increased sedative effect of both drugs.
Antihistamines	Increased sedative effect of both drugs.
Antihypertensives	Excessively low blood pressure.
Cimetidine	Excess sedation.
Disulfiram	Increased clorazepate effect.
MAO inhibitors	Convulsions, deep sedation, rage.
Narcotics	Increased sedative effect of both drugs.
Sedatives	Increased sedative effect of both drugs.
Sleep inducers	Increased sedative effect of both drugs.
Tranquilizers	Increased sedative effect of both drugs.

INTERACTION WITH OTHER SUBSTANCES

INTERACTS WITH	COMBINED EFFECT
Alcohol:	Heavy sedation. Avoid.
Beverages:	None expected.
Cocaine:	Decreased clorazepate effect.
Foods:	None expected.
Marijuana:	Heavy sedation. Avoid.
Tobacco:	Decreased clorazepate effect.

CLORTERMINE

BRAND NAMES

Voranil

GENERAL INFORMATION

Habit forming? Yes
Prescription needed? Yes
Available as generic? Yes
Drug class: Appetite suppressant

 USES

Suppresses appetite.

 DOSAGE & USAGE INFORMATION

How to take:
Extended-release tablets—Swallow each dose whole with liquid.

When to take:
10 to 14 hours before bedtime.

If you forget a dose:
Take as soon as you remember up to 2 hours late. If more than 2 hours, wait for next scheduled dose (don't double this dose).

What drug does:
Apparently stimulates brain's appetite-control center.

Time lapse before drug works:
Begins in 1 hour. Lasts 14 hours.

Don't take with:
- Non-prescription drugs without consulting doctor.
- See Interaction column and consult doctor.

 OVERDOSE

Symptoms:
Irritability, overactivity, trembling, insomnia, mood changes, rapid heartbeat, confusion, disorientation, hallucinations, convulsions, coma.

What to do:
- Dial 0 (operator) or 911 (emergency) for an ambulance or medical help. Then give first aid immediately.
- Additional emergency information on page 886.

POSSIBLE ADVERSE REACTIONS OR SIDE EFFECTS

SYMPTOMS	FREQUENCY	WHAT TO DO
Brain & nervous system:		
• Irritability, nervousness, insomnia.	Common	4
• Mood changes.	Rare	3
Skin:		
• Hair loss.	Rare	4
• Rash or hives.	Rare	3
Eyes:		
Blurred vision.	Infrequent	4
Ears, nose, throat:		
Unpleasant taste or dry mouth.	Infrequent	4
Digestive:		
Constipation or diarrhea, nausea, vomiting, cramps.	Infrequent	4
Heart & lungs:		
• Irregular or pounding heartbeat.	Infrequent	3
• Breathing difficulty.	Rare	3
Blood vessels, muscles, bones, joints, kidneys, liver, allergic, blood:	None expected.	
Genital, urinary:		
Urinary urgency and difficulty.	Infrequent	3
Others:		
• False sense of well-being.	Common	4
• Changes in sex drive.	Infrequent	4
• Sweat increase.	Infrequent	4

1-Life-threatening. Seek emergency treatment immediately.
2-Discontinue. Seek emergency treatment.
3-Discontinue. Call doctor right away.
4-Continue. Call doctor when convenient.

WARNINGS & PRECAUTIONS

Don't take if:
- You are allergic to any sympathomimetic or phenylpropanolamine.
- You have glaucoma.
- You have taken MAO inhibitors within 2 weeks.
- You plan to become pregnant within medication period.
- You have a history of drug abuse.

Before you start, consult your doctor:
- If you have high blood pressure or heart disease.
- If you have an overactive thyroid, nervous tension or "anxiety."
- If you have epilepsy.

Over age 60:
Adverse reactions and side effects may be more frequent and severe than in younger persons.

Pregnancy:
Safety not established. Avoid.

Breast-feeding:
No proven problems. Consult doctor.

Infants & children:
Don't give to children younger than 12.

Prolonged use:
Loses effectiveness. Avoid.

Skin & sunlight:
No problems expected.

Driving, piloting or hazardous work:
Don't drive or pilot aircraft until you learn how medicine affects you. Don't work around dangerous machinery. Don't climb ladders or work in high places. Danger increases if you drink alcohol or take medicine affecting alertness and reflexes, such as antihistamines, tranquilizers, sedatives, pain medicine, narcotics and mind-altering drugs.

Airplane passengers:
No problems expected.

Discontinuing:
Don't discontinue without consulting doctor. Dose may require gradual reduction if you have taken drug for a long time. Doses of other drugs may also require adjustment.

Others:
Don't increase dose.

INTERACTION WITH OTHER DRUGS

GENERIC NAME OR DRUG CLASS	COMBINED EFFECT
Appetite suppressants (other)	Dangerous overstimulation.
Caffeine	Increased stimulant effect of clortermine.
Guanethidine	Decreased guanethidine effect.
Hydralazine	Decreased hydralazine effect.
MAO inhibitors	Dangerous blood-pressure rise.
Methyldopa	Decreased methyldopa effect.
Phenothiazines	Decreased clortermine effect.
Rauwolfia alkaloids	Decreased effect of rauwolfia alkaloids.

INTERACTION WITH OTHER SUBSTANCES

INTERACTS WITH	COMBINED EFFECT
Alcohol: Beer, chianti wines, vermouth.	Dangerous blood-pressure rise.
Beverages: • Caffeine drinks • Drinks containing tyramine (see page 851).	Excessive stimulation. Blood-pressure rise.
Cocaine:	Excessive stimulation.
Foods: Foods containing tyramine (see page 851).	Blood-pressure rise.
Marijuana:	Frequent use—Irregular heartbeat.
Tobacco:	None expected.

CLOXACILLIN

BRAND NAMES

Bactopen
Cloxapen
Novocloxin
Tegopen

GENERAL INFORMATION

Habit forming? No
Prescription needed? Yes
Available as generic? Yes
Drug class: Antibiotic (penicillin)

 USES

Treatment of bacterial infections that are susceptible to cloxacillin.

 DOSAGE & USAGE INFORMATION

How to take:
- Tablets or capsules—Swallow with liquid on an empty stomach 1 hour before or 2 hours after eating.
- Liquid—Take with cold beverage. Liquid form is perishable and effective for only 7 days at room temperature. Effective for 14 days if stored in refrigerator. Don't freeze.

When to take:
Follow instructions on prescription label or side of package. Doses should be evenly spaced. For example, 4 times a day means every 6 hours.

If you forget a dose:
Take as soon as you remember. Continue regular schedule.

What drug does:
Destroys susceptible bacteria. Does not kill viruses.

Time lapse before drug works:
May be several days before medicine affects infection.

Don't take with:
See Interaction column and consult doctor.

 OVERDOSE

Symptoms:
Severe diarrhea, nausea or vomiting.

What to do:
Overdose unlikely to threaten life. If person takes much larger amount than prescribed, call doctor, poison-control center or hospital emergency room for instructions.

 POSSIBLE ADVERSE REACTIONS OR SIDE EFFECTS

SYMPTOMS	FREQUENCY	WHAT TO DO
Brain & nervous system:	None expected.	
Skin: Hives, rash, intense itch soon after a dose.	Rare	1
Eyes:	None expected.	
Ears, nose, throat: Dark or discolored tongue.	Common	5
Digestive: Mild nausea, vomiting, diarrhea.	Infrequent	4
Heart & lungs:	None expected.	
Blood vessels: Unexplained bleeding.	Rare	3
Muscles, bones, joints:	None expected.	
Genital, urinary:	None expected.	
Kidneys:	None expected.	
Liver:	None expected.	
Allergic: Life-threatening anaphylaxis may occur!	Rare	1 See Page 888.
Blood:	None expected.	
Others:	None expected.	

1- Life-threatening. Seek emergency treatment immediately.
2- Discontinue. Seek emergency treatment.
3- Discontinue. Call doctor right away.
4- Continue. Call doctor when convenient.
5- Continue. Tell doctor at next visit.
6- No action necessary.

WARNINGS & PRECAUTIONS

Don't take if:
You are allergic to cloxacillin, cephalosporin antibiotics, other penicillins or penicillamine. Life-threatening reaction may occur.

Before you start, consult your doctor:
If you are allergic to any substance or drug.

Over age 60:
You may have skin reactions, particularly around genitals and anus.

Pregnancy:
Studies inconclusive on harm to unborn child. Animal studies show fetal abnormalities. Decide with your doctor whether drug benefits justify risk to unborn child.

Breast-feeding:
Drug passes into milk. Child may become sensitive to penicillins and have allergic reactions to penicillin drugs. Avoid cloxacillin or discontinue nursing until you finish medicine. Consult doctor for advice on maintaining milk supply.

Infants & children:
No problems expected.

Prolonged use:
You may become more susceptible to infections caused by germs not responsive to cloxacillin.

Skin & sunlight:
No problems expected.

Driving, piloting or hazardous work:
Usually not dangerous. Most hazardous reactions likely to occur a few minutes after taking cloxacillin.

Airplane passengers:
No problems expected.

Discontinuing:
Don't discontinue without doctor's advice until you complete prescribed dose, even though symptoms diminish or disappear.

Others:
No problems expected.

INTERACTION WITH OTHER DRUGS

GENERIC NAME OR DRUG CLASS	COMBINED EFFECT
Chloramphenicol	Decreased effect of both drugs.
Erythromycins	Decreased effect of both drugs.
Paromomycin	Decreased effect of both drugs.
Tetracyclines	Decreased effect of both drugs.
Troleandomycin	Decreased effect of both drugs.

INTERACTION WITH OTHER SUBSTANCES

INTERACTS WITH	COMBINED EFFECT
Alcohol:	Occasional stomach irritation.
Beverages:	None expected.
Cocaine:	No proven problems.
Foods:	None expected.
Marijuana:	No proven problems.
Tobacco:	None expected.

CODEINE

BRAND NAMES

Acetaminophen w/Codeine (M)
Actifed-C Expectorant (M)
A.P.C. w/Codeine
  Phosphate Tablets (M)
Ascriptin w/Codeine (M)

Calcidrine Syrup (M)
Dimetane Expectorant-DC (M)
Empirin w/Codeine (M)
Fiorinal w/Codeine (M)
Novahistine Expectorant (M)

See complete brand names list, page 824.

GENERAL INFORMATION

Habit forming? Yes
Prescription needed? Yes
Available as generic? Yes
Drug class: Narcotic

 ## USES

- Relieves pain.
- Suppresses cough.

 ## DOSAGE & USAGE INFORMATION

How to take:
- Tablet or capsule—Swallow with liquid. If you can't swallow whole, crumble tablet or open capsule and take with liquid or food.
- Drops or liquid—Dilute dose in beverage before swallowing.

When to take:
When needed. No more often than every 4 hours.

If you forget a dose:
Take as soon as you remember. Wait 4 hours for next dose.

What drug does:
- Blocks pain messages to brain and spinal cord.
- Reduces sensitivity of brain's cough-control center.

Time lapse before drug works:
30 minutes.

Don't take with:
See Interaction column and consult doctor.

 ## OVERDOSE

Symptoms:
Deep sleep; slow breathing; slow pulse; flushed, warm skin; constricted pupils.

What to do:
- Dial 0 (operator) or 911 (emergency) for an ambulance or medical help. Then give first aid immediately.
- Additional emergency information on page 886.

 ## POSSIBLE ADVERSE REACTIONS OR SIDE EFFECTS

SYMPTOMS	FREQUENCY	WHAT TO DO
Brain & nervous system:		
• Depression	Rare	4
• Dizziness	Common	4
Skin:		
• Hives, rash, itch, face swelling.	Rare	3
• Flushed face.	Common	4
Eyes: Blurred vision.	Rare	4
Ears, nose, throat:	None expected.	
Digestive: Severe constipation, abdominal pain, vomiting.	Infrequent	3
Heart & lungs: Slow heartbeat, irregular breathing.	Rare	3
Blood vessels:	None expected.	
Muscles, bones, joints:	None expected.	
Genital, urinary: Difficult urination.	Common	4
Kidneys:	None expected.	
Liver:	None expected.	
Allergic:	None expected	
Blood:	None expected.	
Others: Unusual tiredness.	Common	4

1- Life-threatening. Seek emergency treatment immediately.
2- Discontinue. Seek emergency treatment.
3- Discontinue. Call doctor right away.
4- Continue. Call doctor when convenient.
5- Continue. Tell doctor at next visit.
6- No action necessary.

WARNINGS & PRECAUTIONS

Don't take if:
You are allergic to any narcotic.

Before you start, consult your doctor:
If you have impaired liver or kidney function.

Over age 60:
More likely to be drowsy, dizzy, unsteady or constipated. Avoid prolonged use.

Pregnancy:
Studies inconclusive on harm to unborn child. Animal studies show fetal abnormalities. Decide with your doctor whether drug benefits justify risk to unborn child. Abuse by pregnant woman will result in addicted newborn. Withdrawal can be life-threatening.

Breast-feeding:
Drug filters into milk. May depress infant.

Infants & children:
Not recommended.

Prolonged use:
Causes psychological and physical dependence.

Skin & sunlight:
May cause rash, itch or intensify sunburn in areas exposed to sun or sunlamp.

Driving, piloting or hazardous work:
Don't drive or pilot aircraft until you learn how medicine affects you. Don't work around dangerous machinery. Don't climb ladders or work in high places. Danger increases if you drink alcohol or take medicine affecting alertness and reflexes, such as antihistamines, tranquilizers, sedatives, pain medicine, other narcotics and mind-altering drugs.

Airplane passengers:
No proven problems.

Discontinuing:
May be unnecessary to finish medicine. Follow doctor's instructions.

Others:
No problems expected.

INTERACTION WITH OTHER DRUGS

GENERIC NAME OR DRUG CLASS	COMBINED EFFECT
Analgesics	Increased analgesic effect.
Antidepressants	Increased sedative effect.
Antihistamines	Increased sedative effect.
Mind-altering drugs	Increased sedative effect.
Narcotics (other)	Increased narcotic effect.
Phenothiazines	Increased phenothiazine effect.
Sedatives	Increased sedative effect.
Sleep inducers	Increased sedative effect.
Tranquilizers	Increased sedative effect.

INTERACTION WITH OTHER SUBSTANCES

INTERACTS WITH	COMBINED EFFECT
Alcohol:	Increases alcohol's intoxicating effect. Avoid.
Beverages:	None expected.
Cocaine:	Increased cocaine effect.
Foods:	None expected.
Marijuana:	Impairs physical and mental performance.
Tobacco:	None expected.

COLCHICINE

BRAND NAMES

ColBenemid (M)
Novocolchine

GENERAL INFORMATION

Habit forming? No
Prescription needed? Yes
Available as generic? Yes
Drug class: Antigout

 ## USES

Relieves joint pain, inflammation, swelling of gout.

 ## DOSAGE & USAGE INFORMATION

How to take:
- Tablet—Swallow with liquid or food to lessen stomach irritation.
- Granules—Dissolve in 3 oz. of fluid. Drink all fluid.

When to take:
As prescribed. Stop taking when pain stops or at first sign of digestive upset. Wait at least 3 days between treatments.

If you forget a dose:
Don't double next dose. Consult doctor.

What drug does:
Decreases acidity of joint tissues and prevents deposits of uric-acid crystals.

Time lapse before drug works:
12 to 48 hours.

Don't take with:
See Interaction column and consult doctor.

 ## OVERDOSE

Symptoms:
Bloody urine, diarrhea, muscle weakness, fever, shortness of breath, stupor, convulsions, coma.

What to do:
- Dial 0 (operator) or 911 (emergency) for an ambulance or medical help. Then give first aid immediately.
- Additional emergency information on page 886.

POSSIBLE ADVERSE REACTIONS OR SIDE EFFECTS

SYMPTOMS	FREQUENCY	WHAT TO DO
Brain & nervous system:	None expected.	
Skin: Rash, itch.	Infrequent	3
Eyes:	None expected.	
Ears, nose, throat:	None expected.	
Digestive: Diarrhea, nausea, vomiting, abdominal pain.	Common	3
Heart & lungs:	None expected.	
Blood vessels: Unusual bruising.	Infrequent	3
Muscles, bones, joints: Numbness, tingling, pain, weakness in hands or feet.	Infrequent	4
Genital, urinary: Bloody urine.	Infrequent	3
Kidneys:	None expected.	
Liver: Jaundice (yellow eyes and skin).	Rare	3
Allergic: Life-threatening anaphylaxis (with injections).	Rare	1 See page 888.
Blood:	None expected.	
Others: Unusual tiredness or weakness, fever.	Infrequent	4

1- Life-threatening. Seek emergency treatment immediately.
2- Discontinue. Seek emergency treatment.
3- Discontinue. Call doctor right away.
4- Continue. Call doctor when convenient.
5- Continue. Tell doctor at next visit.
6- No action necessary.

WARNINGS & PRECAUTIONS

Don't take if:
You are allergic to colchicine.

Before you start, consult your doctor:
- If you have had peptic ulcers or ulcerative colitis.
- If you have heart, liver or kidney disease.
- If you will have surgery within 2 months, including dental surgery, requiring general or spinal anesthesia.

Over age 60:
Adverse reactions and side effects may be more frequent and severe than in younger persons. Colchicine has a narrow margin of safety for people in this age group.

Pregnancy:
Risk to unborn child outweighs drug benefits. Don't use.

Breast-feeding:
No problems expected, but consult doctor.

Infants & children:
Not recommended.

Prolonged use:
- Permanent hair loss.
- Anemia. Request blood counts.
- Numbness or tingling in hands and feet.

Skin & sunlight:
No problems expected.

Driving, piloting or hazardous work:
Don't drive or pilot aircraft until you learn how medicine affects you. Don't work around dangerous machinery. Don't climb ladders or work in high places. Danger increases if you drink alcohol or take medicine affecting alertness and reflexes, such as antihistamines, tranquilizers, sedatives, pain medicine, narcotics and mind-altering drugs.

Airplane passengers:
Carry drug with you to treat gout attacks while traveling.

Discontinuing:
- May be unnecessary to finish medicine. Follow doctor's instructions.
- Stop taking if digestive upsets occur before symptoms are relieved.

Others:
- Limit each course of treatment to 8 mg. Don't exceed 3 mg. per 24 hours.
- Possible sperm damage. May cause birth defects if child conceived while father taking colchicine.

INTERACTION WITH OTHER DRUGS

GENERIC NAME OR DRUG CLASS	COMBINED EFFECT
Amphetamines	Increased amphetamine effect.
Anticoagulants	Decreased anticoagulant effect.
Antidepressants	Oversedation.
Antihistamines	Oversedation.
Antihypertensives	Decreased antihypertensive effect.
Appetite suppressants	Increased suppressant effect.
Mind-altering drugs	Oversedation.
Narcotics	Oversedation.
Sedatives	Oversedation.
Sleep inducers	Oversedation.
Tranquilizers	Oversedation.

INTERACTION WITH OTHER SUBSTANCES

INTERACTS WITH	COMBINED EFFECT
Alcohol:	No proven problems
Beverages: Herbal teas	Increased colchicine effect. Avoid.
Cocaine:	Overstimulation. Avoid.
Foods:	No proven problems.
Marijuana:	Decreased colchicine effect.
Tobacco:	No proven problems.

CONJUGATED ESTROGENS

BRAND NAMES

Premarin

GENERAL INFORMATION

Habit forming? No
Prescription needed? Yes
Available as generic? Yes
Drug class: Female sex hormone (estrogen)

 ## USES

- Treatment for symptoms of menopause and menstrual-cycle irregularity.
- Replacement for female hormone deficiency.
- Treatment for estrogen-deficiency osteoporosis (bone softening from calcium loss).
- Treatment for cancer of prostate and breast.

 ## DOSAGE & USAGE INFORMATION

How to take:
- Tablet—Swallow with liquid. If you can't swallow whole, crumble tablet and take with liquid or food.
- Vaginal cream—Use as directed on label.

When to take:
At the same time each day.

If you forget a dose:
Take as soon as you remember up to 12 hours late. If more than 12 hours, wait for next scheduled dose (don't double this dose).

What drug does:
Restores normal estrogen level in tissues.

Time lapse before drug works:
10 to 20 days.

Don't take with:
See Interaction column and consult doctor.

 ## OVERDOSE

Symptoms:
Nausea, vomiting, fluid retention, breast enlargement and discomfort, abnormal vaginal bleeding.

What to do:
Overdose unlikely to threaten life. If person takes much larger amount than prescribed, call doctor, poison-control center or hospital emergency room for instructions.

 ## POSSIBLE ADVERSE REACTIONS OR SIDE EFFECTS

SYMPTOMS	FREQUENCY	WHAT TO DO
Brain & nervous system: Depression, dizziness, irritability.	Infrequent	4
Skin:		
• Rash	Infrequent	3
• Brown blotches.	Infrequent	5
• Hair loss.	Infrequent	5
Eyes, ears, nose, throat, heart & lungs, muscles, bones, joints, kidneys, allergic, blood:	None expected.	
Digestive:		
• Stomach or side pain.	Infrequent	3
• Stomach cramps.	Common	3
• Appetite loss.	Common	4
• Nausea, diarrhea.	Common	5
• Vomiting	Infrequent	4
Blood vessels: Swollen ankles, feet.	Common	5
Genital, urinary: Vaginal discharge or bleeding.	Infrequent	5
Liver: Jaundice (yellow skin and eyes).	Rare	3
Others:		
• Breast lumps.	Infrequent	4
• Swollen, tender breasts.	Common	5
• Changes in sex drive.	Infrequent	5

1-Life-threatening. Seek emergency treatment immediately.
2-Discontinue. Seek emergency treatment.
3-Discontinue. Call doctor right away.
4-Continue. Call doctor when convenient.
5-Continue. Tell doctor at next visit.

WARNINGS & PRECAUTIONS

Don't take if:
- You are allergic to any estrogen-containing drugs.
- You have impaired liver function.
- You have had blood clots, stroke or heart attack.
- You have unexplained vaginal bleeding.

Before you start, consult your doctor:
- If you have had cancer of breast or reproductive organs, fibrocystic breast disease, fibroid tumors of the uterus or endometriosis.
- If you have had migraine headaches, epilepsy or porphyria.
- If you have diabetes, high blood pressure, asthma, congestive heart failure, kidney disease or gallstones.
- If you plan to become pregnant within 3 months.

Over age 60:
Controversial. You and your doctor must decide if drug risks outweigh benefits.

Pregnancy:
Risk to unborn child outweighs drug benefits. Don't use.

Breast-feeding:
Drug filters into milk. May harm child. Avoid.

Infants & children:
Not recommended.

Prolonged use:
Increased growth of fibroid tumors of uterus. Possible association with cancer of uterus.

Skin & sunlight:
May cause rash or intensify sunburn in areas exposed to sun or sunlamp.

Driving, piloting or hazardous work:
No problems expected.

Airplane passengers:
No problems expected.

Discontinuing:
You may need to discontinue estrogen periodically. Consult your doctor.

Others:
In rare instances, may cause blood clot in lung, brain or leg. Symptoms are *sudden* severe headache, coordination loss, vision change, chest pain, breathing difficulty, slurred speech, pain in legs or groin. Seek emergency treatment immediately.

INTERACTION WITH OTHER DRUGS

GENERIC NAME OR DRUG CLASS	COMBINED EFFECT
Anticoagulants (oral)	Decreased anticoagulant effect.
Anticonvulsants (hydantoin)	Increased seizures.
Antidiabetics (oral)	Unpredictable increase or decrease in blood sugar.
Clofibrate	Decreased clofibrate effect.
Carbamazepine	Increased seizures.
Meprobamate	Increased effect of conjugated estrogens.
Phenobarbital	Decreased effect of conjugated estrogens.
Primidone	Decreased effect of conjugated estrogens.
Rifampin	Decreased effect of conjugated estrogens.
Thyroid hormones	Decreased thyroid effect.

INTERACTION WITH OTHER SUBSTANCES

INTERACTS WITH	COMBINED EFFECT
Alcohol:	None expected.
Beverages:	None expected.
Cocaine:	No proven problems.
Foods:	None expected.
Marijuana:	Possible menstrual irregularities and bleeding between periods.
Tobacco:	Increased risk of blood clots leading to stroke or heart attack.

CONTRACEPTIVES (ORAL)

BRAND NAMES

Anoryol (M)	Micronor (M)	Nor-Q.D. (M)
Brevicon (M)	Min-Ovral (M)	Ortho-Novum (M)
Demulen (M)	Modacon (M)	Ovcon (M)
Enovid (M)	Modicon (M)	Ovral (M)
Loestrin (M)	Norlestrin (M)	Ovrette (M)
Lo-Ovral (M)	Norlinyl	Ovulen (M)

GENERAL INFORMATION

Habit forming? No
Prescription needed? Yes
Available as generic? Yes
Drug class: Female sex hormone, contraceptive

USES

- Prevents pregnancy.
- Regulates menstrual periods.

DOSAGE & USAGE INFORMATION

How to take:
Tablet or capsule—Swallow with liquid or food to lessen stomach irritation.

When to take:
At same time each day according to prescribed instructions, usually for 21 days of 28-day cycle.

If you forget a dose:
Call doctor's office for advice about additional protection against pregnancy.

What drug does:
- Alters mucus at cervix entrance to prevent sperm entry.
- Alters uterus lining to resist implantation of fertilized egg.
- Creates same chemical atmosphere in blood that exists during pregnancy, suppressing pituitary hormones which stimulate ovulation.

Time lapse before drug works:
10 days or more to provide contraception.

Don't take with:
- Tobacco
- See Interaction column and consult doctor.

OVERDOSE

Symptoms:
Drowsiness

What to do:
Overdose unlikely to threaten life. If person takes much larger amount than prescribed, call doctor, poison-control center or hospital emergency room for instructions.

POSSIBLE ADVERSE REACTIONS OR SIDE EFFECTS

SYMPTOMS	FREQUENCY	WHAT TO DO
Brain & nervous system:		
• Headache, depression.	Infrequent	3
• Stroke	Rare	1
Skin:		
• Brown blotches.	Common	4
• Rash, hives, itch.	Rare	3
Eyes:		
Blue tinge to objects, lights.	Infrequent	4
Ears, nose, throat, kidneys, allergic:	None expected.	
Digestive:		
Appetite change, nausea, bloating, vomiting, pain.	Infrequent	4
Heart & lungs:		
Chest pain.	Rare	1
Blood vessels:		
Blood clots—Pain, swelling in leg.	Infrequent	3
Muscles, bones, joints:		
Muscle, joint pain.	Infrequent	3
Genital, urinary:		
Vaginal discharge, itch.	Common	4
Liver:		
Jaundice (yellow skin and eyes).	Rare	3
Blood:		
Clotting tendency.	Rare	2
Others:		
• Changed sex drive.	Infrequent	4
• Fluid retention.	Common	4

1- Life-threatening. Seek emergency treatment immediately.
2- Discontinue. Seek emergency treatment.
3- Discontinue. Call doctor right away.
4- Continue. Call doctor when convenient.

CONTRACEPTIVES (ORAL)

WARNINGS & PRECAUTIONS

Don't take if:
- You are allergic to any female hormone.
- You have had heart disease, blood clots or stroke.
- You have liver disease.
- You have cancer of breast, uterus or ovaries.
- You have unexplained vaginal bleeding.

Before you start, consult your doctor:
- If you have fibrocystic disease of breast.
- If you have migraine headaches.
- If you have fibroid tumors of uterus.
- If you have epilepsy.
- If you have asthma.
- If you have high blood pressure.
- If you will have surgery within 2 months, including dental surgery, requiring general or spinal anesthesia.
- If you have endometriosis.
- If you have diabetes.
- If you have sickle-cell anemia.
- If you smoke cigarettes.

Over age 60:
Not used.

Pregnancy:
May harm child. Discontinue at first sign of pregnancy.

Breast-feeding:
Drug passes into milk. Avoid drug or discontinue nursing.

Infants & children:
Not recommended.

Prolonged use:
- Gallstones
- Gradual blood-pressure rise.
- Possible difficulty becoming pregnant after discontinuing.

Skin & sunlight:
May cause rash or intensify sunburn in areas exposed to sun or sunlamp.

Driving, piloting or hazardous work:
No problems expected.

Airplane passengers:
No problems expected.

Discontinuing:
Don't become pregnant for 6 months after discontinuing.

Others:
Failure to take oral contraceptives for 1 day may cancel pregnancy protection. If you forget a dose, use other contraceptive measures and call doctor for instructions on re-starting oral contraceptive.

INTERACTION WITH OTHER DRUGS

GENERIC NAME OR DRUG CLASS	COMBINED EFFECT
Ampicillin	Decreased contraceptive effect.
Anticoagulants	Decreased anticoagulant effect.
Anticonvulsants (hydantoin)	Decreased contraceptive effect.
Antidiabetics	Decreased antidiabetic effect.
Antihistamines	Decreased contraceptive effect.
Antiinflammatory drugs (non-steroid)	Decreased contraceptive effect.
Barbiturates	Decreased contraceptive effect.
Chloramphenicol	Decreased contraceptive effect.
Clofibrate	Decreased clofibrate effect.
Guanethidine	Decreased guanethidine effect.
Meperidine	Increased meperidine effect.
Meprobamate	Decreased contraceptive effect.
Mineral oil	Decreased contraceptive effect.

Additional interactions on page 835.

INTERACTION WITH OTHER SUBSTANCES

INTERACTS WITH	COMBINED EFFECT
Alcohol:	No proven problems.
Beverages:	No proven problems.
Cocaine:	No proven problems.
Foods: Salt	Increased edema (fluid retention).
Marijuana:	Increased bleeding between periods. Avoid.
Tobacco:	Possible heart attack, blood clots and stroke.

CORTISONE

BRAND NAMES

Cortone

GENERAL INFORMATION

Habit forming? No
Prescription needed? Yes
Available as generic? Yes
Drug class: Cortisone drug (adrenal corticosteroid)

 USES

- Reduces inflammation caused by many different medical problems.
- Treatment for some allergic diseases, blood disorders, kidney diseases, asthma and emphysema.
- Replaces corticosteroid deficiencies.

 DOSAGE & USAGE INFORMATION

How to take:
Tablet—Swallow with liquid or food to lessen stomach irritation. If you can't swallow whole, crumble tablet and take with liquid or food.

When to take:
At the same times each day. Take once-a-day or once-every-other-day doses in mornings.

If you forget a dose:
- Several-doses-per-day prescription—Take as soon as you remember up to 2 hours late. If more than 2 hours, wait for next scheduled dose (don't double this dose).
- Once-a-day dose or less—Wait for next dose. Double this dose.

What drug does:
Decreases inflammatory responses.

Time lapse before drug works:
2 to 4 days.

Don't take with:
See Interaction column and consult doctor.

 OVERDOSE

Symptoms:
Headache, convulsions, heart failure.

What to do:
- Dial 0 (operator) or 911 (emergency) for an ambulance or medical help. Then give first aid immediately.
- Additional emergency information on page 886.

POSSIBLE ADVERSE REACTIONS OR SIDE EFFECTS

SYMPTOMS	FREQUENCY	WHAT TO DO
Brain & nervous system:		
Mood changes, insomnia, restlessness.	Infrequent	4
Skin:		
• Acne	Common	4
• Rash	Rare	3
• Poor wound healing.	Common	4
Eyes:		
Blurred vision, halos around lights.	Infrequent	3
Ears, nose, throat:		
• Sore throat, fever.	Infrequent	3
• Thirst	Common	4
Digestive:		
• Indigestion, nausea, vomiting.	Common	4
• Bloody or black, tarry stool.	Infrequent	2
Heart & lungs:		
Irregular heartbeat.	Rare	2
Blood vessels, kidneys, liver, allergic, blood:	None expected.	
Muscles, bones, joints:		
Muscle cramps, swollen legs, feet.	Infrequent	3
Genital, urinary:		
Frequent urination.	Infrequent	4
Others:		
• Weight gain, round face.	Infrequent	4
• Fatigue, weakness.	Infrequent	4
• TB recurrence.	Infrequent	4
• Irregular menstrual periods.	Infrequent	4

1- Life-threatening. Seek emergency treatment immediately.
2- Discontinue. Seek emergency treatment.
3- Discontinue. Call doctor right away.
4- Continue. Call doctor when convenient.

CORTISONE

WARNINGS & PRECAUTIONS

Don't take if:
- You are allergic to any cortisone drug.
- You have tuberculosis or fungus infection.
- You have herpes infection of eyes, lips or genitals.

Before you start, consult your doctor:
- If you have had tuberculosis.
- If you have congestive heart failure.
- If you have diabetes.
- If you have peptic ulcer.
- If you have glaucoma.
- If you have underactive thyroid.
- If you have high blood pressure.
- If you have myasthenia gravis.
- If you have blood clots in legs or lungs.

Over age 60:
Adverse reactions and side effects may be more frequent and severe than in younger persons. Likely to aggravate edema, diabetes or ulcers. Likely to cause cataracts and osteoporosis (softening of the bones).

Pregnancy:
Risk to unborn child outweighs drug benefits. Don't use.

Breast-feeding:
Drug passes into milk. Avoid drug or discontinue nursing until you finish medicine. Consult doctor for advice on maintaining milk supply.

Infants & children:
Use only under medical supervision.

Prolonged use:
- Retards growth in children.
- Possible glaucoma, cataracts, diabetes, fragile bones and thin skin.
- Functional dependence.

Skin & sunlight:
No problems expected.

Driving, piloting or hazardous work:
No problems expected.

Airplane passengers:
No problems expected.

Discontinuing:
- Don't discontinue without doctor's advice until you complete prescribed dose, even though symptoms diminish or disappear.
- Drug affects your response to surgery, illness, injury or stress for 2 years after discontinuing. Tell about drug to anyone who takes medical care of you within 2 years.

Others:
Avoid immunizations if possible.

INTERACTION WITH OTHER DRUGS

GENERIC NAME OR DRUG CLASS	COMBINED EFFECT
Amphoterecin B	Potassium depletion.
Anticholinergics	Possible glaucoma.
Anticoagulants (oral)	Decreased anticoagulant effect.
Anticonvulsants (hydantoin)	Decreased cortisone effect.
Antidiabetics (oral)	Decreased antidiabetic effect.
Antihistamines	Decreased cortisone effect.
Aspirin	Increased cortisone effect.
Barbiturates	Decreased cortisone effect. Oversedation.
Beta-adrenergic blockers	Decreased cortisone effect.
Chloral hydrate	Decreased cortisone effect.
Chlorthalidone	Potassium depletion.
Cholinergics	Decreased cholinergic effect.
Contraceptives (oral)	Increased cortisone effect.
Digitalis preparations	Dangerous potassium depletion. Possible digitalis toxicity.
Diuretics (thiazide)	Potassium depletion.

Additional interactions on page 835.

INTERACTION WITH OTHER SUBSTANCES

INTERACTS WITH	COMBINED EFFECT
Alcohol:	Risk of stomach ulcers.
Beverages:	No proven problems.
Cocaine:	Overstimulation. Avoid.
Foods:	No proven problems.
Marijuana:	Decreased immunity.
Tobacco:	Increased cortisone effect. Possible toxicity.

CROMOLYN

BRAND NAMES

Intal
Opticrom
Rynacrom

GENERAL INFORMATION

Habit forming? No
Prescription needed? Yes
Available as generic? No
Drug class: Antiasthmatic

 USES

Prevents asthma attacks. Will not stop an active asthma attack.

 DOSAGE & USAGE INFORMATION

How to take:
Inhaler—Follow instructions enclosed with inhaler. Don't swallow cartridges for inhaler. Gargle and rinse mouth after inhalations.

When to take:
At the same times each day. If you also use a bronchodilator inhaler, use the bronchodilator before the cromolyn.

If you forget a dose:
Take as soon as you remember up to 2 hours late. If more than 2 hours, wait for next scheduled dose (don't double this dose).

What drug does:
Prevents constriction of bronchial tubes by blocking histamine release from mast cells. Has no direct bronchodilator, antihistamine or antiinflammatory action.

Time lapse before drug works:
4 weeks.

Don't take with:
See Interaction column and consult doctor.

 OVERDOSE

Symptoms:
Increased side effects and adverse reactions listed.

What to do:
Overdose unlikely to threaten life. If person inhales much larger amount than prescribed, call doctor, poison-control center or hospital emergency room for instructions.

POSSIBLE ADVERSE REACTIONS OR SIDE EFFECTS

SYMPTOMS	FREQUENCY	WHAT TO DO
Brain & nervous system: Drowsiness, dizziness, headache.	Infrequent	4
Skin: Rash, hives.	Infrequent	3
Eyes: Watering	Infrequent	4
Ears, nose, throat:		
• Swallowing difficulty.	Infrequent	3
• Hoarseness	Common	4
• Stuffy nose, throat irritation.	Infrequent	4
• Nosebleed	Rare	4
Digestive: Nausea, vomiting.	Infrequent	3
Heart & lungs:		
• Increased wheezing.	Infrequent	3
• Cough	Common	4
Blood vessels, kidneys, liver, blood:	None expected.	
Muscles, bones, joints:		
• Joint pain or swelling.	Infrequent	3
• Muscle pain, weakness.	Infrequent	3
Genital, urinary: Difficult or painful urination.	Infrequent	3
Allergic: Life-threatening anaphylaxis may occur.	Rare	1 See page 888.

1- Life-threatening. Seek emergency treatment immediately.
2- Discontinue. Seek emergency treatment.
3- Discontinue. Call doctor right away.
4- Continue. Call doctor when convenient.

CROMOLYN

WARNINGS & PRECAUTIONS

Don't take if:
You are allergic to cromolyn, lactose, milk or milk products.

Before you start, consult your doctor:
- If you plan to become pregnant within medication period.
- If you have kidney or liver disease.

Over age 60:
Adverse reactions and side effects may be more frequent and severe than in younger persons.

Pregnancy:
Risk to unborn child outweighs drug benefits. Don't use.

Breast-feeding:
Drug passes into milk. Avoid drug or discontinue nursing.

Infants & children:
Use only under medical supervision.

Prolonged use:
No problems expected.

Skin & sunlight:
No problems expected.

Driving, piloting or hazardous work:
No problems expected.

Airplane passengers:
No problems expected.

Discontinuing:
No problems expected.

Others:
- Inhaler must be cleaned and work well for drug to be effective.
- This treatment does not stop an acute asthma attack. It may aggravate it.

INTERACTION WITH OTHER DRUGS

GENERIC NAME OR DRUG CLASS	COMBINED EFFECT
Cortisone drugs	Increased cortisone effect in treating asthma. Cortisone dose may be decreased.

INTERACTION WITH OTHER SUBSTANCES

INTERACTS WITH	COMBINED EFFECT
Alcohol:	None expected.
Beverages:	None expected.
Cocaine:	None expected.
Foods:	None expected.
Marijuana:	None expected.
Tobacco:	None expected, but tobacco smoke aggravates asthma. Avoid.

CYCLACILLIN

BRAND NAMES

Cyclapen-W

GENERAL INFORMATION

Habit forming? No
Prescription needed? Yes
Available as generic? Yes
Drug class: Antibiotic (penicillin)

USES

Treatment of bacterial infections that are susceptible to cyclacillin.

DOSAGE & USAGE INFORMATION

How to take:
- Tablets or capsules—Swallow with liquid on an empty stomach 1 hour before or 2 hours after eating.
- Liquid—Take with cold beverage. Liquid form is perishable and effective for only 7 days at room temperature. Effective for 14 days if stored in refrigerator. Don't freeze.

When to take:
Follow instructions on prescription label or side of package. Doses should be evenly spaced. For example, 4 times a day means every 6 hours.

If you forget a dose:
Take as soon as you remember. Continue regular schedule.

What drug does:
Destroys susceptible bacteria. Does not kill viruses.

Time lapse before drug works:
May be several days before medicine affects infection.

Don't take with:
See Interaction column and consult doctor.

OVERDOSE

Symptoms:
Severe diarrhea, nausea or vomiting.

What to do:
Overdose unlikely to threaten life. If person takes much larger amount than prescribed, call doctor, poison-control center or hospital emergency room for instructions.

POSSIBLE ADVERSE REACTIONS OR SIDE EFFECTS

SYMPTOMS	FREQUENCY	WHAT TO DO
Brain & nervous system:	None expected.	
Skin: Hives, rash, intense itch soon after a dose.	Rare	1
Eyes:	None expected.	
Ears, nose, throat: Dark or discolored tongue.	Common	5
Digestive: Mild nausea, vomiting, diarrhea.	Infrequent	4
Heart & lungs:	None expected.	
Blood vessels: Unexplained bleeding.	Rare	3
Muscles, bones, joints:	None expected.	
Genital, urinary:	None expected.	
Kidneys:	None expected.	
Liver:	None expected.	
Allergic: Life-threatening anaphylaxis may occur!	Rare	1 See page 888.
Blood:	None expected.	
Others:	None expected.	

1- Life-threatening. Seek emergency treatment immediately.
2- Discontinue. Seek emergency treatment.
3- Discontinue. Call doctor right away.
4- Continue. Call doctor when convenient.
5- Continue. Tell doctor at next visit.
6- No action necessary.

WARNINGS & PRECAUTIONS

Don't take if:
Your are allergic to cyclacillin, cephalosporin antibiotics, other penicillins or penicillamine. Life-threatening reaction may occur.

Before you start, consult your doctor:
If you are allergic to any substance or drug.

Over age 60:
You may have skin reactions, particularly around genitals and anus.

Pregnancy:
Studies inconclusive on harm to unborn child. Animal studies show fetal abnormalities. Decide with your doctor whether drug benefits justify risk to unborn child.

Breast-feeding:
Drug passes into milk. Child may become sensitive to penicillins and have allergic reactions to penicillin drugs. Avoid cyclacillin or discontinue nursing until you finish medicine. Consult doctor for advice on maintaining milk supply.

Infants & children:
No problems expected.

Prolonged use:
You may become more susceptible to infections caused by germs not responsive to cyclacillin.

Skin & sunlight:
No problems expected.

Driving, piloting or hazardous work:
Usually not dangerous. Most hazardous reactions likely to occur a few minutes after taking cyclacillin.

Airplane passengers:
No problems expected.

Discontinuing:
Don't discontinue without doctor's advice until you complete prescribed dose, even though symptoms diminish or disappear.

Others:
No problems expected.

INTERACTION WITH OTHER DRUGS

GENERIC NAME OR DRUG CLASS	COMBINED EFFECT
Chloramphenicol	Decreased effect of both drugs.
Erythromycins	Decreased effect of both drugs.
Paromomycin	Decreased effect of both drugs.
Tetracyclines	Decreased effect of both drugs.
Troleandomycin	Decreased effect of both drugs.

INTERACTION WITH OTHER SUBSTANCES

INTERACTS WITH	COMBINED EFFECT
Alcohol:	Occasional stomach irritation.
Beverages:	None expected.
Cocaine:	No proven problems.
Foods:	Decreased effect of cyclacillin.
Marijuana:	No proven problems.
Tobacco:	None expected

CYCLANDELATE

BRAND NAMES

Cyclospasmol
Cyraso-400

GENERAL INFORMATION

Habit forming? No
Prescription needed? U.S.: Yes
Canada: No
Available as generic? Yes
Drug class: Vasodilator

 ## USES

Improves poor blood flow to brain and extremities.

 ## DOSAGE & USAGE INFORMATION

How to take:
Tablet or capsule—Swallow with liquid. If you can't swallow whole, crumble tablet or open capsule and take with liquid or food.

When to take:
At the same time each day.

If you forget a dose:
Take as soon as you remember up to 2 hours late. If more than 2 hours, wait for next scheduled dose (don't double this dose).

What drug does:
Increases blood flow by relaxing and expanding blood-vessel walls.

Time lapse before drug works:
3 weeks.

Don't take with:
See Interaction column and consult doctor.

 ## OVERDOSE

Symptoms:
Severe headache, dizziness; nausea, vomiting; flushed, hot face.

What to do:
Overdose unlikely to threaten life. If person takes much larger amount than prescribed, call doctor, poison-control center or hospital emergency room for instructions.

 ## POSSIBLE ADVERSE REACTIONS OR SIDE EFFECTS

SYMPTOMS	FREQUENCY	WHAT TO DO
Brain & nervous system: Dizziness, headache, weakness.	Infrequent	4
Skin: Flushed face.	Infrequent	4
Eyes:	None expected.	
Ears, nose, throat:	None expected.	
Digestive: Belching, heartburn, nausea or stomach pain.	Infrequent	5
Heart & lungs: Rapid heartbeat.	Infrequent	3
Blood vessels:	None expected.	
Muscles, bones, joints: Tingling in face, fingers or toes.	Infrequent	4
Genital, urinary:	None expected.	
Kidneys:	None expected.	
Liver:	None expected.	
Allergic:	None expected.	
Blood:	None expected.	
Others: Unusual sweating.	Infrequent	4

1-Life-threatening. Seek emergency treatment immediately.
2-Discontinue. Seek emergency treatment.
3-Discontinue. Call doctor right away.
4-Continue. Call doctor when convenient.
5-Continue. Tell doctor at next visit.
6-No action necessary.

CYCLANDELATE

WARNINGS & PRECAUTIONS

Don't take if:
You have had allergic reaction to cyclandelate.

Before you start, consult your doctor:
● If you have glaucoma.
● If you have had heart attack or stroke.

Over age 60:
Adverse reactions and side effects may be more frequent and severe than in younger persons.

Pregnancy:
No proven harm to unborn child. Avoid if possible.

Breast-feeding:
No proven problems. Consult doctor.

Infants & children:
Not recommended.

Prolonged use:
No problems expected.

Skin & sunlight:
No problems expected.

Driving, piloting or hazardous work:
Avoid if you feel dizzy or weak. Otherwise, no problems expected.

Airplane passengers:
No problems expected.

Discontinuing:
Don't discontinue without doctor's advice until you complete prescribed dose, even though symptoms diminish or disappear.

Others:
Response to drug varies. If your symptoms don't improve after 3 weeks of use, consult doctor.

INTERACTION WITH OTHER DRUGS

GENERIC NAME OR DRUG CLASS	COMBINED EFFECT
None	

INTERACTION WITH OTHER SUBSTANCES

INTERACTS WITH	COMBINED EFFECT
Alcohol:	None expected.
Beverages:	None expected.
Cocaine:	Decreased cyclandelate effect. Avoid.
Foods:	None expected.
Marijuana:	None expected.
Tobacco:	May decrease cyclandelate effect.

CYCLIZINE

BRAND NAMES

Marezine

USES

Prevents motion sickness.

DOSAGE & USAGE INFORMATION

How to take:
Tablet—Swallow with liquid or food to lessen stomach irritation. If you can't swallow whole, crumble tablet and chew or take with liquid or food.

When to take:
30 minutes to 1 hour before traveling.

If you forget a dose:
Take as soon as you remember. Wait 4 hours for next dose.

What drug does:
Reduces sensitivity of nerve endings in inner ear, blocking messages to brain's vomiting center.

Time lapse before drug works:
30 to 60 minutes.

Don't take with:
See Interaction column and consult doctor.

OVERDOSE

Symptoms:
Drowsiness, confusion, incoordination, stupor, coma, weak pulse, shallow breathing.

What to do:
- Dial 0 (operator) or 911 (emergency) for an ambulance or medical help. Then give first aid immediately.
- Additional emergency information on page 886.

GENERAL INFORMATION

Habit forming? No
Prescription needed? U.S.: No
Canada: Yes
Available as generic? No
Drug class: Antihistamine, antiemetic

POSSIBLE ADVERSE REACTIONS OR SIDE EFFECTS

SYMPTOMS	FREQUENCY	WHAT TO DO
Brain & nervous system:		
● Drowsiness	Common	5
● Headache	Infrequent	4
● Restlessness, excitement, insomnia.	Rare	4
Skin:		
Rash or hives.	Rare	3
Eyes:		
Blurred vision.	Rare	4
Ears, nose, throat:		
Dry mouth, nose, throat.	Infrequent	5
Digestive:		
● Appetite loss, nausea.	Rare	5
● Diarrhea or constipation.	Infrequent	4
Heart & lungs:		
Fast heartbeat.	Infrequent	4
Blood vessels:	None expected.	
Muscles, bones, joints:	None expected.	
Genital, urinary: Urinary frequency, difficult urination.	Rare	4
Kidneys:	None expected.	
Liver: Jaundice (yellow eyes and skin).	Rare	3
Allergic:	None expected.	
Blood:	None expected.	
Others:	None expected.	

1-Life-threatening. Seek emergency treatment immediately.
2-Discontinue. Seek emergency treatment.
3-Discontinue. Call doctor right away.
4-Continue. Call doctor when convenient.
5-Continue. Tell doctor at next visit.

WARNINGS & PRECAUTIONS

Don't take if:
- You are allergic to meclizine, buclizine or cyclizine.
- You have taken MAO inhibitors in the past 2 weeks.

Before you start, consult your doctor:
- If you have glaucoma.
- If you have prostate enlargement.
- If you have reacted badly to any antihistamine.

Over age 60:
Adverse reactions and side effects may be more frequent and severe than in younger persons, especially impaired urination from enlarged prostate gland.

Pregnancy:
Studies inconclusive on harm to unborn child. Animal studies show fetal abnormalities. Decide with your doctor whether drug benefits justify risk to unborn child.

Breast-feeding:
Drug passes into milk. Avoid drug or discontinue nursing until you finish medicine. Consult doctor for advice on maintaining milk supply.

Infants & children:
No problems expected.

Prolonged use:
No problems expected.

Skin & sunlight:
No problems expected.

Driving, piloting or hazardous work:
Don't fly aircraft. Don't drive until you learn how medicine affects you. Don't work around dangerous machinery. Don't climb ladders or work in high places. Danger increases if you drink alcohol or take medicine affecting alertness and reflexes, such as antihistamines, tranquilizers, sedatives, pain medicine, narcotics and mind-altering drugs.

Airplane passengers:
Take 30 minutes before takeoff and every 4 hours while in the air.

Discontinuing:
No problems expected.

Others:
No problems expected.

INTERACTION WITH OTHER DRUGS

GENERIC NAME OR DRUG CLASS	COMBINED EFFECT
Amphetamines	May decrease drowsiness caused by cyclizine.
Anticholinergics	Increased effect of both drugs.
Antidepressants (tricyclic)	Increased effect of both drugs.
MAO inhibitors	Increased cyclizine effect.
Narcotics	Increased effect of both drugs.
Pain relievers	Increased effect of both drugs.
Sedatives	Increased effect of both drugs.
Sleep inducers	Increased effect of both drugs.
Tranquilizers	Increased effect of both drugs.

INTERACTION WITH OTHER SUBSTANCES

INTERACTS WITH	COMBINED EFFECT
Alcohol:	Increased sedation. Avoid.
Beverages: Caffeine drinks	May decrease drowsiness.
Cocaine:	None expected.
Foods:	None expected.
Marijuana:	Increased drowsiness, dry mouth.
Tobacco:	None expected.

CYCLOBENZAPRINE

BRAND NAMES

Flexeril

GENERAL INFORMATION

Habit forming? No
Prescription needed? Yes
Available as generic? No
Drug class: Muscle relaxant (skeletal)

USES

Treatment for pain and limited motion caused by spasms in voluntary muscles.

DOSAGE & USAGE INFORMATION

How to take:
Tablet or capsule—Swallow with liquid.

When to take:
At the same time each day or according to label instructions.

If you forget a dose:
Take as soon as you remember. Wait 4 hours for next dose.

What drug does:
Blocks body's pain messages to brain. May also sedate.

Time lapse before drug works:
30 to 60 minutes.

Don't take with:
- Non-prescription drugs without consulting doctor.
- See Interaction column and consult doctor.

OVERDOSE

Symptoms:
Drowsiness, confusion, difficulty concentrating, visual problems, vomiting, blood-pressure drop, low body temperature, weak and rapid pulse, convulsions, coma.

What to do:
- Dial 0 (operator) or 911 (emergency) for an ambulance or medical help. Then give first aid immediately.
- If patient is unconscious and not breathing, give mouth-to-mouth breathing. If there is no heartbeat, use cardiac massage and mouth-to-mouth breathing (CPR). Don't try to make patient vomit. If you can't get help quickly, take patient to nearest emergency facility.
- Additional emergency information on page 886.

POSSIBLE ADVERSE REACTIONS OR SIDE EFFECTS

SYMPTOMS	FREQUENCY	WHAT TO DO
Brain & nervous system:		
• Drowsiness, dizziness.	Common	4
• Unsteadiness, confusion, depression, hallucinations.	Rare	3
Skin:		
Rash, itch, swelling.	Rare	3
Eyes:		
Blurred vision.	Infrequent	3
Ears, nose, throat:		
• Dry mouth.	Common	4
• Bad taste in mouth.	Infrequent	4
Digestive:	None expected.	
Heart & lungs:		
• Breathing difficulty.	Rare	3
• Fast heartbeat.	Infrequent	3
Blood vessels:	None expected.	
Muscles, bones, joints:	None expected.	
Genital, urinary:		
Difficulty urinating.	Rare	4
Kidneys:	None expected.	
Liver:	None expected.	
Allergic:	None expected.	
Blood:	None expected.	
Others:		
Insomnia, numbness in extremities.	Infrequent	4

1- Life-threatening. Seek emergency treatment immediately.
2- Discontinue. Seek emergency treatment.
3- Discontinue. Call doctor right away.
4- Continue. Call doctor when convenient.
5- Continue. Tell doctor at next visit.
6- No action necessary.

CYCLOBENZAPRINE

WARNINGS & PRECAUTIONS

Don't take if:
- You are allergic to any skeletal-muscle relaxant.
- You have taken MAO inhibitors in last 2 weeks.
- You have had a heart attack within 6 weeks, or suffer from congestive heart failure.
- You have overactive thyroid.

Before you start, consult your doctor:
- If you have a heart problem.
- If you have reacted to tricyclic antidepressants.
- If you have glaucoma.
- If you have a prostate condition and urination difficulty.
- If you intend to pilot aircraft.

Over age 60:
Adverse reactions and side effects may be more frequent and severe than in younger persons. Avoid extremes of heat and cold.

Pregnancy:
Risk to unborn child outweighs drug benefits. Don't use.

Breast-feeding:
Drug passes into milk. Avoid drug or discontinue nursing until you finish medicine. Consult doctor for advice on maintaining milk supply.

Infants & children:
Don't use for children younger than 15.

Prolonged use:
No problems expected.

Skin & sunlight:
May cause rash or intensify sunburn in areas exposed to sun or sunlamp.

Driving, piloting or hazardous work:
Don't drive or pilot aircraft until you learn how medicine affects you. Don't work around dangerous machinery. Don't climb ladders or work in high places. Danger increases if you drink alcohol or take medicine affecting alertness and reflexes.

Airplane passengers:
Possible side effects may make flying difficult. Consult your doctor.

Discontinuing:
May be unnecessary to finish medicine. Follow doctor's instructions.

Others:
No problems expected.

INTERACTION WITH OTHER DRUGS

GENERIC NAME OR DRUG CLASS	COMBINED EFFECT
Anticholinergics	Increased anticholinergic effect.
Antidepressants	Increased sedation.
Antihistamines	Increased antihistamine effect.
Clonidine	Decreased clonidine effect.
Guanethidine	Decreased guanethidine effect.
MAO inhibitors	High fever, convulsions, possible death.
Mind-altering drugs	Increased mind-altering effect.
Narcotics	Increased sedation.
Pain relievers	Increased pain reliever effect.
Rauwolfia alkaloids	Decreased effect of rauwolfia alkaloids.
Sedatives	Increased sedative effect.
Sleep inducers	Increased sedation.
Tranquilizers	Increased tranquilizer effect.

INTERACTION WITH OTHER SUBSTANCES

INTERACTS WITH	COMBINED EFFECT
Alcohol:	Depressed brain function. Avoid.
Beverages:	None expected.
Cocaine:	Decreased cyclobenzaprine effect.
Foods:	None expected.
Marijuana:	Occasional use—Drowsiness. Frequent use—Severe mental and physical impairment.
Tobacco:	None expected.

CYCLOPHOSPHAMIDE

BRAND NAMES

Cytoxan
Procytox

Habit forming? No
Prescription needed? Yes

GENERAL INFORMATION

Available as generic? No
Drug class: Immunosuppressive

USES

- Treatment for cancer.
- Treatment for severe rheumatoid arthritis.
- Treatment for blood-vessel disease.
- Treatment for skin disease.

DOSAGE & USAGE INFORMATION

How to take:
Tablet—Swallow with liquid. If you can't swallow whole, crumble tablet and take with liquid or food.

When to take:
Works best if taken first thing in morning. However, may take with food to lessen stomach irritation. Don't take at bedtime.

If you forget a dose:
Take as soon as you remember up to 12 hours late. If more than 12 hours, wait for next scheduled dose (don't double this dose).

What drug does:
- Kills cancer cells.
- Suppresses spread of cancer cells.
- Suppresses immune system.

Time lapse before drug works:
7 to 10 days continual use.

Don't take with:
See Interaction column and consult doctor.

OVERDOSE

Symptoms:
Bloody urine, water retention, weight gain, severe infection.

What to do:
Overdose unlikely to threaten life. If person takes much larger amount than prescribed, call doctor, poison-control center or hospital emergency room for instructions.

POSSIBLE ADVERSE REACTIONS OR SIDE EFFECTS

SYMPTOMS	FREQUENCY	WHAT TO DO
Brain & nervous system: Confusion, agitation, headache, dizziness.	Infrequent	4
Skin:		
• Rash, hives, itch.	Infrequent	3
• Flushed face.	Infrequent	4
• Dark skin, nails.	Common	4
Eyes: Blurred vision.	Rare	4
Ears, nose, throat:		
• Sore throat, fever.	Common	3
• Mouth, lip sores.	Rare	3
Digestive:		
• Black stool.	Rare	3
• Nausea, appetite loss, vomiting.	Common	4
• Stomach pain.	Infrequent	4
Heart & lungs: Shortness of breath, rapid heartbeat, cough.	Infrequent	3
Blood vessels, allergic, liver:	None expected.	
Muscles, bones, joints: Joint pain.	Infrequent	4
Genital, urinary:		
• Bloody urine, painful urination.	Infrequent	3
• More urination.	Rare	4
Kidneys: Pain in side.	Infrequent	3
Blood: Bleeding, bruising.	Infrequent	3
Others:		
• Missed period.	Common	4
• Fatigue, weakness.	Infrequent	4
• Unusual thirst.	Rare	3
• More sweating.	Infrequent	3

1- Life-threatening. Seek emergency treatment immediately.
2- Discontinue. Seek emergency treatment.
3- Discontinue. Call doctor right away.
4- Continue. Call doctor when convenient.

CYCLOPHOSPHAMIDE

WARNINGS & PRECAUTIONS

Don't take if:
- You are allergic to any alkylating agent.
- You have an infection.
- You have bloody urine.
- You will have surgery within 2 months, including dental surgery, requiring general or spinal anesthesia.

Before you start, consult your doctor:
- If you have impaired liver or kidney function.
- If you have impaired bone-marrow or blood-cell production.
- If you have had chemotherapy or X-ray therapy.
- If you have taken cortisone drugs in the past year.

Over age 60:
Adverse reactions and side effects may be more frequent and severe than in younger persons. To reduce risk of chemical bladder inflammation, drink 8 to 10 glasses of water daily.

Pregnancy:
Risk to unborn child outweighs drug benefits. Don't use.

Breast-feeding:
Drug passes into milk. Avoid drug or discontinue nursing until you finish medicine. Consult doctor for advice on maintaining milk supply.

Infants & children:
Use only under medical supervision.

Prolonged use:
- Development of fibrous lung tissue.
- Possible jaundice (yellow skin and eyes).
- Swelling of feet, lower legs.

Skin & sunlight:
No problems expected.

Driving, piloting or hazardous work:
Avoid if you feel dizzy or have blurred vision. Otherwise, no problems expected.

Airplane passengers:
No problems expected.

Discontinuing:
Don't discontinue without consulting doctor. Dose may require gradual reduction if you have taken drug for a long time. Doses of other drugs may also require adjustment.

Others:
Frequently causes hair loss. After treatment ends, hair should grow back.

INTERACTION WITH OTHER DRUGS

GENERIC NAME OR DRUG CLASS	COMBINED EFFECT
Allopurinol	Possible anemia.
Antidiabetics (oral)	Increased antidiabetic effect.
Insulin	Increased insulin effect.
Phenobarbital	Increased cyclophosphamide effect.

INTERACTION WITH OTHER SUBSTANCES

INTERACTS WITH	COMBINED EFFECT
Alcohol:	No problems expected.
Beverages:	No problems expected. Drink at least 2 quarts fluid every day.
Cocaine:	None expected.
Foods:	None expected.
Marijuana:	Increased impairment of immunity.
Tobacco:	None expected.

CYCLOTHIAZIDE

BRAND NAMES

Anhydron

GENERAL INFORMATION

Habit forming? No
Prescription needed? Yes
Available as generic? Yes
Drug class: Antihypertensive,
diuretic (thiazide)

USES

- Controls, but doesn't cure, high blood pressure.
- Reduces fluid retention (edema) caused by conditions such as heart disorders and liver disease.

DOSAGE & USAGE INFORMATION

How to take:
Tablet or capsule—Swallow with liquid. If you can't swallow whole, crumble tablet or open capsule and take with liquid or food.

When to take:
At the same time each day.

If you forget a dose:
Take as soon as you remember up to 2 hours late. If more than 2 hours, wait for next scheduled dose (don't double this dose).

What drug does:
- Forces sodium and water excretion, reducing body fluid.
- Relaxes muscle cells of small arteries.
- Reduced body fluid and relaxed arteries lower blood pressure.

Time lapse before drug works:
4 to 6 hours. May require several weeks to lower blood pressure.

Don't take with:
- See Interaction column and consult doctor.
- Non-prescription drugs without consulting doctor.

OVERDOSE

Symptoms:
Cramps, weakness, drowsiness, weak pulse, coma.

What to do:
- Dial 0 (operator) or 911 (emergency) for an ambulance or medical help. Then give first aid immediately.
- Additional emergency information on page 886.

POSSIBLE ADVERSE REACTIONS OR SIDE EFFECTS

SYMPTOMS	FREQUENCY	WHAT TO DO
Brain & nervous system:		
● Dizziness	Infrequent	4
● Mood changes.	Infrequent	4
● Headaches	Infrequent	4
Skin: Rash or hives.	Rare	2
Eyes: Blurred vision.	Infrequent	3
Ears, nose, throat:		
● Sore throat, fever.	Rare	3
● Dry mouth, thirst.	Infrequent	5
Digestive: Severe abdominal pain, nausea, vomiting.	Infrequent	3
Heart & lungs: Irregular heartbeat, weak pulse.	Infrequent	3
Blood vessels:	None expected.	
Muscles, bones, joints: Weakness, tiredness.	Infrequent	4
Genital, urinary:	None expected.	
Kidneys:	None expected.	
Liver: Jaundice (yellow skin and eyes).	Rare	3
Blood:	None expected.	
Others: Weight changes.	Infrequent	4

1-Life-threatening. Seek emergency treatment immediately.
2-Discontinue. Seek emergency treatment.
3-Discontinue. Call doctor right away.
4-Continue. Call doctor when convenient.
5-Continue. Tell doctor at next visit.
6-No action necessary.

WARNINGS & PRECAUTIONS

Don't take if:
You are allergic to any thiazide diuretic drugs.

Before you start, consult your doctor:
- If you are allergic to any sulfa drug.
- If you have gout.
- If you have liver, pancreas or kidney disorder.

Over age 60:
Adverse reactions and side effects may be more frequent and severe than in younger persons, especially dizziness and excessive potassium loss.

Pregnancy:
Risk to unborn child outweighs drug benefits. Don't use.

Breast-feeding:
Drug passes into milk. Avoid drug or discontinue nursing.

Infants & children:
No problems expected.

Prolonged use:
You may need medicine to treat high blood pressure for the rest of your life.

Skin & sunlight:
May cause rash or intensify sunburn in areas exposed to sun or sunlamp.

Driving, piloting or hazardous work:
Don't drive or pilot aircraft until you learn how medicine affects you. Don't work around dangerous machinery. Don't climb ladders or work in high places. Danger increases if you drink alcohol or take medicine affecting alertness and reflexes, such as antihistamines, tranquilizers, sedatives, pain medicine, narcotics and mind-altering drugs.

Airplane passengers:
No problems expected.

Discontinuing:
Don't discontinue without medical advice.

Others:
- Hot weather and fever may cause dehydration and drop in blood pressure. Dose may require temporary adjustment. Weigh daily and report any unexpected weight decreases to your doctor.
- May cause rise in uric acid, leading to gout.
- May cause blood-sugar rise in diabetics.

INTERACTION WITH OTHER DRUGS

GENERIC NAME OR DRUG CLASS	COMBINED EFFECT
Allopurinol	Decreased allopurinol effect.
Antidepressants (tricyclic)	Dangerous drop in blood pressure. Avoid combination unless under medical supervision.
Barbiturates	Increased cyclothiazide effect.
Cholestyramine	Decreased cyclothiazide effect.
Cortisone drugs	Excessive potassium loss that causes dangerous heart rhythms.
Digitalis preparations	Excessive potassium loss that causes dangerous heart rhythms.
Diuretics (thiazide)	Increased effect of other thiazide diuretics.
Lithium	Increased effect of lithium.
MAO Inhibitors	Increased cyclothiazide effect.
Probenecid	Decreased probenecid effect.

INTERACTION WITH OTHER SUBSTANCES

INTERACTS WITH	COMBINED EFFECT
Alcohol:	Dangerous blood-pressure drop.
Beverages:	None expected.
Cocaine:	None expected.
Foods: Licorice	Excessive potassium loss that causes dangerous heart rhythms.
Marijuana:	May increase blood pressure.
Tobacco:	None expected.

CYCRIMINE

BRAND NAMES

Pagitane

GENERAL INFORMATION

Habit forming? No
Prescription needed? Yes
Available as generic? No
Drug class: Antidyskinetic, antiparkinsonism

USES

- Treatment of Parkinson's disease.
- Treatment of adverse effects of phenothiazines.

DOSAGE & USAGE INFORMATION

How to take:
Tablets or capsules—Take with food to lessen stomach irritation.

When to take:
At the same times each day.

If you forget a dose:
Take as soon as you remember up to 2 hours late. If more than 2 hours, wait for next scheduled dose (don't double this dose).

What drug does:
- Balances chemical reactions necessary to send nerve impulses within base of brain.
- Improves muscle control and reduces stiffness.

Time lapse before drug works:
1 to 2 hours.

Don't take with:
- Non-prescription drugs for colds, cough or allergy.
- See Interaction column and consult doctor.

OVERDOSE

Symptoms:
Agitation, dilated pupils, hallucinations, dry mouth, rapid heartbeat, sleepiness.

What to do:
- Dial 0 (operator) or 911 (emergency) for an ambulance or medical help. Then give first aid immediately.
- If patient is unconscious and not breathing, give mouth-to-mouth breathing. If there is no heartbeat, use cardiac massage and mouth-to-mouth breathing (CPR). Don't try to make patient vomit. If you can't get help quickly, take patient to nearest emergency facility.
- Additional emergency information on page 886.

POSSIBLE ADVERSE REACTIONS OR SIDE EFFECTS

SYMPTOMS	FREQUENCY	WHAT TO DO
Brain & nervous system: Confusion, dizziness.	Rare	4
Skin: Rash	Rare	3
Eyes:		
• Pain	Rare	3
• Blurred vision, light sensitivity.	Common	4
Ears, nose, throat: Sore mouth or tongue.	Rare	4
Digestive:		
• Constipation	Common	4
• Nausea, vomiting.	Common	4
Heart & lungs:	None expected.	
Blood vessels:	None expected.	
Muscles, bones, joints:		
• Muscle cramps.	Rare	4
• Numbness, weakness in hands or feet.	Rare	4
Genital, urinary: Difficult or painful urination.	Common	5
Kidneys:	None expected.	
Liver:	None expected.	
Allergic:	None expected.	
Blood:	None expected.	
Others:	None expected.	

1- Life-threatening. Seek emergency treatment immediately.
2- Discontinue. Seek emergency treatment.
3- Discontinue. Call doctor right away.
4- Continue. Call doctor when convenient.
5- Continue. Tell doctor at next visit.
6- No action necessary.

WARNINGS & PRECAUTIONS

Don't take if:
You are allergic to any antidyskinetic.

Before you start, consult your doctor:
- If you have had glaucoma.
- If you have had high blood pressure or heart disease.
- If you have had impaired liver function.
- If you have had kidney disease or urination difficulty.

Over age 60:
More sensitive to drug. Aggravates symptoms of enlarged prostate. Causes impaired thinking, hallucinations, nightmares. Consult doctor about any of these.

Pregnancy:
Studies inconclusive on harm to unborn child. Animal studies show fetal abnormalities. Decide with your doctor whether drug benefits justify risk to unborn child.

Breast-feeding:
No problems expected.

Infants & children:
Not recommended for children 3 and younger. Use for older children only under doctor's supervision.

Prolonged use:
Possible glaucoma.

Skin & sunlight:
No problems expected.

Driving, piloting or hazardous work:
Don't drive or pilot aircraft until you learn how medicine affects you. Don't work around dangerous machinery. Don't climb ladders or work in high places. Danger increases if you drink alcohol or take medicine affecting alertness and reflexes, such as antihistamines, tranquilizers, sedatives, pain medicine, narcotics and mind-altering drugs.

Airplane passengers:
No problems expected.

Discontinuing:
Don't discontinue without consulting doctor. Dose may require gradual reduction if you have taken drug for a long time. Doses of other drugs may also require adjustment.

Others:
- Internal eye pressure should be measured regularly.
- Avoid becoming overheated.

INTERACTION WITH OTHER DRUGS

GENERIC NAME OR DRUG CLASS	COMBINED EFFECT
Amantadine	Increased amantadine effect.
Antidepressants (tricyclic)	Increased cycrimine effect. May cause glaucoma.
Antihistamines	Increased cycrimine effect.
Levodopa	Increased levodopa effect. Improved results in treating Parkinson's disease.
Meperidine	Increased cycrimine effect.
MAO inhibitors	Increased cycrimine effect.
Orphenadrine	Increased cycrimine effect.
Phenothiazines	Behavior changes.
Primidone	Excessive sedation.
Procainamide	Increased procainamide effect.
Quinidine	Increased cycrimine effect.
Tranquilizers	Excessive sedation.

INTERACTION WITH OTHER SUBSTANCES

INTERACTS WITH	COMBINED EFFECT
Alcohol:	None expected.
Beverages:	None expected.
Cocaine:	Decreased cycrimine effect. Avoid.
Foods:	None expected.
Marijuana:	None expected.
Tobacco:	None expected.

CYPROHEPTADINE

BRAND NAMES

Cyprodine
Periactin
Vimicon

Habit forming? No
Prescription needed? Yes
Available as generic? Yes
Drug class: Antihistamine

USES

- Reduces allergic symptoms such as hay fever, hives, rash or itching.
- Induces sleep.
- Reduces symptoms of cold urticaria.

DOSAGE & USAGE INFORMATION

How to take:
Tablet or syrup—Swallow with liquid or food to lessen stomach irritation.

When to take:
Varies with form. Follow label directions.

If you forget a dose:
Take as soon as you remember up to 2 hours late. If more than 2 hours, wait for next scheduled dose (don't double this dose).

What drug does:
Blocks action of histamine after an allergic response triggers histamine release in sensitive cells.

Time lapse before drug works:
30 minutes.

Don't take with:
See Interaction column and consult doctor.

OVERDOSE

Symptoms:
Convulsions, red face, hallucinations, coma.

What to do:
- Dial 0 (operator) or 911 (emergency) for an ambulance or medical help. Then give first aid immediately.
- If patient is unconscious and not breathing, give mouth-to-mouth breathing. If there is no heartbeat, use cardiac massage and mouth-to-mouth breathing (CPR). Don't try to make patient vomit. If you can't get help quickly, take patient to nearest emergency facility.
- Additional emergency information on page 886.

POSSIBLE ADVERSE REACTIONS OR SIDE EFFECTS

SYMPTOMS	FREQUENCY	WHAT TO DO
Brain & nervous system:		
• Nightmares, agitation, irritability.	Rare	3
• Drowsiness, dizziness.	Common	5
Skin:	None expected.	
Eyes:		
• Vision changes.	Infrequent	3
• Less tolerance for contact lenses.	Infrequent	4
Ears, nose, throat:		
• Sore throat, fever.	Rare	3
• Dry mouth, nose, throat.	Common	5
Digestive:		
• Nausea	Common	5
• Appetite loss.	Infrequent	5
Heart & lungs:		
Rapid heartbeat.	Rare	3
Blood vessels:		
Unusual bleeding or bruising.	Rare	3
Muscles, bones, joints, kidneys, liver, allergic, blood:	None expected.	
Genital, urinary:		
Urination difficulty.	Infrequent	4
Others:		
Fatigue, weakness.	Rare	3

1 - Life-threatening. Seek emergency treatment immediately.
2 - Discontinue. Seek emergency treatment.
3 - Discontinue. Call doctor right away.
4 - Continue. Call doctor when convenient.
5 - Continue. Tell doctor at next visit.
6 - No action necessary.

WARNINGS & PRECAUTIONS

Don't take if:
You are allergic to any antihistamine.

Before you start, consult your doctor:
- If you have glaucoma.
- If you have enlarged prostate.
- If you have asthma.
- If you have kidney disease.
- If you have peptic ulcer.
- If you will have surgery within 2 months, including dental surgery, requiring general or spinal anesthesia.

Over age 60:
Don't exceed recommended dose. Adverse reactions and side effects may be more frequent and severe than in younger persons, especially urination difficulty, diminished alertness and other brain and nervous-system symptoms.

Pregnancy:
No proven harm to unborn child. Avoid if possible.

Breast-feeding:
Drug passes into milk. Avoid drug or discontinue nursing until you finish medicine. Consult doctor for advice on maintaining milk supply.

Infants & children:
Not recommended for premature or newborn infants. Otherwise, no problems expected.

Prolonged use:
Avoid. May damage bone marrow and nerve cells.

Skin & sunlight:
May cause rash or intensify sunburn in areas exposed to sun or sunlamp.

Driving, piloting or hazardous work:
Don't drive or pilot aircraft until you learn how medicine affects you. Don't work around dangerous machinery. Don't climb ladders or work in high places. Danger increases if you drink alcohol or take medicine affecting alertness and reflexes, such as antihistamines, tranquilizers, sedatives, pain medicine, narcotics and mind-altering drugs.

Airplane passengers:
No problems expected.

Discontinuing:
No problems expected.

Others:
May mask symptoms of hearing damage from aspirin, other salicylates, cisplatin, paromomycin, vancomycin or anticonvulsants. Consult doctor if you use these.

INTERACTION WITH OTHER DRUGS

GENERIC NAME OR DRUG CLASS	COMBINED EFFECT
Anticholinergics	Increased anticholinergic effect.
Antidepressants	Excess sedation. Avoid.
Antihistamines (other)	Excess sedation. Avoid.
Hypnotics	Excess sedation. Avoid.
MAO inhibitors	Increased cyproheptadine effect.
Mind-altering drugs	Excess sedation. Avoid.
Narcotics	Excess sedation. Avoid.
Sedatives	Excess sedation. Avoid.
Sleep inducers	Excess sedation. Avoid.
Tranquilizers	Excess sedation. Avoid.

INTERACTION WITH OTHER SUBSTANCES

INTERACTS WITH	COMBINED EFFECT
Alcohol:	Excess sedation. Avoid.
Beverages: Caffeine drinks	Less cyproheptadine sedation.
Cocaine:	Decreased cyproheptadine effect. Avoid.
Foods:	None expected.
Marijuana:	Excess sedation. Avoid.
Tobacco:	None expected.

DANTHRON

BRAND NAMES

Dorbane
Doxidan (M)
Modane

GENERAL INFORMATION

Habit forming? No
Prescription needed? No
Available as generic? Yes
Drug class: Laxative (stimulant)

 ## USES

Constipation relief.

 ## DOSAGE & USAGE INFORMATION

How to take:
- Tablet—Swallow with liquid or food.
- Liquid—Drink 6 to 8 glasses of water each day, in addition to one taken with each dose.

When to take:
Usually at bedtime with a snack, unless directed otherwise.

If you forget a dose:
Take as soon as you remember.

What drug does:
Acts on smooth muscles of intestine wall to cause vigorous bowel movement.

Time lapse before drug works:
6 to 10 hours.

Don't take with:
- See Interaction column and consult doctor.
- Don't take within 2 hours of taking another medicine. Laxative interferes with medicine absorption.

 ## OVERDOSE

Symptoms:
Vomiting, electrolyte depletion.

What to do:
Overdose unlikely to threaten life. If person takes much larger amount than prescribed, call doctor, poison-control center or hospital emergency room for instructions.

POSSIBLE ADVERSE REACTIONS OR SIDE EFFECTS

SYMPTOMS	FREQUENCY	WHAT TO DO
Brain & nervous system: Irritability, confusion, headache.	Rare	3
Skin: Rash	Rare	3
Eyes:	None expected.	
Ears, nose, throat:	None expected.	
Digestive: Belching, cramps, nausea.	Infrequent	4
Heart & lungs: Breathing difficulty, irregular heartbeat.	Rare	3
Blood vessels:	None expected.	
Muscles, bones, joints: Muscle cramps.	Rare	3
Genital, urinary:	None expected.	
Kidneys: Burning on urination.	Rare	4
Liver:	None expected.	
Allergic:	None expected.	
Blood:	None expected.	
Others: • Rectal irritation.	Common	4
• Dangerous potassium loss.	Infrequent	3
• Unusual tiredness or weakness.	Rare	3

1- Life-threatening. Seek emergency treatment immediately.
2- Discontinue. Seek emergency treatment.
3- Discontinue. Call doctor right away.
4- Continue. Call doctor when convenient.
5- Continue. Tell doctor at next visit.
6- No action necessary.

DANTHRON

WARNINGS & PRECAUTIONS

Don't take if:
- You have symptoms of appendicitis, inflamed bowel or intestinal blockage.
- You are allergic to a stimulant laxative.
- You have missed a bowel movement for only 1 or 2 days.

Before you start, consult your doctor:
- If you have a colostomy or ileostomy.
- If you have congestive heart disease.
- If you have diabetes.
- If you have high blood pressure.
- If you have a laxative habit.
- If you have rectal bleeding.
- If you take other laxatives.

Over age 60:
Adverse reactions and side effects may be more frequent and severe than in younger persons.

Pregnancy:
Risk to mother and unborn child outweighs drug benefits. Don't use.

Breast-feeding:
Drug passes into milk. Avoid drug or discontinue nursing until you finish medicine. Consult doctor for advice on maintaining milk supply.

Infants & children:
Use only under medical supervision.

Prolonged use:
Don't take for more than 1 week unless under a doctor's supervision. May cause laxative dependence.

Skin & sunlight:
No problems expected.

Driving, piloting or hazardous work:
No problems expected.

Airplane passengers:
No problems expected.

Discontinuing:
May be unnecessary to finish medicine. Follow doctor's instructions.

Others:
Don't take to "flush out" your system or as a "tonic."

INTERACTION WITH OTHER DRUGS

GENERIC NAME OR DRUG CLASS	COMBINED EFFECT
Antihypertensives	May cause dangerous low potassium level.
Diuretics	May cause dangerous low potassium level.
Docusate calcium	Liver toxicity.
Docusate sodium	Liver toxicity.

INTERACTION WITH OTHER SUBSTANCES

INTERACTS WITH	COMBINED EFFECT
Alcohol:	None expected.
Beverages:	None expected.
Cocaine:	None expected.
Foods:	None expected.
Marijuana:	None expected.
Tobacco:	None expected.

DEHYDROCHOLIC ACID

BRAND NAMES

Cholan-DH
Cholan-HMB (M)
Decholin
G.B.S. (M)
Hepahydrin
Neocholan

GENERAL INFORMATION

Habit forming? No
Prescription needed? No
Available as generic? Yes
Drug class: Laxative (stimulant)

 USES

Constipation relief.

 DOSAGE & USAGE INFORMATION

How to take:
Tablet—Swallow with liquid.

When to take:
Usually at bedtime with a snack, unless directed otherwise.

If you forget a dose:
Take as soon as you remember.

What drug does:
Acts on smooth muscles of intestine wall to cause vigorous bowel movement.

Time lapse before drug works:
6 to 10 hours.

Don't take with:
- See Interaction column and consult doctor.
- Don't take within 2 hours of taking another medicine. Laxative interferes with medicine absorption.

 OVERDOSE

Symptoms:
Vomiting, electrolyte depletion.

What to do:
Overdose unlikely to threaten life. If person takes much larger amount than prescribed, call doctor, poison-control center or hospital emergency room for instructions.

POSSIBLE ADVERSE REACTIONS OR SIDE EFFECTS

SYMPTOMS	FREQUENCY	WHAT TO DO
Brain & nervous system: Irritability, confusion, headache.	Rare	3
Skin: Rash	Rare	3
Eyes:	None expected.	
Ears, nose, throat:	None expected.	
Digestive: Belching, cramps, nausea.	Infrequent	4
Heart & lungs: Breathing difficulty, irregular heartbeat.	Rare	3
Blood vessels:	None expected.	
Muscles, bones, joints: Muscle cramps.	Rare	3
Genital, urinary:	None expected.	
Kidneys: Burning on urination.	Rare	4
Liver:	None expected.	
Allergic:	None expected.	
Blood:	None expected.	
Others: • Rectal irritation.	Common	4
• Dangerous potassium loss.	Infrequent	3
• Unusual tiredness or weakness.	Rare	3

1- Life-threatening. Seek emergency treatment immediately.
2- Discontinue. Seek emergency treatment.
3- Discontinue. Call doctor right away.
4- Continue. Call doctor when convenient.
5- Continue. Tell doctor at next visit.
6- No action necessary.

DEHYDROCHOLIC ACID

WARNINGS & PRECAUTIONS

Don't take if:
- You have symptoms of appendicitis, inflamed bowel or intestinal blockage.
- You are allergic to a stimulant laxative.
- You have missed a bowel movement for only 1 or 2 days.
- You have liver disease.

Before you start, consult your doctor:
- If you have a colostomy or ileostomy.
- If you have congestive heart disease.
- If you have diabetes.
- If you have enlarged prostate.
- If you have a laxative habit.
- If you have rectal bleeding.
- If you take other laxatives.

Over age 60:
Adverse reactions and side effects may be more frequent and severe than in younger persons.

Pregnancy:
Risk to mother and unborn child outweighs drug benefits. Don't use.

Breast-feeding:
Drug passes into milk. Avoid drug or discontinue nursing until you finish medicine. Consult doctor for advice on maintaining milk supply.

Infants & children:
Use only under medical supervision.

Prolonged use:
Don't take for more than 1 week unless under a doctor's supervision. May cause laxative dependence.

Skin & sunlight:
No problems expected.

Driving, piloting or hazardous work:
No problems expected.

Airplane passengers:
No problems expected.

Discontinuing:
May be unnecessary to finish medicine. Follow doctor's instructions.

Others:
Don't take to "flush out" your system or as a "tonic."

INTERACTION WITH OTHER DRUGS

GENERIC NAME OR DRUG CLASS	COMBINED EFFECT
Antihypertensives	May cause dangerous low potassium level.
Diuretics	May cause dangerous low potassium level.

INTERACTION WITH OTHER SUBSTANCES

INTERACTS WITH	COMBINED EFFECT
Alcohol:	None expected.
Beverages:	None expected.
Cocaine:	None expected.
Foods:	None expected.
Marijuana:	None expected.
Tobacco:	None expected.

DEMECLOCYCLINE

BRAND NAMES

Declomycin

GENERAL INFORMATION

Habit forming? No
Prescription needed? Yes
Available as generic? Yes
Drug class: Antibiotic (tetracycline)

USES

- Treatment for infections susceptible to demeclocycline. Will not cure virus infections such as colds or flu.
- Treatment for acne.

DOSAGE & USAGE INFORMATION

How to take:
Tablet or capsule—Take on empty stomach 1 hour before or 2 hours after eating. If you can't swallow whole, crumble tablet or open capsule and take with liquid or food.

When to take:
At the same times each day, evenly spaced.

If you forget a dose:
Take as soon as you remember up to 2 hours late. If more than 2 hours, wait for next scheduled dose (don't double this dose).

What drug does:
Prevents germ growth and reproduction.

Time lapse before drug works:
- Infections—May require 5 days to affect infection.
- Acne—May require 4 weeks to affect acne.

Don't take with:
- Non-prescription drugs without consulting doctor.
- See Interaction column and consult doctor.

OVERDOSE

Symptoms:
Severe nausea, vomiting, diarrhea.

What to do:
Overdose unlikely to threaten life. If person takes much larger amount than prescribed, call doctor, poison-control center or hospital emergency room for instructions.

POSSIBLE ADVERSE REACTIONS OR SIDE EFFECTS

SYMPTOMS	FREQUENCY	WHAT TO DO
Brain & nervous system:		
Headache	Infrequent	3
Skin:		
• Itching around rectum and genitals.	Common	3
• Rash	Infrequent	3
Eyes:		
Blurred vision.	Rare	3
Ears, nose, throat:		
• Dark tongue.	Common	5
• Sore mouth or tongue.	Common	2
• Excessive thirst.	Infrequent	4
Digestive:		
Nausea, vomiting, diarrhea, abdominal burning.	Common	2
Heart & lungs:	None expected.	
Blood vessels:	None expected.	
Muscles, bones, joints:	None expected.	
Genital, urinary:		
Increased urination.	Infrequent	4
Kidneys:	None expected.	
Liver:		
Jaundice (yellow eyes and skin) in pregnant women.	Rare	3
Allergic:	None expected.	
Blood:	None expected.	
Others:	None expected.	

1- Life-threatening. Seek emergency treatment immediately.
2- Discontinue. Seek emergency treatment.
3- Discontinue. Call doctor right away.
4- Continue. Call doctor when convenient.
5- Continue. Tell doctor at next visit.
6- No action necessary.

DEMECLOCYCLINE

WARNINGS & PRECAUTIONS

Don't take if:
You are allergic to any tetracycline antibiotic.

Before you start, consult your doctor:
- If you have kidney or liver disease.
- If you have lupus.
- If you have myasthenia gravis.

Over age 60:
Dosage usually less than in younger adults. More likely to cause itching around rectum. Ask you doctor how to prevent it.

Pregnancy:
Risk to unborn child outweighs drug benefits. Don't use.

Breast-feeding:
Drug passes into milk. Avoid drug or discontinue nursing until you finish medicine. Consult doctor for advice on maintaining milk supply.

Infants & children:
May cause permanent teeth malformation or discoloration in children less than 8 years old. Don't use.

Prolonged use:
- You may become more susceptible to infections caused by germs not responsive to demeclocycline.
- May cause rare problems in liver, kidney or bone marrow. Periodic laboratory blood studies, liver- and kidney-function tests recommended if you use drug a long time.

Skin & sunlight:
May cause rash or intensify sunburn in areas exposed to sun or sunlamp.

Driving, piloting or hazardous work:
No problems expected.

Airplane passengers:
No problems expected.

Discontinuing:
Don't discontinue without doctor's advice until you complete prescribed dose, even though symptoms diminish or disappear.

Others:
No problems expected.

INTERACTION WITH OTHER DRUGS

GENERIC NAME OR DRUG CLASS	COMBINED EFFECT
Antacids	Decreased demeclocycline effect.
Anticoagulants (oral)	Increased anticoagulant effect.
Contraceptives (oral)	Decreased contraceptive effect.
Digitalis preparations	Increased digitalis effect.
Mineral supplements (iron, calcium, magnesium, zinc)	Decreased demeclocycline absorption. Separate doses by 1 to 2 hours.
Lithium	Increased lithium effect.
Penicillins	Decreased penicillin effect.
Sodium bicarbonate	Decreased demeclocycline effect.

INTERACTION WITH OTHER SUBSTANCES

INTERACTS WITH	COMBINED EFFECT
Alcohol:	Possible liver damage. Avoid.
Beverages: Milk	Decreased demeclocycline absorption. Take dose 2 hours after or 1 hour before drinking.
Cocaine:	No proven problems.
Foods: Dairy products	Decreased demeclocycline absorption. Take dose 2 hours after or 1 hour before eating.
Marijuana:	No interactions expected, but marijuana may slow body's recovery. Avoid.
Tobacco:	None expected.

DESERPIDINE

BRAND NAMES

Harmonyl
Raunormine

GENERAL INFORMATION

Habit forming? No
Prescription needed? Yes
Available as generic? Yes
Drug class: Antihypertensive, tranquilizer
(rauwolfia alkaloid)

 ## USES

- Treatment for high blood pressure.
- Tranquilizer for mental and emotional disturbances.

 ## DOSAGE & USAGE INFORMATION

How to take:
Tablet—Swallow with liquid or food to lessen stomach irritation. If you can't swallow whole, crumble tablet and take with liquid or food.

When to take:
At the same times each day.

If you forget a dose:
Take as soon as you remember up to 2 hours late. If more than 2 hours, wait for next scheduled dose (don't double this dose).

What drug does:
- Interferes with nerve impulses and relaxes blood-vessel muscles, reducing blood pressure.
- Suppresses brain centers that control emotions.

Time lapse before drug works:
3 weeks continual use required to determine effectiveness.

Don't take with:
See Interaction column and consult doctor.

 ## OVERDOSE

Symptoms:
Drowsiness; slow, weak pulse; slow, shallow breathing; diarrhea; coma; flush; low body temperature.

What to do:
- Dial 0 (operator) or 911 (emergency) for an ambulance or medical help. Then give first aid immediately.
- Additional emergency information on page 886.

POSSIBLE ADVERSE REACTIONS OR SIDE EFFECTS

SYMPTOMS	FREQUENCY	WHAT TO DO
Brain & nervous system:		
• Trembling hands.	Infrequent	4
• Headache, drowsiness or faintness, lethargy.	Common	5
• Depression	Common	4
Skin:		
Rash or itch.	Rare	3
Eyes:		
Redness	Common	5
Ears, nose, throat:		
• Sore throat, fever.	Rare	3
• Stuffy nose.	Common	5
Digestive:		
• Stomach pain, nausea, vomiting.	Rare	3
• Black stool, bloody vomit.	Infrequent	3
Heart & lungs:		
Chest pain, shortness of breath, irregular or slow heartbeat.	Infrequent	3
Blood vessels:		
Unusual bleeding or bruising.	Rare	3
Muscles, bones, joints:		
Stiffness	Infrequent	3
Genital, urinary:		
• Painful urination.	Rare	4
• Impotence, lower sex drive.	Common	5
Kidneys, allergic, blood, others:	None expected.	
Liver:		
Jaundice (yellow skin and eyes).	Rare	3

1-Life-threatening. Seek emergency treatment immediately.
2-Discontinue. Seek emergency treatment.
3-Discontinue. Call doctor right away.
4-Continue. Call doctor when convenient.
5-Continue. Tell doctor at next visit.

WARNINGS & PRECAUTIONS

Don't take if:
- You are allergic to any rauwolfia alkaloid.
- You are depressed.
- You have active peptic ulcer.
- You have ulcerative colitis.

Before you start, consult your doctor:
- If you have been depressed.
- If you have had peptic ulcer, ulcerative colitis or gallstones.
- If you have epilepsy.
- If you will have surgery within 2 months, including dental surgery, requiring general or spinal anesthesia.

Over age 60:
Adverse reactions and side effects may be more frequent and severe than in younger persons.

Pregnancy:
Studies inconclusive on harm to unborn child. Animal studies show fetal abnormalities. Decide with your doctor whether drug benefits justify risk to unborn child.

Breast-feeding:
Drug passes into milk. Avoid drug or discontinue nursing until you finish medicine. Consult doctor for advice on maintaining milk supply.

Infants & children:
Not recommended.

Prolonged use:
Causes cancer in laboratory animals. Consult your doctor if you have family or personal history of cancer.

Skin & sunlight:
No problems expected.

Driving, piloting or hazardous work:
Avoid if you feel drowsy, dizzy or faint. Otherwise, no problems expected.

Airplane passengers:
No problems expected.

Discontinuing:
Don't discontinue without consulting doctor. Dose may require gradual reduction if you have taken drug for a long time. Doses of other drugs may also require adjustment.

Others:
Consult your doctor if you do isometric exercises. These raise blood pressure. Drug may intensify blood-pressure rise.

INTERACTION WITH OTHER DRUGS

GENERIC NAME OR DRUG CLASS	COMBINED EFFECT
Anticoagulants (oral)	Unpredictable increased or decreased effect of anticoagulant.
Anticonvulsants	Serious change in seizure pattern.
Antidepressants	Increased antidepressant effect.
Antihistamines	Increased antihistamine effect.
Aspirin	Decreased aspirin effect.
Beta-adrenergic blockers	Increased effect of deserpidine. Excessive sedation.
Digitalis preparations	Irregular heartbeat.
Levodopa	Decreased levodopa effect.
MAO inhibitors	Severe depression.
Mind-altering drugs	Excessive sedation.

Additional interactions on page 835.

INTERACTION WITH OTHER SUBSTANCES

INTERACTS WITH	COMBINED EFFECT
Alcohol:	Increased intoxication. Use with extreme caution.
Beverages: Carbonated drinks	Decreased deserpidine effect.
Cocaine:	Decreased deserpidine effect.
Foods: Spicy foods	Possible digestive upset.
Marijuana:	Occasional use—Mild drowsiness. Daily use—Moderate drowsiness, low blood pressure, depression.
Tobacco:	No problems expected.

DESIPRAMINE

BRAND NAMES

Norpramin
Pertofrane

GENERAL INFORMATION

Habit forming? No
Prescription needed? Yes
Available as generic? Yes
Drug class: Antidepressant (tricyclic)

 ## USES

Gradually relieves, but doesn't cure, symptoms of depression.

 ## DOSAGE & USAGE INFORMATION

How to take:
Tablet or capsule—Swallow with liquid.

When to take:
At the same time each day, usually bedtime.

If you forget a dose:
Bedtime dose—If you forget your once-a-day bedtime dose, don't take it more than 3 hours late. If more than 3 hours, wait for next scheduled dose. Don't double this dose.

What drug does:
Probably affects part of brain that controls messages between nerve cells.

Time lapse before drug works:
Begins in 1 to 2 weeks. May require 4 to 6 weeks for maximum benefit.

Don't take with:
- Non-prescription drugs without consulting doctor.
- See Interaction column and consult doctor.

 ## OVERDOSE

Symptoms:
Hallucinations, convulsions, coma.

What to do:
- Dial 0 (operator) or 911 (emergency) for an ambulance or medical help. Then give first aid immediately.
- If patient is unconscious and not breathing, give mouth-to-mouth breathing. If there is no heartbeat, use cardiac massage and mouth-to-mouth breathing (CPR). Don't try to make patient vomit. If you can't get help quickly, take patient to nearest emergency facility.
- Additional emergency information on page 886.

POSSIBLE ADVERSE REACTIONS OR SIDE EFFECTS

SYMPTOMS	FREQUENCY	WHAT TO DO
Brain & nervous system:		
• Hallucinations, shakiness, dizziness, fainting.	Infrequent	3
• Headache	Common	4
• Seizures	Rare	1
• Insomnia	Common	5
Skin:		
Rash, itch.	Rare	3
Eyes:		
Blurred vision, pain.	Infrequent	3
Ears, nose, throat:		
• Sore throat.	Rare	3
• Dry mouth or unpleasant taste.	Common	4
Digestive:		
• Constipation or diarrhea, nausea, indigestion.	Common	4
• Vomiting	Infrequent	3
• "Sweet tooth"	Common	5
Heart & lungs:		
Irregular heartbeat or slow pulse.	Infrequent	3
Blood vessels, muscles, bones, joints, kidneys, allergic, blood:	None expected.	
Genital, urinary:		
Difficulty urinating.	Infrequent	4
Liver:		
Jaundice (yellow skin and eyes).	Rare	3
Others:		
• Fever	Rare	3
• Fatigue, weakness.	Common	4

1- Life-threatening. Seek emergency treatment immediately.
2- Discontinue. Seek emergency treatment.
3- Discontinue. Call doctor right away.
4- Continue. Call doctor when convenient.
5- Continue. Tell doctor at next visit.

WARNINGS & PRECAUTIONS

Don't take if:
- You are allergic to any tricyclic antidepressant.
- You drink alcohol.
- You have had a heart attack within 6 weeks.
- You have glaucoma.
- You have taken MAO inhibitors within 2 weeks.
- Patient is younger than 12.

Before you start, consult your doctor:
- If you will have surgery within 2 months, including dental surgery, requiring general or spinal anesthesia.
- If you have an enlarged prostate.
- If you have heart disease or high blood pressure.
- If you have stomach or intestinal problems.
- If you have an overactive thyroid.
- If you have asthma.
- If you have liver disease.

Over age 60:
More likely to develop urination difficulty and side effects under *Brain & nervous system*, opposite page.

Pregnancy:
Studies inconclusive on harm to unborn child. Animal studies show fetal abnormalities. Decide with your doctor whether drug benefits justify risk to unborn child.

Breast-feeding:
Drug passes into milk. Avoid drug or discontinue nursing until you finish medicine. Consult doctor on maintaining milk supply.

Infants & children:
Don't give to children younger than 12.

Prolonged use:
No problems expected.

Skin & sunlight:
May cause rash or intensify sunburn in areas exposed to sun or sunlamp.

Driving, piloting or hazardous work:
Don't drive or pilot aircraft until you learn how medicine affects you. Don't work around dangerous machinery. Don't climb ladders or work in high places. Danger increases if you drink alcohol or take medicine affecting alertness and reflexes.

Airplane passengers:
No problems expected.

Discontinuing:
Don't discontinue without consulting doctor. Dose may require gradual reduction if you have taken drug for a long time. Doses of other drugs may also require adjustment.

INTERACTION WITH OTHER DRUGS

GENERIC NAME OR DRUG CLASS	COMBINED EFFECT
Anticoagulants (oral)	Increased anticoagulant effect.
Anticholinergics	Increased sedation.
Antihistamines	Increased antihistamine effect.
Barbiturates	Decreased antidepressant effect.
Clonidine	Decreased clonidine effect.
Diuretics (thiazide)	Increased desipramine effect.
Ethchlorvynol	Delirium
Guanethidine	Decreased guanethidine effect.
MAO inhibitors	Fever, delirium, convulsions.
Methyldopa	Decreased methyldopa effect.
Narcotics	Dangerous oversedation.
Phenytoin	Decreased phenytoin effect.
Quinidine	Irregular heartbeat.
Sedatives	Dangerous oversedation.
Sympathomimetics	Increased sympathomimetic effect.
Thyroid hormones	Irregular heartbeat.

INTERACTION WITH OTHER SUBSTANCES

INTERACTS WITH	COMBINED EFFECT
Alcohol: Beverages or medicines with alcohol.	Excessive intoxication. Avoid.
Beverages:	None expected.
Cocaine:	Excessive intoxication. Avoid.
Foods:	None expected.
Marijuana:	Excessive drowsiness. Avoid.
Tobacco:	None expected.

DEXAMETHASONE

BRAND NAMES

Dalalon L.A.
Decadron
Decadron L.A.
Decadron Respihaler
Decadron with Xylocaine (M)

Dexasone
Dexone
Hexadrol
SK-Dexamethasone
Turbinaire Decadron

GENERAL INFORMATION

Habit forming? No
Prescription needed? Yes
Available as generic? Yes
Drug class: Cortisone drug
(adrenal corticosteroid)

 USES

- Reduces inflammation caused by many different medical problems.
- Treatment for some allergic diseases, blood disorders, kidney diseases, asthma and emphysema.
- Replaces corticosteroid deficiencies.

 DOSAGE & USAGE INFORMATION

How to take:
- Tablet or liquid—Swallow with liquid or food to lessen stomach irritation. If you can't swallow whole, crumble tablet and take with liquid or food.
- Inhaler—Follow label instructions.

When to take:
At the same times each day. Take once-a-day or once-every-other-day doses in mornings.

If you forget a dose:
- Several-doses-per-day prescription—Take as soon as you remember up to 2 hours late. If more than 2 hours, wait for next scheduled dose (don't double this dose).
- Once-a-day dose or less—Wait for next dose. Double this dose.

What drug does:
Decreases inflammatory responses.

Time lapse before drug works:
2 to 4 days.

Don't take with:
See Interaction column and consult doctor.

 OVERDOSE

Symptoms:
Headache, convulsions, heart failure.

What to do:
- Dial 0 (operator) or 911 (emergency) for an ambulance or medical help. Then give first aid immediately.
- Additional emergency information on page 886.

POSSIBLE ADVERSE REACTIONS OR SIDE EFFECTS

SYMPTOMS	FREQUENCY	WHAT TO DO
Brain & nervous system:		
Mood changes, insomnia, restlessness.	Infrequent	4
Skin:		
• Acne	Common	4
• Rash	Rare	3
• Poor wound healing.	Common	4
Eyes:		
Blurred vision, halos around lights.	Infrequent	3
Ears, nose, throat:		
• Sore throat, fever.	Infrequent	3
• Thirst	Common	4
Digestive:		
• Indigestion, nausea, vomiting.	Common	4
• Bloody or black, tarry stool.	Infrequent	2
Heart & lungs:		
Irregular heartbeat.	Rare	2
Blood vessels, kidneys, liver, allergic, blood:	None expected.	
Muscles, bones, joints:		
Muscle cramps, swollen legs, feet.	Infrequent	3
Genital, urinary:		
Frequent urination.	Infrequent	4
Others:		
• Weight gain, round face.	Infrequent	4
• Fatigue, weakness.	Infrequent	4
• TB recurrence.	Infrequent	4
• Irregular menstrual periods.	Infrequent	4

1- Life-threatening. Seek emergency treatment immediately.
2- Discontinue. Seek emergency treatment.
3- Discontinue. Call doctor right away.
4- Continue. Call doctor when convenient.

WARNINGS & PRECAUTIONS

Don't take if:
- You are allergic to any cortisone drug.
- You have tuberculosis or fungus infection.
- You have herpes infection of eyes, lips or genitals.

Before you start, consult your doctor:
- If you have had tuberculosis.
- If you have congestive heart failure.
- If you have diabetes.
- If you have peptic ulcer.
- If you have glaucoma.
- If you have underactive thyroid.
- If you have high blood pressure.
- If you have myasthenia gravis.
- If you have blood clots in legs or lungs.

Over age 60:
Adverse reactions and side effects may be more frequent and severe than in younger persons. Likely to aggravate edema, diabetes or ulcers. Likely to cause cataracts and osteoporosis (softening of the bones).

Pregnancy:
Risk to unborn child outweighs drug benefits. Don't use.

Breast-feeding:
Drug passes into milk. Avoid drug or discontinue nursing until you finish medicine. Consult doctor for advice on maintaining milk supply.

Infants & children:
Use only under medical supervision.

Prolonged use:
- Retards growth in children.
- Possible glaucoma, cataracts, diabetes, fragile bones and thin skin.
- Functional dependence.

Skin & sunlight:
No problems expected.

Driving, piloting or hazardous work:
No problems expected.

Airplane passengers:
No problems expected.

Discontinuing:
- Don't discontinue without doctor's advice until you complete prescribed dose, even though symptoms diminish or disappear.
- Drug affects your response to surgery, illness, injury or stress for 2 years after discontinuing. Tell about drug to anyone who takes medical care of you within 2 years.

Others:
Avoid immunizations if possible.

INTERACTION WITH OTHER DRUGS

GENERIC NAME OR DRUG CLASS	COMBINED EFFECT
Amphoterecin B	Potassium depletion.
Anticholinergics	Possible glaucoma.
Anticoagulants (oral)	Decreased anticoagulant effect.
Anticonvulsants (hydantoin)	Decreased dexamethasone effect.
Antidiabetics (oral)	Decreased antidiabetic effect.
Antihistamines	Decreased dexamethasone effect.
Aspirin	Increased dexamethasone effect.
Barbiturates	Decreased dexamethasone effect. Oversedation.
Beta-adrenergic blockers	Decreased dexamethasone effect.
Chloral hydrate	Decreased dexamethasone effect.
Chlorthalidone	Potassium depletion.
Cholinergics	Decreased cholinergic effect.
Contraceptives (oral)	Increased dexamethasone effect.
Digitalis preparations	Dangerous potassium depletion. Possible digitalis toxicity.

Additional interactions on page 835.

INTERACTION WITH OTHER SUBSTANCES

INTERACTS WITH	COMBINED EFFECT
Alcohol:	Risk of stomach ulcers.
Beverages:	No proven problems.
Cocaine:	Overstimulation. Avoid.
Foods:	No proven problems.
Marijuana:	Decreased immunity.
Tobacco:	Increased dexamethasone effect. Possible toxicity.

DEXCHLORPHENIRAMINE

BRAND NAMES

Polaramine

GENERAL INFORMATION

Habit forming? No
Prescription needed? Yes
Available as generic? No
Drug class: Antihistamine

 ## USES

- Reduces allergic symptoms such as hay fever, hives, rash or itching.
- Induces sleep.

 ## DOSAGE & USAGE INFORMATION

How to take:
- Tablet or syrup—Swallow with liquid or food to lessen stomach irritation.
- Extended-release tablets or capsules—Swallow each dose whole. If you take regular tablets, you may chew or crush them.

When to take:
Varies with form. Follow label directions.

If you forget a dose:
Take as soon as you remember up to 2 hours late. If more than 2 hours, wait for next scheduled dose (don't double this dose).

What drug does:
Blocks action of histamine after an allergic response triggers histamine release in sensitive cells.

Time lapse before drug works:
30 minutes.

Don't take with:
See Interaction column and consult doctor.

 ## OVERDOSE

Symptoms:
Convulsions, red face, hallucinations, coma.

What to do:
- Dial 0 (operator) or 911 (emergency) for an ambulance or medical help. Then give first aid immediately.
- If patient is unconscious and not breathing, give mouth-to-mouth breathing. If there is no heartbeat, use cardiac massage and mouth-to-mouth breathing (CPR). Don't try to make patient vomit. If you can't get help quickly, take patient to nearest emergency facility.
- Additional emergency information on page 886.

POSSIBLE ADVERSE REACTIONS OR SIDE EFFECTS

SYMPTOMS	FREQUENCY	WHAT TO DO
Brain & nervous system:		
• Nightmares, agitation, irritability.	Rare	3
• Drowsiness, dizziness.	Common	5
Skin:	None expected.	
Eyes:		
• Vision changes.	Infrequent	3
• Less tolerance for contact lenses.	Infrequent	4
Ears, nose, throat:		
• Sore throat, fever.	Rare	3
• Dry mouth, nose, throat.	Common	5
Digestive:		
• Nausea	Common	5
• Appetite loss.	Infrequent	5
Heart & lungs:		
Rapid heartbeat.	Rare	3
Blood vessels:		
Unusual bleeding or bruising.	Rare	3
Muscles, bones, joints, kidneys, liver, allergic, blood:	None expected.	
Genital, urinary:		
Urination difficulty.	Infrequent	4
Others:		
Fatigue, weakness.	Rare	3

1- Life-threatening. Seek emergency treatment immediately.
2- Discontinue. Seek emergency treatment.
3- Discontinue. Call doctor right away.
4- Continue. Call doctor when convenient.
5- Continue. Tell doctor at next visit.
6- No action necessary.

DEXCHLORPHENIRAMINE

WARNINGS & PRECAUTIONS

Don't take if:
You are allergic to any antihistamine.

Before you start, consult your doctor:
- If you have glaucoma.
- If you have enlarged prostate.
- If you have asthma.
- If you have kidney disease.
- If you have peptic ulcer.
- If you will have surgery within 2 months, including dental surgery, requiring general or spinal anesthesia.

Over age 60:
Don't exceed recommended dose. Adverse reactions and side effects may be more frequent and severe than in younger persons, especially urination difficulty, diminished alertness and other brain and nervous-system symptoms.

Pregnancy:
No proven harm to unborn child. Avoid if possible.

Breast-feeding:
Drug passes into milk. Avoid drug or discontinue nursing until you finish medicine. Consult doctor for advice on maintaining milk supply.

Infants & children:
Not recommended for premature or newborn infants. Otherwise, no problems expected.

Prolonged use:
Avoid. May damage bone marrow and nerve cells.

Skin & sunlight:
May cause rash or intensify sunburn in areas exposed to sun or sunlamp.

Driving, piloting or hazardous work:
Don't drive or pilot aircraft until you learn how medicine affects you. Don't work around dangerous machinery. Don't climb ladders or work in high places. Danger increases if you drink alcohol or take medicine affecting alertness and reflexes, such as antihistamines, tranquilizers, sedatives, pain medicine, narcotics and mind-altering drugs.

Airplane passengers:
No problems expected.

Discontinuing:
No problems expected.

Others:
May mask symptoms of hearing damage from aspirin, other salicylates, cisplatin, paromomycin, vancomycin or anticonvulsants. Consult doctor if you use these.

INTERACTION WITH OTHER DRUGS

GENERIC NAME OR DRUG CLASS	COMBINED EFFECT
Anticholinergics	Increased anticholinergic effect.
Antidepressants	Excess sedation. Avoid.
Antihistamines (other)	Excess sedation. Avoid.
Hypnotics	Excess sedation. Avoid.
MAO inhibitors	Increased dexchlorpheniramine effect.
Mind-altering drugs	Excess sedation. Avoid.
Narcotics	Excess sedation. Avoid.
Sedatives	Excess sedation. Avoid.
Sleep inducers	Excess sedation. Avoid.
Tranquilizers	Excess sedation. Avoid.

INTERACTION WITH OTHER SUBSTANCES

INTERACTS WITH	COMBINED EFFECT
Alcohol:	Excess sedation. Avoid.
Beverages: Caffeine drinks	Less dexchlorpheniramine sedation.
Cocaine:	Decreased dexchlorpheniramine effect. Avoid.
Foods:	None expected.
Marijuana:	Excess sedation. Avoid.
Tobacco:	None expected.

DEXTROAMPHETAMINE

BRAND NAMES

Amphaplex (M)	Dexedrine	Obotan
Biphetamine (M)	Eskatrol (M)	Oxydess II
Declobese (M)	Ferndex	Spancap No. 1
Dexampex	Obetrol (M)	

GENERAL INFORMATION

Habit forming? Yes
Prescription needed? Yes
Available as generic? Yes
Drug class: Central-nervous-system
stimulant (amphetamine)

 USES

- Prevents narcolepsy (attacks of uncontrollable sleepiness).
- Controls hyperactivity in children.

 DOSAGE & USAGE INFORMATION

How to take:
- Tablet or liquid—Swallow with water.
- Extended-release capsules—Swallow each dose whole with liquid.

When to take:
- At the same times each day.
- Short-acting form—Don't take later than 6 hours before bedtime.
- Long-acting form—Take on awakening.

If you forget a dose:
- Short-acting form—Take up to 2 hours late. If more than 2 hours, wait for next dose (don't double this).
- Long-acting form—Take as soon as you remember. Wait 20 hours for next dose.

What drug does:
- Narcolepsy—Apparently affects brain centers to decrease fatigue or sleepiness and increase alertness and motor activity.
- Hyperactive children—Calms children, opposite to effect on narcoleptic adults.

Time lapse before drug works:
15 to 30 minutes.

Don't take with:
See Interaction column and consult doctor.

 OVERDOSE

Symptoms:
Rapid heartbeat, hyperactivity, high fever, hallucinations, suicidal or homicidal feelings, convulsions, coma.

What to do:
- Dial 0 (operator) or 911 (emergency) for an ambulance or medical help. Then give first aid immediately.
- Additional emergency information on page 886.

POSSIBLE ADVERSE REACTIONS OR SIDE EFFECTS

SYMPTOMS	FREQUENCY	WHAT TO DO
Brain & nervous system:		
• Headache	Infrequent	4
• Dizziness, lack of alertness.	Infrequent	3
• Mood changes.	Rare	4
• Irritability, nervousness, insomnia.	Common	4
Skin:		
Rash, hives.	Rare	3
Eyes:		
Blurred vision.	Infrequent	3
Ears, nose, throat:		
Dry mouth.	Common	5
Digestive:		
Diarrhea or constipation, appetite loss, stomach pain, nausea, vomiting, weight loss.	Infrequent	5
Heart & lungs:		
• Fast, pounding heartbeat.	Infrequent	3
• Chest pain or irregular heartbeat.	Rare	3
Blood vessels, kidneys, liver, allergic, blood:	None expected.	
Muscles, bones, joints:		
Uncontrolled movements of head, neck, arms, legs.	Rare	3
Genital, urinary:		
Decreased sex drive, impotence.	Infrequent	5
Others:		
• Enlarged breasts.	Rare	4
• Unusual sweating.	Infrequent	3

1 - Life-threatening. Seek emergency treatment immediately.
2 - Discontinue. Seek emergency treatment.
3 - Discontinue. Call doctor right away.
4 - Continue. Call doctor when convenient.
5 - Continue. Tell doctor at next visit.

DEXTROAMPHETAMINE

WARNINGS & PRECAUTIONS

Don't take if:
- You are allergic to any dextroamphetamine.
- You will have surgery within 2 months, including dental surgery, requiring general or spinal anesthesia.

Before you start, consult your doctor:
- If you plan to become pregnant within medication period.
- If you have glaucoma.
- If you have heart or blood-vessel disease, or high blood pressure.
- If you have overactive thyroid, anxiety or tension.
- If you have a severe mental illness (especially children).

Over age 60:
Adverse reactions and side effects may be more frequent and severe than in younger persons.

Pregnancy:
Risk to unborn child outweighs drug benefits. Don't use.

Breast-feeding:
Drug passes into milk. Avoid drug or discontinue nursing.

Infants & children:
Not recommended for children under 12.

Prolonged use:
Habit forming.

Skin & sunlight:
No problems expected.

Driving, piloting or hazardous work:
Don't drive or pilot aircraft until you learn how medicine affects you. Don't work around dangerous machinery. Don't climb ladders or work in high places. Danger increases if you drink alcohol or take medicine affecting alertness and reflexes.

Airplane passengers:
No problems expected.

Discontinuing:
May be unnecessary to finish medicine. Follow doctor's instructions.

Others:
- This is a dangerous drug and must be closely supervised. Don't use for appetite control or depression. Potential for damage and abuse.
- During withdrawal phase, may cause prolonged sleep of several days.

INTERACTION WITH OTHER DRUGS

GENERIC NAME OR DRUG CLASS	COMBINED EFFECT
Anesthesias (general)	Irregular heartbeat.
Antidepressants (tricyclic)	Decreased dextroamphetamine effect.
Antihypertensives	Decreased antihypertensive effect.
Carbonic anhydrase inhibitors	Increased dextroamphetamine effect.
Guanethidine	Decreased guanethidine effect.
Haloperidol	Decreased dextroamphetamine effect.
MAO inhibitors	May severely increase blood pressure.
Phenothiazines	Decreased dextroamphetamine effect.
Sodium bicarbonate	Increased dextroamphetamine effect.

INTERACTION WITH OTHER SUBSTANCES

INTERACTS WITH	COMBINED EFFECT
Alcohol:	Decreased dextroamphetamine effect. Avoid.
Beverages: Caffeine drinks	Overstimulation. Avoid.
Cocaine:	Dangerous stimulation of nervous system. Avoid.
Foods:	None expected.
Marijuana:	Frequent use—Severely impaired mental function.
Tobacco:	None expected.

DEXTROMETHORPHAN

BRAND NAMES

Dristan Cough	Nyquil	Silexin
Formula	Robitussin-DM	Trocal
Formula 44-D	Romilar (M)	Tussaminic
Hold Cough	St. Joseph	Vicks Cough Syrup
Suppressant	Cough Syrup	

See complete brand names list, page 825.

See complete brand names list, page 825.

GENERAL INFORMATION

Habit forming? No
Prescription needed? No
Available as generic? Yes
Drug class: Cough suppressant

 ## USES

Suppresses cough associated with allergies or infections such as colds, bronchitis, flu and lung disorders.

 ## DOSAGE & USAGE INFORMATION

How to take:
- Tablet or capsule—Swallow with liquid. If you can't swallow whole, crumble tablet or open capsule and take with liquid or food.
- Lozenges or syrups—Take as directed on label.

When to take:
As needed, no more often than every 3 hours.

If you forget a dose:
Take as soon as you remember. Wait 3 hours for next dose.

What drug does:
Reduces sensitivity of brain's cough-control center, suppressing urge to cough.

Time lapse before drug works:
15 to 30 minutes.

Don't take with:
See Interaction column and consult doctor.

 ## OVERDOSE

Symptoms:
Euphoria, overactivity, sense of intoxication, visual and auditory hallucinations, lack of coordination, stagger, stupor, shallow breathing.

What to do:
- Dial 0 (operator) or 911 (emergency) for an ambulance or medical help. Then give first aid immediately.
- Additional emergency information on page 886.

POSSIBLE ADVERSE REACTIONS OR SIDE EFFECTS

SYMPTOMS	FREQUENCY	WHAT TO DO
Brain & nervous system: Dizziness, drowsiness.	Rare	3
Skin: Rash	Rare	3
Eyes:	None expected.	
Ears, nose, throat:	None expected.	
Digestive: Diarrhea, nausea or vomiting, stomach pain.	Rare	3
Heart & lungs:	None expected.	
Blood vessels:	None expected.	
Muscles, bones, joints:	None expected.	
Genital, urinary:	None expected.	
Kidneys:	None expected.	
Liver:	None expected.	
Allergic:	None expected.	
Blood:	None expected.	
Others:	None expected.	

1- Life-threatening. Seek emergency treatment immediately.
2- Discontinue. Seek emergency treatment.
3- Discontinue. Call doctor right away.
4- Continue. Call doctor when convenient.
5- Continue. Tell doctor at next visit.
6- No action necessary.

WARNINGS & PRECAUTIONS

Don't take if:
You are allergic to any cough syrup containing dextromethorphan.

Before you start, consult your doctor:
- If you have asthma attacks.
- If you have impaired liver function.

Over age 60:
May become constipated, excessively drowsy or unsteady. If drug is used for cough, other treatment may be necessary to liquefy thick mucus in bronchial tubes.

Pregnancy:
No proven harm to unborn child. Avoid if possible.

Breast-feeding:
No proven problems. Consult doctor.

Infants & children:
Use only as label directs.

Prolonged use:
No problems expected.

Skin & sunlight:
No problems expected.

Driving, piloting or hazardous work:
Don't drive or pilot aircraft until you learn how medicine affects you. Don't work around dangerous machinery. Don't climb ladders or work in high places. Danger increases if you drink alcohol or take medicine affecting alertness and reflexes, such as antihistamines, tranquilizers, sedatives, pain medicine, narcotics and mind-altering drugs.

Airplane passengers:
No problems expected.

Discontinuing:
May be unnecessary to finish medicine. Follow doctor's instructions.

Others:
- If cough persists or if you cough blood or brown-yellow, thick mucus, call your doctor.
- Excessive use may lead to functional dependence.

 ## INTERACTION WITH OTHER DRUGS

GENERIC NAME OR DRUG CLASS	COMBINED EFFECT
MAO inhibitors	Disorientation, high fever, drop in blood pressure and loss of consciousness.

 ## INTERACTION WITH OTHER SUBSTANCES

INTERACTS WITH	COMBINED EFFECT
Alcohol:	None expected.
Beverages:	None expected.
Cocaine:	Decreased dextromethorphan effect. Avoid.
Foods:	None expected.
Marijuana:	None expected.
Tobacco:	None expected.

DIAZEPAM

BRAND NAMES

D-Tran   Valium
E-Pam   Vivol
Neo-Calme
Novodipam
Rival
Stress-Pam

GENERAL INFORMATION

Habit forming? Yes
Prescription needed? Yes
Available as generic? No
Drug class: Tranquilizer (benzodiazepine)

 USES

- Treatment for nervousness or tension.
- Treatment for muscle spasm.
- Treatment for convulsive disorders.

 DOSAGE & USAGE INFORMATION

How to take:
Tablet or capsule—Swallow with liquid. If you can't swallow whole, crumble tablet or open capsule and take with liquid or food.

When to take:
At the same time each day, according to instructions on prescription label.

If you forget a dose:
Take as soon as you remember up to 2 hours late. If more than 2 hours, wait for next scheduled dose (don't double this dose).

What drug does:
Affects limbic system of brain—part that controls emotions.

Time lapse before drug works:
2 hours. May take 6 weeks for full benefit.

Don't take with:
See Interaction column and consult doctor.

 OVERDOSE

Symptoms:
Drowsiness, weakness, tremor, stupor, coma.

What to do:
- Dial 0 (operator) or 911 (emergency) for an ambulance or medical help. Then give first aid immediately.
- If patient is unconscious and not breathing, give mouth-to-mouth breathing. If there is no heartbeat, use cardiac massage and mouth-to-mouth breathing (CPR). Don't try to make patient vomit. If you can't get help quickly, take patient to nearest emergency facility.
- Additional emergency information on page 886.

POSSIBLE ADVERSE REACTIONS OR SIDE EFFECTS

SYMPTOMS	FREQUENCY	WHAT TO DO
Brain & nervous system:		
• Clumsiness, drowsiness, dizziness.	Common	4
• Hallucinations, confusion, depression, irritability.	Infrequent	3
Skin: Rash, itch.	Infrequent	3
Eyes: Vision changes.	Infrequent	3
Ears, nose, throat: Mouth, throat ulcers.	Rare	3
Digestive: Constipation or diarrhea, nausea, vomiting.	Infrequent	4
Heart & lungs: Slow heartbeat, breathing difficulty.	Rare	2
Blood vessels:	None expected.	
Muscles, bones, joints:	None expected.	
Genital, urinary: Urination difficulty.	Infrequent	4
Kidneys:	None expected.	
Liver: Jaundice (yellow eyes and skin).	Rare	3
Allergic:	None expected.	
Blood:	None expected.	
Others:	None expected.	

1- Life-threatening. Seek emergency treatment immediately.
2- Discontinue. Seek emergency treatment.
3- Discontinue. Call doctor right away.
4- Continue. Call doctor when convenient.
5- Continue. Tell doctor at next visit.
6- No action necessary.

DIAZEPAM

WARNINGS & PRECAUTIONS

Don't take if:
- You are allergic to any benzodiazepine.
- You have myasthenia gravis.
- You have glaucoma.
- You are active or recovering alcoholic.
- Patient is younger than 6 months.

Before you start, consult your doctor:
- If you have liver, kidney or lung disease.
- If you have diabetes, epilepsy or porphyria.

Over age 60:
Adverse reactions and side effects may be more frequent and severe than in younger persons. You need smaller doses for shorter periods of time. May develop agitation, rage or "hangover effect."

Pregnancy:
Risk to unborn child outweighs drug benefits. Don't use.

Breast-feeding:
Drug passes into milk. Avoid drug or discontinue nursing until you finish medicine. Consult doctor for advice on maintaining milk supply.

Infants & children:
Use only under medical supervision for children older than 6 months.

Prolonged use:
May impair liver function.

Skin & sunlight:
No problems expected.

Driving, piloting or hazardous work:
Don't drive or pilot aircraft until you learn how medicine affects you. Don't work around dangerous machinery. Don't climb ladders or work in high places. Danger increases if you drink alcohol or take medicine affecting alertness and reflexes.

Airplane passengers:
No problems expected.

Discontinuing:
Don't discontinue without consulting doctor. Dose may require gradual reduction if you have taken drug for a long time. Doses of other drugs may also require adjustment.

Others:
- Hot weather, heavy exercise and profuse sweat may reduce excretion and cause overdose.
- Blood sugar may rise in diabetics, requiring insulin adjustment.

INTERACTION WITH OTHER DRUGS

GENERIC NAME OR DRUG CLASS	COMBINED EFFECT
Anticonvulsants	Change in seizure frequency or severity.
Antidepressants	Increased sedative effect of both drugs.
Antihistamines	Increased sedative effect of both drugs.
Antihypertensives	Excessively low blood pressure.
Cimetidine	Excess sedation.
Disulfiram	Increased diazepam effect.
MAO inhibitors	Convulsions, deep sedation, rage.
Narcotics	Increased sedative effect of both drugs.
Sedatives	Increased sedative effect of both drugs.
Sleep inducers	Increased sedative effect of both drugs.
Tranquilizers	Increased sedative effect of both drugs.

INTERACTION WITH OTHER SUBSTANCES

INTERACTS WITH	COMBINED EFFECT
Alcohol:	Heavy sedation. Avoid.
Beverages:	None expected.
Cocaine:	Decreased diazepam effect.
Foods:	None expected.
Marijuana:	Heavy sedation. Avoid.
Tobacco:	Decreased diazepam effect.

DICHLORPHENAMIDE

BRAND NAMES

Daranide
Oratrol

Habit forming? No
Prescription needed? Yes
Available as generic? No

GENERAL INFORMATION

Drug class: Diuretic (carbonic anhydrase inhibitor, sulfonamide), antiglaucoma

 ## USES

Treatment of glaucoma.

 ## DOSAGE & USAGE INFORMATION

How to take:
- Tablets—Swallow whole with liquid or food to lessen stomach irritation.
- Granules—Dissolve in 4 oz. cool water. Drink all water.

When to take:
- 1 dose per day—At the same time each morning.
- More than 1 dose per day—Take last dose several hours before bedtime.

If you forget a dose:
Take as soon as you remember. Continue regular schedule.

What drug does:
- Inhibits action of carbonic anhydrase, an enzyme. This lowers the internal eye pressure by decreasing fluid formation in the eye.
- Forces sodium and water excretion, reducing body fluid.

Time lapse before drug works:
2 hours.

Don't take with:
- Non-prescription drugs without consulting doctor.
- See Interaction column and consult doctor.

 ## OVERDOSE

Symptoms:
Drowsiness, confusion, excitement, nausea, vomiting, numbness in hands and feet, coma.

What to do:
Call your doctor or poison-control center for advice if you suspect overdose, even if not sure. Symptoms may not appear until damage has occurred.

POSSIBLE ADVERSE REACTIONS OR SIDE EFFECTS

SYMPTOMS	FREQUENCY	WHAT TO DO
Brain & nervous system:		
● Headache, mood changes, nervousness, clumsiness, trembling, confusion.	Rare	3
● Convulsions	Rare	1
Skin:		
Hives, itch, rash, or sores.	Rare	3
Ears, nose, throat:		
● Ringing in ears, hoarseness, dry mouth, thirst.	Rare	3
● Sore throat, fever.	Rare	3
Digestive:		
● Appetite change, nausea, vomiting.	Rare	3
● Black, tarry stool.	Rare	3
Heart & lungs:		
Breathing difficulty, irregular or weak heartbeat.	Rare	3
Blood vessels:		
Easy bleeding or bruising.	Rare	3
Muscles, bones, joints:		
Muscle cramps.	Rare	3
Genital, urinary:		
Painful or frequent urination, bloody urine.	Rare	3
Kidneys:		
Back pain.	Infrequent	3
Allergic, blood, liver, eyes:		
None expected.		
Others:		
● Fatigue, weakness.	Infrequent	4
● Tingling or burning in feet or hands.	Infrequent	4

1- Life-threatening. Seek emergency treatment immediately.
2- Discontinue. Seek emergency treatment.
3- Discontinue. Call doctor right away.
4- Continue. Call doctor when convenient.

DICHLORPHENAMIDE

WARNINGS & PRECAUTIONS

Don't take if:
- You are allergic to any carbonic anhydrase inhibitor.
- You have liver or kidney disease.
- You have Addison's disease (adrenal gland failure).
- You have diabetes.

Before you start, consult your doctor:
- If you have gout or lupus.
- If you are allergic to any sulfa drug.

Over age 60:
- Don't exceed recommended dose.
- If you take a digitalis preparation, eat foods high in potassium content or take a potassium supplement.

Pregnancy:
No proven harm to unborn child. Avoid if possible, especially first 3 months.

Breast-feeding:
Avoid drug or don't nurse your infant.

Infants & children:
Not recommended for children younger than 12.

Prolonged use:
May cause kidney stones, vision change, loss of taste and smell, jaundice (yellow skin and eyes) or weight loss.

Skin & sunlight:
No problems expected.

Driving, piloting or hazardous work:
Avoid if you feel drowsy or dizzy. Otherwise, no problems expected.

Airplane passengers:
No problems expected.

Discontinuing:
Don't discontinue without medical advice.

Others:
Medicine may increase sugar levels in blood and urine. Diabetics may need insulin adjustment.

INTERACTION WITH OTHER DRUGS

GENERIC NAME OR DRUG CLASS	COMBINED EFFECT
Amphetamines	Increased amphetamine effect.
Anticonvulsants	Increased loss of bone minerals.
Antidepressants (tricyclic)	Increased antidepressant effect.
Antidiabetics (oral)	Increased potassium loss.
Aspirin	Decreased aspirin effect.
Cortisone drugs	Increased potassium loss.
Digitalis preparations	Possible digitalis toxicity.
Diuretics (other)	Increased potassium loss.
Lithium	Decreased lithium effect.
Methenamine	Decreased methenamine effect.
Quinidine	Increased quinidine effect.
Sympathomimetics	Increased sympathomimetic effect.

INTERACTION WITH OTHER SUBSTANCES

INTERACTS WITH	COMBINED EFFECT
Alcohol:	None expected.
Beverages:	None expected.
Cocaine:	Decreased dichlorphenamide effect.
Foods: Potassium-rich foods.	Eat these to decrease potassium loss. See page 850.
Marijuana:	Increased dichlorphenamide effect.
Tobacco:	None expected.

DICLOXACILLIN

BRAND NAMES

Dycill
Dynapen
Pathocil

GENERAL INFORMATION

Habit forming? No
Prescription needed? Yes
Available as generic? Yes
Drug class: Antibiotic (penicillin)

 USES

Treatment of bacterial infections that are susceptible to dicloxacillin.

 DOSAGE & USAGE INFORMATION

How to take:
- Tablets or capsules—Swallow with liquid on an empty stomach 1 hour before or 2 hours after eating.
- Liquid—Take with cold beverage. Liquid form is perishable and effective for only 7 days at room temperature. Effective for 14 days if stored in refrigerator. Don't freeze.

When to take:
Follow instructions on prescription label or side of package. Doses should be evenly spaced. For example, 4 times a day means every 6 hours.

If you forget a dose:
Take as soon as you remember. Continue regular schedule.

What drug does:
Destroys susceptible bacteria. Does not kill viruses.

Time lapse before drug works:
May be several days before medicine affects infection.

Don't take with:
See Interaction column and consult doctor.

 OVERDOSE

Symptoms:
Severe diarrhea, nausea or vomiting.

What to do:
Overdose unlikely to threaten life. If person takes much larger amount than prescribed, call doctor, poison-control center or hospital emergency room for instructions.

 POSSIBLE ADVERSE REACTIONS OR SIDE EFFECTS

SYMPTOMS	FREQUENCY	WHAT TO DO
Brain & nervous system:	None expected.	
Skin: Hives, rash, intense itch soon after a dose.	Rare	1
Eyes:	None expected.	
Ears, nose, throat: Dark or discolored tongue.	Common	5
Digestive: Mild nausea, vomiting, diarrhea.	Infrequent	4
Heart & lungs:	None expected.	
Blood vessels: Unexplained bleeding.	Rare	3
Muscles, bones, joints:	None expected.	
Genital, urinary:	None expected.	
Kidneys:	None expected.	
Liver:	None expected.	
Allergic: Life-threatening anaphylaxis may occur!	Rare	1 See page 888.
Blood:	None expected.	
Others:	None expected.	

1- Life-threatening. Seek emergency treatment immediately.
2- Discontinue. Seek emergency treatment.
3- Discontinue. Call doctor right away.
4- Continue. Call doctor when convenient.
5- Continue. Tell doctor at next visit.
6- No action necessary.

WARNINGS & PRECAUTIONS

Don't take if:
You are allergic to dicloxacillin, cephalosporin antibiotics, other penicillins or penicillamine. Life-threatening reaction may occur.

Before you start, consult your doctor:
If you are allergic to any substance or drug.

Over age 60:
You may have skin reactions, particularly around genitals and anus.

Pregnancy:
Studies inconclusive on harm to unborn child. Animal studies show fetal abnormalities. Decide with your doctor whether drug benefits justify risk to unborn child.

Breast-feeding:
Drug passes into milk. Child may become sensitive to penicillins and have allergic reactions to penicillin drugs. Avoid dicloxacillin or discontinue nursing until you finish medicine. Consult doctor for advice on maintaining milk supply.

Infants & children:
No problems expected.

Prolonged use:
You may become more susceptible to infections caused by germs not responsive to dicloxacillin.

Skin & sunlight:
No problems expected.

Driving, piloting or hazardous work:
Usually not dangerous. Most hazardous reactions likely to occur a few minutes after taking dicloxacillin.

Airplane passengers:
No problems expected.

Discontinuing:
Don't discontinue without doctor's advice until you complete prescribed dose, even though symptoms diminish or disappear.

Others:
No problems expected.

INTERACTION WITH OTHER DRUGS

GENERIC NAME OR DRUG CLASS	COMBINED EFFECT
Chloramphenicol	Decreased effect of both drugs.
Erythromycins	Decreased effect of both drugs.
Paromomycin	Decreased effect of both drugs.
Tetracyclines	Decreased effect of both drugs.
Troleandomycin	Decreased effect of both drugs.

INTERACTION WITH OTHER SUBSTANCES

INTERACTS WITH	COMBINED EFFECT
Alcohol:	Occasional stomach irritation.
Beverages:	None expected.
Cocaine:	No proven problems.
Foods:	None expected.
Marijuana:	No proven problems.
Tobacco:	None expected.

DICUMAROL

BRAND NAMES

Dufalone
Melitoxin

GENERAL INFORMATION

Habit forming? No
Prescription needed? Yes
Available as generic? Yes
Drug class: Anticoagulant

 ## USES

Reduces blood clots. Used for abnormal clotting inside blood vessels.

 ## DOSAGE & USAGE INFORMATION

How to take:
Tablet—Swallow with liquid. If you can't swallow whole, crumble tablet and take with liquid or food.

When to take:
At the same time each day.

If you forget a dose:
Take as soon as you remember up to 12 hours late. If more than 12 hours, wait for next scheduled dose (don't double this dose). Inform your doctor of any missed doses.

What drug does:
Blocks action of vitamin K necessary for blood clotting.

Time lapse before drug works:
36 to 48 hours.

Don't take with:
See Interaction column and consult doctor.

 ## OVERDOSE

Symptoms:
Bloody vomit and bloody or black stools, red urine.

What to do:
- Dial 0 (operator) or 911 (emergency) for an ambulance or medical help. Then give first aid immediately.
- Additional emergency information on page 886.

POSSIBLE ADVERSE REACTIONS OR SIDE EFFECTS

SYMPTOMS	FREQUENCY	WHAT TO DO
Brain & nervous system: Dizziness, headache.	Rare	3
Skin: Rash, hives, itch.	Infrequent	3
Eyes: Blurred vision.	Infrequent	3
Ears, nose, throat:		
● Sore throat.	Infrequent	3
● Mouth sores.	Rare	3
Digestive:		
● Black stools or bloody vomit.	Infrequent	2
● Diarrhea, cramps, nausea, vomiting.	Infrequent	4
● Bloating, gas.	Common	5
Heart & lungs: Coughing up blood.	Infrequent	2
Blood vessels: Easy bruising, bleeding.	Infrequent	3
Muscles, bones, joints: Swollen feet, legs.	Infrequent	4
Genital, urinary: Cloudy or red urine.	Infrequent	3
Kidneys: Back pain.	Infrequent	3
Liver: Jaundice (yellow skin and eyes).	Infrequent	3
Allergic, blood:	None expected.	
Others:		
● Fever, chills.	Infrequent	3
● Hair loss.	Infrequent	4
● Fatigue, weakness.	Infrequent	3

1- Life-threatening. Seek emergency treatment immediately.
2- Discontinue. Seek emergency treatment.
3- Discontinue. Call doctor right away.
4- Continue. Call doctor when convenient.
5- Continue. Tell doctor at next visit.

WARNINGS & PRECAUTIONS

Don't take if:
- You have been allergic to any oral anticoagulant.
- You have a bleeding disorder.
- You have an active peptic ulcer.
- You have ulcerative colitis.

Before you start, consult your doctor:
- If you take any other drugs, including non-prescription drugs.
- If you have high blood pressure.
- If you have heavy or prolonged menstrual periods.
- If you have diabetes.
- If you have a bladder catheter.
- If you have serious liver or kidney disease.
- If you will have surgery within 2 months, including dental surgery, requiring general or spinal anesthesia.

Over age 60:
Adverse reactions and side effects may be more frequent and severe than in younger persons.

Pregnancy:
Risk to unborn child outweighs drug benefits. Don't use.

Breast-feeding:
Drug filters into milk. May harm child. Avoid.

Infants & children:
Use only under doctor's supervision.

Prolonged use:
No problems expected.

Skin & sunlight:
No problems expected.

Driving, piloting or hazardous work:
- Avoid hazardous activities that could cause injury.
- Don't drive if you feel dizzy or have blurred vision.

Airplane passengers:
No problems expected.

Discontinuing:
Don't discontinue without consulting doctor. Dose may require gradual reduction if you have taken drug for a long time. Doses of other drugs may also require adjustment.

Others:
Carry identification to state you take anticoagulants.

 INTERACTION WITH OTHER DRUGS

GENERIC NAME OR DRUG CLASS	COMBINED EFFECT
Acetaminophen	Increased dicumarol effect.
Allopurinol	Increased dicumarol effect.
Androgens	Increased dicumarol effect.
Antacids (large doses)	Decreased dicumarol effect.
Antibiotics	Increased dicumarol effect.
Anticonvulsants (hydantoin)	Increased effect of both drugs.
Antidepressants (tricyclic)	Increased dicumarol effect.
Antidiabetics (oral)	Increased dicumarol effect.
Antihistamines	Unpredictable increased or decreased anticoagulant effect.
Barbiturates	Decreased dicumarol effect.
Benzodiazepines	Unpredictable increased or decreased anticoagulant effect.
Carbamazepine	Decreased dicumarol effect.

Additional interactions on page 836.

 INTERACTION WITH OTHER SUBSTANCES

INTERACTS WITH	COMBINED EFFECT
Alcohol:	Can increase or decrease effect of anticoagulant. Use with caution.
Beverages:	None expected.
Cocaine:	None expected.
Foods: High in vitamin K such as fish, liver, spinach, cabbage.	May decrease anticoagulant effect.
Marijuana:	None expected.
Tobacco:	None expected.

DICYCLOMINE

BRAND NAMES

Bentyl	Spasmoban
Bentylol	Triactin
Cyclobec	Viscerol
Dyspas	
Formulex	
Menospasm	

 USES

Reduces spasms of digestive system, bladder and urethra.

 DOSAGE & USAGE INFORMATION

How to take:
- Tablet, syrup or capsule—Swallow with liquid or food to lessen stomach irritation.
- Drops—Dilute dose in beverage before swallowing.

When to take:
30 minutes before meals (unless directed otherwise by doctor).

If you forget a dose:
Take as soon as you remember up to 2 hours late. If more than 2 hours, wait for next scheduled dose (don't double this dose).

What drug does:
Blocks nerve impulses at parasympathetic nerve endings, preventing muscle contractions and gland secretions of organs involved.

Time lapse before drug works:
15 to 30 minutes.

Don't take with:
See Interaction column and consult doctor.

 OVERDOSE

Symptoms:
Dilated pupils; rapid pulse and breathing; dizziness; fever; hallucinations; confusion; slurred speech; agitation; flushed face; convulsions; coma.

What to do:
- Dial 0 (operator) or 911 (emergency) for an ambulance or medical help. Then give first aid immediately.
- Additional emergency information on page 886.

POSSIBLE ADVERSE REACTIONS OR SIDE EFFECTS

SYMPTOMS	FREQUENCY	WHAT TO DO
Brain & nervous system:		
● Headache	Infrequent	4
● Confusion, delirium.	Common	3
Skin:		
Rash or hives.	Rare	3
Eyes:		
Pain, blurred vision.	Rare	3
Ears, nose, throat:		
Dryness	Common	6
Digestive:		
● Constipation	Common	5
● Nausea, vomiting.	Common	4
Heart & lungs:		
Rapid heartbeat.	Common	3
Blood vessels:	None expected.	
Muscles, bones, joints:	None expected.	
Genital, urinary:		
Difficult urination.	Infrequent	4
Kidneys:	None expected.	
Liver:	None expected.	
Allergic:	None expected.	
Blood:	None expected.	
Others:		
Less perspiration.	Common	4

1- Life-threatening. Seek emergency treatment immediately.
2- Discontinue. Seek emergency treatment.
3- Discontinue. Call doctor right away.
4- Continue. Call doctor when convenient.
5- Continue. Tell doctor at next visit.
6- No action necessary.

DICYCLOMINE

 WARNINGS & PRECAUTIONS

Don't take if:
- You are allergic to any anticholinergic.
- You have trouble with stomach bloating.
- You have difficulty emptying your bladder completely.
- You have narrow-angle glaucoma.
- You have severe ulcerative colitis.

Before you start, consult your doctor:
- If you have open-angle glaucoma.
- If you have angina.
- If you have chronic bronchitis or asthma.
- If you have hiatal hernia.
- If you have liver disease.
- If you have enlarged prostate.
- If you have myasthenia gravis.
- If you have peptic ulcer.
- If you will have surgery within 2 months, including dental surgery, requiring general or spinal anesthesia.

Over age 60:
Adverse reactions and side effects may be more frequent and severe than in younger persons.

Pregnancy:
Studies inconclusive on harm to unborn child. Animal studies show fetal abnormalities. Decide with your doctor whether drug benefits justify risk to unborn child.

Breast-feeding:
Drug passes into milk and decreases milk flow. Avoid drug or discontinue nursing until you finish medicine. Consult doctor for advice on maintaining milk supply.

Infants & children:
Use only under medical supervision.

Prolonged use:
Chronic constipation, possible fecal impaction. Consult doctor immediately.

Skin & sunlight:
No problems expected.

Driving, piloting or hazardous work:
Use disqualifies you for piloting aircraft. Otherwise, no problems expected.

Airplane passengers:
No problems expected.

Discontinuing:
May be unnecessary to finish medicine. Follow doctor's instructions.

Others:
No problems expected.

 INTERACTION WITH OTHER DRUGS

GENERIC NAME OR DRUG CLASS	COMBINED EFFECT
Amantadine	Increased dicyclomine effect.
Anticholinergics (other)	Increased dicyclomine effect.
Antidepressants (tricyclic)	Increased dicyclomine effect.
Antihistamines	Increased dicyclomine effect.
Cortisone drugs	Increased internal-eye pressure.
Haloperidol	Increased internal-eye pressure.
MAO inhibitors	Increased dicyclomine effect.
Meperidine	Increased dicyclomine effect.
Methylphenidate	Increased dicyclomine effect.
Orphenadrine	Increased dicyclomine effect.
Phenothiazines	Increased dicyclomine effect.
Pilocarpine	Loss of pilocarpine effect in glaucoma treatment.
Vitamin C	Decreased dicyclomine effect. Avoid large doses of vitamin C.

 INTERACTION WITH OTHER SUBSTANCES

INTERACTS WITH	COMBINED EFFECT
Alcohol:	None expected.
Beverages:	None expected.
Cocaine:	Excessively rapid heartbeat. Avoid.
Foods:	None expected.
Marijuana:	Drowsiness and dry mouth.
Tobacco:	None expected.

DIETHYLPROPION

BRAND NAMES

D.E.P.-75	Nobesine-75	Ro-Diet
Depletite	Nu-Dispoz	Tenuate
Dietec	Regibon	Tepanil

GENERAL INFORMATION

Habit forming? Yes
Prescription needed? Yes
Available as generic? Yes
Drug class: Appetite suppressant

USES

Suppresses appetite.

DOSAGE & USAGE INFORMATION

How to take:
- Tablet—Swallow with liquid. You may chew or crush tablet.
- Extended-release tablets or capsules—Swallow each dose whole with liquid.

When to take:
- Long-acting forms—10 to 14 hours before bedtime.
- Short-acting forms—1 hour before meals. Last dose no later than 4 to 6 hours before bedtime.

If you forget a dose:
- Long-acting form—Take as soon as you remember up to 2 hours late. If more than 2 hours, wait for next scheduled dose (don't double this dose).
- Short-acting form—Wait for next scheduled dose. Don't double this dose.

What drug does:
Apparently stimulates brain's appetite-control center.

Time lapse before drug works:
Begins in 1 hour. Short-acting form lasts 4 hours. Long-acting form lasts 14 hours.

Don't take with:
- Non-prescription drugs without consulting doctor.
- See Interaction column and consult doctor.

OVERDOSE

Symptoms:
Irritability, overactivity, trembling, insomnia, mood changes, rapid heartbeat, confusion, disorientation, hallucinations, convulsions, coma.

What to do:
- Dial 0 (operator) or 911 (emergency) for an ambulance or medical help. Then give first aid immediately.
- Additional emergency information on page 886.

POSSIBLE ADVERSE REACTIONS OR SIDE EFFECTS

SYMPTOMS	FREQUENCY	WHAT TO DO
Brain & nervous system:		
● Irritability, nervousness, insomnia.	Common	4
● Mood changes.	Rare	3
Skin:		
● Hair loss.	Rare	4
● Rash or hives.	Rare	3
Eyes:		
Blurred vision.	Infrequent	4
Ears, nose, throat:		
Unpleasant taste or dry mouth.	Infrequent	4
Digestive:		
Constipation or diarrhea, nausea, vomiting, cramps.	Infrequent	4
Heart & lungs:		
● Irregular or pounding heartbeat.	Infrequent	3
● Breathing difficulty.	Rare	3
Blood vessels, muscles, bones, joints, kidneys, liver, allergic, blood:	None expected.	
Genital, urinary:		
Urinary urgency and difficulty.	Infrequent	3
Others:		
● False sense of well-being.	Common	4
● Changes in sex drive.	Infrequent	4
● Sweat increase.	Infrequent	4

1-Life-threatening. Seek emergency treatment immediately.
2-Discontinue. Seek emergency treatment.
3-Discontinue. Call doctor right away.
4-Continue. Call doctor when convenient.

DIETHYLPROPION

WARNINGS & PRECAUTIONS

Don't take if:
- You are allergic to any sympathomimetic or phenylpropanolamine.
- You have glaucoma.
- You have taken MAO inhibitors within 2 weeks.
- You plan to become pregnant within medication period.
- You have a history of drug abuse.

Before you start, consult your doctor:
- If you have high blood pressure or heart disease.
- If you have an overactive thyroid, nervous tension or "anxiety."
- If you have epilepsy.

Over age 60:
Adverse reactions and side effects may be more frequent and severe than in younger persons.

Pregnancy:
Safety not established. Avoid.

Breast-feeding:
No proven problems. Consult doctor.

Infants & children:
Don't give to children younger than 12.

Prolonged use:
Loses effectiveness. Avoid.

Skin & sunlight:
No problems expected.

Driving, piloting or hazardous work:
Don't drive or pilot aircraft until you learn how medicine affects you. Don't work around dangerous machinery. Don't climb ladders or work in high places. Danger increases if you drink alcohol or take medicine affecting alertness and reflexes, such as antihistamines, tranquilizers, sedatives, pain medicine, narcotics and mind-altering drugs.

Airplane passengers:
No problems expected.

Discontinuing:
Don't discontinue without consulting doctor. Dose may require gradual reduction if you have taken drug for a long time. Doses of other drugs may also require adjustment.

Others:
Don't increase dose.

INTERACTION WITH OTHER DRUGS

GENERIC NAME OR DRUG CLASS	COMBINED EFFECT
Appetite suppressants (other)	Dangerous overstimulation.
Caffeine	Increased stimulant effect of diethylpropion.
Guanethidine	Decreased guanethidine effect.
Hydralazine	Decreased hydralazine effect.
MAO inhibitors	Dangerous blood-pressure rise.
Methyldopa	Decreased methyldopa effect.
Phenothiazines	Decreased diethylpropion effect.
Rauwolfia alkaloids	Decreased effect of rauwolfia alkaloids.

INTERACTION WITH OTHER SUBSTANCES

INTERACTS WITH	COMBINED EFFECT
Alcohol: Beer, chianti wines, vermouth.	Dangerous blood-pressure rise.
Beverages: • Caffeine drinks	Excessive stimulation.
• Drinks containing tyramine (see page 851).	Blood-pressure rise.
Cocaine:	Excessive stimulation.
Foods: Foods containing tyramine (see page 851).	Blood-pressure rise.
Marijuana:	Frequent use—Irregular heartbeat.
Tobacco:	None expected.

DIETHYLSTILBESTROL

BRAND NAMES

DES
Stilbestrol
Stilphostrol

GENERAL INFORMATION

Habit forming? No
Prescription needed? Yes
Available as generic? Yes
Drug class: Female sex hormone (estrogen)

USES

- Treatment for symptoms of menopause and menstrual-cycle irregularity.
- Replacement for female hormone deficiency.
- Treatment for cancer of prostate and breast.

DOSAGE & USAGE INFORMATION

How to take:
- Tablet—Swallow with liquid. If you can't swallow whole, crumble tablet and take with liquid or food.
- Vaginal suppositories—Use as directed on label.

When to take:
At the same time each day.

If you forget a dose:
Take as soon as you remember up to 12 hours late. If more than 12 hours, wait for next scheduled dose (don't double this dose).

What drug does:
Restores normal estrogen level in tissues.

Time lapse before drug works:
10 to 20 days.

Don't take with:
See Interaction column and consult doctor.

OVERDOSE

Symptoms:
Nausea, vomiting, fluid retention, breast enlargement and discomfort, abnormal vaginal bleeding.

What to do:
Overdose unlikely to threaten life. If person takes much larger amount than prescribed, call doctor, poison-control center or hospital emergency room for instructions.

POSSIBLE ADVERSE REACTIONS OR SIDE EFFECTS

SYMPTOMS	FREQUENCY	WHAT TO DO
Brain & nervous system:		
Depression, dizziness, irritability.	Infrequent	4
Skin:		
• Rash	Infrequent	3
• Brown blotches.	Infrequent	5
• Hair loss.	Infrequent	5
Eyes, ears, nose, throat, heart & lungs, muscles, bones, joints, kidneys, allergic, blood:	None expected.	
Digestive:		
• Stomach or side pain.	Infrequent	3
• Stomach cramps.	Common	3
• Appetite loss.	Common	4
• Nausea, diarrhea.	Common	5
• Vomiting	Infrequent	4
Blood vessels:		
Swollen ankles, feet.	Common	5
Genital, urinary:		
Vaginal discharge or bleeding.	Infrequent	5
Liver:		
Jaundice (yellow skin and eyes).	Rare	3
Others:		
• Breast lumps.	Infrequent	4
• Swollen, tender breasts.	Common	5
• Changes in sex drive.	Infrequent	5

1- Life-threatening. Seek emergency treatment immediately.
2- Discontinue. Seek emergency treatment.
3- Discontinue. Call doctor right away.
4- Continue. Call doctor when convenient.
5- Continue. Tell doctor at next visit.

DIETHYLSTILBESTROL

WARNINGS & PRECAUTIONS

Don't take if:
- You are allergic to any estrogen-containing drugs.
- You have impaired liver function.
- You have had blood clots, stroke or heart attack.
- You have unexplained vaginal bleeding.

Before you start, consult your doctor:
- If you have had cancer of breast or reproductive organs, fibrocystic breast disease, fibroid tumors of the uterus or endometriosis.
- If you have had migraine headaches, epilepsy or porphyria.
- If you have diabetes, high blood pressure, asthma, congestive heart failure, kidney disease or gallstones.
- If you plan to become pregnant within 3 months.

Over age 60:
Controversial. You and your doctor must decide if drug risks outweigh benefits.

Pregnancy:
Risk to unborn child outweighs drug benefits. Don't use.

Breast-feeding:
Drug filters into milk. May harm child. Avoid.

Infants & children:
Not recommended.

Prolonged use:
Increased growth of fibroid tumors of uterus. Possible association with cancer of uterus.

Skin & sunlight:
May cause rash or intensify sunburn in areas exposed to sun or sunlamp.

Driving, piloting or hazardous work:
No problems expected.

Airplane passengers:
No problems expected.

Discontinuing:
You may need to discontinue diethylstilbestrol periodically. Consult your doctor.

Others:
In rare instances, may cause blood clot in lung, brain or leg. Symptoms are *sudden* severe headache, coordination loss, vision change, chest pain, breathing difficulty, slurred speech, pain in legs or groin. Seek emergency treatment immediately.

INTERACTION WITH OTHER DRUGS

GENERIC NAME OR DRUG CLASS	COMBINED EFFECT
Anticoagulants (oral)	Decreased anticoagulant effect.
Anticonvulsants (hydantoin)	Increased seizures.
Antidiabetics (oral)	Unpredictable increase or decrease in blood sugar.
Clofibrate	Decreased clofibrate effect.
Carbamazepine	Increased seizures.
Meprobamate	Increased diethylstilbestrol effect.
Phenobarbital	Decreased diethylstilbestrol effect.
Primidone	Decreased diethylstilbestrol effect.
Rifampin	Decreased diethylstilbestrol effect.
Thyroid hormones	Decreased thyroid effect.

INTERACTION WITH OTHER SUBSTANCES

INTERACTS WITH	COMBINED EFFECT
Alcohol:	None expected.
Beverages:	None expected.
Cocaine:	No proven problems.
Foods:	None expected.
Marijuana:	Possible menstrual irregularities and bleeding between periods.
Tobacco:	Increased risk of blood clots leading to stroke or heart attack.

DIGITALIS

BRAND NAMES

Digifortis
Pil-Digis

GENERAL INFORMATION

Habit forming? No
Prescription needed? Yes
Available as generic? Yes
Drug class: Digitalis preparation

USES

- Strengthens weak heart-muscle contractions to prevent congestive heart failure.
- Corrects irregular heartbeat.

DOSAGE & USAGE INFORMATION

How to take:
- Tablet or capsule—Swallow with liquid. If you can't swallow whole, crumble tablet or open capsule and take with liquid or food.
- Liquid—Dilute dose in beverage before swallowing.

When to take:
At the same time each day.

If you forget a dose:
Take as soon as you remember up to 12 hours late. If more than 12 hours, wait for next scheduled dose (don't double this dose).

What drug does:
- Strengthens heart-muscle contraction.
- Delays nerve impulses to heart.

Time lapse before drug works:
May require regular use for a week or more.

Don't take with:
- Non-prescription drugs without consulting doctor.
- See Interaction column and consult doctor.

OVERDOSE

Symptoms:
Nausea, vomiting, diarrhea, vision disturbances with halos around lights, irregular heartbeat, confusion, hallucinations, convulsions.

What to do:
- Dial 0 (operator) or 911 (emergency) for an ambulance or medical help. Then give first aid immediately.
- Additional emergency information on page 886.

POSSIBLE ADVERSE REACTIONS OR SIDE EFFECTS

SYMPTOMS	FREQUENCY	WHAT TO DO
Brain & nervous system: Drowsiness, lethargy, disorientation.	Infrequent	3
Skin: Rash, hives.	Rare	3
Eyes: Double or yellow-green vision.	Rare	4
Ears, nose, throat:	None expected.	
Digestive: Appetite loss, diarrhea.	Common	4
Heart & lungs:	None expected.	
Blood vessels:	None expected.	
Muscles, bones, joints:	None expected.	
Genital, urinary:	None expected.	
Kidneys:	None expected.	
Liver:	None expected.	
Allergic:	None expected.	
Blood:	None expected.	
Others: •Enlarged, sensitive male breasts.	Rare	4
•Tiredness, weakness.	Rare	4

1- Life-threatening. Seek emergency treatment immediately.
2- Discontinue. Seek emergency treatment.
3- Discontinue. Call doctor right away.
4- Continue. Call doctor when convenient.
5- Continue. Tell doctor at next visit.
6- No action necessary.

WARNINGS & PRECAUTIONS

Don't take if:
- You are allergic to any digitalis preparation.
- Your heartbeat is slower than 50 beats per minute.

Before you start, consult your doctor:
- If you have taken another digitalis preparation in past 2 weeks.
- If you have taken a diuretic within 2 weeks.
- If you have liver or kidney disease.
- If you have a thyroid disorder.

Over age 60:
Adverse reactions and side effects may be more frequent and severe than in younger persons.

Pregnancy:
Studies inconclusive on harm to unborn child. Consult your doctor.

Breast-feeding:
Drug filters into milk. May harm child. Avoid.

Infants & children:
Use only under medical supervision.

Prolonged use:
No problems expected.

Skin & sunlight:
No problems expected.

Driving, piloting or hazardous work:
Possible vision disturbances. Otherwise, no problems expected.

Airplane passengers:
Nausea more likely.

Discontinuing:
Don't stop without doctor's advice.

Others:
No problems expected.

INTERACTION WITH OTHER DRUGS

GENERIC NAME OR DRUG CLASS	COMBINED EFFECT
Antacids	Decreased digitalis effect.
Anticonvulsants (hydantoin)	Increased digitalis effect at first, then decreased.
Beta-adrenergic blockers	Increased digitalis effect.
Cortisone drugs	Digitalis toxicity.
Diuretics	Digitalis toxicity.
Ephedrine	Disturbs heart rhythm. Avoid.
Epinephrine	Disturbs heart rhythm. Avoid.
Guanethidine	Increased digitalis effect.
Laxatives	Decreased digitalis effect.
Oxyphenbutazone	Decreased digitalis effect.
Phenobarbital	Decreased digitalis effect.
Phenylbutazone	Decreased digitalis effect.
Quinidine	Increased digitalis effect.
Rauwolfia alkaloids	Increased digitalis effect.
Thyroid hormones	Digitalis toxicity.

INTERACTION WITH OTHER SUBSTANCES

INTERACTS WITH	COMBINED EFFECT
Alcohol:	None expected.
Beverages: Caffeine drinks	Irregular heartbeat. Avoid.
Cocaine:	Irregular heartbeat. Avoid.
Foods:	None expected.
Marijuana:	Decreased digitalis effect.
Tobacco:	Irregular heartbeat. Avoid.

DIGITOXIN

BRAND NAMES

Crystodigin
Purodigin

GENERAL INFORMATION

Habit forming? No
Prescription needed? Yes
Available as generic? Yes
Drug class: Digitalis preparation

USES

- Strengthens weak heart-muscle contractions to prevent congestive heart failure.
- Corrects irregular heartbeat.

DOSAGE & USAGE INFORMATION

How to take:
- Tablet or capsule—Swallow with liquid. If you can't swallow whole, crumble tablet or open capsule and take with liquid or food.
- Liquid—Dilute dose in beverage before swallowing.

When to take:
At the same time each day.

If you forget a dose:
Take as soon as you remember up to 12 hours late. If more than 12 hours, wait for next scheduled dose (don't double this dose).

What drug does:
- Strengthens heart-muscle contraction.
- Delays nerve impulses to heart.

Time lapse before drug works:
May require regular use for a week or more.

Don't take with:
- Non-prescription drugs without consulting doctor.
- See Interaction column and consult doctor.

OVERDOSE

Symptoms:
Nausea, vomiting, diarrhea, vision disturbances with halos around lights, irregular heartbeat, confusion, hallucinations, convulsions.

What to do:
- Dial 0 (operator) or 911 (emergency) for an ambulance or medical help. Then give first aid immediately.
- Additional emergency information on page 886.

POSSIBLE ADVERSE REACTIONS OR SIDE EFFECTS

SYMPTOMS	FREQUENCY	WHAT TO DO
Brain & nervous system: Drowsiness, lethargy, disorientation.	Infrequent	3
Skin: Rash, hives.	Rare	3
Eyes: Double or yellow-green vision.	Rare	4
Ears, nose, throat:	None expected.	
Digestive: Appetite loss, diarrhea.	Common	4
Heart & lungs:	None expected.	
Blood vessels:	None expected.	
Muscles, bones, joints:	None expected.	
Genital, urinary:	None expected.	
Kidneys:	None expected.	
Liver:	None expected.	
Allergic:	None expected.	
Blood:	None expected.	
Others: • Enlarged, sensitive male breasts.	Rare	4
• Tiredness, weakness.	Rare	4

1- Life-threatening. Seek emergency treatment immediately.
2- Discontinue. Seek emergency treatment.
3- Discontinue. Call doctor right away.
4- Continue. Call doctor when convenient.
5- Continue. Tell doctor at next visit.
6- No action necessary.

DIGITOXIN

WARNINGS & PRECAUTIONS

Don't take if:
- You are allergic to any digitalis preparation.
- Your heartbeat is slower than 50 beats per minute.

Before you start, consult your doctor:
- If you have taken another digitalis preparation in past 2 weeks.
- If you have taken a diuretic within 2 weeks.
- If you have liver or kidney disease.
- If you have a thyroid disorder.

Over age 60:
Adverse reactions and side effects may be more frequent and severe than in younger persons.

Pregnancy:
Studies inconclusive on harm to unborn child. Consult your doctor.

Breast-feeding:
Drug filters into milk. May harm child. Avoid.

Infants & children:
Use only under medical supervision.

Prolonged use:
No problems expected.

Skin & sunlight:
No problems expected.

Driving, piloting or hazardous work:
Possible vision disturbances. Otherwise, no problems expected.

Airplane passengers:
Nausea more likely.

Discontinuing:
Don't stop without doctor's advice.

Others:
No problems expected.

INTERACTION WITH OTHER DRUGS

GENERIC NAME OR DRUG CLASS	COMBINED EFFECT
Antacids	Decreased digitoxin effect.
Anticonvulsants (hydantoin)	Increased digitoxin effect at first, then decreased.
Beta-adrenergic blockers	Increased digitoxin effect.
Cortisone drugs	Digitoxin toxicity.
Diuretics	Digitoxin toxicity.
Ephedrine	Disturbs heart rhythm. Avoid.
Epinephrine	Disturbs heart rhythm. Avoid.
Guanethidine	Increased digitoxin effect.
Laxatives	Decreased digitoxin effect.
Oxyphenbutazone	Decreased digitoxin effect.
Phenobarbital	Decreased digitoxin effect.
Phenylbutazone	Decreased digitoxin effect.
Quinidine	Increased digitoxin effect.
Rauwolfia alkaloids	Increased digitoxin effect.
Thyroid hormones	Digitoxin toxicity.

INTERACTION WITH OTHER SUBSTANCES

INTERACTS WITH	COMBINED EFFECT
Alcohol:	None expected.
Beverages: Caffeine drinks	Irregular heartbeat. Avoid.
Cocaine:	Irregular heartbeat. Avoid.
Foods:	None expected.
Marijuana:	Increased digitoxin effect.
Tobacco:	Irregular heartbeat. Avoid.

DIGOXIN

BRAND NAMES

Lanoxin

GENERAL INFORMATION

Habit forming? No
Prescription needed? Yes
Available as generic? Yes
Drug class: Digitalis preparation

 USES

- Strengthens weak heart-muscle contractions to prevent congestive heart failure.
- Corrects irregular heartbeat.

 DOSAGE & USAGE INFORMATION

How to take:
- Tablet or capsule—Swallow with liquid. If you can't swallow whole, crumble tablet or open capsule and take with liquid or food.
- Liquid—Dilute dose in beverage before swallowing.

When to take:
At the same time each day.

If you forget a dose:
Take as soon as you remember up to 12 hours late. If more than 12 hours, wait for next scheduled dose (don't double this dose).

What drug does:
- Strengthens heart-muscle contraction.
- Delays nerve impulses to heart.

Time lapse before drug works:
May require regular use for a week or more.

Don't take with:
- Non-prescription drugs without consulting doctor.
- See Interaction column and consult doctor.

 OVERDOSE

Symptoms:
Nausea, vomiting, diarrhea, vision disturbances with halos around lights, irregular heartbeat, confusion, hallucinations, convulsions.

What to do:
- Dial 0 (operator) or 911 (emergency) for an ambulance or medical help. Then give first aid immediately.
- Additional emergency information on page 886.

POSSIBLE ADVERSE REACTIONS OR SIDE EFFECTS

SYMPTOMS	FREQUENCY	WHAT TO DO
Brain & nervous system: Drowsiness, lethargy, disorientation.	Infrequent	3
Skin: Rash, hives.	Rare	3
Eyes: Double or yellow-green vision.	Rare	4
Ears, nose, throat:	None expected.	
Digestive: Appetite loss, diarrhea.	Common	4
Heart & lungs:	None expected.	
Blood vessels:	None expected.	
Muscles, bones, joints:	None expected.	
Genital, urinary:	None expected.	
Kidneys:	None expected.	
Liver:	None expected.	
Allergic:	None expected.	
Blood:	None expected.	
Others: • Enlarged, sensitive male breasts.	Rare	4
• Tiredness, weakness.	Rare	4

1 - Life-threatening. Seek emergency treatment immediately.
2 - Discontinue. Seek emergency treatment.
3 - Discontinue. Call doctor right away.
4 - Continue. Call doctor when convenient.
5 - Continue. Tell doctor at next visit.
6 - No action necessary.

DIGOXIN

WARNINGS & PRECAUTIONS

Don't take if:
- You are allergic to any digitalis preparation.
- Your heartbeat is slower than 50 beats per minute.

Before you start, consult your doctor:
- If you have taken another digitalis preparation in past 2 weeks.
- If you have taken a diuretic within 2 weeks.
- If you have liver or kidney disease.
- If you have a thyroid disorder.

Over age 60:
Adverse reactions and side effects may be more frequent and severe than in younger persons.

Pregnancy:
Studies inconclusive on harm to unborn child. Consult your doctor.

Breast-feeding:
Drug filters into milk. May harm child. Avoid.

Infants & children:
Use only under medical supervision.

Prolonged use:
No problems expected.

Skin & sunlight:
No problems expected.

Driving, piloting or hazardous work:
Possible vision disturbances. Otherwise, no problems expected.

Airplane passengers:
Nausea more likely

Discontinuing:
Don't stop without doctor's advice.

Others:
No problems expected.

INTERACTION WITH OTHER DRUGS

GENERIC NAME OR DRUG CLASS	COMBINED EFFECT
Antacids	Decreased digoxin effect.
Anticonvulsants (hydantoin)	Increased digoxin effect at first, then decreased.
Beta-adrenergic blockers	Increased digoxin effect.
Cortisone drugs	Digoxin toxicity.
Diuretics	Digoxin toxicity.
Ephedrine	Disturbs heart rhythm. Avoid.
Epinephrine	Disturbs heart rhythm. Avoid.
Guanethidine	Increased digoxin effect.
Laxatives	Decreased digoxin effect.
Oxyphenbutazone	Decreased digoxin effect.
Phenobarbital	Decreased digoxin effect.
Phenylbutazone	Decreased digoxin effect.
Quinidine	Increased digoxin effect.
Rauwolfia alkaloids	Increased digoxin effect.
Thyroid hormones	Digoxin toxicity.

INTERACTION WITH OTHER SUBSTANCES

INTERACTS WITH	COMBINED EFFECT
Alcohol:	None expected.
Beverages: Caffeine drinks	Irregular heartbeat. Avoid.
Cocaine:	Irregular heartbeat. Avoid.
Foods:	None expected.
Marijuana:	Decreased digoxin effect.
Tobacco:	Irregular heartbeat. Avoid.

DILTIAZEM

BRAND NAMES

Cardizem

GENERAL INFORMATION

Habit forming? No
Prescription needed? Yes
Available as generic? No
Drug class: Calcium-channel blocker,
antiarrhythmic, antianginal

 ## USES

- Prevents angina attacks.
- Stabilizes irregular heartbeat.

 ## DOSAGE & USAGE INFORMATION

How to take:
Tablet or capsule—Swallow with liquid.

When to take:
At the same times each day 1 hour before or 2 hours after eating.

If you forget a dose:
Take as soon as you remember up to 2 hours late. If more than 2 hours, wait for next scheduled dose (don't double this dose).

What drug does:
- Reduces work that heart must perform.
- Reduces normal artery pressure.
- Increases oxygen to heart muscle.

Time lapse before drug works:
1 to 2 hours.

Don't take with:
See Interaction column and consult doctor.

 ## OVERDOSE

Symptoms:
Unusually fast or unusually slow heartbeat; loss of consciousness, cardiac arrest.

What to do:
- Dial 0 (operator) or 911 (emergency) for an ambulance or medical help. Then give first aid immediately.
- Additional emergency information on page 886.

POSSIBLE ADVERSE REACTIONS OR SIDE EFFECTS

SYMPTOMS	FREQUENCY	WHAT TO DO
Brain & nervous system:		
• Dizziness	Infrequent	4
• Headache	Rare	5
• Fainting	Rare	3
Skin:		
Rash	Rare	3
Eyes, ears, nose, throat, kidneys, blood vessels, allergic, blood:	None expected.	
Digestive:		
Nausea, constipation or diarrhea, vomiting, indigestion.	Infrequent	5
Heart & lungs:		
• Unusually fast or slow heartbeat.	Infrequent	3
• Wheezing, cough, shortness of breath.	Infrequent	3
Muscles, bones, joints:		
• Numbness, tingling in hands and feet.	Infrequent	4
• Swelling of ankles, feet, legs.	Infrequent	4
Genital, urinary:		
Difficult urination.	Infrequent	4
Liver:		
Jaundice (yellow eyes and skin).	Rare	3
Others:		
Tiredness	Common	5

1- Life-threatening. Seek emergency treatment immediately.
2- Discontinue. Seek emergency treatment.
3- Discontinue. Call doctor right away.
4- Continue. Call doctor when convenient.
5- Continue. Tell doctor at next visit.

WARNINGS & PRECAUTIONS

Don't take if:
You are allergic to any calcium-channel blocker.

Before you start, consult your doctor:
- If you have kidney or liver disease.
- If you have high or low blood pressure.
- If you have heart disease other than coronary artery disease.

Over age 60:
Adverse reactions and side effects may be more frequent and severe than in younger persons.

Pregnancy:
No proven harm to unborn child. Avoid if possible.

Breast-feeding:
No problems expected.

Infants & children:
Not recommended.

Prolonged use:
No problems expected.

Skin & sunlight:
May cause rash or intensify sunburn in areas exposed to sun or sunlamp.

Driving, piloting or hazardous work:
Avoid if you feel dizzy. Otherwise, no problems expected.

Airplane passengers:
No problems expected.

Discontinuing:
Don't discontinue without consulting doctor.

Others:
Learn to check your own pulse rate. If it drops to 50 beats per minute or lower, don't take diltiazem until your consult your doctor.

INTERACTION WITH OTHER DRUGS

GENERIC NAME OR DRUG CLASS	COMBINED EFFECT
Antihypertensives	Dangerous blood-pressure drop.
Beta-adrenergic blockers	Decreased angina attacks.
Diuretics	Dangerous blood-pressure drop.
Disopyramide	May cause dangerously slow, fast or irregular heartbeat.
Nitrates	Reduced angina attacks.
Quinidine	Increased quinidine effect.

INTERACTION WITH OTHER SUBSTANCES

INTERACTS WITH	COMBINED EFFECT
Alcohol:	Dangerously low blood pressure.
Beverages:	None expected.
Cocaine:	Possible irregular heartbeat. Avoid.
Foods:	None expected.
Marijuana:	Possible irregular heartbeat. Avoid.
Tobacco:	Possible rapaid heartbeat. Avoid.

DIMENHYDRINATE

BRAND NAMES

Dimentabs	Marine
Dramaban	Novodimenate
Dramamine	Travamine
Eldodram	
Gravol	

GENERAL INFORMATION

Habit forming? No
Prescription needed? High strength: Yes
Low strength: No
Available as generic? Yes
Drug class: Antihistamine

USES

- Reduces allergic symptoms such as hay fever, hives, rash or itching.
- Prevents motion sickness, nausea, vomiting.
- Induces sleep.

DOSAGE & USAGE INFORMATION

How to take:
Tablet or liquid—Swallow with liquid or food to lessen stomach irritation.

When to take:
Varies with form. Follow label directions.

If you forget a dose:
Take as soon as you remember up to 2 hours late. If more than 2 hours, wait for next scheduled dose (don't double this dose).

What drug does:
Blocks action of histamine after an allergic response triggers histamine release in sensitive cells.

Time lapse before drug works:
30 minutes.

Don't take with:
See Interaction column and consult doctor.

OVERDOSE

Symptoms:
Convulsions, red face, hallucinations, coma.

What to do:
- Dial 0 (operator) or 911 (emergency) for an ambulance or medical help. Then give first aid immediately.
- If patient is unconscious and not breathing, give mouth-to-mouth breathing. If there is no heartbeat, use cardiac massage and mouth-to-mouth breathing (CPR). Don't try to make patient vomit. If you can't get help quickly, take patient to nearest emergency facility.
- Additional emergency information on page 886.

POSSIBLE ADVERSE REACTIONS OR SIDE EFFECTS

SYMPTOMS	FREQUENCY	WHAT TO DO
Brain & nervous system:		
• Nightmares, agitation, irritability.	Rare	3
• Drowsiness, dizziness.	Common	5
Skin:	None expected.	
Eyes:		
• Vision changes.	Infrequent	3
• Less tolerance for contact lenses.	Infrequent	4
Ears, nose, throat:		
• Sore throat, fever.	Rare	3
• Dry mouth, nose, throat.	Common	5
Digestive:		
• Nausea	Common	5
• Appetite loss.	Infrequent	5
Heart & lungs:		
Rapid heartbeat.	Rare	3
Blood vessels:		
Unusual bleeding or bruising.	Rare	3
Muscles, bones, joints, kidneys, liver, allergic, blood:	None expected.	
Genital, urinary:		
Urination difficulty.	Infrequent	4
Others:		
Fatigue, weakness.	Rare	3

1 - Life-threatening. Seek emergency treatment immediately.
2 - Discontinue. Seek emergency treatment.
3 - Discontinue. Call doctor right away.
4 - Continue. Call doctor when convenient.
5 - Continue. Tell doctor at next visit.
6 - No action necessary.

DIMENHYDRINATE

 ## WARNINGS & PRECAUTIONS

Don't take if:
You are allergic to any antihistamine.

Before you start, consult your doctor:
- If you have glaucoma.
- If you have enlarged prostate.
- If you have asthma.
- If you have kidney disease.
- If you have peptic ulcer.
- If you will have surgery within 2 months, including dental surgery, requiring general or spinal anesthesia.

Over age 60:
Don't exceed recommended dose. Adverse reactions and side effects may be more frequent and severe than in younger persons, especially urination difficulty, diminished alertness and other brain and nervous-system symptoms.

Pregnancy:
No proven harm to unborn child. Avoid if possible.

Breast-feeding:
Drug passes into milk. Avoid drug or discontinue nursing until you finish medicine. Consult doctor for advice on maintaining milk supply.

Infants & children:
Not recommended for premature or newborn infants. Otherwise, no problems expected.

Prolonged use:
Avoid. May damage bone marrow and nerve cells.

Skin & sunlight:
May cause rash or intensify sunburn in areas exposed to sun or sunlamp.

Driving, piloting or hazardous work:
Don't drive or pilot aircraft until you learn how medicine affects you. Don't work around dangerous machinery. Don't climb ladders or work in high places. Danger increases if you drink alcohol or take medicine affecting alertness and reflexes, such as antihistamines, tranquilizers, sedatives, pain medicine, narcotics and mind-altering drugs.

Airplane passengers:
No problems expected.

Discontinuing:
No problems expected.

Others:
May mask symptoms of hearing damage from aspirin, other salicylates, cisplatin, paromomycin, vancomycin or anticonvulsants. Consult doctor if you use these.

 ## INTERACTION WITH OTHER DRUGS

GENERIC NAME OR DRUG CLASS	COMBINED EFFECT
Anticholinergics	Increased anticholinergic effect.
Antidepressants	Excess sedation. Avoid.
Antihistamines (other)	Excess sedation. Avoid.
Hypnotics	Excess sedation. Avoid.
MAO inhibitors	Increased dimenhydrinate effect.
Mind-altering drugs	Excess sedation. Avoid.
Narcotics	Excess sedation. Avoid.
Sedatives	Excess sedation. Avoid.
Sleep Inducers	Excess sedation. Avoid.
Tranquilizers	Excess sedation. Avoid.

 ## INTERACTION WITH OTHER SUBSTANCES

INTERACTS WITH	COMBINED EFFECT
Alcohol:	Excess sedation. Avoid.
Beverages: Caffeine drinks	Less dimenhydrinate sedation.
Cocaine:	Decreased dimenhydrinate effect. Avoid.
Foods:	None expected.
Marijuana:	Excess sedation. Avoid.
Tobacco:	None expected.

DIMETHINDENE

BRAND NAMES

Forhistal
Triten

GENERAL INFORMATION

Habit forming? No
Prescription needed? Yes
Available as generic? Yes
Drug class: Antihistamine

USES

- Reduces allergic symptoms such as hay fever, hives, rash or itching.
- Induces sleep.

DOSAGE & USAGE INFORMATION

How to take:
Extended-release tablets or capsules—Take with liquid or food. Swallow each dose whole.

When to take:
Varies with form. Follow label directions.

If you forget a dose:
Take as soon as you remember up to 2 hours late. If more than 2 hours, wait for next scheduled dose (don't double this dose).

What drug does:
Blocks action of histamine after an allergic response triggers histamine release in sensitive cells.

Time lapse before drug works:
30 minutes.

Don't take with:
See Interaction column and consult doctor.

OVERDOSE

Symptoms:
Convulsions, red face, hallucinations, coma.

What to do:
- Dial 0 (operator) or 911 (emergency) for an ambulance or medical help. Then give first aid immediately.
- If patient is unconscious and not breathing, give mouth-to-mouth breathing. If there is no heartbeat, use cardiac massage and mouth-to-mouth breathing (CPR). Don't try to make patient vomit. If you can't get help quickly, take patient to nearest emergency facility.
- Additional emergency information on page 886.

POSSIBLE ADVERSE REACTIONS OR SIDE EFFECTS

SYMPTOMS	FREQUENCY	WHAT TO DO
Brain & nervous system:		
● Nightmares, agitation, irritability.	Rare	3
● Drowsiness, dizziness.	Common	5
Skin:	None expected.	
Eyes:		
● Vision changes.	Infrequent	3
● Less tolerance for contact lenses.	Infrequent	4
Ears, nose, throat:		
● Sore throat, fever.	Rare	3
● Dry mouth, nose, throat.	Common	5
Digestive:		
● Nausea	Common	5
● Appetite loss.	Infrequent	5
Heart & lungs:		
Rapid heartbeat.	Rare	3
Blood vessels:		
Unusual bleeding or bruising.	Rare	3
Muscles, bones, joints, kidneys, liver, allergic, blood:	None expected.	
Genital, urinary:		
Urination difficulty.	Infrequent	4
Others:		
Fatigue, weakness.	Rare	3

1- Life-threatening. Seek emergency treatment immediately.
2- Discontinue. Seek emergency treatment.
3- Discontinue. Call doctor right away.
4- Continue. Call doctor when convenient.
5- Continue. Tell doctor at next visit.
6- No action necessary.

DIMETHINDENE

WARNINGS & PRECAUTIONS

Don't take if:
You are allergic to any antihistamine.

Before you start, consult your doctor:
- If you have glaucoma.
- If you have enlarged prostate.
- If you have asthma.
- If you have kidney disease.
- If you have peptic ulcer.
- If you will have surgery within 2 months, including dental surgery, requiring general or spinal anesthesia.

Over age 60:
Don't exceed recommended dose. Adverse reactions and side effects may be more frequent and severe than in younger persons, especially urination difficulty, diminished alertness and other brain and nervous-system symptoms.

Pregnancy:
No proven harm to unborn child. Avoid if possible.

Breast-feeding:
Drug passes into milk. Avoid drug or discontinue nursing until you finish medicine. Consult doctor for advice on maintaining milk supply.

Infants & children:
Not recommended for premature or newborn infants. Otherwise, no problems expected.

Prolonged use:
Avoid. May damage bone marrow and nerve cells.

Skin & sunlight:
May cause rash or intensify sunburn in areas exposed to sun or sunlamp.

Driving, piloting or hazardous work:
Don't drive or pilot aircraft until you learn how medicine affects you. Don't work around dangerous machinery. Don't climb ladders or work in high places. Danger increases if you drink alcohol or take medicine affecting alertness and reflexes, such as antihistamines, tranquilizers, sedatives, pain medicine, narcotics and mind-altering drugs.

Airplane passengers:
No problems expected.

Discontinuing:
No problems expected.

Others:
May mask symptoms of hearing damage from aspirin, other salicylates, cisplatin, paromomycin, vancomycin or anticonvulsants. Consult doctor if you use these.

INTERACTION WITH OTHER DRUGS

GENERIC NAME OR DRUG CLASS	COMBINED EFFECT
Anticholinergics	Increased anticholinergic effect.
Antidepressants	Excess sedation. Avoid.
Antihistamines (other)	Excess sedation. Avoid.
Hypnotics	Excess sedation. Avoid.
MAO inhibitors	Increased dimethindene effect.
Mind-altering drugs	Excess sedation. Avoid.
Narcotics	Excess sedation. Avoid.
Sedatives	Excess sedation. Avoid.
Sleep inducers	Excess sedation. Avoid.
Tranquilizers	Excess sedation. Avoid.

INTERACTION WITH OTHER SUBSTANCES

INTERACTS WITH	COMBINED EFFECT
Alcohol:	Excess sedation. Avoid.
Beverages: Caffeine drinks	Less dimethindene sedation.
Cocaine:	Decreased dimethindene effect. Avoid.
Foods:	None expected.
Marijuana:	Excess sedation. Avoid.
Tobacco:	None expected.

DIPHENHYDRAMINE

BRAND NAMES

Ambenyl
Expectorant (M)
Benadryl
Bendylate
Benylin
Cough Syrup

Eldadryl
Fenylhist
Insomnal
Nordryl
Nytol

SK-
 Diphenhydramine
Sominex
Valdrene

GENERAL INFORMATION

Habit forming? No
Prescription needed? High strength: Yes
Low strength: No
Available as generic? Yes
Drug class: Antihistamine

USES

- Reduces allergic symptoms such as hay fever, hives, rash or itching.
- Prevents motion sickness, nausea, vomiting.
- Induces sleep.
- Reduces stiffness and tremors of Parkinson's disease.

DOSAGE & USAGE INFORMATION

How to take:
- Tablet or capsule—Swallow with liquid or food to lessen stomach irritation.
- Extended-release tablets or capsules—Swallow each dose whole.
- Suppositories—Remove wrapper and moisten suppository with water. Gently insert larger end into rectum. Push well into rectum with finger.

When to take:
Varies with form. Follow label directions.

If you forget a dose:
Take as soon as you remember up to 2 hours late. If more than 2 hours, wait for next scheduled dose (don't double this dose).

What drug does:
Blocks action of histamine after an allergic response triggers histamine release in sensitive cells.

Time lapse before drug works:
30 minutes.

Don't take with:
See Interaction column and consult doctor.

OVERDOSE

Symptoms:
Convulsions, red face, hallucinations, coma.

What to do:
- Dial 0 (operator) or 911 (emergency) for an ambulance or medical help. Then give first aid immediately.
- Additional emergency information on page 886.

POSSIBLE ADVERSE REACTIONS OR SIDE EFFECTS

SYMPTOMS	FREQUENCY	WHAT TO DO
Brain & nervous system:		
• Nightmares, agitation, irritability.	Rare	3
• Drowsiness, dizziness.	Common	5
Skin:	None expected.	
Eyes:		
• Vision changes.	Infrequent	3
• Less tolerance for contact lenses.	Infrequent	4
Ears, nose, throat:		
• Sore throat, fever.	Rare	3
• Dry mouth, nose, throat.	Common	5
Digestive:		
• Nausea	Common	5
• Appetite loss.	Infrequent	5
Heart & lungs: Rapid heartbeat.	Rare	3
Blood vessels: Unusual bleeding or bruising.	Rare	3
Muscles, bones, joints, kidneys, liver, allergic, blood:	None expected.	
Genital, urinary: Urination difficulty.	Infrequent	4
Others: Fatigue, weakness.	Rare	3

1-Life-threatening. Seek emergency treatment immediately.
2-Discontinue. Seek emergency treatment.
3-Discontinue. Call doctor right away.
4-Continue. Call doctor when convenient.
5-Continue. Tell doctor at next visit.
6-No action necessary.

DIPHENYDRAMINE

WARNINGS & PRECAUTIONS

Don't take if:
You are allergic to any antihistamine.

Before you start, consult your doctor:
- If you have glaucoma.
- If you have enlarged prostate.
- If you have asthma.
- If you have kidney disease.
- If you have peptic ulcer.
- If you will have surgery within 2 months, including dental surgery, requiring general or spinal anesthesia.

Over age 60:
Don't exceed recommended dose. Adverse reactions and side effects may be more frequent and severe than in younger persons, especially urination difficulty, diminished alertness and other brain and nervous-system symptoms.

Pregnancy:
No proven harm to unborn child. Avoid if possible.

Breast-feeding:
Drug passes into milk. Avoid drug or discontinue nursing until you finish medicine. Consult doctor for advice on maintaining milk supply.

Infants & children:
Not recommended for premature or newborn infants. Otherwise, no problems expected.

Prolonged use:
Avoid. May damage bone marrow and nerve cells.

Skin & sunlight:
May cause rash or intensify sunburn in areas exposed to sun or sunlamp.

Driving, piloting or hazardous work:
Don't drive or pilot aircraft until you learn how medicine affects you. Don't work around dangerous machinery. Don't climb ladders or work in high places. Danger increases if you drink alcohol or take medicine affecting alertness and reflexes, such as antihistamines, tranquilizers, sedatives, pain medicine, narcotics and mind-altering drugs.

Airplane passengers:
No problems expected.

Discontinuing:
No problems expected.

Others:
May mask symptoms of hearing damage from aspirin, other salicylates, cisplatin, paromomycin, vancomycin or anticonvulsants. Consult doctor if you use these.

INTERACTION WITH OTHER DRUGS

GENERIC NAME OR DRUG CLASS	COMBINED EFFECT
Anticholinergics	Increased anticholinergic effect.
Antidepressants	Excess sedation. Avoid.
Antihistamines (other)	Excess sedation. Avoid.
Hypnotics	Excess sedation. Avoid.
MAO inhibitors	Increased diphenhydramine effect.
Mind-altering drugs	Excess sedation. Avoid.
Narcotics	Excess sedation. Avoid.
Sedatives	Excess sedation. Avoid.
Sleep inducers	Excess sedation. Avoid.
Tranquilizers	Excess sedation Avoid.

INTERACTION WITH OTHER SUBSTANCES

INTERACTS WITH	COMBINED EFFECT
Alcohol:	Excess sedation. Avoid.
Beverages: Caffeine drinks	Less diphenhydramine sedation.
Cocaine:	Decreased diphenhydramine effect. Avoid.
Foods:	None expected.
Marijuana:	Excess sedation. Avoid.
Tobacco:	None expected.

DIPHENOXYLATE & ATROPINE

BRAND NAMES

Colonil
Lomotil
SK-Diphenoxylate

GENERAL INFORMATION

Habit forming? Yes
Prescription needed? Yes
Available as generic? Yes
Drug class: Antidiarrheal

 USES

Relieves diarrhea and intestinal cramps.

 DOSAGE & USAGE INFORMATION

How to take:
- Tablet or capsule—Swallow with liquid or food to lessen stomach irritation.
- Drops or liquid—Follow label instructions and use marked dropper.

When to take:
No more often than directed on label.

If you forget a dose:
Take as soon as you remember up to 2 hours late. If more than 2 hours, wait for next scheduled dose (don't double this dose).

What drug does:
Blocks digestive tract's nerve supply, which reduces propelling movements.

Time lapse before drug works:
May require 12 to 24 hours of regular doses to control diarrhea.

Don't take with:
See Interaction column and consult doctor.

 OVERDOSE

Symptoms:
Excitement, constricted pupils, shallow breathing, coma.

What to do:
- Dial 0 (operator) or 911 (emergency) for an ambulance or medical help. Then give first aid immediately.
- If patient is unconscious and not breathing, give mouth-to-mouth breathing. If there is no heartbeat, use cardiac massage and mouth-to-mouth breathing (CPR). Don't try to make patient vomit. If you can't get help quickly, take patient to nearest emergency facility.
- Additional emergency information on page 886.

POSSIBLE ADVERSE REACTIONS OR SIDE EFFECTS

SYMPTOMS	FREQUENCY	WHAT TO DO
Brain & nervous system:		
• Dizziness, depression, drowsiness.	Infrequent	4
• Restlessness, flush, fever, headache.	Rare	3
Skin: Rash or itch.	Infrequent	4
Eyes: Blurred vision.	Infrequent	4
Ears, nose, throat: Dry mouth or swollen gums.	Infrequent	3
Digestive: Stomach pain, nausea, vomiting, bloating, constipation.	Rare	3
Heart & lungs: Rapid heartbeat.	Infrequent	3
Blood vessels: Numbness of hands or feet.	Rare	3
Muscles, bones, joints:	None expected.	
Genital, urinary: Decreased urination.	Infrequent	4
Kidneys:	None expected.	
Liver:	None expected.	
Allergic:	None expected.	
Blood:	None expected.	
Others:	None expected.	

1- Life-threatening. Seek emergency treatment immediately.
2- Discontinue. Seek emergency treatment.
3- Discontinue. Call doctor right away.
4- Continue. Call doctor when convenient.
5- Continue. Tell doctor at next visit.
6- No action necessary.

DIPHENOXYLATE & ATROPINE

 WARNINGS & PRECAUTIONS

Don't take if:
- You are allergic to diphenoxylate & atropine or any narcotic or anticholinergic.
- You have jaundice (yellow skin and eyes).
- Patient is younger than 2.

Before you start, consult your doctor:
- If you have had liver problems.
- If you have ulcerative colitis.
- If you plan to become pregnant within medication period.
- If you have any medical disorder.
- If you take any medication, including non-prescription drugs.

Over age 60:
Adverse reactions and side effects may be more frequent and severe than in younger persons.

Pregnancy:
No proven harm to unborn child. Avoid because of many side effects.

Breast-feeding:
Drug passes into milk. Avoid drug or discontinue nursing until you finish medicine. Consult doctor for advice on maintaining milk supply.

Infants & children:
Don't give to infants or toddlers. Use only under doctor's supervision for children older than 2.

Prolonged use:
Habit forming.

Skin & sunlight:
No problems expected.

Driving, piloting or hazardous work:
Don't drive or pilot aircraft until you learn how medicine affects you. Don't work around dangerous machinery. Don't climb ladders or work in high places. Danger increases if you drink alcohol or take medicine affecting alertness and reflexes.

Airplane passengers:
No problems expected.

Discontinuing:
- May be unnecessary to finish medicine. Follow doctor's instructions.
- After discontinuing, consult doctor if you experience muscle cramps, nausea, vomiting, trembling, stomach cramps or unusual sweating.

Others:
If diarrhea lasts longer than 4 days, discontinue and call doctor.

 INTERACTION WITH OTHER DRUGS

GENERIC NAME OR DRUG CLASS	COMBINED EFFECT
MAO inhibitors	May increase blood pressure excessively.
Sedatives	Increased effect of both drugs.
Tranquilizers	Increased effect of both drugs.

 INTERACTION WITH OTHER SUBSTANCES

INTERACTS WITH	COMBINED EFFECT
Alcohol:	Depressed brain function. Avoid.
Beverages:	None expected.
Cocaine:	Decreased effect of diphenoxylate and atropine.
Foods:	None expected.
Marijuana:	None expected.
Tobacco:	None expected.

DIPHENYLPYRALINE

BRAND NAMES

Diafen
Hispril

GENERAL INFORMATION

Habit forming? No
Prescription needed? High strength: Yes
Low strength: No
Available as generic? No
Drug class: Antihistamine

USES

- Reduces allergic symptoms such as hay fever, hives, rash or itching.
- Induces sleep.

DOSAGE & USAGE INFORMATION

How to take:
Extended-release capsules—Swallow each dose whole with liquid.

When to take:
Varies with form. Follow label directions.

If you forget a dose:
Take as soon as you remember up to 2 hours late. If more than 2 hours, wait for next scheduled dose (don't double this dose).

What drug does:
Blocks action of histamine after an allergic response triggers histamine release in sensitive cells.

Time lapse before drug works:
30 minutes.

Don't take with:
See Interaction column and consult doctor.

OVERDOSE

Symptoms:
Convulsions, red face, hallucinations, coma.

What to do:
- Dial 0 (operator) or 911 (emergency) for an ambulance or medical help. Then give first aid immediately.
- If patient is unconscious and not breathing, give mouth-to-mouth breathing. If there is no heartbeat, use cardiac massage and mouth-to-mouth breathing (CPR). Don't try to make patient vomit. If you can't get help quickly, take patient to nearest emergency facility.
- Additional emergency information on page 886.

POSSIBLE ADVERSE REACTIONS OR SIDE EFFECTS

SYMPTOMS	FREQUENCY	WHAT TO DO
Brain & nervous system:		
● Nightmares, agitation, irritability.	Rare	3
● Drowsiness, dizziness.	Common	5
Skin:	None expected.	
Eyes:		
● Vision changes.	Infrequent	3
● Less tolerance for contact lenses.	Infrequent	4
Ears, nose, throat:		
● Sore throat, fever.	Rare	3
● Dry mouth, nose, throat.	Common	5
Digestive:		
● Nausea	Common	5
● Appetite loss.	Infrequent	5
Heart & lungs:		
Rapid heartbeat.	Rare	3
Blood vessels:		
Unusual bleeding or bruising.	Rare	3
Muscles, bones, joints, kidneys, liver, allergic, blood:	None expected.	
Genital, urinary:		
Urination difficulty.	Infrequent	4
Others:		
Fatigue, weakness.	Rare	3

1- Life-threatening. Seek emergency treatment immediately.
2- Discontinue. Seek emergency treatment.
3- Discontinue. Call doctor right away.
4- Continue. Call doctor when convenient.
5- Continue. Tell doctor at next visit.
6- No action necessary.

DIPHENYLPYRALINE

WARNINGS & PRECAUTIONS

Don't take if:
You are allergic to any antihistamine.

Before you start, consult your doctor:
- If you have glaucoma.
- If you have enlarged prostate.
- If you have asthma.
- If you have kidney disease.
- If you have peptic ulcer.
- If you will have surgery within 2 months, including dental surgery, requiring general or spinal anesthesia.

Over age 60:
Don't exceed recommended dose. Adverse reactions and side effects may be more frequent and severe than in younger persons, especially urination difficulty, diminished alertness and other brain and nervous-system symptoms.

Pregnancy:
No proven harm to unborn child. Avoid if possible.

Breast-feeding:
Drug passes into milk. Avoid drug or discontinue nursing until you finish medicine. Consult doctor for advice on maintaining milk supply.

Infants & children:
Not recommended for premature or newborn infants. Otherwise, no problems expected.

Prolonged use:
Avoid. May damage bone marrow and nerve cells.

Skin & sunlight:
May cause rash or intensify sunburn in areas exposed to sun or sunlamp.

Driving, piloting or hazardous work:
Don't drive or pilot aircraft until you learn how medicine affects you. Don't work around dangerous machinery. Don't climb ladders or work in high places. Danger increases if you drink alcohol or take medicine affecting alertness and reflexes, such as antihistamines, tranquilizers, sedatives, pain medicine, narcotics and mind-altering drugs.

Airplane passengers:
No problems expected.

Discontinuing:
No problems expected.

Others:
May mask symptoms of hearing damage from aspirin, other salicylates, cisplatin, paromomycin, vancomycin or anticonvulsants. Consult doctor if you use these.

INTERACTION WITH OTHER DRUGS

GENERIC NAME OR DRUG CLASS	COMBINED EFFECT
Anticholinergics	Increased anticholinergic effect.
Antidepressants	Excess sedation. Avoid.
Antihistamines (other)	Excess sedation. Avoid.
Hypnotics	Excess sedation. Avoid.
MAO inhibitors	Increased diphenylpyraline effect.
Mind-altering drugs	Excess sedation. Avoid.
Narcotics	Excess sedation. Avoid.
Sedatives	Excess sedation. Avoid.
Sleep inducers	Excess sedation. Avoid.
Tranquilizers	Excess sedation. Avoid.

INTERACTION WITH OTHER SUBSTANCES

INTERACTS WITH	COMBINED EFFECT
Alcohol:	Excess sedation. Avoid.
Beverages: Caffeine drinks	Less diphenylpyraline sedation.
Cocaine:	Decreased diphenylpyraline effect. Avoid.
Foods:	None expected.
Marijuana:	Excess sedation. Avoid.
Tobacco:	None expected.

DIPYRIDAMOLE

BRAND NAMES

Persantine

GENERAL INFORMATION

Habit forming? No
Prescription needed? U.S.: Yes; Canada: No
Available as generic? No
Drug class: Coronary vasodilator

USES

- Reduces frequency and intensity of angina attacks.
- Prevents blood clots after heart surgery.

DOSAGE & USAGE INFORMATION

How to take:
Tablet or capsule—Swallow with liquid. If you can't swallow whole, crumble tablet or open capsule and take with liquid.

When to take:
1 hour before meals.

If you forget a dose:
Take as soon as you remember up to 2 hours late. If more than 2 hours, wait for next scheduled dose (don't double this dose).

What drug does:
- Probably dilates blood vessels to increase oxygen to heart.
- Prevents platelet clumping, which causes blood clots.

Time lapse before drug works:
3 months of continual use.

Don't take with:
See Interaction column and consult doctor.

OVERDOSE

Symptoms:
Decreased blood pressure; weak, rapid pulse; cold, clammy skin; collapse.

What to do:
- Dial 0 (operator) or 911 (emergency) for an ambulance or medical help. Then give first aid immediately.
- If patient is unconscious and not breathing, give mouth-to-mouth breathing. If there is no heartbeat, use cardiac massage and mouth-to-mouth breathing (CPR). Don't try to make patient vomit. If you can't get help quickly, take patient to nearest emergency facility.
- Additional emergency information on page 886.

POSSIBLE ADVERSE REACTIONS OR SIDE EFFECTS

SYMPTOMS	FREQUENCY	WHAT TO DO
Brain & nervous system: Dizziness, fainting, headache.	Infrequent	3
Skin: Red flush, rash.	Infrequent	4
Eyes:	None expected.	
Ears, nose, throat:	None expected.	
Digestive: Nausea, vomiting, cramps.	Infrequent	4
Heart & lungs:	None expected.	
Blood vessels:	None expected.	
Muscles, bones, joints:	None expected.	
Genital, urinary:	None expected.	
Kidneys:	None expected.	
Liver:	None expected.	
Allergic:	None expected.	
Blood:	None expected.	
Others: Weakness	Infrequent	4

1- Life-threatening. Seek emergency treatment immediately.
2- Discontinue. Seek emergency treatment.
3- Discontinue. Call doctor right away.
4- Continue. Call doctor when convenient.
5- Continue. Tell doctor at next visit.
6- No action necessary.

DIPYRIDAMOLE

 ## WARNINGS & PRECAUTIONS

Don't take if:
- You are allergic to dipyridamole.
- You are recovering from a heart attack.

Before you start, consult your doctor:
- If you have low blood pressure.
- If you have liver disease.

Over age 60:
Begin treatment with small doses.

Pregnancy:
No proven harm to unborn child. Avoid if possible.

Breast-feeding:
No proven problems. Consult doctor.

Infants & children:
Not recommended.

Prolonged use:
No problems expected.

Skin & sunlight:
No problems expected.

Driving, piloting or hazardous work:
Avoid if you feel dizzy. Otherwise, no problems expected.

Airplane passengers:
No problems expected.

Discontinuing:
Don't discontinue without doctor's advice until you complete prescribed dose, even though symptoms diminish or disappear.

Others:
Drug increases your ability to be active without angina pain. Avoid excessive physical exertion that might injure heart.

 ## INTERACTION WITH OTHER DRUGS

GENERIC NAME OR DRUG CLASS	COMBINED EFFECT
Anticoagulants (oral)	Increased anticoagulant effect. Bleeding tendency.
Antihypertensives	Increased antihypertensive effect.
Aspirin	Increased dipyridamole effect. Dose may need adjustment.

 ## INTERACTION WITH OTHER SUBSTANCES

INTERACTS WITH	COMBINED EFFECT
Alcohol:	May lower blood pressure excessively.
Beverages:	None expected.
Cocaine:	No proven problems.
Foods:	Decreased dipyridamole absorption unless taken 1 hour before eating.
Marijuana:	Daily use— Decreased dipyridamole effect.
Tobacco: Nicotine	May decrease dipyridamole effect.

DISOPYRAMIDE

BRAND NAMES

Norpace
Rythmodan

GENERAL INFORMATION

Habit forming? No
Prescription needed? Yes
Available as generic? No
Drug class: Antiarrhythmic

 USES

Corrects heart rhythm disorders.

 DOSAGE & USAGE INFORMATION

How to take:
Tablet or capsule—Swallow with liquid. If you can't swallow whole, crumble tablet or open capsule and take with liquid or food.

When to take:
At the same times each day.

If you forget a dose:
Take as soon as you remember up to 2 hours late. If more than 2 hours, wait for next scheduled dose (don't double this dose).

What drug does:
Delays nerve impulses to heart to regulate heartbeat.

Time lapse before drug works:
Begins in 30 to 60 minutes. Must use for 5 to 7 days to determine effectiveness.

Don't take with:
See Interaction column and consult doctor.

 OVERDOSE

Symptoms:
Blood-pressure drop, irregular heartbeat.

What to do:
- Dial 0 (operator) or 911 (emergency) for an ambulance or medical help. Then give first aid immediately.
- If patient is unconscious and not breathing, give mouth-to-mouth breathing. If there is no heartbeat, use cardiac massage and mouth-to-mouth breathing (CPR). Don't try to make patient vomit. If you can't get help quickly, take patient to nearest emergency facility.
- Additional emergency information on page 886.

POSSIBLE ADVERSE REACTIONS OR SIDE EFFECTS

SYMPTOMS	FREQUENCY	WHAT TO DO
Brain & nervous system: Dizziness, fainting, confusion, nervousness, depression.	Infrequent	3
Skin, blood vessels, kidneys, allergic, blood:	None expected.	
Eyes: Pain	Rare	4
Ears, nose, throat: Sore throat with fever.	Rare	3
Digestive: Dry mouth, constipation.	Common	4
Heart & lungs: Chest pain, very fast or very slow heartbeat.	Infrequent	3
Muscles, bones, joints: Swollen feet.	Infrequent	4
Genital, urinary: Difficult urination.	Common	4
Liver: Jaundice (yellow skin and eyes).	Rare	3
Others: • Hypoglycemia	Common	3
• Lower sex drive.	Rare	4
• Rapid weight gain.	Common	4

1- Life-threatening. Seek emergency treatment immediately.
2- Discontinue. Seek emergency treatment.
3- Discontinue. Call doctor right away.
4- Continue. Call doctor when convenient.

DISOPYRAMIDE

WARNINGS & PRECAUTIONS

Don't take if:
- You are allergic to disopyramide or any antiarrhythmic.
- You have second- or third-degree heart block.

Before you start, consult your doctor:
- If you react unfavorably to other antiarrhythmic drugs.
- If you have had heart disease.
- If you have low blood pressure.
- If you have liver disease.
- If you have glaucoma.
- If you have enlarged prostate.
- If you have myasthenia gravis.
- If you take digitalis preparations or diuretics.

Over age 60:
- May require reduced dose.
- More likely to have difficulty urinating or be constipated.
- More likely to have blood-pressure drop.

Pregnancy:
No proven harm to unborn child. Avoid if possible.

Breast-feeding:
Drug passes into milk. Avoid drug or discontinue nursing until you finish medicine. Consult doctor for advice on maintaining milk supply.

Infants & children:
Safety not established. Don't use.

Prolonged use:
No problems expected.

Skin & sunlight:
No problems expected.

Driving, piloting or hazardous work:
Don't drive or pilot aircraft until you learn how medicine affects you. Don't work around dangerous machinery. Don't climb ladders or work in high places. Danger increases if you drink alcohol or take medicine affecting alertness and reflexes, such as antihistamines, tranquilizers, sedatives, pain medicine, narcotics, or mind-altering drugs.

Airplane passengers:
No problems expected.

Discontinuing:
Don't discontinue without doctor's advice until you complete prescribed dose, even though symptoms diminish or disappear.

Others:
If new illness, injury or surgery occurs, tell doctors of disopyramide use.

INTERACTION WITH OTHER DRUGS

GENERIC NAME OR DRUG CLASS	COMBINED EFFECT
Ambenonium	Decreased ambenonium effect.
Anticholinergics	Increased anticholinergic effect.
Anticoagulants (oral)	Increased anticoagulant effect.
Antihypertensives	Increased antihypertensive effect.
Antimyasthenics	Decreased antimyasthenic effect.

INTERACTION WITH OTHER SUBSTANCES

INTERACTS WITH	COMBINED EFFECT
Alcohol:	Decreased blood pressure and blood sugar. Use caution.
Beverages:	None expected.
Cocaine:	Irregular heartbeat.
Foods:	None expected.
Marijuana:	Unpredictable. May decrease disopyramide effect.
Tobacco:	None expected.

DISULFIRAM

BRAND NAMES

Antabuse

GENERAL INFORMATION

Habit forming? No
Prescription needed? Yes
Available as generic? Yes
Drug class: None

 USES

Treatment for alcoholism. Will not cure alcoholism, but is a powerful deterrent to drinking.

 DOSAGE & USAGE INFORMATION

How to take:
Tablet or capsule—Swallow with liquid.

When to take:
Morning or bedtime. Avoid if you have used within 12 hours *any* alcohol, tonics, cough syrups, fermented vinegar, after-shave lotion or backrub solutions.

If you forget a dose:
Take as soon as you remember up to 12 hours late. If more than 12 hours, wait for next scheduled dose (don't double this dose).

What drug does:
In combination with alcohol, produces a metabolic change that causes severe, temporary toxicity.

Time lapse before drug works:
3 weeks or more.

Don't take with:
- See Interaction column and consult doctor.
- Non-prescription drugs that contain *any* alcohol.

 OVERDOSE

Symptoms:
Memory loss, behavior disturbances, lethargy, confusion and headaches; nausea, vomiting, stomach pain and diarrhea; weakness and unsteady walk; temporary paralysis.

What to do:
- Dial 0 (operator) or 911 (emergency) for an ambulance or medical help. Then give first aid immediately.
- Additional emergency information on page 886.

POSSIBLE ADVERSE REACTIONS OR SIDE EFFECTS

SYMPTOMS	FREQUENCY	WHAT TO DO
Brain & nervous system:		
● Drowsiness	Common	5
● Mood changes.	Infrequent	5
Skin:		
Rash	Rare	3
Eyes:		
Pain, vision changes.	Infrequent	4
Ears, nose, throat:		
Bad taste in mouth (metal or garlic).	Infrequent	6
Digestive:		
Stomach discomfort.	Infrequent	4
Heart & lungs:	None expected.	
Blood vessels:		
Throbbing headache.	Infrequent	4
Muscles, bones, joints:	None expected.	
Genital, urinary:		
Decreased sexual ability in men.	Infrequent	5
Kidneys:	None expected.	
Liver:		
Jaundice (yellow skin and eyes).	Rare	3
Allergic:	None expected.	
Blood:	None expected.	
Others:		
● Tiredness	Infrequent	5
● Numbness in hands and feet.	Infrequent	4

1- Life-threatening. Seek emergency treatment immediately.
2- Discontinue. Seek emergency treatment.
3- Discontinue. Call doctor right away.
4- Continue. Call doctor when convenient.
5- Continue. Tell doctor at next visit.
6- No action necessary.

DISULFIRAM

 ## WARNINGS & PRECAUTIONS

Don't take if:
- You are allergic to disulfiram. (Alcohol-disulfiram combination is not an allergic reaction).
- You have used alcohol in any form or amount within 12 hours.
- You have taken paraldehyde within 1 week.
- You have heart disease.

Before you start, consult your doctor:
- If you have allergies.
- If you plan to become pregnant within medication period.
- If no one has explained to you how disulfiram reacts.
- If you think you cannot avoid drinking.
- If you have diabetes, epilepsy, liver or kidney disease.
- If you take other drugs.

Over age 60:
Adverse reactions and side effects may be more frequent and severe than in younger persons.

Pregnancy:
Risk to unborn child outweighs drug benefits. Don't use.

Breast-feeding:
Studies inconclusive. Consult your doctor.

Infants & children:
Not recommended.

Prolonged use:
Periodic blood-cell counts and liver-function tests recommended if you take this drug a long time.

Skin & sunlight:
No problems expected.

Driving, piloting or hazardous work:
Avoid if you feel drowsy or have vision side effects. Otherwise, no restrictions.

Airplane passengers:
Avoid if you feel drowsy or dizzy. Otherwise, no restrictions.

Discontinuing:
Don't discontinue without consulting doctor. Dose may require gradual reduction if you have taken drug for a long time. Doses of other drugs may also require adjustment. Avoid alcohol at least 14 days following last dose.

Others:
No problems expected.

 ## INTERACTION WITH OTHER DRUGS

GENERIC NAME OR DRUG CLASS	COMBINED EFFECT
Anticoagulants	Possible unexplained bleeding.
Anticonvulsants	Excessive sedation.
Barbiturates	Excessive sedation.
Cephalosporins	Disulfiram reaction, see page 848.
Isoniazid	Unsteady walk and disturbed behavior.
Metronidazole	Disulfiram reaction, see page 848.
Sedatives	Excessive sedation.

 ## INTERACTION WITH OTHER SUBSTANCES

INTERACTS WITH	COMBINED EFFECT
Alcohol: Any form or amount.	Possible life-threatening toxicity. See disulfiram reaction, page 848.
Beverages: Punch or fruit drink that may contain alcohol.	Disulfiram reaction, see page 848.
Cocaine:	Increased disulfiram effect.
Foods: Sauces, fermented vinegar, marinades, desserts or other foods prepared with any alcohol.	Disulfiram reaction, see page 848.
Marijuana:	None expected.
Tobacco:	None expected.

DOCUSATE CALCIUM

BRAND NAMES

Surfak

GENERAL INFORMATION

Habit forming? No
Prescription needed? No
Available as generic? Yes
Drug class: Laxative (emollient)

 USES

Constipation relief.

 DOSAGE & USAGE INFORMATION

How to take:
- Tablet or capsule—Swallow with liquid. Don't open capsules.
- Drops—Dilute dose in beverage before swallowing.
- Syrup—Take as directed on bottle.

When to take:
At the same time each day, preferably bedtime.

If you forget a dose:
Take as soon as you remember. Wait 12 hours for next dose. Return to regular schedule.

What drug does:
Makes stool hold fluid so it is easier to pass.

Time lapse before drug works:
2 to 3 days of continual use.

Don't take with:
- Other medicines at same time. Wait 2 hours.
- See Interaction column and consult doctor.

 OVERDOSE

Symptoms:
Appetite loss, nausea, vomiting, diarrhea.

What to do:
Overdose unlikely to threaten life. If person takes much larger amount than prescribed, call doctor, poison-control center or hospital emergency room for instructions.

POSSIBLE ADVERSE REACTIONS OR SIDE EFFECTS

SYMPTOMS	FREQUENCY	WHAT TO DO
Brain & nervous system:	None expected.	
Skin: Rash	Rare	3
Eyes:	None expected.	
Ears, nose, throat: Throat irritation (liquid only).	Infrequent	4
Digestive: Intestinal and stomach cramps.	Infrequent	4
Heart & lungs:	None expected.	
Blood vessels:	None expected.	
Muscles, bones, joints:	None expected.	
Genital, urinary:	None expected.	
Kidneys:	None expected.	
Liver:	None expected.	
Allergic:	None expected.	
Blood:	None expected.	
Others:	None expected.	

1- Life-threatening. Seek emergency treatment immediately.
2- Discontinue. Seek emergency treatment.
3- Discontinue. Call doctor right away.
4- Continue. Call doctor when convenient.
5- Continue. Tell doctor at next visit.
6- No action necessary.

WARNINGS & PRECAUTIONS

Don't take if:
- You are allergic to any emollient laxative.
- You have abdominal pain and fever that might be appendicitis.

Before you start, consult your doctor:
- If you are taking other laxatives.
- To be sure constipation isn't a sign of a serious disorder.

Over age 60:
You must drink 6 to 8 glasses of fluid every 24 hours for drug to work.

Pregnancy:
No problems expected. Consult doctor.

Breast-feeding:
No problems expected.

Infants & children:
No problems expected.

Prolonged use:
Avoid. Overuse of laxatives may damage intestine lining.

Skin & sunlight:
No problems expected.

Driving, piloting or hazardous work:
No problems expected.

Airplane passengers:
No problems expected.

Discontinuing:
May be unnecessary to finish medicine. Follow doctor's instructions.

Others:
No problems expected.

INTERACTION WITH OTHER DRUGS

GENERIC NAME OR DRUG CLASS	COMBINED EFFECT
Danthron	Possible liver damage.
Digitalis preparations	Toxic absorption of digitalis.
Mineral oil	Increased mineral oil absorption into bloodstream. Avoid.
Phenolphthalein	Increased phenolphthalein absorption. Possible toxicity.

INTERACTION WITH OTHER SUBSTANCES

INTERACTS WITH	COMBINED EFFECT
Alcohol:	None expected.
Beverages:	None expected.
Cocaine:	None expected.
Foods:	None expected.
Marijuana:	None expected.
Tobacco:	None expected.

DOCUSATE POTASSIUM

BRAND NAMES

Kasof

GENERAL INFORMATION

Habit forming? No
Prescription needed? No
Available as generic? Yes
Drug class: Laxative (emollient)

 ## USES

Constipation relief.

 ## DOSAGE & USAGE INFORMATION

How to take:
- Tablet or capsule—Swallow with liquid. Don't open capsules.
- Drops—Dilute dose in beverage before swallowing.
- Syrup—Take as directed on bottle.

When to take:
At the same time each day, preferably bedtime.

If you forget a dose:
Take as soon as you remember. Wait 12 hours for next dose. Return to regular schedule.

What drug does:
Makes stool hold fluid so it is easier to pass.

Time lapse before drug works:
2 to 3 days of continual use.

Don't take with:
- Other medicines at same time. Wait 2 hours.
- See Interaction column and consult doctor.

 ## OVERDOSE

Symptoms:
Appetite loss, nausea, vomiting, diarrhea.

What to do:
Overdose unlikely to threaten life. If person takes much larger amount than prescribed, call doctor, poison-control center or hospital emergency room for instructions.

 ## POSSIBLE ADVERSE REACTIONS OR SIDE EFFECTS

SYMPTOMS	FREQUENCY	WHAT TO DO
Brain & nervous system:	None expected.	
Skin: Rash	Rare	3
Eyes:	None expected.	
Ears, nose, throat: Throat irritation (liquid only).	Infrequent	4
Digestive: Intestinal and stomach cramps.	Infrequent	4
Heart & lungs:	None expected.	
Blood vessels:	None expected.	
Muscles, bones, joints:	None expected.	
Genital, urinary:	None expected.	
Kidneys:	None expected.	
Liver:	None expected.	
Allergic:	None expected.	
Blood:	None expected.	
Others:	None expected.	

1- Life-threatening. Seek emergency treatment immediately.
2- Discontinue. Seek emergency treatment.
3- Discontinue. Call doctor right away.
4- Continue. Call doctor when convenient.
5- Continue. Tell doctor at next visit.
6- No action necessary.

DOCUSATE POTASSIUM

WARNINGS & PRECAUTIONS

Don't take if:
- You are allergic to any emollient laxative.
- You have abdominal pain and fever that might be appendicitis.

Before you start, consult your doctor:
- If you are taking other laxatives.
- To be sure constipation isn't a sign of a serious disorder.

Over age 60:
You must drink 6 to 8 glasses of fluid every 24 hours for drug to work.

Pregnancy:
No problems expected. Consult doctor.

Breast-feeding:
No problems expected.

Infants & children:
No problems expected.

Prolonged use:
Avoid. Overuse of laxatives may damage intestine lining.

Skin & sunlight:
No problems expected.

Driving, piloting or hazardous work:
No problems expected.

Airplane passengers:
No problems expected.

Discontinuing:
May be unnecessary to finish medicine. Follow doctor's instructions.

Others:
No problems expected.

INTERACTION WITH OTHER DRUGS

GENERIC NAME OR DRUG CLASS	COMBINED EFFECT
Danthron	Possible liver damage.
Digitalis preparations	Toxic absorption of digitalis.
Mineral oil	Increased mineral oil absorption into bloodstream. Avoid.
Phenolphthalein	Increased phenolphthalein absorption. Possible toxicity.

INTERACTION WITH OTHER SUBSTANCES

INTERACTS WITH	COMBINED EFFECT
Alcohol:	None expected.
Beverages:	None expected.
Cocaine:	None expected.
Foods:	None expected.
Marijuana:	None expected.
Tobacco:	None expected.

DOCUSATE SODIUM

BRAND NAMES

Afko-Lube
Colace
Colax
Comfolaax
Dioctyl Sodium
 Sulfosuccinate
Dialose
Doxidan (M)
Ferro-sequels (M)
Peri-Colase (M)

GENERAL INFORMATION

Habit forming? No
Prescription needed? No
Available as generic? Yes
Drug class: Laxative (emollient)

 USES

Constipation relief.

 DOSAGE & USAGE INFORMATION

How to take:
- Tablet or capsule—Swallow with liquid. Don't open capsules.
- Drops—Dilute dose in beverage before swallowing.
- Syrup—Take as directed on bottle.

When to take:
At the same time each day, preferably bedtime.

If you forget a dose:
Take as soon as you remember. Wait 12 hours for next dose. Return to regular schedule.

What drug does:
Makes stool hold fluid so it is easier to pass.

Time lapse before drug works:
2 to 3 days of continual use.

Don't take with:
- Other medicines at same time. Wait 2 hours.
- See Interaction column and consult doctor.

 OVERDOSE

Symptoms:
Appetite loss, nausea, vomiting, diarrhea.

What to do:
Overdose unlikely to threaten life. If person takes much larger amount than prescribed, call doctor, poison-control center or hospital emergency room for instructions.

 POSSIBLE ADVERSE REACTIONS OR SIDE EFFECTS

SYMPTOMS	FREQUENCY	WHAT TO DO
Brain & nervous system:	None expected.	
Skin: Rash	Rare	3
Eyes:	None expected.	
Ears, nose, throat: Throat irritation (liquid only).	Infrequent	4
Digestive: Intestinal and stomach cramps.	Infrequent	4
Heart & lungs:	None expected.	
Blood vessels:	None expected.	
Muscles, bones, joints:	None expected.	
Genital, urinary:	None expected.	
Kidneys:	None expected.	
Liver:	None expected.	
Allergic:	None expected.	
Blood:	None expected.	
Others:	None expected.	

1- Life-threatening. Seek emergency treatment immediately.
2- Discontinue. Seek emergency treatment.
3- Discontinue. Call doctor right away.
4- Continue. Call doctor when convenient.
5- Continue. Tell doctor at next visit.
6- No action necessary.

DOCUSATE SODIUM

 WARNINGS & PRECAUTIONS

Don't take if:
- You are allergic to any emollient laxative.
- You have abdominal pain and fever that might be appendicitis.

Before you start, consult your doctor:
- If you are taking other laxatives.
- To be sure constipation isn't a sign of a serious disorder.

Over age 60:
You must drink 6 to 8 glasses of fluid every 24 hours for drug to work.

Pregnancy:
No problems expected. Consult doctor.

Breast-feeding:
No problems expected.

Infants & children:
No problems expected.

Prolonged use:
Avoid. Overuse of laxatives may damage intestine lining.

Skin & sunlight:
No problems expected.

Driving, piloting or hazardous work:
No problems expected.

Airplane passengers:
No special problems.

Discontinuing:
May be unnecessary to finish medicine. Follow doctor's instructions.

Others:
No problems expected.

 INTERACTION WITH OTHER DRUGS

GENERIC NAME OR DRUG CLASS	COMBINED EFFECT
Danthron	Possible liver damage.
Digitalis preparations	Toxic absorption of digitalis.
Mineral oil	Increased mineral oil absorption into bloodstream. Avoid.
Phenolphthalein	Increased phenolphthalein absorption. Possible toxicity.

 INTERACTION WITH OTHER SUBSTANCES

INTERACTS WITH	COMBINED EFFECT
Alcohol:	None expected.
Beverages:	None expected.
Cocaine:	None expected.
Foods:	None expected.
Marijuana:	None expected.
Tobacco:	None expected.

DOXEPIN

BRAND NAMES

Adapin
Sinequan

GENERAL INFORMATION

Habit forming? No
Prescription needed? Yes
Available as generic? Yes
Drug class: Antidepressant (tricyclic)

USES

Gradually relieves, but doesn't cure, symptoms of depression.

DOSAGE & USAGE INFORMATION

How to take:
- Tablet or capsule—Swallow with liquid.
- Oral concentrate—Dilute with liquid.

When to take:
At the same time each day, usually bedtime.

If you forget a dose:
Bedtime dose—If you forget your once-a-day bedtime dose, don't take it more than 3 hours late. If more than 3 hours, wait for next scheduled dose. Don't double this dose.

What drug does:
Probably affects part of brain that controls messages between nerve cells.

Time lapse before drug works:
Begins in 1 to 2 weeks. May require 4 to 6 weeks for maximum benefit.

Don't take with:
- Non-prescription drugs without consulting doctor.
- See Interaction column and consult doctor.

OVERDOSE

Symptoms:
Hallucinations, convulsions, coma.

What to do:
- Dial 0 (operator) or 911 (emergency) for an ambulance or medical help. Then give first aid immediately.
- If patient is unconscious and not breathing, give mouth-to-mouth breathing. If there is no heartbeat, use cardiac massage and mouth-to-mouth breathing (CPR). Don't try to make patient vomit. If you can't get help quickly, take patient to nearest emergency facility.
- Additional emergency information on page 886.

POSSIBLE ADVERSE REACTIONS OR SIDE EFFECTS

SYMPTOMS	FREQUENCY	WHAT TO DO
Brain & nervous system:		
• Hallucinations, shakiness, dizziness, fainting.	Infrequent	3
• Headache	Common	4
• Seizures	Rare	1
• Insomnia	Common	5
Skin:		
Rash, itch.	Rare	3
Eyes:		
Blurred vision, pain.	Infrequent	3
Ears, nose, throat:		
• Sore throat.	Rare	3
• Dry mouth or unpleasant taste.	Common	4
Digestive:		
• Constipation or diarrhea, nausea, indigestion.	Common	4
• Vomiting	Infrequent	3
• "Sweet tooth"	Common	5
Heart & lungs:		
Irregular heartbeat or slow pulse.	Infrequent	3
Blood vessels, muscles, bones, joints, kidneys, allergic, blood:	None expected.	
Genital, urinary:		
Difficulty urinating.	Infrequent	4
Liver:		
Jaundice (yellow skin and eyes).	Rare	3
Others:		
• Fever	Rare	3
• Fatigue, weakness.	Common	4

1- Life-threatening. Seek emergency treatment immediately.
2- Discontinue. Seek emergency treatment.
3- Discontinue. Call doctor right away.
4- Continue. Call doctor when convenient.
5- Continue. Tell doctor at next visit.

WARNINGS & PRECAUTIONS

Don't take if:
- You are allergic to any tricyclic antidepressant.
- You drink alcohol.
- You have had a heart attack within 6 weeks.
- You have glaucoma.
- You have taken MAO inhibitors within 2 weeks.
- Patient is younger than 12.

Before you start, consult your doctor:
- If you will have surgery within 2 months, including dental surgery, requiring general or spinal anesthesia.
- If you have an enlarged prostate.
- If you have heart disease or high blood pressure.
- If you have stomach or intestinal problems.
- If you have an overactive thyroid.
- If you have asthma.
- If you have liver disease.

Over age 60:
More likely to develop urination difficulty and side effects under *Brain & nervous system*, opposite.

Pregnancy:
Studies inconclusive on harm to unborn child. Animal studies show fetal abnormalities. Decide with your doctor whether drug benefits justify risk to unborn child.

Breast-feeding:
Drug passes into milk. Avoid drug or discontinue nursing until you finish medicine. Consult doctor on maintaining milk supply.

Infants & children:
Don't give to children younger than 12.

Prolonged use:
No problems expected.

Skin & sunlight:
May cause rash or intensify sunburn in areas exposed to sun or sunlamp.

Driving, piloting or hazardous work:
Don't drive or pilot aircraft until you learn how medicine affects you. Don't work around dangerous machinery. Don't climb ladders or work in high places. Danger increases if you drink alcohol or take medicine affecting alertness and reflexes.

Airplane passengers:
No problems expected.

Discontinuing:
Don't discontinue without consulting doctor. Dose may require gradual reduction if you have taken drug for a long time. Doses of other drugs may also require adjustment.

INTERACTION WITH OTHER DRUGS

GENERIC NAME OR DRUG CLASS	COMBINED EFFECT
Anticoagulants (oral)	Increased anticoagulant effect.
Anticholinergics	Increased sedation.
Antihistamines	Increased antihistamine effect.
Barbiturates	Decreased antidepressant effect.
Clonidine	Decreased clonidine effect.
Diuretics (thiazide)	Increased doxepin effect.
Ethchlorvynol	Delirium
Guanethidine	Decreased guanethidine effect.
MAO inhibitors	Fever, delirium, convulsions.
Methyldopa	Decreased methyldopa effect.
Narcotics	Dangerous oversedation.
Phenytoin	Decreased phenytoin effect.
Quinidine	Irregular heartbeat.
Sedatives	Dangerous oversedation.
Sympathomimetics	Increased sympathomimetic effect.
Thyroid hormones	Irregular heartbeat.

INTERACTION WITH OTHER SUBSTANCES

INTERACTS WITH	COMBINED EFFECT
Alcohol: Beverages or medicines with alcohol.	Excessive intoxication. Avoid.
Beverages:	None expected.
Cocaine:	Excessive intoxication. Avoid.
Foods:	None expected.
Marijuana:	Excessive drowsiness. Avoid.
Tobacco:	None expected.

DOXYCYCLINE

BRAND NAMES

Doxychel
Doxy-Lemmon
Doxy-Tabs
Vibramycin
Vibra-Tabs

USES

- Treatment for infections susceptible to doxycycline. Will not cure virus infections such as colds or flu.
- Treatment for acne.

DOSAGE & USAGE INFORMATION

How to take:
- Tablet or capsule—Take on empty stomach 1 hour before or 2 hours after eating. If you can't swallow whole, crumble tablet or open capsule and take with liquid or food.
- Liquid—Shake well. Take with measuring spoon.

When to take:
At the same times each day, evenly spaced.

If you forget a dose:
Take as soon as you remember up to 2 hours late. If more than 2 hours, wait for next scheduled dose (don't double this dose).

What drug does:
Prevents germ growth and reproduction.

Time lapse before drug works:
- Infections—May require 5 days to affect infection.
- Acne—May require 4 weeks to affect acne.

Don't take with:
- Non-prescription drugs without consulting doctor.
- See Interaction column and consult doctor.

OVERDOSE

Symptoms:
Severe nausea, vomiting, diarrhea.

What to do:
Overdose unlikely to threaten life. If person takes much larger amount than prescribed, call doctor, poison-control center or hospital emergency room for instructions.

POSSIBLE ADVERSE REACTIONS OR SIDE EFFECTS

SYMPTOMS	FREQUENCY	WHAT TO DO
Brain & nervous system:		
● Dizziness	Common	3
● Headache	Infrequent	3
Skin:		
● Itching around rectum and genitals.	Common	3
● Rash	Infrequent	3
Eyes:		
Blurred vision.	Rare	3
Ears, nose, throat:		
● Dark tongue.	Common	5
● Sore mouth or tongue.	Common	2
● Excessive thirst.	Infrequent	4
Digestive:		
Nausea, vomiting, diarrhea, abdominal burning.	Common	2
Heart & lungs:		
Blurred vision.	Rare	3
Blood vessels:	None expected.	
Muscles, bones, joints:	None expected.	
Genital, urinary:		
Increased urination.	Infrequent	4
Kidneys:	None expected.	
Liver:		
Jaundice (yellow eyes and skin) in pregnant women.	Rare	3
Allergic:	None expected.	
Blood:	None expected.	
Others:	None expected.	

1- Life-threatening. Seek emergency treatment immediately.
2- Discontinue. Seek emergency treatment.
3- Discontinue. Call doctor right away.
4- Continue. Call doctor when convenient.
5- Continue. Tell doctor at next visit.
6- No action necessary.

DOXYCYCLINE

WARNINGS & PRECAUTIONS

Don't take if:
You are allergic to any tetracycline antibiotic.

Before you start, consult your doctor:
• If you have kidney or liver disease.
• If you have lupus.
• If you have myasthenia gravis.

Over age 60:
Dosage usually less than in younger adults. More likely to cause itching around rectum. Ask you doctor how to prevent it.

Pregnancy:
Risk to unborn child outweighs drug benefits. Don't use.

Breast-feeding:
Drug passes into milk. Avoid drug or discontinue nursing until you finish medicine. Consult doctor for advice on maintaining milk supply.

Infants & children:
May cause permanent teeth malformation or discoloration in children less than 8 years old. Don't use.

Prolonged use:
• You may become more susceptible to infections caused by germs not responsive to doxycycline.
• May cause rare problems in liver, kidney or bone marrow. Periodic laboratory blood studies, liver- and kidney-function tests recommended if you use drug a long time.

Skin & sunlight:
May cause rash or intensify sunburn in areas exposed to sun or sunlamp.

Driving, piloting or hazardous work:
No problems expected.

Airplane passengers:
No problems expected.

Discontinuing:
Don't discontinue without doctor's advice until you complete prescribed dose, even though symptoms diminish or disappear.

Others:
No problems expected.

INTERACTION WITH OTHER DRUGS

GENERIC NAME OR DRUG CLASS	COMBINED EFFECT
Antacids	Decreased doxycycline effect.
Anticoagulants (oral)	Increased anticoagulant effect.
Contraceptives (oral)	Decreased contraceptive effect.
Digitalis preparations	Increased digitalis effect.
Mineral supplements (iron, calcium, magnesium, zinc)	Decreased doxycycline absorption. Separate doses by 1 to 2 hours.
Lithium	Increased lithium effect.
Penicillins	Decreased penicillin effect.
Sodium bicarbonate	Decreased doxycycline effect.

INTERACTION WITH OTHER SUBSTANCES

INTERACTS WITH	COMBINED EFFECT
Alcohol:	Possible liver damage. Avoid.
Beverages: Milk	Decreased doxycycline absorption. Take dose 2 hours after or 1 hour before drinking.
Cocaine:	No proven problems.
Foods: Dairy products	Decreased doxycycline absorption. Take dose 2 hours after or 1 hour before eating.
Marijuana:	No interactions expected, but marijuana may slow body's recovery. Avoid.
Tobacco:	None expected.

DOXYLAMINE

BRAND NAMES

Bendectin (M)
Decapryn
Unisom Nighttime Sleep Aid

Habit forming? No
Prescription needed? Yes
Available as generic? No
Drug class: Antihistamine

USES

- Reduces allergic symptoms such as hay fever, hives, rash or itching.
- Prevents motion sickness, nausea, vomiting.
- Induces sleep.

DOSAGE & USAGE INFORMATION

How to take:
- Tablet or syrup—Swallow with liquid or food to lessen stomach irritation.

When to take:
Varies with form. Follow label directions.

If you forget a dose:
Take as soon as you remember up to 2 hours late. If more than 2 hours, wait for next scheduled dose (don't double this dose).

What drug does:
Blocks action of histamine after an allergic response triggers histamine release in sensitive cells.

Time lapse before drug works:
30 minutes.

Don't take with:
See Interaction column and consult doctor.

OVERDOSE

Symptoms:
Convulsions, red face, hallucinations, coma.

What to do:
- Dial 0 (operator) or 911 (emergency) for an ambulance or medical help. Then give first aid immediately.
- If patient is unconscious and not breathing, give mouth-to-mouth breathing. If there is no heartbeat, use cardiac massage and mouth-to-mouth breathing (CPR). Don't try to make patient vomit. If you can't get help quickly, take patient to nearest emergency facility.
- Additional emergency information on page 886.

POSSIBLE ADVERSE REACTIONS OR SIDE EFFECTS

SYMPTOMS	FREQUENCY	WHAT TO DO
Brain & nervous system:		
• Nightmares, agitation, irritability.	Rare	3
• Drowsiness, dizziness.	Common	5
Skin:	None expected.	
Eyes:		
• Vision changes.	Infrequent	3
• Less tolerance for contact lenses.	Infrequent	4
Ears, nose, throat:		
• Sore throat, fever.	Rare	3
• Dry mouth, nose, throat.	Common	5
Digestive:		
• Nausea	Common	5
• Appetite loss.	Infrequent	5
Heart & lungs:		
Rapid heartbeat.	Rare	3
Blood vessels:		
Unusual bleeding or bruising.	Rare	3
Muscles, bones, joints, kidneys, liver, allergic, blood:	None expected.	
Genital, urinary:		
Urination difficulty.	Infrequent	4
Others:		
Fatigue, weakness.	Rare	3

1- Life-threatening. Seek emergency treatment immediately.
2- Discontinue. Seek emergency treatment.
3- Discontinue. Call doctor right away.
4- Continue. Call doctor when convenient.
5- Continue. Tell doctor at next visit.
6- No action necessary.

DOXYLAMINE

WARNINGS & PRECAUTIONS

Don't take if:
You are allergic to any antihistamine.

Before you start, consult your doctor:
- If you have glaucoma.
- If you have enlarged prostate.
- If you have asthma.
- If you have kidney disease.
- If you have peptic ulcer.
- If you will have surgery within 2 months, including dental surgery, requiring general or spinal anesthesia.

Over age 60:
Don't exceed recommended dose. Adverse reactions and side effects may be more frequent and severe than in younger persons, especially urination difficulty, diminished alertness and other brain and nervous-system symptoms.

Pregnancy:
No proven harm to unborn child. Avoid if possible.

Breast-feeding:
Drug passes into milk. Avoid drug or discontinue nursing until you finish medicine. Consult doctor for advice on maintaining milk supply.

Infants & children:
Not recommended for premature or newborn infants. Otherwise, no problems expected.

Prolonged use:
Avoid. May damage bone marrow and nerve cells.

Skin & sunlight:
May cause rash or intensify sunburn in areas exposed to sun or sunlamp.

Driving, piloting or hazardous work:
Don't drive or pilot aircraft until you learn how medicine affects you. Don't work around dangerous machinery. Don't climb ladders or work in high places. Danger increases if you drink alcohol or take medicine affecting alertness and reflexes, such as antihistamines, tranquilizers, sedatives, pain medicine, narcotics and mind-altering drugs.

Airplane passengers:
No problems expected.

Discontinuing:
No problems expected.

Others:
May mask symptoms of hearing damage from aspirin, other salicylates, cisplatin, paromomycin, vancomycin or anticonvulsants. Consult doctor if you use these.

INTERACTION WITH OTHER DRUGS

GENERIC NAME OR DRUG CLASS	COMBINED EFFECT
Anticholinergics	Increased anticholinergic effect.
Antidepressants	Excess sedation. Avoid.
Antihistamines (other)	Excess sedation. Avoid.
Hypnotics	Excess sedation. Avoid.
MAO inhibitors	Increased doxylamine effect.
Mind-altering drugs	Excess sedation. Avoid.
Narcotics	Excess sedation. Avoid.
Sedatives	Excess sedation. Avoid.
Sleep inducers	Excess sedation. Avoid.
Tranquilizers	Excess sedation. Avoid.

INTERACTION WITH OTHER SUBSTANCES

INTERACTS WITH	COMBINED EFFECT
Alcohol:	Excess sedation. Avoid.
Beverages: Caffeine drinks	Less doxylamine sedation.
Cocaine:	Decreased doxylamine effect. Avoid.
Foods:	None expected.
Marijuana:	Excess sedation. Avoid.
Tobacco:	None expected.

DYPHYLLINE

BRAND NAMES

Aerophylline   Neothylline
Airet   Protophylline
Dilin
Dilor
Lufyllin

GENERAL INFORMATION

Habit forming? No
Prescription needed? Canada—No
U.S: High strength—Yes
Low strength—No
Available as generic? Yes
Drug class: Bronchodilator (xanthine)

 ## USES

Treatment for bronchial asthma symptoms.

 ## DOSAGE & USAGE INFORMATION

How to take:
- Tablet or capsule—Swallow with liquid.
- Extended-release tablets or capsules—Swallow each dose whole. If you take regular tablets, you may chew or crush them.
- Suppositories—Remove wrapper and moisten suppository with water. Gently insert larger end into rectum. Push well into rectum with finger.
- Syrup—Take as directed on bottle.
- Enema—Use as directed on label.

When to take:
Most effective taken on empty stomach 1 hour before or 2 hours after eating. However, may take with food to lessen stomach upset.

If you forget a dose:
Take as soon as you remember up to 2 hours late. If more than 2 hours, wait for next scheduled dose (don't double this dose).

What drug does:
Relaxes and expands bronchial tubes.

Time lapse before drug works:
15 to 30 minutes.

Don't take with:
See Interaction column and consult doctor.

 ## OVERDOSE

Symptoms:
Restlessness, irritability, confusion, delirium, convulsions, rapid pulse, coma.

What to do:
- Dial 0 (operator) or 911 (emergency) for an ambulance or medical help. Then give first aid immediately.
- Additional emergency information on page 886.

POSSIBLE ADVERSE REACTIONS OR SIDE EFFECTS

SYMPTOMS	FREQUENCY	WHAT TO DO
Brain & nervous system:		
● Headache, irritability, nervousness, restlessness, insomnia.	Common	4
● Dizziness or lightheadedness.	Infrequent	4
Skin:		
● Rash or hives.	Infrequent	3
● Flushed face.	Infrequent	4
Eyes:	None expected.	
Ears, nose, throat:	None expected.	
Digestive:		
● Nausea, vomiting, stomach pain.	Common	4
● Diarrhea, appetite-loss.	Infrequent	3
Heart & lungs:		
● Rapid breathing.	Infrequent	3
● Irregular heartbeat.	Infrequent	3
Blood vessels:	None expected.	
Muscles, bones, joints:	None expected.	
Genital, urinary:	None expected.	
Kidneys:	None expected.	
Liver:	None expected.	
Allergic:	None expected.	
Blood:	None expected.	
Others:	None expected.	

1- Life-threatening. Seek emergency treatment immediately.
2- Discontinue. Seek emergency treatment.
3- Discontinue. Call doctor right away.
4- Continue. Call doctor when convenient.
5- Continue. Tell doctor at next visit.
6- No action necessary.

WARNINGS & PRECAUTIONS

Don't take if:
- You are allergic to any bronchodilator.
- You have an active peptic ulcer.

Before you start, consult your doctor:
- If you have had impaired kidney or liver function.
- If you have gastritis.
- If you have a peptic ulcer.
- If you have high blood pressure or heart disease.
- If you take medication for gout.

Over age 60:
Adverse reactions and side effects may be more frequent and severe than in younger persons.

Pregnancy:
Risk to unborn child outweighs drug benefits. Don't use.

Breast-feeding:
Drug passes into milk. Avoid drug or discontinue nursing until you finish medicine. Consult doctor for advice on maintaining milk supply.

Infants & children:
Use only under medical supervision.

Prolonged use:
Stomach irritation.

Skin & sunlight:
No problems expected.

Driving, piloting or hazardous work:
Avoid if lightheaded or dizzy. Otherwise, no problems expected.

Airplane passengers:
No problems expected.

Discontinuing:
May be unnecessary to finish medicine. Follow doctor's instructions.

Others:
No problems expected.

INTERACTION WITH OTHER DRUGS

GENERIC NAME OR DRUG CLASS	COMBINED EFFECT
Allopurinol	Decreased allopurinol effect.
Ephedrine	Increased effect of both drugs.
Epinephrine	Increased effect of both drugs.
Erythromycin	Increased dyphylline effect.
Furosemide	Increased furosemide effect.
Lincomycins	Increased dyphylline effect.
Lithium	Decreased lithium effect.
Probenecid	Decreased effect of both drugs.
Propranolol	Decreased dyphylline effect.
Rauwolfia alkaloids	Rapid heartbeat.
Sulfinpyrazone	Decreased sulfinpyrazone effect.
Troleandomycin	Increased dyphylline effect.

INTERACTION WITH OTHER SUBSTANCES

INTERACTS WITH	COMBINED EFFECT
Alcohol:	None expected.
Beverages: Caffeine drinks	Nervousness and insomnia.
Cocaine:	Excess stimulation. Avoid.
Foods:	None expected.
Marijuana:	Slightly increased antiasthmatic effect of dyphylline.
Tobacco:	Decreased dyphylline effect.

EPHEDRINE

BRAND NAMES

Acet-Am (M)	Ectasule Minus	Quadrinal (M)
Amesec (M)	Ephedrol	Quelidrine (M)
Bronkaid (M)	Marax (M)	Quibron Plus (M)
Bronkotabs (M)	Nyquil (M)	Tedral (M)

See complete brand names list, page 825.

GENERAL INFORMATION

Habit forming? No
Prescription needed? Low strength: No
High strength: Yes
Available as generic? Yes
Drug class: Sympathomimetic

 USES

- Relieves bronchial asthma.
- Decreases congestion of breathing passages.
- Suppresses allergic reactions.

 DOSAGE & USAGE INFORMATION

How to take:
- Tablet or capsule—Swallow with liquid. You may chew or crush tablet.
- Extended-release tablets or capsules—Swallow each dose whole.
- Syrup—Take as directed on bottle.
- Drops—Dilute dose in beverage.

When to take:
As needed, no more often than every 4 hours.

If you forget a dose:
Take up to 2 hours late. If more than 2 hours, wait for next dose (don't double this).

What drug does:
- Prevents cells from releasing allergy-causing chemicals (histamines).
- Relaxes muscles of bronchial tubes.
- Decreases blood-vessel size and blood flow, thus causing decongestion.

Time lapse before drug works:
30 to 60 minutes.

Don't take with:
- See Interaction column and consult doctor.
- Non-prescription drugs with ephedrine, pseudoephedrine or epinephrine.
- Non-prescription drugs for cough, cold, allergy or asthma without consulting doctor.

 OVERDOSE

Symptoms:
Severe anxiety, confusion, delirium, muscle tremors, rapid and irregular pulse.

What to do:
- Dial 0 (operator) or 911 (emergency) for an ambulance or medical help. Then give first aid immediately.
- Additional emergency information on page 886.

POSSIBLE ADVERSE REACTIONS OR SIDE EFFECTS

SYMPTOMS	FREQUENCY	WHAT TO DO
Brain & nervous system:		
• Nervousness, headache.	Common	4
• Dizziness	Infrequent	4
Skin:		
Paleness	Common	4
Eyes:	None expected.	
Ears, nose, throat:	None expected.	
Digestive:		
Appetite loss, nausea, vomiting.	Infrequent	4
Heart & lungs:		
• Irregular heartbeat.	Infrequent	3
• Rapid heartbeat.	Common	4
Blood vessels:	None expected.	
Muscles, bones, joints:	None expected.	
Genital, urinary:		
Difficult urination.	Infrequent	4
Kidneys:	None expected.	
Liver:	None expected.	
Allergic:	None expected.	
Blood:	None expected.	
Others:		
Insomnia	Common	5

1- Life-threatening. Seek emergency treatment immediately.
2- Discontinue. Seek emergency treatment.
3- Discontinue. Call doctor right away.
4- Continue. Call doctor when convenient.
5- Continue. Tell doctor at next visit.
6- No action necessary.

WARNINGS & PRECAUTIONS

Don't take if:
You are allergic to ephedrine or any sympathomimetic drug.

Before you start, consult your doctor:
- If you have high blood pressure.
- If you have diabetes.
- If you have overactive thyroid gland.
- If you have difficulty urinating.
- If you have taken any MAO inhibitor in past 2 weeks
- If you have taken digitalis preparations in the last 7 days.
- If you will have surgery within 2 months, including dental surgery, requiring general or spinal anesthesia.

Over age 60:
More likely to develop high blood pressure, heart-rhythm disturbances, angina and to feel drug's stimulant effects.

Pregnancy:
No proven harm to unborn child. Avoid if possible.

Breast-feeding:
Drug passes into milk. Avoid drug or discontinue nursing until you finish medicine. Consult doctor for advice on maintaining milk supply.

Infants & children:
No problems expected.

Prolonged use:
- Excessive doses—Rare toxic psychosis.
- Men with enlarged prostate gland may have more urination difficulty.

Skin & sunlight:
No problems expected.

Driving, piloting or hazardous work:
Avoid if you feel dizzy. Otherwise, no problems expected.

Airplane passengers:
No problems expected.

Discontinuing:
May be unnecessary to finish medicine. Follow doctor's instructions.

Others:
No problems expected.

INTERACTION WITH OTHER DRUGS

GENERIC NAME OR DRUG CLASS	COMBINED EFFECT
Antidepressants (tricyclic)	Increased effect of ephedrine. Excessive stimulation of heart and blood pressure.
Antihypertensives	Decreased antihypertensive effect.
Digitalis preparations	Serious heart-rhythm disturbances.
Epinephrine	Increased epinephrine effect.
Ergot preparations	Serious blood-pressure rise.
Guanethidine	Decreased effect of both drugs.
MAO inhibitors	Increased ephedrine effect. Dangerous blood-pressure rise.
Pseudoephedrine	Increased pseudoephedrine effect.

INTERACTION WITH OTHER SUBSTANCES

INTERACTS WITH	COMBINED EFFECT
Alcohol:	None expected.
Beverages: Caffeine drinks.	Nervousness or insomnia.
Cocaine:	Rapid heartbeat. Avoid.
Foods:	None expected.
Marijuana:	Rapid heartbeat, possible heart-rhythm disturbance.
Tobacco:	None expected.

EPINEPHRINE

BRAND NAMES

Adrenalin	Dysne-Inhal	microNEFRIN
Asmolin	Epifrin	Primatene Mist
Asthma Haler	Epitrate	Simplene
Asthma Nefrin	Eppy	Sus-phrine
Bronitin	Glaucon	Vaponefrin
Bronkaid Mist	Medihaler-Epi	

GENERAL INFORMATION

Habit forming? No
Prescription needed? Yes
Available as generic? Nose drops,
aerosol inhaler—No
Eye drops, injection—Yes
Drug class: Sympathomimetic, antiglaucoma

 ## USES

- Relieves allergic symptoms of anaphylaxis.
- Eases symptoms of acute bronchial spasms.
- Relieves congestion of nose, sinuses and throat.
- Reduces internal eye pressure.

 ## DOSAGE & USAGE INFORMATION

How to take:
Eyedrops, nose drops, aerosol inhaler, injection—Use as directed on labels.

When to take:
As needed, no more often than label directs.

If you forget a dose:
If needed, take when you remember. Wait 3 hours for next dose.

What drug does:
- Contracts blood-vessel walls and raises blood pressure.
- Inhibits release of histamine.
- Dilates constricted bronchial tubes and decreases volume of blood in nasal tissue.
- Reduces fluid formation within the eye.

Time lapse before drug works:
1 to 2 minutes.

Don't take with:
- Non-prescription drugs without consulting doctor.
- See Interaction column and consult doctor.

 ## OVERDOSE

Symptoms:
Tremor, rapid breathing, palpitations, extreme rise in blood pressure, irregular heartbeat, breathing difficulty, convulsions, coma.

What to do:
- Dial 0 (operator) or 911 (emergency) for an ambulance or medical help. Then give first aid immediately.
- Additional emergency information on page 886.

POSSIBLE ADVERSE REACTIONS OR SIDE EFFECTS

SYMPTOMS	FREQUENCY	WHAT TO DO
Brain & nervous system:		
● Headache, agitation, dizziness.	Common	4
● Trembling	Infrequent	4
● Insomnia	Common	4
Skin:		
Flushed face or paleness.	Infrequent	4
Eyes, blood vessels, muscles, bones, joints, genital, urinary, kidneys, liver, allergic, blood:	None expected.	
Ears, nose, throat:		
Dry mouth and throat (inhaler only).	Common	5
Digestive:		
Nausea, vomiting.	Infrequent	4
Heart & lungs:		
● Fast or pounding heartbeat.	Common	4
● Chest pain, irregular heartbeat.	Rare	3
● Breathing difficulty.	Infrequent	3
● Cough or bronchial irritation (inhaler only).	Infrequent	4
Others:		
● Sweating	Rare	3
● Weakness	Infrequent	4

1 - Life-threatening. Seek emergency treatment immediately.
2 - Discontinue. Seek emergency treatment.
3 - Discontinue. Call doctor right away.
4 - Continue. Call doctor when convenient.
5 - Continue. Tell doctor at next visit.

WARNINGS & PRECAUTIONS

Don't take if:
- You are allergic to any sympathomimetic.
- You have narrow-angle glaucoma.
- You have had a stroke or heart attack within 3 weeks.
- You have heart-rhythm disturbance.

Before you start, consult your doctor:
- If you have high blood pressure, heart disease or have had a stroke.
- If you have diabetes.
- If you have overactive thyroid.

Over age 60:
- Use with caution if you have hardening of the arteries.
- If you have enlarged prostate, drug may increase urination difficulty.
- If you have Parkinson's disease, drug may temporarily increase rigidity and tremor.
- If you see "floaters" in field of vision, tell your doctor.

Pregnancy:
No proven harm to unborn child. Avoid if possible.

Breast-feeding:
Drug passes into milk. Avoid drug or discontinue nursing until you finish medicine. Consult doctor for advice on maintaining milk supply.

Infants & children:
Use only under medical supervision.

Prolonged use:
- You may stop responding to drug.
- Drug may reduce blood volume.
- Drug may damage eye retina and impair vision.

Skin & sunlight:
No problems expected.

Driving, piloting or hazardous work:
No problems expected. Use caution if you feel dizzy or nervous.

Airplane passengers:
No problems expected.

Discontinuing:
- May be unnecessary to finish medicine. Follow doctor's instructions.
- If drug fails to provide relief after several doses, discontinue. Don't increase dose or frequency.

Others:
- May temporarily raise blood sugar in diabetics.
- Excessive use can cause sudden death.
- Discard medicine if cloudy or discolored.

INTERACTION WITH OTHER DRUGS

GENERIC NAME OR DRUG CLASS	COMBINED EFFECT
Antidepressants (tricyclic)	Increased epinephrine effect.
Antidiabetics (oral)	Decreased antidiabetic effect.
Antihistamines	Increased epinephrine effect.
Beta-adrenergic blockers	Decreased epinephrine effect.
Carbonic anhydrase inhibitors	Increased epinephrine effect.
Digitalis preparations	Possible irregular heartbeat.
Ephedrine	Increased ephedrine effect.
Guanethidine	Decreased guanethidine effect.
Insulin	Decreased insulin effect.
Isoproterenol	Dangerous to heart.
MAO Inhibitors	Dangerous to heart.
Pilocarpine	Increased pilocarpine effect.
Rauwolfia alkaloids	Increased epinephrine effect.
Thyroid preparations	Increased epinephrine effect.

INTERACTION WITH OTHER SUBSTANCES

INTERACTS WITH	COMBINED EFFECT
Alcohol:	May increase urinary excretion of drug and reduce effectiveness.
Beverages:	None expected.
Cocaine:	Dangerous overstimulation. Avoid.
Foods:	None expected.
Marijuana:	Increase in epinephrine's antiasthmatic effect.
Tobacco:	None expected.

ERGOLOID MESYLATES

BRAND NAMES

Circanol
Deapril-ST
Hydergine

GENERAL INFORMATION

Habit forming? No
Prescription needed? Yes
Available as generic? No
Drug class: Ergot preparation

USES

Treatment for reduced alertness, poor memory, confusion, depression or lack of motivation in the elderly.

DOSAGE & USAGE INFORMATION

How to take:
- Tablet or capsule—Swallow with liquid. If you can't swallow whole, crumble tablet or open capsule and take with liquid or food.
- Liquid—Take as directed on label.
- Sublingual tablets—Dissolve tablet under tongue.

When to take:
At the same times each day.

If you forget a dose:
Take as soon as you remember up to 2 hours late. If more than 2 hours, wait for next scheduled dose (don't double this dose).

What drug does:
Stimulates brain-cell metabolism to increase use of oxygen and nutrients.

Time lapse before drug works:
Gradual improvement over 3 to 4 months.

Don't take with:
- Non-prescription drugs containing alcohol without consulting doctor.
- See Interaction column and consult doctor.

OVERDOSE

Symptoms:
Headache, flushed face, nasal congestion, nausea, vomiting, blood-pressure drop, weakness, collapse, coma.

What to do:
- Dial 0 (operator) or 911 (emergency) for an ambulance or medical help. Then give first-aid immediately.
- Additional emergency information on page 886.

POSSIBLE ADVERSE REACTIONS OR SIDE EFFECTS

SYMPTOMS	FREQUENCY	WHAT TO DO
Brain & nervous system:		
• Dizziness when getting up, drowsiness.	Rare	4
• Nervousness, hostility, confusion, depression.	Infrequent	4
• Fainting	Rare	2
Skin:		
Rash	Rare	3
Eyes:		
Blurred vision.	Infrequent	4
Ears, nose, throat:		
• Soreness under tongue.	Rare	4
• Nasal congestion.	Common	5
Digestive:		
• Appetite loss.	Rare	4
• Nausea, vomiting, stomach cramps.	Rare	3
Heart & lungs:		
Slow heartbeat.	Infrequent	3
Blood vessels:	None expected.	
Muscles, bones, joints:	None expected.	
Genital, urinary:	None expected.	
Kidneys:	None expected.	
Liver:	None expected.	
Allergic:	None expected.	
Blood:	None expected.	
Others:		
• Fever	Rare	4
• Tingling fingers.	Infrequent	3

1 - Life-threatening. Seek emergency treatment immediately.
2 - Discontinue. Seek emergency treatment.
3 - Discontinue. Call doctor right away.
4 - Continue. Call doctor when convenient.
5 - Continue. Tell doctor at next visit.
6 - No action necessary.

WARNINGS & PRECAUTIONS

Don't take if:
- You are allergic to any ergot preparation.
- Your heartbeat is less than 60 beats per minute.
- Your systolic blood pressure is consistently below 100.

Before you start, consult your doctor:
If you have had low blood pressure.

Over age 60:
Primarily used in people older than 60. Results unpredictable, but many patients show improved brain function.

Pregnancy:
Not recommended.

Breast-feeding:
Risk to nursing child outweighs drug benefits. Don't use.

Infants & children:
Not recommended.

Prolonged use:
No problems expected.

Skin & sunlight:
No problems expected.

Driving, piloting or hazardous work:
Avoid if you feel dizzy, faint or have blurred vision. Otherwise, no problems expected.

Airplane passengers:
No problems expected.

Discontinuing:
No problems expected.

Others:
No problems expected.

INTERACTION WITH OTHER DRUGS

GENERIC NAME OR DRUG CLASS	COMBINED EFFECT
Antihypertensives	Increased antihypertensive effect.
Beta-adrenergic blockers	Excessive decrease in heartbeat and/or blood pressure.
Digitalis preparations	Excessively slow heartbeat.

INTERACTION WITH OTHER SUBSTANCES

INTERACTS WITH	COMBINED EFFECT
Alcohol:	Use caution. May drop blood pressure excessively.
Beverages:	None expected.
Cocaine:	Overstimulation. Avoid.
Foods:	None expected.
Marijuana:	Decreased effect of ergot alkaloids.
Tobacco:	None expected.

ERGONOVINE

BRAND NAMES
Ergotrate

GENERAL INFORMATION

Habit forming? No
Prescription needed? Yes
Available as generic? Yes
Drug class: Ergot preparation (uterine stimulant)

 USES

Retards excessive post-delivery bleeding.

 DOSAGE & USAGE INFORMATION

How to take:
Tablet—Swallow with liquid or food to lessen stomach irritation.

When to take:
At the same times each day.

If you forget a dose:
Don't take missed dose and don't double next one. Wait for next scheduled dose.

What drug does:
Causes smooth-muscle cells of uterine wall to contract and surround bleeding blood vessels of relaxed uterus.

Time lapse before drug works:
Tablets—20 to 30 minutes.

Don't take with:
See Interaction column and consult doctor.

 OVERDOSE

Symptoms:
Vomiting, diarrhea, weak pulse, low blood pressure, convulsions.

What to do:
- Dial 0 (operator) or 911 (emergency) for an ambulance or medical help. Then give first aid immediately.
- If patient is unconscious and not breathing, give mouth-to-mouth breathing. If there is no heartbeat, use cardiac massage and mouth-to-mouth breathing (CPR). Don't try to make patient vomit. If you can't get help quickly, take patient to nearest emergency facility.
- Additional emergency information on page 886.

 POSSIBLE ADVERSE REACTIONS OR SIDE EFFECTS

SYMPTOMS	FREQUENCY	WHAT TO DO
Brain & nervous system:		
• Sudden, severe headache.	Rare	2
• Confusion	Infrequent	3
Skin:	None expected.	
Eyes:	None expected.	
Ears, nose, throat: Ringing in ears.	Infrequent	3
Digestive:		
• Nausea, vomiting.	Common	3
• Diarrhea	Infrequent	3
Heart & lungs: Shortness of breath, chest pain.	Rare	2
Blood vessels:	None expected.	
Muscles, bones, joints:		
• Muscle cramps.	Infrequent	3
• Numb, cold hands and feet.	Rare	2
Genital, urinary:	None expected.	
Kidneys:	None expected.	
Liver:	None expected.	
Allergic:	None expected.	
Blood:	None expected.	
Others: Unusual sweating.	Infrequent	4

1-Life-threatening. Seek emergency treatment immediately.
2-Discontinue. Seek emergency treatment.
3-Discontinue. Call doctor right away.
4-Continue. Call doctor when convenient.
5-Continue. Tell doctor at next visit.
6-No action necessary.

ERGONOVINE

WARNINGS & PRECAUTIONS

Don't take if:
You are allergic to any ergot preparation.

Before you start, consult your doctor:
- If you have coronary-artery or blood-vessel disease.
- If you have liver or kidney disease.
- If you have high blood pressure.
- If you have postpartum infection.

Over age 60:
Not recommended.

Pregnancy:
Risk to unborn child outweighs drug benefits. Don't use.

Breast-feeding:
Drug passes into milk. Avoid drug or discontinue nursing until you finish medicine. Consult doctor for advice on maintaining milk supply.

Infants & children:
Not recommended.

Prolonged use:
Not recommended.

Skin & sunlight:
No problems expected.

Driving, piloting or hazardous work:
No problems expected.

Airplane passengers:
No problems expected.

Discontinuing:
May be unnecessary to finish medicine. Follow doctor's instructions.

Others:
Drug should be used for short time only following childbirth or miscarriage.

INTERACTION WITH OTHER DRUGS

GENERIC NAME OR DRUG CLASS	COMBINED EFFECT
Ergot preparations (other)	Increased ergonovine effect.

INTERACTION WITH OTHER SUBSTANCES

INTERACTS WITH	COMBINED EFFECT
Alcohol:	None expected.
Beverages:	None expected.
Cocaine:	None expected.
Foods:	None expected.
Marijuana:	None expected.
Tobacco:	None expected.

ERGOTAMINE

BRAND NAMES

Bellergal (M)
Cafergot (M)
Cafergot-PB (M)
Ergomar
Ergostat

Gynergen
Medihaler-Ergotamine
Migraine (M)
Migrastat (M)

GENERAL INFORMATION

Habit forming? No
Prescription needed? Yes
Available as generic? Yes
Drug class: Vasoconstrictor, ergot preparation

 ## USES

Relieves pain of migraines and other headaches caused by dilated blood vessels. Will not prevent headaches.

 ## DOSAGE & USAGE INFORMATION

How to take:
- Tablet or capsule—Swallow with liquid, or let dissolve under tongue. If you can't swallow whole, crumble tablet or open capsule and take with liquid or food.
- Suppositories—Remove wrapper and moisten suppository with water. Gently insert larger end into rectum. Push well into rectum with finger.
- Aerosol inhaler—Use only as directed on prescription label.
- Lie down in quiet, dark room after taking.

When to take:
At first sign of vascular or migraine headache.

If you forget a dose:
Take as soon as you remember. Wait 4 hours for next dose.

What drug does:
Constricts blood vessels in the head.

Time lapse before drug works:
30 to 60 minutes.

Don't take with:
See Interaction column and consult doctor.

 ## OVERDOSE

Symptoms:
Tingling, cold extremities and muscle pain. Progresses to nausea, vomiting, diarrhea, cold skin, rapid and weak pulse, severe numbness of extremities, confusion, convulsions, coma.

What to do:
- Dial 0 (operator) or 911 (emergency) for an ambulance or medical help. Then give first aid immediately.
- Additional emergency information on page 886.

POSSIBLE ADVERSE REACTIONS OR SIDE EFFECTS

SYMPTOMS	FREQUENCY	WHAT TO DO
Brain & nervous system:		
• Anxiety or confusion.	Rare	3
• Dizziness	Common	4
Skin:		
• Red or purple blisters, especially on hands, feet.	Rare	3
• Itch, swelling.	Infrequent	3
Eyes:		
Vision changes.	Rare	3
Ears, nose, throat:		
Extreme thirst.	Rare	3
Digestive:		
• Stomach pain or bloating.	Rare	3
• Nausea, diarrhea, vomiting.	Common	4
Heart & lungs:		
Unusually fast or slow heartbeat, possible chest pain.	Rare	3
Blood vessels:		
Cold, pale hands or feet.	Infrequent	3
Muscles, bones, joints:		
Pain or weakness in arms, legs, back.	Infrequent	3
Genital, urinary, kidneys, liver, allergic, blood:	None expected.	
Others:		
Numbness or tingling of face, fingers, toes.	Rare	3

1- Life-threatening. Seek emergency treatment immediately.
2- Discontinue. Seek emergency treatment.
3- Discontinue. Call doctor right away.
4- Continue. Call doctor when convenient.

WARNINGS & PRECAUTIONS

Don't take if:
You are allergic to any ergot preparation.

Before you start, consult your doctor:
- If you plan to become pregnant within medication period.
- If you have an infection.
- If you have angina, heart problems, high blood pressure, hardening of the arteries or vein problems.
- If you have kidney or liver disease.
- If you are allergic to other spray inhalants.

Over age 60:
Adverse reactions and side effects may be more frequent and severe than in younger persons.

Pregnancy:
Risk to unborn child outweighs drug benefits. Don't use.

Breast-feeding:
Drug filters into milk. May harm child. Avoid.

Infants & children:
Studies inconclusive on harm to children. Consult your doctor.

Prolonged use:
Cold skin, muscle pain, gangrene of hands and feet. This medicine not intended for uninterrupted use.

Skin & sunlight:
No problems expected.

Driving, piloting or hazardous work:
Don't drive or pilot aircraft until you learn how medicine affects you. Don't work around dangerous machinery. Don't climb ladders or work in high places. Danger increases if you drink alcohol or take medicine affecting alertness and reflexes, such as antihistamines, tranquilizers, sedatives, pain medicine, narcotics and mind-altering drugs.

Airplane passengers:
No problems expected.

Discontinuing:
May be unnecessary to finish medicine. Follow doctor's instructions.

Others:
Impaired blood circulation can lead to gangrene in intestines or extremities. Never exceed recommended dose.

INTERACTION WITH OTHER DRUGS

GENERIC NAME OR DRUG CLASS	COMBINED EFFECT
Amphetamines	Dangerous blood-pressure rise.
Ephedrine	Dangerous blood-pressure rise.
Epinephrine	Dangerous blood-pressure rise.
Pseudoephedrine	Dangerous blood-pressure rise.
Troleandomycin	Increased adverse reactions of ergotamine.

INTERACTION WITH OTHER SUBSTANCES

INTERACTS WITH	COMBINED EFFECT
Alcohol:	Dilates blood vessels. Makes headache worse.
Beverages: Caffeine drinks	May help relieve headache.
Cocaine:	Decreased ergotamine effect.
Foods: Any to which you are allergic.	May make headache worse. Avoid.
Marijuana:	Occasional use—Cool extremities. Regular use—Persistent chill.
Tobacco:	Decreased effect of ergotamine. Makes headache worse.

ERYTHRITYL TETRANITRATE

BRAND NAMES

Cardilate

GENERAL INFORMATION

Habit forming? No
Prescription needed? Yes
Available as generic? No
Drug class: Antianginal (nitrate)

USES

Reduces frequency and severity of angina attacks.

DOSAGE & USAGE INFORMATION

How to take:
- Sublingual tablet—Dissolve under tongue at earliest sign of angina.
- Chewable tablet—Chew tablet at earliest sign of angina, and hold in mouth for 2 minutes.
- Regular tablet—Swallow with liquid. You may chew or crush it.

When to take:
Swallowed tablets—Take at the same times each day, 1 or 2 hours after meals.

If you forget a dose:
Swallowed tablets—Take as soon as you remember up to 2 hours late. If more than 2 hours, wait for next scheduled dose (don't double this dose).

What drug does:
Relaxes blood vessels, increasing blood flow to heart muscle.

Time lapse before drug works:
- Sublingual or chewable tablets—3 to 5 minutes.
- Swallowed tablets—30 minutes.

Don't take with:
See Interaction column and consult doctor.

OVERDOSE

Symptoms:
Vomiting, sweating, shortness of breath, loss of consciousness.

What to do:
- Dial 0 (operator) or 911 (emergency) for an ambulance or medical help. Then give first aid immediately.
- Additional emergency information on page 886.

POSSIBLE ADVERSE REACTIONS OR SIDE EFFECTS

SYMPTOMS	FREQUENCY	WHAT TO DO
Brain & nervous system:		
• Headache	Common	5
• Fainting	Infrequent	3
Skin:		
• Rash	Rare	3
• Flushed face and neck.	Common	5
Eyes:	None expected.	
Ears, nose, throat:	None expected.	
Digestive: Nausea, vomiting.	Common	5
Heart & lungs: Rapid heartbeat.	Common	5
Blood vessels:	None expected.	
Muscles, bones, joints:	None expected.	
Genital, urinary:	None expected.	
Kidneys:	None expected.	
Liver:	None expected.	
Allergic:	None expected.	
Blood:	None expected.	
Others:	None expected.	

1- Life-threatening. Seek emergency treatment immediately.
2- Discontinue. Seek emergency treatment.
3- Discontinue. Call doctor right away.
4- Continue. Call doctor when convenient.
5- Continue. Tell doctor at next visit.
6- No action necessary.

ERYTHRITYL TETRANITRATE

WARNINGS & PRECAUTIONS

Don't take if:
You are allergic to nitrates, including nitroglycerin.

Before you start, consult your doctor:
If you have glaucoma.

Over age 60:
Adverse reactions and side effects may be more frequent and severe than in younger persons.

Pregnancy:
No proven harm to unborn child. Avoid if possible.

Breast-feeding:
No proven problems. Consult your doctor.

Infants & children:
Not recommended.

Prolonged use:
Drug may become less effective and require higher doses.

Skin & sunlight:
No problems expected.

Driving, piloting or hazardous work:
Don't drive or pilot aircraft until you learn how medicine affects you. Don't work around dangerous machinery. Don't climb ladders or work in high places. Danger increases if you drink alcohol or take medicine affecting alertness and reflexes, such as antihistamines, tranquilizers, sedatives, pain medicine, narcotics and mind-altering drugs.

Airplane passengers:
No problems expected.

Discontinuing:
Don't discontinue without doctor's advice until you complete prescribed dose, even though symptoms diminish or disappear.

Others:
Periodic laboratory blood studies recommended if you take erythrityl tetranitrate.

INTERACTION WITH OTHER DRUGS

GENERIC NAME OR DRUG CLASS	COMBINED EFFECT
Anticholinergics	Increased internal eye pressure.
Antidepressants (tricyclic)	Excessive blood-pressure drop.
Antihypertensives	Excessive blood-pressure drop.
Beta-adrenergic blockers	Excessive blood-pressure drop.
Cholinergics	Decreased cholinergic effect.
Ephedrine	Decreased effect of erythrityl tetranitrate.

INTERACTION WITH OTHER SUBSTANCES

INTERACTS WITH	COMBINED EFFECT
Alcohol:	Excessive blood-pressure drop.
Beverages:	None expected.
Cocaine:	Flushed face and headache. Avoid.
Foods:	None expected.
Marijuana:	Decreased effect of erythrityl tetranitrate.
Tobacco:	Decreased effect of erythrityl tetranitrate.

ERYTHROMYCIN

BRAND NAMES

Dowmycin	Erythromid
E-Biotic	Kesso-mycin
E-Mycin	Novorythro
Eryc	Robimycin
Ery-derm	RP-Mycin
Ery-Tab	

GENERAL INFORMATION

Habit forming? No
Prescription needed? Yes
Available as generic? Yes
Drug class: Antibiotic (erythromycin)

 ## USES

Treatment of infections responsive to erythromycin.

 ## DOSAGE & USAGE INFORMATION

How to take:
- Tablet or capsule—Swallow with liquid.
- Extended-release tablets or capsules—Swallow each dose whole. If you take regular tablets, you may chew or crush them.
- Liquid, drops, granules, skin ointment, eye ointment, skin solution—Follow prescription label directions.

When to take:
At the same times each day, 1 hour before or 2 hours after eating.

If you forget a dose:
- If you take 3 or more doses daily—Take as soon as you remember. Return to regular schedule.
- If you take 2 doses daily—Take as soon as you remember. Wait 5 to 6 hours for next dose. Return to regular schedule.

What drug does:
Prevents growth and reproduction of susceptible bacteria.

Time lapse before drug works:
2 to 5 days.

Don't take with:
See Interaction column and consult doctor.

 ## OVERDOSE

Symptoms:
Nausea, vomiting, abdominal discomfort, diarrhea.

What to do:
Overdose unlikely to threaten life. If person takes much larger amount than prescribed, call doctor, poison-control center or hospital emergency room for instructions.

 ## POSSIBLE ADVERSE REACTIONS OR SIDE EFFECTS

SYMPTOMS	FREQUENCY	WHAT TO DO
Brain & nervous system:	None expected.	
Skin: Dryness, irritation, itch, stinging with use of skin solution.	Infrequent	4
Eyes:	None expected.	
Ears, nose, throat: Sore mouth or tongue.	Infrequent	4
Digestive: Diarrhea, nausea, stomach cramps, discomfort, vomiting.	Infrequent	3
Heart & lungs:	None expected.	
Blood vessels:	None expected.	
Muscles, bones, joints:	None expected.	
Genital, urinary:	None expected.	
Kidneys:	None expected.	
Liver: Jaundice (yellow skin and eyes) in adults.	Rare	3
Allergic:	None expected.	
Blood:	None expected.	
Others: Unusual tiredness or weakness.	Rare	4

1- Life-threatening. Seek emergency treatment immediately.
2- Discontinue. Seek emergency treatment.
3- Discontinue. Call doctor right away.
4- Continue. Call doctor when convenient.
5- Continue. Tell doctor at next visit.
6- No action necessary.

WARNINGS & PRECAUTIONS

Don't take if:
- You are allergic to any erythromycin.
- You have had liver disease or impaired liver function.

Before you start, consult your doctor:
If you have taken erythromycin estolate in the past.

Over age 60:
Adverse reactions and side effects may be more frequent and severe than in younger persons, especially skin reactions around genitals and anus.

Pregnancy:
No proven harm to unborn child. Avoid if possible.

Breast-feeding:
Drug passes into milk. Avoid drug or discontinue nursing until you finish medicine. Consult doctor for advice on maintaining milk supply.

Infants & children:
Use only under medical supervision.

Prolonged use:
You may become more susceptible to infections caused by germs not responsive to erythromycin.

Skin & sunlight:
No problems expected.

Driving, piloting or hazardous work:
No problems expected.

Airplane passengers:
No problems expected.

Discontinuing:
You must take full dose at least 10 consecutive days for streptococcal or staphylococcal infections.

Others:
No problems expected.

INTERACTION WITH OTHER DRUGS

GENERIC NAME OR DRUG CLASS	COMBINED EFFECT
Aminophylline	Increased effect of aminophylline in blood.
Lincomycins	Decreased lincomycin effect.
Oxtriphylline	Increased level of oxtriphylline in blood.
Penicillins	Decreased penicillin effect.
Theophylline	Increased level of theophylline in blood.

INTERACTION WITH OTHER SUBSTANCES

INTERACTS WITH	COMBINED EFFECT
Alcohol:	Possible liver damage.
Beverages:	None expected.
Cocaine:	None expected.
Foods:	None expected.
Marijuana:	None expected.
Tobacco:	None expected.

ERYTHROMYCIN ESTOLATE

BRAND NAMES

Ilosone
Novorythro

GENERAL INFORMATION

Habit forming? No
Prescription needed? Yes
Available as generic? Yes
Drug class: Antibiotic (erythromycin)

USES

Treatment of infections responsive to
erythromycin estolate.

DOSAGE & USAGE INFORMATION

How to take:
- Tablet or capsule—Swallow with liquid.
- Extended-release tablets or capsules—Swallow each dose whole. If you take regular tablets, you may chew or crush them.
- Liquid, drops, granules, skin ointment, eye ointment, skin solution—Follow prescription label directions.

When to take:
At the same times each day, 1 hour before or 2 hours after eating.

If you forget a dose:
- If you take 3 or more doses daily—Take as soon as you remember. Return to regular schedule.
- If you take 2 doses daily—Take as soon as you remember. Wait 5 to 6 hours for next dose. Return to regular schedule.

What drug does:
Prevents growth and reproduction of susceptible bacteria.

Time lapse before drug works:
2 to 5 days.

Don't take with:
See Interaction column and consult doctor.

OVERDOSE

Symptoms:
Nausea, vomiting, abdominal discomfort, diarrhea.

What to do:
Overdose unlikely to threaten life. If person takes much larger amount than prescribed, call doctor, poison-control center or hospital emergency room for instructions.

POSSIBLE ADVERSE REACTIONS OR SIDE EFFECTS

SYMPTOMS	FREQUENCY	WHAT TO DO
Brain & nervous system:	None expected.	
Skin: Dryness, irritation, itch, stinging with use of skin solution.	Infrequent	4
Eyes:	None expected.	
Ears, nose, throat: Sore mouth or tongue.	Infrequent	4
Digestive: Diarrhea, nausea, stomach cramps and discomfort, vomiting.	Infrequent	3
Heart & lungs:	None expected.	
Blood vessels:	None expected.	
Muscles, bones, joints:	None expected.	
Genital, urinary:	None expected.	
Kidneys:	None expected.	
Liver: Jaundice (yellow skin and eyes).	Infrequent	3
Allergic:	None expected.	
Blood:	None expected.	
Others: Unusual tiredness or weakness.	Rare	4

1- Life-threatening. Seek emergency treatment immediately.
2- Discontinue. Seek emergency treatment.
3- Discontinue. Call doctor right away.
4- Continue. Call doctor when convenient.
5- Continue. Tell doctor at next visit.
6- No action necessary.

ERYTHROMYCIN ESTOLATE

WARNINGS & PRECAUTIONS

Don't take if:
- You are allergic to any erythromycin.
- You have had liver disease or impaired liver function.

Before you start, consult your doctor:
If you have taken erythromycin estolate in the past.

Over age 60:
Adverse reactions and side effects may be more frequent and severe than in younger persons, especially skin reactions around genitals and anus.

Pregnancy:
No proven harm to unborn child. Avoid if possible.

Breast-feeding:
Drug passes into milk. Avoid drug or discontinue nursing until you finish medicine. Consult doctor for advice on maintaining milk supply.

Infants & children:
Use only under medical supervision.

Prolonged use:
You may become more susceptible to infections caused by germs not responsive to erythromycin estolate.

Skin & sunlight:
No problems expected.

Driving, piloting or hazardous work:
No problems expected.

Airplane passengers.
No problems expected.

Discontinuing:
You must take full dose at least 10 consecutive days for streptococcal or staphylococcal infections.

Others:
Erythromycin estolate more likely to damage liver than other erythromycins. If you drink alcohol or have had liver disease, use a different antibiotic.

INTERACTION WITH OTHER DRUGS

GENERIC NAME OR DRUG CLASS	COMBINED EFFECT
Aminophylline	Increased effect of aminophylline in blood.
Lincomycins	Decreased lincomycin effect.
Oxtriphylline	Increased level of oxtriphylline in blood.
Penicillins	Decreased penicillin effect.
Theophylline	Increased level of theophylline in blood.

INTERACTION WITH OTHER SUBSTANCES

INTERACTS WITH	COMBINED EFFECT
Alcohol:	Possible liver damage.
Beverages:	None expected.
Cocaine:	None expected.
Foods:	None expected.
Marijuana:	None expected.
Tobacco:	None expected.

ERYTHROMYCIN ETHYLSUCCINATE

BRAND NAMES

E.E.S.
E-Mycin E
EryPed
Pediamycin
Wyamycin E

GENERAL INFORMATION

Habit forming? No
Prescription needed? Yes
Available as generic? Yes
Drug class: Antibiotic (erythromycin)

 ## USES

Treatment of infections responsive to
erythromycin ethylsuccinate.

 ## DOSAGE & USAGE INFORMATION

How to take:
- Tablet or capsule—Swallow with liquid.
- Extended-release tablets or
  capsules—Swallow each dose whole. If
  you take regular tablets, you may chew or
  crush them.
- Liquid, drops, granules, skin ointment, eye
  ointment, skin solution—Follow
  prescription label directions.

When to take:
At the same times each day, 1 hour before or
2 hours after eating.

If you forget a dose:
- If you take 3 or more doses daily—Take as
  soon as you remember. Return to regular
  schedule.
- If you take 2 doses daily—Take as soon as
  you remember. Wait 5 to 6 hours for next
  dose. Return to regular schedule.

What drug does:
Prevents growth and reproduction of
susceptible bacteria.

Time lapse before drug works:
2 to 5 days.

Don't take with:
See Interaction column and consult doctor.

 ## OVERDOSE

Symptoms:
Nausea, vomiting, abdominal discomfort,
diarrhea.

What to do:
Overdose unlikely to threaten life. If person
takes much larger amount than prescribed,
call doctor, poison-control center or hospital
emergency room for instructions.

 ## POSSIBLE ADVERSE REACTIONS OR SIDE EFFECTS

SYMPTOMS	FREQUENCY	WHAT TO DO
Brain & nervous system:	None expected.	
Skin: Dryness, irritation, itch, stinging with use of skin solution.	Infrequent	4
Eyes:	None expected.	
Ears, nose, throat: Sore mouth or tongue.	Infrequent	4
Digestive: Diarrhea, nausea, stomach cramps and discomfort, vomiting.	Infrequent	3
Heart & lungs:	None expected.	
Blood vessels:	None expected.	
Muscles, bones, joints:	None expected.	
Genital, urinary:	None expected.	
Kidneys:	None expected.	
Liver: Jaundice (yellow skin and eyes).	Rare	3
Allergic:	None expected.	
Blood:	None expected.	
Others: Unusual tiredness or weakness.	Rare	4

1- Life-threatening. Seek emergency
   treatment immediately.
2- Discontinue. Seek emergency treatment.
3- Discontinue. Call doctor right away.
4- Continue. Call doctor when convenient.
5- Continue. Tell doctor at next visit.
6- No action necessary.

ERYTHROMYCIN ETHYLSUCCINATE

WARNINGS & PRECAUTIONS

Don't take if:
- You are allergic to any erythromycin.
- You have had liver disease or impaired liver function.

Before you start, consult your doctor:
If you have taken erythromycin estolate in the past.

Over age 60:
Adverse reactions and side effects may be more frequent and severe than in younger persons, especially skin reactions around genitals and anus.

Pregnancy:
No proven harm to unborn child. Avoid if possible.

Breast-feeding:
Drug passes into milk. Avoid drug or discontinue nursing until you finish medicine. Consult doctor for advice on maintaining milk supply.

Infants & children:
Use only under medical supervision.

Prolonged use:
You may become more susceptible to infections caused by germs not responsive to erythromycin ethylsuccinate.

Skin & sunlight:
No problems expected.

Driving, piloting or hazardous work:
No problems expected.

Airplane passengers:
No problems expected.

Discontinuing:
You must take full dose at least 10 consecutive days for streptococcal or staphylococcal infections.

Others:
Possible liver damage. If you are alcoholic or have liver disease, use a different antibiotic.

INTERACTION WITH OTHER DRUGS

GENERIC NAME OR DRUG CLASS	COMBINED EFFECT
Aminophylline	Increased effect of aminophylline in blood.
Lincomycins	Decreased lincomycin effect.
Oxtriphylline	Increased level of oxtriphylline in blood.
Penicillins	Decreased penicillin effect.
Theophylline	Increased level of theophylline in blood.

INTERACTION WITH OTHER SUBSTANCES

INTERACTS WITH	COMBINED EFFECT
Alcohol:	Possible liver damage.
Beverages:	None expected.
Cocaine:	None expected.
Foods:	None expected.
Marijuana:	None expected.
Tobacco:	None expected.

ERYTHROMYCIN GLUCEPTATE

BRAND NAMES

Ilotycin

GENERAL INFORMATION

Habit forming? No
Prescription needed? Yes
Available as generic? Yes
Drug class: Antibiotic (erythromycin)

 USES

Treatment of infections responsive to erythromycin gluceptate.

 DOSAGE & USAGE INFORMATION

How to take:
- Tablet or capsule—Swallow with liquid.
- Extended-release tablets or capsules—Swallow each dose whole. If you take regular tablets, you may chew or crush them.
- Liquid, drops, granules, skin ointment, eye ointment, skin solution—Follow prescription label directions.

When to take:
At the same times each day, 1 hour before or 2 hours after eating.

If you forget a dose:
- If you take 3 or more doses daily—Take as soon as you remember. Return to regular schedule.
- If you take 2 doses daily—Take as soon as you remember. Wait 5 to 6 hours for next dose. Return to regular schedule.

What drug does:
Prevents growth and reproduction of susceptible bacteria.

Time lapse before drug works:
2 to 5 days.

Don't take with:
See Interaction column and consult doctor.

 OVERDOSE

Symptoms:
Nausea, vomiting, abdominal discomfort, diarrhea.

What to do:
Overdose unlikely to threaten life. If person takes much larger amount than prescribed, call doctor, poison-control center or hospital emergency room for instructions.

 POSSIBLE ADVERSE REACTIONS OR SIDE EFFECTS

SYMPTOMS	FREQUENCY	WHAT TO DO
Brain & nervous system:	None expected.	
Skin: Dryness, irritation, itch, stinging with use of skin solution.	Infrequent	4
Eyes:	None expected.	
Ears, nose, throat: Sore mouth or tongue.	Infrequent	4
Digestive: Diarrhea, nausea, stomach cramps, discomfort, vomiting.	Infrequent	3
Heart & lungs:	None expected.	
Blood vessels:	None expected.	
Muscles, bones, joints:	None expected.	
Genital, urinary:	None expected.	
Kidneys:	None expected.	
Liver: Jaundice (yellow skin and eyes) in adults.	Rare	3
Allergic:	None expected.	
Blood:	None expected.	
Others: Unusual tiredness or weakness.	Rare	4

1- Life-threatening. Seek emergency treatment immediately.
2- Discontinue. Seek emergency treatment.
3- Discontinue. Call doctor right away.
4- Continue. Call doctor when convenient.
5- Continue. Tell doctor at next visit.
6- No action necessary.

ERYTHROMYCIN GLUCEPTATE

WARNINGS & PRECAUTIONS

Don't take if:
- You are allergic to any erythromycin.
- You have had liver disease or impaired liver function.

Before you start, consult your doctor:
If you have taken erythromycin estolate in the past.

Over age 60:
Adverse reactions and side effects may be more frequent and severe than in younger persons, especially skin reactions around genitals and anus.

Pregnancy:
No proven harm to unborn child. Avoid if possible.

Breast-feeding:
Drug passes into milk. Avoid drug or discontinue nursing until you finish medicine. Consult doctor for advice on maintaining milk supply.

Infants & children:
Use only under medical supervision.

Prolonged use:
You may become more susceptible to infections caused by germs not responsive to erythromycin gluceptate.

Skin & sunlight:
No problems expected.

Driving, piloting or hazardous work:
No problems expected.

Airplane passengers:
No problems expected.

Discontinuing:
You must take full dose at least 10 consecutive days for streptococcal or staphylococcal infections.

Others:
No problems expected.

INTERACTION WITH OTHER DRUGS

GENERIC NAME OR DRUG CLASS	COMBINED EFFECT
Aminophylline	Increased effect of aminophylline in blood.
Lincomycins	Decreased lincomycin effect.
Oxtriphylline	Increased level of oxtriphylline in blood.
Penicillins	Decreased penicillin effect.
Theophylline	Increased level of theophylline in blood.

INTERACTION WITH OTHER SUBSTANCES

INTERACTS WITH	COMBINED EFFECT
Alcohol:	Possible liver damage.
Beverages:	None expected.
Cocaine:	None expected.
Foods:	None expected.
Marijuana:	None expected.
Tobacco:	None expected.

ERYTHROMYCIN LACTOBIONATE

BRAND NAMES

Erythrocin

GENERAL INFORMATION

Habit forming? No
Prescription needed? Yes
Available as generic? Yes
Drug class: Antibiotic (erythromycin)

USES

Treatment of infections responsive to erythromycin lactobionate.

DOSAGE & USAGE INFORMATION

How to take:
- Tablet or capsule—Swallow with liquid.
- Extended-release tablets or capsules—Swallow each dose whole. If you take regular tablets, you may chew or crush them.
- Liquid, drops, granules, skin ointment, eye ointment, skin solution—Follow prescription label directions.

When to take:
At the same times each day, 1 hour before or 2 hours after eating.

If you forget a dose:
- If you take 3 or more doses daily—Take as soon as you remember. Return to regular schedule.
- If you take 2 doses daily—Take as soon as you remember. Wait 5 to 6 hours for next dose. Return to regular schedule.

What drug does:
Prevents growth and reproduction of susceptible bacteria.

Time lapse before drug works:
2 to 5 days.

Don't take with:
See Interaction column and consult doctor.

OVERDOSE

Symptoms:
Nausea, vomiting, abdominal discomfort, diarrhea.

What to do:
Overdose unlikely to threaten life. If person takes much larger amount than prescribed, call doctor, poison-control center or hospital emergency room for instructions.

POSSIBLE ADVERSE REACTIONS OR SIDE EFFECTS

SYMPTOMS	FREQUENCY	WHAT TO DO
Brain & nervous system:	None expected.	
Skin: Dryness, irritation, itch, stinging with use of skin solution.	Infrequent	4
Eyes:	None expected.	
Ears, nose, throat: Sore mouth or tongue.	Infrequent	4
Digestive: Diarrhea, nausea, stomach cramps, discomfort, vomiting.	Infrequent	3
Heart & lungs:	None expected.	
Blood vessels:	None expected.	
Muscles, bones, joints:	None expected.	
Genital, urinary:	None expected.	
Kidneys:	None expected.	
Liver: Jaundice (yellow skin and eyes) in adults.	Rare	3
Allergic:	None expected.	
Blood:	None expected.	
Others: Unusual tiredness or weakness.	Rare	4

1- Life-threatening. Seek emergency treatment immediately.
2- Discontinue. Seek emergency treatment.
3- Discontinue. Call doctor right away.
4- Continue. Call doctor when convenient.
5- Continue. Tell doctor at next visit.
6- No action necessary.

ERYTHROMYCIN LACTOBIONATE

WARNINGS & PRECAUTIONS

Don't take if:
- You are allergic to any erythromycin.
- You have had liver disease or impaired liver function.

Before you start, consult your doctor:
If you have taken erythromycin estolate in the past.

Over age 60:
Adverse reactions and side effects may be more frequent and severe than in younger persons, especially skin reactions around genitals and anus.

Pregnancy:
No proven harm to unborn child. Avoid if possible.

Breast-feeding:
Drug passes into milk. Avoid drug or discontinue nursing until you finish medicine. Consult doctor for advice on maintaining milk supply.

Infants & children:
Use only under medical supervision.

Prolonged use:
You may become more susceptible to infections caused by germs not responsive to erythromycin lactobionate.

Skin & sunlight:
No problems expected.

Driving, piloting or hazardous work:
No problems expected.

Airplane passengers:
No problems expected.

Discontinuing:
You must take full dose at least 10 consecutive days for streptococcal or staphylococcal infections.

Others:
No problems expected.

INTERACTION WITH OTHER DRUGS

GENERIC NAME OR DRUG CLASS	COMBINED EFFECT
Aminophylline	Increased effect of aminophylline in blood.
Lincomycins	Decreased lincomycin effect.
Oxtriphylline	Increased level of oxtriphylline in blood.
Penicillins	Decreased penicillin effect.
Theophylline	Increased level of theophylline in blood.

INTERACTION WITH OTHER SUBSTANCES

INTERACTS WITH	COMBINED EFFECT
Alcohol:	Possible liver damage.
Beverages:	None expected.
Cocaine:	None expected.
Foods:	None expected.
Marijuana:	None expected.
Tobacco:	None expected.

ERYTHROMYCIN STEARATE

BRAND NAMES

Bristamycin   Pfizer-E
Erypar   SK-Erythromycin
Ethril   Wyamycin S

GENERAL INFORMATION

Habit forming? No
Prescription needed? Yes
Available as generic? Yes
Drug class: Antibiotic (erythromycin)

USES

Treatment of infections responsive to erythromycin stearate.

DOSAGE & USAGE INFORMATION

How to take:
- Tablet or capsule—Swallow with liquid.
- Extended-release tablets or capsules—Swallow each dose whole. If you take regular tablets, you may chew or crush them.
- Liquid, drops, granules, skin ointment, eye ointment, skin solution—Follow prescription label directions.

When to take:
At the same times each day, 1 hour before or 2 hours after eating.

If you forget a dose:
- If you take 3 or more doses daily—Take as soon as you remember. Return to regular schedule.
- If you take 2 doses daily—Take as soon as you remember. Wait 5 to 6 hours for next dose. Return to regular schedule.

What drug does:
Prevents growth and reproduction of susceptible bacteria.

Time lapse before drug works:
2 to 5 days.

Don't take with:
See Interaction column and consult doctor.

OVERDOSE

Symptoms:
Nausea, vomiting, abdominal discomfort, diarrhea.

What to do:
Overdose unlikely to threaten life. If person takes much larger amount than prescribed, call doctor, poison-control center or hospital emergency room for instructions.

POSSIBLE ADVERSE REACTIONS OR SIDE EFFECTS

SYMPTOMS	FREQUENCY	WHAT TO DO
Brain & nervous system:	None expected.	
Skin: Dryness, irritation, itch, stinging with use of skin solution.	Infrequent	4
Eyes:	None expected.	
Ears, nose, throat: Sore mouth or tongue.	Infrequent	4
Digestive: Diarrhea, nausea, stomach cramps, discomfort, vomiting.	Infrequent	3
Heart & lungs:	None expected.	
Blood vessels:	None expected.	
Muscles, bones, joints:	None expected.	
Genital, urinary:	None expected.	
Kidneys:	None expected.	
Liver: Jaundice (yellow skin and eyes) in adults.	Rare	3
Allergic:	None expected.	
Blood:	None expected.	
Others: Unusual tiredness or weakness.	Rare	4

1- Life-threatening. Seek emergency treatment immediately.
2- Discontinue. Seek emergency treatment.
3- Discontinue. Call doctor right away.
4- Continue. Call doctor when convenient.
5- Continue. Tell doctor at next visit.
6- No action necessary.

ERYTHROMYCIN STEARATE

WARNINGS & PRECAUTIONS

Don't take if:
- You are allergic to any erythromycin.
- You have had liver disease or impaired liver function.

Before you start, consult your doctor:
If you have taken erythromycin estolate in the past.

Over age 60:
Adverse reactions and side effects may be more frequent and severe than in younger persons, especially skin reactions around genitals and anus.

Pregnancy:
No proven harm to unborn child. Avoid if possible.

Breast-feeding:
Drug passes into milk. Avoid drug or discontinue nursing until you finish medicine. Consult doctor for advice on maintaining milk supply.

Infants & children:
Use only under medical supervision.

Prolonged use:
You may become more susceptible to infections caused by germs not responsive to erythromycin stearate.

Skin & sunlight:
No problems expected.

Driving, piloting or hazardous work:
No problems expected.

Airplane passengers:
No problems expected.

Discontinuing:
You must take full dose at least 10 consecutive days for streptococcal or staphylococcal infections.

Others:
No problems expected.

INTERACTION WITH OTHER DRUGS

GENERIC NAME OR DRUG CLASS	COMBINED EFFECT
Aminophylline	Increased effect of aminophylline in blood.
Lincomycins	Decreased lincomycin effect.
Oxtriphylline	Increased level of oxtriphylline in blood.
Penicillins	Decreased penicillin effect.
Theophylline	Increased level of theophylline in blood.

INTERACTION WITH OTHER SUBSTANCES

INTERACTS WITH	COMBINED EFFECT
Alcohol:	Possible liver damage.
Beverages:	None expected.
Cocaine:	None expected.
Foods:	None expected.
Marijuana:	None expected.
Tobacco:	None expected.

ESTERIFIED ESTROGENS

BRAND NAMES

Amnestrogen
Evex

GENERAL INFORMATION

Habit forming? No
Prescription needed? Yes
Available as generic? Yes
Drug class: Female sex hormone (estrogen)

USES

- Treatment for symptoms of menopause and menstrual-cycle irregularity.
- Replacement for female hormone deficiency.
- Treatment for cancer of prostate and breast.

DOSAGE & USAGE INFORMATION

How to take:
Tablet—Swallow with liquid. If you can't swallow whole, crumble tablet and take with liquid or food.

When to take:
At the same time each day.

If you forget a dose:
Take as soon as you remember up to 12 hours late. If more than 12 hours, wait for next scheduled dose (don't double this dose).

What drug does:
Restores normal estrogen level in tissues.

Time lapse before drug works:
10 to 20 days.

Don't take with:
See Interaction column and consult doctor.

OVERDOSE

Symptoms:
Nausea, vomiting, fluid retention, breast enlargement and discomfort, abnormal vaginal bleeding.

What to do:
Overdose unlikely to threaten life. If person takes much larger amount than prescribed, call doctor, poison-control center or hospital emergency room for instructions.

POSSIBLE ADVERSE REACTIONS OR SIDE EFFECTS

SYMPTOMS	FREQUENCY	WHAT TO DO
Brain & nervous system: Depression, dizziness, irritability.	Infrequent	4
Skin:		
• Rash	Infrequent	3
• Brown blotches.	Infrequent	5
• Hair loss.	Infrequent	5
Eyes, ears, nose, throat, heart & lungs, muscles, bones, joints, kidneys, allergic, blood:	None expected.	
Digestive:		
• Stomach or side pain.	Infrequent	3
• Stomach cramps.	Common	3
• Appetite loss.	Common	4
• Nausea, diarrhea.	Common	5
• Vomiting	Infrequent	4
Blood vessels: Swollen ankles, feet.	Common	5
Genital, urinary: Vaginal discharge or bleeding.	Infrequent	5
Liver: Jaundice (yellow skin and eyes).	Rare	3
Others:		
• Breast lumps.	Infrequent	4
• Swollen, tender breasts.	Common	5
• Changes in sex drive.	Infrequent	5

1- Life-threatening. Seek emergency treatment immediately.
2- Discontinue. Seek emergency treatment.
3- Discontinue. Call doctor right away.
4- Continue. Call doctor when convenient.
5- Continue. Tell doctor at next visit.

ESTERIFIED ESTROGENS

WARNINGS & PRECAUTIONS

Don't take if:
- You are allergic to any estrogen-containing drugs.
- You have impaired liver function.
- You have had blood clots, stroke or heart attack.
- You have unexplained vaginal bleeding.

Before you start, consult your doctor:
- If you have had cancer of breast or reproductive organs, fibrocystic breast disease, fibroid tumors of the uterus or endometriosis.
- If you have had migraine headaches, epilepsy or porphyria.
- If you have diabetes, high blood pressure, asthma, congestive heart failure, kidney disease or gallstones.
- If you plan to become pregnant within 3 months.

Over age 60:
Controversial. You and your doctor must decide if drug risks outweigh benefits.

Pregnancy:
Risk to unborn child outweighs drug benefits. Don't use.

Breast-feeding:
Drug filters into milk. May harm child. Avoid.

Infants & children:
Not recommended.

Prolonged use:
Increased growth of fibroid tumors of uterus. Possible association with cancer of uterus.

Skin & sunlight:
May cause rash or intensify sunburn in areas exposed to sun or sunlamp.

Driving, piloting or hazardous work:
No problems expected.

Airplane passengers:
No problems expected.

Discontinuing:
You may need to discontinue estrogen periodically. Consult your doctor.

Others:
In rare instances, may cause blood clot in lung, brain or leg. Symptoms are *sudden* severe headache, coordination loss, vision change, chest pain, breathing difficulty, slurred speech, pain in legs or groin. Seek emergency treatment immediately.

INTERACTION WITH OTHER DRUGS

GENERIC NAME OR DRUG CLASS	COMBINED EFFECT
Anticoagulants (oral)	Decreased anticoagulant effect.
Anticonvulsants (hydantoin)	Increased seizures.
Antidiabetics (oral)	Unpredictable increase or decrease in blood sugar.
Clofibrate	Decreased clofibrate effect.
Carbamazepine	Increased seizures.
Meprobamate	Increased effect of esterified estrogens.
Phenobarbital	Decreased effect of esterified estrogens.
Primidone	Decreased effect of esterified estrogens.
Rifampin	Decreased effect of esterified estrogens.
Thyroid hormones	Decreased thyroid effect.

INTERACTION WITH OTHER SUBSTANCES

INTERACTS WITH	COMBINED EFFECT
Alcohol:	None expected.
Beverages:	None expected.
Cocaine:	No proven problems.
Foods:	None expected.
Marijuana:	Possible menstrual irregularities and bleeding between periods.
Tobacco:	Increased risk of blood clots leading to stroke or heart attack.

ESTRADIOL

BRAND NAMES

Delestrogen
Estrace

GENERAL INFORMATION

Habit forming? No
Prescription needed? Yes
Available as generic? Yes
Drug class: Female sex hormone (estrogen)

USES

- Treatment for symptoms of menopause and menstrual-cycle irregularity.
- Replacement for female hormone deficiency.
- Treatment for cancer of prostate and breast.

DOSAGE & USAGE INFORMATION

How to take:
Tablet—Swallow with liquid. If you can't swallow whole, crumble tablet and take with liquid or food.

When to take:
At the same time each day.

If you forget a dose:
Take as soon as you remember up to 12 hours late. If more than 12 hours, wait for next scheduled dose (don't double this dose).

What drug does:
Restores normal estrogen level in tissues.

Time lapse before drug works:
10 to 20 days.

Don't take with:
See Interaction column and consult doctor.

OVERDOSE

Symptoms:
Nausea, vomiting, fluid retention, breast enlargement and discomfort, abnormal vaginal bleeding.

What to do:
Overdose unlikely to threaten life. If person takes much larger amount than prescribed, call doctor, poison-control center or hospital emergency room for instructions.

POSSIBLE ADVERSE REACTIONS OR SIDE EFFECTS

SYMPTOMS	FREQUENCY	WHAT TO DO
Brain & nervous system: Depression, dizziness, irritability.	Infrequent	4
Skin:		
• Rash	Infrequent	3
• Brown blotches.	Infrequent	5
• Hair loss.	Infrequent	5
Eyes, ears, nose, throat, heart & lungs, muscles, bones, joints, kidneys, allergic, blood:	None expected.	
Digestive:		
• Stomach or side pain.	Infrequent	3
• Stomach cramps.	Common	3
• Appetite loss.	Common	4
• Nausea, diarrhea.	Common	5
• Vomiting	Infrequent	4
Blood vessels: Swollen ankles, feet.	Common	5
Genital, urinary: Vaginal discharge or bleeding.	Infrequent	5
Liver: Jaundice (yellow skin and eyes).	Rare	3
Others:		
• Breast lumps.	Infrequent	4
• Swollen, tender breasts.	Common	5
• Changes in sex drive.	Infrequent	5

1 - Life-threatening. Seek emergency treatment immediately.
2 - Discontinue. Seek emergency treatment.
3 - Discontinue. Call doctor right away.
4 - Continue. Call doctor when convenient.
5 - Continue. Tell doctor at next visit.

ESTRADIOL

WARNINGS & PRECAUTIONS

Don't take if:
- You are allergic to any estrogen-containing drugs.
- You have impaired liver function.
- You have had blood clots, stroke or heart attack.
- You have unexplained vaginal bleeding.

Before you start, consult your doctor:
- If you have had cancer of breast or reproductive organs, fibrocystic breast disease, fibroid tumors of the uterus or endometriosis.
- If you have had migraine headaches, epilepsy or porphyria.
- If you have diabetes, high blood pressure, asthma, congestive heart failure, kidney disease or gallstones.
- If you plan to become pregnant within 3 months.

Over age 60:
Controversial. You and your doctor must decide if drug risks outweigh benefits.

Pregnancy:
Risk to unborn child outweighs drug benefits. Don't use.

Breast-feeding:
Drug filters into milk. May harm child. Avoid.

Infants & children:
Not recommended.

Prolonged use:
Increased growth of fibroid tumors of uterus. Possible association with cancer of uterus.

Skin & sunlight:
May cause rash or intensify sunburn in areas exposed to sun or sunlamp.

Driving, piloting or hazardous work:
No problems expected.

Airplane passengers:
No problems expected.

Discontinuing:
You may need to discontinue estradiol periodically. Consult your doctor.

Others:
In rare instances, may cause blood clot in lung, brain or leg. Symptoms are *sudden* severe headache, coordination loss, vision change, chest pain, breathing difficulty, slurred speech, pain in legs or groin. Seek emergency treatment immediately.

INTERACTION WITH OTHER DRUGS

GENERIC NAME OR DRUG CLASS	COMBINED EFFECT
Anticoagulants (oral)	Decreased anticoagulant effect.
Anticonvulsants (hydantoin)	Increased seizures.
Antidiabetics (oral)	Unpredictable increase or decrease in blood sugar.
Clofibrate	Decreased clofibrate effect.
Carbamazepine	Increased seizures.
Meprobamate	Increased estradiol effect.
Phenobarbital	Decreased estradiol effect.
Primidone	Decreased estradiol effect.
Rifampin	Decreased estradiol effect.
Thyroid hormones	Decreased thyroid effect.

INTERACTION WITH OTHER SUBSTANCES

INTERACTS WITH	COMBINED EFFECT
Alcohol:	None expected.
Beverages:	None expected.
Cocaine:	No proven problems.
Foods:	None expected.
Marijuana:	Possible menstrual irregularities and bleeding between periods.
Tobacco:	Increased risk of blood clots leading to stroke or heart attack.

ESTROGEN

BRAND NAMES

Amnestrogen	Estomed	Hormonin	Milprem
Clinestrone	Estrovis	Menest	PMB-200
DES	Evex	Menotrol	PMB-400
Delestrogen	Feminone	Menrium	Premarin
Estinyl	Femogen	Oestrilin	Stilphostrol
Estrace	Formatrix	Oagen	Theogen

GENERAL INFORMATION

Habit forming? No
Prescription needed? Yes
Available as generic? Yes
Drug class: Female sex hormone
(estrogen)

USES

- Treatment for symptoms of menopause and menstrual-cycle irregularity.
- Treatment for estrogen-deficiency osteoporosis (bone softening from calcium loss).
- Treatment for DES-induced cancer.

DOSAGE & USAGE INFORMATION

How to take:
- Tablet or capsule—Swallow with liquid. If you can't swallow whole, crumble tablet or open capsule and take with liquid or food.
- Vaginal cream—Use as directed on label.

When to take:
At the same time each day.

If you forget a dose:
Take as soon as you remember up to 12 hours late. If more than 12 hours, wait for next scheduled dose (don't double this dose).

What drug does:
Restores normal estrogen level in tissues.

Time lapse before drug works:
10 to 20 days.

Don't take with:
See Interaction column and consult doctor.

OVERDOSE

Symptoms:
Nausea, vomiting, fluid retention, breast enlargement and discomfort, abnormal vaginal bleeding.

What to do:
Overdose unlikely to threaten life. If person takes much larger amount than prescribed, call doctor, poison-control center or hospital emergency room for instructions.

POSSIBLE ADVERSE REACTIONS OR SIDE EFFECTS

SYMPTOMS	FREQUENCY	WHAT TO DO
Brain & nervous system:		
Depression, dizziness, irritability.	Infrequent	4
Skin:		
• Rash	Infrequent	3
• Brown blotches.	Infrequent	5
• Hair loss.	Infrequent	5
Eyes, ears, nose, throat, heart & lungs, muscles, bones, joints, kidneys, allergic, blood:	None expected.	
Digestive:		
• Stomach or side pain.	Infrequent	3
• Stomach cramps.	Common	3
• Appetite loss.	Common	4
• Nausea, diarrhea.	Common	5
• Vomiting	Infrequent	4
Blood vessels:		
Swollen ankles, feet.	Common	5
Genital, urinary:		
Vaginal discharge or bleeding.	Infrequent	5
Liver:		
Jaundice (yellow skin and eyes).	Rare	3
Others:		
• Breast lumps.	Infrequent	4
• Swollen, tender breasts.	Common	5
• Changes in sex drive.	Infrequent	5

1- Life-threatening. Seek emergency treatment immediately.
2- Discontinue. Seek emergency treatment.
3- Discontinue. Call doctor right away.
4- Continue. Call doctor when convenient.
5- Continue. Tell doctor at next visit.
6- No action necessary.

ESTROGEN

WARNINGS & PRECAUTIONS

Don't take if:
- You are allergic to any estrogen-containing drugs.
- You have impaired liver function.
- You have had blood clots, stroke or heart attack.
- You have unexplained vaginal bleeding.

Before you start, consult your doctor:
- If you have had cancer of breast or reproductive organs, fibrocystic breast disease, fibroid tumors of the uterus or endometriosis.
- If you have had migraine headaches, epilepsy or porphyria.
- If you have diabetes, high blood pressure, asthma, congestive heart failure, kidney disease or gallstones.
- If you plan to become pregnant within 3 months.

Over age 60:
Controversial. You and your doctor must decide if drug risks outweigh benefits.

Pregnancy:
Risk to unborn child outweighs drug benefits. Don't use.

Breast-feeding:
Drug filters into milk. May harm child. Avoid.

Infants & children:
Not recommended.

Prolonged use:
Increased growth of fibroid tumors of uterus. Possible association with cancer of uterus.

Skin & sunlight:
May cause rash or intensify sunburn in areas exposed to sun or sunlamp.

Driving, piloting or hazardous work:
No problems expected.

Airplane passengers:
No problems expected.

Discontinuing:
You may need to discontinue estrogens periodically. Consult your doctor.

Others:
In rare instances, may cause blood clot in lung, brain or leg. Symptoms are *sudden* severe headache, coordination loss, vision change, chest pain, breathing difficulty, slurred speech, pain in legs or groin. Seek emergency treatment immediately.

INTERACTION WITH OTHER DRUGS

GENERIC NAME OR DRUG CLASS	COMBINED EFFECT
Anticoagulants (oral)	Decreased anticoagulant effect.
Anticonvulsants (hydantoin)	Increased seizures.
Antidiabetics (oral)	Unpredictable increase or decrease in blood sugar.
Clofibrate	Decreased clofibrate effect.
Carbamazepine	Increased seizures.
Meprobamate	Increased estrogen effect.
Phenobarbital	Decreased estrogen effect.
Primidone	Decreased estrogen effect.
Rifampin	Decreased estrogen effect.
Thyroid hormones	Decreased thyroid effect.

INTERACTION WITH OTHER SUBSTANCES

INTERACTS WITH	COMBINED EFFECT
Alcohol:	None expected.
Beverages:	None expected.
Cocaine:	No proven problems.
Foods:	None expected.
Marijuana:	Possible menstrual irregularities and bleeding between periods.
Tobacco:	Increased risk of blood clots leading to stroke or heart attack.

ESTRONE

BRAND NAMES

Besterone
Kestrin
Theelin
Theogen

GENERAL INFORMATION

Habit forming? No
Prescription needed? Yes
Available as generic? Yes
Drug class: Female sex hormone (estrogen)

USES

- Treatment for symptoms of menopause and menstrual-cycle irregularity.
- Replacement for female hormone deficiency.
- Treatment for cancer of prostate.

DOSAGE & USAGE INFORMATION

How to take:
By injection under medical supervision.

When to take:
Varies according to doctor's instructions.

If you forget an injection:
Consult doctor.

What drug does:
Restores normal estrogen level in tissues.

Time lapse before drug works:
10 to 20 days.

Don't take with:
See Interaction column and consult doctor.

OVERDOSE

Symptoms:
Nausea, vomiting, fluid retention, breast enlargement and discomfort, abnormal vaginal bleeding.

What to do:
Overdose unlikely to threaten life. If person takes much larger amount than prescribed, call doctor, poison-control center or hospital emergency room for instructions.

POSSIBLE ADVERSE REACTIONS OR SIDE EFFECTS

SYMPTOMS	FREQUENCY	WHAT TO DO
Brain & nervous system: Depression, dizziness, irritability.	Infrequent	4
Skin:		
• Rash	Infrequent	3
• Brown blotches.	Infrequent	5
• Hair loss.	Infrequent	5
Eyes, ears, nose, throat, heart & lungs, muscles, bones, joints, kidneys, allergic, blood:	None expected.	
Digestive:		
• Stomach or side pain.	Infrequent	3
• Stomach cramps.	Common	3
• Appetite loss.	Common	4
• Nausea, diarrhea.	Common	5
• Vomiting	Infrequent	4
Blood vessels: Swollen ankles, feet.	Common	5
Genital, urinary: Vaginal discharge or bleeding.	Infrequent	5
Liver: Jaundice (yellow skin and eyes).	Rare	3
Others:		
• Breast lumps.	Infrequent	4
• Swollen, tender breasts.	Common	5
• Changes in sex drive.	Infrequent	5

1- Life-threatening. Seek emergency treatment immediately.
2- Discontinue. Seek emergency treatment.
3- Discontinue. Call doctor right away.
4- Continue. Call doctor when convenient.
5- Continue. Tell doctor at next visit.

WARNINGS & PRECAUTIONS

Don't take if:
- You are allergic to any estrogen-containing drugs.
- You have impaired liver function.
- You have had blood clots, stroke or heart attack.
- You have unexplained vaginal bleeding.

Before you start, consult your doctor:
- If you have had cancer of breast or reproductive organs, fibrocystic breast disease, fibroid tumors of the uterus or endometriosis.
- If you have had migraine headaches, epilepsy or porphyria.
- If you have diabetes, high blood pressure, asthma, congestive heart failure, kidney disease or gallstones.
- If you plan to become pregnant within 3 months.

Over age 60:
Controversial. You and your doctor must decide if drug risks outweigh benefits.

Pregnancy:
Risk to unborn child outweighs drug benefits. Don't use.

Breast-feeding:
Drug filters into milk. May harm child. Avoid.

Infants & children:
Not recommended.

Prolonged use:
Increased growth of fibroid tumors of uterus. Possible association with cancer of uterus.

Skin & sunlight:
May cause rash or intensify sunburn in areas exposed to sun or sunlamp.

Driving, piloting or hazardous work:
No problems expected.

Airplane passengers:
No problems expected.

Discontinuing:
You may need to discontinue estrone periodically. Consult your doctor.

Others:
In rare instances, may cause blood clot in lung, brain or leg. Symptoms are *sudden* severe headache, coordination loss, vision change, chest pain, breathing difficulty, slurred speech, pain in legs or groin. Seek emergency treatment immediately.

 ## INTERACTION WITH OTHER DRUGS

GENERIC NAME OR DRUG CLASS	COMBINED EFFECT
Anticoagulants (oral)	Decreased anticoagulant effect.
Anticonvulsants (hydantoin)	Increased seizures.
Antidiabetics (oral)	Unpredictable increase or decrease in blood sugar.
Clofibrate	Decreased clofibrate effect.
Carbamazepine	Increased seizures.
Meprobamate	Increased estrone effect.
Phenobarbital	Decreased estrone effect.
Primidone	Decreased estrone effect.
Rifampin	Decreased estrone effect.
Thyroid hormones	Decreased thyroid effect.

 ## INTERACTION WITH OTHER SUBSTANCES

INTERACTS WITH	COMBINED EFFECT
Alcohol:	None expected.
Beverages:	None expected.
Cocaine:	No proven problems.
Foods:	None expected.
Marijuana:	Possible menstrual irregularities and bleeding between periods.
Tobacco:	Increased risk of blood clots leading to stroke or heart attack.

ESTROPIPATE

BRAND NAMES

Ogen
Piperazine Estrone Sulfate

GENERAL INFORMATION

Habit forming? No
Prescription needed? Yes
Available as generic? Yes
Drug class: Female sex hormone (estrogen)

 ## USES

- Treatment for symptoms of menopause and menstrual-cycle irregularity.
- Replacement for female hormone deficiency.

 ## DOSAGE & USAGE INFORMATION

How to take:
- Tablet—Swallow with liquid. If you can't swallow whole, crumble tablet and take with liquid or food.
- Vaginal cream—Use as directed on label.

When to take:
At the same time each day.

If you forget a dose:
Take as soon as you remember up to 12 hours late. If more than 12 hours, wait for next scheduled dose (don't double this dose).

What drug does:
Restores normal estrogen level in tissues.

Time lapse before drug works:
10 to 20 days.

Don't take with:
See Interaction column and consult doctor.

 ## OVERDOSE

Symptoms:
Nausea, vomiting, fluid retention, breast enlargement and discomfort, abnormal vaginal bleeding.

What to do:
Overdose unlikely to threaten life. If person takes much larger amount than prescribed, call doctor, poison-control center or hospital emergency room for instructions.

 ## POSSIBLE ADVERSE REACTIONS OR SIDE EFFECTS

SYMPTOMS	FREQUENCY	WHAT TO DO
Brain & nervous system: Depression, dizziness, irritability.	Infrequent	4
Skin:		
• Rash	Infrequent	3
• Brown blotches.	Infrequent	5
• Hair loss.	Infrequent	5
Eyes, ears, nose, throat, heart & lungs, muscles, bones, joints, kidneys, allergic, blood:	None expected.	
Digestive:		
• Stomach or side pain.	Infrequent	3
• Stomach cramps.	Common	3
• Appetite loss.	Common	4
• Nausea, diarrhea.	Common	5
• Vomiting	Infrequent	4
Blood vessels: Swollen ankles, feet.	Common	5
Genital, urinary: Vaginal discharge or bleeding.	Infrequent	5
Liver: Jaundice (yellow skin and eyes).	Rare	3
Others:		
• Breast lumps.	Infrequent	4
• Swollen, tender breasts.	Common	5
• Changes in sex drive.	Infrequent	5

1- Life-threatening. Seek emergency treatment immediately.
2- Discontinue. Seek emergency treatment.
3- Discontinue. Call doctor right away.
4- Continue. Call doctor when convenient.
5- Continue. Tell doctor at next visit.

WARNINGS & PRECAUTIONS

Don't take if:
- You are allergic to any estrogen-containing drugs.
- You have impaired liver function.
- You have had blood clots, stroke or heart attack.
- You have unexplained vaginal bleeding.

Before you start, consult your doctor:
- If you have had cancer of breast or reproductive organs, fibrocystic breast disease, fibroid tumors of the uterus or endometriosis.
- If you have had migraine headaches, epilepsy or porphyria.
- If you have diabetes, high blood pressure, asthma, congestive heart failure, kidney disease or gallstones.
- If you plan to become pregnant within 3 months.

Over age 60:
Controversial. You and your doctor must decide if drug risks outweigh benefits.

Pregnancy:
Risk to unborn child outweighs drug benefits. Don't use.

Breast-feeding:
Drug filters into milk. May harm child. Avoid.

Infants & children:
Not recommended.

Prolonged use:
Increased growth of fibroid tumors of uterus. Possible association with cancer of uterus.

Skin & sunlight:
May cause rash or intensify sunburn in areas exposed to sun or sunlamp.

Driving, piloting or hazardous work:
No problems expected.

Airplane passengers:
No problems expected.

Discontinuing:
You may need to discontinue estropipate periodically. Consult your doctor.

Others:
In rare instances, may cause blood clot in lung, brain or leg. Symptoms are *sudden* severe headache, coordination loss, vision change, chest pain, breathing difficulty, slurred speech, pain in legs or groin. Seek emergency treatment immediately.

INTERACTION WITH OTHER DRUGS

GENERIC NAME OR DRUG CLASS	COMBINED EFFECT
Anticoagulants (oral)	Decreased anticoagulant effect.
Anticonvulsants (hydantoin)	Increased seizures.
Antidiabetics (oral)	Unpredictable increase or decrease in blood sugar.
Clofibrate	Decreased clofibrate effect.
Carbamazepine	Increased seizures.
Meprobamate	Increased estropipate effect.
Phenobarbital	Decreased estropipate effect.
Primidone	Decreased estropipate effect.
Rifampin	Decreased estropipate effect.
Thyroid hormones	Decreased thyroid effect.

INTERACTION WITH OTHER SUBSTANCES

INTERACTS WITH	COMBINED EFFECT
Alcohol:	None expected.
Beverages:	None expected.
Cocaine:	No proven problems.
Foods:	None expected.
Marijuana:	Possible menstrual irregularities and bleeding between periods.
Tobacco:	Increased risk of blood clots leading to stroke or heart attack.

ETHCHLORVYNOL

BRAND NAMES

Placidyl

GENERAL INFORMATION

Habit forming? Yes
Prescription needed? Yes
Available as generic? No
Drug class: Sleep inducer (hypnotic)

 ## USES

Treatment of insomnia.

 ## DOSAGE & USAGE INFORMATION

How to take:
With food or milk to lessen side effects.

When to take:
At or near bedtime.

If you forget a dose:
Bedtime dose—If you forget your once-a-day bedtime dose, don't take it more than 3 hours late.

What drug does:
Affects brain centers that control waking and sleeping.

Time lapse before drug works:
30 to 60 minutes.

Don't take with:
See Interaction column and consult doctor.

 ## OVERDOSE

Symptoms:
Excitement, delirium, incoordination, excessive drowsiness, deep coma.

What to do:
- Dial 0 (operator) or 911 (emergency) for an ambulance or medical help. Then give first aid immediately.
- If patient is unconscious and not breathing, give mouth-to-mouth breathing. If there is no heartbeat, use cardiac massage and mouth-to-mouth breathing (CPR). Don't try to make patient vomit. If you can't get help quickly, take patient to nearest emergency facility.
- Additional emergency information on page 886.

POSSIBLE ADVERSE REACTIONS OR SIDE EFFECTS

SYMPTOMS	FREQUENCY	WHAT TO DO
Brain & nervous system:		
• Jitters, clumsiness, unsteadiness.	Infrequent	3
• Dizziness	Common	4
• Drowsiness, confusion.	Infrequent	3
Skin:		
Rash, hives.	Infrequent	3
Eyes:		
Blurred vision.	Common	4
Ears, nose, throat:		
Unpleasant taste in mouth.	Common	5
Digestive:		
Indigestion, nausea, vomiting, stomach pain.	Common	3
Heart & lungs:		
Slow heartbeat, breathing difficulty.	Rare	3
Blood vessels:		
Unusual bleeding or bruising.	Infrequent	3
Muscles, bones, joints:	None expected.	
Genital, urinary:	None expected.	
Kidneys:	None expected.	
Liver:		
Jaundice (yellow skin and eyes).	Rare	3
Allergic:	None expected.	
Blood:	None expected.	
Others:		
Fatigue, weakness.	Common	5

1- Life-threatening. Seek emergency treatment immediately.
2- Discontinue. Seek emergency treatment.
3- Discontinue. Call doctor right away.
4- Continue. Call doctor when convenient.
5- Continue. Tell doctor at next visit.

WARNINGS & PRECAUTIONS

Don't take if:
- You are allergic to any hypnotic.
- You have porphyria.
- Patient is younger than 12.

Before you start, consult your doctor:
- If you plan to become pregnant within medication period.
- If you have kidney or liver disease.

Over age 60:
Adverse reactions and side effects, especially a "hangover" effect, may be more frequent and severe than in younger persons.

Pregnancy:
Risk to unborn child outweighs drug benefits. Don't use.

Breast-feeding:
No problems expected, but observe child and ask doctor for guidance.

Infants & children:
Not recommended.

Prolonged use:
Impaired vision.

Skin & sunlight:
No problems expected.

Driving, piloting or hazardous work:
Don't drive or pilot aircraft until you learn how medicine affects you. Don't work around dangerous machinery. Don't climb ladders or work in high places. Danger increases if you drink alcohol or take medicine affecting alertness and reflexes.

Airplane passengers:
No problems expected, except altitude makes "hangover" effect more likely.

Discontinuing:
- Don't discontinue without consulting doctor. Dose may require gradual reduction if you have taken drug for a long time. Doses of other drugs may also require adjustment.
- Many of side effects, plus irritability, muscle twitching, trembling, hallucinations or seizures, may occur when you stop taking this drug. Consult your doctor if so.

Others:
No problems expected.

INTERACTION WITH OTHER DRUGS

GENERIC NAME OR DRUG CLASS	COMBINED EFFECT
Anticoagulants (oral)	Decreased anticoagulant effect.
Antidepressants (tricyclic)	Delirium and deep sedation.
Antihistamines	Increased antihistamine effect.
Narcotics	Increased narcotic effect.
Pain relievers	Increased effect of pain reliever.
Sedatives	Increased sedative effect.
Tranquilizers	Increased tranquilizer effect.

INTERACTION WITH OTHER SUBSTANCES

INTERACTS WITH	COMBINED EFFECT
Alcohol:	Excessive depressant and sedative effect. Avoid.
Beverages:	None expected.
Cocaine:	Decreased ethchlorvynol effect.
Foods:	None expected.
Marijuana:	Occasional use—Drowsiness, unsteadiness, depressed function. Frequent use—Severe drowsiness, impaired physical and mental function.
Tobacco:	None expected.

ETHINYL ESTRADIOL

BRAND NAMES

Brevicon (M)   Lo/Ovral (M)   Ovcon (M)
Demulen (M)   Modicon (M)   Ovral (M)
Estinyl   Norinyl
Feminone   Norlestrin (M)
Loestrin (M)   Ortho-Novum (M)

GENERAL INFORMATION

Habit forming? No
Prescription needed? Yes
Available as generic? Yes
Drug class: Female sex hormone (estrogen)

 USES

- Treatment for symptoms of menopause and menstrual-cycle irregularity.
- Replacement for female hormone deficiency.
- Prevention of pregnancy.
- Treatment for cancer of breast and prostate.

 DOSAGE & USAGE INFORMATION

How to take:
- Tablet—Swallow with liquid. If you can't swallow whole, crumble tablet and take with liquid or food.

When to take:
At the same time each day.

If you forget a dose:
Take as soon as you remember up to 12 hours late. If more than 12 hours, wait for next scheduled dose (don't double this dose).

What drug does:
- Restores normal estrogen level in tissues.
- Prevents pituitary gland from secreting hormone that causes ovary to ripen and release egg.

Time lapse before drug works:
10 to 20 days.

Don't take with:
See Interaction column and consult doctor.

 OVERDOSE

Symptoms:
Nausea, vomiting, fluid retention, breast enlargement and discomfort, abnormal vaginal bleeding.

What to do:
Overdose unlikely to threaten life. If person takes much larger amount than prescribed, call doctor, poison-control center or hospital emergency room for instructions.

 POSSIBLE ADVERSE REACTIONS OR SIDE EFFECTS

SYMPTOMS	FREQUENCY	WHAT TO DO
Brain & nervous system:		
Depression, dizziness, irritability.	Infrequent	4
Skin:		
• Rash	Infrequent	3
• Brown blotches.	Infrequent	5
• Hair loss.	Infrequent	5
Eyes, ears, nose, throat, heart & lungs, muscles, bones, joints, kidneys, allergic, blood:	None expected.	
Digestive:		
• Stomach or side pain.	Infrequent	3
• Stomach cramps.	Common	3
• Appetite loss.	Common	4
• Nausea, diarrhea.	Common	5
• Vomiting	Infrequent	4
Blood vessels:		
Swollen ankles, feet.	Common	5
Genital, urinary:		
Vaginal discharge or bleeding.	Infrequent	5
Liver:		
Jaundice (yellow skin and eyes).	Rare	3
Others:		
• Breast lumps.	Infrequent	4
• Swollen, tender breasts.	Common	5
• Changes in sex drive.	Infrequent	5

1- Life-threatening. Seek emergency treatment immediately.
2- Discontinue. Seek emergency treatment.
3- Discontinue. Call doctor right away.
4- Continue. Call doctor when convenient.
5- Continue. Tell doctor at next visit.

ETHINYL ESTRADIOL

WARNINGS & PRECAUTIONS

Don't take if:
- You are allergic to any estrogen-containing drugs.
- You have impaired liver function.
- You have had blood clots, stroke or heart attack.
- You have unexplained vaginal bleeding.

Before you start, consult your doctor:
- If you have had cancer of breast or reproductive organs, fibrocystic breast disease, fibroid tumors of the uterus or endometriosis.
- If you have had migraine headaches, epilepsy or porphyria.
- If you have diabetes, high blood pressure, asthma, congestive heart failure, kidney disease or gallstones.
- If you plan to become pregnant within 3 months.

Over age 60:
Controversial. You and your doctor must decide if drug risks outweigh benefits.

Pregnancy:
Risk to unborn child outweighs drug benefits. Don't use.

Breast-feeding:
Drug filters into milk. May harm child. Avoid.

Infants & children:
Not recommended.

Prolonged use:
Increased growth of fibroid tumors of uterus. Possible association with cancer of uterus.

Skin & sunlight:
May cause rash or intensify sunburn in areas exposed to sun or sunlamp.

Driving, piloting or hazardous work:
No problems expected.

Airplane passengers:
No problems expected.

Discontinuing:
You may need to discontinue ethinyl estradiol periodically. Consult your doctor.

Others:
In rare instances, may cause blood clot in lung, brain or leg. Symptoms are *sudden* severe headache, coordination loss, vision change, chest pain, breathing difficulty, slurred speech, pain in legs or groin. Seek emergency treatment immediately.

INTERACTION WITH OTHER DRUGS

GENERIC NAME OR DRUG CLASS	COMBINED EFFECT
Anticoagulants (oral)	Decreased anticoagulant effect.
Anticonvulsants (hydantoin)	Increased seizures.
Antidiabetics (oral)	Unpredictable increase or decrease in blood sugar.
Clofibrate	Decreased clofibrate effect.
Carbamazepine	Increased seizures.
Meprobamate	Increased effect of ethinyl estradiol.
Phenobarbital	Decreased effect of ethinyl estradiol.
Primidone	Decreased effect of ethinyl estradiol.
Rifampin	Decreased effect of ethinyl estradiol.
Thyroid hormones	Decreased thyroid effect.

INTERACTION WITH OTHER SUBSTANCES

INTERACTS WITH	COMBINED EFFECT
Alcohol:	None expected.
Beverages:	None expected.
Cocaine:	No proven problems.
Foods:	None expected.
Marijuana:	Possible menstrual irregularities and bleeding between periods.
Tobacco:	Increased risk of blood clots leading to stroke or heart attack.

ETHOPROPAZINE

BRAND NAMES

Parsidol
Parsitan

GENERAL INFORMATION

Habit forming? No
Prescription needed? Yes
Available as generic? No
Drug class: Antidyskinetic, antiparkinsonism

USES

- Treatment of Parkinson's disease.
- Treatment of adverse effects of phenothiazines.

DOSAGE & USAGE INFORMATION

How to take:
Tablets or capsules—Take with food to lessen stomach irritation.

When to take:
At the same times each day.

If you forget a dose:
Take as soon as you remember up to 2 hours late. If more than 2 hours, wait for next scheduled dose (don't double this dose).

What drug does:
- Balances chemical reactions necessary to send nerve impulses within base of brain.
- Improves muscle control and reduces stiffness.

Time lapse before drug works:
1 to 2 hours.

Don't take with:
- Non-prescription drugs for colds, cough or allergy.
- See Interaction column and consult doctor.

OVERDOSE

Symptoms:
Agitation, dilated pupils, hallucinations, dry mouth, rapid heartbeat, sleepiness.

What to do:
- Dial 0 (operator) or 911 (emergency) for an ambulance or medical help. Then give first aid immediately.
- If patient is unconscious and not breathing, give mouth-to-mouth breathing. If there is no heartbeat, use cardiac massage and mouth-to-mouth breathing (CPR). Don't try to make patient vomit. If you can't get help quickly, take patient to nearest emergency facility.
- Additional emergency information on page 886.

POSSIBLE ADVERSE REACTIONS OR SIDE EFFECTS

SYMPTOMS	FREQUENCY	WHAT TO DO
Brain & nervous system:		
Confusion, dizziness.	Rare	4
Skin:		
Rash	Rare	3
Eyes:		
• Pain	Rare	3
• Blurred vision, light sensitivity.	Common	4
Ears, nose, throat:		
Sore mouth or tongue.	Rare	4
Digestive:		
• Constipation	Common	4
• Nausea, vomiting.	Common	4
Heart & lungs:	None expected.	
Blood vessels:	None expected.	
Muscles, bones, joints:		
• Muscle cramps.	Rare	4
• Numbness, weakness in hands or feet.	Rare	4
Genital, urinary:		
Difficult or painful urination.	Common	5
Kidneys:	None expected.	
Liver:	None expected.	
Allergic:	None expected.	
Blood:	None expected.	
Others:	None expected.	

1 - Life-threatening. Seek emergency treatment immediately.
2 - Discontinue. Seek emergency treatment.
3 - Discontinue. Call doctor right away.
4 - Continue. Call doctor when convenient.
5 - Continue. Tell doctor at next visit.
6 - No action necessary.

ETHOPROPAZINE

 **WARNINGS &
PRECAUTIONS**

Don't take if:
You are allergic to any antidyskinetic.

Before you start, consult your doctor:
● If you have had glaucoma.
● If you have had high blood pressure or
heart disease.
● If you have had impaired liver function.
● If you have had kidney disease or urination
difficulty.

Over age 60:
More sensitive to drug. Aggravates
symptoms of enlarged prostate. Causes
impaired thinking, hallucinations,
nightmares. Consult doctor about any of
these.

Pregnancy:
Studies inconclusive on harm to unborn
child. Animal studies show fetal
abnormalities. Decide with your doctor
whether drug benefits justify risk to unborn
child.

Breast-feeding:
No problems expected.

Infants & children:
Not recommended for children 3 and
younger. Use for older children only under
doctor's supervision.

Prolonged use:
Possible glaucoma.

Skin & sunlight:
No problems expected.

Driving, piloting or hazardous work:
Don't drive or pilot aircraft until you learn how
medicine affects you. Don't work around
dangerous machinery. Don't climb ladders or
work in high places. Danger increases if you
drink alcohol or take medicine affecting
alertness and reflexes, such as
antihistamines, tranquilizers, sedatives, pain
medicine, narcotics and mind-altering drugs.

Airplane passengers:
No problems expected.

Discontinuing:
Don't discontinue without consulting doctor.
Dose may require gradual reduction if you
have taken drug for a long time. Doses of
other drugs may also require adjustment.

Others:
● Internal eye pressure should be measured
regularly.
● Avoid becoming overheated.

 **INTERACTION WITH
OTHER DRUGS**

GENERIC NAME OR DRUG CLASS	COMBINED EFFECT
Amantadine	Increased amantadine effect.
Antidepressants (tricyclic)	Increased ethopropazine effect. May cause glaucoma.
Antihistamines	Increased ethopropazine effect.
Levodopa	Increased levodopa effect. Improved results in treating Parkinson's disease.
Meperidine	Increased ethopropazine effect.
MAO inhibitors	Increased ethopropazine effect.
Orphenadrine	Increased ethopropazine effect.
Phenothiazines	Behavior changes.
Primidone	Excessive sedation.
Procainamide	Increased procainamide effect.
Quinidine	Increased ethopropazine effect.
Tranquilizers	Excessive sedation.

 **INTERACTION WITH
OTHER SUBSTANCES**

INTERACTS WITH	COMBINED EFFECT
Alcohol:	None expected.
Beverages:	None expected.
Cocaine:	Decreased ethopropazine effect. Avoid.
Foods:	None expected.
Marijuana:	None expected.
Tobacco:	None expected.

ETHOSUXIMIDE

BRAND NAMES

Zarontin

GENERAL INFORMATION

Habit forming? No
Prescription needed? Yes
Available as generic? No
Drug class: Anticonvulsant (succinimide)

 ## USES

Controls seizures in treatment of epilepsy.

 ## DOSAGE & USAGE INFORMATION

How to take:
Capsule—Swallow with liquid or food to lessen stomach irritation.

When to take:
Every day in regularly-spaced doses, according to prescription.

If you forget a dose:
Take as soon as you remember up to 2 hours late. If more than 2 hours, wait for next scheduled dose (don't double this dose).

What drug does:
Depresses nerve transmissions in part of brain that controls muscles.

Time lapse before drug works:
3 hours.

Don't take with:
See Interaction column and consult doctor.

 ## OVERDOSE

Symptoms:
Coma

What to do:
- Dial 0 (operator) or 911 (emergency) for an ambulance or medical help. Then give first aid immediately.
- If patient is unconscious and not breathing, give mouth-to-mouth breathing. If there is no heartbeat, use cardiac massage and mouth-to-mouth breathing (CPR). Don't try to make patient vomit. If you can't get help quickly, take patient to nearest emergency facility.
- Additional emergency information on page 886.

POSSIBLE ADVERSE REACTIONS OR SIDE EFFECTS

SYMPTOMS	FREQUENCY	WHAT TO DO
Brain & nervous system: Dizziness, drowsiness, headache, irritability, mood changes.	Infrequent	4
Skin: Rash	Rare	3
Eyes:	None expected.	
Ears, nose, throat: Sore throat, fever.	Rare	3
Digestive: Nausea, vomiting, stomach cramps, appetite loss.	Common	4
Heart & lungs:	None expected.	
Blood vessels:	None expected.	
Muscles, bones, joints:	None expected.	
Genital, urinary:	None expected.	
Kidneys:	None expected.	
Liver:	None expected.	
Allergic:	None expected.	
Blood: Unusual bleeding or bruising.	Rare	3
Others: Swollen lymph glands.	Rare	4

1- Life-threatening. Seek emergency treatment immediately.
2- Discontinue. Seek emergency treatment.
3- Discontinue. Call doctor right away.
4- Continue. Call doctor when convenient.
5- Continue. Tell doctor at next visit.
6- No action necessary.

WARNINGS & PRECAUTIONS

Don't take if:
You are allergic to any succinimide anticonvulsant.

Before you start, consult your doctor:
- If you plan to become pregnant within medication period.
- If you take other anticonvulsants.
- If you have blood disease.
- If you have kidney or liver disease.

Over age 60:
Adverse reactions and side effects may be more frequent and severe than in younger persons.

Pregnancy:
Risk to unborn child outweighs drug benefits. Don't use.

Breast-feeding:
Drug passes into milk. Avoid drug or discontinue nursing.

Infants & children:
Use only under medical supervision.

Prolonged use:
No problems expected.

Skin & sunlight:
No problems expected.

Driving, piloting or hazardous work:
Don't drive or pilot aircraft until you learn how medicine affects you. Don't work around dangerous machinery. Don't climb ladders or work in high places. Danger increases if you drink alcohol or take medicine affecting alertness and reflexes, such as antihistamines, tranquilizers, sedatives, pain medicine, narcotics and mind-altering drugs.

Airplane passengers:
No problems expected.

Discontinuing:
Don't discontinue without doctor's advice until you complete prescribed dose, even though symptoms diminish or disappear.

Others:
- Your response to medicine should be checked regularly by your doctor. Dose and schedule may have to be altered frequently to fit individual needs.
- Periodic blood-cell counts, kidney- and liver-function studies recommended.

INTERACTION WITH OTHER DRUGS

GENERIC NAME OR DRUG CLASS	COMBINED EFFECT
Anticonvulsants (other)	Increased effect of both drugs.
Antidepressants (tricyclic)	May provoke seizures.
Antipsychotics	May provoke seizures.

INTERACTION WITH OTHER SUBSTANCES

INTERACTS WITH	COMBINED EFFECT
Alcohol:	May provoke seizures.
Beverages:	None expected.
Cocaine:	May provoke seizures.
Foods:	None expected.
Marijuana:	May provoke seizures.
Tobacco:	None expected.

ETHOTOIN

BRAND NAMES

Peganone

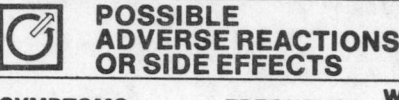

GENERAL INFORMATION

Habit forming? No
Prescription needed? Yes
Available as generic? Yes
Drug class: Anticonvulsant (hydantoin)

USES

- Prevents epileptic seizures.
- Stabilizes irregular heartbeat.

DOSAGE & USAGE INFORMATION

How to take:
- Tablet or capsule—Swallow with liquid.
- Extended-release tablets or capsules—Swallow each dose whole. If you take regular tablets, you may chew or crush them.

When to take:
At the same time each day.

If you forget a dose:
- If drug taken 1 time per day—Take as soon as you remember up to 12 hours late. If more than 12 hours, wait for next scheduled dose (don't double this dose).
- If taken several times per day—Take as soon as possible, then return to regular schedule.

What drug does:
Promotes sodium loss from nerve fibers. This lessens excitability and inhibits spread of nerve impulses.

Time lapse before drug works:
7 to 10 days continual use.

Don't take with:
See Interaction column and consult doctor.

OVERDOSE

Symptoms:
Jerky eye movements; stagger; slurred speech; imbalance; drowsiness; blood-pressure drop; slow, shallow breathing; coma.

What to do:
- Dial 0 (operator) or 911 (emergency) for an ambulance or medical help. Then give first aid immediately.
- Additional emergency information on page 886.

POSSIBLE ADVERSE REACTIONS OR SIDE EFFECTS

SYMPTOMS	FREQUENCY	WHAT TO DO
Brain & nervous system:		
● Mild dizziness, drowsiness.	Common	4
● Headache, sleeplessness.	Infrequent	4
● Hallucinations, confusion, slurred speech, stagger.	Infrequent	3
Skin:		
Rash	Infrequent	3
Eyes:		
Vision changes.	Infrequent	3
Ears, nose, throat:		
Sore throat, fever.	Rare	3
Digestive:		
● Stomach pain.	Rare	3
● Constipation, nausea, vomiting.	Common	4
● Diarrhea	Infrequent	4
Heart & lungs, genital, urinary, kidneys, allergic blood:	None expected.	
Blood vessels:		
Unusual bleeding or bruising.	Rare	3
Muscles, bones, joints:		
Muscle twitching.	Infrequent	4
Liver:		
Jaundice (yellow skin and eyes).	Rare	3
Others:		
Increased body and facial hair.	Infrequent	5

1- Life-threatening. Seek emergency treatment immediately.
2- Discontinue. Seek emergency treatment.
3- Discontinue. Call doctor right away.
4- Continue. Call doctor when convenient.
5- Continue. Tell doctor at next visit.

ETHOTOIN

WARNINGS & PRECAUTIONS

Don't take if:
You are allergic to any hydantoin anticonvulsant.

Before you start, consult your doctor:
- If you have had impaired liver function or disease.
- If you will have surgery within 2 months, including dental surgery, requiring general or spinal anesthesia.

Over age 60:
Adverse reactions and side effects may be more frequent and severe than in younger persons.

Pregnancy:
Risk to unborn child outweighs drug benefits. Don't use.

Breast-feeding:
Drug passes into milk. Avoid drug or discontinue nursing until you finish medicine. Consult doctor for advice on maintaining milk supply.

Infants & children:
Use only under medical supervision.

Prolonged use:
- Weakened bones.
- Lymph gland enlargement.
- Possible liver damage.
- Numbness and tingling of hands and feet.
- Continual back-and-forth eye movements.
- Bleeding, swollen or tender gums.

Skin & sunlight:
May cause rash or intensify sunburn in areas exposed to sun or sunlamp.

Driving, piloting or hazardous work:
Don't drive or pilot aircraft until you learn how medicine affects you. Don't work around dangerous machinery. Don't climb ladders or work in high places. Danger increases if you drink alcohol or take medicine affecting alertness and reflexes.

Airplane passengers:
No problems expected.

Discontinuing:
Don't discontinue without consulting doctor. Dose may require gradual reduction if you have taken drug for a long time. Doses of other drugs may also require adjustment.

INTERACTION WITH OTHER DRUGS

GENERIC NAME OR DRUG CLASS	COMBINED EFFECT
Anticoagulants	Increased effect of both drugs.
Antidepressants (tricyclic)	Need to adjust ethotoin dose.
Antihypertensives	Increased effect of antihypertensive.
Aspirin	Increased ethotoin effect.
Barbiturates	Changed seizure pattern.
Carbonic anhydrase inhibitors	Increased chance of bone disease.
Chloramphenicol	Increased ethotoin effect.
Contraceptives (oral)	Increased seizures.
Cortisone drugs	Decreased cortisone effect.
Digitalis preparations	Decreased digitalis effect.
Disulfiram	Increased ethotoin effect.
Estrogens	Increased ethotoin effect.
Furosemide	Decreased furosemide effect.
Glutethimide	Decreased ethotoin effect.

Additional interactions on page 837.

INTERACTION WITH OTHER SUBSTANCES

INTERACTS WITH	COMBINED EFFECT
Alcohol:	Possible decreased anticonvulsant effect. Use with caution.
Beverages:	None expected.
Cocaine:	Possible seizures.
Foods:	None expected.
Marijuana:	Drowsiness, unsteadiness, decreased anti-convulsant effect.
Tobacco:	None expected.

ETHYLESTRENOL

BRAND NAMES

Maxibolin

Habit forming? No
Prescription needed? Yes

Available as generic? Yes
Drug class: Androgen (male sex hormone)

USES

- Corrects male hormone deficiency.
- Reduces "male menopause" symptoms (loss of sex drive, depression, anxiety).
- Decreases calcium loss of osteoporosis (softened bones).
- Blocks growth of breast-cancer cells in females.
- Corrects undescended testicles in male children.
- Reduces breast pain and fullness following childbirth.
- Augments treatment of aplastic anemia.
- Stimulates weight gain after illness, injury or for chronically underweight persons.
- Stimulates growth in treatment of dwarfism.

DOSAGE & USAGE INFORMATION

How to take:
- Tablets—With food to lessen stomach irritation.
- Injection—Once or twice a month.

When to take:
At the same time each day.

If you forget a dose:
Take as soon as you remember up to 2 hours late. If more than 2 hours, wait for next scheduled dose (don't double this dose).

What drug does:
- Stimulates cells that produce male sex characteristics.
- Replaces hormone deficiencies.
- Stimulates red-blood-cell production.
- Suppresses production of estrogen (female sex hormone).

Time lapse before drug works:
Varies with problems treated. May require 2 or 3 months of regular use for desired effects.

Don't take with:
See Interaction column and consult doctor.

OVERDOSE

Overdose unlikely to threaten life. If person takes much larger amount than prescribed, call doctor, poison-control center or hospital emergency room for instructions.

POSSIBLE ADVERSE REACTIONS OR SIDE EFFECTS

SYMPTOMS	FREQUENCY	WHAT TO DO
Brain & nervous system:		
Depression or confusion.	Infrequent	3
Skin:		
• Flushed face.	Infrequent	3
• Rash or itch.	Infrequent	3
• Hives	Rare	2
• Acne or oily skin in females.	Common	4
Eyes, heart & lungs, blood vessels, kidneys, blood:	None expected.	
Ears, nose, throat:		
• Deep voice.	Common	4
• Sore mouth.	Common	5
• Sore throat, fever.	Rare	3
Digestive:		
• Nausea, vomiting, diarrhea.	Infrequent	3
• Abdominal pain.	Rare	3
• Black stool.	Rare	2
Muscles, bones, joints:		
Swollen feet or legs.	Infrequent	3
Genital, urinary:		
• Enlarged clitoris or frequent erections.	Common	4
• Vaginal bleeding.	Infrequent	3
Liver:		
Jaundice (yellow skin and eyes).	Infrequent	2
Allergic:		
Intense itching, weakness, loss of consciousness.	Rare	1
Others:		
• Higher sex drive.	Common	5
• Swollen breasts in men.	Common	4

1- Life-threatening. Seek emergency treatment immediately.
2- Discontinue. Seek emergency treatment.
3- Discontinue. Call doctor right away.
4- Continue. Call doctor when convenient.
5- Continue. Tell doctor at next visit.

ETHYLESTRENOL

WARNINGS & PRECAUTIONS

Don't take if:
You are allergic to any male hormone.

Before you start, consult your doctor:
- If you might be pregnant.
- If you have cancer of prostate.
- If you have heart disease or arteriosclerosis.
- If you have kidney or liver disease.
- If you have breast cancer (males).
- If you have high blood pressure.
- If you have migraine attacks.
- If you have high level of blood calcium.
- If you have epilepsy.

Over age 60:
- May stimulate sexual activity.
- Can make high blood pressure or heart disease worse.
- Can enlarge prostate and cause urinary retention.

Pregnancy:
Risk to unborn child outweighs drug benefits. Don't use.

Breast-feeding:
Drug passes into milk. Avoid drug or discontinue nursing until you finish medicine. Consult doctor for advice on maintaining milk supply.

Infants & children:
Don't give to children younger than 2. Use with older children only under medical supervision.

Prolonged use:
- Reduces sperm count and volume of semen.
- Possible kidney stones.
- Unnatural hair growth and deep voice in women.

Skin & sunlight:
No problems expected.

Driving, piloting or hazardous work:
No problems expected.

Airplane passengers:
No problems expected.

Discontinuing:
No problems expected.

Others:
- May cause atrophy of testicles.
- Will not increase strength in athletes.

INTERACTION WITH OTHER DRUGS

GENERIC NAME OR DRUG CLASS	COMBINED EFFECT
Anticoagulants	Increased anticoagulant effect.
Antidiabetics (oral)	Increased antidiabetic effect.
Chlorzoxazone	Decreased ethylestrenol effect.
Oxyphenbutazone	Decreased ethylestrenol effect.
Phenobarbital	Decreased ethylestrenol effect.
Phenylbutazone	Decreased ethylestrenol effect.

INTERACTION WITH OTHER SUBSTANCES

INTERACTS WITH	COMBINED EFFECT
Alcohol:	None expected.
Beverages:	None expected.
Cocaine:	No proven problems.
Foods: Salt	Excessive fluid retention (edema). Decrease salt intake while taking male hormones.
Marijuana:	Decreased blood levels of ethylestrenol.
Tobacco:	No proven problems.

FENFLURAMINE

BRAND NAMES

Pondimin

GENERAL INFORMATION

Habit forming? Yes
Prescription needed? Yes
Available as generic? Yes
Drug class: Appetite suppressant

USES

Treatment for overweight. Suppresses appetite.

DOSAGE & USAGE INFORMATION

How to take:
Tablet—Swallow with liquid.

When to take:
1 hour before meals. Last dose no later than 4 to 6 hours before bedtime.

If you forget a dose:
Wait for next scheduled dose. Don't double this dose.

What drug does:
Apparently alters nerve impulses to brain's appetite-control center.

Time lapse before drug works:
1 hour.

Don't take with:
- Non-prescription drugs without consulting doctor.
- See Interaction column and consult doctor.

OVERDOSE

Symptoms:
Agitation, flushing, tremor, dilated pupils, drowsiness, coma.

What to do:
- Dial 0 (operator) or 911 (emergency) for an ambulance or medical help. Then give first aid immediately.
- Additional emergency information on page 886.

POSSIBLE ADVERSE REACTIONS OR SIDE EFFECTS

SYMPTOMS	FREQUENCY	WHAT TO DO
Brain & nervous system:		
• Drowsiness	Common	4
• Headache, nightmares, insomnia, dizziness, depression, clumsiness, speech difficulty.	Infrequent	4
Skin: Rash or hives.	Rare	3
Eyes: Blurred vision.	Infrequent	4
Ears, nose, throat: Unpleasant taste, dry mouth.	Infrequent	4
Digestive: Constipation or diarrhea, nausea, vomiting, cramps.	Infrequent	4
Heart & lungs: Irregular or pounding heartbeat.	Infrequent	3
Blood vessels, muscles, bones, joints, kidneys, liver, allergic, blood:	None expected.	
Genital, urinary: Urinary urgency and difficulty.	Infrequent	3
Others:		
• False sense of well-being.	Common	4
• Changed sex drive.	Infrequent	4
• More sweating.	Infrequent	4

1- Life-threatening. Seek emergency treatment immediately.
2- Discontinue. Seek emergency treatment.
3- Discontinue. Call doctor right away.
4- Continue. Call doctor when convenient.

WARNINGS & PRECAUTIONS

Don't take if:
- You are allergic to any sympathomimetics or phenylpropanolamine.
- You have glaucoma.
- You have taken MAO inhibitors within 2 weeks.
- You plan to become pregnant within medication period.
- You have a history of drug abuse.

Before you start, consult your doctor:
- If you have high blood pressure or heart disease.
- If you have overactive thyroid, nervous tension or "anxiety."
- If you have epilepsy.
- If you have diabetes.

Over age 60:
Adverse reactions and side effects may be more frequent and severe than in younger persons.

Pregnancy:
No proven harm to unborn child. Animal studies show fetal abnormalities. Avoid if possible.

Breast-feeding:
No proven problems. Consult doctor.

Infants & children:
Don't give to children younger than 12.

Prolonged use:
Loses effectiveness. Avoid.

Skin & sunlight:
No problems expected.

Driving, piloting or hazardous work:
Don't drive or pilot aircraft until you learn how medicine affects you. Don't work around dangerous machinery. Don't climb ladders or work in high places. Danger increases if you drink alcohol or take medicine affecting alertness and reflexes, such as antihistamines, tranquilizers, sedatives, pain medicine, narcotics and mind-altering drugs.

Airplane passengers:
No problems expected.

Discontinuing:
Don't discontinue without consulting doctor. Dose may require gradual reduction if you have taken drug for a long time. Doses of other drugs may also require adjustment.

Others:
Don't increase dose.

 ## INTERACTION WITH OTHER DRUGS

GENERIC NAME OR DRUG CLASS	COMBINED EFFECT
Antidepressants (tricyclic)	Increased effect of both drugs.
Caffeine	Increased stimulant effect of fenfluramine.
Guanethidine	Increased guanethidine effect.
Hydralazine	Decreased hydralazine effect.
MAO inhibitors	Dangerous blood-pressure rise.
Methyldopa	Increased methyldopa effect.
Rauwolfia alkaloids	Increased effect of rauwolfia alkaloids.

 ## INTERACTION WITH OTHER SUBSTANCES

INTERACTS WITH	COMBINED EFFECT
Alcohol: Beer, chianti wines, vermouth.	Dangerous blood-pressure rise.
Beverages: • Coffee	Excessive stimulation.
• Drinks containing tyramine (see page 851)	Dangerous blood-pressure rise.
Cocaine:	Excessive stimulation.
Foods: Foods containing tyramine (see page 851)	Dangerous blood-pressure rise.
Marijuana:	Frequent use—Irregular heartbeat.
Tobacco:	None expected.

FENOPROFEN

BRAND NAMES

Nalfon

Habit forming? No
Prescription needed? Yes

GENERAL INFORMATION

Available as generic? No
Drug class: Antiinflammatory (non-steroid)

 USES

- Treatment for joint pain, stiffness, inflammation and swelling of arthritis and gout.
- Pain reliever.
- Treatment for dysmenorrhea (painful or difficult menstruation).

DOSAGE & USAGE INFORMATION

How to take:
Tablet or capsule—Swallow with liquid or food to lessen stomach irritation. If you can't swallow whole, crumble tablet or open capsule and take with liquid or food.

When to take:
At the same times each day.

If you forget a dose:
Take as soon as you remember up to 2 hours late. If more than 2 hours, wait for next scheduled dose (don't double this dose).

What drug does:
Reduces tissue concentration of prostaglandins (hormones which produce inflammation and pain).

Time lapse before drug works:
Begins in 4 to 24 hours. May require 3 weeks regular use for maximum benefit.

Don't take with:
See Interaction column and consult doctor.

 OVERDOSE

Symptoms:
Confusion, agitation, incoherence, convulsions, possible hemorrhage from stomach or intestine, coma.

What to do:
- Dial 0 (operator) or 911 (emergency) for an ambulance or medical help. Then give first aid immediately.
- Additional emergency information on page 886.

 POSSIBLE ADVERSE REACTIONS OR SIDE EFFECTS

SYMPTOMS	FREQUENCY	WHAT TO DO
Brain & nervous system:		
• Depression, drowsiness.	Infrequent	4
• Convulsions, confusion.	Rare	3
• Dizziness	Common	4
• Headache	Common	5
Skin:		
Rash, hives or itch.	Rare	3
Eyes:		
Blurred vision.	Rare	3
Ears, nose, throat:		
Ringing in ears.	Infrequent	4
Digestive:		
• Bloody or black, tarry stools.	Rare	3
• Nausea, pain.	Common	4
• Constipation or diarrhea, vomiting.	Infrequent	4
Heart & lungs:		
Breathing difficulty, tightness in chest, rapid heartbeat.	Rare	3
Blood vessels:		
Unusual bleeding or bruising.	Rare	3
Muscles, bones, joints:		
Swollen feet, legs.	Infrequent	4
Genital, urinary:		
• Bloody urine.	Rare	3
• Difficult, painful or frequent urination.	Rare	4
Kidneys, allergic, blood:	None expected.	
Liver:		
Jaundice (yellow skin and eyes).	Rare	3
Others:		
Fatigue, weakness.	Rare	4

1 - Life-threatening. Seek emergency treatment immediately.
2 - Discontinue. Seek emergency treatment.
3 - Discontinue. Call doctor right away.
4 - Continue. Call doctor when convenient.
5 - Continue. Tell doctor at next visit.

WARNINGS & PRECAUTIONS

Don't take if:
- You are allergic to aspirin or any non-steroid, antiinflammatory drug.
- You have gastritis, peptic ulcer, enteritis, ileitis, ulcerative colitis, asthma, heart faiiure, high blood pressure or bleeding problems.
- Patient is younger than 15.

Before you start, consult your doctor:
- If you have epilepsy.
- If you have Parkinson's disease.
- If you have been mentally ill.
- If you have had kidney disease or impaired kidney function.

Over age 60:
Adverse reactions and side effects may be more frequent and severe than in younger persons.

Pregnancy:
Studies inconclusive on harm to unborn child. Decide with your doctor whether drug benefits justify risk to unborn child.

Breast-feeding:
May harm child. Avoid.

Infants & children:
Not recommended for anyone younger than 15. Use only under medical supervision.

Prolonged use:
- Eye damage.
- Reduced hearing.
- Sore throat, fever.
- Weight gain.

Skin & sunlight:
No problems expected.

Driving, piloting or hazardous work:
Don't drive or pilot aircraft until you learn how medicine affects you. Don't work around dangerous machinery. Don't climb ladders or work in high places. Danger increases if you drink alcohol or take medicine affecting alertness and reflexes, such as antihistamines, tranquilizers, sedatives, pain medicine, narcotics and mind-altering drugs.

Airplane passengers:
No problems expected.

Discontinuing:
Don't discontinue without consulting doctor. Dose may require gradual reduction if you have taken drug for a long time. Doses of other drugs may also require adjustment.

Others:
No problems expected.

 ## INTERACTION WITH OTHER DRUGS

GENERIC NAME OR DRUG CLASS	COMBINED EFFECT
Anticoagulants (oral)	Increased risk of bleeding.
Aspirin	Increased risk of stomach ulcer.
Cortisone drugs	Increased risk of stomach ulcer.
Furosemide	Decreased diuretic effect of furosemide.
Oxyphenbutazone	Possible stomach ulcer.
Phenylbutazone	Possible stomach ulcer.
Probenecid	Increased fenoprofen effect.
Thyroid hormones	Rapid heartbeat, blood-pressure rise.

 ## INTERACTION WITH OTHER SUBSTANCES

INTERACTS WITH	COMBINED EFFECT
Alcohol:	Possible stomach ulcer or bleeding.
Beverages:	None expected.
Cocaine:	None expected.
Foods:	None expected.
Marijuana:	Increased pain relief from fenoprofen.
Tobacco:	None expected.

FERROUS FUMARATE

BRAND NAMES

Feco-T	Fumasorb	Toleron
Femiron	Fumerin	Tolfrinic
Feostat	Ircon	Tolifer
Ferrofume	Laud-Iron	Vitron C
Ferro-sequels (M)	Maniron	
Fersamal	Palafer	

GENERAL INFORMATION

Habit forming? No
Prescription needed? With folic acid: Yes
Without folic acid: No
Available as generic? Yes
Drug class: Mineral supplement (iron)

USES

Treatment for dietary iron deficiency or iron-deficiency anemia from other causes.

DOSAGE & USAGE INFORMATION

How to take:
- Tablet, capsule or liquid—Swallow with liquid or food to lessen stomach irritation. If you can't swallow whole, crumble tablet or open capsule and take with liquid or food. Place medicine far back on tongue to avoid staining teeth.
- Drops—Dilute dose in beverage before swallowing and drink through a straw.

When to take:
1 hour before or 2 hours after meals.

If you forget a dose:
Take up to 2 hours late. If more than 2 hours, wait for next dose (don't double this).

What drug does:
Stimulates bone-marrow production of hemoglobin (red-blood-cell pigment that carries oxygen to body cells).

Time lapse before drug works:
3 to 7 days. May require 3 weeks for maximum benefit.

Don't take with:
- Multiple vitamin and mineral supplements.
- See Interaction column and consult doctor.

OVERDOSE

Symptoms:
Weakness, collapse; pallor, blue lips, hands and fingernails; weak, rapid heartbeat; shallow breathing; convulsions; coma.

What to do:
- Dial 0 (operator) or 911 (emergency) for an ambulance or medical help. Then give first aid immediately.
- Additional emergency information on page 886.

POSSIBLE ADVERSE REACTIONS OR SIDE EFFECTS

SYMPTOMS	FREQUENCY	WHAT TO DO
Brain & nervous system:		
Drowsiness	Rare	4
Skin, eyes, blood vessels, muscles, bones, joints, kidneys, liver, allergic, blood:	None expected.	
Ears, nose, throat:		
Throat or chest pain on swallowing.	Rare	3
Digestive:		
• Gray or black stool.	Always	6
• Constipation or diarrhea, heartburn, nausea, vomiting.	Infrequent	3
• Pain, cramps, blood in stool.	Rare	3
Heart & lungs:		
Weak, rapid heartbeat.	Rare	1
Genital, urinary:		
Dark urine.	Infrequent	5
Others:		
• Stained teeth with liquid iron.	Common	6
• Fatigue, weakness.	Infrequent	4

1- Life-threatening. Seek emergency treatment immediately.
2- Discontinue. Seek emergency treatment.
3- Discontinue. Call doctor right away.
4- Continue. Call doctor when convenient.
5- Continue. Tell doctor at next visit.
6- No action necessary.

FERROUS FUMARATE

WARNINGS & PRECAUTIONS

Don't take if:
- You are allergic to any iron supplement.
- You take iron injections.
- Your daily iron intake is high.
- You plan to take this supplement for a long time.
- You have acute hepatitis.
- You have hemosiderosis or hemochromatosis (conditions involving excess iron in body).
- You have hemolytic anemia.

Before you start, consult your doctor:
- If you plan to become pregnant within medication period.
- If you have had stomach surgery.
- If you have had peptic ulcer disease, enteritis or colitis.
- If you have had pancreatitis or hepatitis.

Over age 60:
May cause hemochromatosis (iron storage disease) with bronze skin, liver damage, diabetes, heart problems and impotence.

Pregnancy:
No proven harm to unborn child. Avoid if possible. Take only if your doctor prescribes supplement during last half of pregnancy.

Breast-feeding:
No problems expected. Take only if your doctor confirms you have a dietary deficiency or an iron-deficiency anemia.

Infants & children:
Use only under medical supervision. Overdose common and dangerous. Keep out of children's reach.

Prolonged use:
May cause hemochromatosis (iron storage disease) with bronze skin, liver damage, diabetes, heart problems and impotence.

Skin & sunlight:
No problems expected.

Driving, piloting or hazardous work:
No problems expected.

Airplane passengers:
No problems expected.

Discontinuing:
May be unnecessary to finish medicine. Follow doctor's instructions.

Others:
Liquid form stains teeth. Mix with water or juice to lessen the effect. Brush with baking soda or hydrogen peroxide to help remove stain.

INTERACTION WITH OTHER DRUGS

GENERIC NAME OR DRUG CLASS	COMBINED EFFECT
Allopurinol	Possible excess iron storage in liver.
Antacids	Poor iron absorption.
Chloramphenicol	Decreased effect of iron. Interferes with red-blood-cell and hemoglobin formation.
Cholestyramine	Decreased iron effect.
Iron supplements (other)	Possible excess iron storage in liver.
Penicillamine	Decreased penicillamine effect.
Sulfasalazine	Decreased iron effect.
Tetracyclines	Decreased tetracycline effect. Take iron 3 hours before or 2 hours after taking tetracycline.
Vitamin C	Increased iron effect. Contributes to red-blood-cell and hemoglobin formation.
Vitamin E	Decreased iron effect.

INTERACTION WITH OTHER SUBSTANCES

INTERACTS WITH	COMBINED EFFECT
Alcohol:	Increased iron absorption. May cause organ damage. Avoid or use in moderation.
Beverages: Milk, tea	Decreased iron effect.
Cocaine:	None expected.
Foods: Dairy foods, eggs, whole-grain bread and cereal.	Decreased iron effect.
Marijuana:	None expected.
Tobacco:	None expected.

FERROUS GLUCONATE

BRAND NAMES

Fergon
Ferralet
Ferralet Plus
Ferrous-G

GENERAL INFORMATION

Habit forming? No
Prescription needed? With folic acid—Yes
Without folic acid—No
Available as generic? Yes
Drug class: Mineral supplement (iron)

 USES

Treatment for dietary iron deficiency or iron-deficiency anemia from other causes.

 DOSAGE & USAGE INFORMATION

How to take:
- Tablet or capsule—Swallow with liquid or food to lessen stomach irritation. If you can't swallow whole, crumble tablet or open capsule and take with liquid or food. Place medicine far back on tongue to avoid staining teeth.
- Drops—Dilute dose in beverage before swallowing and drink through a straw.

When to take:
1 hour before or 2 hours after eating.

If you forget a dose:
Take up to 2 hours late. If more than 2 hours, wait for next dose (don't double this).

What drug does:
Stimulates bone-marrow production of hemoglobin (red-blood-cell pigment that carries oxygen to body cells).

Time lapse before drug works:
3 to 7 days. May require 3 weeks for maximum benefit.

Don't take with:
- Multiple vitamin and mineral supplements.
- See Interaction column and consult doctor.

 OVERDOSE

Symptoms:
- Moderate overdose—Stomach pain, vomiting, diarrhea, black stools, lethargy.
- Serious overdose—Weakness and collapse; pallor, weak and rapid heartbeat; shallow breathing; convulsions and coma.

What to do:
- Dial 0 (operator) or 911 (emergency) for an ambulance or medical help. Then give first aid immediately.
- Additional emergency information on page 886.

POSSIBLE ADVERSE REACTIONS OR SIDE EFFECTS

SYMPTOMS	FREQUENCY	WHAT TO DO
Brain & nervous system: Drowsiness	Rare	4
Skin: Blue lips, fingernails, palms of hands; pale, clammy skin.	Rare	2
Ears, nose, throat:		
• Stained teeth with liquid iron.	Common	6
• Throat pain on swallowing.	Rare	3
Digestive:		
• Gray or black stool.	Always	6
• Constipation or diarrhea, heartburn, nausea, vomiting.	Infrequent	3
• Pain, cramps, blood in stool.	Rare	3
Heart & lungs: Weak, rapid heartbeat.	Rare	1
Eyes, blood vessels, muscles, bones, joints, genital, urinary, kidneys, liver, allergic, blood:	None expected.	
Others: Fatigue, weakness.	Infrequent	4

1- Life-threatening. Seek emergency treatment immediately.
2- Discontinue. Seek emergency treatment.
3- Discontinue. Call doctor right away.
4- Continue. Call doctor when convenient.
5- Continue. Tell doctor at next visit.
6- No action necessary.

FERROUS GLUCONATE

WARNINGS & PRECAUTIONS

Don't take if:
- You are allergic to any iron supplement.
- You take iron injections.
- You have acute hepatitis, hemosiderosis or hemochromatosis (conditions involving excess iron in body).
- You have hemolytic anemia.

Before you start, consult your doctor:
- If you plan to become pregnant within medication period.
- If you have had stomach surgery.
- If you have had peptic ulcer, enteritis or colitis.

Over age 60:
May cause hemochromatosis (iron storage disease) with bronze skin, liver damage, diabetes, heart problems and impotence.

Pregnancy:
No proven harm to unborn child. Avoid if possible. Take only if your doctor advises supplement during last half of pregnancy.

Breast-feeding:
No problems expected. Take only if your doctor confirms you have a dietary deficiency or an iron-deficiency anemia.

Infants & children:
Use only under medical supervision. Overdose common and dangerous. Keep out of children's reach.

Prolonged use:
May cause hemochromatosis (iron storage disease) with bronze skin, liver damage, diabetes, heart problems and impotence.

Skin & sunlight:
No problems expected.

Driving, piloting or hazardous work:
No problems expected.

Airplane passengers:
No problems expected.

Discontinuing:
May be unnecessary to finish medicine. Follow doctor's instructions.

Others:
Liquid form stains teeth. Mix with water or juice to lessen the effect. Brush with baking soda or hydrogen peroxide to help remove.

INTERACTION WITH OTHER DRUGS

GENERIC NAME OR DRUG CLASS	COMBINED EFFECT
Allopurinol	Possible excess iron storage in liver.
Antacids	Poor iron absorption.
Chloramphenicol	Decreased effect of iron. Interferes with red-blood-cell and hemoglobin formation.
Cholestyramine	Decreased iron effect.
Iron supplements (other)	Possible excess iron storage in liver.
Sulfasalazine	Decreased iron effect.
Tetracyclines	Decreased tetracycline effect. Take iron 3 hours before or 2 hours after taking tetracycline.
Vitamin C	Increased iron effect. Contributes to red-blood-cell and hemoglobin formation.
Vitamin E	Decreased iron effect.

INTERACTION WITH OTHER SUBSTANCES

INTERACTS WITH	COMBINED EFFECT
Alcohol:	Increased iron absorption. May cause organ damage. Avoid or use in moderation.
Beverages: Milk, tea	Decreased iron effect.
Cocaine:	None expected.
Foods: Dairy foods, eggs, whole-grain bread and cereal	Decreased iron effect.
Marijuana:	None expected.
Tobacco:	None expected.

FERROUS SULFATE

BRAND NAMES

Feosol	Fesofor
Fer-In-Sol	Geritol Tablets (M)
Fero-folic-500 (M)	Iberet (M)
Fero-Grad-500 (M)	Iberet-500 (M)
Fero-Gradumet	Iberet-Folic-500 (M)
Ferralyn	Mol-Iron

Novoferrosulfa
Slow-Fe

GENERAL INFORMATION

Habit forming? No
Prescription needed?
With folic acid: Yes
Without folic acid: No
Available as generic? Yes
Drug class: Mineral supplement (iron)

 ## USES

Treatment for dietary iron deficiency or iron-deficiency anemia from other causes.

 ## DOSAGE & USAGE INFORMATION

How to take:
- Tablet, capsule, or liquid—Swallow with liquid or food to lessen stomach irritation. Place medicine far back on tongue to avoid staining teeth.
- Drops—Dilute dose in beverage before swallowing and drink through a straw.
- Extended release tablet or capsule—Swallow whole with liquid.

When to take:
1 hour before or 2 hours after meals.

If you forget a dose:
Take up to 2 hours late. If more than 2 hours, wait for next dose (don't double this).

What drug does:
Stimulates bone-marrow production of hemoglobin (red-blood-cell pigment that carries oxygen to body cells).

Time lapse before drug works:
3 to 7 days. May require 3 weeks for maximum benefit.

Don't take with:
- Multiple vitamin and mineral supplements.
- See Interaction column and consult doctor.

 ## OVERDOSE

Symptoms:
Weakness, collapse; pallor, blue lips, hands and fingernails; weak, rapid heartbeat; shallow breathing; convulsions; coma.

What to do:
- Dial 0 (operator) or 911 (emergency) for an ambulance or medical help. Then give first aid immediately.
- Additional information on page 886.

 ## POSSIBLE ADVERSE REACTIONS OR SIDE EFFECTS

SYMPTOMS	FREQUENCY	WHAT TO DO
Brain & nervous system: Drowsiness	Rare	4
Skin, eyes, blood vessels, muscles, bones, joints, kidneys, liver, allergic, blood:	None expected.	
Ears, nose, throat: Throat or chest pain on swallowing.	Rare	3
Digestive:		
• Gray or black stool.	Always	6
• Constipation or diarrhea, heartburn, nausea, vomiting.	Infrequent	3
• Pain, cramps, blood in stool.	Rare	3
Heart & lungs: Weak, rapid heartbeat.	Rare	1
Genital, urinary: Dark urine.	Infrequent	5
Others:		
• Stained teeth with liquid iron.	Common	6
• Fatigue, weakness.	Infrequent	4

1-Life-threatening. Seek emergency treatment immediately.
2-Discontinue. Seek emergency treatment.
3-Discontinue. Call doctor right away.
4-Continue. Call doctor when convenient.
5-Continue. Tell doctor at next visit.
6-No action necessary.

WARNINGS & PRECAUTIONS

Don't take if:
- You are allergic to any iron supplement.
- You take iron injections.
- Your daily iron intake is high.
- You plan to take this supplement for a long time.
- You have acute hepatitis.
- You have hemosiderosis or hemochromatosis (conditions involving excess iron in body).
- You have hemolytic anemia.

Before you start, consult your doctor:
- If you plan to become pregnant within medication period.
- If you have had stomach surgery.
- If you have had peptic ulcer disease, enteritis or colitis.
- If you have had pancreatitis or hepatitis.

Over age 60:
May cause hemochromatosis (iron storage disease) with bronze skin, liver damage, diabetes, heart problems and impotence.

Pregnancy:
No proven harm to unborn child. Avoid if possible. Take only if your doctor prescribes supplement during last half of pregnancy.

Breast-feeding:
No problems expected. Take only if your doctor confirms you have a dietary deficiency or an iron-deficiency anemia.

Infants & children:
Use only under medical supervision. Overdose common and dangerous. Keep out of children's reach.

Prolonged use:
May cause hemochromatosis (iron storage disease) with bronze skin, liver damage, diabetes, heart problems and impotence.

Skin & sunlight:
No problems expected.

Driving, piloting or hazardous work:
No problems expected.

Airplane passengers:
No problems expected.

Discontinuing:
May be unnecessary to finish medicine. Follow doctor's instructions.

Others:
Liquid form stains teeth. Mix with water or juice to lessen the effect. Brush with baking soda or hydrogen peroxide to help remove stain.

INTERACTION WITH OTHER DRUGS

GENERIC NAME OR DRUG CLASS	COMBINED EFFECT
Allopurinol	Possible excess iron storage in liver.
Antacids	Poor iron absorption.
Chloramphenicol	Decreased effect of iron. Interferes with red-blood-cell and hemoglobin formation.
Cholestyramine	Decreased iron effect.
Iron supplements (other)	Possible excess iron storage in liver.
Penicillamine	Decreased penicillamine effect.
Sulfasalazine	Decreased iron effect.
Tetracyclines	Decreased tetracycline effect. Take iron 3 hours before or 2 hours after taking tetracycline.
Vitamin C	Increased iron effect. Contributes to red-blood-cell and hemoglobin formation.
Vitamin E	Decreased iron effect.

INTERACTION WITH OTHER SUBSTANCES

INTERACTS WITH	COMBINED EFFECT
Alcohol:	Increased iron absorption. May cause organ damage. Avoid or use in moderation.
Beverages: Milk, tea	Decreased iron effect.
Cocaine:	None expected.
Foods: Dairy foods, eggs, whole-grain bread and cereal.	Decreased iron effect.
Marijuana:	None expected.
Tobacco:	None expected.

FLUOXYMESTERONE

BRAND NAMES

Halotestin
Oratestin
Ora-Testryl

Habit forming? No
Prescription needed? Yes

Available as generic? Yes
Drug class: Androgen (male sex hormone)

USES

- Corrects male hormone deficiency.
- Reduces "male menopause" symptoms (loss of sex drive, depression, anxiety).
- Decreases calcium loss of osteoporosis (softened bones).
- Blocks growth of breast-cancer cells in females.
- Corrects undescended testicles in male children.
- Reduces breast pain and fullness following childbirth.
- Augments treatment of aplastic anemia.
- Stimulates weight gain after illness, injury or for chronically underweight persons.
- Stimulates growth in treatment of dwarfism.

DOSAGE & USAGE INFORMATION

How to take:
- Tablets—With food to lessen stomach irritation.
- Injection—Once or twice a month.

When to take:
At the same time each day.

If you forget a dose:
Take as soon as you remember up to 2 hours late. If more than 2 hours, wait for next scheduled dose (don't double this dose).

What drug does:
- Stimulates cells that produce male sex characteristics.
- Replaces hormone deficiencies.
- Stimulates red-blood-cell production.
- Suppresses production of estrogen (female sex hormone).

Time lapse before drug works:
Varies with problems treated. May require 2 or 3 months of regular use for desired effects.

Don't take with:
See Interaction column and consult doctor.

OVERDOSE

Overdose unlikely to threaten life. If person takes much larger amount than prescribed, call doctor, poison-control center or hospital emergency room for instructions.

POSSIBLE ADVERSE REACTIONS OR SIDE EFFECTS

SYMPTOMS	FREQUENCY	WHAT TO DO
Brain & nervous system:		
Depression or confusion.	Infrequent	3
Skin:		
• Flushed face.	Infrequent	3
• Rash or itch.	Infrequent	3
• Hives	Rare	2
• Acne or oily skin in females.	Common	4
Eyes, heart & lungs, blood vessels, kidneys, blood:	None expected.	
Ears, nose, throat:		
• Deep voice.	Common	4
• Sore mouth.	Common	5
• Sore throat, fever.	Rare	3
Digestive:		
• Nausea, vomiting, diarrhea.	Infrequent	3
• Abdominal pain.	Rare	3
• Black stool.	Rare	2
Muscles, bones, joints:		
Swollen feet or legs.	Infrequent	3
Genital, urinary:		
• Enlarged clitoris or frequent erections.	Common	4
• Vaginal bleeding.	Infrequent	3
Liver:		
Jaundice (yellow skin and eyes).	Infrequent	2
Allergic:		
Intense itching, weakness, loss of consciousness.	Rare	1
Others:		
• Higher sex drive.	Common	5
• Swollen breasts in men.	Common	4

1 - Life-threatening. Seek emergency treatment immediately.
2 - Discontinue. Seek emergency treatment.
3 - Discontinue. Call doctor right away.
4 - Continue. Call doctor when convenient.
5 - Continue. Tell doctor at next visit.

WARNINGS & PRECAUTIONS

Don't take if:
You are allergic to any male hormone.

Before you start, consult your doctor:
- If you might be pregnant.
- If you have cancer of prostate.
- If you have heart disease or arteriosclerosis.
- If you have kidney or liver disease.
- If you have breast cancer (males).
- If you have high blood pressure.
- If you have migraine attacks.
- If you have high level of blood calcium.
- If you have epilepsy.

Over age 60:
- May stimulate sexual activity.
- Can make high blood pressure or heart disease worse.
- Can enlarge prostate and cause urinary retention.

Pregnancy:
Risk to unborn child outweighs drug benefits. Don't use.

Breast-feeding:
Drug passes into milk. Avoid drug or discontinue nursing until you finish medicine. Consult doctor for advice on maintaining milk supply.

Infants & children:
Don't give to children younger than 2. Use with older children only under medical supervision.

Prolonged use:
- Reduces sperm count and volume of semen.
- Possible kidney stones.
- Unnatural hair growth and deep voice in women.

Skin & sunlight:
No problems expected.

Driving, piloting or hazardous work:
No problems expected.

Airplane passengers:
No problems expected.

Discontinuing:
No problems expected.

Others:
- May cause atrophy of testicles.
- Will not increase strength in athletes.

 ## INTERACTION WITH OTHER DRUGS

GENERIC NAME OR DRUG CLASS	COMBINED EFFECT
Anticoagulants	Increased anticoagulant effect.
Antidiabetics (oral)	Increased antidiabetic effect.
Chlorzoxazone	Decreased fluoxymesterone effect.
Oxyphenbutazone	Decreased fluoxymesterone effect.
Phenobarbital	Decreased fluoxymesterone effect.
Phenylbutazone	Decreased fluoxymesterone effect.

 ## INTERACTION WITH OTHER SUBSTANCES

INTERACTS WITH	COMBINED EFFECT
Alcohol:	None expected.
Beverages:	None expected.
Cocaine:	No proven problems.
Foods: Salt	Excessive fluid retention (edema). Decrease salt intake while taking male hormones.
Marijuana:	Decreased blood levels of fluoxymesterone.
Tobacco:	No proven problems.

FLUPHENAZINE

BRAND NAMES

Modecate
Moditen
Permitil
Prolixin

GENERAL INFORMATION

Habit forming? No
Prescription needed? Yes
Available as generic? Yes
Drug class: Tranquilizer, antiemetic (phenothiazine)

 USES

- Stops nausea, vomiting.
- Reduces anxiety, agitation.

 DOSAGE & USAGE INFORMATION

How to take:
- Tablet or capsule—Swallow with liquid or food to lessen stomach irritation.
- Suppositories—Remove wrapper and moisten suppository with water. Gently insert into rectum, large end first.
- Drops or liquid—Dilute dose in beverage.

When to take:
- Nervous and mental disorders—Take at the same times each day.
- Nausea and vomiting—Take as needed, no more often than every 4 hours.

If you forget a dose:
- Nervous and mental disorders—Take up to 2 hours late. If more than 2 hours, wait for next scheduled dose (don't double this).
- Nausea and vomiting—Take as soon as you remember. Wait 4 hours for next dose.

What drug does:
- Suppresses brain's vomiting center.
- Suppresses brain centers that control abnormal emotions and behavior.

Time lapse before drug works:
- Nausea and vomiting—1 hour or less.
- Nervous and mental disorders—4-6 weeks.

Don't take with:
- Antacid or medicine for diarrhea.
- Non-prescription drug for cough, cold or allergy.
- See Interaction column and consult doctor.

 OVERDOSE

Symptoms:
Stupor, convulsions, coma.

What to do:
- Dial 0 (operator) or 911 (emergency) for an ambulance or medical help. Then give first aid immediately.
- Additional emergency information on page 886.

 POSSIBLE ADVERSE REACTIONS OR SIDE EFFECTS

SYMPTOMS	FREQUENCY	WHAT TO DO
Brain & nervous system:		
• Restlessness, tremor.	Common	3
• Fainting	Infrequent	2
• Drowsiness	Common	3
Skin:		
• Rash	Infrequent	3
• Less perspiration.	Common	4
Eyes:		
Vision changes.	Rare	3
Ears, nose, throat:		
• Sore throat, fever.	Rare	3
• Dry mouth, nasal congestion.	Common	4
Digestive:		
Constipation	Common	4
Heart & lungs, blood vessels, kidneys, allergic, blood:	None expected.	
Muscles, bones, joints:		
Muscle spasms of face and neck, unsteady gait.	Common	2
Genital, urinary:		
Urination difficulty.	Infrequent	4
Liver:		
Jaundice (yellow eyes and skin).	Rare	3
Others:		
Less interest in sex, breast swelling, change in menstrual pattern.	Infrequent	4

1- Life-threatening. Seek emergency treatment immediately.
2- Discontinue. Seek emergency treatment.
3- Discontinue. Call doctor right away.
4- Continue. Call doctor when convenient.
5- Continue. Tell doctor at next visit.
6- No action necessary.

WARNINGS & PRECAUTIONS

Don't take if:
- You are allergic to any phenothiazine.
- You have a blood or bone-marrow disease.

Before you start, consult your doctor:
- If you will have surgery within 2 months, including dental surgery, requiring general or spinal anesthesia.
- If you have asthma, emphysema or other lung disorder.
- If you take non-prescription ulcer medicine, asthma medicine or amphetamines.

Over age 60:
Adverse reactions and side effects may be more frequent and severe than in younger persons. More likely to develop involuntary movement of jaws, lips, tongue, chewing. Report this to your doctor immediately. Early treatment can help.

Pregnancy:
Risk to unborn child outweighs drug benefits. Don't use.

Breast-feeding:
Drug passes into milk. Avoid drug or discontinue nursing until you finish medicine. Consult doctor for advice on maintaining milk supply.

Infants & children:
Don't give to children younger than 2.

Prolonged use:
May lead to tardive dyskinesia (involuntary movement of jaws, lips, tongue, chewing).

Skin & sunlight:
May cause rash or intensify sunburn in areas exposed to sun or sunlamp. Skin may remain sensitive for 3 months after discontinuing.

Driving, piloting or hazardous work:
Don't drive or pilot aircraft until you learn how medicine affects you. Don't work around dangerous machinery. Don't climb ladders or work in high places. Danger increases if you drink alcohol or take medicine affecting alertness and reflexes.

Airplane passengers:
No problems expected.

Discontinuing:
- Nervous and mental disorders—Don't discontinue without doctor's advice until you complete prescribed dose, even though symptoms diminish or disappear.
- Nausea and vomiting—May be unnecessary to finish medicine. Follow doctor's instructions.

INTERACTION WITH OTHER DRUGS

GENERIC NAME OR DRUG CLASS	COMBINED EFFECT
Anticholinergics	Increased anticholinergic effect.
Antidepressants (tricyclic)	Increased fluphenazine effect.
Antihistamines	Increased antihistamine effect.
Appetite suppressants	Decreased suppressant effect.
Levodopa	Decreased levodopa effect.
Mind-altering drugs	Increased effect of mind-altering drugs.
Narcotics	Increased narcotic effect.
Phenytoin	Increased phenytoin effect.
Quinidine	Impaired heart function. Dangerous mixture.
Sedatives	Increased sedative effect.
Tranquilizers (other)	Increased tranquilizer effect.

INTERACTION WITH OTHER SUBSTANCES

INTERACTS WITH	COMBINED EFFECT
Alcohol:	Dangerous oversedation.
Beverages:	None expected.
Cocaine:	Decreased fluphenazine effect. Avoid.
Foods:	None expected.
Marijuana:	Drowsiness. May increase antinausea effect.
Tobacco:	None expected.

FLUPREDNISOLONE

BRAND NAMES

Alphadrol

GENERAL INFORMATION

Habit forming? No
Prescription needed? Yes
Available as generic? No
Drug class: Cortisone drug (adrenal corticosteroid)

 USES

- Reduces inflammation caused by many different medical problems.
- Treatment for some allergic diseases, blood disorders, kidney diseases, asthma and emphysema.
- Replaces corticosteroid deficiencies.

 DOSAGE & USAGE INFORMATION

How to take:
Tablet—Swallow with liquid or food to lessen stomach irritation. If you can't swallow whole, crumble tablet.

When to take:
At the same times each day. Take once-a-day or once-every-other-day doses in mornings.

If you forget a dose:
- Several-doses-per-day prescription—Take as soon as you remember up to 2 hours late. If more than 2 hours, wait for next scheduled dose (don't double this dose).
- Once-a-day dose or less—Wait for next dose. Double this dose.

What drug does:
Decreases inflammatory responses.

Time lapse before drug works:
2 to 4 days.

Don't take with:
See Interaction column and consult doctor.

 OVERDOSE

Symptoms:
Headache, convulsions, heart failure.

What to do:
- Dial 0 (operator) or 911 (emergency) for an ambulance or medical help. Then give first aid immediately.
- Additional emergency information on page 886.

 POSSIBLE ADVERSE REACTIONS OR SIDE EFFECTS

SYMPTOMS	FREQUENCY	WHAT TO DO
Brain & nervous system:		
Mood changes, insomnia, restlessness.	Infrequent	4
Skin:		
• Acne	Common	4
• Rash	Rare	3
• Poor wound healing.	Common	4
Eyes:		
Blurred vision, halos around lights.	Infrequent	3
Ears, nose, throat:		
• Sore throat, fever.	Infrequent	3
• Thirst	Common	4
Digestive:		
• Indigestion, nausea, vomiting.	Common	4
• Bloody or black, tarry stool.	Infrequent	2
Heart & lungs:		
Irregular heartbeat.	Rare	2
Blood vessels, kidneys, liver, allergic, blood:	None expected.	
Muscles, bones, joints:		
Muscle cramps, swollen legs, feet.	Infrequent	3
Genital, urinary:		
Frequent urination.	Infrequent	4
Others:		
• Weight gain, round face.	Infrequent	4
• Fatigue, weakness.	Infrequent	4
• TB recurrence.	Infrequent	4
• Irregular menstrual periods.	Infrequent	4

1- Life-threatening. Seek emergency treatment immediately.
2- Discontinue. Seek emergency treatment.
3- Discontinue. Call doctor right away.
4- Continue. Call doctor when convenient.

FLUPREDNISOLONE

WARNINGS & PRECAUTIONS

Don't take if:
- You are allergic to any cortisone drug.
- You have tuberculosis or fungus infection.
- You have herpes infection of eyes, lips or genitals.

Before you start, consult your doctor:
- If you have had tuberculosis.
- If you have congestive heart failure.
- If you have diabetes.
- If you have peptic ulcer.
- If you have glaucoma.
- If you have underactive thyroid.
- If you have high blood pressure.
- If you have myasthenia gravis.
- If you have blood clots in legs or lungs.

Over age 60:
Adverse reactions and side effects may be more frequent and severe than in younger persons. Likely to aggravate edema, diabetes or ulcers. Likely to cause cataracts and osteoporosis (softening of the bones).

Pregnancy:
Risk to unborn child outweighs drug benefits. Don't use.

Breast-feeding:
Drug passes into milk. Avoid drug or discontinue nursing until you finish medicine. Consult doctor for advice on maintaining milk supply.

Infants & children:
Use only under medical supervision.

Prolonged use:
- Retards growth in children.
- Possible glaucoma, cataracts, diabetes, fragile bones and thin skin.
- Functional dependence.

Skin & sunlight:
No problems expected.

Driving, piloting or hazardous work:
No problems expected.

Airplane passengers:
No problems expected.

Discontinuing:
- Don't discontinue without doctor's advice until you complete prescribed dose, even though symptoms diminish or disappear.
- Drug affects your response to surgery, illness, injury or stress for 2 years after discontinuing. Tell about drug to anyone who takes medical care of you within 2 years.

Others:
Avoid immunizations if possible.

INTERACTION WITH OTHER DRUGS

GENERIC NAME OR DRUG CLASS	COMBINED EFFECT
Amphoterecin B	Potassium depletion.
Anticholinergics	Possible glaucoma.
Anticoagulants (oral)	Decreased anticoagulant effect.
Anticonvulsants (hydantoin)	Decreased fluprednisolone effect.
Antidiabetics (oral)	Decreased antidiabetic effect.
Antihistamines	Decreased fluprednisolone effect.
Aspirin	Increased fluprednisolone effect.
Barbiturates	Decreased fluprednisolone effect. Oversedation.
Beta-adrenergic blockers	Decreased fluprednisolone effect.
Chloral hydrate	Decreased fluprednisolone effect.
Chlorthalidone	Potassium depletion.
Cholinergics	Decreased cholinergic effect.
Contraceptives (oral)	Increased fluprednisolone effect.
Digitalis preparations	Dangerous potassium depletion. Possible digitalis toxicity.

Additional interactions on page 837.

INTERACTION WITH OTHER SUBSTANCES

INTERACTS WITH	COMBINED EFFECT
Alcohol:	Risk of stomach ulcers.
Beverages:	No proven problems.
Cocaine:	Overstimulation. Avoid.
Foods:	No proven problems.
Marijuana:	Decreased immunity.
Tobacco:	Increased fluprednisolone effect. Possible toxicity.

FLURAZEPAM

BRAND NAMES

Dalmane
Novoflupam

GENERAL INFORMATION

Habit forming? Yes
Prescription needed? Yes
Available as generic? No
Drug class: Tranquilizer (benzodiazepine)

USES

Treatment for insomnia and tension.

DOSAGE & USAGE INFORMATION

How to take:
Tablet or capsule—Swallow with liquid. If you can't swallow whole, crumble tablet or open capsule and take with liquid or food.

When to take:
At the same time each day, according to instructions on prescription label.

If you forget a dose:
Take as soon as you remember up to 2 hours late. If more than 2 hours, wait for next scheduled dose (don't double this dose).

What drug does:
Affects limbic system of brain—part that controls emotions. Induces near-normal sleep pattern.

Time lapse before drug works:
30 minutes.

Don't take with:
See Interaction column and consult doctor.

OVERDOSE

Symptoms:
Drowsiness, weakness, tremor, stupor, coma.

What to do:
- Dial 0 (operator) or 911 (emergency) for an ambulance or medical help. Then give first aid immediately.
- If patient is unconscious and not breathing, give mouth-to-mouth breathing. If there is no heartbeat, use cardiac massage and mouth-to-mouth breathing (CPR). Don't try to make patient vomit. If you can't get help quickly, take patient to nearest emergency facility.
- Additional emergency information on page 886.

POSSIBLE ADVERSE REACTIONS OR SIDE EFFECTS

SYMPTOMS	FREQUENCY	WHAT TO DO
Brain & nervous system:		
• Clumsiness, drowsiness, dizziness.	Common	4
• Hallucinations, confusion, depression, irritability.	Infrequent	3
Skin:		
Rash, itch.	Infrequent	3
Eyes:		
Vision changes.	Infrequent	3
Ears, nose, throat:		
Mouth, throat ulcers.	Rare	3
Digestive:		
Constipation or diarrhea, nausea, vomiting.	Infrequent	4
Heart & lungs:		
Slow heartbeat, breathing difficulty.	Rare	2
Blood vessels:	None expected.	
Muscles, bones, joints:	None expected.	
Genital, urinary:		
Urination difficulty.	Infrequent	4
Kidneys:	None expected.	
Liver:		
Jaundice (yellow eyes and skin).	Rare	3
Allergic:	None expected.	
Blood:	None expected.	
Others:	None expected.	

1- Life-threatening. Seek emergency treatment immediately.
2- Discontinue. Seek emergency treatment.
3- Discontinue. Call doctor right away.
4- Continue. Call doctor when convenient.
5- Continue. Tell doctor at next visit.
6- No action necessary.

WARNINGS & PRECAUTIONS

Don't take if:
- You are allergic to any benzodiazepine.
- You have myasthenia gravis.
- You have glaucoma.
- You are active or recovering alcoholic.
- Patient is younger than 6 months.

Before you start, consult your doctor:
- If you have liver, kidney or lung disease.
- If you have diabetes, epilepsy or porphyria.

Over age 60:
Adverse reactions and side effects may be more frequent and severe than in younger persons. May develop agitation, rage or "hangover effect."

Pregnancy:
Risk to unborn child outweighs drug benefits. Don't use.

Breast-feeding:
Drug passes into milk. Avoid drug or discontinue nursing until you finish medicine. Consult doctor for advice on maintaining milk supply.

Infants & children:
Use only under medical supervision for children older than 6 months.

Prolonged use:
May impair liver function.

Skin & sunlight:
No problems expected.

Driving, piloting or hazardous work:
Don't drive or pilot aircraft until you learn how medicine affects you. Don't work around dangerous machinery. Don't climb ladders or work in high places. Danger increases if you drink alcohol or take medicine affecting alertness and reflexes.

Airplane passengers:
No problems expected.

Discontinuing:
Don't discontinue without doctor's advice until you complete prescribed dose, even though symptoms diminish or disappear.

Others:
- Hot weather, heavy exercise and profuse sweat may reduce excretion and cause overdose.
- "Hangover effect" may occur.
- Blood sugar may rise in diabetics, requiring insulin adjustment.

INTERACTION WITH OTHER DRUGS

GENERIC NAME OR DRUG CLASS	COMBINED EFFECT
Anticonvulsants	Change in seizure frequency or severity.
Antidepressants	Increased sedative effect of both drugs.
Antihistamines	Increased sedative effect of both drugs.
Antihypertensives	Excessively low blood pressure.
Cimetidine	Excess sedation.
Disulfiram	Increased flurazepam effect.
MAO inhibitors	Convulsions, deep sedation, rage.
Narcotics	Increased sedative effect of both drugs.
Sedatives	Increased sedative effect of both drugs.
Sleep inducers	Increased sedative effect of both drugs.
Tranquilizers	Increased sedative effect of both drugs.

INTERACTION WITH OTHER SUBSTANCES

INTERACTS WITH	COMBINED EFFECT
Alcohol:	Heavy sedation. Avoid.
Beverages:	None expected.
Cocaine:	Decreased flurazepam effect.
Foods:	None expected.
Marijuana:	Heavy sedation. Avoid.
Tobacco:	Decreased flurazepam effect.

FOLIC ACID (VITAMIN B-9)

BRAND NAMES

Folvite
Novofolacid
Numerous other multiple vitamin-mineral supplements.

GENERAL INFORMATION

Habit forming? No
Prescription needed? High strength: Yes
Vitamin mixtures: No
Available as generic? Yes
Drug class: Vitamin supplement

 ## USES

- Dietary supplement to promote normal growth, development and good health.
- Treatment for anemias due to folic-acid deficiency occurring from alcoholism, liver disease, hemolytic anemia, sprue, infants on artificial formula, pregnancy, breast-feeding and oral-contraceptive use.

 ## DOSAGE & USAGE INFORMATION

How to take:
Tablet—Swallow with liquid or food to lessen stomach irritation. If you can't swallow whole, crumble tablet and take with liquid or food.

When to take:
At the same time each day.

If you forget a dose:
Take when you remember. Don't double next dose. Resume regular schedule.

What drug does:
Essential to normal red-blood-cell formation.

Time lapse before drug works:
Not determined.

Don't take with:
See Interaction column and consult doctor.

 ## OVERDOSE

Symptoms:
None expected.

What to do:
Overdose unlikely to threaten life.

 ## POSSIBLE ADVERSE REACTIONS OR SIDE EFFECTS

SYMPTOMS	FREQUENCY	WHAT TO DO
Brain & nervous system:	None expected.	
Skin:	None expected.	
Eyes:	None expected.	
Ears, nose, throat:	None expected.	
Digestive:	None expected.	
Heart & lungs:	None expected.	
Blood vessels:	None expected.	
Muscles, bones, joints:	None expected.	
Genital, urinary: Large dose may produce yellow urine.	Common	5
Kidneys:	None expected.	
Liver:	None expected.	
Allergic:	None expected.	
Blood:	None expected.	
Others:	None expected.	

1- Life-threatening. Seek emergency treatment immediately.
2- Discontinue. Seek emergency treatment.
3- Discontinue. Call doctor right away.
4- Continue. Call doctor when convenient.
5- Continue. Tell doctor at next visit.
6- No action necessary.

FOLIC ACID (VITAMIN B-9)

 WARNINGS & PRECAUTIONS

Don't take if:
You are allergic to any B vitamin.

Before you start, consult your doctor:
- If you have liver disease.
- If you have pernicious anemia. (Folic acid corrects anemia, but nerve damage of pernicious anemia continues.)

Over age 60:
No problems expected.

Pregnancy:
No problems expected.

Breast-feeding:
No problems expected.

Infants & children:
No problems expected.

Prolonged use:
No problems expected.

Skin & sunlight:
No problems expected.

Driving, piloting or hazardous work:
No problems expected.

Airplane passengers:
No problems expected.

Discontinuing:
Don't discontinue without doctor's advice until you complete prescribed dose, even though symptoms diminish or disappear.

Others:
- Folic acid removed by kidney dialysis. Dialysis patients should increase intake to 300% of RDA.
- A balanced diet should provide all the folic acid a healthy person needs and make supplements unnecessary. Best sources are green, leafy vegetables, fruits, liver and kidney.

 INTERACTION WITH OTHER DRUGS

GENERIC NAME OR DRUG CLASS	COMBINED EFFECT
Analgesics	Decreased effect of folic acid.
Anticonvulsants	Decreased effect of folic acid.
Contraceptives (oral)	Decreased effect of folic acid.
Cortisone drugs	Decreased effect of folic acid.
Methotrexate	Decreased effect of folic acid.
Pyrimethamine	Decreased effect of folic acid.
Quinine	Decreased effect of folic acid.
Triamterene	Decreased effect of folic acid.
Trimethoprim	Decreased effect of folic acid.

 INTERACTION WITH OTHER SUBSTANCES

INTERACTS WITH	COMBINED EFFECT
Alcohol:	None expected.
Beverages:	None expected.
Cocaine:	None expected.
Foods:	None expected.
Marijuana:	None expected.
Tobacco:	None expected.

FUROSEMIDE

BRAND NAMES

Furoside	Novosemide
Lasix	SK-Furosemide
Neo-Renal	Uritol

GENERAL INFORMATION

Habit forming? No
Prescription needed? Yes
Available as generic? No
Drug class: Diuretic, antihypertensive

 USES

- Lowers high blood pressure.
- Decreases fluid retention.

 DOSAGE & USAGE INFORMATION

How to take:
Tablet, liquid or capsule—Swallow with liquid. If you can't swallow whole, crumble tablet or open capsule and take with liquid or food.

When to take:
- 1 dose a day—Take after breakfast.
- More than 1 dose a day—Take last dose no later than 6 p.m. unless otherwise directed.

If you forget a dose:
- 1 dose a day—Take as soon as you remember up to 12 hours late. If more than 12 hours, wait for next scheduled dose (don't double this dose).
- More than 1 dose a day—Take as soon as you remember up to 2 hours late. If more than 2 hours, wait for next scheduled dose (don't double this dose).

What drug does:
Increases elimination of sodium and water from body. Decreased body fluid reduces blood pressure.

Time lapse before drug works:
1 hour to increase water loss. Requires 2 to 3 weeks to lower blood pressure.

Don't take with:
- Non-prescription drugs with aspirin.
- See Interaction column and consult doctor.

 OVERDOSE

Symptoms:
Weakness, lethargy, dizziness, confusion, nausea, vomiting, leg-muscle cramps, thirst, stupor, deep sleep, weak and rapid pulse, cardiac arrest.

What to do:
- Dial 0 (operator) or 911 (emergency) for an ambulance or medical help. Then give first aid immediately.
- Additional emergency information on page 886.

 POSSIBLE ADVERSE REACTIONS OR SIDE EFFECTS

SYMPTOMS	FREQUENCY	WHAT TO DO
Brain & nervous system:		
• Dizziness	Common	4
• Mood changes.	Infrequent	3
Skin:		
Rash or hives.	Rare	3
Eyes:		
Yellow vision.	Rare	3
Ears, nose, throat:		
• Ringing in ears, hearing loss.	Rare	3
• Sore throat, fever.	Rare	3
• Dry mouth, thirst.	Rare	3
Digestive:		
• Side or stomach pain, nausea, vomiting.	Rare	3
• Appetite loss, diarrhea.	Infrequent	3
Heart & lungs:		
Irregular heartbeat.	Infrequent	3
Blood vessels:		
Unusual bleeding or bruising.	Rare	3
Muscles, bones, joints:		
• Joint pain.	Rare	3
• Muscle cramps.	Infrequent	3
Genital, urinary, kidneys, allergic, blood:	None expected.	
Liver:		
Jaundice (yellow skin and eyes).	Rare	3
Others:		
Fatigue, weakness.	Infrequent	3

1- Life-threatening. Seek emergency treatment immediately.
2- Discontinue. Seek emergency treatment.
3- Discontinue. Call doctor right away.
4- Continue. Call doctor when convenient.

WARNINGS & PRECAUTIONS

Don't take if:
You are allergic to furosemide.

Before you start, consult your doctor:
- If you are allergic to any sulfa drug.
- If you have liver or kidney disease.
- If you have gout.
- If you have diabetes.
- If you have impaired hearing.
- If you will have surgery within 2 months, including dental surgery, requiring general or spinal anesthesia.

Over age 60:
Adverse reactions and side effects may be more frequent and severe than in younger persons.

Pregnancy:
Risk to unborn child outweighs drug benefits. Don't use.

Breast-feeding:
Drug filters into milk. May harm child. Avoid.

Infants & children:
Use only under medical supervision.

Prolonged use:
- Impaired balance of water, salt and potassium in blood and body tissues.
- Possible diabetes.

Skin & sunlight:
May cause rash or intensify sunburn in areas exposed to sun or sunlamp.

Driving, piloting or hazardous work.
No problems expected.

Airplane passengers:
No problems expected.

Discontinuing:
Don't discontinue without doctor's advice until you complete prescribed dose, even though symptoms diminish or disappear.

Others:
Frequent laboratory studies to monitor potassium level in blood recommended. Eat foods rich in potassium (see page 850) or take potassium supplements. Consult doctor.

 ## INTERACTION WITH OTHER DRUGS

GENERIC NAME OR DRUG CLASS	COMBINED EFFECT
Allopurinol	Decreased allopurinol effect.
Anticoagulants	Abnormal clotting.
Antidepressants (tricyclic)	Excessive blood-pressure drop.
Antidiabetics (oral)	Decreased antidiabetic effect.
Antiinflammatory drugs (non-steroid)	Decreased furosemide effect.
Antihypertensives	Increased antihypertensive effect.
Barbiturates	Low blood pressure.
Cortisone drugs	Excessive potassium loss.
Digitalis preparations	Serious heart-rhythm disorders.
Insulin	Decreased insulin effect.
Lithium	Increased lithium toxicity.
MAO inhibitors	Increased furosemide effect.
Narcotics	Dangerous low blood pressure. Avoid.
Phenothiazines	Increased phenothiazine effect.

Additional interactions on page 837.

 ## INTERACTION WITH OTHER SUBSTANCES

INTERACTS WITH	COMBINED EFFECT
Alcohol:	Blood-pressure drop. Avoid.
Beverages:	None expected.
Cocaine:	Dangerous blood-pressure drop. Avoid.
Foods:	None expected.
Marijuana:	Increased thirst and urinary frequency, fainting.
Tobacco:	Decreased furosemide effect.

GITALIN

BRAND NAMES

Gitaligin

GENERAL INFORMATION

Habit forming? No
Prescription needed? Yes
Available as generic? Yes
Drug class: Digitalis preparation

USES

- Strengthens weak heart-muscle contractions to prevent congestive heart failure.
- Corrects irregular heartbeat.

DOSAGE & USAGE INFORMATION

How to take:
- Tablet or capsule—Swallow with liquid. If you can't swallow whole, crumble tablet or open capsule and take with liquid or food.
- Liquid—Dilute dose in beverage before swallowing.

When to take:
At the same time each day.

If you forget a dose:
Take as soon as you remember up to 12 hours late. If more than 12 hours, wait for next scheduled dose (don't double this dose).

What drug does:
- Strengthens heart-muscle contraction.
- Delays nerve impulses to heart.

Time lapse before drug works:
May require regular use for a week or more.

Don't take with:
- Non-prescription drugs without consulting doctor.
- See Interaction column and consult doctor.

OVERDOSE

Symptoms:
Nausea, vomiting, diarrhea, vision disturbances with halos around lights, irregular heartbeat, confusion, hallucinations, convulsions.

What to do:
- Dial 0 (operator) or 911 (emergency) for an ambulance or medical help. Then give first aid immediately.
- Additional emergency information on page 886.

POSSIBLE ADVERSE REACTIONS OR SIDE EFFECTS

SYMPTOMS	FREQUENCY	WHAT TO DO
Brain & nervous system: Drowsiness, lethargy, disorientation.	Infrequent	3
Skin: Rash, hives.	Rare	3
Eyes: Double or yellow-green vision.	Rare	4
Ears, nose, throat:	None expected.	
Digestive: Appetite loss, diarrhea.	Common	4
Heart & lungs:	None expected.	
Blood vessels:	None expected.	
Muscles, bones, joints:	None expected.	
Genital, urinary:	None expected.	
Kidneys:	None expected.	
Liver:	None expected.	
Allergic:	None expected.	
Blood:	None expected.	
Others: ● Enlarged, sensitive male breasts.	Rare	4
● Tiredness, weakness.	Rare	4

1- Life-threatening. Seek emergency treatment immediately.
2- Discontinue. Seek emergency treatment.
3- Discontinue. Call doctor right away.
4- Continue. Call doctor when convenient.
5- Continue. Tell doctor at next visit.
6- No action necessary.

WARNINGS & PRECAUTIONS

Don't take if:
- You are allergic to any digitalis preparation.
- Your heartbeat is slower than 50 beats per minute.

Before you start, consult your doctor:
- If you have taken another digitalis preparation in past 2 weeks.
- If you have taken a diuretic within 2 weeks.
- If you have liver or kidney disease.
- If you have a thyroid disorder.

Over age 60:
Adverse reactions and side effects may be more frequent and severe than in younger persons.

Pregnancy:
Studies inconclusive on harm to unborn child. Consult your doctor.

Breast-feeding:
Drug filters into milk. May harm child. Avoid.

Infants & children:
Use only under medical supervision.

Prolonged use:
No problems expected.

Skin & sunlight:
No problems expected.

Driving, piloting or hazardous work:
Possible vision disturbances. Otherwise, no problems expected.

Airplane passengers:
Nausea more likely.

Discontinuing:
Don't stop without doctor's advice.

Others:
No problems expected.

INTERACTION WITH OTHER DRUGS

GENERIC NAME OR DRUG CLASS	COMBINED EFFECT
Antacids	Decreased gitalin effect.
Anticonvulsants (hydantoin)	Increased gitalin effect at first, then decreased.
Beta-adrenergic blockers	Increased gitalin effect.
Cortisone drugs	Gitalin toxicity.
Diuretics	Gitalin toxicity.
Ephedrine	Disturbs heart rhythm. Avoid.
Epinephrine	Disturbs heart rhythm. Avoid.
Guanethidine	Increased gitalin effect.
Laxatives	Decreased gitalin effect.
Oxyphenbutazone	Decreased gitalin effect.
Phenobarbital	Decreased gitalin effect.
Phenylbutazone	Decreased gitalin effect.
Quinidine	Increased gitalin effect.
Rauwolfia alkaloids	Increased gitalin effect.
Thyroid hormones	Gitalin toxicity.

INTERACTION WITH OTHER SUBSTANCES

INTERACTS WITH	COMBINED EFFECT
Alcohol:	None expected.
Beverages: Caffeine drinks	Irregular heartbeat. Avoid.
Cocaine:	Irregular heartbeat. Avoid.
Foods:	None expected.
Marijuana:	Decreased gitalin effect.
Tobacco:	Irregular heartbeat. Avoid.

GRISEOFULVIN

BRAND NAMES

Fulvicin P/G   Gris-PEG
Fulvicin U/F   grisOwen
Grifulvin V
Grisactin
Grisovin-FP

GENERAL INFORMATION

Habit forming? No
Prescription needed? Yes
Available as generic? Yes
Drug class: Antibiotic (antifungal)

 ## USES

Treatment for fungal infections susceptible
to griseofulvin.

 ## DOSAGE & USAGE INFORMATION

How to take:
- Tablet or capsule—Swallow with liquid or
  food to lessen stomach irritation. If you
  can't swallow whole, crumble tablet or
  open capsule and take with liquid or food.
- Liquid—Follow label instructions.

When to take:
With or immediately after meals.

If you forget a dose:
Take as soon as you remember up to 2 hours
late. If more than 2 hours, wait for next
scheduled dose (don't double this dose).

What drug does:
Prevents fungi from growing and reproducing.

Time lapse before drug works:
2 to 10 days for skin infections. 2 to 4 weeks
for infections of fingernails or toenails.
Complete cure of either may require several
months.

Don't take with:
See Interaction column and consult doctor.

 ## OVERDOSE

Symptoms:
Nausea, vomiting, diarrhea. In sensitive
individuals, severe diarrhea may occur
without overdosing.

What to do:
Overdose unlikely to threaten life. If person
takes much larger amount than prescribed,
call doctor, poison-control center or hospital
emergency room for instructions.

 ## POSSIBLE ADVERSE REACTIONS OR SIDE EFFECTS

SYMPTOMS	FREQUENCY	WHAT TO DO
Brain & nervous system:		
• Insomnia	Infrequent	4
• Confusion	Infrequent	3
• Headache	Common	5
Skin:		
Rash, hives, itch.	Infrequent	3
Eyes:	None expected.	
Ears, nose, throat:		
• Sore throat, fever.	Rare	3
• Mouth or tongue irritation, soreness.	Infrequent	3
Digestive:		
Nausea, vomiting, diarrhea, stomach pain.	Infrequent	3
Heart & lungs:	None expected.	
Blood vessels:	None expected.	
Muscles, bones, joints:	None expected.	
Genital, urinary:	None expected.	
Kidneys:	None expected.	
Liver:	None expected.	
Allergic:	None expected.	
Blood:	None expected.	
Others:		
• Tiredness	Infrequent	4
• Numbness, tingling, pain or weakness in extremities.	Rare	3

1- Life-threatening. Seek emergency
   treatment immediately.
2- Discontinue. Seek emergency treatment.
3- Discontinue. Call doctor right away.
4- Continue. Call doctor when convenient.
5- Continue. Tell doctor at next visit.
6- No action necessary.

WARNINGS & PRECAUTIONS

Don't take if:
- You are allergic to any antifungal medicine.
- You have liver disease.
- You have porphyria.
- The infection is minor and will respond to less-potent drugs.

Before you start, consult your doctor:
- If you plan to become pregnant within medication period.
- If you have liver disease.
- If you have lupus.

Over age 60:
Adverse reactions and side effects may be more frequent and severe than in younger persons.

Pregnancy:
Risk to unborn child outweighs drug benefits. Don't use.

Breast-feeding:
No problems expected, but consult your doctor.

Infants & children:
Not recommended for children younger than 2.

Prolonged use:
You may become susceptible to infections caused by germs not responsive to griseofulvin.

Skin & sunlight:
May cause rash or intensify sunburn in areas exposed to sun or sunlamp.

Driving, piloting or hazardous work:
- Don't drive if you feel dizzy or have vision problems.
- Don't pilot aircraft.

Airplane passengers:
No problems expected.

Discontinuing:
Don't discontinue without doctor's advice until you complete prescribed dose, even though symptoms diminish or disappear.

Others:
Periodic laboratory blood studies and liver- and kidney-function tests recommended.

INTERACTION WITH OTHER DRUGS

GENERIC NAME OR DRUG CLASS	COMBINED EFFECT
Anticoagulants (oral)	Decreased anticoagulant effect.
Barbiturates	Decreased griseofulvin effect.

INTERACTION WITH OTHER SUBSTANCES

INTERACTS WITH	COMBINED EFFECT
Alcohol:	Increased intoxication. Possible disulfiram reaction (see page 848).
Beverages:	None expected.
Cocaine:	None expected.
Foods:	None expected, but foods high in fat will improve drug absorption.
Marijuana:	None expected.
Tobacco:	None expected.

GUAIFENESIN

BRAND NAMES

Ambenyl
Expectorant (M)
Cheracol Cough
Syrup (M)
Chlor-Trimeton
Expectorant (M)

Dimetane
Expectorant (M)
Dristan Cough
Formula (M)
Formula 44-D (M)

Vicks Cough
Syrup (M)

See complete brand names list, page 826.

GENERAL INFORMATION

Habit forming? No
Prescription needed? No
Available as generic? Yes
Drug class: Cough/cold preparation

 ## USES

Loosens mucus in respiratory passages from allergies and infections (hay fever, cough, cold).

 ## DOSAGE & USAGE INFORMATION

How to take:
- Tablet or capsule—Swallow with liquid. If you can't swallow whole, crumble tablet or open capsule and take with liquid or food.
- Syrup or lozenge—Take as directed on label. Follow with 8 oz. water.

When to take:
As needed, no more often than every 3 hours.

If you forget a dose:
Take as soon as you remember. Wait 3 hours for next dose.

What drug does:
Increases production of watery fluids to thin mucus so it can be coughed out or absorbed.

Time lapse before drug works:
15 to 30 minutes. Regular use for 5 to 7 days necessary for maximum benefit.

Don't take with:
See Interaction column and consult doctor.

 ## OVERDOSE

Symptoms:
Drowsiness, mild weakness, nausea, vomiting.

What to do:
Overdose unlikely to threaten life. If person takes much larger amount than prescribed, call doctor, poison-control center or hospital emergency room for instructions.

 ## POSSIBLE ADVERSE REACTIONS OR SIDE EFFECTS

SYMPTOMS	FREQUENCY	WHAT TO DO
Brain & nervous system: Drowsiness	Infrequent	4
Skin: Rash	Infrequent	3
Eyes:	None expected.	
Ears, nose, throat:	None expected.	
Digestive:		
• Stomach pain, diarrhea.	Infrequent	3
• Nausea, vomiting.	Infrequent	3
Heart & lungs:	None expected.	
Blood vessels:	None expected.	
Muscles, bones, joints:	None expected.	
Genital, urinary:	None expected.	
Kidneys:	None expected.	
Liver:	None expected.	
Allergic:	None expected.	
Blood:	None expected.	
Others:	None expected.	

1- Life-threatening. Seek emergency treatment immediately.
2- Discontinue. Seek emergency treatment.
3- Discontinue. Call doctor right away.
4- Continue. Call doctor when convenient.
5- Continue. Tell doctor at next visit.
6- No action necessary.

WARNINGS & PRECAUTIONS

Don't take if:
You are allergic to any cough or cold preparation containing guaifenesin.

Before you start, consult your doctor:
See Interaction column and consult doctor.

Over age 60:
Adverse reactions and side effects may be more frequent and severe than in younger persons. For drug to work, you must drink 8 to 10 glasses of fluid per day.

Pregnancy:
No proven harm to unborn child. Avoid if possible.

Breast-feeding:
No proven problems. Consult your doctor.

Infants & children:
No problems expected.

Prolonged use:
No problems expected.

Skin & sunlight:
No problems expected.

Driving, piloting or hazardous work:
Avoid if you feel drowsy. Otherwise, no problems expected.

Airplane passengers:
No problems expected.

Discontinuing:
May be unnecessary to finish medicine. Discontinue when symptoms disappear. If symptoms persist more than 1 week, consult doctor.

Others:
No problems expected.

 ## INTERACTION WITH OTHER DRUGS

GENERIC NAME OR DRUG CLASS	COMBINED EFFECT
Anticoagulants	Risk of bleeding.

 ## INTERACTION WITH OTHER SUBSTANCES

INTERACTS WITH	COMBINED EFFECT
Alcohol:	No proven problems.
Beverages:	You must drink 8 to 10 glasses of fluid per day for drug to work.
Cocaine:	No proven problems.
Foods:	None expected.
Marijuana:	No proven problems.
Tobacco:	No proven problems.

GUANETHIDINE

BRAND NAMES

Esimil (M)
Ismelin
Ismelin-Esidrix (M)

GENERAL INFORMATION

Habit forming? No
Prescription needed? Yes
Available as generic? No
Drug class: Antihypertensive

 USES

Reduces high blood pressure.

 DOSAGE & USAGE INFORMATION

How to take:
Tablet or capsule—Swallow with liquid. If you can't swallow tablet or capsule whole, crumble or open and take with liquid or food.

When to take:
At the same time each day.

If you forget a dose:
Take as soon as you remember up to 2 hours late. If more than 2 hours, wait for next scheduled dose (don't double this dose).

What drug does:
Displaces norepinephrine—hormone necessary to maintain small blood-vessel tone. Blood vessels relax and high blood pressure drops.

Time lapse before drug works:
Regular use for several weeks may be necessary to determine effectiveness.

Don't take with:
- Non-prescription drugs containing alcohol without consulting doctor.
- See Interaction column and consult doctor.

 OVERDOSE

Symptoms:
Severe blood-pressure drop; fainting; slow, weak pulse; cold, sweaty skin; loss of consciousness.

What to do:
- Dial 0 (operator) or 911 (emergency) for an ambulance or medical help. Then give first aid immediately.
- Additional emergency information on page 886.

POSSIBLE ADVERSE REACTIONS OR SIDE EFFECTS

SYMPTOMS	FREQUENCY	WHAT TO DO
Brain & nervous system: Dizziness, headache.	Common	5
Skin: Rash	Infrequent	3
Eyes: Blurred vision, drooping eyelids.	Infrequent	3
Ears, nose, throat: Stuffy nose, dry mouth.	Common	6
Digestive: • Diarrhea, more bowel movements.	Common	4
• Nausea or vomiting.	Infrequent	4
Heart & lungs: • Chest pains or shortness of breath.	Infrequent	3
• Unusually slow heartbeat.	Common	3
Blood vessels, kidneys, liver, allergic, blood:	None expected.	
Muscles, bones, joints: • Muscle pain or tremors.	Infrequent	3
• Swollen feet, legs.	Common	4
Genital, urinary: • Impotence	Infrequent	5
• Nighttime urination.	Infrequent	5
Others: • Fatigue, weakness.	Common	4
• Lower sex drive.	Common	5

1- Life-threatening. Seek emergency treatment immediately.
2- Discontinue. Seek emergency treatment.
3- Discontinue. Call doctor right away.
4- Continue. Call doctor when convenient.
5- Continue. Tell doctor at next visit.

WARNINGS & PRECAUTIONS

Don't take if:
- You are allergic to guanethidine.
- You have taken MAO inhibitors within 2 weeks.

Before you start, consult your doctor:
- If you have had stroke or heart disease.
- If you have asthma.
- If you have had kidney disease.
- If you have peptic ulcer or chronic acid indigestion.
- If you will have surgery within 2 months, including dental surgery, requiring general or spinal anesthesia.

Over age 60:
Adverse reactions and side effects may be more frequent and severe than in younger persons. Start with small doses and monitor blood pressure frequently.

Pregnancy:
No proven harm to unborn child. Avoid if possible.

Breast-feeding:
No proven harm to nursing infant. Avoid if possible.

Infants & children:
Not recommended.

Prolonged use:
Due to drug's cumulative effect, dose will require adjustment to prevent wide fluctuations in blood pressure.

Skin & sunlight:
No problems expected.

Driving, piloting or hazardous work:
Don't drive or pilot aircraft until you learn how medicine affects you. Don't work around dangerous machinery. Don't climb ladders or work in high places. Danger increases if you drink alcohol or take medicine affecting alertness and reflexes, such as antihistamines, tranquilizers, sedatives, pain medicine, narcotics and mind-altering drugs.

Airplane passengers:
No problems expected.

Discontinuing:
Don't discontinue without consulting doctor. Dose may require gradual reduction if you have taken drug for a long time. Doses of other drugs may also require adjustment.

Others:
Hot weather further lowers blood pressure.

 ## INTERACTION WITH OTHER DRUGS

GENERIC NAME OR DRUG CLASS	COMBINED EFFECT
Amphetamines	Decreased guanethidine effect.
Antidepressants (tricyclic)	Decreased guanethidine effect.
Antihistamines	Decreased guanethidine effect.
Contraceptives (oral)	Decreased guanethidine effect.
Digitalis preparations	Slower heartbeat.
Diuretics (thiazide)	Increased guanethidine effect.
Rauwolfia alkaloids	Increased guanethidine effect.

 ## INTERACTION WITH OTHER SUBSTANCES

INTERACTS WITH	COMBINED EFFECT
Alcohol:	Use caution. Decreases blood pressure.
Beverages: Carbonated drinks	Use sparingly. Sodium content increases blood pressure.
Cocaine:	Raises blood pressure. Avoid.
Foods: Spicy or acid foods	Avoid if subject to indigestion or peptic ulcer.
Marijuana:	Excessively low blood pressure. Avoid.
Tobacco:	Possible blood-pressure rise. Avoid.

HALAZEPAM

BRAND NAMES

Paxipam

GENERAL INFORMATION

Habit forming? Yes
Prescription needed? Yes
Available as generic? No
Drug class: Tranquilizer (benzodiazepine)

 USES

Treatment for nervousness or tension.

 DOSAGE & USAGE INFORMATION

How to take:
Tablet or capsule—Swallow with liquid. If you can't swallow whole, crumble tablet or open capsule and take with liquid or food.

When to take:
At the same time each day, according to instructions on prescription label.

If you forget a dose:
Take as soon as you remember up to 2 hours late. If more than 2 hours, wait for next scheduled dose (don't double this dose).

What drug does:
Affects limbic system of brain—part that controls emotions.

Time lapse before drug works:
2 hours. May take 6 weeks for full benefit.

Don't take with:
See Interaction column and consult doctor.

 OVERDOSE

Symptoms:
Drowsiness, weakness, tremor, stupor, coma.

What to do:
- Dial 0 (operator) or 911 (emergency) for an ambulance or medical help. Then give first aid immediately.
- If patient is unconscious and not breathing, give mouth-to-mouth breathing. If there is no heartbeat, use cardiac massage and mouth-to-mouth breathing (CPR). Don't try to make patient vomit. If you can't get help quickly, take patient to nearest emergency facility.
- Additional emergency information on page 886.

POSSIBLE ADVERSE REACTIONS OR SIDE EFFECTS

SYMPTOMS	FREQUENCY	WHAT TO DO
Brain & nervous system:		
● Clumsiness, drowsiness, dizziness.	Common	4
● Hallucinations, confusion, depression, irritability.	Infrequent	3
Skin: Rash, itch.	Infrequent	3
Eyes: Vision changes.	Infrequent	3
Ears, nose, throat: Mouth, throat ulcers.	Rare	3
Digestive: Constipation or diarrhea, nausea, vomiting.	Infrequent	4
Heart & lungs: Slow heartbeat, breathing difficulty.	Rare	2
Blood vessels:	None expected.	
Muscles, bones, joints:	None expected.	
Genital, urinary: Urination difficulty.	Infrequent	4
Kidneys:	None expected.	
Liver: Jaundice (yellow eyes and skin).	Rare	3
Allergic:	None expected.	
Blood:	None expected.	
Others:	None expected.	

1- Life-threatening. Seek emergency treatment immediately.
2- Discontinue. Seek emergency treatment.
3- Discontinue. Call doctor right away.
4- Continue. Call doctor when convenient.
5- Continue. Tell doctor at next visit.
6- No action necessary.

WARNINGS & PRECAUTIONS

Don't take if:
- You are allergic to any benzodiazepine.
- You have myasthenia gravis.
- You have glaucoma.
- You are active or recovering alcoholic.
- Patient is younger than 6 months.

Before you start, consult your doctor:
- If you have liver, kidney or lung disease.
- If you have diabetes, epilepsy or porphyria.

Over age 60:
Adverse reactions and side effects may be more frequent and severe than in younger persons. You need smaller doses for shorter periods of time. May develop agitation, rage or "hangover effect."

Pregnancy:
Risk to unborn child outweighs drug benefits. Don't use.

Breast-feeding:
Drug passes into milk. Avoid drug or discontinue nursing until you finish medicine. Consult doctor for advice on maintaining milk supply.

Infants & children:
Use only under medical supervision for children older than 6 months.

Prolonged use:
May impair liver function.

Skin & sunlight:
No problems expected.

Driving, piloting or hazardous work:
Don't drive or pilot aircraft until you learn how medicine affects you. Don't work around dangerous machinery. Don't climb ladders or work in high places. Danger increases if you drink alcohol or take medicine affecting alertness and reflexes.

Airplane passengers:
No problems expected.

Discontinuing:
Don't discontinue without consulting doctor. Dose may require gradual reduction if you have taken drug for a long time. Doses of other drugs may also require adjustment.

Others:
- Hot weather, heavy exercise and profuse sweat may reduce excretion and cause overdose.
- Blood sugar may rise in diabetics, requiring insulin adjustment.

INTERACTION WITH OTHER DRUGS

GENERIC NAME OR DRUG CLASS	COMBINED EFFECT
Anticonvulsants	Change in seizure frequency or severity.
Antidepressants	Increased sedative effect of both drugs.
Antihistamines	Increased sedative effect of both drugs.
Antihypertensives	Excessively low blood pressure.
Cimetidine	Excess sedation.
Disulfiram	Increased halazepam effect.
MAO inhibitors	Convulsions, deep sedation, rage.
Narcotics	Increased sedative effect of both drugs.
Sedatives	Increased sedative effect of both drugs.
Sleep Inducers	Increased sedative effect of both drugs.
Tranquilizers	Increased sedative effect of both drugs.

INTERACTION WITH OTHER SUBSTANCES

INTERACTS WITH	COMBINED EFFECT
Alcohol:	Heavy sedation. Avoid.
Beverages:	None expected.
Cocaine:	Decreased halazepam effect.
Foods:	None expected.
Marijuana:	Heavy sedation. Avoid.
Tobacco:	Decreased halazepam effect.

HALOPERIDOL

BRAND NAMES

Haldol

GENERAL INFORMATION

Habit forming? No
Prescription needed? Yes
Available as generic? No
Drug class: Tranquilizer (antipsychotic)

 ## USES

Reduces severe anxiety, agitation and psychotic behavior.

DOSAGE & USAGE INFORMATION

How to take:
- Tablet or capsule—Swallow with liquid. If you can't swallow whole, crumble tablet or open capsule and take with liquid or food.
- Drops—Dilute dose in beverage before swallowing.

When to take:
At the same times each day.

If you forget a dose:
Take as soon as you remember up to 2 hours late. If more than 2 hours, wait for next scheduled dose (don't double this dose).

What drug does:
Corrects an imbalance in nerve impulses from brain.

Time lapse before drug works:
3 weeks to 2 months for maximum benefit.

Don't take with:
- Non-prescription drugs without consulting doctor.
- See Interaction column and consult doctor.

 ## OVERDOSE

Symptoms:
Weak, rapid pulse; shallow, slow breathing; very low blood pressure; convulsions; deep sleep ending in coma.

What to do:
- Dial O (operator) or 911 (emergency) for an ambulance or medical help. Then give first aid immediately.
- If patient is unconscious and not breathing, give mouth-to-mouth breathing. If there is no heartbeat, use cardiac massage and mouth-to-mouth breathing (CPR). Don't try to make patient vomit. If you can't get help quickly, take patient to nearest emergency facility.
- Additional emergency information on page 886.

POSSIBLE ADVERSE REACTIONS OR SIDE EFFECTS

SYMPTOMS	FREQUENCY	WHAT TO DO
Brain & nervous system:		
• Shuffling, stiffness, jerkiness, trembling.	Common	4
• Dizziness, faintness, drowsiness.	Infrequent	4
Skin:		
Rash	Infrequent	3
Eyes:		
Blurred vision.	Common	3
Ears, nose, throat:		
• Dry mouth.	Common	6
• Circling motions of tongue.	Infrequent	3
• Sore throat, fever.	Rare	3
Digestive:		
• Constipation	Common	4
• Nausea or vomiting.	Infrequent	4
Heart & lungs, blood vessels, muscles, bones, joints, kidneys, allergic, blood:	None expected.	
Genital, urinary:		
• Urination difficulty.	Infrequent	4
• Decreased sexual ability.	Infrequent	4
Liver:		
Jaundice (yellow skin and eyes).	Rare	3

1- Life-threatening. Seek emergency treatment immediately.
2- Discontinue. Seek emergency treatment.
3- Discontinue. Call doctor right away.
4- Continue. Call doctor when convenient.
5- Continue. Tell doctor at next visit.
6- No action necessary.

HALOPERIDOL

WARNINGS & PRECAUTIONS

Don't take if:
- You have ever been allergic to haloperidol.
- You are depressed.
- You have Parkinson's disease.
- Patient is younger than 3 years old.

Before you start, consult your doctor:
- If you take sedatives, sleeping pills, tranquilizers, antidepressants, antihistamines, narcotics or mind-altering drugs.
- If you have a history of mental depression.
- If you have had kidney or liver problems.
- If you have diabetes, epilepsy, glaucoma, high blood pressure or heart disease.
- If you drink alcoholic beverages frequently.

Over age 60:
Adverse reactions and side effects may be more frequent and severe than in younger persons.

Pregnancy:
Risk to unborn child outweighs drug benefits. Don't use.

Breast-feeding:
No proven harm to nursing infant. Avoid if possible.

Infants & children:
Not recommended.

Prolonged use:
May develop tardive dyskinesia (involuntary movements of jaws, lips and tongue).

Skin & sunlight:
May cause rash or intensify sunburn in areas exposed to sun or sunlamp.

Driving, piloting or hazardous work:
Don't drive or pilot aircraft until you learn how medicine affects you. Don't work around dangerous machinery. Don't climb ladders or work in high places. Danger increases if you drink alcohol or take medicine affecting alertness and reflexes.

Airplane passengers:
Don't fly without medical advice.

Discontinuing:
Don't discontinue without consulting doctor. Dose may require gradual reduction if you have taken drug for a long time. Doses of other drugs may also require adjustment.

Others:
No problems expected.

INTERACTION WITH OTHER DRUGS

GENERIC NAME OR DRUG CLASS	COMBINED EFFECT
Anticholinergics	Increased anticholinergic effect. May cause pressure within the eye.
Anticoagulants (oral)	Decreased anticoagulant effect.
Anticonvulsants	Changed seizure pattern.
Antidepressants	Excessive sedation.
Antihistamines	Excessive sedation.
Antihypertensives	May cause severe blood-pressure drop.
Barbiturates	Excessive sedation.
Bethanidine	Decreased bethanidine effect.
Guanethidine	Decreased guanethidine effect.
Levodopa	Decreased levodopa effect.
Methyldopa	Possible psychosis.
Narcotics	Excessive sedation.
Sedatives	Excessive sedation.
Tranquilizers	Excessive sedation.

INTERACTION WITH OTHER SUBSTANCES

INTERACTS WITH	COMBINED EFFECT
Alcohol:	Excessive sedation and depressed brain function. Avoid.
Beverages:	None expected.
Cocaine:	Decreased effect of haloperidol. Avoid.
Foods:	None expected.
Marijuana:	Occasional use—Increased sedation. Frequent use—Possible toxic psychosis.
Tobacco:	None expected.

HETACILLIN

BRAND NAMES

Versapen
Versapen-K

Habit forming? No
Prescription needed? Yes
Available as generic? Yes
Drug class: Antibiotic (penicillin)

 USES

Treatment of bacterial infections that are susceptible to hetacillin.

 DOSAGE & USAGE INFORMATION

How to take:
- Tablets or capsules—Swallow with liquid on an empty stomach 1 hour before or 2 hours after eating.
- Liquid—Take with cold beverage. Liquid form is perishable and effective for only 7 days at room temperature. Effective for 14 days if stored in refrigerator. Don't freeze.

When to take:
Follow instructions on prescription label or side of package. Doses should be evenly spaced. For example, 4 times a day means every 6 hours.

If you forget a dose:
Take as soon as you remember. Continue regular schedule.

What drug does:
Destroys susceptible bacteria. Does not kill viruses.

Time lapse before drug works:
May be several days before medicine affects infection.

Don't take with:
See Interaction column and consult doctor.

 OVERDOSE

Symptoms:
Severe diarrhea, nausea or vomiting.

What to do:
Overdose unlikely to threaten life. If person takes much larger amount than prescribed, call doctor, poison-control center or hospital emergency room for instructions.

 POSSIBLE ADVERSE REACTIONS OR SIDE EFFECTS

SYMPTOMS	FREQUENCY	WHAT TO DO
Brain & nervous system:	None expected.	
Skin: Hives, rash, intense itch soon after a dose.	Rare	1
Eyes:	None expected.	
Ears, nose, throat: Dark or discolored tongue.	Common	5
Digestive: Nausea, vomiting, diarrhea.	Infrequent	4
Heart & lungs:	None expected.	
Blood vessels: Unexplained bleeding.	Rare	3
Muscles, bones, joints:	None expected.	
Genital, urinary:	None expected.	
Kidneys:	None expected.	
Liver:	None expected.	
Allergic: Life-threatening anaphylaxis may occur!	Rare	1 See page 888.
Blood:	None expected.	
Others:	None expected.	

1- Life-threatening. Seek emergency treatment immediately.
2- Discontinue. Seek emergency treatment.
3- Discontinue. Call doctor right away.
4- Continue. Call doctor when convenient.
5- Continue. Tell doctor at next visit.
6- No action necessary.

WARNINGS & PRECAUTIONS

Don't take if:
You are allergic to hetacillin, cephalosporin antibiotics, other penicillins or penicillamine. Life-threatening reaction may occur.

Before you start, consult your doctor:
If you are allergic to any substance or drug.

Over age 60:
You may have skin reactions, particularly around genitals and anus.

Pregnancy:
Studies inconclusive on harm to unborn child. Animal studies show fetal abnormalities. Decide with your doctor whether drug benefits justify risk to unborn child.

Breast-feeding:
Drug passes into milk. Child may become sensitive to penicillins and have allergic reactions to penicillin drugs. Avoid hetacillin or discontinue nursing until you finish medicine. Consult doctor for advice on maintaining milk supply.

Infants & children:
No problems expected.

Prolonged use:
You may become more susceptible to infections caused by germs not responsive to hetacillin.

Skin & sunlight:
No problems expected.

Driving, piloting or hazardous work:
Usually not dangerous. Most hazardous reactions likely to occur a few minutes after taking hetacillin.

Airplane passengers:
No problems expected.

Discontinuing:
Don't discontinue without doctor's advice until you complete prescribed dose, even though symptoms diminish or disappear.

Others:
Urine sugar test for diabetes may show false positive result.

INTERACTION WITH OTHER DRUGS

GENERIC NAME OR DRUG CLASS	COMBINED EFFECT
Chloramphenicol	Decreased effect of both drugs.
Erythromycins	Decreased effect of both drugs.
Paromomycin	Decreased effect of both drugs.
Tetracyclines	Decreased effect of both drugs.
Troleandomycin	Decreased effect of both drugs.

INTERACTION WITH OTHER SUBSTANCES

INTERACTS WITH	COMBINED EFFECT
Alcohol:	Occasional stomach irritation.
Beverages:	None expected.
Cocaine:	No proven problems.
Foods:	None expected.
Marijuana:	No proven problems.
Tobacco:	None expected.

HEXOBARBITAL

BRAND NAMES

Sombulex

GENERAL INFORMATION

Habit forming? Yes
Prescription needed? Yes
Available as generic? Yes
Drug class: Sedative, hypnotic (barbiturate)

 USES

- Reduces anxiety or nervous tension (low dose).
- Relieves insomnia (higher bedtime dose).

 DOSAGE & USAGE INFORMATION

How to take:
Tablet—Swallow with liquid or food to lessen stomach irritation. If you can't swallow whole, crumble tablet and take with liquid or food.

When to take:
At the same times each day.

If you forget a dose:
Take as soon as you remember up to 2 hours late. If more than 2 hours, wait for next scheduled dose (don't double this dose).

What drug does:
May partially block nerve impulses at nerve-cell connections.

Time lapse before drug works:
60 minutes.

Don't take with:
- Non-prescription drugs without consulting doctor.
- See Interaction column and consult doctor.

 OVERDOSE

Symptoms:
Deep sleep, weak pulse, coma.

What to do:
- Dial 0 (operator) or 911 (emergency) for an ambulance or medical help. Then give first aid immediately.
- If patient is unconscious and not breathing, give mouth-to-mouth breathing. If there is no heartbeat use cardiac massage and mouth-to-mouth breathing (CPR). Don't try to make patient vomit. If you can't help quickly, take patient to nearest emergency facility.
- Additional emergency information on page 886.

 POSSIBLE ADVERSE REACTIONS OR SIDE EFFECTS

SYMPTOMS	FREQUENCY	WHAT TO DO
Brain & nervous system:		
• Dizziness, drowsiness, "hangover effect."	Common	4
• Depression, confusion, slurred speech.	Infrequent	4
• Agitation	Rare	3
Skin:		
• Rash or hives.	Infrequent	3
• Face, lip swelling.	Infrequent	3
Eyes:		
Eyelid swelling.	Infrequent	3
Ears, nose, throat:		
Sore throat, fever.	Infrequent	3
Digestive:		
Diarrhea, nausea, vomiting.	Infrequent	4
Heart & lungs:		
• Slow heartbeat.	Rare	3
• Breathing difficulty.	Rare	3
Blood vessels:		
Unexplained bleeding or bruising.	Rare	4
Muscles, bones, joints:		
Joint or muscle pain.	Infrequent	4
Genital, urinary:	None expected.	
Kidneys:	None expected.	
Liver:		
Jaundice (yellow skin and eyes).	Rare	3
Allergic:	None expected.	
Blood:	None expected.	
Others:	None expected.	

1 - Life-threatening. Seek emergency treatment immediately.
2 - Discontinue. Seek emergency treatment.
3 - Discontinue. Call doctor right away.
4 - Continue. Call doctor when convenient.

HEXOBARBITAL

WARNINGS & PRECAUTIONS

Don't take if:
- You are allergic to any barbiturate.
- You have porphyria.

Before you start, consult your doctor:
- If you have epilepsy.
- If you have kidney or liver damage.
- If you have asthma.
- If you have anemia.
- If you have chronic pain.
- If you will have surgery within 2 months, including dental surgery, requiring general or spinal anesthesia.

Over age 60:
Adverse reactions and side effects may be more frequent and severe than in younger persons. Use small doses.

Pregnancy:
Risk to unborn child outweighs drug benefits. Don't use.

Breast-feeding:
Drug passes into milk. Avoid drug or discontinue nursing until you finish medicine. Consult doctor for advice on maintaining milk supply.

Infants & children:
Use only under doctor's supervision.

Prolonged use:
- May cause addiction, anemia, chronic intoxication.
- May lower body temperature, making exposure to cold temperatures hazardous.

Skin & sunlight:
May cause rash or intensify sunburn in areas exposed to sun or sunlamp.

Driving, piloting or hazardous work:
Don't drive or pilot aircraft until you learn how medicine affects you. Don't work around dangerous machinery. Don't climb ladders or work in high places. Danger increases if you drink alcohol or take medicine affecting alertness and reflexes.

Airplane passengers:
No problems expected.

Discontinuing:
May be unnecessary to finish medicine. Follow doctor's instructions. If you develop withdrawal symptoms of hallucinations, agitation or sleeplessness after discontinuing, call doctor right away.

Others:
No problems expected.

INTERACTION WITH OTHER DRUGS

GENERIC NAME OR DRUG CLASS	COMBINED EFFECT
Anticoagulants (oral)	Decreased anticoagulant effect.
Anticonvulsants	Changed seizure patterns.
Antidepressants (tricyclic)	Decreased antidepressant effect.
Antidiabetics (oral)	Increased hexobarbital effect.
Antihistamines	Dangerous sedation. Avoid.
Antiinflammatory drugs (non-steroidal)	Decreased antiinflammatory effect.
Aspirin	Decreased aspirin effect.
Beta-adrenergic blockers	Decreased effect of beta-adrenergic blocker.
Contraceptives (oral)	Decreased contraceptive effect.
Cortisone drugs	Decreased cortisone effect.
Digitoxin	Decreased digitoxin effect.
Doxycycline	Decreased doxycycline effect.
Griseofulvin	Decreased griseofulvin effect.

Additional interactions on page 837.

INTERACTION WITH OTHER SUBSTANCES

INTERACTS WITH	COMBINED EFFECT
Alcohol:	Possible fatal oversedation. Avoid.
Beverages:	None expected.
Cocaine:	Decreased hexobarbital effect.
Foods:	None expected.
Marijuana:	Excessive sedation. Avoid.
Tobacco:	None expected.

HYDRALAZINE

BRAND NAMES

Apresazide (M)
Apresoline
Dralserp (M)
Dralzine
Hydralazide (M)

Rolazine
Ser-Ap-Es (M)
Serpasil-Apresoline (M)
Uniserp

GENERAL INFORMATION

Habit forming? No
Prescription needed? Yes
Available as generic? Yes
Drug class: Antihypertensive

 USES

Treatment for high blood pressure and congestive heart failure.

 DOSAGE & USAGE INFORMATION

How to take:
Tablet or capsule—Swallow with liquid. If you can't swallow whole, crumble tablet or open capsule and take with liquid or food.

When to take:
At the same time each day.

If you forget a dose:
Take as soon as you remember up to 2 hours late. If more than 2 hours, wait for next scheduled dose (don't double this dose).

What drug does:
Relaxes and expands blood-vessel walls, lowering blood pressure.

Time lapse before drug works:
Regular use for several weeks may be necessary to determine drug's effectiveness.

Don't take with:
- Non-prescription drugs containing alcohol without consulting doctor.
- See Interaction column and consult doctor.

 OVERDOSE

Symptoms:
Rapid and weak heartbeat, fainting, extreme weakness, cold and sweaty skin.

What to do:
- Dial 0 (operator) or 911 (emergency) for an ambulance or medical help. Then give first aid immediately.
- If patient is unconscious and not breathing, give mouth-to-mouth breathing. If there is no heartbeat, use cardiac massage and mouth-to-mouth breathing (CPR). Don't try to make patient vomit. If you can't get help quickly, take patient to nearest emergency facility.
- Additional emergency information on page 886.

POSSIBLE ADVERSE REACTIONS OR SIDE EFFECTS

SYMPTOMS	FREQUENCY	WHAT TO DO
Brain & nervous system:		
● Headache	Common	5
● Confusion, dizziness.	Infrequent	4
Skin:		
● Hives or rash.	Infrequent	3
● Flushed face.	Infrequent	3
Eyes:		
Watering, irritation.	Infrequent	5
Ears, nose, throat:		
Sore throat, fever.	Infrequent	3
Digestive:		
● Diarrhea, appetite loss.	Common	5
● Nausea or vomiting.	Common	3
● Constipation	Infrequent	5
Heart & lungs:		
● Chest pain.	Infrequent	3
● Rapid or irregular heartbeat.	Common	3
Blood vessels, kidneys, allergic, blood:	None expected.	
Muscles, bones, joints:		
Joint pain.	Infrequent	4
Genital, urinary:		
Difficult urination.	Common	5
Liver:		
Jaundice (yellow skin and eyes).	Rare	3
Others:		
● Swelling of lymph glands.	Infrequent	3
● General discomfort or weakness.	Infrequent	4

1- Life-threatening. Seek emergency treatment immediately.
2- Discontinue. Seek emergency treatment.
3- Discontinue. Call doctor right away.
4- Continue. Call doctor when convenient.
5- Continue. Tell doctor at next visit.

WARNINGS & PRECAUTIONS

Don't take if:
- You are allergic to hydralazine.
- You have history of coronary-artery disease or rheumatic heart disease.

Before you start, consult your doctor:
- If you feel pain in chest, neck or arms on physical exertion.
- If you have had lupus.
- If you have had a stroke.
- If you have had kidney disease or impaired kidney function.
- If you will have surgery within 2 months, including dental surgery, requiring general or spinal anesthesia.

Over age 60:
Adverse reactions and side effects may be more frequent and severe than in younger persons.

Pregnancy:
Risk to unborn child outweighs drug benefits. Don't use.

Breast-feeding:
Drug filters into milk. May harm child. Avoid.

Infants & children:
Not recommended.

Prolonged use:
- May cause lupus (arthritis-like illness).
- Possible psychosis.
- May cause numbness, tingling in hands or feet.

Skin & sunlight:
No problems expected.

Driving, piloting or hazardous work:
Don't drive or pilot aircraft until you learn how medicine affects you. Don't work around dangerous machinery. Don't climb ladders or work in high places. Danger increases if you drink alcohol or take medicine affecting alertness and reflexes, such as antihistamines, tranquilizers, sedatives, pain medicine, narcotics and mind-altering drugs.

Airplane passengers:
No problems expected.

Discontinuing:
Don't discontinue without doctor's advice until you complete prescribed dose, even though symptoms diminish or disappear.

Others:
Vitamin B-6 diet supplement may be advisable. Consult doctor.

INTERACTION WITH OTHER DRUGS

GENERIC NAME OR DRUG CLASS	COMBINED EFFECT
Amphetamines	Decreased hydralazine effect.
Antidepressants (tricyclic)	Increased hydralazine effect.
Antihypertensives (other)	Increased antihypertensive effect.
Diuretics (oral)	Increased hydralazine effect.
MAO inhibitors	Increased hydralazine effect.

INTERACTION WITH OTHER SUBSTANCES

INTERACTS WITH	COMBINED EFFECT
Alcohol:	May lower blood pressure excessively. Use extreme caution.
Beverages:	None expected.
Cocaine:	Dangerous blood-pressure rise. Avoid.
Foods:	Increased hydralazine absorption.
Marijuana:	Weakness on standing.
Tobacco:	Possible angina attacks.

HYDROCHLOROTHIAZIDE

BRAND NAMES

Aldactazide (M)
Apresazide (M)
Diuchlor H
Esidrix
Hydrid

Hydro-Aquil
HydroDIURIL
Hydrozide-Z-50
Hyperetic
Inderide (M)

Neo-Codema
Novohydrazide
Oretic
Thiuretic
Urozide

Zide

See complete brand names list, page 826.

GENERAL INFORMATION

Habit forming? No
Prescription needed? Yes
Available as generic? Yes
Drug class: Antihypertensive,
diuretic (thiazide)

USES

- Controls, but doesn't cure, high blood pressure.
- Reduces fluid retention (edema).

DOSAGE & USAGE INFORMATION

How to take:
Tablet or capsule—Swallow with liquid. If you can't swallow whole, crumble tablet or open capsule and take with liquid or food.

When to take:
At the same time each day.

If you forget a dose:
Take as soon as you remember up to 2 hours late. If more than 2 hours, wait for next scheduled dose (don't double this dose).

What drug does:
- Forces sodium and water excretion, reducing body fluid.
- Relaxes muscle cells of small arteries.
- Reduced body fluid and relaxed arteries lower blood pressure.

Time lapse before drug works:
4 to 6 hours. May require several weeks to lower blood pressure.

Don't take with:
- See Interaction column and consult doctor.
- Non-prescription drugs without consulting doctor.

OVERDOSE

Symptoms:
Cramps, weakness, drowsiness, weak pulse, coma.

What to do:
- Dial 0 (operator) or 911 (emergency) for an ambulance or medical help. Then give first aid immediately.
- Additional emergency information on page 886.

POSSIBLE ADVERSE REACTIONS OR SIDE EFFECTS

SYMPTOMS	FREQUENCY	WHAT TO DO
Brain & nervous system:		
● Dizziness	Infrequent	4
● Mood changes.	Infrequent	4
● Headaches	Infrequent	4
Skin:		
Rash or hives.	Rare	2
Eyes:		
Blurred vision.	Infrequent	3
Ears, nose, throat:		
● Sore throat, fever.	Rare	3
● Dry mouth, thirst.	Infrequent	5
Digestive:		
Severe abdominal pain, nausea, vomiting.	Infrequent	3
Heart & lungs:		
Irregular heartbeat, weak pulse.	Infrequent	3
Blood vessels:	None expected.	
Muscles, bones, joints:		
Weakness, tiredness.	Infrequent	4
Genital, urinary:	None expected.	
Kidneys:	None expected.	
Liver:		
Jaundice (yellow skin and eyes).	Rare	3
Allergic:	None expected.	
Blood:	None expected.	
Others:		
Weight changes.	Infrequent	4

1- Life-threatening. Seek emergency treatment immediately.
2- Discontinue. Seek emergency treatment.
3- Discontinue. Call doctor right away.
4- Continue. Call doctor when convenient.
5- Continue. Tell doctor at next visit.
6- No action necessary.

HYDROCHLOROTHIAZIDE

WARNINGS & PRECAUTIONS

Don't take if:
You are allergic to any thiazide diuretic drug.

Before you start, consult your doctor:
- If you are allergic to any sulfa drug.
- If you have gout.
- If you have liver, pancreas or kidney disorder.

Over age 60:
Adverse reactions and side effects may be more frequent and severe than in younger persons, especially dizziness and excessive potassium loss.

Pregnancy:
Risk to unborn child outweighs drug benefits. Don't use.

Breast-feeding:
Drug passes into milk. Avoid drug or discontinue nursing.

Infants & children:
No problems expected.

Prolonged use:
You may need medicine to treat high blood pressure for the rest of your life.

Skin & sunlight:
May cause rash or intensify sunburn in areas exposed to sun or sunlamp.

Driving, piloting or hazardous work:
Don't drive or pilot aircraft until you learn how medicine affects you. Don't work around dangerous machinery. Don't climb ladders or work in high places. Danger increases if you drink alcohol or take medicine affecting alertness and reflexes, such as antihistamines, tranquilizers, sedatives, pain medicine, narcotics and mind-altering drugs.

Airplane passengers:
No problems expected.

Discontinuing:
Don't discontinue without medical advice.

Others:
- Hot weather and fever may cause dehydration and drop in blood pressure. Dose may require temporary adjustment. Weigh daily and report any unexpected weight decreases to your doctor.
- May cause rise in uric acid, leading to gout.
- May cause blood-sugar rise in diabetics.

INTERACTION WITH OTHER DRUGS

GENERIC NAME OR DRUG CLASS	COMBINED EFFECT
Allopurinol	Decreased allopurinol effect.
Antidepressants (tricyclic)	Dangerous drop in blood pressure. Avoid combination unless under medical supervision.
Barbiturates	Increased hydrochlorothiazide effect.
Cholestyramine	Decreased hydrochlorothiazide effect.
Cortisone drugs	Excessive potassium loss that causes dangerous heart rhythms.
Digitalis preparations	Excessive potassium loss that causes dangerous heart rhythms.
Diuretics (thiazide)	Increased effect of other thiazide diuretics.
Lithium	Increased effect of lithium.
MAO inhibitors	Increased hydrochlorothiazide effect.
Probenecid	Decreased probenecid effect.

INTERACTION WITH OTHER SUBSTANCES

INTERACTS WITH	COMBINED EFFECT
Alcohol:	Dangerous blood-pressure drop.
Beverages:	None expected.
Cocaine:	None expected.
Foods: Licorice	Excessive potassium loss that causes dangerous heart rhythms.
Marijuana:	May increase blood pressure.
Tobacco:	None expected.

HYDROCODONE

BRAND NAMES

Codone
Corutol DH
Dicodid
Hycodan (M)
Robidone

GENERAL INFORMATION

Habit forming? Yes
Prescription needed? Yes
Available as generic? Yes
Drug class: Narcotic

USES

- Relieves pain.
- Suppresses cough.

DOSAGE & USAGE INFORMATION

How to take:
- Tablet or capsule—Swallow with liquid. If you can't swallow whole, crumble tablet or open capsule and take with liquid or food.
- Drops or liquid—Dilute dose in beverage before swallowing.

When to take:
When needed. No more often the every 4 hours.

If you forget a dose:
Take as soon as you remember. Wait 4 hours for next dose.

What drug does:
- Reduces sensitivity of brain's cough-control center.
- Blocks pain messages to brain and spinal cord.

Time lapse before drug works:
30 minutes.

Don't take with:
See Interaction column and consult doctor.

OVERDOSE

Symptoms:
Deep sleep; slow breathing; slow pulse; flushed, warm skin; constricted pupils.

What to do:
- Dial 0 (operator) or 911 (emergency) for an ambulance or medical help. Then give first aid immediately.
- If patient is unconscious and not breathing, give mouth-to-mouth breathing. If there is no heartbeat, use cardiac massage and mouth-to-mouth breathing (CPR). Don't try to make patient vomit. If you can't get help quickly, take patient to nearest emergency facility.
- Additional emergency information on page 886.

POSSIBLE ADVERSE REACTIONS OR SIDE EFFECTS

SYMPTOMS	FREQUENCY	WHAT TO DO
Brain & nervous system: Depression, confusion, hallucinations.	Infrequent	4
Skin:		
• Hives, rash, itch, face swelling.	Rare	3
• Flushed face.	Common	4
Eyes: Blurred vision.	Rare	4
Ears, nose, throat:	None expected.	
Digestive: Severe constipation, abdominal pain, vomiting.	Infrequent	3
Heart & lungs: Slow heartbeat, irregular breathing.	Rare	3
Blood vessels:	None expected.	
Muscles, bones, joints:	None expected.	
Genital, urinary: Difficult urination.	Common	4
Kidneys: Less urine.	Common	4
Liver:	None expected.	
Allergic:	None expected.	
Blood:	None expected.	
Others: Unusual tiredness.	Common	4

1- Life-threatening. Seek emergency treatment immediately.
2- Discontinue. Seek emergency treatment.
3- Discontinue. Call doctor right away.
4- Continue. Call doctor when convenient.
5- Continue. Tell doctor at next visit.
6- No action necessary.

HYDROCODONE

 WARNINGS & PRECAUTIONS

Don't take if:
You are allergic to any narcotic.

Before you start, consult your doctor:
If you have impaired liver or kidney function.

Over age 60:
More likely to be drowsy, dizzy, unsteady or constipated. Avoid prolonged used.

Pregnancy:
Studies inconclusive on harm to unborn child. Animal studies show fetal abnormalities. Decide with your doctor whether drug benefits justify risk to unborn child. Abuse by pregnant woman will result in addicted newborn. Withdrawal can be life-threatening.

Breast-feeding:
Drug filters into milk. May depress infant. Avoid.

Infants & children:
Not recommended.

Prolonged use:
Causes psychological and physical dependence.

Skin & sunlight:
May cause rash, itch or intensify sunburn in areas exposed to sun or sunlamp.

Driving, piloting or hazardous work:
Don't drive or pilot aircraft until you learn how medicine affects you. Don't work around dangerous machinery. Don't climb ladders or work in high places. Danger increases if you drink alcohol or take medicine affecting alertness and reflexes, such as antihistamines, tranquilizers, sedatives, pain medicine, other narcotics and mind-altering drugs.

Airplane passengers:
No proven problems.

Discontinuing:
May be unnecessary to finish medicine. Follow doctor's instructions.

Others:
No problems expected.

 INTERACTION WITH OTHER DRUGS

GENERIC NAME OR DRUG CLASS	COMBINED EFFECT
Analgesics	Increased analgesic effect.
Antidepressants	Increased sedative effect.
Antihistamines	Increased sedative effect.
Mind-altering drugs	Increased sedative effect.
Narcotics (other)	Increased narcotic effect.
Phenothiazines	Increased phenothiazine effect.
Sedatives	Increased sedative effect.
Sleep inducers	Increased sedative effect.
Tranquilizers	Increased sedative effect.

 INTERACTION WITH OTHER SUBSTANCES

INTERACTS WITH	COMBINED EFFECT
Alcohol:	Increases alcohol's intoxicating effect. Avoid.
Beverages:	None expected.
Cocaine:	Increased cocaine effect.
Foods:	None expected.
Marijuana:	Impairs physical and mental performance.
Tobacco:	None expected.

HYDROCORTISONE (CORTISOL)

BRAND NAMES

A-hydroCort	Cortifoam
Biosone	Fernisone
Cortef	Hydrocortone
Cortef Fluid	Rectoid
Cortenema	Solu-Cortef

GENERAL INFORMATION

Habit forming? No
Prescription needed? Yes
Available as generic? Yes
Drug class: Cortisone drug (adrenal corticosteroid)

USES

- Reduces inflammation caused by many different medical problems.
- Treatment for some allergic diseases, blood disorders, kidney diseases, asthma and emphysema.
- Replaces corticosteroid deficiencies.

DOSAGE & USAGE INFORMATION

How to take:
- Tablet or liquid—Swallow with liquid or food to lessen stomach irritation. If you can't swallow whole, crumble tablet.
- Other forms—Follow label instructions.

When to take:
At the same times each day. Take once-a-day or once-every-other-day doses in mornings.

If you forget a dose:
- Several-doses-per-day prescription—Take as soon as you remember up to 2 hours late. If more than 2 hours, wait for next scheduled dose (don't double this dose).
- Once-a-day dose or less—Wait for next dose. Double this dose.

What drug does:
Decreases inflammatory responses.

Time lapse before drug works:
2 to 4 days.

Don't take with:
See Interaction column and consult doctor.

OVERDOSE

Symptoms:
Headache, convulsions, heart failure.

What to do:
- Dial 0 (operator) or 911 (emergency) for an ambulance or medical help. Then give first aid immediately.
- Additional emergency information on page 886.

POSSIBLE ADVERSE REACTIONS OR SIDE EFFECTS

SYMPTOMS	FREQUENCY	WHAT TO DO
Brain & nervous system:		
Mood changes, insomnia, restlessness.	Infrequent	4
Skin:		
● Acne	Common	4
● Rash	Rare	3
● Poor wound healing.	Common	4
Eyes:		
Blurred vision, halos around lights.	Infrequent	3
Ears, nose, throat:		
● Sore throat, fever.	Infrequent	3
● Thirst	Common	4
Digestive:		
● Indigestion, nausea, vomiting.	Common	4
● Bloody or black, tarry stool.	Infrequent	2
Heart & lungs:		
Irregular heartbeat.	Rare	2
Blood vessels, kidneys, liver, allergic, blood:	None expected.	
Muscles, bones, joints:		
Muscle cramps, swollen legs, feet.	Infrequent	3
Genital, urinary:		
Frequent urination.	Infrequent	4
Others:		
● Weight gain, round face.	Infrequent	4
● Fatigue, weakness.	Infrequent	4
● TB recurrence.	Infrequent	4
● Irregular menstrual periods.	Infrequent	4

1-Life-threatening. Seek emergency treatment immediately.
2-Discontinue. Seek emergency treatment.
3-Discontinue. Call doctor right away.
4-Continue. Call doctor when convenient.

HYDROCORTISONE (CORTISOL)

WARNINGS & PRECAUTIONS

Don't take if:
- You are allergic to any cortisone drug.
- You have tuberculosis or fungus infection.
- You have herpes infection of eyes, lips or genitals.

Before you start, consult your doctor:
- If you have had tuberculosis.
- If you have congestive heart failure.
- If you have diabetes.
- If you have peptic ulcer.
- If you have glaucoma.
- If you have underactive thyroid.
- If you have high blood pressure.
- If you have myasthenia gravis.
- If you have blood clots in legs or lungs.

Over age 60:
Adverse reactions and side effects may be more frequent and severe than in younger persons. Likely to aggravate edema, diabetes or ulcers. Likely to cause cataracts and osteoporosis (softening of the bones).

Pregnancy:
Risk to unborn child outweighs drug benefits. Don't use.

Breast-feeding:
Drug passes into milk. Avoid drug or discontinue nursing until you finish medicine. Consult doctor for advice on maintaining milk supply.

Infants & children:
Use only under medical supervision.

Prolonged use:
- Retards growth in children.
- Possible glaucoma, cataracts, diabetes, fragile bones and thin skin.
- Functional dependence.

Skin & sunlight:
No problems expected.

Driving, piloting or hazardous work:
No problems expected.

Airplane passengers:
No problems expected.

Discontinuing:
- Don't discontinue without doctor's advice until you complete prescribed dose, even though symptoms diminish or disappear.
- Drug affects your response to surgery, illness, injury or stress for 2 years after discontinuing. Tell about drug to anyone who takes medical care of you within 2 years.

Others:
Avoid immunizations if possible.

INTERACTION WITH OTHER DRUGS

GENERIC NAME OR DRUG CLASS	COMBINED EFFECT
Amphoterecin B	Potassium depletion.
Anticholinergics	Possible glaucoma.
Anticoagulants (oral)	Decreased anticoagulant effect.
Anticonvulsants (hydantoin)	Decreased hydrocortisone effect.
Antidiabetics (oral)	Decreased antidiabetic effect.
Antihistamines	Decreased hydrocortisone effect.
Aspirin	Increased hydrocortisone effect.
Barbiturates	Decreased hydrocortisone effect. Oversedation.
Beta-adrenergic blockers	Decreased hydrocortisone effect.
Chloral hydrate	Decreased hydrocortisone effect.
Chlorthalidone	Potassium depletion.
Cholinergics	Decreased cholinergic effect.
Contraceptives (oral)	Increased hydrocortisone effect.
Digitalis preparations	Dangerous potassium depletion. Possible digitalis toxicity.
Diuretics (thiazide)	Potassium depletion.

Additional interactions on page 838.

INTERACTION WITH OTHER SUBSTANCES

INTERACTS WITH	COMBINED EFFECT
Alcohol:	Risk of stomach ulcers.
Beverages:	No proven problems.
Cocaine:	Overstimulation. Avoid.
Foods:	No proven problems.
Marijuana:	Decreased immunity.
Tobacco:	Increased hydrocortisone effect. Possible toxicity.

HYDROFLUMETHIAZIDE

BRAND NAMES

Diucardin
Saluron
Salutensin (M)

GENERAL INFORMATION

Habit forming? No
Prescription needed? Yes
Available as generic? Yes
Drug class: Antihypertensive,
diuretic (thiazide)

USES

- Controls, but doesn't cure, high blood pressure.
- Reduces fluid retention (edema) caused by conditions such as heart disorders and liver disease.

DOSAGE & USAGE INFORMATION

How to take:
Tablet or capsule—Swallow with liquid. If you can't swallow whole, crumble tablet or open capsule and take with liquid or food. Don't exceed dose.

When to take:
At the same time each day.

If you forget a dose:
Take as soon as you remember up to 2 hours late. If more than 2 hours, wait for next scheduled dose (don't double this dose).

What drug does:
- Forces sodium and water excretion, reducing body fluid.
- Relaxes muscle cells of small arteries.
- Reduced body fluid and relaxed arteries lower blood pressure.

Time lapse before drug works:
4 to 6 hours. May require several weeks to lower blood pressure.

Don't take with:
- See Interaction column and consult doctor.
- Non-prescription drugs without consulting doctor.

OVERDOSE

Symptoms:
Cramps, weakness, drowsiness, weak pulse, coma.

What to do:
- Dial 0 (operator) or 911 (emergency) for an ambulance or medical help. Then give first aid immediately.
- Additional emergency information on page 886.

POSSIBLE ADVERSE REACTIONS OR SIDE EFFECTS

SYMPTOMS	FREQUENCY	WHAT TO DO
Brain & nervous system:		
• Dizziness	Infrequent	4
• Mood changes.	Infrequent	4
• Headaches	Infrequent	4
Skin:		
Rash or hives.	Rare	2
Eyes:		
Blurred vision.	Infrequent	3
Ears, nose, throat:		
• Sore throat, fever.	Rare	3
• Dry mouth, thirst.	Infrequent	5
Digestive:		
Severe abdominal pain, nausea, vomiting.	Infrequent	3
Heart & lungs:		
Irregular heartbeat, weak pulse.	Infrequent	3
Blood vessels:	None expected.	
Muscles, bones, joints:		
Weakness, tiredness.	Infrequent	4
Genital, urinary:	None expected.	
Kidneys:	None expected.	
Liver:		
Jaundice (yellow skin and eyes).	Rare	3
Allergic:	None expected.	
Blood:	None expected.	
Others:		
Weight changes.	Infrequent	4

1- Life-threatening. Seek emergency treatment immediately.
2- Discontinue. Seek emergency treatment.
3- Discontinue. Call doctor right away.
4- Continue. Call doctor when convenient.
5- Continue. Tell doctor at next visit.
6- No action necessary.

HYDROFLUMETHIAZIDE

WARNINGS & PRECAUTIONS

Don't take if:
You are allergic to any thiazide diuretic drug.

Before you start, consult your doctor:
- If you are allergic to any sulfa drug.
- If you have gout.
- If you have liver, pancreas or kidney disorder.

Over age 60:
Adverse reactions and side effects may be more frequent and severe than in younger persons, especially dizziness and excessive potassium loss.

Pregnancy:
Risk to unborn child outweighs drug benefits. Don't use.

Breast-feeding:
Drug passes into milk. Avoid drug or discontinue nursing.

Infants & children:
No problems expected.

Prolonged use:
You may need medicine to treat high blood pressure for the rest of your life.

Skin & sunlight:
May cause rash or intensify sunburn in areas exposed to sun or sunlamp.

Driving, piloting or hazardous work:
Don't drive or pilot aircraft until you learn how medicine affects you. Don't work around dangerous machinery. Don't climb ladders or work in high places. Danger increases if you drink alcohol or take medicine affecting alertness and reflexes, such as antihistamines, tranquilizers, sedatives, pain medicine, narcotics and mind-altering drugs.

Airplane passengers:
No problems expected.

Discontinuing:
Don't discontinue without medical advice.

Others:
- Hot weather and fever may cause dehydration and drop in blood pressure. Dose may require temporary adjustment. Weigh daily and report any unexpected weight decreases to your doctor.
- May cause rise in uric acid, leading to gout.
- May cause blood-sugar rise in diabetics.

INTERACTION WITH OTHER DRUGS

GENERIC NAME OR DRUG CLASS	COMBINED EFFECT
Allopurinol	Decreased allopurinol effect.
Antidepressants (tricyclic)	Dangerous drop in blood pressure. Avoid combination unless under medical supervision.
Barbiturates	Increased hydroflumethiazide effect.
Cholestyramine	Decreased hydroflumethiazide effect.
Cortisone drugs	Excessive potassium loss that causes dangerous heart rhythms.
Digitalis preparations	Excessive potassium loss that causes dangerous heart rhythms.
Diuretics (thiazide)	Increased effect of other thiazide diuretics.
Lithium	Increased effect of lithium.
MAO inhibitors	Increased hydroflumethiazide effect.
Probenecid	Decreased probenecid effect.

INTERACTION WITH OTHER SUBSTANCES

INTERACTS WITH	COMBINED EFFECT
Alcohol:	Dangerous blood-pressure drop.
Beverages:	None expected.
Cocaine:	None expected.
Foods: Licorice	Excessive potassium loss that causes dangerous heart rhythms.
Marijuana:	May increase blood pressure.
Tobacco:	None expected.

HYDROMORPHONE

BRAND NAMES

Dilaudid

GENERAL INFORMATION

Habit forming? Yes
Prescription needed? Yes
Available as generic? Yes
Drug class: Narcotic

USES

Relieves pain.

DOSAGE & USAGE INFORMATION

How to take:
- Tablet or capsule—Swallow with liquid. If you can't swallow whole, crumble tablet or open capsule and take with liquid or food.
- Drops or liquid—Dilute dose in beverage before swallowing.

When to take:
When needed. No more often than every 4 hours.

If you forget a dose:
Take as soon as you remember. Wait 4 hours for next dose.

What drug does:
Blocks pain messages to brain and spinal cord.

Time lapse before drug works:
30 minutes.

Don't take with:
See Interaction column and consult doctor.

OVERDOSE

Symptoms:
Deep sleep; slow breathing; slow pulse; flushed, warm skin; constricted pupils.

What to do:
- Dial 0 (operator) or 911 (emergency) for an ambulance or medical help. Then give first aid immediately.
- If patient is unconscious and not breathing, give mouth-to-mouth breathing. If there is no heartbeat, use cardiac massage and mouth-to-mouth breathing (CPR). Don't try to make patient vomit. If you can't get help quickly, take patient to nearest emergency facility.
- Additional emergency information on page 886.

POSSIBLE ADVERSE REACTIONS OR SIDE EFFECTS

SYMPTOMS	FREQUENCY	WHAT TO DO
Brain & nervous system: Depression, confusion, hallucinations.	Infrequent	4
Skin:		
• Hives, rash, itch, face swelling.	Rare	3
• Flushed face.	Common	4
Eyes: Blurred vision.	Rare	4
Ears, nose, throat:	None expected.	
Digestive: Severe constipation, abdominal pain, vomiting.	Infrequent	3
Heart & lungs: Slow heartbeat, irregular breathing.	Rare	3
Blood vessels:	None expected.	
Muscles, bones, joints:	None expected.	
Genital, urinary: Difficult urination.	Common	4
Kidneys: Less urine.	Common	4
Liver:	None expected.	
Allergic:	None expected.	
Blood:	None expected.	
Others: Unusual tiredness.	Common	4

1- Life-threatening. Seek emergency treatment immediately.
2- Discontinue. Seek emergency treatment.
3- Discontinue. Call doctor right away.
4- Continue. Call doctor when convenient.
5- Continue. Tell doctor at next visit.
6- No action necessary.

HYDROMORPHONE

WARNINGS & PRECAUTIONS

Don't take if:
You are allergic to any narcotic.

Before you start, consult your doctor:
If you have impaired liver or kidney function.

Over age 60:
More likely to be drowsy, dizzy, unsteady or constipated. Avoid prolonged use.

Pregnancy:
Studies inconclusive on harm to unborn child. Animal studies show fetal abnormalities. Decide with your doctor whether drug benefits justify risk to unborn child. Abuse by pregnant woman will result in addicted newborn. Withdrawal can be life-threatening.

Breast-feeding:
Drug filters into milk. May depress infant. Avoid.

Infants & children:
Not recommended.

Prolonged use:
Causes psychological and physical dependence.

Skin & sunlight:
No problems expected.

Driving, piloting or hazardous work:
Don't drive or pilot aircraft until you learn how medicine affects you. Don't work around dangerous machinery. Don't climb ladders or work in high places. Danger increases if you drink alcohol or take medicine affecting alertness and reflexes, such as antihistamines, tranquilizers, sedatives, pain medicine, other narcotics and mind-altering drugs.

Airplane passengers:
No proven problems.

Discontinuing:
May be unnecessary to finish medicine. Follow doctor's instructions.

Others:
No problems expected.

INTERACTION WITH OTHER DRUGS

GENERIC NAME OR DRUG CLASS	COMBINED EFFECT
Analgesics	Increased analgesic effect.
Antidepressants	Increased sedative effect.
Antihistamines	Increased sedative effect.
Mind-altering drugs	Increased sedative effect.
Narcotics (other)	Increased narcotic effect.
Phenothiazines	Increased phenothiazine effect.
Sedatives	Increased sedative effect.
Sleep inducers	Increased sedative effect.
Tranquilizers	Increased sedative effect.

INTERACTION WITH OTHER SUBSTANCES

INTERACTS WITH	COMBINED EFFECT
Alcohol:	Increases alcohol's intoxicating effect. Avoid.
Beverages:	None expected.
Cocaine:	Increased cocaine effect.
Foods:	None expected.
Marijuana:	Impairs physical and mental performance.
Tobacco:	None expected.

HYDROXYCHLOROQUINE

BRAND NAMES

Plaquenil

GENERAL INFORMATION

Habit forming? No
Prescription needed? Yes
Available as generic? Yes
Drug class: Antiprotozoal, antirheumatic

USES

Treatment for protozoal infections, such as malaria and amebiasis.
Treatment for some forms of arthritis and lupus.

DOSAGE & USAGE INFORMATION

How to take:
Tablet—Swallow with food or milk to lessen stomach irritation.

When to take:
- Depends on condition. Is adjusted during treatment.
- Malaria prevention—Begin taking medicine 2 weeks before entering areas with malaria.

If you forget a dose:
- 1 or more doses a day—Take as soon as you remember up to 2 hours late. If more than 2 hours, wait for next scheduled dose (don't double this dose).
- 1 dose weekly—Take as soon as possible, then return to regular dosing schedule.

What drug does:
- Inhibits parasite multiplication.
- Decreases inflammatory response in diseased joint.

Time lapse before drug works:
1 to 2 hours.

Don't take with:
See Interaction column and consult doctor.

OVERDOSE

Symptoms:
Severe breathing difficulty, drowsiness, faintness.

What to do:
- Dial 0 (operator) or 911 (emergency) for an ambulance or medical help. Then give first aid immediately.
- Additional emergency information on page 886.

POSSIBLE ADVERSE REACTIONS OR SIDE EFFECTS

SYMPTOMS	FREQUENCY	WHAT TO DO
Brain & nervous system:		
• Mood or mental changes, seizures.	Rare	3
• Headache	Common	5
Skin:		
Rash or itch.	Infrequent	4
Eyes:		
Blurred or changed vision.	Infrequent	3
Ears, nose, throat:		
• Ringing or buzzing in ears, hearing loss.	Rare	4
• Sore throat, fever.	Rare	3
Digestive:		
Diarrhea, nausea, vomiting.	Infrequent	4
Heart & lungs:	None expected.	
Blood vessels:		
Unusual bleeding or bruising.	Rare	3
Muscles, bones, joints:		
Muscle weakness.	Rare	3
Genital, urinary:	None expected.	
Kidneys:	None expected.	
Liver:	None expected.	
Allergic:	None expected.	
Blood:	None expected.	
Others:	None expected.	

1- Life threatening. Seek emergency treatment immediately.
2- Discontinue. Seek emergency treatment.
3- Discontinue. Call doctor right away.
4- Continue. Call doctor when convenient.
5- Continue. Tell doctor at next visit.
6- No action necessary.

HYDROXYCHLOROQUINE

WARNINGS & PRECAUTIONS

Don't take if:
You are allergic to chloroquine or hydroxychloroquine.

Before you start, consult your doctor:
- If you plan to become pregnant within the medication period.
- If you have blood disease.
- If you have eye or vision problems.
- If you have a G6PD deficiency.
- If you have liver disease.
- If you have nerve or brain disease (including seizure disorders).
- If you have porphyria.
- If you have psoriasis.
- If you have stomach or intestinal disease.
- If you drink more than 3 oz. of alcohol daily.

Over age 60:
Adverse reactions and side effects may be more frequent and severe than in younger persons.

Pregnancy:
Risk to unborn child outweighs drug benefits. Don't use.

Breast-feeding:
Drug passes into milk. Avoid drug or discontinue nursing.

Infants & children:
Not recommended. Dangerous.

Prolonged use:
Permanent damage to the retina (back part of the eye) or nerve deafness.

Skin & sunlight:
May cause rash or intensify sunburn in areas exposed to sun or sunlamp.

Driving, piloting or hazardous work:
Don't drive or pilot aircraft until you learn how medicine affects you. Don't work around dangerous machinery. Don't climb ladders or work in high places. Danger increases if you drink alcohol or take medicine affecting alertness and reflexes.

Airplane passengers:
No problems expected.

Discontinuing:
Don't discontinue without doctor's advice until you complete prescribed dose, even though symptoms diminish or disappear.

Others:
- Periodic physical and blood examinations recommended.
- If you are in a malaria area for a long time, you may need to change to another preventive drug every 2 years.

INTERACTION WITH OTHER DRUGS

GENERIC NAME OR DRUG CLASS	COMBINED EFFECT
Estrogens	Possible liver toxicity.
Gold compounds	Risk of severe rash and itch.
Oxyphenbutazone	Risk of severe rash and itch.
Penicillamine	Possible blood or kidney toxicity.
Phenylbutazone	Risk of severe rash and itch.
Sulfa drugs	Possible liver toxicity.

INTERACTION WITH OTHER SUBSTANCES

INTERACTS WITH	COMBINED EFFECT
Alcohol:	Possible liver toxicity. Avoid.
Beverages:	None expected.
Cocaine:	None expected.
Foods:	None expected.
Marijuana:	None expected.
Tobacco:	None expected.

HYDROXYZINE

BRAND NAMES

Atarax   Vistaril
Ataraxoid (M)   Vistrax (M)
Cartrax (M)
Enarax (M)
Marax (M)

GENERAL INFORMATION

Habit forming? No
Prescription needed? Yes
Available as generic? No
Drug class: Tranquilizer, antihistamine

 ## USES

- Treatment for anxiety, tension and agitation.
- Relieves itching from allergic reactions.

 ## DOSAGE & USAGE INFORMATION

How to take:
- Tablet or capsule—Swallow with liquid. If you can't swallow whole, crumble tablet or open capsule and take with liquid or food.
- Liquid—If desired, dilute dose in beverage before swallowing.

When to take:
At the same times each day.

If you forget a dose:
Take as soon as you remember up to 2 hours late. If more than 2 hours, wait for next scheduled dose (don't double this dose).

What drug does:
May reduce activity in areas of the brain that influence emotional stability.

Time lapse before drug works:
15 to 30 minutes.

Don't take with:
- Non-prescription drugs without consulting doctor.
- See Interaction column and consult doctor.

 ## OVERDOSE

Symptoms:
Drowsiness, unsteadiness, agitation, purposeless movements, tremor, convulsions.

What to do:
- Dial 0 (operator) or 911 (emergency) for an ambulance or medical help. Then give first aid immediately.
- Additional emergency information on page 886.

 ## POSSIBLE ADVERSE REACTIONS OR SIDE EFFECTS

SYMPTOMS	FREQUENCY	WHAT TO DO
Brain & nervous system:		
● Headache	Infrequent	5
● Tremor	Rare	3
● Drowsiness	Common	5
Skin:		
Rash	Rare	3
Eyes:	None expected.	
Ears, nose, throat:		
Dry mouth.	Common	5
Digestive:	None expected.	
Heart & lungs:	None expected.	
Blood vessels:	None expected.	
Muscles, bones, joints:	None expected.	
Genital, urinary:		
Difficult urination.	Common	5
Kidneys:	None expected.	
Liver:	None expected.	
Allergic:	None expected.	
Blood:	None expected.	
Others:	None expected.	

1- Life-threatening. Seek emergency treatment immediately.
2- Discontinue. Seek emergency treatment.
3- Discontinue. Call doctor right away.
4- Continue. Call doctor when convenient.
5- Continue. Tell doctor at next visit.
6- No action necessary.

WARNINGS & PRECAUTIONS

Don't take if:
You are allergic to any antihistamine.

Before you start, consult your doctor:
- If you have epilepsy.
- If you will have surgery within 2 months, including dental surgery, requiring general or spinal anesthesia.

Over age 60:
Adverse reactions and side effects may be more frequent and severe than in younger persons. Drug likely to increase urination difficulty caused by enlarged prostate gland.

Pregnancy:
Studies inconclusive on harm to unborn child. Animal studies show fetal abnormalities. Decide with your doctor whether drug benefits justify risk to unborn child.

Breast-feeding:
Drug passes into milk. Avoid drug or discontinue nursing until you finish medicine. Consult doctor for advice on maintaining milk supply.

Infants & children:
Use only under medical supervision.

Prolonged use:
Tolerance develops and reduces effectiveness.

Skin & sunlight:
No problems expected.

Driving, piloting or hazardous work:
Don't drive or pilot aircraft until you learn how medicine affects you. Don't work around dangerous machinery. Don't climb ladders or work in high places. Danger increases if you drink alcohol or take medicine affecting alertness and reflexes, such as antihistamines, tranquilizers, sedatives, pain medicine, narcotics and mind-altering drugs.

Airplane passengers:
No problems expected.

Discontinuing:
Don't discontinue without consulting doctor. Dose may require gradual reduction if you have taken drug for a long time. Doses of other drugs may also require adjustment.

Others:
No problems expected.

INTERACTION WITH OTHER DRUGS

GENERIC NAME OR DRUG CLASS	COMBINED EFFECT
Anticoagulants (oral)	Increased anticoagulant effect.
Anticonvulsants (hydantoin)	Decreased anticonvulsant effect.
Antidepressants (tricyclic)	Increased effect of both drugs.
Antihistamines	Increased hydroxyzine effect.
Narcotics	Increased effect of both drugs.
Pain relievers	Increased effect of both drugs.
Sedatives	Increased effect of both drugs.
Sleep inducers	Increased effect of both drugs.
Tranquilizers	Increased effect of both drugs.

INTERACTION WITH OTHER SUBSTANCES

INTERACTS WITH	COMBINED EFFECT
Alcohol:	Increased sedation and intoxication. Use with caution.
Beverages: Caffeine drinks	Decreased tranquilizer effect of hydroxyzine.
Cocaine:	Decreased hydroxyzine effect. Avoid.
Foods:	None expected.
Marijuana:	None expected.
Tobacco:	None expected.

HYOSCYAMINE

BRAND NAMES

Anaspaz
Barbidonna-CR (M)
Cystospaz
Donnatal (M)

Ergobel (M)
Floramine
Levsin
Omnibel (M)

See complete brand names list, page 827.

GENERAL INFORMATION

Habit forming? No
Prescription needed? Low strength: No
High strength: Yes
Available as generic? Yes
Drug class: Antispasmodic, anticholinergic

 USES

Reduces spasms of digestive system, bladder and urethra.

 DOSAGE & USAGE INFORMATION

How to take:
- Tablet or liquid—Swallow with liquid or food to lessen stomach irritation.
- Extended-release tablets or capsules—Swallow each dose whole. If you take regular tablets, you may chew or crush them.
- Drops—Dilute dose in beverage before swallowing.

When to take:
30 minutes before meals (unless directed otherwise by doctor).

If you forget a dose:
Take as soon as you remember up to 2 hours late. If more than 2 hours, wait for next scheduled dose (don't double this dose).

What drug does:
Blocks nerve impulses at parasympathetic nerve endings, preventing muscle contractions and gland secretions of organs involved.

Time lapse before drug works:
15 to 30 minutes.

Don't take with:
See Interaction column and consult doctor.

 OVERDOSE

Symptoms:
Dilated pupils; rapid pulse and breathing; dizziness; fever; hallucinations; confusion; slurred speech; agitation; flushed face; convulsions; coma.

What to do:
- Dial 0 (operator) or 911 (emergency) for an ambulance or medical help. Then give first aid immediately.
- Additional emergency information on page 886.

POSSIBLE ADVERSE REACTIONS OR SIDE EFFECTS

SYMPTOMS	FREQUENCY	WHAT TO DO
Brain & nervous system:		
● Headache	Infrequent	4
● Confusion, delirium.	Common	3
Skin:		
Rash or hives.	Rare	3
Eyes:		
Pain, blurred vision.	Rare	3
Ears, nose, throat:		
Dryness	Common	6
Digestive:		
● Constipation	Common	5
● Nausea, vomiting.	Common	4
Heart & lungs:		
Rapid heartbeat.	Common	3
Blood vessels:	None expected.	
Muscles, bones, joints:	None expected.	
Genital, urinary:		
Difficult urination.	Infrequent	4
Kidneys:	None expected.	
Liver:	None expected.	
Allergic:	None expected.	
Blood:	None expected.	
Others:		
Less perspiration.	Common	4

1- Life-threatening. Seek emergency treatment immediately.
2- Discontinue. Seek emergency treatment.
3- Discontinue. Call doctor right away.
4- Continue. Call doctor when convenient.
5- Continue. Tell doctor at next visit.
6- No action necessary.

WARNINGS & PRECAUTIONS

Don't take if:
- You are allergic to any anticholinergic.
- You have trouble with stomach bloating.
- You have difficulty emptying your bladder completely.
- You have narrow-angle glaucoma.
- You have severe ulcerative colitis.

Before you start, consult your doctor:
- If you have open-angle glaucoma.
- If you have angina.
- If you have chronic bronchitis or asthma.
- If you have hiatal hernia.
- If you have liver disease.
- If you have enlarged prostate.
- If you have myasthenia gravis.
- If you have peptic ulcer.
- If you will have surgery within 2 months, including dental surgery, requiring general or spinal anesthesia.

Over age 60:
Adverse reactions and side effects may be more frequent and severe than in younger persons.

Pregnancy:
Studies inconclusive on harm to unborn child. Animal studies show fetal abnormalities. Decide with your doctor whether drug benefits justify risk to unborn child.

Breast-feeding:
Drug passes into milk and decreases milk flow. Avoid drug or discontinue nursing until you finish medicine. Consult doctor for advice on maintaining milk supply.

Infants & children:
Use only under medical supervision.

Prolonged use:
Chronic constipation, possible fecal impaction. Consult doctor immediately.

Skin & sunlight:
No problems expected.

Driving, piloting or hazardous work:
Use disqualifies you for piloting aircraft. Otherwise, no problems expected.

Airplane passengers:
No problems expected.

Discontinuing:
May be unnecessary to finish medicine. Follow doctor's instructions.

Others:
No problems expected.

INTERACTION WITH OTHER DRUGS

GENERIC NAME OR DRUG CLASS	COMBINED EFFECT
Amantadine	Increased hyoscyamine effect.
Anticholinergics (other)	Increased hyoscyamine effect.
Antidepressants (tricyclic)	Increased hyoscyamine effect.
Antihistamines	Increased hyoscyamine effect.
Cortisone drugs	Increased internal-eye pressure.
Haloperidol	Increased internal-eye pressure.
MAO inhibitors	Increased hyoscyamine effect.
Meperidine	Increased hyoscyamine effect.
Methylphenidate	Increased hyoscyamine effect.
Orphenadrine	Increased hyoscyamine effect.
Phenothiazines	Increased hyoscyamine effect.
Pilocarpine	Loss of pilocarpine effect in glaucoma treatment.
Vitamin C	Decreased hyoscyamine effect. Avoid large doses of vitamin C.

INTERACTION WITH OTHER SUBSTANCES

INTERACTS WITH	COMBINED EFFECT
Alcohol:	None expected.
Beverages:	None expected.
Cocaine:	Excessively rapid heartbeat. Avoid.
Foods:	None expected.
Marijuana:	Drowsiness and dry mouth.
Tobacco:	None expected.

IBUPROFEN

BRAND NAMES

Motrin
Rufen

Habit forming? No
Prescription needed? Yes

GENERAL INFORMATION

Available as generic? Yes
Drug class: Antiinflammatory (non-steroid)

 USES

- Treatment for joint pain, stiffness, inflammation and swelling of arthritis and gout.
- Pain reliever.
- Treatment for dysmenorrhea (painful or difficult menstruation).

 DOSAGE & USAGE INFORMATION

How to take:
Tablet—Swallow with liquid or food to lessen stomach irritation. If you can't swallow whole, crumble tablet and take with liquid or food.

When to take:
At the same times each day.

If you forget a dose:
Take as soon as you remember up to 2 hours late. If more than 2 hours, wait for next scheduled dose (don't double this dose).

What drug does:
Reduces tissue concentration of prostaglandins (hormones which produce inflammation and pain).

Time lapse before drug works:
Begins in 4 to 24 hours. May require 3 weeks regular use for maximum benefit.

Don't take with:
See Interaction column and consult doctor.

 OVERDOSE

Symptoms:
Confusion, agitation, incoherence, convulsions, possible hemorrhage from stomach or intestine, coma.

What to do:
- Dial 0 (operator) or 911 (emergency) for an ambulance or medical help. Then give first aid immediately.
- Additional emergency information on page 886.

POSSIBLE ADVERSE REACTIONS OR SIDE EFFECTS

SYMPTOMS	FREQUENCY	WHAT TO DO
Brain & nervous system:		
• Depression, drowsiness.	Infrequent	4
• Convulsions, confusion.	Rare	3
• Dizziness	Common	4
• Headache	Common	5
Skin:		
Rash, hives or itch.	Rare	3
Eyes:		
Blurred vision.	Rare	3
Ears, nose, throat:		
Ringing in ears.	Infrequent	4
Digestive:		
• Bloody or black, tarry stools.	Rare	3
• Nausea, pain.	Common	4
• Constipation or diarrhea, vomiting.	Infrequent	4
Heart & lungs:		
Breathing difficulty, tightness in chest, rapid heartbeat.	Rare	3
Blood vessels:		
Unusual bleeding or bruising.	Rare	3
Muscles, bones, joints:		
Swollen feet, legs.	Infrequent	4
Genital, urinary:		
• Bloody urine.	Rare	3
• Difficult, painful or frequent urination.	Rare	4
Kidneys, allergic, blood:		
	None expected.	
Liver:		
Jaundice (yellow skin and eyes).	Rare	3
Others:		
Fatigue, weakness.	Rare	4

1 - Life-threatening. Seek emergency treatment immediately.
2 - Discontinue. Seek emergency treatment.
3 - Discontinue. Call doctor right away.
4 - Continue. Call doctor when convenient.
5 - Continue. Tell doctor at next visit.

IBUPROFEN

WARNINGS & PRECAUTIONS

Don't take if:
- You are allergic to aspirin or any non-steroid, antiinflammatory drug.
- You have gastritis, peptic ulcer, enteritis, ileitis, ulcerative colitis, asthma, heart failure, high blood pressure or bleeding problems.
- Patient is younger than 15.

Before you start, consult your doctor:
- If you have epilepsy.
- If you have Parkinson's disease.
- If you have been mentally ill.
- If you have had kidney disease or impaired kidney function.

Over age 60:
Adverse reactions and side effects may be more frequent and severe than in younger persons.

Pregnancy:
Studies inconclusive on harm to unborn child. Decide with your doctor whether drug benefits justify risk to unborn child.

Breast-feeding:
May harm child. Avoid.

Infants & children:
Not recommended for anyone younger than 15. Use only under medical supervision.

Prolonged use:
- Eye damage.
- Reduced hearing.
- Sore throat, fever.
- Weight gain.

Skin & sunlight:
No problems expected.

Driving, piloting or hazardous work:
Don't drive or pilot aircraft until you learn how medicine affects you. Don't work around dangerous machinery. Don't climb ladders or work in high places. Danger increases if you drink alcohol or take medicine affecting alertness and reflexes, such as antihistamines, tranquilizers, sedatives, pain medicine, narcotics and mind-altering drugs.

Airplane passengers:
No problems expected.

Discontinuing:
Don't discontinue without consulting doctor. Dose may require gradual reduction if you have taken drug for a long time. Doses of other drugs may also require adjustment.

Others:
No problems expected.

INTERACTION WITH OTHER DRUGS

GENERIC NAME OR DRUG CLASS	COMBINED EFFECT
Anticoagulants (oral)	Increased risk of bleeding.
Aspirin	Increased risk of stomach ulcer.
Cortisone drugs	Increased risk of stomach ulcer.
Furosemide	Decreased diuretic effect of furosemide.
Oxyphenbutazone	Possible stomach ulcer.
Phenylbutazone	Possible stomach ulcer.
Probenecid	Increased ibuprofen effect.
Thyroid hormones	Rapid heartbeat, blood pressure rise.

INTERACTION WITH OTHER SUBSTANCES

INTERACTS WITH	COMBINED EFFECT
Alcohol:	Possible stomach ulcer or bleeding.
Beverages:	None expected.
Cocaine:	None expected.
Foods:	None expected.
Marijuana:	Increased pain relief from ibuprofen.
Tobacco:	None expected.

IMIPRAMINE

BRAND NAMES

Imavate
Janimine
Presamine
SK-Pramine
Tofranil
Tofranil-PM

GENERAL INFORMATION

Habit forming? No
Prescription needed? Yes
Available as generic? Yes
Drug class: Antidepressant (tricyclic)

USES

- Gradually relieves, but doesn't cure, symptoms of depression.
- Decreases bed-wetting.

DOSAGE & USAGE INFORMATION

How to take:
Tablet or capsule—Swallow with liquid.

When to take:
At the same time each day, usually bedtime.

If you forget a dose:
Bedtime dose—If you forget your once-a-day bedtime dose, don't take it more than 3 hours late. If more than 3 hours, wait for next scheduled dose. Don't double this dose.

What drug does:
Probably affects part of brain that controls messages between nerve cells.

Time lapse before drug works:
Begins in 1 to 2 weeks. May require 4 to 6 weeks for maximum benefit.

Don't take with:
- Non-prescription drugs without consulting doctor.
- See Interaction column and consult doctor.

OVERDOSE

Symptoms:
Hallucinations, convulsions, coma.

What to do:
- Dial 0 (operator) or 911 (emergency) for an ambulance or medical help. Then give first aid immediately.
- If patient is unconscious and not breathing, give mouth-to-mouth breathing. If there is no heartbeat, use cardiac massage and mouth-to-mouth breathing (CPR). Don't try to make patient vomit. If you can't get help quickly, take patient to nearest emergency facility.
- Additional emergency information on page 886.

POSSIBLE ADVERSE REACTIONS OR SIDE EFFECTS

SYMPTOMS	FREQUENCY	WHAT TO DO
Brain & nervous system:		
• Hallucinations, shakiness, dizziness, fainting.	Infrequent	3
• Headache	Common	4
• Seizures	Rare	1
• Insomnia	Common	5
Skin:		
Rash, itch.	Rare	3
Eyes:		
Blurred vision, pain.	Infrequent	3
Ears, nose, throat:		
• Sore throat.	Rare	3
• Dry mouth or unpleasant taste.	Common	4
Digestive:		
• Constipation or diarrhea, nausea, indigestion.	Common	4
• Vomiting	Infrequent	3
• "Sweet tooth"	Common	5
Heart & lungs:		
Irregular heartbeat or slow pulse.	Infrequent	3
Blood vessels, muscles, bones, joints, kidneys, allergic, blood:	None expected.	
Genital, urinary:		
Difficulty urinating.	Infrequent	4
Liver:		
Jaundice (yellow skin and eyes).	Rare	3
Others:		
• Fever	Rare	3
• Fatigue, weakness.	Common	4

1 - Life-threatening. Seek emergency treatment immediately.
2 - Discontinue. Seek emergency treatment.
3 - Discontinue. Call doctor right away.
4 - Continue. Call doctor when convenient.
5 - Continue. Tell doctor at next visit.

IMIPRAMINE

WARNINGS & PRECAUTIONS

Don't take if:
- You are allergic to any tricyclic antidepressant.
- You drink alcohol.
- You have had a heart attack within 6 weeks.
- You have glaucoma.
- You have taken MAO inhibitors within 2 weeks.
- Patient is younger than 12.

Before you start, consult your doctor:
- If you will have surgery within 2 months, including dental surgery, requiring general or spinal anesthesia.
- If you have an enlarged prostate.
- If you have heart disease or high blood pressure.
- If you have stomach or intestinal problems.
- If you have an overactive thyroid.
- If you have asthma.
- If you have liver disease.

Over age 60:
More likely to develop urination difficulty and side effects under *Brain & nervous system,* opposite.

Pregnancy:
Studies inconclusive on harm to unborn child. Animal studies show fetal abnormalities. Decide with your doctor whether drug benefits justify risk to unborn child.

Breast-feeding:
Drug passes into milk. Avoid drug or discontinue nursing until you finish medicine. Consult doctor on maintaining milk supply.

Infants & children:
Don't give to children younger than 12.

Prolonged use:
No problems expected.

Skin & sunlight:
May cause rash or intensify sunburn in areas exposed to sun or sunlamp.

Driving, piloting or hazardous work:
Don't drive or pilot aircraft until you learn how medicine affects you. Don't work around dangerous machinery. Don't climb ladders or work in high places. Danger increases if you drink alcohol or take medicine affecting alertness and reflexes.

Airplane passengers:
No problems expected.

Discontinuing:
Don't discontinue without consulting doctor. Dose may require gradual reduction if you have taken drug for a long time. Doses of other drugs may also require adjustment.

INTERACTION WITH OTHER DRUGS

GENERIC NAME OR DRUG CLASS	COMBINED EFFECT
Anticoagulants (oral)	Increased anticoagulant effect.
Anticholinergics	Increased sedation.
Antihistamines	Increased antihistamine effect.
Barbiturates	Decreased antidepressant effect.
Clonidine	Decreased clonidine effect.
Diuretics (thiazide)	Increased imipramine effect.
Ethchlorvynol	Delirium
Guanethidine	Decreased guanethidine effect.
MAO inhibitors	Fever, delirium, convulsions.
Methyldopa	Decreased methyldopa effect.
Narcotics	Dangerous oversedation.
Phenytoin	Decreased phenytoin effect.
Quinidine	Irregular heartbeat.
Sedatives	Dangerous oversedation.
Sympathomimetics	Increased sympathomimetic effect.
Thyroid hormones	Irregular heartbeat.

INTERACTION WITH OTHER SUBSTANCES

INTERACTS WITH	COMBINED EFFECT
Alcohol: Beverages or medicines with alcohol.	Excessive intoxication. Avoid.
Beverages:	None expected.
Cocaine:	Excessive intoxication. Avoid.
Foods:	None expected.
Marijuana:	Excessive drowsiness. Avoid.
Tobacco:	None expected.

INDOMETHACIN

BRAND NAMES

Indocid
Indocin

Habit forming? No
Prescription needed? Yes

Available as generic? No
Drug class: Antiinflammatory (non-steroid)

USES

- Treatment for joint pain, stiffness, inflammation and swelling of arthritis and gout.
- Pain reliever.
- Treatment for dysmenorrhea (painful or difficult menstruation).

DOSAGE & USAGE INFORMATION

How to take:
- Tablet or capsule—Swallow with liquid or food to lessen stomach irritation. If you can't swallow whole, crumble tablet or open capsule and take with liquid or food.
- Extended release tablets or capsules—Swallow whole with liquid or food to lessen stomach irritation.

When to take:
At the same times each day.

If you forget a dose:
Take as soon as you remember up to 2 hours late. If more than 2 hours, wait for next scheduled dose (don't double this dose).

What drug does:
Reduces tissue concentration of prostaglandins (hormones which produce inflammation and pain).

Time lapse before drug works:
Begins in 4 to 24 hours. May require 3 weeks regular use for maximum benefit.

Don't take with:
See Interaction column and consult doctor.

OVERDOSE

Symptoms:
Confusion, agitation, incoherence, convulsions, possible hemorrhage from stomach or intestine, coma.

What to do:
- Dial 0 (operator) or 911 (emergency) for an ambulance or medical help. Then give first aid immediately.
- Additional emergency information on page 886.

POSSIBLE ADVERSE REACTIONS OR SIDE EFFECTS

SYMPTOMS	FREQUENCY	WHAT TO DO
Brain & nervous system:		
• Depression, drowsiness.	Infrequent	4
• Convulsions, confusion.	Rare	3
• Dizziness	Common	4
• Headache	Common	5
Skin:		
Rash, hives or itch.	Rare	3
Eyes:		
Blurred vision.	Rare	3
Ears, nose, throat:		
Ringing in ears.	Infrequent	4
Digestive:		
• Bloody or black, tarry stools.	Rare	3
• Nausea, pain.	Common	4
• Constipation or diarrhea, vomiting.	Infrequent	4
Heart & lungs:		
Breathing difficulty, tightness in chest, rapid heartbeat.	Rare	3
Blood vessels:		
Unusual bleeding or bruising.	Rare	3
Muscles, bones, joints:		
Swollen feet, legs.	Infrequent	4
Genital, urinary:		
• Bloody urine.	Rare	3
• Difficult, painful or frequent urination.	Rare	4
Kidneys, allergic, blood:		
	None expected.	
Liver:		
Jaundice (yellow skin and eyes).	Rare	3
Others:		
Fatigue, weakness.	Rare	4

1- Life-threatening. Seek emergency treatment immediately.
2- Discontinue. Seek emergency treatment.
3- Discontinue. Call doctor right away.
4- Continue. Call doctor when convenient.
5- Continue. Tell doctor at next visit.

WARNINGS & PRECAUTIONS

Don't take if:
- You are allergic to aspirin or any non-steroid, antiinflammatory drug.
- You have gastritis, peptic ulcer, enteritis, ileitis, ulcerative colitis, asthma, heart failure, high blood pressure or bleeding problems.
- Patient is younger than 15.

Before you start, consult your doctor:
- If you have epilepsy.
- If you have Parkinson's disease.
- If you have been mentally ill.
- If you have had kidney disease or impaired kidney function.

Over age 60:
Adverse reactions and side effects may be more frequent and severe than in younger persons.

Pregnancy:
Studies inconclusive on harm to unborn child. Decide with your doctor whether drug benefits justify risk to unborn child.

Breast-feeding:
May harm child. Avoid.

Infants & children:
Not recommended for anyone younger than 15. Use only under medical supervision.

Prolonged use:
- Eye damage.
- Reduced hearing.
- Sore throat, fever.
- Weight gain.

Skin & sunlight:
No problems expected.

Driving, piloting or hazardous work:
Don't drive or pilot aircraft until you learn how medicine affects you. Don't work around dangerous machinery. Don't climb ladders or work in high places. Danger increases if you drink alcohol or take medicine affecting alertness and reflexes, such as antihistamines, tranquilizers, sedatives, pain medicine, narcotics and mind-altering drugs.

Airplane passengers:
No problems expected.

Discontinuing:
Don't discontinue without consulting doctor. Dose may require gradual reduction if you have taken drug for a long time. Doses of other drugs may also require adjustment.

Others:
No problems expected.

INTERACTION WITH OTHER DRUGS

GENERIC NAME OR DRUG CLASS	COMBINED EFFECT
Anticoagulants (oral)	Increased risk of bleeding.
Aspirin	Increased risk of stomach ulcer.
Cortisone drugs	Increased risk of stomach ulcer.
Furosemide	Decreased diuretic effect of furosemide.
Lithium	Increased lithium effect.
Oxyphenbutazone	Possible stomach ulcer.
Phenylbutazone	Possible stomach ulcer.
Probenecid	Increased indomethacin effect.
Thyroid hormones	Rapid heartbeat, blood-pressure rise.

INTERACTION WITH OTHER SUBSTANCES

INTERACTS WITH	COMBINED EFFECT
Alcohol:	Possible stomach ulcer or bleeding.
Beverages:	None expected.
Cocaine:	None expected.
Foods:	None expected.
Marijuana:	Increased pain relief from indomethacin.
Tobacco:	None expected.

INSULIN

BRAND NAMES

Actrapid	Lente Insulin	PZI
Globin Insulin	Mixtard	Protamine Zinc
Insulatard	Monotard	& Iletin II
Lentard	NPH	Regular Iletin II
Lente Iletin II	NPH Iletin II	Regular Insulin

See complete brand names list, page 827.

USES

Controls diabetes, a complex metabolic disorder, in which the body does not manufacture insulin.

DOSAGE & USAGE INFORMATION

How to take:
Must be taken by injection under the skin. Use disposable, sterile needles. Rotate injection sites.

When to take:
At the same time each day.

If you forget a dose:
Take as soon as you remember. Wait at least 4 hours for next dose. Resume regular schedule.

What drug does:
Facilitates passage of blood sugar through cell membranes so sugar is usable.

Time lapse before drug works:
30 minutes to 8 hours, depending on type of insulin used.

Don't take with:
See Interaction column and consult doctor.

OVERDOSE

Symptoms:
Low blood sugar (hypoglycemia) — Anxiety; chills, cold sweats, pale skin; drowsiness; excess hunger; headache; nausea; nervousness; fast heartbeat; shakiness; unusual tiredness or weakness.

What to do:
- Eat some type of sugar immediately, such as orange juice, honey, sugar cubes, crackers, sandwich.
- If patient loses consciousness, give glucagon if you have it and know how to use it.
- Otherwise, dial 0 (operator) or 911 (emergency) for an ambulance or medical help. Then give first aid immediately.
- Additional emergency information on page 886.

GENERAL INFORMATION

Habit forming? No
Prescription needed? No
Available as generic? Yes
Drug class: Antidiabetic

POSSIBLE ADVERSE REACTIONS OR SIDE EFFECTS

SYMPTOMS	FREQUENCY	WHAT TO DO
Brain & nervous system:	None expected.	
Skin:		
• Swelling, redness, itch at injection site.	Infrequent	4
• Hives	Infrequent	3
Eyes:	None expected.	
Ears, nose, throat:	None expected.	
Digestive:	None expected.	
Heart & lungs:	None expected.	
Blood vessels:	None expected.	
Muscles, bones, joints:	None expected.	
Genital, urinary:	None expected.	
Kidneys:	None expected.	
Liver:	None expected.	
Allergic: Life-threatening anaphylaxis may occur.	Rare	1 See Page 888.
Blood:	None expected.	
Others:	None expected.	

1- Life-threatening. Seek emergency treatment immediately.
2- Discontinue. Seek emergency treatment.
3- Discontinue. Call doctor right away.
4- Continue. Call doctor when convenient.
5- Continue. Tell doctor at next visit.
6- No action necessary.

WARNINGS & PRECAUTIONS

Don't take if:
- Your diagnosis and dose schedule is not established.
- You don't know how to deal with overdose emergencies.

Before you start, consult your doctor:
- If you are allergic to insulin.
- If you take MAO inhibitors.
- If you have liver or kidney disease or low thyroid function.

Over age 60:
Guard against hypoglycemia. Repeated episodes can cause permanent confusion and abnormal behavior.

Pregnancy:
Possible drug benefits outweigh risk to unborn child. Adhere rigidly to diabetes treatment program.

Breast-feeding:
No problems expected.

Infants & children:
Use only under medical supervision.

Prolonged use:
No problems expected.

Skin & sunlight:
No problems expected.

Driving, piloting or hazardous work:
No problems expected after dose is established.

Airplane passengers:
No problems expected.

Discontinuing:
Don't discontinue without doctor's advice until you complete prescribed dose, even though symptoms diminish or disappear.

Others:
- Diet and exercise affect how much insulin you need. Work with your doctor to determine accurate dose.
- Notify your doctor if you skip a dose, overeat, have fever or infection.
- Notify doctor if you develop symptoms of high blood sugar: drowsiness, dry skin, orange fruit-like odor to breath, increased urination, appetite loss, unusual thirst.

INTERACTION WITH OTHER DRUGS

GENERIC NAME OR DRUG CLASS	COMBINED EFFECT
Anticoagulants (oral)	Increased anticoagulant effect.
Anticonvulsants (hydantoin)	Decreased insulin effect.
Antidiabetics (oral)	Increased antibiabetic effect.
Beta-adrenergic blockers	Can mask symptoms of low blood sugar.
Contraceptives (oral)	Decreased insulin effect.
Cortisone drugs	Decreased insulin effect.
Diuretics	Decreased insulin effect.
Furosemide	Decreased insulin effect.
MAO inhibitors	Increased insulin effect.
Oxyphenbutazone	Increased insulin effect.
Phenylbutazone	Increased insulin effect.
Salicylates	Increased insulin effect.
Sulfa drugs	Increased insulin effect.

Additional interactions on page 838.

INTERACTION WITH OTHER SUBSTANCES

INTERACTS WITH	COMBINED EFFECT
Alcohol:	Increased insulin effect. May cause hypoglycemia and brain damage.
Beverages:	None expected.
Cocaine:	May cause brain damage.
Foods:	None expected.
Marijuana:	Possible increase in blood sugar.
Tobacco:	None expected.

IRON-POLYSACCHARIDE

BRAND NAMES

Hytinic
Niferex
Nu-Iron

GENERAL INFORMATION

Habit forming? No
Prescription needed? With folic acid: Yes
Without folic acid: No
Available as generic? Yes
Drug class: Mineral supplement (iron)

USES

Treatment for dietary iron deficiency or iron-deficiency anemia from other causes.

DOSAGE & USAGE INFORMATION

How to take:
Tablet, capsule or liquid—Swallow with liquid or food to lessen stomach irritation. If you can't swallow whole, crumble tablet or open capsule and take with liquid or food. Place medicine far back on tongue to avoid staining teeth.

When to take:
1 hour before or 2 hours after meals.

If you forget a dose:
Take up to 2 hours late. If more than 2 hours, wait for next dose (don't double this).

What drug does:
Stimulates bone-marrow production of hemoglobin (red-blood-cell pigment that carries oxygen to body cells).

Time lapse before drug works:
3 to 7 days. May require 3 weeks for maximum benefit.

Don't take with:
- Multiple vitamin and mineral supplements.
- See Interaction column and consult doctor.

OVERDOSE

Symptoms:
Weakness, collapse; pallor, blue lips, hands and fingernails; weak, rapid heartbeat; shallow breathing; convulsions; coma.

What to do:
- Dial 0 (operator) or 911 (emergency) for an ambulance or medical help. Then give first aid immediately.
- Additional emergency information on page 886.

POSSIBLE ADVERSE REACTIONS OR SIDE EFFECTS

SYMPTOMS	FREQUENCY	WHAT TO DO
Brain & nervous system:		
Drowsiness	Rare	4
Skin, eyes, blood vessels, muscles, bones, joints, kidneys, liver, allergic, blood:	None expected.	
Ears, nose, throat:		
Throat or chest pain on swallowing.	Rare	3
Digestive:		
• Gray or black stool.	Always	6
• Constipation or diarrhea, heartburn, nausea, vomiting.	Infrequent	3
• Pain, cramps, blood in stool.	Rare	3
Heart & lungs:		
Weak, rapid heartbeat.	Rare	1
Genital, urinary:		
Dark urine.	Infrequent	5
Others:		
• Stained teeth with liquid iron.	Common	6
• Fatigue, weakness.	Infrequent	4

1- Life-threatening. Seek emergency treatment immediately.
2- Discontinue. Seek emergency treatment.
3- Discontinue. Call doctor right away.
4- Continue. Call doctor when convenient.
5- Continue. Tell doctor at next visit.
6- No action necessary.

IRON-POLYSACCHARIDE

WARNINGS & PRECAUTIONS

Don't take if:
- You are allergic to any iron supplement.
- You take iron injections.
- Your daily iron intake is high.
- You plan to take this supplement for a long time.
- You have acute hepatitis.
- You have hemosiderosis or hemochromatosis (conditions involving excess iron in body).
- You have hemolytic anemia.

Before you start, consult your doctor:
- If you plan to become pregnant within medication period.
- If you have had stomach surgery.
- If you have had peptic ulcer disease, enteritis or colitis.
- If you have had pancreatitis or hepatitis.

Over age 60:
May cause hemochromatosis (iron storage disease) with bronze skin, liver damage, diabetes, heart problems and impotence.

Pregnancy:
No proven harm to unborn child. Avoid if possible. Take only if your doctor prescribes supplement during last half of pregnancy.

Breast-feeding:
No problems expected. Take only if your doctor confirms you have a dietary deficiency or an iron-deficiency anemia.

Infants & children:
Use only under medical supervision. Overdose common and dangerous. Keep out of children's reach.

Prolonged use:
May cause hemochromatosis (iron storage disease) with bronze skin, liver damage, diabetes, heart problems and impotence.

Skin & sunlight:
No problems expected.

Driving, piloting or hazardous work:
No problems expected.

Airplane passengers:
No problems expected.

Discontinuing:
May be unnecessary to finish medicine. Follow doctor's instructions.

Others:
Liquid form stains teeth. Mix with water or juice to lessen the effect. Brush with baking soda or hydrogen peroxide to help remove stain.

INTERACTION WITH OTHER DRUGS

GENERIC NAME OR DRUG CLASS	COMBINED EFFECT
Allopurinol	Possible excess iron storage in liver.
Antacids	Poor iron absorption.
Chloramphenicol	Decreased effect of iron. Interferes with red-blood-cell and hemoglobin formation.
Cholestyramine	Decreased iron effect.
Iron supplements (other)	Possible excess iron storage in liver.
Penicillamine	Decreased penicillamine effect.
Sulfasalazine	Decreased iron effect.
Tetracyclines	Decreased tetracycline effect. Take iron 3 hours before or 2 hours after taking tetracycline.
Vitamin C	Increased iron effect. Contributes to red-blood-cell and hemoglobin formation.
Vitamin E	Decreased iron effect.

INTERACTION WITH OTHER SUBSTANCES

INTERACTS WITH	COMBINED EFFECT
Alcohol:	Increased iron absorption. May cause organ damage. Avoid or use in moderation.
Beverages: Milk, tea	Decreased iron effect.
Cocaine:	None expected.
Foods: Dairy foods, eggs, whole-grain bread and cereal.	Decreased iron effect.
Marijuana:	None expected.
Tobacco:	None expected.

ISOCARBOXAZID

BRAND NAMES

Marplan

Habit forming? No
Prescription needed? Yes
Available as generic? No

GENERAL INFORMATION

Drug class: MAO inhibitor
(monamine oxidase inhibitor),
antidepressant

USES

Treatment for depression.

DOSAGE & USAGE INFORMATION

How to take:
Tablet—Swallow with liquid. If you can't swallow whole, crumble tablet and take with liquid or food.

When to take:
At the same times each day.

If you forget a dose:
Take as soon as you remember up to 2 hours late. If more than 2 hours, wait for next scheduled dose (don't double this dose).

What drug does:
Inhibits nerve transmissions in brain that may cause depression.

Time lapse before drug works:
4 to 6 weeks for maximum effect.

Don't take with:
- Non-prescription diet pills, nose drops, medicine for asthma, cough, cold or allergy, or medicine containing caffeine or alcohol.
- See Interaction column and consult doctor.

OVERDOSE

Symptoms:
Restlessness, agitation, fever, convulsions, coma.

What to do:
- Dial 0 (operator) or 911 (emergency) for an ambulance or medical help. Then give first aid immediately.
- Additional emergency information on page 886.

POSSIBLE ADVERSE REACTIONS OR SIDE EFFECTS

SYMPTOMS	FREQUENCY	WHAT TO DO
Brain & nervous system:		
• Fainting	Infrequent	2
• Severe headache.	Infrequent	3
• Dizziness when changing position.	Common	5
• Hallucinations, insomnia, nightmares.	Infrequent	4
Skin:		
Rash	Rare	3
Eyes, blood vessels, kidneys, allergic, blood:	None expected.	
Ears, nose, throat:		
Dry mouth.	Common	5
Digestive:		
• Diarrhea	Infrequent	4
• Constipation	Common	5
• Nausea, vomiting.	Rare	3
Heart & lungs:		
• Rapid or pounding heartbeat.	Infrequent	4
• Chest pain.	Infrequent	3
Muscles, bones, joints:		
Stiff neck.	Rare	3
Genital, urinary:		
Difficult urination.	Common	5
Liver:		
Jaundice (yellow skin and eyes).	Rare	3
Others:		
• Swollen feet, legs.	Infrequent	4
• Fever	Rare	3
• Lower sex drive.	Infrequent	5
• Fatigue, weakness.	Common	4

1 - Life-threatening. Seek emergency treatment immediately.
2 - Discontinue. Seek emergency treatment.
3 - Discontinue. Call doctor right away.
4 - Continue. Call doctor when convenient.
5 - Continue. Tell doctor at next visit.

WARNINGS & PRECAUTIONS

Don't take if:
- You are allergic to any MAO inhibitor.
- You have heart disease, congestive heart failure, heart-rhythm irregularities or high blood pressure.
- You have liver or kidney disease.

Before you start, consult your doctor:
- If you are alcoholic.
- If you have asthma.
- If you have had a stroke.
- If you have diabetes or epilepsy.
- If you have overactive thyroid.
- If you have schizophrenia.
- If you have Parkinson's disease.
- If you have adrenal-gland tumor.
- If you will have surgery within 2 months, including dental surgery, requiring general or spinal anesthesia.

Over age 60:
Not recommended.

Pregnancy:
No proven harm to unborn child. Avoid if possible.

Breast-feeding:
Safety not established. Consult doctor.

Infants & children:
Not recommended.

Prolonged use:
May be toxic to liver.

Skin & sunlight:
May cause rash or intensify sunburn in areas exposed to sun or sunlamp.

Driving, piloting or hazardous work:
Don't drive or pilot aircraft until you learn how medicine affects you. Don't work around dangerous machinery. Don't climb ladders or work in high places. Danger increases if you drink alcohol or take medicine affecting alertness and reflexes.

Airplane passengers:
No problems expected.

Discontinuing:
- Don't discontinue without doctor's advice until you complete prescribed dose, even though symptoms diminish or disappear.
- Follow precautions regarding foods, drinks and other medicines for 2 weeks after discontinuing.

Others:
- May affect blood-sugar levels in patients with diabetes.
- Fever may indicate that MAO inhibitor dose requires adjustment.

INTERACTION WITH OTHER DRUGS

GENERIC NAME OR DRUG CLASS	COMBINED EFFECT
Amphetamines	Blood-pressure rise to life-threatening level.
Anticonvulsants	Changed seizure pattern.
Antidepressants (tricyclic)	Blood-pressure rise to life-threatening level.
Antidiabetics (oral and insulin)	Excessively low blood sugar.
Antihypertensives	Excessively low blood pressure.
Caffeine	Irregular heartbeat or high blood pressure.
Carbamazepine	Fever, seizures. Avoid.
Cyclobenzaprine	Fever, seizures. Avoid.
Diuretics	Excessively low blood pressure.
Guanethidine	Blood-pressure rise to life-threatening level.
Levodopa	Sudden, severe blood-pressure rise.
MAO inhibitors (other)	High fever, convulsions, death.

Additional interactions on page 838.

INTERACTION WITH OTHER SUBSTANCES

INTERACTS WITH	COMBINED EFFECT
Alcohol:	Increased sedation to dangerous level.
Beverages: Caffeine drinks	Irregular heartbeat or high blood pressure.
Drinks containing tyramine (see page 851).	Blood-pressure rise to life-threatening level.
Cocaine:	Overstimulation. Possibly fatal.
Foods: Foods containing tyramine (see page 851).	Blood-pressure rise to life-threatening level.
Marijuana:	Overstimulation. Avoid.
Tobacco:	No proven problems.

ISOETHARINE

BRAND NAMES

Bronkometer (M)
Bronkosol (M)
Dilabron

GENERAL INFORMATION

Habit forming? No
Prescription needed? Yes
Available as generic? No
Drug class: Sympathomimetic (bronchodilator)

 USES

Eases breathing difficulty from bronchial asthma attacks, bronchitis and emphysema.

 DOSAGE & USAGE INFORMATION

How to take:
Aerosol—Use only as directed on label. Don't inhale medicine more than twice per dose unless otherwise directed by doctor.

When to take:
As needed, no more often than every 3 hours.

If you forget a dose:
Take as soon as you remember if you need it. Never double dose.

What drug does:
Dilates constricted bronchial tubes so air can pass.

Time lapse before drug works:
1 to 2 minutes.

Don't take with:
- Non-prescription drugs containing caffeine without consulting doctor.
- See Interaction column and consult doctor.

 OVERDOSE

Symptoms:
Nervousness, anxiety, dizziness, palpitations, tremor, rapid heartbeat, spasm of bronchial tubes, cardiac arrest.

What to do:
- Dial 0 (operator) or 911 (emergency) for an ambulance or medical help. Then give first aid immediately.
- If patient is unconscious and not breathing, give mouth-to-mouth breathing. If there is no heartbeat, use cardiac massage and mouth-to-mouth breathing (CPR). Don't try to make patient vomit. If you can't get help quickly, take patient to nearest emergency facility.
- Additional emergency information on page 886.

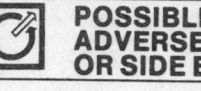 **POSSIBLE ADVERSE REACTIONS OR SIDE EFFECTS**

SYMPTOMS	FREQUENCY	WHAT TO DO
Brain & nervous system: Dizziness, agitation, headache, insomnia.	Common	4
Skin:	None expected.	
Eyes:	None expected.	
Ears, nose, throat:	None expected.	
Digestive: Nausea	Common	4
Heart & lungs:		
● Fast or pounding heartbeat.	Common	4
● Constriction of bronchial tubes, particularly after overuse.	Infrequent	3
Blood vessels:	None expected.	
Muscles, bones, joints:	None expected.	
Genital, urinary:	None expected.	
Kidneys:	None expected.	
Liver:	None expected.	
Allergic:	None expected.	
Blood:	None expected.	
Others: Weakness	Infrequent	4

1 - Life-threatening. Seek emergency treatment immediately.
2 - Discontinue. Seek emergency treatment.
3 - Discontinue. Call doctor right away.
4 - Continue. Call doctor when convenient.
5 - Continue. Tell doctor at next visit.
6 - No action necessary.

ISOETHARINE

WARNINGS & PRECAUTIONS

Don't take if:
- You are allergic to any sympathomimetic drug.
- You have a heart-rhythm disorder.
- You have taken MAO inhibitors in past 2 weeks.

Before you start, consult your doctor:
- If you use epinephrine for asthma.
- If you have diabetes.
- If you have an overactive thyroid gland.
- If you take a digitalis preparation, have high blood pressure or heart disease.

Over age 60:
- If you have hardening of the arteries, use with caution.
- If you have enlarged prostate gland, drug may increase urination difficulty.
- If you have Parkinson's disease, drug may temporarily increase rigidity and tremor in extremities.

Pregnancy:
No proven harm to unborn child. Avoid if possible.

Breast-feeding:
No problems expected, but consult doctor.

Infants & children:
Don't give to infants younger than 2. For older children, use only under medical supervision.

Prolonged use:
No problems expected.

Skin & sunlight:
No problems expected.

Driving, piloting or hazardous work:
No problems expected. Use caution if you feel nervous or dizzy.

Airplane passengers:
No problems expected.

Discontinuing:
Discontinue if drug fails to provide relief. Don't increase dose or frequency.

Others:
May increase blood- and urine-sugar levels, particularly in diabetics.

INTERACTION WITH OTHER DRUGS

GENERIC NAME OR DRUG CLASS	COMBINED EFFECT
Beta-adrenergic blockers	Decreased isoetharine effect.
Ephedrine	Increased ephedrine effect. Excessive heart stimulation.
Epinephrine	Excessive heart stimulation.
Isoproterenol	Excessive heart stimulation.
MAO inhibitors	Dangerous mixture. Avoid.

INTERACTION WITH OTHER SUBSTANCES

INTERACTS WITH	COMBINED EFFECT
Alcohol:	None expected.
Beverages: Caffeine drinks	May cause irregular or fast heartbeat.
Cocaine:	Excessive stimulation. Avoid.
Foods: Chocolates	May cause irregular or fast heartbeat.
Marijuana:	Improves drug's antiasthmatic effect.
Tobacco:	None expected.

ISONIAZID

BRAND NAMES

INH
Laniazid C.P.
Nydrazid

GENERAL INFORMATION

Habit forming? No
Prescription needed? Yes
Available as generic? Yes
Drug class: Antitubercular (antimicrobial)

 USES

Kills tuberculosis germs.

 DOSAGE & USAGE INFORMATION

How to take:
- Tablet or capsule—Swallow with liquid to lessen stomach irritation.
- Syrup—Follow label directions.

When to take:
At the same time each day.

If you forget a dose:
Take as soon as you remember up to 12 hours late. If more than 12 hours, wait for next scheduled dose (don't double this dose).

What drug does:
Interferes with TB germ metabolism. Eventually destroys the germ.

Time lapse before drug works:
3 to 6 months. You may need to take drug as long as 2 years.

Don't take with:
See Interaction column and consult doctor.

 OVERDOSE

Symptoms:
Difficult breathing, convulsions, coma.

What to do:
- Dial 0 (operator) or 911 (emergency) for an ambulance or medical help. Then give first aid immediately.
- If patient is unconscious and not breathing, give mouth-to-mouth breathing. If there is no heartbeat, use cardiac massage and mouth-to-mouth breathing (CPR). Don't try to make patient vomit. If you can't get help quickly, take patient to nearest emergency facility.
- Additional emergency information on page 886.

POSSIBLE ADVERSE REACTIONS OR SIDE EFFECTS

SYMPTOMS	FREQUENCY	WHAT TO DO
Brain & nervous system:		
• Confusion, unsteady walk.	Common	4
• Dizziness	Infrequent	4
Skin:		
Rash, fever.	Rare	3
Eyes:		
Impaired vision.	Rare	3
Ears, nose, throat:		
Swollen glands.	Infrequent	3
Digestive:		
Nausea, indigestion, vomiting, appetite loss.	Infrequent	3
Heart & lungs, blood vessels, genital, urinary, kidneys, allergic:	None expected.	
Muscles, bones, joints:		
Pain in muscles and joints, tingling or numbness in extremities.	Common	3
Liver:		
Jaundice (yellow skin and eyes).	Common	3
Blood:		
• Anemia with fatigue, weakness, fever, sore throat, unusual bruising or bleeding.	Rare	3
• Increase in blood sugar.	Infrequent	4
Others:		
Breast enlargement or discomfort.	Rare	5

1-Life-threatening. Seek emergency treatment immediately.
2-Discontinue. Seek emergency treatment.
3-Discontinue. Call doctor right away.
4-Continue. Call doctor when convenient.
5-Continue. Tell doctor at next visit.

WARNINGS & PRECAUTIONS

Don't take if:
You are allergic to isoniazid.

Before you start, consult your doctor:
- If you plan to become pregnant within medication period.
- If you are allergic to athionamide, pyrazinamide or nicotinic acid.
- If you drink alcohol.
- If you have liver or kidney disease.
- If you have epilepsy, diabetes or lupus.

Over age 60:
Adverse reactions and side effects, especially jaundice, may be more frequent and severe than in younger persons. Kidneys may be less efficient.

Pregnancy:
No proven harm to unborn child. Avoid if possible, especially in the first 6 months of pregnancy. Consult doctor about use in last 3 months.

Breast-feeding:
Drug passes into milk. Avoid drug or discontinue nursing until you finish medicine. Consult doctor for advice on maintaining milk supply.

Infants & children:
Use only under medical supervision.

Prolonged use:
Numbness and tingling of hands and feet.

Skin & sunlight:
No problems expected.

Driving, piloting or hazardous work:
Avoid if you feel dizzy. Otherwise, no problems expected.

Airplane passengers:
Avoid if you feel dizzy. Otherwise, no problems expected.

Discontinuing:
Don't discontinue without doctor's advice until you complete prescribed dose, even though symptoms diminish or disappear.

Others:
- Diabetic patients may have false blood-sugar tests.
- Periodic liver-function tests and laboratory blood studies recommended.
- Prescription for vitamin B-6 (pyridoxine) recommended to prevent nerve damage.

INTERACTION WITH OTHER DRUGS

GENERIC NAME OR DRUG CLASS	COMBINED EFFECT
Antacids	Decreased absorption of isoniazid.
Anticholinergics	May increase pressure within eyeball.
Anticoagulants	Increased anticoagulant effect.
Antidiabetics	Increased antidiabetic effect.
Antihypertensives	Increased antihypertensive effect.
Disulfiram	Increased effect of disulfiram.
Laxatives	Decreased absorption and effect of isoniazid.
Narcotics	Increased narcotic effect.
Phenytoin	Increased phenytoin effect.
Pyridoxine (Vitamin B-6)	Decreased chance of nerve damage in extremities.
Rifampin	Increased isoniazid toxicity to liver.
Sedatives	Increased sedative effect.
Stimulants	Increased stimulant effect.

INTERACTION WITH OTHER SUBSTANCES

INTERACTS WITH	COMBINED EFFECT
Alcohol:	Decreased isoniazid effect. Avoid.
Beverages:	None expected.
Cocaine:	None expected.
Foods:	Decreased absorption of isoniazid.
Marijuana:	No interactions expected, but marijuana may slow body's recovery.
Tobacco:	No interactions expected, but tobacco may slow body's recovery.

ISOPROPAMIDE

BRAND NAMES

Allernade
Capade
Combid (M)
Darbid
Ornade (M)

GENERAL INFORMATION

Habit forming? No
Prescription needed? Low strength: No
High strength: Yes
Available as generic? Yes
Drug class: Antispasmodic, anticholinergic

USES

Reduces spasms of digestive system, bladder and urethra.

DOSAGE & USAGE INFORMATION

How to take:
- Tablet or capsule—Swallow with liquid or food to lessen stomach irritation.
- Extended-release tablets or capsules—Swallow each dose whole. If you take regular tablets, you may chew or crush them.

When to take:
30 minutes before meals (unless directed otherwise by doctor).

If you forget a dose:
Take as soon as you remember up to 2 hours late. If more than 2 hours, wait for next scheduled dose (don't double this dose).

What drug does:
Blocks nerve impulses at parasympathetic nerve endings, preventing muscle contractions and gland secretions of organs involved.

Time lapse before drug works:
15 to 30 minutes.

Don't take with:
See Interaction column and consult doctor.

OVERDOSE

Symptoms:
Dilated pupils; rapid pulse and breathing; dizziness; fever; hallucinations; confusion; slurred speech; agitation; flushed face; convulsions; coma.

What to do:
- Dial 0 (operator) or 911 (emergency) for an ambulance or medical help. Then give first aid immediately.
- Additional emergency information on page 886.

POSSIBLE ADVERSE REACTIONS OR SIDE EFFECTS

SYMPTOMS	FREQUENCY	WHAT TO DO
Brain & nervous system:		
• Headache	Infrequent	4
• Confusion, delirium.	Common	3
Skin:		
Rash or hives.	Rare	3
Eyes:		
Pain, blurred vision.	Rare	3
Ears, nose, throat:		
Dryness	Common	6
Digestive:		
• Constipation	Common	5
• Nausea, vomiting.	Common	4
Heart & lungs:		
Rapid heartbeat.	Common	3
Blood vessels:	None expected.	
Muscles, bones, joints:	None expected.	
Genital, urinary:		
Difficult urination.	Infrequent	4
Kidneys:	None expected.	
Liver:	None expected.	
Allergic:	None expected.	
Blood:	None expected.	
Others:		
Less perspiration.	Common	4

1- Life-threatening. Seek emergency treatment immediately.
2- Discontinue. Seek emergency treatment.
3- Discontinue. Call doctor right away.
4- Continue. Call doctor when convenient.
5- Continue. Tell doctor at next visit.
6- No action necessary.

ISOPROPAMIDE

WARNINGS & PRECAUTIONS

Don't take if:
- You are allergic to any anticholinergic.
- You have trouble with stomach bloating.
- You have difficulty emptying your bladder completely.
- You have narrow-angle glaucoma.
- You have severe ulcerative colitis.

Before you start, consult your doctor:
- If you have open-angle glaucoma.
- If you have angina.
- If you have chronic bronchitis or asthma.
- If you have hiatal hernia.
- If you have liver disease.
- If you have enlarged prostate.
- If you have myasthenia gravis.
- If you have peptic ulcer.
- If you will have surgery within 2 months, including dental surgery, requiring general or spinal anesthesia.

Over age 60:
Adverse reactions and side effects may be more frequent and severe than in younger persons.

Pregnancy:
Studies inconclusive on harm to unborn child. Animal studies show fetal abnormalities. Decide with your doctor whether drug benefits justify risk to unborn child.

Breast-feeding:
Drug passes into milk and decreases milk flow. Avoid drug or discontinue nursing until you finish medicine. Consult doctor for advice on maintaining milk supply.

Infants & children:
Use only under medical supervision.

Prolonged use:
Chronic constipation, possible fecal impaction. Consult doctor immediately.

Skin & sunlight:
No problems expected.

Driving, piloting or hazardous work:
Use disqualifies you for piloting aircraft. Otherwise, no problems expected.

Airplane passengers:
No problems expected.

Discontinuing:
May be unnecessary to finish medicine. Follow doctor's instructions.

Others:
No problems expected.

INTERACTION WITH OTHER DRUGS

GENERIC NAME OR DRUG CLASS	COMBINED EFFECT
Amantadine	Increased isopropamide effect.
Anticholinergics (other)	Increased isopropamide effect
Antidepressants (tricyclic)	Increased isopropamide effect.
Antihistamines	Increased isopropamide effect.
Cortisone drugs	Increased internal-eye pressure.
Haloperidol	Increased internal-eye pressure.
MAO inhibitors	Increased isopropamide effect.
Meperidine	Increased isopropamide effect
Methylphenidate	Increased isopropamide effect.
Orphenadrine	Increased isopropamide effect.
Phenothiazines	Increased isopropamide effect.
Pilocarpine	Loss of pilocarpine effect in glaucoma treatment.
Vitamin C	Decreased isopropamide effect. Avoid large doses of vitamin C.

INTERACTION WITH OTHER SUBSTANCES

INTERACTS WITH	COMBINED EFFECT
Alcohol:	None expected.
Beverages:	None expected.
Cocaine:	Excessively rapid heartbeat. Avoid.
Foods:	None expected.
Marijuana:	Drowsiness and dry mouth.
Tobacco:	None expected.

ISOPROTERENOL

BRAND NAMES

Aerolone
Brondilate (M)
Duo-Medihaler (M)
Iprenol
Isuprel

Medihaler-Iso
Norisodrine Aerotrol
Proternol
Vapo-Iso

GENERAL INFORMATION

Habit forming? No
Prescription needed? Yes
Available as generic? No
Drug class: Sympathomimetic, bronchodilator

 ## USES

Treatment for breathing difficulty from acute asthma, bronchitis and emphysema.

 ## DOSAGE & USAGE INFORMATION

How to take:
- Tablet—Swallow with liquid or food to lessen stomach irritation.
- Extended-release tablets—Swallow each dose whole.
- Sublingual tablets—Dissolve under tongue.
- Aerosol inhaler—Don't inhale more than twice per dose.

When to take:
As needed, no more often than every 4 hours.

If you forget a dose:
Take as soon as you remember. Wait 4 hours for next dose.

What drug does:
- Dilates constricted bronchial tubes, improving air flow.
- Stimulates heart muscle and dilates blood vessels.

Time lapse before drug works:
2 to 4 minutes.

Don't take with:
See Interaction column and consult doctor.

 ## OVERDOSE

Symptoms:
Nervousness, rapid or irregular heartbeat, fainting, sweating, headache, tremor, vomiting, chest pain, blood-pressure drop.

What to do:
- Dial 0 (operator) or 911 (emergency) for an ambulance or medical help. Then give first aid immediately.
- Additional emergency information on page 886.

POSSIBLE ADVERSE REACTIONS OR SIDE EFFECTS

SYMPTOMS	FREQUENCY	WHAT TO DO
Brain & nervous system:		
• Nervousness, insomnia.	Common	4
• Dizziness, headache, trembling, weakness.	Infrequent	4
Skin: Flushed face.	Infrequent	4
Eyes:	None expected.	
Ears, nose, throat: Dry mouth, throat.	Common	5
Digestive: Nausea, vomiting.	Infrequent	4
Heart & lungs: Chest pain; irregular, fast or pounding heartbeat.	Infrequent	3
Blood vessels:	None expected.	
Muscles, bones, joints:	None expected.	
Genital, urinary:	None expected.	
Kidneys:	None expected.	
Liver:	None expected.	
Allergic:	None expected.	
Blood:	None expected.	
Others: Unusual sweating.	Infrequent	3

1 - Life-threatening. Seek emergency treatment immediately.
2 - Discontinue. Seek emergency treatment.
3 - Discontinue. Call doctor right away.
4 - Continue. Call doctor when convenient.
5 - Continue. Tell doctor at next visit.
6 - No action necessary.

WARNINGS & PRECAUTIONS

Don't take if:
- You are allergic to any sympathomimetic, including some diet pills.
- You have serious heart-rhythm disorder.
- You have taken MAO inhibitors in past 2 weeks.

Before you start, consult your doctor:
- If you are sensitive to sympathomimetics.
- If you use epinephrine.
- If you have high blood pressure, heart disease, or take a digitalis preparation.
- If you have diabetes.
- If you have overactive thyroid.
- If your heartbeat is faster than 100 beats per minute.

Over age 60:
You may be more sensitive to drug's stimulant effects. Use with caution if you have hardening of the arteries.

Pregnancy:
Studies inconclusive on harm to unborn child. Animal studies show fetal abnormalities. Decide with your doctor whether drug benefits justify risk to unborn child.

Breast-feeding:
Drug does not appear in milk. Consult doctor.

Infants & children:
Not recommended.

Prolonged use:
- Salivary glands may swell.
- Mouth ulcers (sublingual tablets).

Skin & sunlight:
No problems expected.

Driving, piloting or hazardous work:
Use caution if you feel dizzy or nervous.

Airplane passengers:
No problems expected.

Discontinuing:
Discontinue if drug fails to provide relief after 2 or 3 days. Consult doctor.

Others:
No problems expected.

INTERACTION WITH OTHER DRUGS

GENERIC NAME OR DRUG CLASS	COMBINED EFFECT
Antidepressants (tricyclic)	Increased effect of both drugs.
Beta-adrenergic blockers	Decreased isoproterenol effect.
Ephedrine	Increased ephedrine effect.
Epinephrine	Increased chance of serious heart disturbances.
Sympathomimetics (other)	Increased effect of both drugs, especially harmful side effects.

INTERACTION WITH OTHER SUBSTANCES

INTERACTS WITH	COMBINED EFFECT
Alcohol:	Decreased isoproterenol effect.
Beverages: Caffeine drinks	Overstimulation. Avoid.
Cocaine:	Overstimulation of brain and heart. Avoid.
Foods:	None expected.
Marijuana:	Increased antiasthmatic effect of isoproterenol.
Tobacco:	None expected.

ISOSORBIDE DINITRATE

BRAND NAMES

Coronex
Dilatrate-SR
Iso-Bid
Isogard

Isordil
Isptrate
Onset

Sorate
Sorbide
Sorbitrate

GENERAL INFORMATION

Habit forming? No
Prescription needed? Yes
Available as generic? Yes
Drug class: Antianginal (nitrate)

USES

Reduces frequency and severity of angina attacks.

DOSAGE & USAGE INFORMATION

How to take:
- Sublingual tablet—Dissolve under tongue at earliest sign of angina.
- Chewable tablet—Chew tablet at earliest sign of angina, and hold in mouth for 2 minutes.
- Regular tablet—Swallow with liquid. You may chew or crush it.
- Extended-release tablets or capsules—Swallow each dose whole with liquid.

When to take:
Swallowed tablets—Take at the same times each day, 1 or 2 hours after meals.

If you forget a dose:
Swallowed tablets or capsules—Take as soon as you remember up to 2 hours late. If more than 2 hours, wait for next scheduled dose (don't double this dose).

What drug does:
Relaxes blood vessels, increasing blood flow to heart muscle.

Time lapse before drug works:
- Sublingual or chewable tablets—3 to 5 minutes.
- Swallowed tablets or capsules—30 minutes.

Don't take with:
See Interaction column and consult doctor.

OVERDOSE

Symptoms:
Vomiting, sweating, shortness of breath, loss of consciousness.

What to do:
- Dial 0 (operator) or 911 (emergency) for an ambulance or medical help. Then give first aid immediately.
- Additional emergency information on page 886.

POSSIBLE ADVERSE REACTIONS OR SIDE EFFECTS

SYMPTOMS	FREQUENCY	WHAT TO DO
Brain & nervous system:		
• Headache	Common	5
• Fainting	Infrequent	3
Skin:		
• Rash	Rare	3
• Flushed face and neck.	Common	5
Eyes:	None expected.	
Ears, nose, throat:	None expected.	
Digestive: Nausea, vomiting.	Common	5
Heart & lungs: Rapid heartbeat.	Common	5
Blood vessels:	None expected.	
Muscles, bones, joints:	None expected.	
Genital, urinary:	None expected.	
Kidneys:	None expected.	
Liver:	None expected.	
Allergic:	None expected.	
Blood:	None expected.	
Others:	None expected.	

1- Life-threatening. Seek emergency treatment immediately.
2- Discontinue. Seek emergency treatment.
3- Discontinue. Call doctor right away.
4- Continue. Call doctor when convenient.
5- Continue. Tell doctor at next visit.
6- No action necessary.

WARNINGS & PRECAUTIONS

Don't take if:
You are allergic to nitrates, including nitroglycerin.

Before you start, consult your doctor:
If you have glaucoma.

Over age 60:
Adverse reactions and side effects may be more frequent and severe than in younger persons.

Pregnancy:
No proven harm to unborn child. Avoid if possible.

Breast-feeding:
No proven problems. Consult your doctor.

Infants & children:
Not recommended.

Prolonged use:
Drug may become less effective and require higher doses.

Skin & sunlight:
No problems expected.

Driving, piloting or hazardous work:
Don't drive or pilot aircraft until you learn how medicine affects you. Don't work around dangerous machinery. Don't climb ladders or work in high places. Danger increases if you drink alcohol or take medicine affecting alertness and reflexes, such as antihistamines, tranquilizers, sedatives, pain medicine, narcotics and mind-altering drugs.

Airplane passengers:
No problems expected.

Discontinuing:
Don't discontinue without doctor's advice until you complete prescribed dose, even though symptoms diminish or disappear.

Others:
Periodic laboratory blood studies recommended if you take isosorbide dinitrate.

INTERACTION WITH OTHER DRUGS

GENERIC NAME OR DRUG CLASS	COMBINED EFFECT
Anticholinergics	Increased internal eye pressure.
Antidepressants (tricyclic)	Excessive blood-pressure drop.
Antihypertensives	Excessive blood-pressure drop.
Beta-adrenergic blockers	Excessive blood-pressure drop.
Cholinergics	Decreased cholinergic effect.
Ephedrine	Decreased effect of isosorbide dinitrate.

INTERACTION WITH OTHER SUBSTANCES

INTERACTS WITH	COMBINED EFFECT
Alcohol:	Excessive blood-pressure drop.
Beverages:	None expected.
Cocaine:	Flushed face and headache. Avoid.
Foods:	None expected.
Marijuana:	Decreased effect of isosorbide dinitrate.
Tobacco:	Decreased effect of isosorbide dinitrate.

ISOXSUPRINE

BRAND NAMES

Vasodilan
Vasoprine

GENERAL INFORMATION

Habit forming? No
Prescription needed? Yes
Available as generic? Yes
Drug class: Vasodilator

 USES

Improves poor blood circulation.

 DOSAGE & USAGE INFORMATION

How to take:
Tablet—Swallow with liquid or food to lessen stomach irritation. If you can't swallow whole, crumble tablet and take with liquid or food.

When to take:
At the same times each day.

If you forget a dose:
Take as soon as you remember up to 2 hours late. If more than 2 hours, wait for next scheduled dose (don't double this dose).

What drug does:
Expands blood vessels, increasing flow and permitting distribution of oxygen and nutrients.

Time lapse before drug works:
1 hour.

Don't take with:
See Interaction column and consult doctor.

 OVERDOSE

Symptoms:
Headache, dizziness, flush, vomiting, weakness, sweating, fainting, shortness of breath, coma.

What to do:
- Dial 0 (operator) or 911 (emergency) for an ambulance or medical help. Then give first aid immediately.
- If patient is unconscious and not breathing, give mouth-to-mouth breathing. If there is no heartbeat, use cardiac massage and mouth-to-mouth breathing (CPR). Don't try to make patient vomit. If you can't get help quickly, take patient to nearest emergency facility.
- Additional emergency information on page 886.

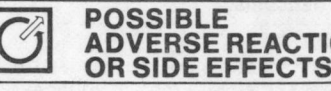 **POSSIBLE ADVERSE REACTIONS OR SIDE EFFECTS**

SYMPTOMS	FREQUENCY	WHAT TO DO
Brain & nervous system: Dizziness, faintness.	Common	4
Skin: Rash	Infrequent	3
Eyes:	None expected.	
Ears, nose, throat:	None expected.	
Digestive: Appetite loss, nausea, vomiting.	Common	3
Heart & lungs: Rapid or irregular heartbeat.	Rare	3
Blood vessels:	None expected.	
Muscles, bones, joints:	None expected.	
Genital, urinary:	None expected.	
Kidneys:	None expected.	
Liver:	None expected.	
Allergic:	None expected.	
Blood:	None expected.	
Others: Weakness, lethargy.	Common	5

1- Life-threatening. Seek emergency treatment immediately.
2- Discontinue. Seek emergency treatment.
3- Discontinue. Call doctor right away.
4- Continue. Call doctor when convenient.
5- Continue. Tell doctor at next visit.
6- No action necessary.

WARNINGS & PRECAUTIONS

Don't take if:
- You are allergic to any vasodilator.
- You have any bleeding disease.

Before you start, consult your doctor:
- If you have high blood pressure, hardening of the arteries or heart disease.
- If you plan to become pregnant within medication period.
- If you have glaucoma.

Over age 60:
Adverse reactions and side effects may be more frequent and severe than in younger persons.

Pregnancy:
Studies inconclusive on harm to unborn child. Decide with your doctor whether drug benefits justify risk to unborn child.

Breast-feeding:
No problems expected, but consult doctor.

Infants & children:
Not recommended.

Prolonged use:
No problems expected.

Skin & sunlight:
No problems expected.

Driving, piloting or hazardous work:
Avoid if you feel dizzy or faint. Otherwise, no problems expected.

Airplane passengers:
No problems expected.

Discontinuing:
Don't discontinue without doctor's advice until you complete prescribed dose, even though symptoms diminish or disappear.

Others:
Be cautious when arising from lying or sitting position, when climbing stairs, or if dizziness occurs.

INTERACTION WITH OTHER DRUGS

GENERIC NAME OR DRUG CLASS	COMBINED EFFECT
None	

INTERACTION WITH OTHER SUBSTANCES

INTERACTS WITH	COMBINED EFFECT
Alcohol:	None expected.
Beverages: Milk	Decreased stomach irritation.
Cocaine:	Decreased blood circulation to extremities. Avoid.
Foods:	None expected.
Marijuana:	Rapid heartbeat.
Tobacco:	Decreased isoxsuprine effect.

LACTULOSE

BRAND NAMES

Cephalac
Chronulac

GENERAL INFORMATION

Habit forming? No
Prescription needed? No
Available as generic? No
Drug class: Laxative (hyperosmotic)

USES

Constipation relief.

DOSAGE & USAGE INFORMATION

How to take:
Liquid—Dilute dose in beverage before swallowing.

When to take:
Usually once a day, preferably in the morning.

If you forget a dose:
Take as soon as you remember up to 8 hours before bedtime. If later, wait for next scheduled dose (don't double this dose). Don't take at bedtime.

What drug does:
Draws water into bowel from other body tissues. Causes distention through fluid accumulation, which promotes soft stool and accelerates bowel motion.

Time lapse before drug works:
30 minutes to 3 hours.

Don't take with:
Another medicine. Space 2 hours apart.

OVERDOSE

Symptoms:
Fluid depletion, weakness, vomiting, fainting.

What to do:
Overdose unlikely to threaten life. If person takes much larger amount than prescribed, call doctor, poison-control center or hospital emergency room for instructions.

POSSIBLE ADVERSE REACTIONS OR SIDE EFFECTS

SYMPTOMS	FREQUENCY	WHAT TO DO
Brain & nervous system: Dizziness, confusion.	Rare	4
Skin:	None expected.	
Eyes:	None expected.	
Ears, nose, throat: Increased thirst.	Infrequent	5
Digestive: Cramps, nausea, diarrhea, gas.	Infrequent	5
Heart & lungs: Irregular heartbeat.	Infrequent	3
Blood vessels:	None expected.	
Muscles, bones, joints:	None expected.	
Genital, urinary:	None expected.	
Kidneys:	None expected.	
Liver:	None expected.	
Allergic:	None expected.	
Blood:	None expected.	
Others: Fatigue, weakness.	Rare	4

1-Life-threatening. Seek emergency treatment immediately.
2-Discontinue. Seek emergency treatment.
3-Discontinue. Call doctor right away.
4-Continue. Call doctor when convenient.
5-Continue. Tell doctor at next visit.
6-No action necessary.

LACTULOSE

WARNINGS & PRECAUTIONS

Don't take if:
- You are allergic to any hyperosmotic laxative.
- You have symptoms of appendicitis, inflamed bowel or intestinal blockage.
- You have missed a bowel movement for only 1 or 2 days.

Before you start, consult your doctor:
- If you have congestive heart disease.
- If you have diabetes.
- If you have high blood pressure.
- If you have a colostomy or ileostomy.
- If you have kidney disease.
- If you have a laxative habit.
- If you have rectal bleeding.
- If you take another laxative.
- If you require a low-galactose diet.

Over age 60:
Adverse reactions and side effects may be more frequent and severe than in younger persons.

Pregnancy:
No proven problems. Avoid if possible.

Breast-feeding:
No problems expected.

Infants & children:
Use only under medical supervision.

Prolonged use:
Don't take for more than 1 week unless under a doctor's supervision. May cause laxative dependence

Skin & sunlight:
No problems expected.

Driving, piloting or hazardous work:
No problems expected.

Airplane passengers:
No problems expected.

Discontinuing:
May be unnecessary to finish medicine. Follow doctor's instructions.

Others:
Don't take to "flush out" your system or as a "tonic."

INTERACTION WITH OTHER DRUGS

GENERIC NAME OR DRUG CLASS	COMBINED EFFECT
None	

INTERACTION WITH OTHER SUBSTANCES

INTERACTS WITH	COMBINED EFFECT
Alcohol:	None expected.
Beverages:	None expected.
Cocaine:	None expected.
Foods:	None expected.
Marijuana:	None expected.
Tobacco:	None expected.

LEVODOPA

BRAND NAMES

Bendopa
Dopar
Larodopa
Levopa

GENERAL INFORMATION

Habit forming? No
Prescription needed? Yes
Available as generic? Yes
Drug class: Antiparkinsonism

USES

Controls Parkinson's disease symptoms such as rigidity, tremor and unsteady gait.

DOSAGE & USAGE INFORMATION

How to take:
Tablet or capsule—Swallow with liquid or food to lessen stomach irritation. If you can't swallow whole, crumble tablet or open capsule and take with liquid or food.

When to take:
At the same times each day.

If you forget a dose:
Take as soon as you remember up to 2 hours late. If more than 2 hours, wait for next scheduled dose (don't double this dose).

What drug does:
Restores chemical balance necessary for normal nerve impulses.

Time lapse before drug works:
2 to 3 weeks to improve; 6 weeks or longer for maximum benefit.

Don't take with:
See Interaction column and consult doctor.

OVERDOSE

Symptoms:
Muscle twitch, spastic eyelid closure, nausea, vomiting, diarrhea, irregular and rapid pulse, weakness, fainting, confusion, agitation, hallucination, coma.

What to do:
- Dial 0 (operator) or 911 (emergency) for an ambulance or medical help. Then give first aid immediately.
- If patient is unconscious and not breathing, give mouth-to-mouth breathing. If there is no heartbeat, use cardiac massage and mouth-to-mouth breathing (CPR). Don't try to make patient vomit. If you can't get help quickly, take patient to nearest emergency facility.
- Additional emergency information on page 886.

POSSIBLE ADVERSE REACTIONS OR SIDE EFFECTS

SYMPTOMS	FREQUENCY	WHAT TO DO
Brain & nervous system:		
• Fainting, severe dizziness, headache, insomnia, nightmares.	Infrequent	3
• Mood changes, uncontrolled body movements.	Common	4
Skin:		
• Flushed face.	Infrequent	4
• Rash, itch.	Infrequent	3
Eyes:		
Blurred vision.	Infrequent	4
Ears, nose, throat:		
Dry mouth.	Common	6
Digestive:		
• Duodenal ulcer.	Rare	4
• Diarrhea	Common	4
• Constipation	Infrequent	5
• Nausea, vomiting.	Infrequent	3
Heart & lungs:		
Irregular heartbeat.	Infrequent	3
Blood vessels:		
High blood pressure.	Rare	3
Muscles, bones, joints:		
Muscle twitching.	Infrequent	4
Genital, urinary:		
• Discolored or dark urine.	Infrequent	4
• Difficult urination.	Infrequent	4
Kidneys, liver, allergic:	None expected.	
Blood:		
Anemia	Rare	4
Others:		
• Tiredness	Infrequent	5
• Body odor.	Common	6

1- Life-threatening. Seek emergency treatment immediately.
2- Discontinue. Seek emergency treatment.
3- Discontinue. Call doctor right away.
4- Continue. Call doctor when convenient.
5- Continue. Tell doctor at next visit.
6- No action necessary.

WARNINGS & PRECAUTIONS

Don't take if:
- You are allergic to levodopa or carbidopa.
- You have taken MAO inhibitors in past 2 weeks.
- You have glaucoma (narrow-angle type).

Before you start, consult your doctor:
- If you have diabetes or epilepsy.
- If you have had high blood pressure, heart or lung disease.
- If you have had liver or kidney disease.
- If you have a peptic ulcer.
- If you have malignant melanoma.
- If you will have surgery within 2 months, including dental surgery, requiring general or spinal anesthesia.

Over age 60:
Adverse reactions and side effects may be more frequent and severe than in younger persons.

Pregnancy:
Risk to unborn child outweighs drug benefits. Don't use.

Breast-feeding:
Drug filters into milk. May harm child. Avoid.

Infants & children:
Not recommended.

Prolonged use:
May lead to uncontrolled movements of head, face, mouth, tongue, arms or legs.

Skin & sunlight:
No problems expected.

Driving, piloting or hazardous work:
Don't drive or pilot aircraft until you learn how medicine affects you. Don't work around dangerous machinery. Don't climb ladders or work in high places. Danger increases if you drink alcohol or take medicine affecting alertness and reflexes, such as antihistamines, tranquilizers, sedatives, pain medicine, narcotics and mind-altering drugs.

Airplane passengers:
No problems expected.

Discontinuing:
Don't discontinue without doctor's advice until you complete prescribed dose, even though symptoms diminish or disappear.

Others:
Expect to start with small dose and increase gradually to lessen frequency and severity of adverse reactions.

INTERACTION WITH OTHER DRUGS

GENERIC NAME OR DRUG CLASS	COMBINED EFFECT
Antiparkinsonism drugs (other)	Increased levodopa effect.
Haloperidol	Decreased levodopa effect.
MAO inhibitors	Dangerous rise in blood pressure.
Methyldopa	Decreased levodopa effect.
Papaverine	Decreased levodopa effect.
Phenothiazines	Decreased levodopa effect.
Pyridoxine (Vitamin B-6)	Decreased levodopa effect.
Rauwolfia alkaloids	Decreased levodopa effect.

INTERACTION WITH OTHER SUBSTANCES

INTERACTS WITH	COMBINED EFFECT
Alcohol:	None expected.
Beverages:	None expected.
Cocaine:	Decreased levodopa effect.
Foods:	None expected.
Marijuana:	Increased fatigue, lethargy, fainting.
Tobacco:	None expected.

LEVORPHANOL

BRAND NAMES

Levo-Dromoran

GENERAL INFORMATION

Habit forming? Yes
Prescription needed? Yes
Available as generic? Yes
Drug class: Narcotic

 ## USES

- Relieves pain.
- Suppresses cough.

 ## DOSAGE & USAGE INFORMATION

How to take:
- Tablet or capsule—Swallow with liquid. If you can't swallow whole, crumble tablet or open capsule and take with liquid or food.
- Drops or liquid—Dilute dose in beverage before swallowing.

When to take:
When needed. No more often than every 4 hours.

If you forget a dose:
Take as soon as you remember. Wait 4 hours for next dose.

What drug does:
- Reduces sensitivity of brain's cough-control center.
- Blocks pain messages to brain and spinal cord.

Time lapse before drug works:
30 minutes.

Don't take with:
See Interaction column and consult doctor.

 ## OVERDOSE

Symptoms:
Deep sleep; slow breathing; slow pulse; flushed, warm skin; constricted pupils.

What to do:
- Dial 0 (operator) or 911 (emergency) for an ambulance or medical help. Then give first aid immediately.
- If patient is unconscious and not breathing, give mouth-to-mouth breathing. If there is no heartbeat, use cardiac massage and mouth-to-mouth breathing (CPR). Don't try to make patient vomit. If you can't get help quickly, take patient to nearest emergency facility.
- Additional emergency information on page 886.

POSSIBLE ADVERSE REACTIONS OR SIDE EFFECTS

SYMPTOMS	FREQUENCY	WHAT TO DO
Brain & nervous system: Depression, confusion, hallucinations.	Infrequent	4
Skin:		
• Hives, rash, itch, face swelling.	Rare	3
• Flushed face.	Common	4
Eyes: Blurred vision.	Rare	4
Ears, nose, throat:	None expected.	
Digestive: Severe constipation, abdominal pain, vomiting.	Infrequent	3
Heart & lungs: Slow heartbeat, irregular breathing.	Rare	3
Blood vessels:	None expected.	
Muscles, bones, joints:	None expected.	
Genital, urinary: Difficult urination.	Common	4
Kidneys: Less urine.	Common	4
Liver:	None expected.	
Allergic:	None expected.	
Blood:	None expected.	
Others: Unusual tiredness.	Common	4

1- Life-threatening. Seek emergency treatment immediately.
2- Discontinue. Seek emergency treatment.
3- Discontinue. Call doctor right away.
4- Continue. Call doctor when convenient.
5- Continue. Tell doctor at next visit.
6- No action necessary.

WARNINGS & PRECAUTIONS

Don't take if:
You are allergic to any narcotic.

Before you start, consult your doctor:
If you have impaired liver or kidney function.

Over age 60:
More likely to be drowsy, dizzy, unsteady or constipated. Avoid prolonged use.

Pregnancy:
Studies inconclusive on harm to unborn child. Animal studies show fetal abnormalities. Decide with your doctor whether drug benefits justify risk to unborn child. Abuse by pregnant woman will result in addicted newborn. Withdrawal can be life-threatening.

Breast-feeding:
Drug filters into milk. May depress infant. Avoid.

Infants & children:
Not recommended.

Prolonged use:
Causes psychological and physical dependence.

Skin & sunlight:
No problems expected.

Driving, piloting or hazardous work:
Don't drive or pilot aircraft until you learn how medicine affects you. Don't work around dangerous machinery. Don't climb ladders or work in high places. Danger increases if you drink alcohol or take medicine affecting alertness and reflexes, such as antihistamines, tranquilizers, sedatives, pain medicine, other narcotics and mind-altering drugs.

Airplane passengers:
No proven problems.

Discontinuing:
May be unnecessary to finish medicine. Follow doctor's instructions.

Others:
No problems expected.

INTERACTION WITH OTHER DRUGS

GENERIC NAME OR DRUG CLASS	COMBINED EFFECT
Analgesics	Increased analgesic effect.
Antidepressants	Increased sedative effect.
Antihistamines	Increased sedative effect.
Mind-altering drugs	Increased sedative effect.
Narcotics (other)	Increased narcotic effect.
Phenothiazines	Increased phenothiazine effect.
Sedatives	Increased sedative effect.
Sleep inducers	Increased sedative effect.
Tranquilizers	Increased sedative effect.

INTERACTION WITH OTHER SUBSTANCES

INTERACTS WITH	COMBINED EFFECT
Alcohol:	Increases alcohol's intoxicating effect. Avoid.
Beverages:	None expected.
Cocaine:	Increased cocaine effect.
Foods:	None expected
Marijuana:	Impaired physical and mental performance.
Tobacco:	None expected.

LINCOMYCIN

BRAND NAMES

Lincocin

GENERAL INFORMATION

Habit forming? No
Prescription needed? Yes
Available as generic? No
Drug class: Antibiotic (lincomycin)

USES

Treatment of bacterial infections that are susceptible to lincomycin.

DOSAGE & USAGE INFORMATION

How to take:
Capsule or liquid—Swallow with liquid 1 hour before or 2 hours after eating.

When to take:
At the same times each day.

If you forget a dose:
Take as soon as you remember up to 2 hours late. If more than 2 hours, wait for next scheduled dose (don't double this dose).

What drug does:
Destroys susceptible bacteria. Does not kill viruses.

Time lapse before drug works:
3 to 5 days.

Don't take with:
See Interaction column and consult doctor.

OVERDOSE

Symptoms:
Severe nausea, vomiting, diarrhea.

What to do:
Overdose unlikely to threaten life. If person takes much larger amount than prescribed, call doctor, poison-control center or hospital emergency room for instructions.

POSSIBLE ADVERSE REACTIONS OR SIDE EFFECTS

SYMPTOMS	FREQUENCY	WHAT TO DO
Brain & nervous system:	None expected.	
Skin: Rash, itch around groin, rectum or armpits.	Infrequent	4
Eyes:	None expected.	
Ears, nose, throat:		
• Unusual thirst.	Infrequent	3
• White patches in mouth.	Infrequent	4
Digestive: Vomiting, stomach cramps, severe and watery diarrhea with blood or mucus.	Infrequent	3
Heart & lungs:	None expected.	
Blood vessels:	None expected.	
Muscles, bones, joints: Painful, swollen joints.	Infrequent	3
Genital, urinary: Vaginal discharge, itching.	Infrequent	4
Kidneys:	None expected.	
Liver: Jaundice (yellow skin and eyes).	Infrequent	3
Allergic:	None expected.	
Blood:	None expected.	
Others:		
• Fever	Infrequent	3
• Tiredness, weakness, weight loss.	Infrequent	3

1-Life-threatening. Seek emergency treatment immediately.
2-Discontinue. Seek emergency treatment.
3-Discontinue. Call doctor right away.
4-Continue. Call doctor when convenient.

WARNINGS & PRECAUTIONS

Don't take if:
- You are allergic to lincomycins.
- You have had ulcerative colitis.
- Prescribed for infant under 1 month old.

Before you start, consult your doctor:
- If you have had yeast infections of mouth, skin or vagina.
- If you will have surgery within 2 months, including dental surgery, requiring general or spinal anesthesia.
- If you have kidney or liver disease.
- If you have allergies of any kind.

Over age 60:
Adverse reactions and side effects may be more frequent and severe than in younger persons.

Pregnancy:
Risk to unborn child outweighs drug benefits. Don't use.

Breast-feeding:
Drug passes into milk. Avoid drug or discontinue nursing until you finish medicine. Consult doctor for advice on maintaining milk supply.

Infants & children:
Don't give to infants younger than 1 month. Use for children only under medical supervision.

Prolonged use:
- Severe colitis with diarrhea and bleeding.
- You may become more susceptible to infections caused by germs not responsive to lincomycin.

Skin & sunlight:
No problems expected.

Driving, piloting or hazardous work:
No problems expected.

Airplane passengers:
No problems expected.

Discontinuing:
Don't discontinue without doctor's advice until you complete prescribed dose, even though symptoms diminish or disappear.

Others:
No problems expected.

INTERACTION WITH OTHER DRUGS

GENERIC NAME OR DRUG CLASS	COMBINED EFFECT
Antidiarrheal preparations	Decreased lincomycin effect.
Chloramphenicol	Decreased lincomycin effect.
Erythromycin	Decreased lincomycin effect.

INTERACTION WITH OTHER SUBSTANCES

INTERACTS WITH	COMBINED EFFECT
Alcohol:	None expected.
Beverages:	None expected.
Cocaine:	None expected.
Foods:	None expected.
Marijuana:	None expected.
Tobacco:	None expected.

LIOTHYRONINE

BRAND NAMES

Cytomel
Ro-Thyronine
Tertroxin

GENERAL INFORMATION

Habit forming? No
Prescription needed? Yes
Available as generic? Yes
Drug class: Thyroid hormone

 USES

Replacement for thyroid hormone deficiency.

 DOSAGE & USAGE INFORMATION

How to take:
- Tablet or capsule—Swallow with liquid.
- Extended-release tablets or capsules—Swallow each dose whole. If you take regular tablets, you may chew or crush them.

When to take:
At the same time each day before a meal or on awakening.

If you forget a dose:
Take as soon as you remember up to 12 hours late. If more than 12 hours, wait for next scheduled dose (don't double this dose).

What drug does:
Increases cell metabolism rate.

Time lapse before drug works:
48 hours.

Don't take with:
See Interaction column and consult doctor.

 OVERDOSE

Symptoms:
"Hot" feeling, heart palpitations, nervousness, sweating, hand tremors, insomnia, rapid and irregular pulse, headache, irritability, diarrhea, weight loss, muscle cramps.

What to do:
Overdose unlikely to threaten life. If person takes much larger amount than prescribed, call doctor, poison-control center or hospital emergency room for instructions.

POSSIBLE ADVERSE REACTIONS OR SIDE EFFECTS

SYMPTOMS	FREQUENCY	WHAT TO DO
Brain & nervous system: Tremor, headache, irritability, insomnia.	Common	3
Skin: Hives, rash.	Infrequent	3
Eyes:	None expected.	
Ears, nose, throat:	None expected.	
Digestive:		
• Appetite change.	Common	4
• Diarrhea	Common	4
• Vomiting	Infrequent	3
Heart & lungs: Chest pain, rapid and irregular heartbeat, shortness of breath.	Infrequent	3
Blood vessels:	None expected.	
Muscles, bones, joints: Leg cramps.	Common	4
Genital, urinary:	None expected.	
Kidneys:	None expected.	
Liver:	None expected.	
Allergic:	None expected.	
Blood:	None expected.	
Others:		
• Change in menstrual periods.	Common	4
• Fever, heat sensitivity, unusual sweating.	Common	4
• Weight loss.	Common	4

1 - Life-threatening. Seek emergency treatment immediately.
2 - Discontinue. Seek emergency treatment.
3 - Discontinue. Call doctor right away.
4 - Continue. Call doctor when convenient.
5 - Continue. Tell doctor at next visit.
6 - No action necessary.

WARNINGS & PRECAUTIONS

Don't take if:
- You have had a heart attack within 6 weeks.
- You have no thyroid deficiency, but use this to lose weight.

Before you start, consult your doctor:
- If you have heart disease or high blood pressure.
- If you have diabetes.
- If you have Addison's disease, have had adrenal gland deficiency or use epinephrine, ephedrine or isoproterenol for asthma.

Over age 60:
More sensitive to thyroid hormone. May need smaller doses.

Pregnancy:
Considered safe if for thyroid deficiency only.

Breast-feeding:
Present in milk. Considered safe if dose is correct.

Infants & children:
Use only under medical supervision.

Prolonged use:
No problems expected, if dose is correct.

Skin & sunlight:
No problems expected.

Driving, piloting or hazardous work:
No problems expected.

Airplane passengers:
No problems expected.

Discontinuing:
Don't discontinue without consulting doctor. Dose may require gradual reduction if you have taken drug for a long time. Doses of other drugs may also require adjustment.

Others:
Digestive upsets, tremors, cramps, nervousness, insomnia or diarrhea may indicate need for dose adjustment.

INTERACTION WITH OTHER DRUGS

GENERIC NAME OR DRUG CLASS	COMBINED EFFECT
Amphetamines	Increased amphetamine effect.
Anticoagulants (oral)	Increased anticoagulant effect.
Antidepressants (tricyclic)	Increased antidepressant effect.
Antidiabetics	Antidiabetic may require adjustment.
Aspirin (large doses, continuous use)	Increased liothyronine effect.
Barbiturates	Decreased barbiturate effect.
Cholestyramine	Decreased liothyronine effect.
Contraceptives (oral)	Decreased liothyronine effect.
Cortisone drugs	Requires dose adjustment to prevent cortisone deficiency.
Digitalis preparations	Increased digitalis effect.
Ephedrine	Increased ephedrine effect.
Epinephrine	Increased epinephrine effect.
Methylphenidate	Increased methylphenidate effect.
Phenytoin	Increased liothyronine effect.

INTERACTION WITH OTHER SUBSTANCES

INTERACTS WITH	COMBINED EFFECT
Alcohol:	None expected.
Beverages:	None expected.
Cocaine:	Excess stimulation. Avoid.
Foods: Soybeans	Heavy consumption interferes with thyroid function.
Marijuana:	None expected.
Tobacco:	None expected.

LIOTRIX

BRAND NAMES

Euthroid
Thyrolar

GENERAL INFORMATION

Habit forming? No
Prescription needed? Yes
Available as generic? Yes
Drug class: Thyroid hormone

USES

Replacement for thyroid hormone deficiency.

DOSAGE & USAGE INFORMATION

How to take:
- Tablet or capsule—Swallow with liquid.
- Extended-release tablets or capsules—Swallow each dose whole. If you take regular tablets, you may chew or crush them.

When to take:
At the same time each day before a meal or on awakening.

If you forget a dose:
Take as soon as you remember up to 12 hours late. If more than 12 hours, wait for next scheduled dose (don't double this dose).

What drug does:
Increases cell metabolism rate.

Time lapse before drug works:
48 hours.

Don't take with:
See Interaction column and consult doctor.

OVERDOSE

Symptoms:
"Hot" feeling, heart palpitations, nervousness, sweating, hand tremors, insomnia, rapid and irregular pulse, headache, irritability, diarrhea, weight loss, muscle cramps.

What to do:
Overdose unlikely to threaten life. If person takes much larger amount than prescribed, call doctor, poison-control center or hospital emergency room for instructions.

POSSIBLE ADVERSE REACTIONS OR SIDE EFFECTS

SYMPTOMS	FREQUENCY	WHAT TO DO
Brain & nervous system: Tremor, headache, irritability, insomnia.	Common	3
Skin: Hives, rash.	Infrequent	3
Eyes:	None expected.	
Ears, nose, throat:	None expected.	
Digestive:		
• Appetite change.	Common	4
• Diarrhea	Common	4
• Vomiting	Infrequent	3
Heart & lungs: Chest pain, rapid and irregular heartbeat, shortness of breath.	Infrequent	3
Blood vessels:	None expected.	
Muscles, bones, joints: Leg cramps.	Common	4
Genital, urinary:	None expected.	
Kidneys:	None expected.	
Liver:	None expected.	
Allergic:	None expected.	
Blood:	None expected.	
Others:		
• Change in menstrual periods.	Common	4
• Fever, heat sensitivity, unusual sweating.	Common	4
• Weight loss.	Common	4

1- Life-threatening. Seek emergency treatment immediately.
2- Discontinue. Seek emergency treatment.
3- Discontinue. Call doctor right away.
4- Continue. Call doctor when convenient.
5- Continue. Tell doctor at next visit.
6- No action necessary.

LIOTRIX

WARNINGS & PRECAUTIONS

Don't take if:
- You have had a heart attack within 6 weeks.
- You have no thyroid deficiency, but use this to lose weight.

Before you start, consult your doctor:
- If you have heart disease or high blood pressure.
- If you have diabetes.
- If you have Addison's disease, have had adrenal gland deficiency or use epinephrine, ephedrine or isoproterenol for asthma.

Over age 60:
More sensitive to thyroid hormone. May need smaller doses.

Pregnancy:
Considered safe if for thyroid deficiency only.

Breast-feeding:
Present in milk. Considered safe if dose is correct.

Infants & children:
Use only under medical supervision.

Prolonged use:
No problems expected, if dose is correct.

Skin & sunlight:
No problems expected.

Driving, piloting or hazardous work:
No problems expected.

Airplane passengers:
No problems expected.

Discontinuing:
Don't discontinue without consulting doctor. Dose may require gradual reduction if you have taken drug for a long time. Doses of other drugs may also require adjustment.

Others:
Digestive upsets, tremors, cramps, nervousness, insomnia or diarrhea may indicate need for dose adjustment.

INTERACTION WITH OTHER DRUGS

GENERIC NAME OR DRUG CLASS	COMBINED EFFECT
Amphetamines	Increased amphetamine effect.
Anticoagulants (oral)	Increased anticoagulant effect.
Antidepressants (tricyclic)	Increased antidepressant effect.
Antidiabetics	Antidiabetic may require adjustment.
Aspirin (large doses, continuous use)	Increased liotrix effect.
Barbiturates	Decreased barbiturate effect.
Cholestyramine	Decreased liotrix effect.
Contraceptives (oral)	Decreased liotrix effect.
Cortisone drugs	Requires dose adjustment to prevent cortisone deficiency.
Digitalis preparations	Increased digitalis effect.
Ephedrine	Increased ephedrine effect.
Epinephrine	Increased epinephrine effect.
Methylphenidate	Increased methylphenidate effect.
Phenytoin	Increased liotrix effect.

INTERACTION WITH OTHER SUBSTANCES

INTERACTS WITH	COMBINED EFFECT
Alcohol:	None expected.
Beverages:	None expected.
Cocaine:	Excess stimulation. Avoid.
Foods: Soybeans	Heavy consumption interferes with thyroid function.
Marijuana:	None expected.
Tobacco:	None expected.

LITHIUM

BRAND NAMES

Carbolith	Lithobid
Eskalith	Lithonate
Lithane	Lithotabs
Lithizine	Pfi-Lithium

GENERAL INFORMATION

Habit forming? No
Prescription needed? Yes
Available as generic? Yes
Drug class: Tranquilizer

 USES

Normalizes mood and behavior in manic-depressive illness.

 DOSAGE & USAGE INFORMATION

How to take:
- Tablet or capsule—Swallow with liquid or food to lessen stomach irritation. If you can't swallow whole, crumble tablet or open capsule and take with liquid or food. Drink 2 or 3 quarts liquid per day.
- Extended-release tablets or capsules—Swallow each dose whole.
- Syrup—Take at mealtime. Follow with 8 oz. water.

When to take:
At the same times each day, preferably mealtime.

If you forget a dose:
Take as soon as you remember up to 2 hours late. If more than 2 hours, wait for next scheduled dose (don't double this dose).

What drug does:
May correct chemical imbalance in brain's transmission of nerve impulses that influence mood and behavior.

Time lapse before drug works:
1 to 3 weeks. May require 3 months before depressive phase of illness improves.

Don't take with:
See Interaction column and consult doctor.

 OVERDOSE

Symptoms:
Moderate overdose increases some side effects. Large overdose may cause convulsions, stupor and coma.

What to do:
- Dial 0 (operator) or 911 (emergency) for an ambulance or medical help. Then give first aid immediately.
- Additional emergency information on page 886.

 POSSIBLE ADVERSE REACTIONS OR SIDE EFFECTS

SYMPTOMS	FREQUENCY	WHAT TO DO
Brain & nervous system:		
• Dizziness	Common	4
• Drowsiness, confusion.	Infrequent	5
Skin:		
Rash	Infrequent	3
Eyes:		
Blurred vision.	Rare	3
Ears, nose, throat:		
Dry mouth, thirst.	Common	5
Digestive:		
• Diarrhea, nausea, vomiting.	Common	4
• Stomach pain.	Infrequent	3
Heart & lungs, blood vessels, kidneys, liver, allergic, blood:	None expected.	
Muscles, bones, joints:		
• Shakiness, tremor.	Common	4
• Weakness	Infrequent	5
• Jerking of arms and legs.	Rare	4
• Swollen hands, feet.	Infrequent	4
Genital, urinary:		
Decreased sexual ability, increased urination.	Common	5
Others:		
• Slurred speech.	Infrequent	4
• Thyroid impairment—coldness; dry, puffy skin; muscle aches; headaches; weight gain; fatigue; menstrual changes.	Infrequent	4

1- Life-threatening. Seek emergency treatment immediately.
2- Discontinue. Seek emergency treatment.
3- Discontinue. Call doctor right away.
4- Continue. Call doctor when convenient.
5- Continue. Tell doctor at next visit.

WARNINGS & PRECAUTIONS

Don't take if:
- You are allergic to lithium.
- You have kidney or heart disease.
- Patient is younger than 12.

Before you start, consult your doctor:
- About all medications you take.
- If you plan to become pregnant within medication period.
- If you have diabetes, low thyroid function, epilepsy or any significant medical problem.
- If you are on a low-salt diet or drink more than 4 cups of coffee per day.
- If you plan surgery within 2 months.

Over age 60:
Adverse reactions and side effects may be more frequent and severe than in younger persons.

Pregnancy:
Risk to unborn child outweighs drug benefits. Don't use.

Breast-feeding:
Drug passes into milk. Avoid drug or discontinue nursing until you finish medicine. Consult doctor for advice on maintaining milk supply.

Infants & children:
Don't give to children younger than 12.

Prolonged use:
Enlarged thyroid with possible impaired function.

Skin & sunlight:
No problems expected.

Driving, piloting or hazardous work:
Don't drive or pilot aircraft until you learn how medicine affects you. Don't work around dangerous machinery. Don't climb ladders or work in high places. Danger increases if you drink alcohol or take medicine affecting alertness and reflexes.

Airplane passengers:
Consult doctor.

Discontinuing:
Don't discontinue without consulting doctor. Dose may require gradual reduction if you have taken drug for a long time. Doses of other drugs may also require adjustment.

Others:
- Regular checkups, periodic blood tests, and tests of lithium levels and thyroid function recommended.
- Avoid exercise in hot weather and other activities that cause heavy sweating. This contributes to lithium poisoning.

INTERACTION WITH OTHER DRUGS

GENERIC NAME OR DRUG CLASS	COMBINED EFFECT
Acetazolamide	Decreased lithium effect.
Aminophylline	Decreased lithium effect.
Diuretics	Increased lithium effect.
Haloperidol	Increased toxicity of both drugs.
Indomethacin	Increased lithium effect.
Methyldopa	Increased lithium effect.
Muscle relaxants (skeletal)	Increased skeletal-muscle relaxation.
Oxyphenbutazone	Increased lithium effect.
Phenothiazines	Decreased lithium effect.
Phentyoin	Increased lithium effect.
Phenylbutazone	Increased lithium effect.
Potassium iodide	Increased potassium iodide effect.
Sodium bicarbonate	Decreased lithium effect.
Tetracyclines	Increased lithium effect.

INTERACTION WITH OTHER SUBSTANCES

INTERACTS WITH	COMBINED EFFECT
Alcohol:	Possible lithium poisoning.
Beverages: Caffeine drinks	Increased lithium effect.
Cocaine:	Possible psychosis.
Foods: Salt	*Don't* restrict intake.
Marijuana:	Increased tremor and possible psychosis.
Tobacco:	None expected.

LORAZEPAM

BRAND NAMES

Ativan

GENERAL INFORMATION

Habit forming? Yes
Prescription needed? Yes
Available as generic? No
Drug class: Tranquilizer (benzodiazepine)

USES

Treatment for nervousness or tension.

DOSAGE & USAGE INFORMATION

How to take:
Tablet or capsule—Swallow with liquid. If you can't swallow whole, crumble tablet or open capsule and take with liquid or food.

When to take:
At the same time each day, according to instructions on prescription label.

If you forget a dose:
Take as soon as you remember up to 2 hours late. If more than 2 hours, wait for next scheduled dose (don't double this dose).

What drug does:
Affects limbic system of brain—part that controls emotions.

Time lapse before drug works:
2 hours. May take 6 weeks for full benefit.

Don't take with:
See Interaction column and consult doctor.

OVERDOSE

Symptoms:
Drowsiness, weakness, tremor, stupor, coma.

What to do:
- Dial 0 (operator) or 911 (emergency) for an ambulance or medical help. Then give first aid immediately.
- If patient is unconscious and not breathing, give mouth-to-mouth breathing. If there is no heartbeat, use cardiac massage and mouth-to-mouth breathing (CPR). Don't try to make patient vomit. If you can't get help quickly, take patient to nearest emergency facility.
- Additional emergency information on page 886.

POSSIBLE ADVERSE REACTIONS OR SIDE EFFECTS

SYMPTOMS	FREQUENCY	WHAT TO DO
Brain & nervous system:		
• Clumsiness, drowsiness, dizziness.	Common	4
• Hallucinations, confusion, depression, irritability.	Infrequent	3
Skin:		
Rash, itch.	Infrequent	3
Eyes:		
Vision changes.	Infrequent	3
Ears, nose, throat:		
Mouth, throat ulcers.	Rare	3
Digestive:		
Constipation or diarrhea, nausea, vomiting.	Infrequent	4
Heart & lungs:		
Slow heartbeat, breathing difficulty.	Rare	2
Blood vessels:	None expected.	
Muscles, bones, joints:	None expected.	
Genital, urinary:		
Urination difficulty.	Infrequent	4
Kidneys:	None expected.	
Liver:		
Jaundice (yellow eyes and skin).	Rare	3
Allergic:	None expected.	
Blood:	None expected.	
Others:	None expected.	

1- Life-threatening. Seek emergency treatment immediately.
2- Discontinue. Seek emergency treatment.
3- Discontinue. Call doctor right away.
4- Continue. Call doctor when convenient.
5- Continue. Tell doctor at next visit.
6- No action necessary.

LORAZEPAM

WARNINGS & PRECAUTIONS

Don't take if:
- You are allergic to any benzodiazepine.
- You have myasthenia gravis.
- You have glaucoma.
- You are active or recovering alcoholic.
- Patient is younger than 6 months.

Before you start, consult your doctor:
- If you have liver, kidney or lung disease.
- If you have diabetes, epilepsy or porphyria.

Over age 60:
Adverse reactions and side effects may be more frequent and severe than in younger persons. You need smaller doses for shorter periods of time. May develop agitation, rage or "hangover effect."

Pregnancy:
Risk to unborn child outweighs drug benefits. Don't use.

Breast-feeding:
Drug passes into milk. Avoid drug or discontinue nursing until you finish medicine. Consult doctor for advice on maintaining milk supply.

Infants & children:
Use only under medical supervision for children older than 6 months.

Prolonged use:
May impair liver function.

Skin & sunlight:
No problems expected.

Driving, piloting or hazardous work:
Don't drive or pilot aircraft until you learn how medicine affects you. Don't work around dangerous machinery. Don't climb ladders or work in high places. Danger increases if you drink alcohol or take medicine affecting alertness and reflexes.

Airplane passengers:
No problems expected.

Discontinuing:
Don't discontinue without consulting doctor. Dose may require gradual reduction if you have taken drug for a long time. Doses of other drugs may also require adjustment.

Others:
- Hot weather, heavy exercise and profuse sweat may reduce excretion and cause overdose.
- Blood sugar may rise in diabetics, requiring insulin adjustment.

INTERACTION WITH OTHER DRUGS

GENERIC NAME OR DRUG CLASS	COMBINED EFFECT
Anticonvulsants	Change in seizure frequency or severity.
Antidepressants	Increased sedative effect of both drugs.
Antihistamines	Increased sedative effect of both drugs.
Antihypertensives	Excessively low blood pressure.
Cimetidine	Excess sedation.
Disulfiram	Increased lorazepam effect.
MAO inhibitors	Convulsions, deep sedation, rage.
Narcotics	Increased sedative effect of both drugs.
Sedatives	Increased sedative effect of both drugs.
Sleep inducers	Increased sedative effect of both drugs.
Tranquilizers	Increased sedative effect of both drugs.

INTERACTION WITH OTHER SUBSTANCES

INTERACTS WITH	COMBINED EFFECT
Alcohol:	Heavy sedation. Avoid.
Beverages:	None expected.
Cocaine:	Decreased lorazepam effect.
Foods:	None expected.
Marijuana:	Heavy sedation. Avoid.
Tobacco:	Decreased lorazepam effect.

MAGNESIUM CARBONATE

BRAND NAMES

Alkets (M)
Di-Gel (M)
Marblen
Silain-Gel (M)

GENERAL INFORMATION

Habit forming? No
Prescription needed? No
Available as generic? Yes
Drug class: Antacid, laxative

 USES

- Treatment for hyperacidity in upper gastrointestinal tract, including stomach and esophagus. Symptoms may be heartburn or acid indigestion. Diseases include peptic ulcer, gastritis, esophagitis, hiatal hernia.
- Constipation relief.

 DOSAGE & USAGE INFORMATION

How to take:
- Tablet or capsule—Swallow with liquid.
- Chewable tablets or wafers—Chew well before swallowing.
- Liquid—Shake well and take undiluted.
- Powder—Mix with water and drink all liquid.

When to take:
1 to 3 hours after meals unless directed otherwise by your doctor.

If you forget a dose:
Take as soon as you remember.

What drug does:
- Neutralizes some of the hydrochloric acid in the stomach.
- Reduces action of pepsin, a digestive enzyme.
- Stimulates muscles in lower bowel wall.

Time lapse before drug works:
15 minutes.

Don't take with:
Other medicines at the same time. Decreases absorption of other drugs.

 OVERDOSE

Symptoms:
Dry mouth, diarrhea, shallow breathing, stupor.

What to do:
- Dial 0 (operator) or 911 (emergency) for an ambulance or medical help. Then give first aid immediately.
- Additional emergency information on page 886.

POSSIBLE ADVERSE REACTIONS OR SIDE EFFECTS

SYMPTOMS	FREQUENCY	WHAT TO DO
Brain & nervous system: Mood changes.	Infrequent	4
Skin:	None expected.	
Eyes:	None expected.	
Ears, nose, throat:	None expected.	
Digestive:		
• Constipation, appetite loss.	Common	4
• Nausea, vomiting.	Infrequent	4
• Lower abdominal pain and swelling.	Infrequent	3
Heart & lungs:	None expected.	
Blood vessels:	None expected.	
Muscles, bones, joints: Bone pain, muscle weakness.	Infrequent	3
Genital, urinary:	None expected.	
Kidneys:	None expected.	
Liver:	None expected.	
Allergic:	None expected.	
Blood:	None expected.	
Others:		
• Swelling of wrists or ankles.	Infrequent	3
• Unusual weakness or tiredness.	Rare	3
• Weight loss.	Infrequent	4

1- Life-threatening. Seek emergency treatment immediately.
2- Discontinue. Seek emergency treatment.
3- Discontinue. Call doctor right away.
4- Continue. Call doctor when convenient.
5- Continue. Tell doctor at next visit.
6- No action necessary.

MAGNESIUM CARBONATE

WARNINGS & PRECAUTIONS

Don't take if:
You are allergic to any antacid.

Before you start, consult your doctor:
• If you have kidney disease.
• If you have chronic constipation, colitis or diarrhea.
• If you have symptoms of appendicitis.
• If you have stomach or intestinal bleeding.

Over age 60:
Adverse reactions and side effects may be more frequent and severe than in younger persons. Diarrhea or constipation particularly likely.

Pregnancy:
Risk to unborn child outweighs drug benefits. Don't use.

Breast-feeding:
Drug passes into milk. Avoid drug or discontinue nursing until you finish medicine. Consult doctor for advice on maintaining milk supply.

Infants & children:
Use only under medical supervision.

Prolonged use:
No problems expected.

Skin & sunlight:
No problems expected.

Driving, piloting or hazardous work:
No problems expected.

Airplane passengers:
No problems expected.

Discontinuing:
May be unnecessary to finish medicine. Follow doctor's instructions.

Others:
Don't take longer than 2 weeks unless under medical supervision.

INTERACTION WITH OTHER DRUGS

GENERIC NAME OR DRUG CLASS	COMBINED EFFECT
Anticoagulants	Decreased anticoagulant effect.
Chlorpromazine	Decreased chlorpromazine effect.
Digitalis preparations	Decreased digitalis effect.
Iron supplements	Decreased iron effect.
Isoniazid	Decreased isoniazid effect.
Levodopa	Increased levodopa effect.
Meperidine	Increased meperidine effect.
Nalidixic acid	Decreased effect of nalidixic acid.
Oxyphenbutazone	Decreased oxyphenbutazone effect.
Para-aminosalicylic acid (PAS)	Decreased PAS effect.
Penicillins	Decreased penicillin effect.
Pentobarbital	Decreased pentobarbital effect.
Phenylbutazone	Decreased phenylbutazone effect.
Pseudoephedrine	Increased pseudoephedrine effect.

Additional interactions on page 838.

INTERACTION WITH OTHER SUBSTANCES

INTERACTS WITH	COMBINED EFFECT
Alcohol:	Decreased antacid effect.
Beverages:	No proven problems.
Cocaine:	No proven problems.
Foods:	Decreased antacid effect if taken with food. Wait 1 hour after eating.
Marijuana:	No proven problems.
Tobacco:	Decreased antacid effect.

MAGNESIUM CITRATE

BRAND NAMES

Citrate of Magnesia
Citroma
Citro-Nesia

GENERAL INFORMATION

Habit forming? No
Prescription needed? No
Available as generic? Yes
Drug class: Laxative (hyperosmotic)

 USES

Constipation relief.

 DOSAGE & USAGE INFORMATION

How to take:
Liquid—Dilute dose in beverage before swallowing.

When to take:
Usually once a day, preferably in the morning.

If you forget a dose:
Take as soon as you remember up to 8 hours before bedtime. If later, wait for next scheduled dose (don't double this dose). Don't take at bedtime.

What drug does:
Draws water into bowel from other body tissues. Causes distention through fluid accumulation, which promotes soft stool and accelerates bowel motion.

Time lapse before drug works:
30 minutes to 3 hours.

Don't take with:
See Interaction column and consult doctor.

 OVERDOSE

Symptoms:
Fluid depletion, weakness, vomiting, fainting.

What to do:
Overdose unlikely to threaten life. If person takes much larger amount than prescribed, call doctor, poison-control center or hospital emergency room for instructions.

 POSSIBLE ADVERSE REACTIONS OR SIDE EFFECTS

SYMPTOMS	FREQUENCY	WHAT TO DO
Brain & nervous system: Dizziness, confusion.	Rare	4
Skin:	None expected.	
Eyes:	None expected.	
Ears, nose, throat: Increased thirst.	Infrequent	5
Digestive: Cramps, nausea, diarrhea, gas.	Infrequent	5
Heart & lungs: Irregular heartbeat.	Infrequent	3
Blood vessels:	None expected.	
Muscles, bones, joints:	None expected.	
Genital, urinary:	None expected.	
Kidneys:	None expected.	
Liver:	None expected.	
Allergic:	None expected.	
Blood:	None expected.	
Others: Tiredness or weakness.	Rare	4

1- Life-threatening. Seek emergency treatment immediately.
2- Discontinue. Seek emergency treatment.
3- Discontinue. Call doctor right away.
4- Continue. Call doctor when convenient.
5- Continue. Tell doctor at next visit.
6- No action necessary.

WARNINGS & PRECAUTIONS

Don't take if:
- You are allergic to any hyperosmotic laxative.
- You have symptoms of appendicitis, inflamed bowel or intestinal blockage.
- You have missed a bowel movement for only 1 or 2 days.

Before you start, consult your doctor:
- If you have congestive heart disease.
- If you have diabetes.
- If you have high blood pressure.
- If you have a colostomy or ileostomy.
- If you have kidney disease.
- If you have a laxative habit.
- If you have rectal bleeding.
- If you take another laxative.

Over age 60:
Adverse reactions and side effects may be more frequent and severe than in younger persons.

Pregnancy:
Salt content may cause fluid retention and swelling. Avoid if possible.

Breast-feeding:
No problems expected.

Infants & children:
Use only under medical supervision.

Prolonged use:
Don't take for more than 1 week unless under a doctor's supervision. May cause laxative dependence.

Skin & sunlight:
No problems expected.

Driving, piloting or hazardous work:
No problems expected.

Airplane passengers:
No problems expected.

Discontinuing:
May be unnecessary to finish medicine. Follow doctor's instructions.

Others:
- Don't take to "flush out" your system or as a "tonic."
- Don't take within 2 hours of taking another medicine.

INTERACTION WITH OTHER DRUGS

GENERIC NAME OR DRUG CLASS	COMBINED EFFECT
Chlordiazepoxide	Decreased chlordiazepoxide effect.
Chlorpromazine	Decreased chlorpromazine effect.
Dicumarol	Decreased dicumarol effect.
Digoxin	Decreased digoxin effect.
Isoniazid	Decreased isoniazid effect.
Tetracyclines	Possible intestinal blockage.

INTERACTION WITH OTHER SUBSTANCES

INTERACTS WITH	COMBINED EFFECT
Alcohol:	None expected.
Beverages:	None expected.
Cocaine:	None expected.
Foods:	None expected.
Marijuana:	None expected.
Tobacco:	None expected.

MAGNESIUM HYDROXIDE

BRAND NAMES

Aludrox (M)
Camalox (M)
Creamalin (M)
Delcid (M)
Di-Gel (M)
Ducon (M)

Kolantyl (M)
Maalox (M)
Magnatril (M)
Maxamag (M)
Milk of Magnesia
Mucotin (M)

Mylanta (M)
Silain-Gel (M)
Univol
Win-Gel (M)

GENERAL INFORMATION

Habit forming? No
Prescription needed? No
Available as generic? Yes
Drug class: Antacid, laxative

 ## USES

- Treatment for hyperacidity in upper gastrointestinal tract, including stomach and esophagus. Symptoms may be heartburn or acid indigestion. Diseases include peptic ulcer, gastritis, esophagitis, hiatal hernia.
- Constipation relief.

 ## DOSAGE & USAGE INFORMATION

How to take:
- Tablet—Swallow with liquid.
- Liquid—Shake well and take undiluted.

When to take:
1 to 3 hours after meals unless directed otherwise by your doctor.

If you forget a dose:
Take as soon as you remember.

What drug does:
- Neutralizes some of the hydrochloric acid in the stomach.
- Reduces action of pepsin, a digestive enzyme.
- Stimulates muscles in lower bowel wall.

Time lapse before drug works:
15 minutes.

Don't take with:
Other medicines at the same time. Decreases absorption of other drugs.

 ## OVERDOSE

Symptoms:
Dry mouth, shallow breathing, diarrhea, stupor.

What to do:
- Dial 0 (operator) or 911 (emergency) for an ambulance or medical help. Then give first aid immediately.
- Additional emergency information on page 886.

 ## POSSIBLE ADVERSE REACTIONS OR SIDE EFFECTS

SYMPTOMS	FREQUENCY	WHAT TO DO
Brain & nervous system: Mood changes.	Infrequent	4
Skin:	None expected.	
Eyes:	None expected.	
Ears, nose, throat:	None expected.	
Digestive:		
• Constipation, appetite loss.	Common	4
• Nausea, vomiting.	Infrequent	4
• Lower abdominal pain and swelling.	Infrequent	3
Heart & lungs:	None expected.	
Blood vessels:	None expected.	
Muscles, bones, joints: Bone pain, muscle weakness.	Infrequent	3
Genital, urinary:	None expected.	
Kidneys:	None expected.	
Liver:	None expected.	
Allergic:	None expected.	
Blood:	None expected.	
Others:		
• Swelling of wrists or ankles.	Infrequent	3
• Weight loss.	Infrequent	4

1- Life-threatening. Seek emergency treatment immediately.
2- Discontinue. Seek emergency treatment.
3- Discontinue. Call doctor right away.
4- Continue. Call doctor when convenient.
5- Continue. Tell doctor at next visit.
6- No action necessary.

MAGNESIUM HYDROXIDE

WARNINGS & PRECAUTIONS

Don't take if:
You are allergic to any antacid.

Before you start, consult your doctor:
- If you have kidney disease.
- If you have chronic constipation, colitis or diarrhea.
- If you have symptoms of appendicitis.
- If you have stomach or intestinal bleeding.

Over age 60:
Adverse reactions and side effects may be more frequent and severe than in younger persons. Diarrhea or constipation particularly likely.

Pregnancy:
Risk to unborn child outweighs drug benefits. Don't use.

Breast-feeding:
Drug passes into milk. Avoid drug or discontinue nursing until you finish medicine. Consult doctor for advice on maintaining milk supply.

Infants & children:
Use only under medical supervision.

Prolonged use:
No problems expected.

Skin & sunlight:
No problems expected.

Driving, piloting or hazardous work:
No problems expected.

Airplane passengers:
No problems expected.

Discontinuing:
May be unnecessary to finish medicine. Follow doctor's instructions.

Others:
Don't take longer than 2 weeks unless under medical supervision.

INTERACTION WITH OTHER DRUGS

GENERIC NAME OR DRUG CLASS	COMBINED EFFECT
Anticoagulants	Decreased anticoagulant effect.
Chlorpromazine	Decreased chlorpromazine effect.
Digitalis preparations	Decreased digitalis effect.
Iron supplements	Decreased iron effect.
Isoniazid	Decreased isoniazid effect.
Levodopa	Increased levodopa effect.
Meperidine	Increased meperidine effect.
Nalidixic acid	Decreased effect of nalidixic acid.
Oxyphenbutazone	Decreased oxyphenbutazone effect.
Para-aminosalicylic acid (PAS)	Decreased PAS effect.
Penicillins	Decreased penicillin effect
Pentobarbital	Decreased pentobarbital effect.
Phenylbutazone	Decreased phenylbutazone effect.
Pseudoephedrine	Increased pseudoephedrine effect.

Additional interactions on page 838.

INTERACTION WITH OTHER SUBSTANCES

INTERACTS WITH	COMBINED EFFECT
Alcohol:	Decreased antacid effect.
Beverages:	No proven problems.
Cocaine:	No proven problems.
Foods:	Decreased antacid effect if taken with food. Wait 1 hour after eating.
Marijuana:	No proven problems.
Tobacco:	Decreased antacid effect.

MAGNESIUM SULFATE

BRAND NAMES

Epsom Salts

GENERAL INFORMATION

Habit forming? No
Prescription needed? No
Available as generic? Yes
Drug class: Laxative (hyperosmotic)

 ## USES

Constipation relief.

 ## DOSAGE & USAGE INFORMATION

How to take:
Powder or solid form—Dilute dose in beverage before swallowing. Solid form must be dissolved.

When to take:
Usually once a day, preferably in the morning.

If you forget a dose:
Take as soon as you remember up to 8 hours before bedtime. If later, wait for next scheduled dose (don't double this dose). Don't take at bedtime.

What drug does:
Draws water into bowel from other body tissues. Causes distention through fluid accumulation, which promotes soft stool and accelerates bowel motion.

Time lapse before drug works:
30 minutes to 3 hours.

Don't take with:
See Interaction column and consult doctor.

 ## OVERDOSE

Symptoms:
Fluid depletion, weakness, vomiting, fainting.

What to do:
Overdose unlikely to threaten life. If person takes much larger amount than prescribed, call doctor, poison-control center or hospital emergency room for instructions.

 ## POSSIBLE ADVERSE REACTIONS OR SIDE EFFECTS

SYMPTOMS	FREQUENCY	WHAT TO DO
Brain & nervous system: Dizziness, confusion.	Rare	4
Skin:	None expected.	
Eyes:	None expected.	
Ears, nose, throat: Increased thirst.	Infrequent	5
Digestive: Cramps, nausea, diarrhea, gas.	Infrequent	5
Heart & lungs: Irregular heartbeat.	Infrequent	3
Blood vessels:	None expected.	
Muscles, bones, joints:	None expected.	
Genital, urinary:	None expected.	
Kidneys:	None expected.	
Liver:	None expected.	
Allergic:	None expected.	
Blood:	None expected.	
Others: Tiredness or weakness.	Rare	4

1- Life-threatening. Seek emergency treatment immediately.
2- Discontinue. Seek emergency treatment.
3- Discontinue. Call doctor right away.
4- Continue. Call doctor when convenient.
5- Continue. Tell doctor at next visit.
6- No action necessary.

WARNINGS & PRECAUTIONS

Don't take if:
- You are allergic to any hyperosmotic laxative.
- You have symptoms of appendicitis, inflamed bowel or intestinal blockage.
- You have missed a bowel movement for only 1 or 2 days.

Before you start, consult your doctor:
- If you have congestive heart disease.
- If you have diabetes.
- If you have high blood pressure.
- If you have a colostomy or ileostomy.
- If you have kidney disease.
- If you have a laxative habit.
- If you have rectal bleeding.
- If you take another laxative.

Over age 60:
Adverse reactions and side effects may be more frequent and severe than in younger persons.

Pregnancy:
Salt content may cause fluid retention and swelling. Avoid if possible.

Breast-feeding:
No problems expected.

Infants & children:
Use only under medical supervision.

Prolonged use:
Don't take for more than 1 week unless under a doctor's supervision. May cause laxative dependence.

Skin & sunlight:
No problems expected.

Driving, piloting or hazardous work:
No problems expected.

Airplane passengers:
No problems expected.

Discontinuing:
May be unnecessary to finish medicine. Follow doctor's instructions.

Others:
- Don't take to "flush out" your system or as a "tonic."
- Don't take within 2 hours of taking another medicine.

 ## INTERACTION WITH OTHER DRUGS

GENERIC NAME OR DRUG CLASS	COMBINED EFFECT
Chlordiazepoxide	Decreased chlordiazepoxide effect.
Chlorpromazine	Decreased chlorpromazine effect.
Dicumarol	Decreased dicumarol effect.
Digoxin	Decreased digoxin effect.
Isoniazid	Decreased isoniazid effect.
Tetracyclines	Possible intestinal blockage.

 ## INTERACTION WITH OTHER SUBSTANCES

INTERACTS WITH	COMBINED EFFECT
Alcohol:	None expected.
Beverages:	None expected.
Cocaine:	None expected.
Foods:	None expected.
Marijuana:	None expected.
Tobacco:	None expected.

MAGNESIUM TRISILICATE

BRAND NAMES

A-M-T (M)   Mucotin (M)
Gaviscon (M)   Sterazolidin (M)
Gelusil (M)   Trisogel (M)
Gelusil-M (M)
Magnatril (M)

GENERAL INFORMATION

Habit forming? No
Prescription needed? No
Available as generic? Yes
Drug class: Antacid, laxative

USES

- Treatment for hyperacidity in upper gastrointestinal tract, including stomach and esophagus. Symptoms may be heartburn or acid indigestion. Diseases include peptic ulcer, gastritis, esophagitis, hiatal hernia.
- Constipation relief.

DOSAGE & USAGE INFORMATION

How to take:
- Tablet or capsule—Swallow with liquid.
- Chewable tablets or wafers—Chew well before swallowing.
- Liquid—Shake well and take undiluted.

When to take:
1 to 3 hours after meals unless directed otherwise by your doctor.

If you forget a dose:
Take as soon as you remember.

What drug does:
- Neutralizes some of the hydrochloric acid in the stomach.
- Reduces action of pepsin, a digestive enzyme.
- Stimulates muscles in lower bowel wall.

Time lapse before drug works:
15 minutes.

Don't take with:
Other medicines at the same time. Decreases absorption of other drugs.

OVERDOSE

Symptoms:
Dry mouth, diarrhea, shallow breathing, stupor.

What to do:
- Dial 0 (operator) or 911 (emergency) for an ambulance or medical help. Then give first aid immediately.
- Additional emergency information on page 886.

POSSIBLE ADVERSE REACTIONS OR SIDE EFFECTS

SYMPTOMS	FREQUENCY	WHAT TO DO
Brain & nervous system: Mood changes.	Infrequent	4
Skin:	None expected.	
Eyes:	None expected.	
Ears, nose, throat:	None expected.	
Digestive:		
• Constipation, appetite loss.	Common	4
• Nausea, vomiting.	Infrequent	4
• Lower abdominal pain and swelling.	Infrequent	3
Heart & lungs:	None expected.	
Blood vessels:	None expected.	
Muscles, bones, joints: Bone pain, muscle weakness.	Infrequent	3
Genital, urinary:	None expected.	
Kidneys:	None expected.	
Liver:	None expected.	
Allergic:	None expected.	
Blood:	None expected.	
Others:		
• Swelling of wrists or ankles.	Infrequent	3
• Weight loss.	Infrequent	4

1- Life-threatening. Seek emergency treatment immediately.
2- Discontinue. Seek emergency treatment.
3- Discontinue. Call doctor right away.
4- Continue. Call doctor when convenient.
5- Continue. Tell doctor at next visit.
6- No action necessary.

MAGNESIUM TRISILICATE

WARNINGS & PRECAUTIONS

Don't take if:
You are allergic to any antacid.

Before you start, consult your doctor:
- If you have kidney disease.
- If you have chronic constipation, colitis or diarrhea.
- If you have symptoms of appendicitis.
- If you have stomach or intestinal bleeding.

Over age 60:
Adverse reactions and side effects may be more frequent and severe than in younger persons. Diarrhea or constipation particularly likely.

Pregnancy:
Risk to unborn child outweighs drug benefits. Don't use.

Breast-feeding:
Drug passes into milk. Avoid drug or discontinue nursing until you finish medicine. Consult doctor for advice on maintaining milk supply.

Infants & children:
Use only under medical supervision.

Prolonged use:
No problems expected.

Skin & sunlight:
No problems expected.

Driving, piloting or hazardous work:
No problems expected.

Airplane passengers:
No problems expected.

Discontinuing:
May be unnecessary to finish medicine. Follow doctor's instructions.

Others:
Don't take longer than 2 weeks unless under medical supervision.

INTERACTION WITH OTHER DRUGS

GENERIC NAME OR DRUG CLASS	COMBINED EFFECT
Anticoagulants	Decreased anticoagulant effect.
Chlorpromazine	Decreased chlorpromazine effect.
Digitalis preparations	Decreased digitalis effect.
Iron supplements	Decreased iron effect.
Isoniazid	Decreased isoniazid effect.
Levodopa	Increased levodopa effect.
Meperidine	Increased meperidine effect.
Nalidixic acid	Decreased effect of nalidixic acid.
Oxyphenbutazone	Decreased oxyphenbutazone effect.
Para-aminosalicylic acid (PAS)	Decreased PAS effect.
Penicillins	Decreased penicillin effect.
Pentobarbital	Decreased pentobarbital effect.
Phenylbutazone	Decreased phenylbutazone effect.
Pseudoephedrine	Increased pseudoephedrine effect.

Additional interactions on page 838.

INTERACTION WITH OTHER SUBSTANCES

INTERACTS WITH	COMBINED EFFECT
Alcohol:	Decreased antacid effect.
Beverages:	No proven problems.
Cocaine:	No proven problems.
Foods:	Decreased antacid effect if taken with food. Wait 1 hour after eating.
Marijuana:	No proven problems.
Tobacco:	Decreased antacid effect.

MALT SOUP EXTRACT

BRAND NAMES

Maltsupex

GENERAL INFORMATION

Habit forming? No
Prescription needed? No
Available as generic? Yes
Drug class: Laxative (bulk-forming)

 USES

Relieves constipation and prevents straining for bowel movement.

 DOSAGE & USAGE INFORMATION

How to take:
- Liquid or powder—Dilute dose in 8 oz. cold water or fruit juice.
- Tablets—Swallow with 8 oz. cold liquid. Drink 6 to 8 glasses of water each day in addition to the one with each dose.

When to take:
At the same time each day, preferably morning.

If you forget a dose:
Take as soon as you remember. Resume regular schedule.

What drug does:
Absorbs water, stimulating the bowel to form a soft, bulky stool.

Time lapse before drug works:
May require 2 or 3 days to begin, then works in 12 to 24 hours.

Don't take with:
- See Interaction column and consult doctor.
- Don't take within 2 hours of taking another medicine.

 OVERDOSE

Symptoms:
None expected.

What to do:
Overdose unlikely to threaten life. If person takes much larger amount than prescribed, call doctor, poison-control center or hospital emergency room for instructions.

 POSSIBLE ADVERSE REACTIONS OR SIDE EFFECTS

SYMPTOMS	FREQUENCY	WHAT TO DO
Brain & nervous system:	None expected.	
Skin: Itch, rash.	Rare	3
Eyes:	None expected.	
Ears, nose, throat: Swallowing difficulty, "lump in throat" sensation.	Infrequent	4
Digestive:		
• Intestinal blockage.	Rare	3
• Nausea, vomiting, diarrhea.	Infrequent	4
Heart & lungs: Asthma	Rare	3
Blood vessels:	None expected.	
Muscles, bones, joints:	None expected.	
Genital, urinary:	None expected.	
Kidneys:	None expected.	
Liver:	None expected.	
Allergic:	None expected.	
Blood:	None expected.	
Others:	None expected.	

1- Life-threatening. Seek emergency treatment immediately.
2- Discontinue. Seek emergency treatment.
3- Discontinue. Call doctor right away.
4- Continue. Call doctor when convenient.
5- Continue. Tell doctor at next visit.
6- No action necessary.

MALT SOUP EXTRACT

 WARNINGS & PRECAUTIONS

Don't take if:
- You are allergic to any bulk-forming laxative.
- You have symptoms of appendicitis, inflamed bowel or intestinal blockage.
- You have missed a bowel movement for only 1 or 2 days.

Before you start, consult your doctor:
- If you have diabetes.
- If you have a laxative habit.
- If you have rectal bleeding.
- If you have difficulty swallowing.
- If you take other laxatives.

Over age 60:
Adverse reactions and side effects may be more frequent and severe than in younger persons.

Pregnancy:
Most bulk-forming laxatives contain sodium or sugars which may cause fluid retention. Avoid if possible.

Breast-feeding:
No problems expected.

Infants & children:
Use only under medical supervision.

Prolonged use:
Don't take for more than 1 week unless under a doctor's supervision. May cause laxative dependence.

Skin & sunlight:
No problems expected.

Driving, piloting or hazardous work:
No problems expected.

Airplane passengers:
No problems expected.

Discontinuing:
May be unnecessary to finish medicine. Follow doctor's instructions.

Others:
Don't take to "flush out" your system or as a "tonic."

 INTERACTION WITH OTHER DRUGS

GENERIC NAME OR DRUG CLASS	COMBINED EFFECT
Antibiotics	Decreased antibiotic effect.
Anticoagulants	Decreased anticoagulant effect.
Digitalis preparations	Decreased digitalis effect.
Salicylates (including aspirin)	Decreased salicylate effect.

INTERACTION WITH OTHER SUBSTANCES

INTERACTS WITH	COMBINED EFFECT
Alcohol:	None expected.
Beverages:	None expected.
Cocaine:	None expected.
Foods:	None expected.
Marijuana:	None expected.
Tobacco:	None expected.

MAZINDOL

BRAND NAMES

Mazinor
Sanorex

GENERAL INFORMATION

Habit forming? Yes
Prescription needed? Yes
Available as generic? Yes
Drug class: Appetite suppressant

 USES

Suppresses appetite.

 DOSAGE & USAGE INFORMATION

How to take:
Tablet—Swallow with liquid.

When to take:
1 hour before meals. Last dose no later than 4 to 6 hours before bedtime.

If you forget a dose:
Wait for next scheduled dose. Don't double this dose.

What drug does:
Apparently stimulates brain's appetite-control center.

Time lapse before drug works:
Begins in 1 hour. Lasts 4 hours.

Don't take with:
- Non-prescription drugs without consulting doctor.
- See Interaction column and consult doctor.

 OVERDOSE

Symptoms:
Irritability, overactivity, trembling, insomnia, mood changes, rapid heartbeat, confusion, disorientation, hallucinations, convulsions, coma.

What to do:
- Dial 0 (operator) or 911 (emergency) for an ambulance or medical help. Then give first aid immediately.
- Additional emergency information on page 886.

POSSIBLE ADVERSE REACTIONS OR SIDE EFFECTS

SYMPTOMS	FREQUENCY	WHAT TO DO
Brain & nervous system:		
• Irritability, nervousness, insomnia.	Common	4
• Mood changes.	Rare	3
Skin:		
• Hair loss.	Rare	4
• Rash or hives.	Rare	3
Eyes:		
Blurred vision.	Infrequent	4
Ears, nose, throat:		
Unpleasant taste or dry mouth.	Infrequent	4
Digestive:		
Constipation or diarrhea, nausea, vomiting, cramps.	Infrequent	4
Heart & lungs:		
• Irregular or pounding heartbeat.	Infrequent	3
• Breathing difficulty.	Rare	3
Blood vessels, muscles, bones, joints, kidneys, liver, allergic, blood:	None expected.	
Genital, urinary:		
Urinary urgency and difficulty.	Infrequent	3
Others:		
• False sense of well-being.	Common	4
• Changes in sex drive.	Infrequent	4
• Sweat increase.	Infrequent	4

1- Life-threatening. Seek emergency treatment immediately.
2- Discontinue. Seek emergency treatment.
3- Discontinue. Call doctor right away.
4- Continue. Call doctor when convenient.

MAZINDOL

WARNINGS & PRECAUTIONS

Don't take if:
- You are allergic to any sympathomimetic or phenylpropanolamine.
- You have glaucoma.
- You have taken MAO inhibitors within 2 weeks.
- You plan to become pregnant within medication period.
- You have a history of drug abuse.

Before you start, consult your doctor:
- If you have high blood pressure or heart disease.
- If you have an overactive thyroid, nervous tension or "anxiety."
- If you have epilepsy.

Over age 60:
Adverse reactions and side effects may be more frequent and severe than in younger persons.

Pregnancy:
Safety not established. Avoid.

Breast-feeding:
No proven problems. Consult doctor.

Infants & children:
Don't give to children younger than 12.

Prolonged use:
Loses effectiveness. Avoid.

Skin & sunlight:
No problems expected.

Driving, piloting or hazardous work:
Don't drive or pilot aircraft until you learn how medicine affects you. Don't work around dangerous machinery. Don't climb ladders or work in high places. Danger increases if you drink alcohol or take medicine affecting alertness and reflexes, such as antihistamines, tranquilizers, sedatives, pain medicine, narcotics and mind-altering drugs.

Airplane passengers:
No problems expected.

Discontinuing:
Don't discontinue without consulting doctor. Dose may require gradual reduction if you have taken drug for a long time. Doses of other drugs may also require adjustment.

Others:
Don't increase dose.

INTERACTION WITH OTHER DRUGS

GENERIC NAME OR DRUG CLASS	COMBINED EFFECT
Appetite suppressants (other)	Dangerous overstimulation.
Caffeine	Increased stimulant effect of mazindol.
Guanethidine	Decreased guanethidine effect.
Hydralazine	Decreased hydralazine effect.
MAO inhibitors	Dangerous blood-pressure rise.
Methyldopa	Decreased methyldopa effect.
Phenothiazines	Decreased mazindol effect.
Rauwolfia alkaloids	Decreased effect of rauwolfia alkaloids.

INTERACTION WITH OTHER SUBSTANCES

INTERACTS WITH	COMBINED EFFECT
Alcohol: Beer, chianti wines, vermouth.	Dangerous blood-pressure rise.
Beverages: • Caffeine drinks • Drinks containing tyramine (see page 851).	Excessive stimulation. Blood-pressure rise.
Cocaine:	Excessive stimulation.
Foods: Foods containing tyramine (see page 851).	Blood-pressure rise.
Marijuana:	Frequent use—Irregular heartbeat.
Tobacco:	None expected.

MECLIZINE

BRAND NAMES

Antivert
Bonine
Motion Cure
Wehvert

GENERAL INFORMATION

Habit forming? No
Prescription needed? U.S.—Tablets: No
Liquid: Yes
Canada: Yes
Available as generic? No
Drug class: Antihistamine, antiemetic

 ## USES

Prevents motion sickness.

 ## DOSAGE & USAGE INFORMATION

How to take:
Tablet—Swallow with liquid or food to lessen stomach irritation. If you can't swallow whole, crumble tablet and chew or take with liquid or food.

When to take:
30 minutes to 1 hour before traveling.

If you forget a dose:
Take as soon as you remember. Wait 4 hours for next dose.

What drug does:
Reduces sensitivity of nerve endings in inner ear, blocking messages to brain's vomiting center.

Time lapse before drug works:
30 to 60 minutes.

Don't take with:
See Interaction column and consult doctor.

 ## OVERDOSE

Symptoms:
Drowsiness, confusion, incoordination, stupor, coma, weak pulse, shallow breathing.

What to do:
- Dial 0 (operator) or 911 (emergency) for an ambulance or medical help. Then give first aid immediately.
- Additional emergency information on page 886.

 ## POSSIBLE ADVERSE REACTIONS OR SIDE EFFECTS

SYMPTOMS	FREQUENCY	WHAT TO DO
Brain & nervous system:		
● Drowsiness	Common	5
● Headache	Infrequent	4
● Restlessness, excitement, insomnia.	Rare	4
Skin: Rash or hives.	Rare	3
Eyes: Blurred vision.	Rare	4
Ears, nose, throat: Dry mouth, nose, throat.	Infrequent	5
Digestive:		
● Appetite loss, nausea.	Rare	5
● Diarrhea or constipation.	Infrequent	4
Heart & lungs: Fast heartbeat.	Infrequent	4
Blood vessels:	None expected.	
Muscles, bones, joints:	None expected.	
Genital, urinary: Urinary frequency, difficult urination.	Rare	4
Kidneys:	None expected.	
Liver:	None expected.	
Allergic:	None expected.	
Blood:	None expected.	
Others:	None expected.	

1- Life-threatening. Seek emergency treatment immediately.
2- Discontinue. Seek emergency treatment.
3- Discontinue. Call doctor right away.
4- Continue. Call doctor when convenient.
5- Continue. Tell doctor at next visit.

WARNINGS & PRECAUTIONS

Don't take if:
- You are allergic to meclizine, buclizine or cyclizine.
- You have taken MAO inhibitors in the past 2 weeks.

Before you start, consult your doctor:
- If you have glaucoma.
- If you have prostate enlargement.
- If you have reacted badly to any antihistamine.

Over age 60:
Adverse reactions and side effects may be more frequent and severe than in younger persons, especially impaired urination from enlarged prostate gland.

Pregnancy:
Studies inconclusive on harm to unborn child. Animal studies show fetal abnormalities. Decide with your doctor whether drug benefits justify risk to unborn child.

Breast-feeding:
Drug passes into milk. Avoid drug or discontinue nursing until you finish medicine. Consult doctor for advice on maintaining milk supply.

Infants & children:
No problems expected.

Prolonged use:
No problems expected.

Skin & sunlight:
No problems expected.

Driving, piloting or hazardous work:
Don't fly aircraft. Don't drive until you learn how medicine affects you. Don't work around dangerous machinery. Don't climb ladders or work in high places. Danger increases if you drink alcohol or take medicine affecting alertness and reflexes, such as antihistamines, tranquilizers, sedatives, pain medicine, narcotics and mind-altering drugs.

Airplane passengers:
Take 30 minutes before takeoff and every 4 hours while in the air.

Discontinuing:
No problems expected.

Others:
No problems expected.

INTERACTION WITH OTHER DRUGS

GENERIC NAME OR DRUG CLASS	COMBINED EFFECT
Amphetamines	May decrease drowsiness caused by meclizine.
Anticholinergics	Increased effect of both drugs.
Antidepressants (tricyclic)	Increased effect of both drugs.
MAO inhibitors	Increased meclizine effect.
Narcotics	Increased effect of both drugs.
Pain relievers	Increased effect of both drugs.
Sedatives	Increased effect of both drugs.
Sleep inducers	Increased effect of both drugs.
Tranquilizers	Increased effect of both drugs.

INTERACTION WITH OTHER SUBSTANCES

INTERACTS WITH	COMBINED EFFECT
Alcohol:	Increased sedation. Avoid
Beverages: Caffeine drinks	May decrease drowsiness.
Cocaine:	None expected.
Foods:	None expected.
Marijuana:	Increased drowsiness, dry mouth.
Tobacco:	None expected.

MECLOFENAMATE

BRAND NAMES

Meclomen

Habit forming? No
Prescription needed? Yes

 USES

Treatment for joint pain, stiffness, inflammation and swelling of arthritis and gout.

 DOSAGE & USAGE INFORMATION

How to take:
Capsule—Swallow with liquid or food to lessen stomach irritation. If you can't swallow whole, open capsule and take with liquid or food.

When to take:
At the same times each day.

If you forget a dose:
Take as soon as you remember up to 2 hours late. If more than 2 hours, wait for next scheduled dose (don't double this dose).

What drug does:
Reduces tissue concentration of prostaglandins (hormones which produce inflammation and pain).

Time lapse before drug works:
Begins in 4 to 24 hours. May require 3 weeks regular use for maximum benefit.

Don't take with:
See Interaction column and consult doctor.

 OVERDOSE

Symptoms:
Confusion, agitation, incoherence, convulsions, possible hemorrhage from stomach or intestine, coma.

What to do:
- Dial 0 (operator) or 911 (emergency) for an ambulance or medical help. Then give first aid immediately.
- Additional emergency information on page 886.

GENERAL INFORMATION

Available as generic? No
Drug class: Antiinflammatory (non-steroid)

 POSSIBLE ADVERSE REACTIONS OR SIDE EFFECTS

SYMPTOMS	FREQUENCY	WHAT TO DO
Brain & nervous system:		
• Depression, drowsiness.	Infrequent	4
• Convulsions, confusion.	Rare	3
• Dizziness	Common	4
• Headache	Common	5
Skin:		
Rash, hives or itch.	Rare	3
Eyes:		
Blurred vision.	Rare	3
Ears, nose, throat:		
Ringing in ears.	Infrequent	4
Digestive:		
• Bloody or black, tarry stools.	Rare	3
• Nausea, pain.	Common	4
• Constipation or diarrhea, vomiting.	Infrequent	4
Heart & lungs:		
Breathing difficulty, tightness in chest, rapid heartbeat.	Rare	3
Blood vessels:		
Unusual bleeding or bruising.	Rare	3
Muscles, bones, joints:		
Swollen feet, legs.	Infrequent	4
Genital, urinary:		
• Bloody urine.	Rare	3
• Difficult, painful or frequent urination.	Rare	4
Kidneys, allergic, blood:	None expected.	
Liver:		
Jaundice (yellow skin and eyes).	Rare	3
Others:		
Fatigue, weakness.	Rare	4

1- Life-threatening. Seek emergency treatment immediately.
2- Discontinue. Seek emergency treatment.
3- Discontinue. Call doctor right away.
4- Continue. Call doctor when convenient.
5- Continue. Tell doctor at next visit.

MECLOFENAMATE

WARNINGS & PRECAUTIONS

Don't take if:
- You are allergic to aspirin or any non-steroid, antiinflammatory drug.
- You have gastritis, peptic ulcer, enteritis, ileitis, ulcerative colitis, asthma, heart failure, high blood pressure or bleeding problems.
- Patient is younger than 15.

Before you start, consult your doctor:
- If you have epilepsy.
- If you have Parkinson's disease.
- If you have been mentally ill.
- If you have had kidney disease or impaired kidney function.

Over age 60:
Adverse reactions and side effects may be more frequent and severe than in younger persons.

Pregnancy:
Studies inconclusive on harm to unborn child. Decide with your doctor whether drug benefits justify risk to unborn child.

Breast-feeding:
May harm child. Avoid.

Infants & children:
Not recommended for anyone younger than 15. Use only under medical supervision.

Prolonged use:
- Eye damage.
- Reduced hearing.
- Sore throat, fever.
- Weight gain.

Skin & sunlight:
No problems expected.

Driving, piloting or hazardous work:
Don't drive or pilot aircraft until you learn how medicine affects you. Don't work around dangerous machinery. Don't climb ladders or work in high places. Danger increases if you drink alcohol or take medicine affecting alertness and reflexes, such as antihistamines, tranquilizers, sedatives, pain medicine, narcotics and mind-altering drugs.

Airplane passengers:
No problems expected.

Discontinuing:
Don't discontinue without consulting doctor. Dose may require gradual reduction if you have taken drug for a long time. Doses of other drugs may also require adjustment.

Others:
No problems expected.

INTERACTION WITH OTHER DRUGS

GENERIC NAME OR DRUG CLASS	COMBINED EFFECT
Anticoagulants (oral)	Increased risk of bleeding.
Aspirin	Increased risk of stomach ulcer.
Cortisone drugs	Increased risk of stomach ulcer.
Furosemide	Decreased diuretic effect of furosemide.
Oxyphenbutazone	Possible stomach ulcer.
Phenylbutazone	Possible stomach ulcer.
Probenecid	Increased meclofenamate effect.
Thyroid hormones	Rapid heartbeat, blood-pressure rise.

INTERACTION WITH OTHER SUBSTANCES

INTERACTS WITH	COMBINED EFFECT
Alcohol:	Possible stomach ulcer or bleeding.
Beverages:	None expected.
Cocaine:	None expected.
Foods:	None expected.
Marijuana:	Increased pain relief from meclofenamate.
Tobacco:	None expected.

MEDROXYPROGESTERONE

BRAND NAMES

Amen
Depo-Provera
Provera

GENERAL INFORMATION

Habit forming? No
Prescription needed? Yes
Available as generic? No
Drug class: Female sex hormone (progestin)

 ## USES

- Treatment for menstrual or uterine disorders caused by progestin imbalance.
- Contraceptive
- Treatment for cancer of breast and uterus.

 ## DOSAGE & USAGE INFORMATION

How to take:
- Tablet or capsule—Swallow with liquid or food to lessen stomach irritation. You may crumble tablet or open capsule.
- Injection—Take under doctor's supervision.

When to take:
Tablet, capsule—At the same time each day.

If you forget a dose:
- Menstrual disorders—Take up to 2 hours late. If more than 2 hours, wait for next dose (don't double this).
- Contraceptive—Consult your doctor. You may need to use another birth-control method until next period.

What drug does:
- Creates a uterine lining similar to pregnancy that prevents bleeding.
- Suppresses a pituitary gland hormone responsible for ovulation.
- Stimulates cervical mucus, which stops sperm penetration and prevents pregnancy.

Time lapse before drug works:
- Menstrual disorders—24 to 48 hours.
- Contraception—3 weeks.
- Cancer—May require 2 to 3 months regular use for maximum benefit.

Don't take with:
See Interaction column and consult doctor.

 ## OVERDOSE

Symptoms:
Nausea, vomiting, fluid retention, breast discomfort or enlargement, vaginal bleeding.

What to do:
Overdose unlikely to threaten life. If person takes much larger amount than prescribed, call doctor, poison-control center or hospital emergency room for instructions.

POSSIBLE ADVERSE REACTIONS OR SIDE EFFECTS

SYMPTOMS	FREQUENCY	WHAT TO DO
Brain & nervous system:		
Depression	Infrequent	4
Skin:		
• Rash	Rare	3
• Acne, increased facial or body hair.	Infrequent	5
Eyes, ears, nose, throat, heart & lungs, muscles, bones, joints, kidneys, allergic, blood:	None expected.	
Digestive:		
• Stomach or side pain.	Rare	3
• Appetite or weight changes.	Common	5
• Nausea	Infrequent	5
Blood vessels:		
Blood clot in leg, brain or lung.	Rare	1
Muscles, bones, joints:		
Ankle, foot swelling.	Common	5
Genital, urinary:		
Prolonged vaginal bleeding.	Infrequent	3
Liver:		
Jaundice (yellow skin and eyes).	Rare	3
Others:		
• Breast tenderness.	Infrequent	5
• Unusual tiredness or weakness.	Common	5

1- Life-threatening. Seek emergency treatment immediately.
2- Discontinue. Seek emergency treatment.
3- Discontinue. Call doctor right away.
4- Continue. Call doctor when convenient.
5- Continue. Tell doctor at next visit.

MEDROXYPROGESTERONE

WARNINGS & PRECAUTIONS

Don't take if:
- You are allergic to any progestin hormone.
- You may be pregnant.
- You have liver or gallbladder disease.
- You have had thrombophlebitis, embolism or stroke.
- You have unexplained vaginal bleeding.
- You have had breast or uterine cancer.

Before you start, consult your doctor:
- If you have heart or kidney disease.
- If you have diabetes.
- If you have a seizure disorder.
- If you suffer migraines.
- If you are easily depressed.

Over age 60:
Not recommended.

Pregnancy:
May harm child. Discontinue at first sign of pregnancy.

Breast-feeding:
Drug passes into milk. Avoid drug or discontinue nursing until you finish medicine. Consult doctor for advice on maintaining milk supply.

Infants & children:
Use only for female children under medical supervision.

Prolonged use:
No problems expected.

Skin & sunlight:
No problems expected.

Driving, piloting or hazardous work:
No problems expected.

Airplane passengers:
No problems expected.

Discontinuing:
Consult doctor. This medicine stays in the body and causes fetal abnormalities. Wait at least 3 months before becoming pregnant.

Others:
- Patients with diabetes must be monitored closely.
- Symptoms of blood clot in leg, brain or lung are: chest, groin, leg pain; sudden, severe headache; loss of coordination; vision change; shortness of breath; slurred speech.

INTERACTION WITH OTHER DRUGS

GENERIC NAME OR DRUG CLASS	COMBINED EFFECT
Antihistamines	Decreased medroxyprogesterone effect.
Oxyphenbutazone	Decreased medroxyprogesterone effect.
Phenobarbital	Decreased medroxyprogesterone effect.
Phenothiazines	Increased phenothiazine effect.
Phenylbutazone	Decreased medroxyprogesterone effect.
Rifampin	Decreased contraceptive effect.

INTERACTION WITH OTHER SUBSTANCES

INTERACTS WITH	COMBINED EFFECT
Alcohol:	None expected.
Beverages:	None expected.
Cocaine:	Decreased medroxyprogesterone effect.
Foods: Salt	Fluid retention.
Marijuana:	Possible menstrual irregularities or bleeding between periods.
Tobacco: All forms.	Possible blood clots in lung, brain, legs. Avoid.

MEFENAMIC ACID

BRAND NAMES

Ponstan
Ponstel

Habit forming? No
Prescription needed? Yes

USES

- Pain reliever.
- Treatment for dysmenorrhea (painful or difficult menstruation).

DOSAGE & USAGE INFORMATION

How to take:
Capsule—Swallow with liquid or food to lessen stomach irritation. If you can't swallow whole, open capsule and take with liquid or food.

When to take:
At the same times each day.

If you forget a dose:
Take as soon as you remember up to 2 hours late. If more than 2 hours, wait for next scheduled dose (don't double this dose).

What drug does:
Reduces tissue concentration of prostaglandins (hormones which produce inflammation and pain).

Time lapse before drug works:
Begins in 4 to 24 hours. May require 3 weeks regular use for maximum benefit.

Don't take with:
See Interaction column and consult doctor.

OVERDOSE

Symptoms:
Confusion, agitation, incoherence, convulsions, possible hemorrhage from stomach or intestine, coma.

What to do:
- Dial 0 (operator) or 911 (emergency) for an ambulance or medical help. Then give first aid immediately.
- Additional emergency information on page 886.

GENERAL INFORMATION

Available as generic? No
Drug class: Antiinflammatory (non-steroid)

POSSIBLE ADVERSE REACTIONS OR SIDE EFFECTS

SYMPTOMS	FREQUENCY	WHAT TO DO
Brain & nervous system:		
• Depression, drowsiness.	Infrequent	4
• Convulsions, confusion.	Rare	3
• Dizziness	Common	4
• Headache	Common	5
Skin:		
Rash, hives or itch.	Rare	3
Eyes:		
Blurred vision.	Rare	3
Ears, nose, throat:		
Ringing in ears.	Infrequent	4
Digestive:		
• Bloody or black, tarry stools.	Rare	3
• Nausea, pain.	Common	4
• Constipation or diarrhea, vomiting.	Infrequent	4
Heart & lungs:		
Breathing difficulty, tightness in chest, rapid heartbeat.	Rare	3
Blood vessels:		
Unusual bleeding or bruising.	Rare	3
Muscles, bones, joints:		
Swollen feet, legs.	Infrequent	4
Genital, urinary:		
• Bloody urine.	Rare	3
• Difficult, painful or frequent urination.	Rare	4
Kidneys, allergic, blood:		
	None expected.	
Liver:		
Jaundice (yellow skin and eyes).	Rare	3
Others:		
Fatigue, weakness.	Rare	4

1- Life-threatening. Seek emergency treatment immediately.
2- Discontinue. Seek emergency treatment.
3- Discontinue. Call doctor right away.
4- Continue. Call doctor when convenient.
5- Continue. Tell doctor at next visit.

MEFENAMIC ACID

WARNINGS & PRECAUTIONS

Don't take if:
- You are allergic to aspirin or any non-steroid, antiinflammatory drug.
- You have gastritis, peptic ulcer, enteritis, ileitis, ulcerative colitis, asthma, heart failure, high blood pressure or bleeding problems.
- Patient is younger than 15.

Before you start, consult your doctor:
- If you have epilepsy.
- If you have Parkinson's disease.
- If you have been mentally ill.
- If you have had kidney disease or impaired kidney function.

Over age 60:
Adverse reactions and side effects may be more frequent and severe than in younger persons.

Pregnancy:
Studies inconclusive on harm to unborn child. Decide with your doctor whether drug benefits justify risk to unborn child.

Breast-feeding:
May harm child. Avoid.

Infants & children:
Not recommended for anyone younger than 15. Use only under medical supervision.

Prolonged use:
- Eye damage.
- Reduced hearing.
- Sore throat, fever.
- Weight gain.

Skin & sunlight:
No problems expected.

Driving, piloting or hazardous work:
Don't drive or pilot aircraft until you learn how medicine affects you. Don't work around dangerous machinery. Don't climb ladders or work in high places. Danger increases if you drink alcohol or take medicine affecting alertness and reflexes, such as antihistamines, tranquilizers, sedatives, pain medicine, narcotics and mind-altering drugs.

Airplane passengers:
No problems expected.

Discontinuing:
Don't discontinue without consulting doctor. Dose may require gradual reduction if you have taken drug for a long time. Doses of other drugs may also require adjustment.

Others:
Don't take for more than 1 week.

INTERACTION WITH OTHER DRUGS

GENERIC NAME OR DRUG CLASS	COMBINED EFFECT
Anticoagulants (oral)	Increased risk of bleeding.
Aspirin	Increased risk of stomach ulcer.
Cortisone drugs	Increased risk of stomach ulcer.
Furosemide	Decreased diuretic effect of furosemide.
Oxyphenbutazone	Possible stomach ulcer.
Phenylbutazone	Possible stomach ulcer.
Probenecid	Increased effect of mefenamic acid.
Thyroid hormones	Rapid heartbeat, blood-pressure rise.

INTERACTION WITH OTHER SUBSTANCES

INTERACTS WITH	COMBINED EFFECT
Alcohol:	Possible stomach ulcer or bleeding.
Beverages:	None expected.
Cocaine:	None expected.
Foods:	None expected.
Marijuana:	Increased pain relief from mefenamic acid.
Tobacco:	None expected.

MEPERIDINE

BRAND NAMES

A.P.C.-Demerol (M)
Demer-Idine
Demerol
Mepergan Fortis (M)
Pethadol

GENERAL INFORMATION

Habit forming? Yes
Prescription needed? Yes
Available as generic? Yes
Drug class: Narcotic

USES

Relieves pain.

DOSAGE & USAGE INFORMATION

How to take:
- Tablet or capsule—Swallow with liquid. If you can't swallow tablet or capsule whole, crumble or open and take with liquid or food.
- Drops or liquid—Dilute dose in beverage before swallowing.

When to take:
When needed. No more often than every 4 hours.

If you forget a dose:
Take as soon as you remember. Wait 4 hours for next dose.

What drug does:
Blocks pain messages to brain and spinal cord.

Time lapse before drug works:
30 minutes.

Don't take with:
See Interaction column and consult doctor.

OVERDOSE

Symptoms:
Deep sleep; slow breathing; slow pulse; flushed, warm skin; constricted pupils.

What to do:
- Dial 0 (operator) or 911 (emergency) for an ambulance or medical help. Then give first aid immediately.
- If patient is unconscious and not breathing, give mouth-to-mouth breathing. If there is no heartbeat, use cardiac massage and mouth-to-mouth breathing (CPR). Don't try to make patient vomit. If you can't get help quickly, take patient to nearest emergency facility.
- Additional emergency information on page 886.

POSSIBLE ADVERSE REACTIONS OR SIDE EFFECTS

SYMPTOMS	FREQUENCY	WHAT TO DO
Brain & nervous system: Depression, confusion, hallucinations.	Infrequent	4
Skin:		
• Hives, rash, itch, face swelling.	Rare	4
• Flushed face.	Common	4
Eyes: Blurred vision.	Rare	4
Ears, nose, throat:	None expected.	
Digestive: Severe constipation, abdominal pain, vomiting.	Infrequent	3
Heart & lungs: Slow heartbeat, irregular breathing.	Rare	3
Blood vessels:	None expected.	
Muscles, bones, joints:	None expected.	
Genital, urinary: Difficult urination.	Common	4
Kidneys: Less urine.	Common	4
Liver:	None expected.	
Allergic:	None expected.	
Blood:	None expected.	
Others: Unusual tiredness.	Common	4

1- Life-threatening. Seek emergency treatment immediately.
2- Discontinue. Seek emergency treatment.
3- Discontinue. Call doctor right away.
4- Continue. Call doctor when convenient.
5- Continue. Tell doctor at next visit.
6- No action necessary.

WARNINGS & PRECAUTIONS

Don't take if:
You are allergic to any narcotic.

Before you start, consult your doctor:
If you have impaired liver or kidney function.

Over age 60:
More likely to be drowsy, dizzy, unsteady or constipated. Avoid prolonged use.

Pregnancy:
Studies inconclusive on harm to unborn child. Animal studies show fetal abnormalities. Decide with your doctor whether drug benefits justify risk to unborn child. Abuse by pregnant woman will result in addicted newborn. Withdrawal can be life-threatening.

Breast-feeding:
Drug filters into milk. May depress infant. Avoid.

Infants & children:
Not recommended.

Prolonged use:
Causes psychological and physical dependence.

Skin & sunlight:
No problems expected.

Driving, piloting or hazardous work:
Don't drive or pilot aircraft until you learn how medicine affects you. Don't work around dangerous machinery. Don't climb ladders or work in high places. Danger increases if you drink alcohol or take medicine affecting alertness and reflexes, such as antihistamines, tranquilizers, sedatives, pain medicine, other narcotics and mind-altering drugs.

Airplane passengers:
No proven problems.

Discontinuing:
May be unnecessary to finish medicine. Follow doctor's instructions.

Others:
No problems expected.

INTERACTION WITH OTHER DRUGS

GENERIC NAME OR DRUG CLASS	COMBINED EFFECT
Analgesics	Increased analgesic effect.
Antidepressants	Increased sedative effect.
Antihistamines	Increased sedative effect.
Mind-altering drugs	Increased sedative effect.
Narcotics (other)	Increased narcotic effect.
Phenothiazines	Increased phenothiazine effect.
Sedatives	Increased sedative effect.
Sleep inducers	Increased sedative effect.
Tranquilizers	Increased sedative effect.

INTERACTION WITH OTHER SUBSTANCES

INTERACTS WITH	COMBINED EFFECT
Alcohol:	Increases alcohol's intoxicating effect. Avoid.
Beverages:	None expected.
Cocaine:	Increased cocaine effect.
Foods:	None expected.
Marijuana:	Impairs physical and mental performance.
Tobacco:	None expected.

MEPHENYTOIN

BRAND NAMES

Mesantoin
Methoin

Habit forming? No
Prescription needed? Yes
Available as generic? Yes
Drug class: Anticonvulsant (hydantoin)

USES

- Prevents epileptic seizures.
- Stabilizes irregular heartbeat.

DOSAGE & USAGE INFORMATION

How to take:
- Tablet or capsule—Swallow with liquid.
- Extended-release tablets or capsules—Swallow each dose whole. If you take regular tablets, you may chew or crush them.

When to take:
At the same time each day.

If you forget a dose:
- If drug taken 1 time per day—Take as soon as you remember up to 12 hours late. If more than 12 hours, wait for next scheduled dose (don't double this dose).
- If taken several times per day—Take as soon as possible, then return to regular schedule.

What drug does:
Promotes sodium loss from nerve fibers. This lessens excitability and inhibits spread of nerve impulses.

Time lapse before drug works:
7 to 10 days continual use.

Don't take with:
See Interaction column and consult doctor.

OVERDOSE

Symptoms:
Jerky eye movements; stagger; slurred speech; imbalance; drowsiness; blood-pressure drop; slow, shallow breathing; coma.

What to do:
- Dial 0 (operator) or 911 (emergency) for an ambulance or medical help. Then give first aid immediately.
- Additional emergency information on page 886.

POSSIBLE ADVERSE REACTIONS OR SIDE EFFECTS

SYMPTOMS	FREQUENCY	WHAT TO DO
Brain & nervous system:		
Mild dizziness, drowsiness.	Common	4
Headache, sleeplessness.	Infrequent	4
Hallucinations, confusion, slurred speech, stagger.	Infrequent	3
Skin:		
Rash	Infrequent	3
Eyes:		
Vision changes.	Infrequent	3
Ears, nose, throat:		
Sore throat, fever.	Rare	3
Digestive:		
Stomach pain.	Rare	3
Constipation, nausea, vomiting.	Common	4
Diarrhea	Infrequent	4
Heart & lungs, genital, urinary, kidneys, allergic blood:	None expected.	
Blood vessels:		
Unusual bleeding or bruising.	Rare	3
Muscles, bones, joints:		
Muscle twitching.	Infrequent	4
Liver:		
Jaundice (yellow skin and eyes).	Rare	3
Others:		
Increased body and facial hair.	Infrequent	5

1-Life-threatening. Seek emergency treatment immediately.
2-Discontinue. Seek emergency treatment.
3-Discontinue. Call doctor right away.
4-Continue. Call doctor when convenient.
5-Continue. Tell doctor at next visit.

WARNINGS & PRECAUTIONS

Don't take if:
You are allergic to any hydantoin anticonvulsant.

Before you start, consult your doctor:
- If you have had impaired liver function or disease.
- If you will have surgery within 2 months, including dental surgery, requiring general or spinal anesthesia.

Over age 60:
Adverse reactions and side effects may be more frequent and severe than in younger persons.

Pregnancy:
Risk to unborn child outweighs drug benefits. Don't use.

Breast-feeding:
Drug passes into milk. Avoid drug or discontinue nursing until you finish medicine. Consult doctor for advice on maintaining milk supply.

Infants & children:
Use only under medical supervision.

Prolonged use:
- Weakened bones.
- Lymph gland enlargement.
- Possible liver damage.
- Numbness and tingling of hands and feet.
- Continual back-and forth eye movements.
- Bleeding, swollen or tender gums.

Skin & sunlight:
May cause rash or intensify sunburn in areas exposed to sun or sunlamp.

Driving, piloting or hazardous work:
Don't drive or pilot aircraft until you learn how medicine affects you. Don't work around dangerous machinery. Don't climb ladders or work in high places. Danger increases if you drink alcohol or take medicine affecting alertness and reflexes.

Airplane passengers:
No problems expected.

Discontinuing:
Don't discontinue without consulting doctor. Dose may require gradual reduction if you have taken drug for a long time. Doses of other drugs may also require adjustment.

 INTERACTION WITH OTHER DRUGS

GENERIC NAME OR DRUG CLASS	COMBINED EFFECT
Anticoagulants	Increased effect of both drugs.
Antidepressants (tricyclic)	Need to adjust mephenytoin dose.
Antihypertensives	Increased effect of antihypertensive.
Aspirin	Increased mephenytoin effect.
Barbiturates	Changed seizure pattern.
Carbonic anhydrase inhibitors	Increased chance of bone disease.
Chloramphenicol	Increased mephenytoin effect.
Contraceptives (oral)	Increased seizures.
Cortisone drugs	Decreased cortisone effect.
Digitalis preparations	Decreased digitalis effect.
Disulfiram	Increased mephenytoin effect.
Estrogens	Increased mephenytoin effect.
Furosemide	Decreased furosemide effect.
Glutethimide	Decreased mephenytoin effect.
Griseofulvin	Increased griseofulvin effect.

Additional interactions on page 838.

 INTERACTION WITH OTHER SUBSTANCES

INTERACTS WITH	COMBINED EFFECT
Alcohol:	Possible decreased anticonvulsant effect. Use with caution.
Beverages:	None expected.
Cocaine:	Possible seizures.
Foods:	None expected.
Marijuana:	Drowsiness, unsteadiness, decreased anti-convulsant effect.
Tobacco:	None expected.

MEPHOBARBITAL

BRAND NAMES

Mebaral

GENERAL INFORMATION

Habit forming? Yes
Prescription needed? Yes
Available as generic? Yes
Drug class: Sedative, hypnotic (barbiturate)

 USES

- Reduces anxiety or nervous tension (low dose).
- Relieves insomnia (higher bedtime dose).
- Prevents seizures in epilepsy.

 DOSAGE & USAGE INFORMATION

How to take:
Tablet—Swallow with liquid or food to lessen stomach irritation. If you can't swallow whole, crumble tablet and take with liquid or food.

When to take:
At the same times each day.

If you forget a dose:
Take as soon as you remember up to 2 hours late. If more than 2 hours, wait for next scheduled dose (don't double this dose).

What drug does:
May partially block nerve impulses at nerve-cell connections.

Time lapse before drug works:
60 minutes.

Don't take with:
- Non-prescription drugs without consulting doctor.
- See Interaction column and consult doctor.

 OVERDOSE

Symptoms:
Deep sleep, weak pulse, coma.

What to do:
- Dial 0 (operator) or 911 (emergency) for an ambulance or medical help. Then give first aid immediately.
- If patient is unconscious and not breathing, give mouth-to-mouth breathing. If there is no heartbeat use cardiac massage and mouth-to-mouth breathing (CPR). Don't try to make patient vomit. If you can't help quickly, take patient to nearest emergency facility.
- Additional emergency information on page 886.

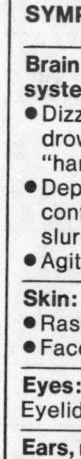 POSSIBLE ADVERSE REACTIONS OR SIDE EFFECTS

SYMPTOMS	FREQUENCY	WHAT TO DO
Brain & nervous system:		
● Dizziness, drowsiness, "hangover effect."	Common	4
● Depression, confusion, slurred speech.	Infrequent	4
● Agitation	Rare	3
Skin:		
● Rash or hives.	Infrequent	3
● Face, lip swelling.	Infrequent	3
Eyes:		
Eyelid swelling.	Infrequent	3
Ears, nose, throat:		
Sore throat, fever.	Infrequent	3
Digestive:		
Diarrhea, nausea, vomiting.	Infrequent	4
Heart & lungs:		
● Slow heartbeat.	Rare	3
● Breathing difficulty.	Rare	3
Blood vessels:		
Unexplained bleeding or bruising.	Rare	4
Muscles, bones, joints:		
Joint or muscle pain.	Infrequent	4
Genital, urinary:	None expected.	
Kidneys:	None expected.	
Liver:		
Jaundice (yellow skin and eyes).	Rare	3
Allergic:	None expected.	
Blood:	None expected.	
Others:	None expected.	

1-Life-threatening. Seek emergency treatment immediately.
2-Discontinue. Seek emergency treatment.
3-Discontinue. Call doctor right away.
4-Continue. Call doctor when convenient.

WARNINGS & PRECAUTIONS

Don't take if:
- You are allergic to any barbiturate.
- You have porphyria.

Before you start, consult your doctor:
- If you have epilepsy.
- If you have kidney or liver damage.
- If you have asthma.
- If you have anemia.
- If you have chronic pain.
- If you will have surgery within 2 months, including dental surgery, requiring general or spinal anesthesia.

Over age 60:
Adverse reactions and side effects may be more frequent and severe than in younger persons. Use small doses.

Pregnancy:
Risk to unborn child outweighs drug benefits. Don't use.

Breast-feeding:
Drug passes into milk. Avoid drug or discontinue nursing until you finish medicine. Consult doctor for advice on maintaining milk supply.

Infants & children:
Use only under doctor's supervision.

Prolonged use:
- May cause addiction, anemia, chronic intoxication.
- May lower body temperature, making exposure to cold temperatures hazardous.

Skin & sunlight:
May cause rash or intensify sunburn in areas exposed to sun or sunlamp.

Driving, piloting or hazardous work:
Don't drive or pilot aircraft until you learn how medicine affects you. Don't work around dangerous machinery. Don't climb ladders or work in high places. Danger increases if you drink alcohol or take medicine affecting alertness and reflexes.

Airplane passengers:
No problems expected.

Discontinuing:
May be unnecessary to finish medicine. Follow doctor's instructions. If you develop withdrawal symptoms of hallucinations, agitation or sleeplessness after discontinuing, call doctor right away.

Others:
No problems expected.

INTERACTION WITH OTHER DRUGS

GENERIC NAME OR DRUG CLASS	COMBINED EFFECT
Anticoagulants (oral)	Decreased anticoagulant effect.
Anticonvulsants	Changed seizure patterns.
Antidepressants (tricyclic)	Decreased antidepressant effect.
Antidiabetics (oral)	Increased mephobarbital effect.
Antihistamines	Dangerous sedation. Avoid.
Antiinflammatory drugs (non-steroidal)	Decreased antiinflammatory effect.
Aspirin	Decreased aspirin effect.
Beta-adrenergic blockers	Decreased effect of beta-adrenergic blocker.
Contraceptives (oral)	Decreased contraceptive effect.
Cortisone drugs	Decreased cortisone effect.
Digitoxin	Decreased digitoxin effect.
Doxycycline	Decreased doxycycline effect.
Griseofulvin	Decreased griseofulvin effect.

Additional interactions on page 839.

INTERACTION WITH OTHER SUBSTANCES

INTERACTS WITH	COMBINED EFFECT
Alcohol:	Possible fatal oversedation. Avoid.
Beverages:	None expected.
Cocaine:	Decreased mephobarbital effect.
Foods:	None expected.
Marijuana:	Excessive sedation. Avoid.
Tobacco:	None expected.

MEPROBAMATE

BRAND NAMES

Arcoban	Kalmn	Meprospan	Novo-Mepro
Bamate	Lan-Dol	Meprotabs	Pax 400
Bamo 400	Medi-Tran	Meribam	Quietal
Coprobate	Mep-E	Miltown	Robamate
Deprol (M)	Meprocon	Neo-Tran	SK-Bamate
Equanil			

GENERAL INFORMATION

Habit forming? Yes
Prescription needed? Yes
Available as generic? Yes
Drug class: Tranquilizer

 ## USES

Reduces mild anxiety, tension and insomnia.

 ## DOSAGE & USAGE INFORMATION

How to take:
- Tablet or capsule—Swallow with liquid.
- Extended-release tablets or capsules—Swallow each dose whole. If you take regular tablets, you may chew or crush them.
- Liquid—Take as directed on label.

When to take:
At the same time each day.

If you forget a dose:
Take as soon as you remember up to 2 hours late. If more than 2 hours, wait for next scheduled dose (don't double this dose).

What drug does:
Sedates brain centers which control behavior and emotions.

Time lapse before drug works:
1 to 2 hours.

Don't take with:
- Non-prescription drugs containing alcohol or caffeine without consulting doctor.
- See Interaction column and consult doctor.

 ## OVERDOSE

Symptoms:
Dizziness, slurred speech, stagger, depressed breathing and heart function, stupor, coma.

What to do:
- Dial 0 (operator) or 911 (emergency) for an ambulance or medical help. Then give first aid immediately.
- Additional emergency information on page 886.

 ## POSSIBLE ADVERSE REACTIONS OR SIDE EFFECTS

SYMPTOMS	FREQUENCY	WHAT TO DO
Brain & nervous system:		
• Dizziness, confusion, agitation, drowsiness, unsteadiness.	Common	5
• False sense of well-being, headache, slurred speech.	Infrequent	4
Skin:		
Rash, hives, itch.	Infrequent	3
Eyes:		
Vision changes.	Infrequent	3
Ears, nose, throat:		
Sore throat, fever.	Rare	3
Digestive:		
Diarrhea, nausea or vomiting.	Infrequent	3
Heart & lungs:		
Rapid, pounding, unusually slow or irregular heartbeat, breathing difficulty.	Rare	3
Blood vessels, muscles, bones, joints, genital, urinary, kidneys, liver, allergic:	None expected.	
Blood:		
Unusual bleeding or bruising.	Rare	3
Others:		
Fatigue, weakness.	Common	5

1 - Life-threatening. Seek emergency treatment immediately.
2 - Discontinue. Seek emergency treatment.
3 - Discontinue. Call doctor right away.
4 - Continue. Call doctor when convenient.
5 - Continue. Tell doctor at next visit.

MEPROBAMATE

WARNINGS & PRECAUTIONS

Don't take if:
- You are allergic to meprobamate, tybanate, carbromal or carisoprodol.
- You have had porphyria.
- Patient is younger than 6.

Before you start, consult your doctor:
- If you have epilepsy.
- If you have impaired liver or kidney function.

Over age 60:
Adverse reactions and side effects may be more frequent and severe than in younger persons.

Pregnancy:
Risk to unborn child outweighs drug benefits. Don't use.

Breast-feeding:
Drug filters into milk. May harm child. Avoid.

Infants & children:
Not recommended.

Prolonged use:
- Habit forming.
- May impair blood-cell production.

Skin & sunlight:
No problems expected.

Driving, piloting or hazardous work:
Don't drive or pilot aircraft until you learn how medicine affects you. Don't work around dangerous machinery. Don't climb ladders or work in high places. Danger increases if you drink alcohol or take medicine affecting alertness and reflexes, such as antihistamines, tranquilizers, sedatives, pain medicine, narcotics and mind-altering drugs.

Airplane passengers:
No problems expected.

Discontinuing:
Don't discontinue without consulting doctor. Dose may require gradual reduction if you have taken drug for a long time. Doses of other drugs may also require adjustment.

Others:
No problems expected.

INTERACTION WITH OTHER DRUGS

GENERIC NAME OR DRUG CLASS	COMBINED EFFECT
Anticoagulants	Decreased anticoagulant effect.
Anticonvulsants	Change in seizure pattern.
Antidepressants	Increased antidepressant effect.
Contraceptives (oral)	Decreased contraceptive effect.
Estrogens	Decreased estrogen effect.
MAO inhibitors	Increased meprobamate effect.
Narcotics	Increased narcotic effect.
Sedatives	Increased sedative effect.
Sleep inducers	Increased effect of sleep inducer.
Tranquilizers	Increased tranquilizer effect.

INTERACTION WITH OTHER SUBSTANCES

INTERACTS WITH	COMBINED EFFECT
Alcohol:	Dangerous increased effect of meprobamate.
Beverages: Caffeine drinks	Decreased calming effect of meprobamate.
Cocaine:	Decreased meprobamate effect.
Foods:	None expected.
Marijuana:	Increased sedative effect of meprobamate.
Tobacco:	None expected.

MESORIDAZINE

BRAND NAMES

Serentil

GENERAL INFORMATION

Habit forming? No
Prescription needed? Yes
Available as generic? Yes
Drug class: Tranquilizer, antiemetic (phenothiazine)

USES

- Stops nausea, vomiting.
- Reduces anxiety, agitation.

DOSAGE & USAGE INFORMATION

How to take:
- Tablet or capsule—Swallow with liquid or food to lessen stomach irritation.
- Suppositories—Remove wrapper and moisten suppository with water. Gently insert into rectum, large end first.
- Drops or liquid—Dilute dose in beverage.

When to take:
- Nervous and mental disorders—Take at the same times each day.
- Nausea and vomiting—Take as needed, no more often than every 4 hours.

If you forget a dose:
- Nervous and mental disorders—Take up to 2 hours late. If more than 2 hours, wait for next scheduled dose (don't double this).
- Nausea and vomiting—Take as soon as you remember. Wait 4 hours for next dose.

What drug does:
- Suppresses brain's vomiting center.
- Suppresses brain centers that control abnormal emotions and behavior.

Time lapse before drug works:
- Nausea and vomiting—1 hour or less.
- Nervous and mental disorders—4-6 weeks.

Don't take with:
- Antacid or medicine for diarrhea.
- Non-prescription drug for cough, cold or allergy.
- See Interaction column and consult doctor.

OVERDOSE

Symptoms:
Stupor, convulsions, coma.

What to do:
- Dial 0 (operator) or 911 (emergency) for an ambulance or medical help. Then give first aid immediately.
- Additional emergency information on page 886.

POSSIBLE ADVERSE REACTIONS OR SIDE EFFECTS

SYMPTOMS	FREQUENCY	WHAT TO DO
Brain & nervous system:		
• Restlessness, tremor.	Common	3
• Fainting	Infrequent	2
• Drowsiness	Common	3
Skin:		
• Rash	Infrequent	3
• Less perspiration.	Common	4
Eyes:		
Vision changes.	Rare	3
Ears, nose, throat:		
• Sore throat, fever.	Rare	3
• Dry mouth, nasal congestion.	Common	4
Digestive:		
Constipation	Common	4
Heart & lungs, blood vessels, kidneys, allergic, blood:	None expected.	
Muscles, bones, joints:		
Muscle spasms of face and neck, unsteady gait.	Common	2
Genital, urinary:		
Urination difficulty.	Infrequent	4
Liver:		
Jaundice (yellow eyes and skin).	Rare	3
Others:		
Less interest in sex, breast swelling, change in menstrual pattern.	Infrequent	4

1- Life-threatening. Seek emergency treatment immediately.
2- Discontinue. Seek emergency treatment.
3- Discontinue. Call doctor right away.
4- Continue. Call doctor when convenient.
5- Continue. Tell doctor at next visit.
6- No action necessary.

MESORIDAZINE

WARNINGS & PRECAUTIONS

Don't take if:
- You are allergic to any phenothiazine.
- You have a blood or bone-marrow disease.

Before you start, consult your doctor:
- If you will have surgery within 2 months, including dental surgery, requiring general or spinal anesthesia.
- If you have asthma, emphysema or other lung disorder.
- If you take non-prescription ulcer medicine, asthma medicine or amphetamines.

Over age 60:
Adverse reactions and side effects may be more frequent and severe than in younger persons. More likely to develop involuntary movement of jaws, lips, tongue, chewing. Report this to your doctor immediately. Early treatment can help.

Pregnancy:
Risk to unborn child outweighs drug benefits. Don't use.

Breast-feeding:
Drug passes into milk. Avoid drug or discontinue nursing until you finish medicine. Consult doctor for advice on maintaining milk supply.

Infants & children:
Don't give to children younger than 2.

Prolonged use:
May lead to tardive dyskinesia (Involuntary movement of jaws, lips, tongue, chewing).

Skin & sunlight:
May cause rash or intensify sunburn in areas exposed to sun or sunlamp. Skin may remain sensitive for 3 months after discontinuing.

Driving, piloting or hazardous work:
Don't drive or pilot aircraft until you learn how medicine affects you. Don't work around dangerous machinery. Don't climb ladders or work in high places. Danger increases if you drink alcohol or take medicine affecting alertness and reflexes.

Airplane passengers:
No problems expected.

Discontinuing:
- Nervous and mental disorders—Don't discontinue without doctor's advice until you complete prescribed dose, even though symptoms diminish or disappear.
- Nausea and vomiting—May be unnecessary to finish medicine. Follow doctor's instructions.

INTERACTION WITH OTHER DRUGS

GENERIC NAME OR DRUG CLASS	COMBINED EFFECT
Anticholinergics	Increased anticholinergic effect.
Antidepressants (tricyclic)	Increased mesoridazine effect.
Antihistamines	Increased antihistamine effect.
Appetite suppressants	Decreased suppressant effect.
Levodopa	Decreased levodopa effect.
Mind-altering drugs	Increased effect of mind-altering drugs.
Narcotics	Increased narcotic effect.
Phenytoin	Increased phenytoin effect.
Quinidine	Impaired heart function. Dangerous mixture.
Sedatives	Increased sedative effect.
Tranquilizers (other)	Increased tranquilizer effect.

INTERACTION WITH OTHER SUBSTANCES

INTERACTS WITH	COMBINED EFFECT
Alcohol:	Dangerous oversedation.
Beverages:	None expected.
Cocaine:	Decreased effect of mesoridazine. Avoid.
Foods:	None expected.
Marijuana:	Drowsiness. May increase antinausea effect.
Tobacco:	None expected.

METAPROTERENOL

BRAND NAMES

Alupent
Metaprel

GENERAL INFORMATION

Habit forming? No
Prescription needed? Yes
Available as generic? No
Drug class: Bronchodilator, sympathomimetic

 USES

Relieves wheezing and shortness of breath in bronchial asthma attacks, bronchitis and emphysema.

 DOSAGE & USAGE INFORMATION

How to take:
- Tablet or liquid—Swallow with liquid or food to lessen stomach irritation.
- Inhaler—Follow instructions on package.

When to take:
When needed, according to doctor's instructions. Don't take more than 2 doses 1 hour apart.

If you forget a dose:
Take when you remember. Wait 2 hours for next dose.

What drug does:
Relaxes smooth muscles to relieve constriction of bronchial tubes.

Time lapse before drug works:
5 to 30 minutes.

Don't take with:
See Interaction column and consult doctor.

 OVERDOSE

Symptoms:
Chest pain, irregular heartbeat, convulsions, coma.

What to do:
- Dial 0 (operator) or 911 (emergency) for an ambulance or medical help. Then give first aid immediately.
- If patient is unconscious and not breathing, give mouth-to-mouth breathing. If there is no heartbeat, use cardiac massage and mouth-to-mouth breathing (CPR). Don't try to make patient vomit. If you can't get help quickly, take patient to nearest emergency facility.
- Additional emergency information on page 886.

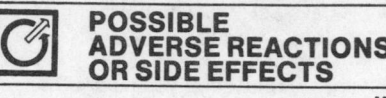 **POSSIBLE ADVERSE REACTIONS OR SIDE EFFECTS**

SYMPTOMS	FREQUENCY	WHAT TO DO
Brain & nervous system: Nervousness, restlessness, dizziness, weakness, headache, trembling.	Common	4
Skin: Paleness	Infrequent	4
Eyes:	None expected.	
Ears, nose, throat: Bad taste in mouth.	Infrequent	4
Digestive: Nausea or vomiting.	Infrequent	4
Heart & lungs: • Rapid or pounding heartbeat.	Common	3
• Chest pain.	Infrequent	3
Blood vessels:	None expected.	
Muscles, bones, joints: Muscle cramps in arms, hands, legs.	Infrequent	3
Genital, urinary:	None expected.	
Kidneys:	None expected.	
Liver:	None expected.	
Allergic:	None expected.	
Blood:	None expected.	
Others: Unusual sweating.	Infrequent	3

1- Life-threatening. Seek emergency treatment immediately.
2- Discontinue. Seek emergency treatment.
3- Discontinue. Call doctor right away.
4- Continue. Call doctor when convenient.
5- Continue. Tell doctor at next visit.
6- No action necessary.

WARNINGS & PRECAUTIONS

Don't take if:
You are allergic to any sympathomimetic.

Before you start, consult your doctor:
- If you have irregular or rapid heartbeat, congestive heart failure, coronary-artery disease or high blood pressure.
- If you have diabetes.
- If you have overactive thyroid.

Over age 60:
Adverse reactions and side effects may be more frequent and severe than in younger persons.

Pregnancy:
Risk to unborn child outweighs drug benefits. Don't use.

Breast-feeding:
Drug passes into milk. Avoid drug or discontinue nursing until you finish medicine. Consult doctor for advice on maintaining milk supply.

Infants & children:
Use only under medical supervision.

Prolonged use:
No problems expected.

Skin & sunlight:
No problems expected.

Driving, piloting or hazardous work:
Don't drive or pilot aircraft until you learn how medicine affects you. Don't work around dangerous machinery. Don't climb ladders or work in high places. Danger increases if you drink alcohol or take medicine affecting alertness and reflexes, such as antihistamines, tranquilizers, sedatives, pain medicine, narcotics and mind-altering drugs.

Airplane passengers:
No problems expected.

Discontinuing:
No problems expected.

Others:
Consult doctor immediately if breathing difficulty continues or worsens after using metaproterenol.

INTERACTION WITH OTHER DRUGS

GENERIC NAME OR DRUG CLASS	COMBINED EFFECT
Antidepressants (tricyclic)	Increased effect of both drugs.
Beta-adrenergic blockers	Decreased metaproterenol effect.
Hydralazine	Decreased hydralazine effect.
Sympathomimetics (other)	Increased effect of both drugs, especially harmful side effects.

INTERACTION WITH OTHER SUBSTANCES

INTERACTS WITH	COMBINED EFFECT
Alcohol:	Decreased metaproterenol effect.
Beverages:	None expected.
Cocaine:	Possible metaproterenol toxicity.
Foods:	None expected.
Marijuana:	Overstimulation. Avoid.
Tobacco:	No proven problems.

METHACYCLINE

BRAND NAMES

Rondomycin

GENERAL INFORMATION

Habit forming? No
Prescription needed? Yes
Available as generic? No
Drug class: Antibiotic (tetracycline)

USES

- Treatment for infections susceptible to methacycline. Will not cure virus infections such as colds or flu.
- Treatment for acne.

DOSAGE & USAGE INFORMATION

How to take:
Capsule—Take on empty stomach 1 hour before or 2 hours after eating. If you can't swallow whole, open capsule and take with liquid or food.

When to take:
At the same times each day, evenly spaced.

If you forget a dose:
Take as soon as you remember up to 2 hours late. If more than 2 hours, wait for next scheduled dose (don't double this dose).

What drug does:
Prevents germ growth and reproduction.

Time lapse before drug works:
- Infections—May require 5 days to affect infection.
- Acne—May require 4 weeks to affect acne.

Don't take with:
- Non-prescription drugs without consulting doctor.
- See Interaction column and consult doctor.

OVERDOSE

Symptoms:
Severe nausea, vomiting, diarrhea.

What to do:
Overdose unlikely to threaten life. If person takes much larger amount than prescribed, call doctor, poison-control center or hospital emergency room for instructions.

POSSIBLE ADVERSE REACTIONS OR SIDE EFFECTS

SYMPTOMS	FREQUENCY	WHAT TO DO
Brain & nervous system:		
Headache	Infrequent	3
Skin:		
• Itching around rectum and genitals.	Common	3
• Rash	Infrequent	3
Eyes:		
Blurred vision.	Rare	3
Ears, nose, throat:		
• Dark tongue.	Common	5
• Sore mouth or tongue.	Common	2
• Excessive thirst.	Infrequent	4
Digestive:		
Nausea, vomiting, diarrhea, abdominal burning.	Common	2
Heart & lungs:	None expected.	
Blood vessels:	None expected.	
Muscles, bones, joints:	None expected.	
Genital, urinary:		
Increased urination.	Infrequent	4
Kidneys:	None expected.	
Liver:		
Jaundice (yellow eyes and skin) in pregnant women.	Rare	3
Allergic:	None expected.	
Blood:	None expected.	
Others:	None expected.	

1- Life-threatening. Seek emergency treatment immediately.
2- Discontinue. Seek emergency treatment.
3- Discontinue. Call doctor right away.
4- Continue. Call doctor when convenient.
5- Continue. Tell doctor at next visit.
6- No action necessary.

WARNINGS & PRECAUTIONS

Don't take if:
You are allergic to any tetracycline antibiotic.

Before you start, consult your doctor:
● If you have kidney or liver disease.
● If you have lupus.
● If you have myasthenia gravis.

Over age 60:
Dosage usually less than in younger adults. More likely to cause itching around rectum. Ask you doctor how to prevent it.

Pregnancy:
Risk to unborn child outweighs drug benefits. Don't use.

Breast-feeding:
Drug passes into milk. Avoid drug or discontinue nursing until you finish medicine. Consult doctor for advice on maintaining milk supply.

Infants & children:
May cause permanent teeth malformation or discoloration in children less than 8 years old. Don't use.

Prolonged use:
● You may become more susceptible to infections caused by germs not responsive to methacycline.
● May cause rare problems in liver, kidney or bone marrow. Periodic laboratory blood studies, liver- and kidney-function tests recommended if you use drug a long time.

Skin & sunlight:
May cause rash or intensify sunburn in areas exposed to sun or sunlamp.

Driving, piloting or hazardous work:
No problems expected.

Airplane passengers:
No problems expected.

Discontinuing:
Don't discontinue without doctor's advice until you complete prescribed dose, even though symptoms diminish or disappear.

Others:
No problems expected.

INTERACTION WITH OTHER DRUGS

GENERIC NAME OR DRUG CLASS	COMBINED EFFECT
Antacids	Decreased methacycline effect.
Anticoagulants (oral)	Increased anticoagulant effect.
Contraceptives (oral)	Decreased contraceptive effect.
Digitalis preparations	Increased digitalis effect.
Mineral supplements (iron, calcium, magnesium, zinc)	Decreased methacycline absorption. Separate doses by 1 to 2 hours.
Lithium	Increased lithium effect.
Penicillins	Decreased penicillin effect.
Sodium bicarbonate	Decreased methacycline effect.

INTERACTION WITH OTHER SUBSTANCES

INTERACTS WITH	COMBINED EFFECT
Alcohol:	Possible liver damage. Avoid.
Beverages: Milk	Decreased methacycline absorption. Take dose 2 hours after or 1 hour before drinking.
Cocaine:	No proven problems.
Foods: Dairy products	Decreased methacycline absorption. Take dose 2 hours after or 1 hour before eating.
Marijuana:	No interactions expected, but marijuana may slow body's recovery. Avoid.
Tobacco:	None expected.

METHADONE

BRAND NAMES

Dolophine

GENERAL INFORMATION

Habit forming? Yes
Prescription needed? Yes
Available as generic? Yes
Drug class: Narcotic

USES

Relieves pain.

DOSAGE & USAGE INFORMATION

How to take:
- Tablet or capsule—Swallow with liquid. If you can't swallow whole, crumble tablet or open capsule and take with liquid or food.
- Drops or liquid—Dilute dose in beverage before swallowing.

When to take:
When needed. No more often than every 4 hours.

If you forget a dose:
Take as soon as you remember. Wait 4 hours for next dose.

What drug does:
Blocks pain messages to brain and spinal cord.

Time lapse before drug works:
30 minutes.

Don't take with:
See Interaction column and consult doctor.

OVERDOSE

Symptoms:
Deep sleep; slow breathing; slow pulse; flushed, warm skin; constricted pupils.

What to do:
- Dial 0 (operator) or 911 (emergency) for an ambulance or medical help. Then give first aid immediately.
- If patient is unconscious and not breathing, give mouth-to-mouth breathing. If there is no heartbeat, use cardiac massage and mouth-to-mouth breathing (CPR). Don't try to make patient vomit. If you can't get help quickly, take patient to nearest emergency facility.
- Additional emergency information on page 886.

POSSIBLE ADVERSE REACTIONS OR SIDE EFFECTS

SYMPTOMS	FREQUENCY	WHAT TO DO
Brain & nervous system: Depression, confusion, hallucinations.	Infrequent	4
Skin: • Hives, rash, itch, face swelling.	Rare	3
• Flushed face.	Common	4
Eyes: Blurred vision.	Rare	4
Ears, nose, throat:	None expected.	
Digestive: Severe constipation, abdominal pain, vomiting.	Infrequent	3
Heart & lungs: Slow heartbeat, irregular breathing.	Rare	3
Blood vessels:	None expected.	
Muscles, bones, joints:	None expected.	
Genital, urinary: Difficult urination.	Common	4
Kidneys: Less urine.	Common	4
Liver:	None expected.	
Allergic:	None expected.	
Blood:	None expected.	
Others: Unusual tiredness.	Common	4

1- Life-threatening. Seek emergency treatment immediately.
2- Discontinue. Seek emergency treatment.
3- Discontinue. Call doctor right away.
4- Continue. Call doctor when convenient.
5- Continue. Tell doctor at next visit.
6- No action necessary.

WARNINGS & PRECAUTIONS

Don't take if:
You are allergic to any narcotic.

Before you start, consult your doctor:
If you have impaired liver or kidney function.

Over age 60:
More likely to be drowsy, dizzy, unsteady or constipated. Avoid prolonged use.

Pregnancy:
Studies inconclusive on harm to unborn child. Animal studies show fetal abnormalities. Decide with your doctor whether drug benefits justify risk to unborn child. Abuse by pregnant woman will result in addicted newborn. Withdrawal can be life-threatening.

Breast-feeding:
Drug filters into milk. May depress infant. Avoid.

Infants & children:
Not recommended.

Prolonged use:
Causes psychological and physical dependence.

Skin & sunlight:
No problems expected.

Driving, piloting or hazardous work:
Don't drive or pilot aircraft until you learn how medicine affects you. Don't work around dangerous machinery. Don't climb ladders or work in high places. Danger increases if you drink alcohol or take medicine affecting alertness and reflexes, such as antihistamines, tranquilizers, sedatives, pain medicine, other narcotics and mind-altering drugs.

Airplane passengers:
No problems expected.

Discontinuing:
May be unnecessary to finish medicine. Follow doctor's instructions.

Others:
No problems expected.

INTERACTION WITH OTHER DRUGS

GENERIC NAME OR DRUG CLASS	COMBINED EFFECT
Analgesics	Increased analgesic effect.
Antidepressants	Increased sedative effect.
Antihistamines	Increased sedative effect.
Mind-altering drugs	Increased sedative effect.
Narcotics (other)	Increased narcotic effect.
Phenothiazines	Increased phenothiazine effect.
Sedatives	Increased sedative effect.
Sleep inducers	Increased sedative effect.
Tranquilizers	Increased sedative effect.

INTERACTION WITH OTHER SUBSTANCES

INTERACTS WITH	COMBINED EFFECT
Alcohol:	Increases alcohol's intoxicating effect. Avoid.
Beverages:	None expected.
Cocaine:	Increased cocaine effect.
Foods:	None expected.
Marijuana:	Impairs physical and mental performance.
Tobacco:	None expected.

METHAMPHETAMINE

BRAND NAMES

Desoxyn
Methampex

GENERAL INFORMATION

Habit forming? Yes
Prescription needed? Yes
Available as generic? Yes
Drug class: Central-nervous-system stimulant (amphetamine)

 USES

- Prevents narcolepsy (attacks of uncontrollable sleepiness).
- Controls hyperactivity in children.

 DOSAGE & USAGE INFORMATION

How to take:
- Tablet—Swallow with liquid.
- Extended-release tablets—Swallow each dose whole with liquid.

When to take:
- At the same times each day.
- Short-acting form—Don't take later than 6 hours before bedtime.
- Long-acting form—Take on awakening.

If you forget a dose:
- Short-acting form—Take up to 2 hours late. If more than 2 hours, wait for next dose (don't double this).
- Long-acting form—Take as soon as you remember. Wait 20 hours for next dose.

What drug does:
- Narcolepsy—Apparently affects brain centers to decrease fatigue or sleepiness and increase alertness and motor activity.
- Hyperactive children—Calms children, opposite to effect on narcoleptic adults.

Time lapse before drug works:
15 to 30 minutes.

Don't take with:
See Interaction column and consult doctor.

 OVERDOSE

Symptoms:
Rapid heartbeat, hyperactivity, high fever, hallucinations, suicidal or homicidal feelings, convulsions, coma.

What to do:
- Dial 0 (operator) or 911 (emergency) for an ambulance or medical help. Then give first aid immediately.
- Additional emergency information on page 886.

POSSIBLE ADVERSE REACTIONS OR SIDE EFFECTS

SYMPTOMS	FREQUENCY	WHAT TO DO
Brain & nervous system:		
● Headache	Infrequent	4
● Dizziness, lack of alertness.	Infrequent	3
● Mood changes.	Rare	4
● Irritability, nervousness, insomnia.	Common	4
Skin:		
Rash, hives.	Rare	3
Eyes:		
Blurred vision.	Infrequent	3
Ears, nose, throat:		
Dry mouth.	Common	5
Digestive:		
Diarrhea or constipation, appetite loss, stomach pain, nausea, vomiting, weight loss.	Infrequent	5
Heart & lungs:		
● Fast, pounding heartbeat.	Infrequent	3
● Chest pain or irregular heartbeat.	Rare	3
Blood vessels, kidneys, liver, allergic, blood:	None expected.	
Muscles, bones, joints:		
Uncontrolled movements of head, neck, arms, legs.	Rare	3
Genital, urinary:		
Decreased sex drive, impotence.	Infrequent	5
Others:		
● Enlarged breasts.	Rare	4
● Unusual sweating.	Infrequent	3

1-Life-threatening. Seek emergency treatment immediately.
2-Discontinue. Seek emergency treatment.
3-Discontinue. Call doctor right away.
4-Continue. Call doctor when convenient.
5-Continue. Tell doctor at next visit.

METHAMPHETAMINE

WARNINGS & PRECAUTIONS

Don't take if:
- You are allergic to any methamphetamine.
- You will have surgery within 2 months, including dental surgery, requiring general or spinal anesthesia.

Before you start, consult your doctor:
- If you plan to become pregnant within medication period.
- If you have glaucoma.
- If you have heart or blood-vessel disease, or high blood pressure.
- If you have overactive thyroid, anxiety or tension.
- If you have a severe mental illness (especially children).

Over age 60:
Adverse reactions and side effects may be more frequent and severe than in younger persons.

Pregnancy:
Risk to unborn child outweighs drug benefits. Don't use.

Breast-feeding:
Drug passes into milk. Avoid drug or discontinue nursing.

Infants & children:
Not recommended for children under 12.

Prolonged use:
Habit forming.

Skin & sunlight:
No problems expected.

Driving, piloting or hazardous work:
Don't drive or pilot aircraft until you learn how medicine affects you. Don't work around dangerous machinery. Don't climb ladders or work in high places. Danger increases if you drink alcohol or take medicine affecting alertness and reflexes.

Airplane passengers:
No problems expected.

Discontinuing:
May be unnecessary to finish medicine. Follow doctor's instructions.

Others:
- This is a dangerous drug and must be closely supervised. Don't use for appetite control or depression. Potential for damage and abuse.
- During withdrawal phase, may cause prolonged sleep of several days.

INTERACTION WITH OTHER DRUGS

GENERIC NAME OR DRUG CLASS	COMBINED EFFECT
Anesthesias (general)	Irregular heartbeat.
Antidepressants (tricyclic)	Decreased methamphetamine effect.
Antihypertensives	Decreased antihypertensive effect.
Carbonic anhydrase inhibitors	Increased methamphetamine effect.
Guanethidine	Decreased guanethidine effect.
Haloperidol	Decreased methamphetamine effect.
MAO inhibitors	May severely increase blood pressure.
Phenothiazines	Decreased methamphetamine effect.
Sodium bicarbonate	Increased methamphetamine effect.

INTERACTION WITH OTHER SUBSTANCES

INTERACTS WITH	COMBINED EFFECT
Alcohol:	Decreased methamphetamine effect. Avoid.
Beverages: Caffeine drinks	Overstimulation. Avoid.
Cocaine:	Dangerous stimulation of nervous system. Avoid.
Foods:	None expected.
Marijuana:	Frequent use—Severely impaired mental function.
Tobacco:	None expected.

METHANDROSTENOLONE

BRAND NAMES

Danabol
Dianabol

Habit forming? No
Prescription needed? Yes

Available as generic? Yes
Drug class: Androgen (male sex hormone)

USES

- Corrects male hormone deficiency.
- Reduces "male menopause" symptoms (loss of sex drive, depression, anxiety).
- Decreases calcium loss of osteoporosis (softened bones).
- Blocks growth of breast-cancer cells in females.
- Corrects undescended testicles in male children.
- Reduces breast pain and fullness following childbirth.
- Augments treatment of aplastic anemia.
- Stimulates weight gain after illness, injury or for chronically underweight persons.
- Stimulates growth in treatment of dwarfism.

DOSAGE & USAGE INFORMATION

How to take:
- Tablets—With food to lessen stomach irritation.
- Injection—Once or twice a month.

When to take:
At the same time each day.

If you forget a dose:
Take as soon as you remember up to 2 hours late. If more than 2 hours, wait for next scheduled dose (don't double this dose).

What drug does:
- Stimulates cells that produce male sex characteristics.
- Replaces hormone deficiencies.
- Stimulates red-blood-cell production.
- Suppresses production of estrogen (female sex hormone).

Time lapse before drug works:
Varies with problems treated. May require 2 or 3 months of regular use for desired effects.

Don't take with:
See Interaction column and consult doctor.

OVERDOSE

Overdose unlikely to threaten life. If person takes much larger amount than prescribed, call doctor, poison-control center or hospital emergency room for instructions.

POSSIBLE ADVERSE REACTIONS OR SIDE EFFECTS

SYMPTOMS	FREQUENCY	WHAT TO DO
Brain & nervous system:		
Depression or confusion.	Infrequent	3
Skin:		
• Flushed face.	Infrequent	3
• Rash or itch.	Infrequent	3
• Hives	Rare	2
• Acne or oily skin in females.	Common	4
Eyes, heart & lungs, blood vessels, kidneys, blood:	None expected.	
Ears, nose, throat:		
• Deep voice.	Common	4
• Sore mouth.	Common	5
• Sore throat, fever.	Rare	3
Digestive:		
• Nausea, vomiting, diarrhea.	Infrequent	3
• Abdominal pain.	Rare	3
• Black stool.	Rare	2
Muscles, bones, joints:		
Swollen feet or legs.	Infrequent	3
Genital, urinary:		
• Enlarged clitoris or frequent erections.	Common	4
• Vaginal bleeding.	Infrequent	3
Liver:		
Jaundice (yellow skin and eyes).	Infrequent	2
Allergic:		
Intense itching, weakness, loss of consciousness.	Rare	1
Others:		
• Higher sex drive.	Common	5
• Swollen breasts in men.	Common	4

1- Life-threatening. Seek emergency treatment immediately.
2- Discontinue. Seek emergency treatment.
3- Discontinue. Call doctor right away.
4- Continue. Call doctor when convenient.
5- Continue. Tell doctor at next visit.

WARNINGS & PRECAUTIONS

Don't take if:
You are allergic to any male hormone.

Before you start, consult your doctor:
- If you might be pregnant.
- If you have cancer of prostate.
- If you have heart disease or arteriosclerosis.
- If you have kidney or liver disease.
- If you have breast cancer (males).
- If you have high blood pressure.
- If you have migraine attacks.
- If you have high level of blood calcium.
- If you have epilepsy.

Over age 60:
- May stimulate sexual activity.
- Can make high blood pressure or heart disease worse.
- Can enlarge prostate and cause urinary retention.

Pregnancy:
Risk to unborn child outweighs drug benefits. Don't use.

Breast-feeding:
Drug passes into milk. Avoid drug or discontinue nursing until you finish medicine. Consult doctor for advice on maintaining milk supply.

Infants & children:
Don't give to children younger than 2. Use with older children only under medical supervision.

Prolonged use:
- Reduces sperm count and volume of semen.
- Possible kidney stones.
- Unnatural hair growth and deep voice in women.

Skin & sunlight:
No problems expected.

Driving, piloting or hazardous work:
No problems expected.

Airplane passengers:
No problems expected.

Discontinuing:
No problems expected.

Others:
- May cause atrophy of testicles.
- Will not increase strength in athletes.

INTERACTION WITH OTHER DRUGS

GENERIC NAME OR DRUG CLASS	COMBINED EFFECT
Anticoagulants	Increased anticoagulant effect.
Antidiabetics (oral)	Increased antidiabetic effect.
Chlorzoxazone	Decreased methandrostenolone effect.
Oxyphenbutazone	Decreased methandrostenolone effect.
Phenobarbital	Decreased methandrostenolone effect.
Phenylbutazone	Decreased methandrostenolone effect.

INTERACTION WITH OTHER SUBSTANCES

INTERACTS WITH	COMBINED EFFECT
Alcohol:	None expected.
Beverages:	None expected.
Cocaine:	No proven problems.
Foods: Salt	Excessive fluid retention (edema). Decrease salt intake while taking male hormones.
Marijuana:	Decreased blood levels of methandrostenolone.
Tobacco:	No proven problems.

METHAQUALONE

BRAND NAMES

Mandrax	Quaalude	Tualone
Mequelon	Rouqualone-300	Vitalone
Mequin	Sedalone	
Methadorm	Sopor	
Parest	Triador	

GENERAL INFORMATION

Habit forming? Yes
Prescription needed? Yes
Available as generic? No
Drug class: Hypnotic

USES

Decreases anxiety, tension or insomnia.

DOSAGE & USAGE INFORMATION

How to take:
Tablet or capsule—Swallow with liquid. If you can't swallow whole, crumble tablet or open capsule and take with liquid or food.

When to take:
At the same time each day.

If you forget a dose:
Don't take missed dose. Wait for next scheduled dose. Don't double this dose.

What drug does:
Undetermined.

Time lapse before drug works:
20 to 30 minutes.

Don't take with:
- Alcohol or mind-altering drugs. Combinations can be fatal.
- Non-prescription drugs without consulting doctor.
- See Interaction column and consult doctor.

OVERDOSE

Symptoms:
Drowsiness, confusion, delirium, incoordination, vomiting, convulsions, abnormal bleeding, stupor, coma.

What to do:
- Dial 0 (operator) or 911 (emergency) for an ambulance or medical help. Then give first aid immediately.
- If patient is unconscious and not breathing, give mouth-to-mouth breathing. If there is no heartbeat, use cardiac massage and mouth-to-mouth breathing (CPR). Don't try to make patient vomit. If you can't get help quickly, take patient to nearest emergency facility.
- Additional emergency information on page 886.

POSSIBLE ADVERSE REACTIONS OR SIDE EFFECTS

SYMPTOMS	FREQUENCY	WHAT TO DO
Brain & nervous system:		
• Agitation	Infrequent	3
• Drowsiness	Common	4
• "Hangover-effect."	Common	6
Skin:		
Rash or hives.	Infrequent	3
Eyes:	None expected.	
Ears, nose, throat:	None expected.	
Digestive:		
Diarrhea, nausea, vomiting, stomach pain.	Common	3
Heart & lungs:		
Unusually slow heartbeat, breathing difficulty.	Infrequent	2
Blood vessels:	None expected.	
Muscles, bones, joints:		
Numbness, tingling, pain or weakness in hands or feet.	Infrequent	3
Genital, urinary:	None expected.	
Kidneys:	None expected.	
Liver:	None expected.	
Allergic:	None expected.	
Blood:	None expected.	
Others:		
• Sweating	Infrequent	3
• Tiredness or weakness.	Common	5

1 - Life-threatening. Seek emergency treatment immediately.
2 - Discontinue. Seek emergency treatment.
3 - Discontinue. Call doctor right away.
4 - Continue. Call doctor when convenient.
5 - Continue. Tell doctor at next visit.
6 - No action necessary.

WARNINGS & PRECAUTIONS

Don't take if:
- You are allergic to any hypnotic drug.
- You plan to become pregnant within medication period.
- Patient is younger than 12.

Before you start, consult your doctor:
- If you have had liver disease or impaired liver function.
- If you will have surgery within 2 months, including dental surgery, requiring general or spinal anesthesia.

Over age 60:
Adverse reactions and side effects may be more frequent and severe than in younger persons.

Pregnancy:
Risk to unborn child outweighs drug benefits. Don't use.

Breast-feeding:
Drug may filter into milk and harm child. Don't use.

Infants & children:
Not recommended.

Prolonged use:
Psychological and physical dependence.

Skin & sunlight:
No problems expected.

Driving, piloting or hazardous work:
Don't drive or pilot aircraft until you learn how medicine affects you. Don't work around dangerous machinery. Don't climb ladders or work in high places. Danger increases if you drink alcohol or take medicine affecting alertness and reflexes, such as antihistamines, tranquilizers, sedatives, pain medicine, narcotics and mind-altering drugs.

Airplane passengers:
Not recommended.

Discontinuing:
Don't discontinue without consulting doctor. Dose may require gradual reduction if you have taken drug for a long time. Doses of other drugs may also require adjustment.

Others:
No problems expected.

INTERACTION WITH OTHER DRUGS

GENERIC NAME OR DRUG CLASS	COMBINED EFFECT
Anticoagulants	Decreased anticoagulant effect.
Antihistamines	Increased sedation.
Narcotics	Increased narcotic effect.
Pain relievers	Increased effect of pain reliever.
Sedatives	Increased sedative effect.
Sleep inducers	Increased effect of sleep inducer.
Tranquilizers	Increased tranquilizer effect.

INTERACTION WITH OTHER SUBSTANCES

INTERACTS WITH	COMBINED EFFECT
Alcohol:	Dangerous depression of brain function. Avoid.
Beverages:	None expected.
Cocaine:	Decreased effect of both drugs. Avoid.
Foods:	None expected.
Marijuana:	Impairs physical performance. Avoid.
Tobacco:	None expected.

METHARBITAL

BRAND NAMES

Gemonil

GENERAL INFORMATION

Habit forming? Yes
Prescription needed? Yes
Available as generic? Yes
Drug class: Sedative, hypnotic (barbiturate)

USES

Prevents convulsions.

DOSAGE & USAGE INFORMATION

How to take:
Tablet—Swallow with liquid or food to lessen stomach irritation. If you can't swallow whole, crumble tablet and take with liquid or food.

When to take:
At the same times each day.

If you forget a dose:
Take as soon as you remember up to 2 hours late. If more than 2 hours, wait for next scheduled dose (don't double this dose).

What drug does:
May partially block nerve impulses at nerve-cell connections.

Time lapse before drug works:
60 minutes.

Don't take with:
- Non-prescription drugs without consulting doctor.
- See Interaction column and consult doctor.

OVERDOSE

Symptoms:
Deep sleep, weak pulse, coma.

What to do:
- Dial 0 (operator) or 911 (emergency) for an ambulance or medical help. Then give first aid immediately.
- If patient is unconscious and not breathing, give mouth-to-mouth breathing. If there is no heartbeat use cardiac massage and mouth-to-mouth breathing (CPR). Don't try to make patient vomit. If you can't help quickly, take patient to nearest emergency facility.
- Additional emergency information on page 886.

POSSIBLE ADVERSE REACTIONS OR SIDE EFFECTS

SYMPTOMS	FREQUENCY	WHAT TO DO
Brain & nervous system:		
● Dizziness, drowsiness, "hangover effect."	Common	4
● Depression, confusion, slurred speech.	Infrequent	4
● Agitation	Rare	3
Skin:		
● Rash or hives.	Infrequent	3
● Face, lip swelling.	Infrequent	3
Eyes:		
Eyelid swelling.	Infrequent	3
Ears, nose, throat:		
Sore throat, fever.	Infrequent	3
Digestive:		
Diarrhea, nausea, vomiting.	Infrequent	4
Heart & lungs:		
● Slow heartbeat.	Rare	3
● Breathing difficulty.	Rare	3
Blood vessels:		
Unexplained bleeding or bruising.	Rare	4
Muscles, bones, joints:		
Joint or muscle pain.	Infrequent	4
Genital, urinary:	None expected.	
Kidneys:	None expected.	
Liver:		
Jaundice (yellow skin and eyes).	Rare	3
Allergic:	None expected.	
Blood:	None expected.	
Others:	None expected.	

1- Life-threatening. Seek emergency treatment immediately.
2- Discontinue. Seek emergency treatment.
3- Discontinue. Call doctor right away.
4- Continue. Call doctor when convenient.

WARNINGS & PRECAUTIONS

Don't take if:
- You are allergic to any barbiturate.
- You have porphyria.

Before you start, consult your doctor:
- If you have epilepsy.
- If you have kidney or liver damage.
- If you have asthma.
- If you have anemia.
- If you have chronic pain.
- If you will have surgery within 2 months, including dental surgery, requiring general or spinal anesthesia.

Over age 60:
Adverse reactions and side effects may be more frequent and severe than in younger persons. Use small doses.

Pregnancy:
Risk to unborn child outweighs drug benefits. Don't use.

Breast-feeding:
Drug passes into milk. Avoid drug or discontinue nursing until you finish medicine. Consult doctor for advice on maintaining milk supply.

Infants & children:
Use only under doctor's supervision.

Prolonged use:
- May cause addiction, anemia, chronic intoxication.
- May lower body temperature, making exposure to cold temperatures hazardous.

Skin & sunlight:
May cause rash or intensify sunburn in areas exposed to sun or sunlamp.

Driving, piloting or hazardous work:
Don't drive or pilot aircraft until you learn how medicine affects you. Don't work around dangerous machinery. Don't climb ladders or work in high places. Danger increases if you drink alcohol or take medicine affecting alertness and reflexes.

Airplane passengers:
No problems expected.

Discontinuing:
May be unnecessary to finish medicine. Follow doctor's instructions. If you develop withdrawal symptoms of hallucinations, agitation or sleeplessness after discontinuing, call doctor right away.

Others:
No problems expected.

INTERACTION WITH OTHER DRUGS

GENERIC NAME OR DRUG CLASS	COMBINED EFFECT
Anticoagulants (oral)	Decreased anticoagulant effect.
Anticonvulsants	Changed seizure patterns.
Antidepressants (tricyclic)	Decreased antidepressant effect.
Antidiabetics (oral)	Increased metharbital effect.
Antihistamines	Dangerous sedation. Avoid.
Antiinflammatory drugs (non-steroidal)	Decreased antiinflammatory effect.
Aspirin	Decreased aspirin effect.
Beta-adrenergic blockers	Decreased effect of beta-adrenergic blocker.
Contraceptives (oral)	Decreased contraceptive effect.
Cortisone drugs	Decreased cortisone effect.
Digitoxin	Decreased digitoxin effect.
Doxycycline	Decreased doxycycline effect.
Griseofulvin	Decreased griseofulvin effect.

Additional interactions on page 839.

INTERACTION WITH OTHER SUBSTANCES

INTERACTS WITH	COMBINED EFFECT
Alcohol:	Possible fatal oversedation. Avoid.
Beverages:	None expected.
Cocaine:	Decreased metharbital effect.
Foods:	None expected.
Marijuana:	Excessive sedation. Avoid.
Tobacco:	None expected.

METHAZOLAMIDE

BRAND NAMES

Neptazane

Habit forming? No
Prescription needed? Yes
Available as generic? No

GENERAL INFORMATION

Drug class: Diuretic (carbonic anhydrase inhibitor, sulfonamide), antiglaucoma

USES

Treatment of glaucoma.

DOSAGE & USAGE INFORMATION

How to take:
Tablets—Swallow whole with liquid or food to lessen stomach irritation.

When to take:
- 1 dose per day—At the same time each morning.
- More than 1 dose per day—Take last dose several hours before bedtime.

If you forget a dose:
Take as soon as you remember. Continue regular schedule.

What drug does:
- Inhibits action of carbonic anhydrase, an enzyme. This lowers the internal eye pressure by decreasing fluid formation in the eye.
- Forces sodium and water excretion, reducing body fluid.

Time lapse before drug works:
2 hours.

Don't take with:
- Non-prescription drugs without consulting doctor.
- See Interaction column and consult doctor.

OVERDOSE

Symptoms:
Drowsiness, confusion, excitement, nausea, vomiting, numbness in hands and feet, coma.

What to do:
Call your doctor or poison-control center for advice if you suspect overdose, even if not sure. Symptoms may not appear until damage has occurred.

POSSIBLE ADVERSE REACTIONS OR SIDE EFFECTS

SYMPTOMS	FREQUENCY	WHAT TO DO
Brain & nervous system:		
• Headache, mood changes, nervousness, clumsiness, trembling, confusion.	Rare	3
• Convulsions	Rare	1
Skin:		
Hives, itch, rash, or sores.	Rare	3
Ears, nose, throat:		
• Ringing in ears, hoarseness, dry mouth, thirst.	Rare	3
• Sore throat, fever.	Rare	3
Digestive:		
• Appetite change, nausea, vomiting.	Rare	3
• Black, tarry stool.	Rare	3
Heart & lungs:		
Breathing difficulty, irregular or weak heartbeat.	Rare	3
Blood vessels:		
Easy bleeding or bruising.	Rare	3
Muscles, bones, joints:		
Muscle cramps.	Rare	3
Genital, urinary:		
Painful or frequent urination, bloody urine.	Rare	3
Kidneys:		
Back pain.	Infrequent	3
Allergic, blood, liver, eyes:	None expected.	
Others:		
• Fatigue, weakness.	Infrequent	4
• Tingling or burning in feet or hands.	Infrequent	4

1-Life-threatening. Seek emergency treatment immediately.
2-Discontinue. Seek emergency treatment.
3-Discontinue. Call doctor right away.
4-Continue. Call doctor when convenient.

METHAZOLAMIDE

WARNINGS & PRECAUTIONS

Don't take if:
- You are allergic to any carbonic anhydrase inhibitor.
- You have liver or kidney disease.
- You have Addison's disease (adrenal gland failure).
- You have diabetes.

Before you start, consult your doctor:
- If you have gout or lupus.
- If you are allergic to any sulfa drug.

Over age 60:
- Don't exceed recommended dose.
- If you take a digitalis preparation, eat foods high in potassium content or take a potassium supplement.

Pregnancy:
No proven harm to unborn child. Avoid if possible, especially first 3 months.

Breast-feeding:
Avoid drug or don't nurse your infant.

Infants & children:
Not recommended for children younger than 12.

Prolonged use:
May cause kidney stones, vision change, loss of taste and smell, jaundice (yellow skin and eyes) or weight loss.

Skin & sunlight:
No problems expected.

Driving, piloting or hazardous work:
Avoid if you feel drowsy or dizzy. Otherwise, no problems expected.

Airplane passengers:
No problems expected.

Discontinuing:
Don't discontinue without medical advice.

Others:
Medicine may increase sugar levels in blood and urine. Diabetics may need insulin adjustment.

INTERACTION WITH OTHER DRUGS

GENERIC NAME OR DRUG CLASS	COMBINED EFFECT
Amphetamines	Increased amphetamine effect.
Anticonvulsants	Increased loss of bone minerals.
Antidepressants (tricyclic)	Increased antidepressant effect.
Antidiabetics (oral)	Increased potassium loss.
Aspirin	Decreased aspirin effect.
Cortisone drugs	Increased potassium loss.
Digitalis preparations	Possible digitalis toxicity.
Diuretics (other)	Increased potassium loss.
Lithium	Decreased lithium effect.
Methenamine	Decreased methenamine effect.
Quinidine	Increased quinidine effect.
Sympathomimetics	Increased sympathomimetic effect.

INTERACTION WITH OTHER SUBSTANCES

INTERACTS WITH	COMBINED EFFECT
Alcohol:	None expected.
Beverages:	None expected.
Cocaine:	Decreased methazolamide effect.
Foods: Potassium-rich foods.	Eat these to decrease potassium loss. See page 850.
Marijuana:	Increased methazolamide effect.
Tobacco:	None expected.

METHENAMINE

BRAND NAMES

Azo-Mandelamine
Hiprex
Mandelamine
Mandelets
Prov-U-Sep
Renalgin (M)

Urex
Urised (M)
Uro-phosphate (M)
Uroquid-Acid (M)

GENERAL INFORMATION

Habit forming? No
Prescription needed? Yes
Available as generic? Yes
Drug class: Antiinfective (urinary)

 ## USES

Suppresses chronic urinary-tract infections.

 ## DOSAGE & USAGE INFORMATION

How to take:
- Tablet—Swallow with liquid or food to lessen stomach irritation. If you can't swallow whole, crumble tablet and take with liquid or food.
- Liquid form—Use a measuring spoon to ensure correct dose.
- Granules—Dissolve dose in 4 oz. of water. Drink all the liquid.

When to take:
At the same times each day.

If you forget a dose:
Take as soon as you remember up to 8 hours late. If more than 8 hours, wait for next scheduled dose (don't double this dose).

What drug does:
A chemical reaction in the urine changes methenamine into formaldehyde, which destroys certain bacteria.

Time lapse before drug works:
Continual use for 3 to 6 months.

Don't take with:
See Interaction column and consult doctor.

 ## OVERDOSE

Symptoms:
Bloody urine, weakness, deep breathing, stupor, coma.

What to do:
- Dial 0 (operator) or 911 (emergency) for an ambulance or medical help. Then give first aid immediately.
- Additional emergency information on page 886.

 ## POSSIBLE ADVERSE REACTIONS OR SIDE EFFECTS

SYMPTOMS	FREQUENCY	WHAT TO DO
Brain & nervous system:	None expected.	
Skin: Rash	Common	3
Eyes:	None expected.	
Ears, nose, throat:	None expected.	
Digestive: Nausea	Common	4
Heart & lungs:	None expected.	
Blood vessels:	None expected.	
Muscles, bones, joints:	None expected.	
Genital, urinary:		
• Urination difficulty.	Common	4
• Bloody urine.	Rare	3
• Burning on urination.	Rare	4
Kidneys: Lower back pain.	Rare	4
Liver:	None expected.	
Allergic:	None expected.	
Blood:	None expected.	
Others:	None expected.	

1 - Life-threatening. Seek emergency treatment immediately.
2 - Discontinue. Seek emergency treatment.
3 - Discontinue. Call doctor right away.
4 - Continue. Call doctor when convenient.
5 - Continue. Tell doctor at next visit.
6 - No action necessary.

WARNINGS & PRECAUTIONS

Don't take if:
- You are allergic to methenamine.
- You have a severe impairment of kidney or liver function.
- The urine cannot or should not be acidified (check with your doctor).

Before you start, consult your doctor:
- If you have had kidney or liver disease.
- If you plan to become pregnant within medication period.
- If you have had gout.

Over age 60:
Don't exceed recommended dose.

Pregnancy:
Studies inconclusive on harm to unborn child. Avoid if possible, especially first 3 months.

Breast-feeding:
Drug passes into milk in small amounts. Consult doctor.

Infants & children:
Use only under medical supervision.

Prolonged use:
No problems expected.

Skin & sunlight:
No problems expected.

Driving, piloting or hazardous work:
No problems expected.

Airplane passengers:
No problems expected.

Discontinuing:
Don't discontinue without doctor's advice until you complete prescribed dose, even though symptoms diminish or disappear.

Others:
Requires an acid urine to be effective. Eat more protein foods, cranberries, cranberry juice with vitamin C, plums, prunes.

INTERACTION WITH OTHER DRUGS

GENERIC NAME OR DRUG CLASS	COMBINED EFFECT
Antacids	Decreased methenamine effect.
Carbonic anhydrase inhibitors	Decreased methenamine effect.
Diuretics (thiazide)	Decreased urine acidity.
Sodium bicarbonate	Decreased methenamine effect.
Sulfa drugs	Possible kidney damage.
Vitamin C (1 to 4 grams per day)	Increased effect of methenamine, contributing to urine's acidity.

INTERACTION WITH OTHER SUBSTANCES

INTERACTS WITH	COMBINED EFFECT
Alcohol:	Possible brain depression. Avoid or use with caution.
Beverages: Milk	Decreased methenamine effect.
Cocaine:	None expected.
Foods:	None expected.
Marijuana:	Drowsiness, muscle weakness or blood-pressure drop.
Tobacco:	None expected.

METHICILLIN

BRAND NAMES

Azapen
Celbenin
Staphcillin

GENERAL INFORMATION

Habit forming? No
Prescription needed? Yes
Available as generic? Yes
Drug class: Antibiotic (penicillin)

 ## USES

Treatment of bacterial infections that are susceptible to methicillin.

 ## DOSAGE & USAGE INFORMATION

How to take:
By injection only.

When to take:
Follow doctor's instructions.

If you forget a dose:
Consult doctor.

What drug does:
Destroys susceptible bacteria. Does not kill viruses.

Time lapse before drug works:
May be several days before medicine affects infection.

Don't take with:
See Interaction column and consult doctor.

 ## OVERDOSE

Symptoms:
Severe diarrhea, nausea or vomiting.

What to do:
Overdose unlikely to threaten life. If person takes much larger amount than prescribed, call doctor, poison-control center or hospital emergency room for instructions.

 ## POSSIBLE ADVERSE REACTIONS OR SIDE EFFECTS

SYMPTOMS	FREQUENCY	WHAT TO DO
Brain & nervous system:	None expected.	
Skin: Hives, rash, intense itch soon after a dose.	Rare	1
Eyes:	None expected.	
Ears, nose, throat: Dark or discolored tongue.	Common	5
Digestive: Mild nausea, vomiting, diarrhea.	Infrequent	4
Heart & lungs:	None expected.	
Blood vessels: Unexplained bleeding.	Rare	3
Muscles, bones, joints:	None expected.	
Genital, urinary:	None expected.	
Kidneys:	None expected.	
Liver:	None expected.	
Allergic: Life-threatening anaphylaxis may occur!	Rare	1 See page 888.
Blood:	None expected.	
Others:	None expected.	

1- Life-threatening. Seek emergency treatment immediately.
2- Discontinue. Seek emergency treatment.
3- Discontinue. Call doctor right away.
4- Continue. Call doctor when convenient.
5- Continue. Tell doctor at next visit.
6- No action necessary.

WARNINGS & PRECAUTIONS

Don't take if:
You are allergic to methicillin, cephalosporin antibiotics, other penicillins or penicillamine. Life-threatening reaction may occur.

Before you start, consult your doctor:
If you are allergic to any substance or drug.

Over age 60:
You may have skin reactions, particularly around genitals and anus.

Pregnancy:
Studies inconclusive on harm to unborn child. Animal studies show fetal abnormalities. Decide with your doctor whether drug benefits justify risk to unborn child.

Breast-feeding:
Drug passes into milk. Child may become sensitive to penicillins and have allergic reactions to penicillin drugs. Avoid methicillin or discontinue nursing until you finish medicine. Consult doctor for advice on maintaining milk supply.

Infants & children:
No problems expected.

Prolonged use:
- You may become more susceptible to infections caused by germs not responsive to methicillin.
- May cause kidney damage. Laboratory studies to detect damage recommended if you take for a long time.

Skin & sunlight:
No problems expected.

Driving, piloting or hazardous work:
Usually not dangerous. Most hazardous reactions likely to occur a few minutes after taking methicillin.

Airplane passengers:
No problems expected.

Discontinuing:
Don't discontinue without doctor's advice until you complete prescribed dose, even though symptoms diminish or disappear.

Others:
No problems expected.

INTERACTION WITH OTHER DRUGS

GENERIC NAME OR DRUG CLASS	COMBINED EFFECT
Chloramphenicol	Decreased effect of both drugs.
Erythromycins	Decreased effect of both drugs.
Paromomycin	Decreased effect of both drugs.
Tetracyclines	Decreased effect of both drugs.
Troleandomycin	Decreased effect of both drugs.

INTERACTION WITH OTHER SUBSTANCES

INTERACTS WITH	COMBINED EFFECT
Alcohol:	Occasional stomach irritation.
Beverages:	None expected.
Cocaine:	No proven problems.
Foods:	None expected.
Marijuana:	No proven problems.
Tobacco:	None expected.

METHOCARBAMOL

BRAND NAMES

Delaxin	Robaxin
Forbaxin	Robaxisal
Marbaxin-750	Spinaxin
Metho-500	Tumol
Robamol	

GENERAL INFORMATION

Habit forming? No
Prescription needed? Yes
Available as generic? Yes
Drug class: Muscle relaxant (skeletal)

 ## USES

Pain reliever for skeletal-muscle spasms.

 ## DOSAGE & USAGE INFORMATION

How to take:
Tablet—Swallow with liquid. If you can't swallow whole, crumble tablet and take with liquid or food.

When to take:
As directed on label.

If you forget a dose:
Take as soon as you remember up to 2 hours late. If more than 2 hours, wait for next scheduled dose (don't double this dose).

What drug does:
Blocks reflex nerve impulses in brain and spinal cord.

Time lapse before drug works:
30 to 45 minutes.

Don't take with:
- Non-prescription drugs containing alcohol without consulting doctor.
- See Interaction column and consult doctor.

 ## OVERDOSE

Symptoms:
Unsteadiness, lack of coordination, extreme weakness, paralysis, weak and rapid pulse, shallow breathing, cold and sweaty skin.

What to do:
- Dial 0 (operator) or 911 (emergency) for an ambulance or medical help. Then give first aid immediately.
- If patient is unconscious and not breathing, give mouth-to-mouth breathing. If there is no heartbeat, use cardiac massage and mouth-to-mouth breathing (CPR). Don't try to make patient vomit. If you can't get help quickly, take patient to nearest emergency facility.
- Additional emergency information on page 886.

 ## POSSIBLE ADVERSE REACTIONS OR SIDE EFFECTS

SYMPTOMS	FREQUENCY	WHAT TO DO
Brain & nervous system:		
● Dizziness, drowsiness, lightheadedness.	Common	4
● Headache	Infrequent	4
Skin:		
Rash or itch.	Infrequent	3
Eyes:		
● Bloodshot eyes.	Infrequent	4
● Blurred or double vision.	Common	3
Ears, nose, throat:		
● Stuffy nose.	Infrequent	5
● Metallic taste.	Infrequent	4
Digestive:		
Nausea	Infrequent	5
Heart & lungs:	None expected.	
Blood vessels:	None expected.	
Muscles, bones, joints:	None expected.	
Genital, urinary:	None expected.	
Kidneys:	None expected.	
Liver:	None expected.	
Allergic:	None expected.	
Blood:	None expected.	
Others:		
Fever	Infrequent	4

1- Life-threatening. Seek emergency treatment immediately.
2- Discontinue. Seek emergency treatment.
3- Discontinue. Call doctor right away.
4- Continue. Call doctor when convenient.
5- Continue. Tell doctor at next visit.
6- No action necessary.

METHOCARBAMOL

WARNINGS & PRECAUTIONS

Don't take if:
You are allergic to any muscle relaxant.

Before you start, consult your doctor:
● If you have epilepsy.
● If you have myasthenia gravis.
● If you have impaired kidney function.

Over age 60:
Adverse reactions and side effects may be more frequent and severe than in younger persons.

Pregnancy:
No proven harm to unborn child. Avoid if possible.

Breast-feeding:
Drug filters into milk. May harm child. Avoid.

Infants & children:
Not recommended.

Prolonged use:
No problems expected.

Skin & sunlight:
No problems expected.

Driving, piloting or hazardous work:
Don't drive or pilot aircraft until you learn how medicine affects you. Don't work around dangerous machinery. Don't climb ladders or work in high places. Danger increases if you drink alcohol or take medicine affecting alertness and reflexes, such as antihistamines, tranquilizers, sedatives, pain medicine, narcotics and mind-altering drugs.

Airplane passengers:
No problems expected.

Discontinuing:
May be unnecessary to finish medicine. Follow doctor's instructions.

Others:
No problems expected.

INTERACTION WITH OTHER DRUGS

GENERIC NAME OR DRUG CLASS	COMBINED EFFECT
Antidepressants (tricyclic)	Increased effect of both drugs.
Antimyasthenics	Decreased antimyasthenic effect.
Narcotics	Increased sedative effect.
Sedatives	Increased sedative effect.
Sleep inducers	Increased effect of sleep inducer.
Tranquilizers	Increased tranquilizer effect.

INTERACTION WITH OTHER SUBSTANCES

INTERACTS WITH	COMBINED EFFECT
Alcohol:	Depressed brain function. Avoid.
Beverages:	None expected.
Cocaine:	May increase muscle spasms.
Foods:	None expected.
Marijuana:	Drowsiness, muscle weakness, lack of coordination, fainting.
Tobacco:	None expected.

METHOTREXATE

BRAND NAMES

Mexate

GENERAL INFORMATION

Habit forming? No
Prescription needed? Yes
Available as generic? Yes
Drug class: Antimetabolite, antipsoriatic

 ## USES

- Treatment for some kinds of cancer.
- Treatment for psoriasis in patients with severe problems.

 ## DOSAGE & USAGE INFORMATION

How to take:
Tablet—Swallow with liquid.

When to take:
At the same time each day.

If you forget a dose:
Skip the missed dose. Don't double the next dose.

What drug does:
Inhibits abnormal-cell reproduction.

Time lapse before drug works:
May require 6 weeks for maximum effect.

Don't take with:
See Interaction column and consult doctor.

 ## OVERDOSE

Symptoms:
Headache, stupor, seizures.

What to do:
- Dial 0 (operator) or 911 (emergency) for an ambulance or medical help. Then give first aid immediately.
- If patient is unconscious and not breathing, give mouth-to-mouth breathing. If there is no heartbeat, use cardiac massage and mouth-to-mouth breathing (CPR). Don't try to make patient vomit. If you can't get help quickly, take patient to nearest emergency facility.
- Additional emergency information on page 886.

POSSIBLE ADVERSE REACTIONS OR SIDE EFFECTS

SYMPTOMS	FREQUENCY	WHAT TO DO
Brain & nervous system:		
• Seizures	Infrequent	2
• Dizziness, drowsiness, headache, confusion.	Infrequent	3
Skin:		
Acne, boils, hair loss, itch.	Infrequent	5
Eyes:		
Blurred vision.	Infrequent	3
Ears, nose, throat:		
Mouth sores, sore throat, fever, chills.	Common	3
Digestive:		
• Black stools or bloody vomit.	Common	2
• Stomach pain, nausea, vomiting.	Common	4
Heart & lungs:		
• Shortness of breath.	Infrequent	3
• Cough	Infrequent	4
Blood vessels:		
Unusual bleeding or bruising.	Common	3
Muscles, bones, joints:		
Joint pain.	Infrequent	3
Genital, urinary:		
Bloody urine.	Infrequent	3
Kidneys, allergic, blood. others:	None expected.	
Liver:		
Jaundice (yellow skin and eyes).	Infrequent	3

1- Life-threatening. Seek emergency treatment immediately.
2- Discontinue. Seek emergency treatment.
3- Discontinue. Call doctor right away.
4- Continue. Call doctor when convenient.
5- Continue. Tell doctor at next visit.

METHOTREXATE

WARNINGS & PRECAUTIONS

Don't take if:
You are allergic to any antimetabolite.

Before you start, consult your doctor:
- If you are alcoholic.
- If you have blood, liver or kidney disease.
- If you have colitis or peptic ulcer.
- If you have gout.
- If you have an infection.
- If you plan to become pregnant within 3 months.

Over age 60:
Adverse reactions and side effects may be more frequent and severe than in younger persons.

Pregnancy:
- Psoriasis—Risk to unborn child outweighs drug benefits. Don't use.
- Cancer—Consult doctor.

Breast-feeding:
Drug passes into milk. Avoid drug or discontinue nursing.

Infants & children:
Use only under special medical supervision.

Prolonged use:
Adverse reactions more likely the longer drug is required.

Skin & sunlight:
No problems expected.

Driving, piloting or hazardous work:
Avoid if you feel dizzy, drowsy or confused. Otherwise, no problems expected.

Airplane passengers:
No problems expected.

Discontinuing:
Don't discontinue without doctor's advice until you complete prescribed dose, even though symptoms diminish or disappear. Some side effects may follow discontinuing. Report to doctor blurred vision, convulsions, confusion, persistent headache.

Others:
- Drink more water than usual to cause frequent urination.
- Don't give this medicine to anyone else for any purpose. It is a strong drug that requires close medical supervision.
- Report for frequent medical follow-up and laboratory studies.

INTERACTION WITH OTHER DRUGS

GENERIC NAME OR DRUG CLASS	COMBINED EFFECT
Anticoagulants (oral)	Increased anticoagulant effect.
Anticonvulsants (hydantoin)	Possible methotrexate toxicity.
Antigout drugs	Decreased antigout effect.
Asparaginase	Decreased methotrexate effect.
Flurouracil	Decreased methotrexate effect.
Oxyphenbutazone	Possible methotrexate toxicity.
Phenylbutazone	Possible methotrexate toxicity.
Probenecid	Possible methotrexate toxicity.
Pyrimethamine	Increased toxic effect of methotrexate.
Salicylates (including aspirin)	Possible methotrexate toxicity.
Sulfa drugs	Possible methotrexate toxicity.
Tetracyclines	Possible methotrexate toxicity.

INTERACTION WITH OTHER SUBSTANCES

INTERACTS WITH	COMBINED EFFECT
Alcohol:	Likely liver damage. Avoid.
Beverages:	Extra fluid intake decreases chance of methotrexate toxicity.
Cocaine:	Increased chance of methotrexate adverse reactions. Avoid.
Foods:	None expected.
Marijuana:	None expected.
Tobacco:	None expected.

METHSUXIMIDE

BRAND NAMES

Celontin

GENERAL INFORMATION

Habit forming? No
Prescription needed? Yes
Available as generic? No
Drug class: Anticonvulsant (succinimide)

 ## USES

Controls seizures in treatment of epilepsy.

 ## DOSAGE & USAGE INFORMATION

How to take:
Capsule—Swallow with liquid or food to lessen stomach irritation.

When to take:
Every day in regularly spaced doses, according to prescription.

If you forget a dose:
Take as soon as you remember up to 2 hours late. If more than 2 hours, wait for next scheduled dose (don't double this dose).

What drug does:
Depresses nerve transmissions in part of brain that controls muscles.

Time lapse before drug works:
3 hours.

Don't take with:
See Interaction column and consult doctor.

 ## OVERDOSE

Symptoms:
Coma

What to do:
- Dial 0 (operator) or 911 (emergency) for an ambulance or medical help. Then give first aid immediately.
- If patient is unconscious and not breathing, give mouth-to-mouth breathing. If there is no heartbeat, use cardiac massage and mouth-to-mouth breathing (CPR). Don't try to make patient vomit. If you can't get help quickly, take patient to nearest emergency facility.
- Additional emergency information on page 886.

POSSIBLE ADVERSE REACTIONS OR SIDE EFFECTS

SYMPTOMS	FREQUENCY	WHAT TO DO
Brain & nervous system: Dizziness, drowsiness, headache, irritability, mood changes.	Infrequent	4
Skin: Rash	Rare	3
Eyes:	None expected.	
Ears, nose, throat: Sore throat, fever.	Rare	3
Digestive: Nausea, vomiting, stomach cramps, appetite loss.	Common	4
Heart & lungs:	None expected.	
Blood vessels:	None expected.	
Muscles, bones, joints:	None expected.	
Genital, urinary:	None expected.	
Kidneys:	None expected.	
Liver:	None expected.	
Allergic:	None expected.	
Blood: Unusual bleeding or bruising.	Rare	3
Others: Swollen lymph glands.	Rare	4

1- Life-threatening. Seek emergency treatment immediately.
2- Discontinue. Seek emergency treatment.
3- Discontinue. Call doctor right away.
4- Continue. Call doctor when convenient.
5- Continue. Tell doctor at next visit.
6- No action necessary.

WARNINGS & PRECAUTIONS

Don't take if:
You are allergic to any succinimide anticonvulsant.

Before you start, consult your doctor:
- If you plan to become pregnant within medication period.
- If you take other anticonvulsants.
- If you have blood disease.
- If you have kidney or liver disease.

Over age 60:
Adverse reactions and side effects may be more frequent and severe than in younger persons.

Pregnancy:
Risk to unborn child outweighs drug benefits. Don't use.

Breast-feeding:
Drug passes into milk. Avoid drug or discontinue nursing.

Infants & children:
Use only under medical supervision.

Prolonged use:
No problems expected.

Skin & sunlight:
No problems expected.

Driving, piloting or hazardous work:
Don't drive or pilot aircraft until you learn how medicine affects you. Don't work around dangerous machinery. Don't climb ladders or work in high places. Danger increases if you drink alcohol or take medicine affecting alertness and reflexes, such as antihistamines, tranquilizers, sedatives, pain medicine, narcotics and mind-altering drugs.

Airplane passengers:
No problems expected.

Discontinuing:
Don't discontinue without doctor's advice until you complete prescribed dose, even though symptoms diminish or disappear.

Others:
- Your response to medicine should be checked regularly by your doctor. Dose and schedule may have to be altered frequently to fit individual needs.
- Periodic blood-cell counts, kidney- and liver-function studies recommended.

INTERACTION WITH OTHER DRUGS

GENERIC NAME OR DRUG CLASS	COMBINED EFFECT
Anticonvulsants (other)	Increased effect of both drugs.
Antidepressants (tricyclic)	May provoke seizures.
Antipsychotics	May provoke seizures.

INTERACTION WITH OTHER SUBSTANCES

INTERACTS WITH	COMBINED EFFECT
Alcohol:	May provoke seizures.
Beverages:	None expected.
Cocaine:	May provoke seizures.
Foods:	None expected.
Marijuana:	May provoke seizures.
Tobacco:	None expected.

METHYCLOTHIAZIDE

BRAND NAMES

Aquatensen
Duretic
Enduron

GENERAL INFORMATION

Habit forming? No
Prescription needed? Yes
Available as generic? Yes
Drug class: Antihypertensive,
diuretic (thiazide)

USES

- Controls, but doesn't cure, high blood pressure.
- Reduces fluid retention (edema) caused by conditions such as heart disorders and liver disease.

DOSAGE & USAGE INFORMATION

How to take:
Tablet or capsule—Swallow with liquid. If you can't swallow whole, crumble tablet or open capsule and take with liquid or food. Don't exceed dose.

When to take:
At the same time each day.

If you forget a dose:
Take as soon as you remember up to 2 hours late. If more than 2 hours, wait for next scheduled dose (don't double this dose).

What drug does:
- Forces sodium and water excretion, reducing body fluid.
- Relaxes muscle cells of small arteries.
- Reduced body fluid and relaxed arteries lower blood pressure.

Time lapse before drug works:
4 to 6 hours. May require several weeks to lower blood pressure.

Don't take with:
- See Interaction column and consult doctor.
- Non-prescription drugs without consulting doctor.

OVERDOSE

Symptoms:
Cramps, weakness, drowsiness, weak pulse, coma.

What to do:
- Dial 0 (operator) or 911 (emergency) for an ambulance or medical help. Then give first aid immediately.
- Additional emergency information on page 886.

POSSIBLE ADVERSE REACTIONS OR SIDE EFFECTS

SYMPTOMS	FREQUENCY	WHAT TO DO
Brain & nervous system:		
• Dizziness	Infrequent	4
• Mood changes.	Infrequent	4
• Headaches	Infrequent	4
Skin:		
Rash or hives.	Rare	2
Eyes:		
Blurred vision.	Infrequent	3
Ears, nose, throat:		
• Sore throat, fever.	Rare	3
• Dry mouth, thirst.	Infrequent	5
Digestive:		
Severe abdominal pain, nausea, vomiting.	Infrequent	3
Heart & lungs:		
Irregular heartbeat, weak pulse.	Infrequent	3
Blood vessels:	None expected.	
Muscles, bones, joints:		
Weakness, tiredness.	Infrequent	4
Genital, urinary:	None expected.	
Kidneys:	None expected.	
Liver:		
Jaundice (yellow skin and eyes).	Rare	3
Allergic:	None expected.	
Blood:	None expected.	
Others:		
Weight changes.	Infrequent	4

1-Life-threatening. Seek emergency treatment immediately.
2-Discontinue. Seek emergency treatment.
3-Discontinue. Call doctor right away.
4-Continue. Call doctor when convenient.
5-Continue. Tell doctor at next visit.
6-No action necessary.

METHYCLOTHIAZIDE

WARNINGS & PRECAUTIONS

Don't take if:
You are allergic to any thiazide diuretic drug.

Before you start, consult your doctor:
- If you are allergic to any sulfa drug.
- If you have gout.
- If you have liver, pancreas or kidney disorder.

Over age 60:
Adverse reactions and side effects may be more frequent and severe than in younger persons, especially dizziness and excessive potassium loss.

Pregnancy:
Risk to unborn child outweighs drug benefits. Don't use.

Breast-feeding:
Drug passes into milk. Avoid drug or discontinue nursing.

Infants & children:
No problems expected.

Prolonged use:
You may need medicine to treat high blood pressure for the rest of your life.

Skin & sunlight:
May cause rash or intensify sunburn in areas exposed to sun or sunlamp.

Driving, piloting or hazardous work:
Don't drive or pilot aircraft until you learn how medicine affects you. Don't work around dangerous machinery. Don't climb ladders or work in high places. Danger increases if you drink alcohol or take medicine affecting alertness and reflexes, such as antihistamines, tranquilizers, sedatives, pain medicine, narcotics and mind-altering drugs.

Airplane passengers:
No problems expected.

Discontinuing:
Don't discontinue without medical advice.

Others:
- Hot weather and fever may cause dehydration and drop in blood pressure. Dose may require temporary adjustment. Weigh daily and report any unexpected weight decreases to your doctor.
- May cause rise in uric acid, leading to gout.
- May cause blood-sugar rise in diabetics.

INTERACTION WITH OTHER DRUGS

GENERIC NAME OR DRUG CLASS	COMBINED EFFECT
Allopurinol	Decreased allopurinol effect.
Antidepressants (tricyclic)	Dangerous drop in blood pressure. Avoid combination unless under medical supervision.
Barbiturates	Increased methyclothiazide effect.
Cholestyramine	Decreased methyclothiazide effect.
Cortisone drugs	Excessive potassium loss that causes dangerous heart rhythms.
Digitalis preparations	Excessive potassium loss that causes dangerous heart rhythms.
Diuretics (thiazide)	Increased effect of other thiazide diuretics.
Lithium	Increased effect of lithium.
MAO Inhibitors	Increased methyclothiazide effect.
Probenecid	Decreased probenecid effect.

INTERACTION WITH OTHER SUBSTANCES

INTERACTS WITH	COMBINED EFFECT
Alcohol:	Dangerous blood-pressure drop.
Beverages:	None expected.
Cocaine:	None expected.
Foods: Licorice	Excessive potassium loss that causes dangerous heart rhythms.
Marijuana:	May increase blood pressure.
Tobacco:	None expected.

METHYLCELLULOSE

BRAND NAMES

Cellothyl
Cologel
Hydrolose

GENERAL INFORMATION

Habit forming? No
Prescription needed? No
Available as generic? Yes
Drug class: Laxative (bulk-forming)

 USES

Relieves constipation and prevents straining for bowel movement.

 DOSAGE & USAGE INFORMATION

How to take:
- Liquid, powder, flakes, granules—Dilute dose in 8 oz. cold water or fruit juice.
- Capsules—Swallow with 8 oz. cold liquid. Drink 6 to 8 glasses of water each day in addition to the one with each dose.

When to take:
At the same time each day, preferably morning.

If you forget a dose:
Take as soon as you remember. Resume regular schedule.

What drug does:
Absorbs water, stimulating the bowel to form a soft, bulky stool.

Time lapse before drug works:
May require 2 or 3 days to begin, then works in 12 to 24 hours.

Don't take with:
- See Interaction column and consult doctor.
- Don't take within 2 hours of taking another medicine. Laxative interferes with medicine absorption.

 OVERDOSE

Symptoms:
None expected.

What to do:
Overdose unlikely to threaten life. If person takes much larger amount than prescribed, call doctor, poison-control center or hospital emergency room for instructions.

 POSSIBLE ADVERSE REACTIONS OR SIDE EFFECTS

SYMPTOMS	FREQUENCY	WHAT TO DO
Brain & nervous system:	None expected.	
Skin: Itch, rash.	Rare	3
Eyes:	None expected.	
Ears, nose, throat: Swallowing difficulty, "lump in throat" sensation.	Infrequent	4
Digestive:		
• Intestinal blockage.	Rare	3
• Nausea, vomiting, diarrhea.	Infrequent	4
Heart & lungs: Asthma	Rare	3
Blood vessels:	None expected.	
Muscles, bones, joints:	None expected.	
Genital, urinary:	None expected.	
Kidneys:	None expected.	
Liver:	None expected.	
Allergic:	None expected.	
Blood:	None expected.	
Others:	None expected.	

1 - Life-threatening. Seek emergency treatment immediately.
2 - Discontinue. Seek emergency treatment.
3 - Discontinue. Call doctor right away.
4 - Continue. Call doctor when convenient.
5 - Continue. Tell doctor at next visit.
6 - No action necessary.

METHYLCELLULOSE

WARNINGS & PRECAUTIONS

Don't take if:
- You are allergic to any bulk-forming laxative.
- You have symptoms of appendicitis, inflamed bowel or intestinal blockage.
- You have missed a bowel movement for only 1 or 2 days.

Before you start, consult your doctor:
- If you have diabetes.
- If you have a laxative habit.
- If you have rectal bleeding.
- If you have difficulty swallowing.
- If you take other laxatives.

Over age 60:
Adverse reactions and side effects may be more frequent and severe than in younger persons.

Pregnancy:
Most bulk-forming laxatives contain sodium or sugars which may cause fluid retention. Avoid if possible.

Breast-feeding:
No problems expected.

Infants & children:
Use only under medical supervision.

Prolonged use:
Don't take for more than 1 week unless under a doctor's supervision. May cause laxative dependence.

Skin & sunlight:
No problems expected.

Driving, piloting or hazardous work:
No problems expected.

Airplane passengers:
No problems expected.

Discontinuing:
May be unnecessary to finish medicine. Follow doctor's instructions.

Others:
Don't take to "flush out" your system or as a "tonic."

INTERACTION WITH OTHER DRUGS

GENERIC NAME OR DRUG CLASS	COMBINED EFFECT
Antibiotics	Decreased antibiotic effect.
Anticoagulants	Decreased anticoagulant effect.
Digitalis preparations	Decreased digitalis effect.
Salicylates (including aspirin)	Decreased salicylate effect.

INTERACTION WITH OTHER SUBSTANCES

INTERACTS WITH	COMBINED EFFECT
Alcohol:	None expected.
Beverages:	None expected.
Cocaine:	None expected.
Foods:	None expected.
Marijuana:	None expected.
Tobacco:	None expected.

METHYLDOPA

BRAND NAMES

Aldomet
Aldoclor (M)
Aldoril-15 (M)
Aldoril-25
Aldoril D30 (M)

Aldoril D50 (M)
Dopamet
Medimet-250
Novomedopa

GENERAL INFORMATION

Habit forming? No
Prescription needed? Yes
Available as generic? No
Drug class: Antihypertensive

USES

Reduces high blood pressure.

DOSAGE & USAGE INFORMATION

How to take:
Liquid or tablet—Swallow with liquid. If you can't swallow whole, crumble tablet and take with liquid or food.

When to take:
At the same times each day.

If you forget a dose:
Take as soon as you remember up to 2 hours late. If more than 2 hours, wait for next scheduled dose (don't double this dose).

What drug does:
Relaxes walls of small arteries to decrease blood pressure.

Time lapse before drug works:
Continual use for 2 to 4 weeks may be necessary to determine effectiveness.

Don't take with:
See Interaction column and consult doctor.

OVERDOSE

Symptoms:
Drowsiness; exhaustion; stupor; confusion; slow, weak pulse.

What to do:
- Dial 0 (operator) or 911 (emergency) for an ambulance or medical help. Then give first aid immediately.
- If patient is unconscious and not breathing, give mouth-to-mouth breathing. If there is no heartbeat, use cardiac massage and mouth-to-mouth breathing (CPR). Don't try to make patient vomit. If you can't get help quickly, take patient to nearest emergency facility.
- Additional emergency information on page 886.

POSSIBLE ADVERSE REACTIONS OR SIDE EFFECTS

SYMPTOMS	FREQUENCY	WHAT TO DO
Brain & nervous system:		
• Depression, nightmares, drowsiness, weakness.	Common	4
• Insomnia	Infrequent	4
Skin: Rash	Rare	3
Eyes:	None expected.	
Ears, nose, throat: Stuffy nose, dry mouth.	Common	4
Digestive: Nausea, vomiting, diarrhea.	Infrequent	4
Heart & lungs: Fast heartbeat.	Infrequent	3
Blood vessels:	None expected.	
Muscles, bones, joints: Swollen feet or legs.	Common	4
Genital, urinary:	None expected.	
Kidneys:	None expected.	
Liver: Jaundice (yellow skin and eyes).	Rare	3
Allergic:	None expected.	
Blood:	None expected.	
Others:		
• Unexplained fever.	Rare	3
• Fluid retention.	Common	4
• Breast swelling.	Infrequent	5
• Lower sex drive.	Infrequent	5

1- Life-threatening. Seek emergency treatment immediately.
2- Discontinue. Seek emergency treatment.
3- Discontinue. Call doctor right away.
4- Continue. Call doctor when convenient.
5- Continue. Tell doctor at next visit.
6- No action necessary.

WARNINGS & PRECAUTIONS

Don't take if:
You will have surgery within 2 months, including dental surgery, requiring general or spinal anesthesia.

Before you start, consult your doctor:
If you have liver disease.

Over age 60:
- Increased susceptibility to dizziness, unsteadiness, fainting, falling.
- Drug can produce or intensify Parkinson's disease.

Pregnancy:
No proven problems. Consult doctor.

Breast-feeding:
No proven problems. Consult doctor.

Infants & children:
Not used.

Prolonged use:
- May cause anemia.
- Severe edema (fluid retention).

Skin & sunlight:
No problems expected.

Driving, piloting or hazardous work:
Don't drive or pilot aircraft until you learn how medicine affects you. Don't work around dangerous machinery. Don't climb ladders or work in high places. Danger increases if you drink alcohol or take medicine affecting alertness and reflexes, such as antihistamines, tranquilizers, sedatives, pain medicine, narcotics and mind-altering drugs.

Airplane passengers:
No problems expected.

Discontinuing:
Don't discontinue without consulting doctor. Dose may require gradual reduction if you have taken drug for a long time. Doses of other drugs may also require adjustment.

Others:
Avoid heavy exercise, exertion, sweating.

INTERACTION WITH OTHER DRUGS

GENERIC NAME OR DRUG CLASS	COMBINED EFFECT
Amphetamines	Decreased methyldopa effect.
Anticoagulants (oral)	Increased anticoagulant effect.
Antidepressants (tricyclic)	Dangerous blood-pressure rise.
Antihypertensives	Increased antihypertensive effect.
Digitalis preparations	Excessively slow heartbeat.
Diuretics (thiazide)	Increased methyldopa effect.
Levodopa	Decreased levodopa effect.
MAO inhibitors	Dangerous blood-pressure rise.

INTERACTION WITH OTHER SUBSTANCES

INTERACTS WITH	COMBINED EFFECT
Alcohol:	Increased sedation. Excessive blood-pressure drop. Avoid.
Beverages:	None expected.
Cocaine:	Decreased methyldopa effect.
Foods:	None expected.
Marijuana:	Possible fainting.
Tobacco:	Possible increased blood pressure.

METHYLERGONOVINE

BRAND NAMES

Methergine

GENERAL INFORMATION

Habit forming? No
Prescription needed? Yes
Available as generic? Yes
Drug class: Ergot preparation (uterine stimulant)

USES

Retards excessive post-delivery bleeding.

DOSAGE & USAGE INFORMATION

How to take:
Tablet—Swallow with liquid or food to lessen stomach irritation.

When to take:
At the same times each day.

If you forget a dose:
Don't take missed dose and don't double next one. Wait for next scheduled dose.

What drug does:
Causes smooth-muscle cells of uterine wall to contract and surround bleeding blood vessels of relaxed uterus.

Time lapse before drug works:
Tablets—20 to 30 minutes.

Don't take with:
See Interaction column and consult doctor.

OVERDOSE

Symptoms:
Vomiting, diarrhea, weak pulse, low blood pressure, convulsions.

What to do:
- Dial 0 (operator) or 911 (emergency) for an ambulance or medical help. Then give first aid immediately.
- If patient is unconscious and not breathing, give mouth-to-mouth breathing. If there is no heartbeat, use cardiac massage and mouth-to-mouth breathing (CPR). Don't try to make patient vomit. If you can't get help quickly, take patient to nearest emergency facility.
- Additional emergency information on page 886.

POSSIBLE ADVERSE REACTIONS OR SIDE EFFECTS

SYMPTOMS	FREQUENCY	WHAT TO DO
Brain & nervous system:		
• Sudden, severe headache.	Rare	2
• Confusion	Infrequent	3
Skin:	None expected.	
Eyes:	None expected.	
Ears, nose, throat:		
Ringing in ears.	Infrequent	3
Digestive:		
• Nausea, vomiting.	Common	3
• Diarrhea	Infrequent	3
Heart & lungs:		
Shortness of breath, chest pain.	Rare	2
Blood vessels:	None expected.	
Muscles, bones, joints:		
• Muscle cramps.	Infrequent	3
• Numb, cold hands and feet.	Rare	2
Genital, urinary:	None expected.	
Kidneys:	None expected.	
Liver:	None expected.	
Allergic:	None expected.	
Blood:	None expected.	
Others:		
Unusual sweating.	Infrequent	4

1- Life-threatening. Seek emergency treatment immediately.
2- Discontinue. Seek emergency treatment.
3- Discontinue. Call doctor right away.
4- Continue. Call doctor when convenient.
5- Continue. Tell doctor at next visit.
6- No action necessary.

METHYLERGONOVINE

WARNINGS & PRECAUTIONS

Don't take if:
You are allergic to any ergot preparation.

Before you start, consult your doctor:
- If you have coronary-artery or blood-vessel disease.
- If you have liver or kidney disease.
- If you have high blood pressure.
- If you have postpartum infection.

Over age 60:
Not recommended.

Pregnancy:
Risk to unborn child outweighs drug benefits. Don't use.

Breast-feeding:
Drug passes into milk. Avoid drug or discontinue nursing until you finish medicine. Consult doctor for advice on maintaining milk supply.

Infants & children:
Not recommended.

Prolonged use:
Not recommended.

Skin & sunlight:
No problems expected.

Driving, piloting or hazardous work:
No problems expected.

Airplane passengers:
No problems expected.

Discontinuing:
May be unnecessary to finish medicine. Follow doctor's instructions.

Others:
Drug should be used for short time only following childbirth or miscarriage.

INTERACTION WITH OTHER DRUGS

GENERIC NAME OR DRUG CLASS	COMBINED EFFECT
Ergot preparations (other)	Increased methylergonovine effect.

INTERACTION WITH OTHER SUBSTANCES

INTERACTS WITH	COMBINED EFFECT
Alcohol:	None expected.
Beverages:	None expected.
Cocaine:	None expected.
Foods:	None expected.
Marijuana:	None expected.
Tobacco:	None expected.

METHYLPHENIDATE

BRAND NAMES

Methidate
Ritalin

Habit forming? Yes
Prescription needed? Yes

GENERAL INFORMATION

Available as generic? Yes
Drug class: Sympathomimetic

USES

- Treatment for hyperactive children.
- Treatment for drowsiness and fatigue in adults.
- Treatment for narcolepsy (uncontrollable attacks of sleepiness).

DOSAGE & USAGE INFORMATION

How to take:
Tablet or capsule—Swallow with liquid or food to lessen stomach irritation. If you can't swallow whole, crumble tablet or open capsule and take with liquid or food.

When to take:
At the same times each day.

If you forget a dose:
Take as soon as you remember up to 2 hours late. If more than 2 hours, wait for next scheduled dose (don't double this dose).

What drug does:
Stimulates brain to improve alertness, concentration and attention span. Calms the hyperactive child.

Time lapse before drug works:
- 1 month or more for maximum effect on child.
- 30 minutes to stimulate adults.

Don't take with:
See Interaction column and consult doctor.

OVERDOSE

Symptoms:
Rapid heartbeat; fever; confusion, hallucinations; convulsions; coma.

What to do:
- Dial 0 (operator) or 911 (emergency) for an ambulance or medical help. Then give first aid immediately.
- If patient is unconscious and not breathing, give mouth-to-mouth breathing. If there is no heartbeat, use cardiac massage and mouth-to-mouth breathing (CPR). Don't try to make patient vomit. If you can't get help quickly, take patient to nearest emergency facility.
- Additional emergency information on page 886.

POSSIBLE ADVERSE REACTIONS OR SIDE EFFECTS

SYMPTOMS	FREQUENCY	WHAT TO DO
Brain & nervous system:		
• Mood changes.	Common	4
• Nervousness, insomnia, dizziness, headache.	Common	5
Skin:		
Rash or hives.	Infrequent	3
Eyes:		
Blurred vision.	Rare	3
Ears, nose, throat:		
Sore throat, fever.	Rare	3
Digestive:		
• Appetite loss.	Common	5
• Nausea, abdominal pain.	Infrequent	4
Heart & lungs:		
Chest pain; fast, irregular heartbeat.	Infrequent	3
Blood vessels:		
Unusual bruising.	Infrequent	3
Muscles, bones, joints:		
Joint pain, uncontrolled movements.	Infrequent	3
Genital, urinary:	None expected.	
Kidneys:	None expected.	
Liver:	None expected.	
Allergic:	None expected.	
Blood:	None expected.	
Others:		
• Unexplained fever.	Infrequent	3
• Unusual tiredness.	Rare	4

1- Life-threatening. Seek emergency treatment immediately.
2- Discontinue. Seek emergency treatment.
3- Discontinue. Call doctor right away.
4- Continue. Call doctor when convenient.
5- Continue. Tell doctor at next visit.
6- No action necessary.

WARNINGS & PRECAUTIONS

Don't take if:
- You are allergic to methylphenidate.
- You have glaucoma.
- Patient is younger than 6.

Before you start, consult your doctor:
- If you have epilepsy.
- If you have high blood pressure.
- If you take MAO inhibitors.

Over age 60:
Adverse reactions and side effects may be more frequent and severe than in younger persons.

Pregnancy:
No proven harm to unborn child. Avoid if possible.

Breast-feeding:
No proven problems. Consult doctor.

Infants & children:
Use only under medical supervision for children 6 or older.

Prolonged use:
Rare possibility of physical growth retardation.

Skin & sunlight:
No problems expected.

Driving, piloting or hazardous work:
No problems expected.

Airplane passengers:
No problems expected.

Discontinuing:
Don't discontinue abruptly. Don't discontinue without doctor's advice until you complete prescribed dose, even though symptoms diminish or disappear.

Others:
Dose must be carefully adjusted by doctor.

INTERACTION WITH OTHER DRUGS

GENERIC NAME OR DRUG CLASS	COMBINED EFFECT
Anticholinergics	Increased anticholinergic effect.
Anticoagulants (oral)	Increased anticoagulant effect.
Anticonvulsants	Increased anticonvulsant effect.
Antidepressants (tricyclic)	Increased antidepressant effect.
Guanethidine	Decreased guanethidine effect.
MAO inhibitors	Dangerous rise in blood pressure.
Oxyphenbutazone	Increased oxyphenbutazone effect.
Phenylbutazone	Increased phenylbutazone effect.

INTERACTION WITH OTHER SUBSTANCES

INTERACTS WITH	COMBINED EFFECT
Alcohol:	None expected.
Beverages: Caffeine drinks	May raise blood pressure.
Cocaine:	Overstimulation. Avoid.
Foods: Foods containing tyramine (see page 851).	May raise blood pressure.
Marijuana:	None expected.
Tobacco:	None expected.

METHYLPREDNISOLONE

BRAND NAMES

A-methaPred	Duralone-80	Medrone-80
Depo-Medrol	Medralone	Mepred-40
Depo-Pred-40	Medralone-40	Methylone
Depo-Pred-80	Medralone-80	Pro-Dep-40
Duralone	Medrol	Pro-Dep-80
Duralone-40	Medrol Enpak	

GENERAL INFORMATION

Habit forming? No
Prescription needed? Yes
Available as generic? Yes
Drug class: Cortisone drug
(adrenal corticosteroid)

USES

- Reduces inflammation caused by many different medical problems.
- Treatment for some allergic diseases, blood disorders, kidney diseases, asthma and emphysema.
- Replaces corticosteroid deficiencies.

DOSAGE & USAGE INFORMATION

How to take:
Tablet—Swallow with liquid or food to lessen stomach irritation. If you can't swallow whole, crumble tablet and take with liquid or food.

When to take:
At the same times each day. Take once-a-day or once-every-other-day doses in mornings.

If you forget a dose:
- Several-doses-per-day prescription—Take as soon as you remember up to 2 hours late. If more than 2 hours, wait for next scheduled dose (don't double this dose).
- Once-a-day dose or less—Wait for next dose. Double this dose.

What drug does:
Decreases inflammatory responses.

Time lapse before drug works:
2 to 4 days.

Don't take with:
See Interaction column and consult doctor.

OVERDOSE

Symptoms:
Headache, convulsions, heart failure.

What to do:
- Dial 0 (operator) or 911 (emergency) for an ambulance or medical help. Then give first aid immediately.
- Additional emergency information on page 886.

POSSIBLE ADVERSE REACTIONS OR SIDE EFFECTS

SYMPTOMS	FREQUENCY	WHAT TO DO
Brain & nervous system: Mood changes, insomnia, restlessness.	Infrequent	4
Skin:		
• Acne	Common	4
• Rash	Rare	3
• Poor wound healing.	Common	4
Eyes: Blurred vision, halos around lights.	Infrequent	3
Ears, nose, throat:		
• Sore throat, fever.	Infrequent	3
• Thirst	Common	4
Digestive:		
• Indigestion, nausea, vomiting.	Common	4
• Bloody or black, tarry stool.	Infrequent	2
Heart & lungs: Irregular heartbeat.	Rare	2
Blood vessels, kidneys, liver, allergic, blood:	None expected.	
Muscles, bones, joints: Muscle cramps, swollen legs, feet.	Infrequent	3
Genital, urinary: Frequent urination.	Infrequent	4
Others:		
• Weight gain, round face.	Infrequent	4
• Fatigue, weakness.	Infrequent	4
• TB recurrence.	Infrequent	4
• Irregular menstrual periods.	Infrequent	4

1- Life-threatening. Seek emergency treatment immediately.
2- Discontinue. Seek emergency treatment.
3- Discontinue. Call doctor right away.
4- Continue. Call doctor when convenient.

METHYLPREDNISOLONE

WARNINGS & PRECAUTIONS

Don't take if:
- You are allergic to any cortisone drug.
- You have tuberculosis or fungus infection.
- You have herpes infection of eyes, lips or genitals.

Before you start, consult your doctor:
- If you have had tuberculosis.
- If you have congestive heart failure.
- If you have diabetes.
- If you have peptic ulcer.
- If you have glaucoma.
- If you have underactive thyroid.
- If you have high blood pressure.
- If you have myasthenia gravis.
- If you have blood clots in legs or lungs.

Over age 60:
Adverse reactions and side effects may be more frequent and severe than in younger persons. Likely to aggravate edema, diabetes or ulcers. Likely to cause cataracts and osteoporosis (softening of the bones).

Pregnancy:
Risk to unborn child outweighs drug benefits. Don't use.

Breast-feeding:
Drug passes into milk. Avoid drug or discontinue nursing until you finish medicine. Consult doctor for advice on maintaining milk supply.

Infants & children:
Use only under medical supervision.

Prolonged use:
- Retards growth in children.
- Possible glaucoma, cataracts, diabetes, fragile bones and thin skin.
- Functional dependence.

Skin & sunlight:
No problems expected.

Driving, piloting or hazardous work:
No problems expected.

Airplane passengers:
No problems expected.

Discontinuing:
- Don't discontinue without doctor's advice until you complete prescribed dose, even though symptoms diminish or disappear.
- Drug affects your response to surgery, illness, injury or stress for 2 years after discontinuing. Tell about drug to anyone who takes medical care of you within 2 years.

Others:
Avoid immunizations if possible.

INTERACTION WITH OTHER DRUGS

GENERIC NAME OR DRUG CLASS	COMBINED EFFECT
Amphotericin B	Potassium depletion.
Anticholinergics	Possible glaucoma.
Anticoagulants (oral)	Decreased anticoagulant effect.
Anticonvulsants (hydantoin)	Decreased methylprednisolone effect.
Antidiabetics (oral)	Decreased antidiabetic effect.
Antihistamines	Decreased methylprednisolone effect.
Aspirin	Increased methylprednisolone effect.
Barbiturates	Decreased methylprednisolone effect. Oversedation.
Beta-adrenergic blockers	Decreased methylprednisolone effect.
Chloral hydrate	Decreased methylprednisolone effect.
Chlorthalidone	Potassium depletion.
Cholinergics	Decreased cholinergic effect.

Additional interactions on page 839.

INTERACTION WITH OTHER SUBSTANCES

INTERACTS WITH	COMBINED EFFECT
Alcohol:	Risk of stomach ulcers.
Beverages:	No proven problems.
Cocaine:	Overstimulation. Avoid.
Foods:	No proven problems.
Marijuana:	Decreased immunity.
Tobacco:	Increased methylprednisolone effect. Possible toxicity.

METHYLTESTOSTERONE

BRAND NAMES

Android   Testred
Metandren
Oreton Methyl

Habit forming? No
Prescription needed? Yes

GENERAL INFORMATION

Available as generic? Yes
Drug class: Androgen (male sex hormone)

 USES

- Corrects male hormone deficiency.
- Reduces "male menopause" symptoms (loss of sex drive, depression, anxiety).
- Decreases calcium loss of osteoporosis (softened bones).
- Blocks growth of breast-cancer cells in females.
- Corrects undescended testicles in male children.
- Reduces breast pain and fullness following childbirth.
- Augments treatment of aplastic anemia.
- Stimulates weight gain after illness, injury or for chronically underweight persons.
- Stimulates growth in treatment of dwarfism.

 DOSAGE & USAGE INFORMATION

How to take:
- Tablets—With food to lessen stomach irritation.
- Injection—Once or twice a month.

When to take:
At the same time each day.

If you forget a dose:
Take as soon as you remember up to 2 hours late. If more than 2 hours, wait for next scheduled dose (don't double this dose).

What drug does:
- Stimulates cells that produce male sex characteristics.
- Replaces hormone deficiencies.
- Stimulates red-blood-cell production.
- Suppresses production of estrogen (female sex hormone).

Time lapse before drug works:
Varies with problems treated. May require 2 or 3 months of regular use for desired effects.

Don't take with:
See Interaction column and consult doctor.

 OVERDOSE

Overdose unlikely to threaten life. If person takes much larger amount than prescribed, call doctor, poison-control center or hospital emergency room for instructions.

POSSIBLE ADVERSE REACTIONS OR SIDE EFFECTS

SYMPTOMS	FREQUENCY	WHAT TO DO
Brain & nervous system:		
Depression or confusion.	Infrequent	3
Skin:		
• Flushed face.	Infrequent	3
• Rash or itch.	Infrequent	3
• Hives	Rare	2
• Acne or oily skin in females.	Common	4
Eyes, heart & lungs, blood vessels, kidneys, blood:	None expected.	
Ears, nose, throat:		
• Deep voice.	Common	4
• Sore mouth.	Common	5
• Sore throat, fever.	Rare	3
Digestive:		
• Nausea, vomiting, diarrhea.	Infrequent	3
• Abdominal pain.	Rare	3
• Black stool.	Rare	2
Muscles, bones, joints:		
Swollen feet or legs.	Infrequent	3
Genital, urinary:		
• Enlarged clitoris or frequent erections.	Common	4
• Vaginal bleeding.	Infrequent	3
Liver:		
Jaundice (yellow skin and eyes).	Infrequent	2
Allergic:		
Intense itching, weakness, loss of consciousness.	Rare	1
Others:		
• Higher sex drive.	Common	5
• Swollen breasts in men.	Common	4

1-Life-threatening. Seek emergency treatment immediately.
2-Discontinue. Seek emergency treatment.
3-Discontinue. Call doctor right away.
4-Continue. Call doctor when convenient.
5-Continue. Tell doctor at next visit.

METHYLTESTOSTERONE

WARNINGS & PRECAUTIONS

Don't take if:
You are allergic to any male hormone.

Before you start, consult your doctor:
- If you might be pregnant.
- If you have cancer of prostate.
- If you have heart disease or arteriosclerosis.
- If you have kidney or liver disease.
- If you have breast cancer (males).
- If you have high blood pressure.
- If you have migraine attacks.
- If you have high level of blood calcium.
- If you have epilepsy.

Over age 60:
- May stimulate sexual activity.
- Can make high blood pressure or heart disease worse.
- Can enlarge prostate and cause urinary retention.

Pregnancy:
Risk to unborn child outweighs drug benefits. Don't use.

Breast-feeding:
Drug passes into milk. Avoid drug or discontinue nursing until you finish medicine. Consult doctor for advice on maintaining milk supply.

Infants & children:
Don't give to children younger than 2. Use with older children only under medical supervision.

Prolonged use:
- Reduces sperm count and volume of semen.
- Possible kidney stones.
- Unnatural hair growth and deep voice in women.

Skin & sunlight:
No problems expected.

Driving, piloting or hazardous work:
No problems expected.

Airplane passengers:
No problems expected.

Discontinuing:
No problems expected.

Others:
- May cause atrophy of testicles.
- Will not increase strength in athletes.

INTERACTION WITH OTHER DRUGS

GENERIC NAME OR DRUG CLASS	COMBINED EFFECT
Anticoagulants	Increased anticoagulant effect.
Antidiabetics (oral)	Increased antidiabetic effect.
Chlorzoxazone	Decreased methyltestosterone effect.
Oxyphenbutazone	Decreased methyltestosterone effect.
Phenobarbital	Decreased methyltestosterone effect.
Phenylbutazone	Decreased methyltestosterone effect.

INTERACTION WITH OTHER SUBSTANCES

INTERACTS WITH	COMBINED EFFECT
Alcohol:	None expected.
Beverages:	None expected.
Cocaine:	No proven problems.
Foods: Salt	Excessive fluid retention (edema). Decrease salt intake while taking male hormones.
Marijuana:	Decreased blood levels of methyltestosterone.
Tobacco:	No proven problems.

METHYSERGIDE

BRAND NAMES

Sansert

Habit forming? No
Prescription needed? Yes

USES

Prevents migraine and other recurring vascular headaches.

DOSAGE & USAGE INFORMATION

How to take:
Tablet—Swallow with liquid or with food to lessen stomach irritation. If you can't swallow whole, crumble tablet and take with liquid or food.

When to take:
At the same times each day.

If you forget a dose:
Don't take missed dose. Wait for next scheduled dose (don't double this dose).

What drug does:
Blocks the action of serotonin, a chemical that constricts blood vessels.

Time lapse before drug works:
About 3 weeks.

Don't take with:
See Interaction column and consult doctor.

OVERDOSE

Symptoms:
Nausea, vomiting, abdominal pain, severe diarrhea, lack of coordination, extreme thirst.

What to do:
Overdose unlikely to threaten life. If person takes much larger amount than prescribed, call doctor, poison-control center or hospital emergency room for instructions.

GENERAL INFORMATION

Available as generic? No
Drug class: Vasoconstrictor (antiserotonin)

POSSIBLE ADVERSE REACTIONS OR SIDE EFFECTS

SYMPTOMS	FREQUENCY	WHAT TO DO
Brain & nervous system:		
● Drowsiness	Common	5
● Anxiety, agitation hallucinations.	Infrequent	3
Skin:		
Itching	Common	3
Eyes:		
Vision changes.	Infrequent	4
Ears, nose, throat:		
Extreme thirst.	Rare	3
Digestive:		
● Appetite loss.	Rare	3
● Nausea, vomiting, diarrhea.	Common	4
Heart & lungs:		
● Chest pain, shortness of breath.	Rare	3
● Unusually fast or slow heartbeat.	Infrequent	3
Blood vessels:		
● Fever, pale or swollen extremities.	Rare	3
● Numbness or tingling of extremities.	Common	4
Muscles, bones, joints:		
● Leg cramps, lower back pain.	Rare	3
● Leg weakness.	Common	4
Genital, urinary:		
Difficult or painful urination.	Rare	4
Kidneys:		
Side or groin pain.	Rare	3
Liver, allergic, blood:	None expected.	
Others:		
Weight change, hair loss.	Rare	5

1 - Life-threatening. Seek emergency treatment immediately.
2 - Discontinue. Seek emergency treatment.
3 - Discontinue. Call doctor right away.
4 - Continue. Call doctor when convenient.
5 - Continue. Tell doctor at next visit.

METHYSERGIDE

WARNINGS & PRECAUTIONS

Don't take if:
- You are allergic to any antiserotonin.
- You plan to become pregnant within medication period.
- You have an infection.
- You have a heart or blood-vessel disease.
- You have a chronic lung disease.
- You have a collagen (connective tissue) disorder.
- You have impaired liver or kidney function.

Before you start, consult your doctor:
- If you have been allergic to any ergot preparation.
- If you have had a peptic ulcer.

Over age 60:
Adverse reactions and side effects may be more frequent and severe than in younger persons.

Pregnancy:
Manufacturer suggests risk to unborn child outweighs drug benefits, even though studies are inconclusive.

Breast-feeding:
Drug probably passes into milk. Avoid drug or discontinue nursing until you finish medicine. Consult doctor for advice on maintaining milk supply.

Infants & children:
Not recommended.

Prolonged use:
Possible fibrosis, a condition in which scar tissue is deposited on heart valves, in lung tissue, blood vessels and internal organs. After 6 months, decrease dose over 2 to 3 weeks. Then discontinue for at least 2 months for re-evaluation.

Skin & sunlight:
No problems expected.

Driving, piloting or hazardous work:
Avoid if you feel drowsy or dizzy. Otherwise, no problems expected.

Airplane passengers:
No problems expected.

Discontinuing:
- Don't discontinue without consulting doctor. Dose may require gradual reduction if you have taken drug for a long time. Doses of other drugs may also require adjustment.
- Probably should discontinue drug if you don't improve after 3 weeks' use.

Others:
Periodic laboratory tests for liver function and blood counts recommended.

INTERACTION WITH OTHER DRUGS

GENERIC NAME OR DRUG CLASS	COMBINED EFFECT
Ergot preparations	Unpredictable increased or decreased effect of either drug.
Narcotics	Decreased narcotic effect.

INTERACTION WITH OTHER SUBSTANCES

INTERACTS WITH	COMBINED EFFECT
Alcohol:	None expected. However, alcohol may trigger a migraine headache.
Beverages: Caffeine drinks	Decreased methysergide effect.
Cocaine:	May make headache worse.
Foods:	None expected. Avoid foods to which you are allergic.
Marijuana:	No proven problems.
Tobacco:	Blood-vessel constriction. Makes headache worse.

METOLAZONE

BRAND NAMES

Diulo
Zaroxolyn

GENERAL INFORMATION

Habit forming? No
Prescription needed? Yes
Available as generic? Yes
Drug class: Antihypertensive,
diuretic (thiazide)

USES

- Controls, but doesn't cure, high blood pressure.
- Reduces fluid retention (edema) caused by conditions such as heart disorders and liver disease.

DOSAGE & USAGE INFORMATION

How to take:
Tablet or capsule—Swallow with 8 oz. of liquid. If you can't swallow whole, crumble tablet or open capsule and take with liquid or food. Don't exceed dose.

When to take:
At the same time each day.

If you forget a dose:
Take as soon as you remember up to 2 hours late. If more than 2 hours, wait for next scheduled dose (don't double this dose).

What drug does:
- Forces sodium and water excretion, reducing body fluid.
- Relaxes muscle cells of small arteries.
- Reduced body fluid and relaxed arteries lower blood pressure.

Time lapse before drug works:
4 to 6 hours. May require several weeks to lower blood pressure.

Don't take with:
- See Interaction column and consult doctor.
- Non-prescription drugs without consulting doctor.

OVERDOSE

Symptoms:
Cramps, weakness, drowsiness, weak pulse, coma.

What to do:
- Dial O (operator) or 911 (emergency) for an ambulance or medical help. Then give first aid immediately.
- Additional emergency information on page 886.

POSSIBLE ADVERSE REACTIONS OR SIDE EFFECTS

SYMPTOMS	FREQUENCY	WHAT TO DO
Brain & nervous system:		
• Dizziness	Infrequent	4
• Mood changes.	Infrequent	4
• Headaches	Infrequent	4
Skin:		
Rash or hives.	Rare	2
Eyes:		
Blurred vision.	Infrequent	3
Ears, nose, throat:		
• Sore throat, fever.	Rare	3
• Dry mouth, thirst.	Infrequent	5
Digestive:		
Severe abdominal pain, nausea, vomiting.	Infrequent	3
Heart & lungs:		
Irregular heartbeat, weak pulse.	Infrequent	3
Blood vessels:	None expected.	
Muscles, bones, joints:		
Weakness, tiredness.	Infrequent	4
Genital, urinary:	None expected.	
Kidneys:	None expected.	
Liver:		
Jaundice (yellow skin and eyes).	Rare	3
Allergic:	None expected.	
Blood:	None expected.	
Others:		
Weight changes.	Infrequent	4

1- Life-threatening. Seek emergency treatment immediately.
2- Discontinue. Seek emergency treatment.
3- Discontinue. Call doctor right away.
4- Continue. Call doctor when convenient.
5- Continue. Tell doctor at next visit.
6- No action necessary.

WARNINGS & PRECAUTIONS

Don't take if:
You are allergic to any thiazide diuretic drug.

Before you start, consult your doctor:
- If you are allergic to any sulfa drug.
- If you have gout.
- If you have liver, pancreas or kidney disorder.

Over age 60:
Adverse reactions and side effects may be more frequent and severe than in younger persons, especially dizziness and excessive potassium loss.

Pregnancy:
Risk to unborn child outweighs drug benefits. Don't use.

Breast-feeding:
Drug passes into milk. Avoid this medicine or discontinue nursing.

Infants & children:
No problems expected.

Prolonged use:
You may need medicine to treat high blood pressure for the rest of your life.

Skin & sunlight:
May cause rash or intensify sunburn in areas exposed to sun or sunlamp.

Driving, piloting or hazardous work:
Don't drive or pilot aircraft until you learn how medicine affects you. Don't work around dangerous machinery. Don't climb ladders or work in high places. Danger increases if you drink alcohol or take medicine affecting alertness and reflexes, such as antihistamines, tranquilizers, sedatives, pain medicine, narcotics and mind-altering drugs.

Airplane passengers:
No problems expected.

Discontinuing:
Don't discontinue without medical advice.

Others:
- Hot weather and fever may cause dehydration and drop in blood pressure. Dose may require temporary adjustment. Weigh daily and report any unexpected weight decreases to your doctor.
- May cause rise in uric acid, leading to gout.
- May cause blood-sugar rise in diabetics.

INTERACTION WITH OTHER DRUGS

GENERIC NAME OR DRUG CLASS	COMBINED EFFECT
Allopurinol	Decreased allopurinol effect.
Antidepressants (tricyclic)	Dangerous drop in blood pressure. Avoid combination unless under medical supervision.
Barbiturates	Increased metolazone effect.
Cholestyramine	Decreased metolazone effect.
Cortisone drugs	Excessive potassium loss that causes dangerous heart rhythms.
Digitalis preparations	Excessive potassium loss that causes dangerous heart rhythms.
Diuretics (thiazide)	Increased effect of other thiazide diuretics.
Lithium	Increased effect of lithium.
MAO inhibitors	Increased metolazone effect.
Probenecid	Decreased probenecid effect.

INTERACTIONS WITH OTHER SUBSTANCES

INTERACTS WITH	COMBINED EFFECT
Alcohol:	Dangerous blood-pressure drop.
Beverages:	None expected.
Cocaine:	None expected.
Foods: Licorice	Excessive potassium loss that causes dangerous heart rhythms.
Marijuana:	May increase blood pressure.
Tobacco:	None expected.

METOPROLOL

BRAND NAMES

Lopressor

GENERAL INFORMATION

Habit forming? No
Prescription needed? Yes
Available as generic? No
Drug class: Beta-adrenergic blocker

 ## USES

- Reduces angina attacks.
- Stabilizes irregular heartbeat.
- Lowers blood pressure.
- Reduces frequency of migraine headaches. (Does not relieve headache pain.)
- Other uses prescribed by your doctor.

 ## DOSAGE & USAGE INFORMATION

How to take:
Tablet or capsule—Swallow with liquid. If you can't swallow whole, crumble tablet or open capsule and take with liquid or food.

When to take:
With meals or immediately after.

If you forget a dose:
Take as soon as you remember. Return to regular schedule, but allow 3 hours between doses.

What drug does:
- Blocks certain actions of sympathetic nervous system.
- Lowers heart's oxygen requirements.
- Slows nerve impulses through heart.
- Reduces blood vessel contraction in heart, scalp and other body parts.

Time lapse before drug works:
1 to 4 hours.

Don't take with:
Non-prescription drugs or drugs in Interaction column without consulting doctor.

 ## OVERDOSE

Symptoms:
Weakness, slow or weak pulse, blood pressure drop, fainting, convulsions, cold and sweaty skin.

What to do:
- Dial O (operator) or 911 (emergency) for an ambulance or medical help. Then give first aid immediately.
- Additional emergency information on page 886.

POSSIBLE ADVERSE REACTIONS OR SIDE EFFECTS

SYMPTOMS	FREQUENCY	WHAT TO DO
Brain & nervous system:		
● Hallucinations, nightmares, insomnia, headache.	Infrequent	3
● Confusion, depression, reduced alertness.	Infrequent	4
● Drowsiness, numbness or tingling of fingers or toes, dizziness.	Common	4
Skin: Rash	Rare	3
Eyes:	None expected.	
Ears, nose, throat: Sore throat, fever.	Rare	3
Digestive:		
● Diarrhea, nausea.	Common	4
● Constipation	Infrequent	5
Heart & lungs:		
● Pulse slower than 50 beats per minute.	Common	3
● Breathing difficulty.	Infrequent	3
Blood vessels: Cold hands, feet.	Common	5
Muscles, bones, joints, genital, urinary, kidneys, liver, allergic:	None expected.	
Blood: Unusual bleeding and bruising.	Rare	4
Others:		
● Fatigue, weakness.	Common	4
● Dry mouth, eyes, skin.	Common	5

1-Life-threatening. Seek emergency treatment immediately.
2-Discontinue. Seek emergency treatment.
3-Discontinue. Call doctor right away.
4-Continue. Call doctor when convenient.
5-Continue. Tell doctor at next visit.

METOPROLOL

 ## WARNINGS & PRECAUTIONS

Don't take if:
- You are allergic to any beta-adrenergic blocker.
- You have asthma.
- You have hay fever symptoms.
- You have taken MAO inhibitors in past 2 weeks.

Before you start, consult your doctor:
- If you have heart disease or poor circulation to the extremities.
- If you have hay fever, asthma, chronic bronchitis, emphysema.
- If you have overactive thyroid function.
- If you have impaired liver or kidney function.
- If you will have surgery within 2 months, including dental surgery, requiring general or spinal anesthesia.
- If you have diabetes or hypoglycemia.

Over age 60:
Adverse reactions and side effects may be more frequent and severe than in younger persons.

Pregnancy:
Risk to unborn child outweighs drug benefits. Don't use.

Breast-feeding:
Drug passes into milk. Avoid drug or discontinue nursing until you finish medicine. Consult doctor for advice on maintaining milk supply.

Infants & children:
Not recommended.

Prolonged use:
Weakens heart muscle contractions.

Skin & sunlight:
No problems expected.

Driving, piloting or hazardous work:
Don't drive or pilot aircraft until you learn how medicine affects you. Don't work around dangerous machinery. Don't climb ladders or work in high places. Danger increases if you drink alcohol or take medicine affecting alertness and reflexes.

Airplane passengers:
No problems expected.

Discontinuing:
Don't discontinue without consulting doctor. Dose may require gradual reduction if you have taken drug for a long time. Doses of other drugs may also require adjustment.

Others:
May mask hypoglycemia.

 ## INTERACTION WITH OTHER DRUGS

GENERIC NAME OR DRUG CLASS	COMBINED EFFECT
Antidiabetics	Increased antidiabetic effect.
Antihistamines	Decreased antihistamine effect.
Antihypertensives	Increased antihypertensive effect.
Antiinflammatory drugs	Decreased antiinflammatory effect.
Barbiturates	Increased barbiturate effect. Dangerous sedation.
Digitalis preparations	Can either increase or decrease heart rate. Improves irregular heartbeat.
Narcotics	Increased narcotic effect. Dangerous sedation.
Phenytoin	Increased metoprolol effect.
Quinidine	Slows heart excessively.
Reserpine	Increased reserpine effect. Excessive sedation and depression.

 ## INTERACTION WITH OTHER SUBSTANCES

INTERACTS WITH	COMBINED EFFECT
Alcohol:	Excessive blood pressure drop. Avoid.
Beverages:	None expected.
Cocaine:	Irregular heartbeat. Avoid.
Foods:	None expected.
Marijuana:	Daily use—Impaired circulation to hands and feet.
Tobacco:	Possible irregular heartbeat.

METRONIDAZOLE

BRAND NAMES

Flagyl	Novonidazol
Metryl	Satric
Neo-Tric	Trikacide

GENERAL INFORMATION

Habit forming? No
Prescription needed? Yes
Available as generic? No
Drug class: Antiprotozoal

USES

Treatment for infections susceptible to metronidazole, such as trichomoniasis and amoebiasis.

DOSAGE & USAGE INFORMATION

How to take:
- Tablet or capsule—Swallow with liquid or food to lessen stomach irritation. If you can't swallow whole, crumble tablet or open capsule and take with liquid or food.
- Suppositories—Remove wrapper and moisten suppository with water. Gently insert larger end into vagina. Push well into vagina with finger or applicator.

When to take:
At the same times each day.

If you forget a dose:
Take as soon as you remember up to 2 hours late. If more than 2 hours, wait for next scheduled dose (don't double this dose).

What drug does:
Kills organisms causing the infection.

Time lapse before drug works:
Begins in 1 hour. May require regular use for 10 days to cure infection.

Don't take with:
- See Interaction column and consult doctor.
- Non-prescription medicines containing alcohol.

OVERDOSE

Symptoms:
Weakness, nausea, vomiting, diarrhea, confusion, seizures.

What to do:
Overdose unlikely to threaten life. If person takes much larger amount than prescribed, call doctor, poison-control center or hospital emergency room for instructions.

POSSIBLE ADVERSE REACTIONS OR SIDE EFFECTS

SYMPTOMS	FREQUENCY	WHAT TO DO
Brain & nervous system:		
● Mood changes, unsteadiness.	Rare	3
● Dizziness	Infrequent	3
● Headache	Infrequent	3
Skin:		
Rash, hives, redness, itch.	Infrequent	3
Eyes, heart & lungs, blood vessels, muscles, bones, joints, kidneys, liver, allergic, blood:	None expected.	
Ears, nose, throat:		
● Unpleasant taste.	Common	5
● Mouth irritation, soreness or infection.	Infrequent	3
● Sore throat, fever.	Infrequent	3
Digestive:		
● Appetite loss, nausea, stomach pain, diarrhea, vomiting.	Common	3
● Constipation	Infrequent	5
Genital, urinary:		
Vaginal irritation, discharge, dryness.	Infrequent	4
Others:		
● Numbness, tingling, weakness or pain in hands or feet.	Rare	3
● Fatigue, weakness.	Infrequent	4

1- Life-threatening. Seek emergency treatment immediately.
2- Discontinue. Seek emergency treatment.
3- Discontinue. Call doctor right away.
4- Continue. Call doctor when convenient.
5- Continue. Tell doctor at next visit.

WARNINGS & PRECAUTIONS

Don't take if:
- You are allergic to metronidazole.
- You have had a blood-cell or bone-marrow disorder.

Before you start, consult your doctor:
- If you plan to become pregnant within medication period.
- If you have a brain or nervous-system disorder.
- If you have liver or heart disease.
- If you drink alcohol.

Over age 60:
Adverse reactions and side effects may be more frequent and severe than in younger persons.

Pregnancy:
Risk to unborn child outweighs drug benefits. Manufacturer advises against use during first 3 months and only limited use after that. Don't use.

Breast-feeding:
Drug passes into milk. Avoid drug or discontinue nursing until you finish medicine. Consult doctor for advice on maintaining milk supply.

Infants & children:
Use in children for amoeba infection only under close medical supervision.

Prolonged use:
No problems expected.

Skin & sunlight:
No problems expected.

Driving, piloting or hazardous work:
Avoid if you feel dizzy or unsteady. Otherwise, no problems expected.

Airplane passengers:
No problems expected.

Discontinuing:
Don't discontinue without doctor's advice until you complete prescribed dose, even though symptoms diminish or disappear.

Others:
No problems expected.

INTERACTION WITH OTHER DRUGS

GENERIC NAME OR DRUG CLASS	COMBINED EFFECT
Anticoagulants (oral)	Decreased anticoagulant effect. Possible bleeding or bruising.
Disulfiram	Disulfiram reaction (see page 848). Avoid.
Oxytetracycline	Decreased metronidazole effect.

INTERACTION WITH OTHER SUBSTANCES

INTERACTS WITH	COMBINED EFFECT
Alcohol:	Possible disulfiram reaction (see page 848). Avoid alcohol in *any* form or amount.
Beverages:	None expected.
Cocaine:	Decreased metronidazole effect. Avoid.
Foods:	None expected.
Marijuana:	None expected.
Tobacco:	None expected.

MINOCYCLINE

BRAND NAMES

Minocin
Ultramycin

GENERAL INFORMATION

Habit forming? No
Prescription needed? Yes
Available as generic? Yes
Drug class: Antibiotic (tetracycline)

USES

- Treatment for infections susceptible to minocycline. Will not cure virus infections such as colds or flu.
- Treatment for acne.

DOSAGE & USAGE INFORMATION

How to take:
- Tablet or capsule—Take on empty stomach 1 hour before or 2 hours after eating. If you can't swallow whole, crumble tablet or open capsule and take with liquid or food.
- Liquid—Shake well. Take with measuring spoon.

When to take:
At the same times each day, evenly spaced.

If you forget a dose:
Take as soon as you remember up to 2 hours late. If more than 2 hours, wait for next scheduled dose (don't double this dose).

What drug does:
Prevents germ growth and reproduction.

Time lapse before drug works:
- Infections—May require 5 days to affect infection.
- Acne—May require 4 weeks to affect acne.

Don't take with:
- Non-prescription drugs without consulting doctor.
- See Interaction column and consult doctor.

OVERDOSE

Symptoms:
Severe nausea, vomiting, diarrhea.

What to do:
Overdose unlikely to threaten life. If person takes much larger amount than prescribed, call doctor, poison-control center or hospital emergency room for instructions.

POSSIBLE ADVERSE REACTIONS OR SIDE EFFECTS

SYMPTOMS	FREQUENCY	WHAT TO DO
Brain & nervous system:		
Headache	Infrequent	3
Skin:		
• Itching around rectum and genitals.	Common	3
• Rash	Infrequent	3
Eyes:		
Blurred vision.	Rare	3
Ears, nose, throat:		
• Dark tongue.	Common	5
• Sore mouth or tongue.	Common	2
• Excessive thirst.	Infrequent	4
Digestive:		
Nausea, vomiting, diarrhea, abdominal burning.	Common	2
Heart & lungs:	None expected.	
Blood vessels:	None expected.	
Muscles, bones, joints:	None expected.	
Genital, urinary:		
Increased urination.	Infrequent	4
Kidneys:	None expected.	
Liver:		
Jaundice (yellow eyes and skin) in pregnant women.	Rare	3
Allergic:	None expected.	
Blood:	None expected.	
Others:	None expected.	

1 - Life-threatening. Seek emergency treatment immediately.
2 - Discontinue. Seek emergency treatment.
3 - Discontinue. Call doctor right away.
4 - Continue. Call doctor when convenient.
5 - Continue. Tell doctor at next visit.
6 - No action necessary.

WARNINGS & PRECAUTIONS

Don't take if:
You are allergic to any tetracycline antibiotic.

Before you start, consult your doctor:
- If you have kidney or liver disease.
- If you have lupus.
- If you have myasthenia gravis.

Over age 60:
Dosage usually less than in younger adults. More likely to cause itching around rectum. Ask you doctor how to prevent it.

Pregnancy:
Risk to unborn child outweighs drug benefits. Don't use.

Breast-feeding:
Drug passes into milk. Avoid drug or discontinue nursing until you finish medicine. Consult doctor for advice on maintaining milk supply.

Infants & children:
May cause permanent teeth malformation or discoloration in children less than 8 years old. Don't use.

Prolonged use:
- You may become more susceptible to infections caused by germs not responsive to minocycline.
- May cause rare problems in liver, kidney or bone marrow. Periodic laboratory blood studies, liver- and kidney-function tests recommended if you use drug a long time.

Skin & sunlight:
May cause rash or intensify sunburn in areas exposed to sun or sunlamp.

Driving, piloting or hazardous work:
Avoid if you feel dizzy. Otherwise, no problems expected.

Airplane passengers:
No problems expected.

Discontinuing:
Don't discontinue without doctor's advice until you complete prescribed dose, even though symptoms diminish or disappear.

Others:
No problems expected.

INTERACTION WITH OTHER DRUGS

GENERIC NAME OR DRUG CLASS	COMBINED EFFECT
Antacids	Decreased minocycline effect.
Anticoagulants (oral)	Increased anticoagulant effect.
Contraceptives (oral)	Decreased contraceptive effect.
Digitalis preparations	Increased digitalis effect.
Mineral supplements (iron, calcium, magnesium, zinc)	Decreased minocycline absorption. Separate doses by 1 to 2 hours.
Lithium	Increased lithium effect.
Penicillins	Decreased penicillin effect.
Sodium bicarbonate	Decreased minocycline effect.

INTERACTION WITH OTHER SUBSTANCES

INTERACTS WITH	COMBINED EFFECT
Alcohol:	Possible liver damage. Avoid.
Beverages: Milk	Decreased minocycline absorption. Take dose 2 hours after or 1 hour before drinking.
Cocaine:	No proven problems.
Foods: Dairy products	Decreased minocycline absorption. Take dose 2 hours after or 1 hour before eating.
Marijuana:	No interactions expected, but marijuana may slow body's recovery. Avoid.
Tobacco:	None expected.

MORPHINE

BRAND NAMES

None

GENERAL INFORMATION

Habit forming? Yes
Prescription needed? Yes
Available as generic? Yes
Drug class: Narcotic

 USES

Relieves pain.

 DOSAGE & USAGE INFORMATION

How to take:
- Tablet or capsule—Swallow with liquid. If you can't swallow whole, crumble tablet or open capsule and take with liquid or food.
- Drops or liquid—Dilute dose in beverage before swallowing.

When to take:
When needed. No more often than every 4 hours.

If you forget a dose:
Take as soon as you remember. Wait 4 hours for next dose.

What drug does:
Blocks pain messages to brain and spinal cord.

Time lapse before drug works:
30 minutes.

Don't take with:
See Interaction column and consult doctor.

 OVERDOSE

Symptoms:
Deep sleep; slow breathing; slow pulse; flushed, warm skin; constricted pupils.

What to do:
- Dial 0 (operator) or 911 (emergency) for an ambulance or medical help. Then give first aid immediately.
- If patient is unconscious and not breathing, give mouth-to-mouth breathing. If there is no heartbeat, use cardiac massage and mouth-to-mouth breathing (CPR). Don't try to make patient vomit. If you can't get help quickly, take patient to nearest emergency facility.
- Additional emergency information on page 886.

POSSIBLE ADVERSE REACTIONS OR SIDE EFFECTS

SYMPTOMS	FREQUENCY	WHAT TO DO
Brain & nervous system: Depression, confusion, hallucinations.	Infrequent	4
Skin:		
• Hives, rash, itch, face swelling.	Rare	3
• Flushed face.	Common	4
Eyes: Blurred vision.	Rare	4
Ears, nose, throat:	None expected.	
Digestive: Severe constipation, abdominal pain, vomiting.	Infrequent	3
Heart & lungs: Slow heartbeat, irregular breathing.	Rare	3
Blood vessels:	None expected.	
Muscles, bones, joints:	None expected.	
Genital, urinary: Difficult urination.	Common	4
Kidneys: Less urine.	Common	4
Liver:	None expected.	
Allergic:	None expected.	
Blood:	None expected.	
Others: Unusual tiredness.	Common	4

1- Life-threatening. Seek emergency treatment immediately.
2- Discontinue. Seek emergency treatment.
3- Discontinue. Call doctor right away.
4- Continue. Call doctor when convenient.
5- Continue. Tell doctor at next visit.
6- No action necessary.

WARNINGS & PRECAUTIONS

Don't take if:
You are allergic to any narcotic.

Before you start, consult your doctor:
If you have impaired liver or kidney function.

Over age 60:
More likely to be drowsy, dizzy, unsteady or constipated. Avoid prolonged use.

Pregnancy:
Studies inconclusive on harm to unborn child. Animal studies show fetal abnormalities. Decide with your doctor whether drug benefits justify risk to unborn child. Abuse by pregnant woman will result in addicted newborn. Withdrawal can be life-threatening.

Breast-feeding:
Drug filters into milk. May depress infant. Avoid.

Infants & children:
Not recommended.

Prolonged use:
Causes psychological and physical dependence.

Skin & sunlight:
No problems expected.

Driving, piloting or hazardous work:
Don't drive or pilot aircraft until you learn how medicine affects you. Don't work around dangerous machinery. Don't climb ladders or work in high places. Danger increases if you drink alcohol or take medicine affecting alertness and reflexes, such as antihistamines, tranquilizers, sedatives, pain medicine, other narcotics and mind-altering drugs.

Airplane passengers:
No proven problems.

Discontinuing:
May be unnecessary to finish medicine. Follow doctor's instructions.

Others:
No problems expected.

INTERACTION WITH OTHER DRUGS

GENERIC NAME OR DRUG CLASS	COMBINED EFFECT
Analgesics	Increased analgesic effect.
Antidepressants	Increased sedative effect.
Antihistamines	Increased sedative effect.
Mind-altering drugs	Increased sedative effect.
Narcotics (other)	Increased narcotic effect.
Phenothiazines	Increased phenothiazine effect.
Sedatives	Increased sedative effect.
Sleep inducers	Increased sedative effect.
Tranquilizers	Increased sedative effect.

INTERACTION WITH OTHER SUBSTANCES

INTERACTS WITH	COMBINED EFFECT
Alcohol:	Increases alcohol's intoxicating effect. Avoid.
Beverages:	None expected.
Cocaine:	Increased cocaine effect.
Foods:	None expected.
Marijuana:	Impairs physical and mental performance.
Tobacco:	None expected.

NADOLOL

BRAND NAMES

Corgard

GENERAL INFORMATION

Habit forming? No
Prescription needed? Yes
Available as generic? No
Drug class: Beta-adrenergic blocker

USES

- Reduces angina attacks.
- Stabilizes irregular heartbeat.
- Lowers blood pressure.
- Reduces frequency of migraine headaches. (Does not relieve headache pain.)
- Other uses prescribed by your doctor.

DOSAGE & USAGE INFORMATION

How to take:
Tablet or capsule—Swallow with liquid. If you can't swallow whole, crumble tablet or open capsule and take with liquid or food.

When to take:
With meals or immediately after.

If you forget a dose:
Take as soon as you remember. Return to regular schedule, but allow 3 hours between doses.

What drug does:
- Blocks certain actions of sympathetic nervous system.
- Lowers heart's oxygen requirements.
- Slows nerve impulses through heart.
- Reduces blood vessel contraction in heart, scalp and other body parts.

Time lapse before drug works:
1 to 4 hours.

Don't take with:
Non-prescription drugs or drugs in Interaction column without consulting doctor.

OVERDOSE

Symptoms:
Weakness, slow or weak pulse, blood pressure drop, fainting, convulsions, cold and sweaty skin.

What to do:
- Dial O (operator) or 911 (emergency) for an ambulance or medical help. Then give first aid immediately.
- Additional emergency information on page 886.

POSSIBLE ADVERSE REACTIONS OR SIDE EFFECTS

SYMPTOMS	FREQUENCY	WHAT TO DO
Brain & nervous system:		
● Hallucinations, nightmares, insomnia, headache.	Infrequent	3
● Confusion, depression, reduced alertness.	Infrequent	4
● Drowsiness, numbness or tingling of fingers or toes, dizziness.	Common	4
Skin: Rash	Rare	3
Eyes:	None expected.	
Ears, nose, throat: Sore throat, fever.	Rare	3
Digestive:		
● Diarrhea, nausea.	Common	4
● Constipation	Infrequent	5
Heart & lungs:		
● Pulse slower than 50 beats per minute.	Common	3
● Breathing difficulty.	Infrequent	3
Blood vessels: Cold hands, feet.	Common	5
Muscles, bones, joints, genital, urinary, kidneys, liver, allergic:	None expected.	
Blood: Unusual bleeding and bruising.	Rare	4
Others:		
● Fatigue, weakness.	Common	4
● Dry mouth, eyes, skin.	Common	5

1-Life-threatening. Seek emergency treatment immediately.
2-Discontinue. Seek emergency treatment.
3-Discontinue. Call doctor right away.
4-Continue. Call doctor when convenient.
5-Continue. Tell doctor at next visit.

NADOLOL

WARNINGS & PRECAUTIONS

Don't take if:
- You are allergic to any beta-adrenergic blocker.
- You have asthma.
- You have hay fever symptoms.
- You have taken MAO inhibitors in past 2 weeks.

Before you start, consult your doctor:
- If you have heart disease or poor circulation to the extremities.
- If you have hay fever, asthma, chronic bronchitis, emphysema.
- If you have overactive thyroid function.
- If you have impaired liver or kidney function.
- If you will have surgery within 2 months, including dental surgery, requiring general or spinal anesthesia.
- If you have diabetes or hypoglycemia.

Over age 60:
Adverse reactions and side effects may be more frequent and severe than in younger persons.

Pregnancy:
Risk to unborn child outweighs drug benefits. Don't use.

Breast-feeding:
Drug passes into milk. Avoid drug or discontinue nursing until you finish medicine. Consult doctor for advice on maintaining milk supply.

Infants & children:
Not recommended.

Prolonged use:
Weakens heart muscle contractions.

Skin & sunlight:
No problems expected.

Driving, piloting or hazardous work:
Don't drive or pilot aircraft until you learn how medicine affects you. Don't work around dangerous machinery. Don't climb ladders or work in high places. Danger increases if you drink alcohol or take medicine affecting alertness and reflexes.

Airplane passengers:
No problems expected.

Discontinuing:
Don't discontinue without consulting doctor. Dose may require gradual reduction if you have taken drug for a long time. Doses of other drugs may also require adjustment.

Others:
May mask hypoglycemia.

INTERACTION WITH OTHER DRUGS

GENERIC NAME OR DRUG CLASS	COMBINED EFFECT
Antidiabetics	Increased antidiabetic effect.
Antihistamines	Decreased antihistamine effect.
Antihypertensives	Increased antihypertensive effect.
Antiinflammatory drugs	Decreased antiinflammatory effect.
Barbiturates	Increased barbiturate effect. Dangerous sedation.
Digitalis preparations	Can either increase or decrease heart rate. Improves irregular heartbeat.
Narcotics	Increased narcotic effect. Dangerous sedation.
Phenytoin	Increased nadolol effect.
Quinidine	Slows heart excessively.
Reserpine	Increased reserpine effect. Excessive sedation and depression.

INTERACTION WITH OTHER SUBSTANCES

INTERACTS WITH	COMBINED EFFECT
Alcohol:	Excessive blood-pressure drop. Avoid.
Beverages:	None expected.
Cocaine:	Irregular heartbeat. Avoid.
Foods:	None expected.
Marijuana:	Daily use—Impaired circulation to hands and feet.
Tobacco:	Possible irregular heartbeat.

NAFCILLIN

BRAND NAMES

Nafcil
Unipen

GENERAL INFORMATION

Habit forming? No
Prescription needed? Yes
Available as generic? Yes
Drug class: Antibiotic (penicillin)

USES

Treatment of bacterial infections that are susceptible to nafcillin.

DOSAGE & USAGE INFORMATION

How to take:
- Tablets or capsules—Swallow with liquid on an empty stomach 1 hour before or 2 hours after eating.
- Liquid—Take with cold beverage. Liquid form is perishable and effective for only 7 days at room temperature. Effective for 14 days if stored in refrigerator. Don't freeze.

When to take:
Follow instructions on prescription label or side of package. Doses should be evenly spaced. For example, 4 times a day means every 6 hours.

If you forget a dose:
Take as soon as you remember. Continue regular schedule.

What drug does:
Destroys susceptible bacteria. Does not kill viruses.

Time lapse before drug works:
May be several days before medicine affects infection.

Don't take with:
See Interaction column and consult doctor.

OVERDOSE

Symptoms:
Severe diarrhea, nausea or vomiting.

What to do:
Overdose unlikely to threaten life. If person takes much larger amount than prescribed, call doctor, poison-control center or hospital emergency room for instructions.

POSSIBLE ADVERSE REACTIONS OR SIDE EFFECTS

SYMPTOMS	FREQUENCY	WHAT TO DO
Brain & nervous system:	None expected.	
Skin: Hives, rash, intense itch soon after a dose.	Rare	1
Eyes:	None expected.	
Ears, nose, throat: Dark or discolored tongue.	Common	5
Digestive: Mild nausea, vomiting, diarrhea.	Infrequent	4
Heart & lungs:	None expected.	
Blood vessels: Unexplained bleeding.	Rare	3
Muscles, bones, joints:	None expected.	
Genital, urinary:	None expected.	
Kidneys:	None expected.	
Liver:	None expected.	
Allergic: Life-threatening anaphylaxis may occur!	Rare	1 See page 888.
Blood:	None expected.	
Others:	None expected.	

1- Life-threatening. Seek emergency treatment immediately.
2- Discontinue. Seek emergency treatment.
3- Discontinue. Call doctor right away.
4- Continue. Call doctor when convenient.
5- Continue. Tell doctor at next visit.
6- No action necessary.

WARNINGS & PRECAUTIONS

Don't take if:
You are allergic to nafcillin, cephalosporin antibiotics, other penicillins or penicillamine. Life-threatening reaction may occur.

Before you start, consult your doctor:
If you are allergic to any substance or drug.

Over age 60:
You may have skin reactions, particularly around genitals and anus.

Pregnancy:
Studies inconclusive on harm to unborn child. Animal studies show fetal abnormalities. Decide with your doctor whether drug benefits justify risk to unborn child.

Breast-feeding:
Drug passes into milk. Child may become sensitive to penicillins and have allergic reactions to penicillin drugs. Avoid nafcillin or discontinue nursing until you finish medicine. Consult doctor for advice on maintaining milk supply.

Infants & children:
No problems expected.

Prolonged use:
You may become more susceptible to infections caused by germs not responsive to nafcillin.

Skin & sunlight:
No problems expected.

Driving, piloting or hazardous work:
Usually not dangerous. Most hazardous reactions likely to occur a few minutes after taking nafcillin.

Airplane passengers:
No problems expected.

Discontinuing:
Don't discontinue without doctor's advice until you complete prescribed dose, even though symptoms diminish or disappear.

Others:
Absorption of this drug in oral form is unpredictable. Injections are more reliable.

INTERACTION WITH OTHER DRUGS

GENERIC NAME OR DRUG CLASS	COMBINED EFFECT
Chloramphenicol	Decreased effect of both drugs.
Erythromycins	Decreased effect of both drugs.
Paromomycin	Decreased effect of both drugs.
Tetracyclines	Decreased effect of both drugs.
Troleandomycin	Decreased effect of both drugs.

INTERACTION WITH OTHER SUBSTANCES

INTERACTS WITH	COMBINED EFFECT
Alcohol:	Occasional stomach irritation.
Beverages:	None expected.
Cocaine:	No proven problems.
Foods:	None expected.
Marijuana:	No proven problems.
Tobacco:	None expected.

NALBUPHINE

BRAND NAMES

Nubain

GENERAL INFORMATION

Habit forming? Yes
Prescription needed? Yes
Available as generic? Yes
Drug class: Narcotic

 USES

Relieves pain.

 DOSAGE & USAGE INFORMATION

How to take:
- Tablet or capsule—Swallow with liquid. If you can't swallow whole, crumble tablet or open capsule and take with liquid or food.
- Drops or liquid—Dilute dose in beverage before swallowing.

When to take:
When needed. No more often than every 4 hours.

If you forget a dose:
Take as soon as you remember. Wait 4 hours for next dose.

What drug does:
Blocks pain messages to brain and spinal cord.

Time lapse before drug works:
30 minutes.

Don't take with:
See Interaction column and consult doctor.

 OVERDOSE

Symptoms:
Deep sleep; slow breathing; slow pulse; flushed, warm skin; constricted pupils.

What to do:
- Dial 0 (operator) or 911 (emergency) for an ambulance or medical help. Then give first aid immediately.
- If patient is unconscious and not breathing, give mouth-to-mouth breathing. If there is no heartbeat, use cardiac massage and mouth-to-mouth breathing (CPR). Don't try to make patient vomit. If you can't get help quickly, take patient to nearest emergency facility.
- Additional emergency information on page 886.

POSSIBLE ADVERSE REACTIONS OR SIDE EFFECTS

SYMPTOMS	FREQUENCY	WHAT TO DO
Brain & nervous system: Depression, confusion, hallucinations.	Infrequent	4
Skin: • Hives, rash, itch, face swelling.	Rare	3
• Flushed face.	Common	4
Eyes: Blurred vision.	Rare	4
Ears, nose, throat:	None expected.	
Digestive: Severe constipation, abdominal pain, vomiting.	Infrequent	3
Heart & lungs: Slow heartbeat, irregular breathing.	Rare	3
Blood vessels:	None expected.	
Muscles, bones, joints:	None expected.	
Genital, urinary: Difficult urination.	Common	4
Kidneys: Less urine.	Common	4
Liver:	None expected.	
Allergic:	None expected.	
Blood:	None expected.	
Others: Unusual tiredness.	Common	4

1- Life-threatening. Seek emergency treatment immediately.
2- Discontinue. Seek emergency treatment.
3- Discontinue. Call doctor right away.
4- Continue. Call doctor when convenient.
5- Continue. Tell doctor at next visit.
6- No action necessary.

WARNINGS & PRECAUTIONS

Don't take if:
You are allergic to any narcotic.

Before you start, consult your doctor:
If you have impaired liver or kidney function.

Over age 60:
More likely to be drowsy, dizzy, unsteady or constipated. Avoid prolonged use.

Pregnancy:
Studies inconclusive on harm to unborn child. Animal studies show fetal abnormalities. Decide with your doctor whether drug benefits justify risk to unborn child. Abuse by pregnant woman will result in addicted newborn. Withdrawal can be life-threatening.

Breast-feeding:
Drug filters into milk. May depress infant. Avoid.

Infants & children:
Not recommended.

Prolonged use:
Causes psychological and physical dependence.

Skin & sunlight:
No problems expected.

Driving, piloting or hazardous work:
Don't drive or pilot aircraft until you learn how medicine affects you. Don't work around dangerous machinery. Don't climb ladders or work in high places. Danger increases if you drink alcohol or take medicine affecting alertness and reflexes, such as antihistamines, tranquilizers, sedatives, pain medicine, other narcotics and mind-altering drugs.

Airplane passengers:
No proven problems.

Discontinuing:
May be unnecessary to finish medicine. Follow doctor's instructions.

Others:
No problems expected.

INTERACTION WITH OTHER DRUGS

GENERIC NAME OR DRUG CLASS	COMBINED EFFECT
Analgesics	Increased analgesic effect.
Antidepressants	Increased sedative effect.
Antihistamines	Increased sedative effect.
Mind-altering drugs	Increased sedative effect.
Narcotics (other)	Increased narcotic effect.
Phenothiazines	Increased phenothiazine effect.
Sedatives	Increased sedative effect.
Sleep inducers	Increased sedative effect.
Tranquilizers	Increased sedative effect.

INTERACTION WITH OTHER SUBSTANCES

INTERACTS WITH	COMBINED EFFECT
Alcohol:	Increases alcohol's intoxicating effect. Avoid.
Beverages:	None expected.
Cocaine:	Increased cocaine effect.
Foods:	None expected.
Marijuana:	Impairs physical and mental performance.
Tobacco:	None expected.

NALIDIXIC ACID

BRAND NAMES

NegGram

GENERAL INFORMATION

Habit forming? No
Prescription needed? Yes
Available as generic? No
Drug class: Antimicrobial

USES

Treatment for urinary-tract infections.

DOSAGE & USAGE INFORMATION

How to take:
- Tablet—Swallow with food or milk to lessen stomach irritation. If you can't swallow whole, crumble tablet and take with liquid or food.
- Liquid—Take with liquid or food.

When to take:
At the same times each day.

If you forget a dose:
Take as soon as you remember up to 2 hours late. If more than 2 hours, wait for next scheduled dose (don't double this dose).

What drug does:
Destroys bacteria susceptible to nalidixic acid.

Time lapse before drug works:
1 to 2 weeks.

Don't take with:
See Interaction column and consult doctor.

OVERDOSE

Symptoms:
Lethargy, stomach upset, behavioral changes, convulsions and stupor.

What to do:
- Dial 0 (operator) or 911 (emergency) for an ambulance or medical help. Then give first aid immediately.
- If patient is unconscious and not breathing, give mouth-to-mouth breathing. If there is no heartbeat, use cardiac massage and mouth-to-mouth breathing (CPR). Don't try to make patient vomit. If you can't get help quickly, take patient to nearest emergency facility.
- Additional emergency information on page 886.

POSSIBLE ADVERSE REACTIONS OR SIDE EFFECTS

SYMPTOMS	FREQUENCY	WHAT TO DO
Brain & nervous system: Dizziness, drowsiness.	Infrequent	4
Skin:		
• Rash, itch.	Common	3
• Paleness	Rare	3
Eyes: Decreased, blurred, or double vision; halos around lights or excess brightness; changes in color vision.	Common	3
Ears, nose, throat: Sore throat or fever.	Rare	3
Digestive:		
• Severe stomach pain, pale stool.	Rare	3
• Nausea, vomiting, diarrhea.	Common	3
Heart & lungs, muscles, bones, joints, genital, urinary, kidneys, allergic, blood:	None expected.	
Blood vessels: Unusual bruising or bleeding.	Rare	3
Liver: Jaundice (yellow skin and eyes).	Rare	3
Others: Fatigue, weakness.	Rare	3

1- Life-threatening. Seek emergency treatment immediately.
2- Discontinue. Seek emergency treatment.
3- Discontinue. Call doctor right away.
4- Continue. Call doctor when convenient.

NALIDIXIC ACID

 ## WARNINGS & PRECAUTIONS

Don't take if:
- You are allergic to nalidixic acid.
- You have a seizure disorder (epilepsy, convulsions).

Before you start, consult your doctor:
- If you plan to become pregnant within medication period.
- If you have or have had kidney or liver disease.
- If you have impaired circulation of the brain (hardened arteries).
- If you have Parkinson's disease.
- If you have diabetes (it may affect urine-sugar tests).

Over age 60:
Adverse reactions and side effects may be more frequent and severe than in younger persons.

Pregnancy:
Risk to unborn child outweighs drug benefits. Don't use, especially during first 3 months.

Breast-feeding:
No problems expected, unless you have impaired kidney function. Consult doctor.

Infants & children:
Don't give to infants younger than 3 months.

Prolonged use:
No problems expected.

Skin & sunlight:
May cause rash or intensify sunburn in areas exposed to sun or sunlamp.

Driving, piloting or hazardous work:
Avoid if you feel drowsy, dizzy or have vision problems. Otherwise, no problems expected.

Airplane passengers:
No problems expected.

Discontinuing:
Don't discontinue without consulting doctor. Dose may require gradual reduction if you have taken drug for a long time. Doses of other drugs may also require adjustment.

Others:
Periodic blood counts and liver- and kidney-function tests recommended.

 ## INTERACTION WITH OTHER DRUGS

GENERIC NAME OR DRUG CLASS	COMBINED EFFECT
Antacids	Decreased absorption of nalidixic acid.
Anticoagulants (oral)	Increased anticoagulant effect.
Nitrofurantoin	Decreased effect of nalidixic acid.
Probenecid	Decreased effect of nalidixic acid.
Vitamin C (in large doses)	Increased effect of nalidixic acid.

 ## INTERACTION WITH OTHER SUBSTANCES

INTERACTS WITH	COMBINED EFFECT
Alcohol:	Impaired alertness, judgment and coordination.
Beverages:	None expected.
Cocaine:	Impaired judgment and coordination.
Foods:	None expected.
Marijuana:	Impaired alertness, judgment and coordination.
Tobacco:	None expected.

NANDROLONE

BRAND NAMES

Anabolin LA 100
Androlone
Deca-Durabolin
Durabolin

GENERAL INFORMATION

Habit forming? No
Prescription needed? Yes
Available as generic? Yes
Drug class: Androgen (male sex hormone)

 USES

- Corrects male hormone deficiency.
- Reduces "male menopause" symptoms (loss of sex drive, depression, anxiety).
- Decreases calcium loss of osteoporosis (softened bones).
- Blocks growth of breast-cancer cells in females.
- Corrects undescended testicles in male children.
- Reduces breast pain and fullness following childbirth.
- Augments treatment of aplastic anemia.
- Stimulates weight gain after illness, injury or for chronically underweight persons.
- Stimulates growth in treatment of dwarfism.

 DOSAGE & USAGE INFORMATION

How to take:
- Tablets—With food to lessen stomach irritation.
- Injection—Once or twice a month.

When to take:
At the same time each day.

If you forget a dose:
Take as soon as you remember up to 2 hours late. If more than 2 hours, wait for next scheduled dose (don't double this dose).

What drug does:
- Stimulates cells that produce male sex characteristics.
- Replaces hormone deficiencies.
- Stimulates red-blood-cell production.
- Suppresses production of estrogen (female sex hormone).

Time lapse before drug works:
Varies with problems treated. May require 2 or 3 months of regular use for desired effects.

Don't take with:
See Interaction column and consult doctor.

 OVERDOSE

Overdose unlikely to threaten life. If person takes much larger amount than prescribed, call doctor, poison-control center or hospital emergency room for instructions.

 POSSIBLE ADVERSE REACTIONS OR SIDE EFFECTS

SYMPTOMS	FREQUENCY	WHAT TO DO
Brain & nervous system:		
Depression or confusion.	Infrequent	3
Skin:		
• Flushed face.	Infrequent	3
• Rash or itch.	Infrequent	3
• Hives	Rare	2
• Acne or oily skin in females.	Common	4
Eyes, heart & lungs, blood vessels, kidneys, blood:	None expected.	
Ears, nose, throat:		
• Deep voice.	Common	4
• Sore mouth.	Common	5
• Sore throat, fever.	Rare	3
Digestive:		
• Nausea, vomiting, diarrhea.	Infrequent	3
• Abdominal pain.	Rare	3
• Black stool.	Rare	2
Muscles, bones, joints:		
Swollen feet or legs.	Infrequent	3
Genital, urinary:		
• Enlarged clitoris or frequent erections.	Common	4
• Vaginal bleeding.	Infrequent	3
Liver:		
Jaundice (yellow skin and eyes).	Infrequent	2
Allergic:		
Intense itching, weakness, loss of consciousness.	Rare	1
Others:		
• Higher sex drive.	Common	5
• Swollen breasts in men.	Common	4

1 - Life-threatening. Seek emergency treatment immediately.
2 - Discontinue. Seek emergency treatment.
3 - Discontinue. Call doctor right away.
4 - Continue. Call doctor when convenient.
5 - Continue. Tell doctor at next visit.

WARNINGS & PRECAUTIONS

Don't take if:
You are allergic to any male hormone.

Before you start, consult your doctor:
- If you might be pregnant.
- If you have cancer of prostate.
- If you have heart disease or arteriosclerosis.
- If you have kidney or liver disease.
- If you have breast cancer (males).
- If you have high blood pressure.
- If you have migraine attacks.
- If you have high level of blood calcium.
- If you have epilepsy.

Over age 60:
- May stimulate sexual activity.
- Can make high blood pressure or heart disease worse.
- Can enlarge prostate and cause urinary retention.

Pregnancy:
Risk to unborn child outweighs drug benefits. Don't use.

Breast-feeding:
Drug passes into milk. Avoid drug or discontinue nursing until you finish medicine. Consult doctor for advice on maintaining milk supply.

Infants & children:
Don't give to children younger than 2. Use with older children only under medical supervision.

Prolonged use:
- Reduces sperm count and volume of semen.
- Possible kidney stones.
- Unnatural hair growth and deep voice in women.

Skin & sunlight:
No problems expected.

Driving, piloting or hazardous work:
No problems expected.

Airplane passengers:
No problems expected.

Discontinuing:
No problems expected.

Others:
- May cause atrophy of testicles.
- Will not increase strength in athletes.

INTERACTION WITH OTHER DRUGS

GENERIC NAME OR DRUG CLASS	COMBINED EFFECT
Anticoagulants	Increased anticoagulant effect.
Antidiabetics (oral)	Increased antidiabetic effect.
Chlorzoxazone	Decreased nandrolone effect.
Oxyphenbutazone	Decreased nandrolone effect.
Phenobarbital	Decreased nandrolone effect.
Phenylbutazone	Decreased nandrolone effect.

INTERACTION WITH OTHER SUBSTANCES

INTERACTS WITH	COMBINED EFFECT
Alcohol:	None expected.
Beverages:	None expected.
Cocaine:	No proven problems.
Foods: Salt	Excessive fluid retention (edema). Decrease salt intake while taking male hormone.
Marijuana:	Decreased blood levels of nandrolone.
Tobacco:	No proven problems.

NAPROXEN

BRAND NAMES

Anaprox
Naprosyn

Habit forming? No
Prescription needed? Yes

USES

- Treatment for joint pain, stiffness, inflammation and swelling of arthritis and gout.
- Pain reliever.
- Treatment for dysmenorrhea (painful or difficult menstruation).

DOSAGE & USAGE INFORMATION

How to take:
Tablet—Swallow with liquid or food to lessen stomach irritation. If you can't swallow whole, crumble tablet and take with liquid or food.

When to take:
At the same times each day.

If you forget a dose:
Take as soon as you remember up to 2 hours late. If more than 2 hours, wait for next scheduled dose (don't double this dose).

What drug does:
Reduces tissue concentration of prostaglandins (hormones which produce inflammation and pain).

Time lapse before drug works:
Begins in 4 to 24 hours. May require 3 weeks regular use for maximum benefit.

Don't take with:
See Interaction column and consult doctor.

OVERDOSE

Symptoms:
Confusion, agitation, incoherence, convulsions, possible hemorrhage from stomach or intestine, coma.

What to do:
- Dial 0 (operator) or 911 (emergency) for an ambulance or medical help. Then give first aid immediately.
- Additional emergency information on page 886.

GENERAL INFORMATION

Available as generic? No
Drug class: Antiinflammatory (non-steroid)

POSSIBLE ADVERSE REACTIONS OR SIDE EFFECTS

SYMPTOMS	FREQUENCY	WHAT TO DO
Brain & nervous system:		
• Depression, drowsiness.	Infrequent	4
• Convulsions, confusion.	Rare	3
• Dizziness	Common	4
• Headache	Common	5
Skin:		
Rash, hives or itch.	Rare	3
Eyes:		
Blurred vision.	Rare	3
Ears, nose, throat:		
Ringing in ears.	Infrequent	4
Digestive:		
• Bloody or black, tarry stools.	Rare	3
• Nausea, pain.	Common	4
• Constipation or diarrhea, vomiting.	Infrequent	4
Heart & lungs:		
Breathing difficulty, tightness in chest, rapid heartbeat.	Rare	3
Blood vessels:		
Unusual bleeding or bruising.	Rare	3
Muscles, bones, joints:		
Swollen feet, legs.	Infrequent	4
Genital, urinary:		
• Bloody urine.	Rare	3
• Difficult, painful or frequent urination.	Rare	4
Kidneys, allergic, blood:		
	None expected.	
Liver:		
Jaundice (yellow skin and eyes).	Rare	3
Others:		
Fatigue, weakness.	Rare	4

1- Life-threatening. Seek emergency treatment immediately.
2- Discontinue. Seek emergency treatment.
3- Discontinue. Call doctor right away.
4- Continue. Call doctor when convenient.
5- Continue. Tell doctor at next visit.

WARNINGS & PRECAUTIONS

Don't take if:
- You are allergic to aspirin or any non-steroid, antiinflammatory drug.
- You have gastritis, peptic ulcer, enteritis, ileitis, ulcerative colitis, asthma, heart failure, high blood pressure or bleeding problems.
- You have had recent rectal bleeding and suppository form has been prescribed.
- Patient is younger than 15.

Before you start, consult your doctor:
- If you have epilepsy.
- If you have Parkinson's disease.
- If you have been mentally ill.
- If you have had kidney disease or impaired kidney function.

Over age 60:
Adverse reactions and side effects may be more frequent and severe than in younger persons.

Pregnancy:
Studies inconclusive on harm to unborn child. Decide with your doctor whether drug benefits justify risk to unborn child.

Breast-feeding:
May harm child. Avoid.

Infants & children:
Not recommended for anyone younger than 15. Use only under medical supervision.

Prolonged use:
- Eye damage.
- Reduced hearing.
- Sore throat, fever.
- Weight gain.

Skin & sunlight:
No problems expected.

Driving, piloting or hazardous work:
Don't drive or pilot aircraft until you learn how medicine affects you. Don't work around dangerous machinery. Don't climb ladders or work in high places. Danger increases if you drink alcohol or take medicine affecting alertness and reflexes, such as antihistamines, tranquilizers, sedatives, pain medicine, narcotics and mind-altering drugs.

Airplane passengers:
No problems expected.

Discontinuing:
Don't discontinue without consulting doctor. Dose may require gradual reduction if you have taken drug for a long time. Doses of other drugs may also require adjustment.

Others:
No problems expected.

INTERACTION WITH OTHER DRUGS

GENERIC NAME OR DRUG CLASS	COMBINED EFFECT
Anticoagulants, (oral)	Increased risk of bleeding.
Aspirin	Increased risk of stomach ulcer.
Cortisone drugs	Increased risk of stomach ulcer.
Furosemide	Decreased diuretic effect of furosemide.
Oxyphenbutazone	Possible stomach ulcer.
Phenylbutazone	Possible stomach ulcer.
Probenecid	Increased naproxen effect.
Thyroid hormones	Rapid heartbeat, blood pressure rise.

INTERACTION WITH OTHER SUBSTANCES

INTERACTS WITH	COMBINED EFFECT
Alcohol:	Possible stomach ulcer or bleeding.
Beverages:	None expected.
Cocaine:	None expected.
Foods:	None expected.
Marijuana:	Increased pain relief from naproxen.
Tobacco:	None expected.

NEOSTIGMINE

BRAND NAMES

Prostigmin

GENERAL INFORMATION

Habit forming? No
Prescription needed? Yes
Available as generic? Yes
Drug class: Cholinergic (anticholinesterase)

 USES

- Treatment of myasthenia gravis.
- Treatment of urinary retention and abdominal distention.
- Antidote to adverse effects of muscle relaxants used in surgery.

 DOSAGE & USAGE INFORMATION

How to take:
Tablet—Swallow with liquid or food to lessen stomach irritation.

When to take:
As directed, usually 3 or 4 times a day.

If you forget a dose:
Take as soon as you remember up to 2 hours late. If more than 2 hours, wait for next scheduled dose (don't double this dose).

What drug does:
Inhibits the chemical activity of an enzyme (cholinesterase) so nerve impulses can cross the junction of nerves and muscles.

Time lapse before drug works:
3 hours.

Don't take with:
See Interaction column and consult doctor.

 OVERDOSE

Symptoms:
Muscle weakness, cramps, twitching or clumsiness; severe diarrhea, nausea, vomiting, stomach cramps or pain; breathing difficulty; confusion, irritability, nervousness, restlessness, fear; unusually slow heartbeat; seizures.

What to do:
- Dial 0 (operator) or 911 (emergency) for an ambulance or medical help. Then give first aid immediately.
- Additional emergency information on page 886.

POSSIBLE ADVERSE REACTIONS OR SIDE EFFECTS

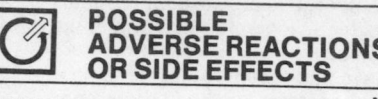

SYMPTOMS	FREQUENCY	WHAT TO DO
Brain & nervous system: Confusion, irritability.	Infrequent	2
Skin:	None expected.	
Eyes: Constricted pupils, watery eyes.	Infrequent	4
Ears, nose, throat: Excess saliva.	Common	4
Digestive: Mild diarrhea, nausea, vomiting, stomach cramps or pain.	Common	3
Heart & lungs: Lung congestion.	Infrequent	4
Blood vessels:	None expected.	
Muscles, bones, joints:	None expected.	
Genital, urinary: Frequent urge to urinate.	Infrequent	4
Kidneys:	None expected.	
Liver:	None expected.	
Allergic:	None expected.	
Blood:	None expected.	
Others: Unusual sweating.	Common	4

1- Life-threatening. Seek emergency treatment immediately.
2- Discontinue. Seek emergency treatment.
3- Discontinue. Call doctor right away.
4- Continue. Call doctor when convenient.
5- Continue. Tell doctor at next visit.
6- No action necessary.

WARNINGS & PRECAUTIONS

Don't take if:
- You are allergic to any cholinergic or bromide.
- You take mecamylamine.

Before you start, consult your doctor:
- If you plan to become pregnant within medication period.
- If you have bronchial asthma.
- If you have heartbeat irregularities.
- If you have urinary obstruction or urinary-tract infection.

Over age 60:
Adverse reactions and side effects may be more frequent and severe than in younger persons.

Pregnancy:
No proven harm to unborn child. Avoid if possible. May increase uterus contractions close to delivery.

Breast-feeding:
No problems expected, but consult doctor.

Infants & children:
Not recommended.

Prolonged use:
Medication may lose effectiveness. Discontinuing for a few days may restore effect.

Skin & sunlight:
No problems expected.

Driving, piloting or hazardous work:
Don't drive or pilot aircraft until you learn how medicine affects you. Don't work around dangerous machinery. Don't climb ladders or work in high places. Danger increases if you drink alcohol or take medicine affecting alertness and reflexes, such as antihistamines, tranquilizers, sedatives, pain medicine, narcotics and mind-altering drugs.

Airplane passengers:
No problems expected.

Discontinuing:
Don't discontinue without doctor's advice until you complete prescribed dose, even though symptoms diminish or disappear.

Others:
No problems expected.

INTERACTION WITH OTHER DRUGS

GENERIC NAME OR DRUG CLASS	COMBINED EFFECT
Anesthetics (local or general)	Decreased neostigmine effect.
Antiarrhythmics	Decreased neostigmine effect.
Antibiotics	Decreased neostigmine effect.
Anticholinergics	Decreased neostigmine effect. May mask severe side effects.
Cholinergics (other)	Reduced intestinal-tract function. Possible brain and nervous-system toxicity.
Mecamylamine	Decreased neostigmine effect.
Quinidine	Decreased neostigmine effect.

INTERACTION WITH OTHER SUBSTANCES

INTERACTS WITH	COMBINED EFFECT
Alcohol:	No proven problems with small doses.
Beverages:	None expected.
Cocaine:	Decreased neostigmine effect. Avoid.
Foods:	None expected.
Marijuana:	No proven problems.
Tobacco:	No proven problems.

NIACIN (NICOTINIC ACID)

BRAND NAMES

Diacin	Nico-Span	Novoniacin
N-Caps	Nicobid	Span-Niacin
Niac	Nicocap	SK-Niacin
Niacin	Nicolar	Tega-Span
Nicalex	Nicotinex	Vasotherm
Nico-400	Nicotym	

Numerous other multiple vitamin-mineral supplements.

GENERAL INFORMATION

Habit forming? No
Prescription needed? Tablets: No
Liquid, capsules: Yes
Available as generic? Yes
Drug class: Vitamin supplement, vasodilator, antihyperlipidemic

USES

- Replacement for niacin deficiency caused by inadequate diet.
- Treatment for vertigo (dizziness) and ringing in ears.
- Prevention of premenstrual headache.
- Reduction of blood levels of cholesterol and triglycerides.
- Treatment for pellagra.

DOSAGE & USAGE INFORMATION

How to take:
- Tablet, capsule or liquid—Swallow with liquid or food to lessen stomach irritation.
- Extended-release tablets or capsules—Swallow each dose whole.

When to take:
At the same times each day.

If you forget a dose:
Take as soon as you remember. Wait 4 hours for next dose.

What drug does:
- Corrects niacin deficiency.
- Dilates blood vessels.
- In large doses, decreases cholesterol production.

Time lapse before drug works:
15 to 20 minutes.

Don't take with:
See Interaction column and consult doctor.

OVERDOSE

Symptoms:
Body flush, nausea, vomiting, abdominal cramps, diarrhea, weakness, lightheadedness, fainting, sweating.

What to do:
Overdose unlikely to threaten life. If person takes much larger amount than prescribed, call doctor, poison-control center or hospital emergency room for instructions.

POSSIBLE ADVERSE REACTIONS OR SIDE EFFECTS

SYMPTOMS	FREQUENCY	WHAT TO DO
Brain & nervous system: Headache, dizziness, faintness.	Infrequent	4
Skin: "Hot" feeling, flush.	Infrequent	6
Eyes:	None expected.	
Ears, nose, throat:	None expected.	
Digestive:	None expected.	
Heart & lungs:	None expected.	
Blood vessels:	None expected.	
Muscles, bones, joints: Temporary numbness and tingling in hands and feet.	Infrequent	4
Genital, urinary:	None expected.	
Kidneys:	None expected.	
Liver: Jaundice (yellow skin and eyes).	Rare	3
Allergic:	None expected.	
Blood:	None expected.	
Others:	None expected.	

1 - Life-threatening. Seek emergency treatment immediately.
2 - Discontinue. Seek emergency treatment.
3 - Discontinue. Call doctor right away.
4 - Continue. Call doctor when convenient.
5 - Continue. Tell doctor at next visit.
6 - No action necessary.

NIACIN (NICOTINIC ACID)

 ## WARNINGS & PRECAUTIONS

Don't take if:
- You are allergic to niacin or any niacin-containing vitamin mixtures.
- You have impaired liver function.
- You have active peptic ulcer.

Before you start, consult your doctor:
- If you have diabetes.
- If you have gout.
- If you have gallbladder or liver disease.

Over age 60:
Response to drug cannot be predicted. Dose must be individualized.

Pregnancy:
Risk to unborn child outweighs drug benefits. Don't use.

Breast-feeding:
Studies inconclusive. Consult doctor.

Infants & children:
- Use only under supervision.
- Keep vitamin-mineral supplements out of children's reach.

Prolonged use:
Possible impaired liver function.

Skin & sunlight:
No problems expected.

Driving, piloting or hazardous work:
Avoid if you feel dizzy or faint. Otherwise, no problems expected.

Airplane passengers:
No problems expected.

Discontinuing:
May be unnecessary to finish medicine. Follow doctor's instructions.

Others:
- A balanced diet should provide all the niacin a healthy person needs and make supplements unnecessary. Best sources are meat, eggs and dairy products.
- Store in original container in cool, dry, dark place. Bathroom medicine chest too moist.
- Obesity reduces effectiveness.

 ## INTERACTION WITH OTHER DRUGS

GENERIC NAME OR DRUG CLASS	COMBINED EFFECT
Antidiabetics	Decreased antidiabetic effect.
Beta-adrenergic blockers	Excessively low blood pressure.
Guanethidine	Increased guanethidine effect.
Isoniazid	Decreased niacin effect.
Mecamylamine	Excessively low blood pressure.
Methyldopa	Excessively low blood pressure.
Pargyline	Excessively low blood pressure.

 ## INTERACTION WITH OTHER SUBSTANCES

INTERACTS WITH	COMBINED EFFECT
Alcohol:	Excessively low blood pressure. Use caution.
Beverages:	None expected.
Cocaine:	Increased flushing.
Foods:	None expected.
Marijuana:	None expected.
Tobacco:	Decreased niacin effect.

NIFEDIPINE

BRAND NAMES

Procardia

GENERAL INFORMATION

Habit forming? No
Prescription needed? Yes
Available as generic? No
Drug class: Calcium-channel blocker, antiarrhythmic, antianginal

USES

Prevents angina attacks.

DOSAGE & USAGE INFORMATION

How to take:
Capsule—Swallow with liquid.

When to take:
At the same times each day 1 hour before or 2 hours after eating.

If you forget a dose:
Take as soon as you remember up to 2 hours late. If more than 2 hours, wait for next scheduled dose (don't double this dose).

What drug does:
- Reduces work that heart must perform.
- Reduces normal artery pressure.
- Increases oxygen to heart muscle.

Time lapse before drug works:
1 to 2 hours.

Don't take with:
See Interaction column and consult doctor.

OVERDOSE

Symptoms:
Unusually fast or unusually slow heartbeat, loss of consciousness, cardiac arrest.

What to do:
- Dial 0 (operator) or 911 (emergency) for an ambulance or medical help. Then give first aid immediately.
- If patient is unconscious and not breathing, give mouth-to-mouth breathing. If there is no heartbeat, use cardiac massage and mouth-to-mouth breathing (CPR). Don't try to make patient vomit. If you can't get help quickly, take patient to nearest emergency facility.
- Additional emergency information on page 886.

POSSIBLE ADVERSE REACTIONS OR SIDE EFFECTS

SYMPTOMS	FREQUENCY	WHAT TO DO
Brain & nervous system:		
● Dizziness	Infrequent	4
● Headache	Rare	5
● Fainting	Rare	3
Skin:	None expected.	
Eyes:	None expected.	
Ears, nose, throat:	None expected.	
Digestive:		
Nausea, constipation.	Infrequent	5
Heart & lungs:		
● Unusually fast or unusually slow heartbeat.	Infrequent	3
● Wheezing, cough, shortness of breath.	Infrequent	3
● Chest pain.	Rare	3
Blood vessels:	None expected.	
Muscles, bones, joints:		
● Numbness, tingling in hands and feet.	Infrequent	4
● Swelling of ankles, feet, legs.	Infrequent	4
Genital, urinary:		
Difficult urination.	Infrequent	4
Kidneys:	None expected.	
Liver:	None expected.	
Allergic:	None expected.	
Blood:	None expected.	
Others:		
Tiredness	Common	5

1-Life-threatening. Seek emergency treatment immediately.
2-Discontinue. Seek emergency treatment.
3-Discontinue. Call doctor right away.
4-Continue. Call doctor when convenient.
5-Continue. Tell doctor at next visit.
6-No action necessary.

WARNINGS & PRECAUTIONS

Don't take if:
- You are allergic to nifedipine.
- You have very low blood pressure.

Before you start, consult your doctor:
- If you have kidney or liver disease.
- If you have high blood pressure.
- If you have heart disease other than coronary-artery disease.

Over age 60:
Adverse reactions and side effects may be more frequent and severe than in younger persons.

Pregnancy:
No proven harm to unborn child. Avoid if possible.

Breast-feeding:
Safety not established. Avoid if possible.

Infants & children:
Not recommended.

Prolonged use:
No problems expected.

Skin & sunlight:
No problems expected.

Driving, piloting or hazardous work:
Avoid if you feel dizzy. Otherwise, no problems expected.

Airplane passengers:
No problems expected.

Discontinuing:
Don't discontinue without doctor's advice until you complete prescribed dose, even though symptoms diminish or disappear.

Others:
- Learn to check your own pulse rate. If it drops to 50 beats per minute or lower, don't take nifedipine until your consult your doctor.
- Drug may lower blood-sugar level if daily dose is more than 60 mg.

INTERACTION WITH OTHER DRUGS

GENERIC NAME OR DRUG CLASS	COMBINED EFFECT
Anticoagulants (oral)	Increased anticoagulant effect.
Anticonvulsants (hydantoin)	Increased anticonvulsant effect.
Antihypertensives	Dangerous blood-pressure drop.
Beta-adrenergic blockers	Possible irregular heartbeat.
Calcium (large doses)	Decreased nifedipine effect.
Diuretics	Dangerous blood-pressure drop.
Digitalis preparations	Increased digitalis effect. May need to reduce dose.
Disopyramide	May cause dangerously slow, fast or irregular heartbeat.
Nitrates	Reduced angina attacks.
Quinidine	Increased quinidine effect.
Vitamin D (large doses)	Decreased nifedipine effect.

INTERACTION WITH OTHER SUBSTANCES

INTERACTS WITH	COMBINED EFFECT
Alcohol:	Dangerously low blood pressure. Avoid.
Beverages:	None expected.
Cocaine:	Possible irregular heartbeat. Avoid.
Foods:	None expected.
Marijuana:	Possible irregular heartbeat. Avoid.
Tobacco:	Possible rapid heartbeat. Avoid.

NITROFURANTOIN

BRAND NAMES

Cyantin	Furantoin	Sarodant
Furadantin	Macrodantin	Trantoin
Furalan	Nitrex	Urotoin
Furaloid	Nitrodan	

USES

Treatment for urinary-tract infections.

DOSAGE & USAGE INFORMATION

How to take:
- Tablet or capsule—Swallow with food or milk to lessen stomach irritation. If you can't swallow whole, crumble tablet or open capsule and take with liquid or food.
- Liquid—Shake well and take with food. Use a measuring spoon to ensure accuracy.

When to take:
At the same times each day.

If you forget a dose:
Take as soon as you remember up to 2 hours late. If more than 2 hours, wait for next scheduled dose (don't double this dose).

What drug does:
Prevents susceptible bacteria in the urinary tract from growing and multiplying.

Time lapse before drug works:
1 to 2 weeks.

Don't take with:
See Interaction column and consult doctor.

OVERDOSE

Symptoms:
Nausea, vomiting, abdominal pain, diarrhea.

What to do:
Overdose unlikely to threaten life. If person takes much larger amount than prescribed, call doctor, poison-control center or hospital emergency room for instructions.

GENERAL INFORMATION

Habit forming? No
Prescription needed? Yes
Available as generic? Yes
Drug class: Antimicrobial

POSSIBLE ADVERSE REACTIONS OR SIDE EFFECTS

SYMPTOMS	FREQUENCY	WHAT TO DO
Brain & nervous system: Dizziness, drowsiness, headache.	Infrequent	4
Skin:		
• Rash, itch.	Infrequent	3
• Numbness, tingling or burning of face or mouth.	Infrequent	3
• Paleness	Infrequent	4
Ears, nose, throat: In children, discolored teeth (liquid).	Infrequent	4
Digestive: Diarrhea, appetite loss, nausea, vomiting.	Common	3
Heart & lungs: Chest pain, cough, breathing difficulty.	Common	3
Eyes, blood vessels, muscles, bones, joints, kidneys, blood:	None expected.	
Genital, urinary: Rusty-color or brown urine.	Common	6
Liver: Jaundice (yellow skin and eyes).	Rare	3
Allergic: Life-threatening anaphylaxis may occur!	Rare	1 See page 888.
Others:		
• Chills or unexplained fever.	Common	3
• Fatigue, weakness	Infrequent	3

1- Life-threatening. Seek emergency treatment immediately.
2- Discontinue. Seek emergency treatment.
3- Discontinue. Call doctor right away.
4- Continue. Call doctor when convenient.
5- Continue. Tell doctor at next visit.
6- No action necessary.

NITROFURANTOIN

 **WARNINGS &
PRECAUTIONS**

Don't take if:
- You are allergic to nitrofurantoin.
- You have impaired kidney function.
- You drink alcohol.

Before you start, consult your doctor:
- If you are prone to allergic reactions.
- If you are pregnant and within 2 weeks of delivery.
- If you have had kidney disease, lung disease, anemia, nerve damage, or G6PD deficiency (a metabolic deficiency).
- If you have diabetes. Drug may affect urine sugar tests.

Over age 60:
Adverse reactions and side effects may be more frequent and severe than in younger persons.

Pregnancy:
Risk to unborn child outweighs drug benefits, especially in last month of pregnancy. Don't use.

Breast-feeding:
Drug passes into milk. Avoid drug or discontinue nursing until you finish medicine. Consult doctor for advice on maintaining milk supply.

Infants & children:
Don't give to infants younger than 1 month. Use only under medical supervision for older children.

Prolonged use:
Chest pain, cough, shortness of breath.

Skin & sunlight:
No problems expected.

Driving, piloting or hazardous work:
Avoid if you feel dizzy or drowsy. Otherwise, no problems expected.

Airplane passengers:
No problems expected.

Discontinuing:
Don't discontinue without consulting doctor. Dose may require gradual reduction if you have taken drug for a long time. Doses of other drugs may also require adjustment.

Others:
Periodic blood counts, liver-function tests, and chest X-rays recommended.

 **INTERACTION WITH
OTHER DRUGS**

GENERIC NAME OR DRUG CLASS	COMBINED EFFECT
Nalidixic acid	Decreased nitrofurantoin effect.
Phenobarbital	Decreased nitrofurantoin effect.
Probenecid	Increased nitrofurantoin effect.
Sulfinpyrazone	Possible nitrofurantoin toxicity.

 **INTERACTION WITH
OTHER SUBSTANCES**

INTERACTS WITH	COMBINED EFFECT
Alcohol:	Possible disulfiram reaction (see page 848). Avoid.
Beverages:	None expected.
Cocaine:	No proven problems.
Foods:	None expected.
Marijuana:	None expected.
Tobacco:	None expected.

NITROGLYCERIN (GLYCERYL TRINITRATE)

BRAND NAMES

Nitro-Bid	Nitrol	Nitrostat
Nitro-Dur	Nitrong	Susadrin
Nitrodisc	Nitrospan	Transderm-Nitro
Nitroglyn	Nitrostabilin	Vasoglyn

GENERAL INFORMATION

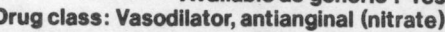

Habit forming? No
Prescription needed? Yes
Available as generic? Yes
Drug class: Vasodilator, antianginal (nitrate)

 ## USES

Treatment for angina pain caused by temporary lack of oxygen to heart muscle.

 ## DOSAGE & USAGE INFORMATION

How to take:
- Tablet or capsule—Swallow whole with liquid. Don't crush, chew or open.
- Ointment—Apply as directed.
- Sublingual tablets—Place under tongue every 3 to 5 minutes at earliest sign of angina. If discomfort is not angina, nitroglycerin will not bring relief. If you don't have complete relief with 3 or 4 tablets, call doctor.

When to take:
Swallowed tablets or capsules—Take at the same time every day.

If you forget a dose:
Swallowed tablets or capsules—Take up to 2 hours late. If more than 2 hours, wait for next dose (don't double this).

What drug does:
Relaxes and expands muscles of arteries to heart, increasing blood and oxygen supply.

Time lapse before drug works:
- Sublingual tablets—1 to 3 minutes.
- Other forms—15 to 30 minutes. Will not stop an attack, but may prevent attacks.

Don't take with:
See Interaction column and consult doctor.

 ## OVERDOSE

Symptoms:
Flushed face, vomiting, weakness, sweating, fainting, shortness of breath, coma.

What to do:
- Dial 0 (operator) or 911 (emergency) for an ambulance or medical help. Then give first aid immediately.
- Additional emergency information on page 886.

POSSIBLE ADVERSE REACTIONS OR SIDE EFFECTS

SYMPTOMS	FREQUENCY	WHAT TO DO
Brain & nervous system: Faintness, dizziness, headache.	Common	5
Skin:		
• Flushed or pale face	Common	5
• Rash	Infrequent	3
• Severe irritation, peeling.	Rare	4
Eyes:	None expected.	
Ears, nose, throat:	None expected.	
Digestive: Nausea, vomiting.	Common	3
Heart & lungs: Rapid heartbeat.	Common	5
Blood vessels:	None expected.	
Muscles, bones, joints:	None expected.	
Genital, urinary:	None expected.	
Kidneys:	None expected.	
Liver:	None expected.	
Allergic:	None expected.	
Blood:	None expected.	
Others:	None expected.	

1- Life-threatening. Seek emergency treatment immediately.
2- Discontinue. Seek emergency treatment.
3- Discontinue. Call doctor right away.
4- Continue. Call doctor when convenient.
5- Continue. Tell doctor at next visit.
6- No action necessary.

NITROGLYCERIN (GLYCERYL TRINITRATE)

 WARNINGS & PRECAUTIONS

Don't take if:
You are allergic to any nitrate.

Before you start, consult your doctor:
- If you are taking non-prescription drugs.
- If you plan to become pregnant within medication period.
- If you have glaucoma.
- If you have reacted badly to any vasodilator drug.
- If you drink alcoholic beverages or smoke marijuana.

Over age 60:
Adverse reactions and side effects may be more frequent and severe than in younger persons. Likely to lower blood pressure excessively.

Pregnancy:
No proven harm to unborn child. Avoid if possible.

Breast-feeding:
No problems expected, but consult doctor.

Infants & children:
Not recommended.

Prolonged use:
No problems expected.

Skin & sunlight:
No problems expected.

Driving, piloting or hazardous work:
Avoid if you feel dizzy or faint. Otherwise, no problems expected.

Airplane passengers:
No problems expected.

Discontinuing:
Don't discontinue without doctor's advice (except sublingual tablets) until you complete prescribed dose, even though symptoms diminish or disappear.

Others:
Keep sublingual tablets in original container. Always carry them with you, but keep from body heat if possible.

 INTERACTION WITH OTHER DRUGS

GENERIC NAME OR DRUG CLASS	COMBINED EFFECT
Anticholinergics	Increased pressure within the eye.
Antidepressants (tricyclic)	Severe blood-pressure drop.
Antihypertensives	Severe blood-pressure drop.
Beta-adrenergic blockers	Dangerous blood-pressure drop.
Cholinergics	Decreased cholinergic effect.
Ephedrine	Decreased nitroglycerin effect.

 INTERACTION WITH OTHER SUBSTANCES

INTERACTS WITH	COMBINED EFFECT
Alcohol:	Increased headache severity and likely fainting. Avoid.
Beverages:	None expected.
Cocaine:	Flushed face and headache. Avoid.
Foods:	None expected.
Marijuana:	Decreased nitroglycerin effect, increased angina pain. Avoid.
Tobacco:	Decreased nitroglycerin effect.

NORETHINDRONE

BRAND NAMES

Micronor
Norlutin
Nor-Q.D.

GENERAL INFORMATION

Habit forming? No
Prescription needed? Yes
Available as generic? No
Drug class: Female sex hormone (progestin)

 USES

- Treatment for menstrual or uterine disorders caused by progestin imbalance.
- Contraceptive

 DOSAGE & USAGE INFORMATION

How to take:
Tablet or capsule—Swallow with liquid or food to lessen stomach irritation. You may crumble tablet or open capsule.

When to take:
At the same time each day.

If you forget a dose:
- Menstrual disorders—Take up to 2 hours late. If more than 2 hours, wait for next dose (don't double this).
- Contraceptive—Consult your doctor. You may need to use another birth-control method until next period.

What drug does:
- Creates a uterine lining similar to pregnancy that prevents bleeding.
- Suppresses a pituitary gland hormone responsible for ovulation.
- Stimulates cervical mucus, which stops sperm penetration and prevents pregnancy.

Time lapse before drug works:
- Menstrual disorders—24 to 48 hours.
- Contraception—3 weeks.

Don't take with:
See Interaction column and consult doctor.

 OVERDOSE

Symptoms:
Nausea, vomiting, fluid retention, breast discomfort or enlargement, vaginal bleeding.

What to do:
Overdose unlikely to threaten life. If person takes much larger amount than prescribed, call doctor, poison-control center or hospital emergency room for instructions.

POSSIBLE ADVERSE REACTIONS OR SIDE EFFECTS

SYMPTOMS	FREQUENCY	WHAT TO DO
Brain & nervous system:		
Depression	Infrequent	4
Skin:		
• Rash	Rare	3
• Acne, increased facial or body hair.	Infrequent	5
Eyes, ears, nose, throat, heart & lungs, muscles, bones, joints, kidneys, allergic, blood:	None expected.	
Digestive:		
• Stomach or side pain.	Rare	3
• Appetite or weight changes.	Common	5
• Nausea	Infrequent	5
Blood vessels:		
Blood clot in leg, brain or lung.	Rare	1
Muscles, bones, joints:		
Ankle, foot swelling.	Common	5
Genital, urinary:		
Prolonged vaginal bleeding.	Infrequent	3
Liver:		
Jaundice (yellow skin and eyes).	Rare	3
Others:		
• Breast tenderness.	Infrequent	5
• Unusual tiredness or weakness.	Common	5

1- Life-threatening. Seek emergency treatment immediately.
2- Discontinue. Seek emergency treatment.
3- Discontinue. Call doctor right away.
4- Continue. Call doctor when convenient.
5- Continue. Tell doctor at next visit.

WARNINGS & PRECAUTIONS

Don't take if:
- You are allergic to any progestin hormone.
- You may be pregnant.
- You have liver or gallbladder disease.
- You have had thrombophlebitis, embolism or stroke.
- You have unexplained vaginal bleeding.
- You have had breast or uterine cancer.

Before you start, consult your doctor:
- If you have heart or kidney disease.
- If you have diabetes.
- If you have a seizure disorder.
- If you suffer migraines.
- If you are easily depressed.

Over age 60:
Not recommended.

Pregnancy:
May harm child. Discontinue at first sign of pregnancy.

Breast-feeding:
Drug passes into milk. Avoid drug or discontinue nursing until you finish medicine. Consult doctor for advice on maintaining milk supply.

Infants & children:
Use only for female children under medical supervision.

Prolonged use:
No problems expected.

Skin & sunlight:
No problems expected.

Driving, piloting or hazardous work:
No problems expected.

Airplane passengers:
No problems expected.

Discontinuing:
Consult doctor. This medicine stays in the body and causes fetal abnormalities. Wait at least 3 months before becoming pregnant.

Others:
- Patients with diabetes must be monitored closely.
- Symptoms of blood clot in leg, brain or lung are: chest, groin, leg pain; sudden, severe headache; loss of coordination; vision change; shortness of breath; slurred speech.

INTERACTION WITH OTHER DRUGS

GENERIC NAME OR DRUG CLASS	COMBINED EFFECT
Antihistamines	Decreased norethindrone effect.
Oxyphenbutazone	Decreased norethindrone effect.
Phenobarbital	Decreased norethindrone effect.
Phenothiazines	Increased phenothiazine effect.
Phenylbutazone	Decreased norethindrone effect.

INTERACTION WITH OTHER SUBSTANCES

INTERACTS WITH	COMBINED EFFECT
Alcohol:	None expected.
Beverages:	None expected.
Cocaine:	Decreased norethindrone effect.
Foods: Salt	Fluid retention.
Marijuana:	Possible menstrual irregularities or bleeding between periods.
Tobacco:	Possible blood clots in lung, brain, legs. Avoid.

NORETHINDRONE ACETATE

BRAND NAMES

Norlutate

GENERAL INFORMATION

Habit forming? No
Prescription needed? Yes
Available as generic? No
Drug class: Female sex hormone (progestin)

 ## USES

- Treatment for menstrual or uterine disorders caused by progestin imbalance.
- Contraceptive
- Treatment for cancer of breast and uterus.

 ## DOSAGE & USAGE INFORMATION

How to take:
Tablet or capsule—Swallow with liquid or food to lessen stomach irritation. You may crumble tablet or open capsule.

When to take:
At the same time each day.

If you forget a dose:
- Menstrual disorders—Take up to 2 hours late. If more than 2 hours, wait for next dose (don't double this).
- Contraceptive—Consult your doctor. You may need to use another birth-control method until next period.

What drug does:
- Creates a uterine lining similar to pregnancy that prevents bleeding.
- Suppresses a pituitary gland hormone responsible for ovulation.
- Stimulates cervical mucus, which stops sperm penetration and prevents pregnancy.

Time lapse before drug works:
- Menstrual disorders—24 to 48 hours.
- Contraception—3 weeks.
- Cancer—May require 2 to 3 months.

Don't take with:
See Interaction column and consult doctor.

 ## OVERDOSE

Symptoms:
Nausea, vomiting, fluid retention, breast discomfort or enlargement, vaginal bleeding.

What to do:
Overdose unlikely to threaten life. If person takes much larger amount than prescribed, call doctor, poison-control center or hospital emergency room for instructions.

POSSIBLE ADVERSE REACTIONS OR SIDE EFFECTS

SYMPTOMS	FREQUENCY	WHAT TO DO
Brain & nervous system:		
Depression	Infrequent	4
Skin:		
• Rash	Rare	3
• Acne, increased facial or body hair.	Infrequent	5
Eyes, ears, nose, throat, heart & lungs, muscles, bones, joints, kidneys, allergic, blood:	None expected.	
Digestive:		
• Stomach or side pain.	Rare	3
• Appetite or weight changes.	Common	5
• Nausea	Infrequent	5
Blood vessels:		
Blood clot in leg, brain or lung.	Rare	1
Muscles, bones, joints:		
Ankle, foot swelling.	Common	5
Genital, urinary:		
Prolonged vaginal bleeding.	Infrequent	3
Liver:		
Jaundice (yellow skin and eyes).	Rare	3
Others:		
• Breast tenderness.	Infrequent	5
• Unusual tiredness or weakness.	Common	5

1- Life-threatening. Seek emergency treatment immediately.
2- Discontinue. Seek emergency treatment.
3- Discontinue. Call doctor right away.
4- Continue. Call doctor when convenient.
5- Continue. Tell doctor at next visit.

NORETHINDRONE ACETATE

WARNINGS & PRECAUTIONS

Don't take if:
- You are allergic to any progestin hormone.
- You may be pregnant.
- You have liver or gallbladder disease.
- You have had thrombophlebitis, embolism or stroke.
- You have unexplained vaginal bleeding.
- You have had breast or uterine cancer.

Before you start, consult your doctor:
- If you have heart or kidney disease.
- If you have diabetes.
- If you have a seizure disorder.
- If you suffer migraines.
- If you are easily depressed.

Over age 60:
Not recommended.

Pregnancy:
May harm child. Discontinue at first sign of pregnancy.

Breast-feeding:
Drug passes into milk. Avoid drug or discontinue nursing until you finish medicine. Consult doctor for advice on maintaining milk supply.

Infants & children:
Use only for female children under medical supervision.

Prolonged use:
No problems expected.

Skin & sunlight:
No problems expected.

Driving, piloting or hazardous work:
No problems expected.

Airplane passengers:
No problems expected.

Discontinuing:
Consult doctor. This medicine stays in the body and causes fetal abnormalities. Wait at least 3 months before becoming pregnant.

Others:
- Patients with diabetes must be monitored closely.
- Symptoms of blood clot in leg, brain or lung are: chest, groin, leg pain; sudden, severe headache; loss of coordination; vision change; shortness of breath; slurred speech.

INTERACTION WITH OTHER DRUGS

GENERIC NAME OR DRUG CLASS	COMBINED EFFECT
Antihistamines	Decreased norethindrone acetate effect.
Oxyphenbutazone	Decreased norethindrone acetate effect.
Phenobarbital	Decreased norethindrone acetate effect.
Phenothiazines	Increased phenothiazine effect.
Phenylbutazone	Decreased norethindrone acetate effect.

INTERACTION WITH OTHER SUBSTANCES

INTERACTS WITH	COMBINED EFFECT
Alcohol:	None expected.
Beverages:	None expected.
Cocaine:	Decreased norethindrone acetate effect.
Foods: Salt	Fluid retention.
Marijuana:	Possible menstrual irregularities or bleeding between periods.
Tobacco:	Possible blood clots in lung, brain, legs. Avoid.

NORGESTREL

BRAND NAMES

Ovrette

GENERAL INFORMATION

Habit forming? No
Prescription needed? Yes
Available as generic? No
Drug class: Female sex hormone (progestin)

USES

Contraceptive

DOSAGE & USAGE INFORMATION

How to take:
Tablet or capsule—Swallow with liquid or food to lessen stomach irritation. You may crumble tablet or open capsule.

When to take:
At the same time each day.

If you forget a dose:
Consult your doctor. You may need to use another birth-control method until next period, then resume norgestrel.

What drug does:
- Creates a uterine lining similar to pregnancy that prevents bleeding.
- Suppresses a pituitary gland hormone responsible for ovulation.
- Stimulates cervical mucus, which stops sperm penetration and prevents pregnancy.

Time lapse before drug works:
3 weeks. Use another method of birth control until then.

Don't take with:
See Interaction column and consult doctor.

OVERDOSE

Symptoms:
Nausea, vomiting, fluid retention, breast discomfort or enlargement, vaginal bleeding.

What to do:
Overdose unlikely to threaten life. If person takes much larger amount than prescribed, call doctor, poison-control center or hospital emergency room for instructions.

POSSIBLE ADVERSE REACTIONS OR SIDE EFFECTS

SYMPTOMS	FREQUENCY	WHAT TO DO
Brain & nervous system:		
Depression	Infrequent	4
Skin:		
• Rash	Rare	3
• Acne, increased facial or body hair.	Infrequent	5
Eyes, ears, nose, throat, heart & lungs, muscles, bones, joints, kidneys, allergic, blood:	None expected.	
Digestive:		
• Stomach or side pain.	Rare	3
• Appetite or weight changes.	Common	5
• Nausea	Infrequent	5
Blood vessels:		
Blood clot in leg, brain or lung.	Rare	1
Muscles, bones, joints:		
Ankle, foot swelling.	Common	5
Genital, urinary:		
Prolonged vaginal bleeding.	Infrequent	3
Liver:		
Jaundice (yellow skin and eyes).	Rare	3
Others:		
• Breast tenderness.	Infrequent	5
• Unusual tiredness or weakness.	Common	5

1-Life-threatening. Seek emergency treatment immediately.
2-Discontinue. Seek emergency treatment.
3-Discontinue. Call doctor right away.
4-Continue. Call doctor when convenient.
5-Continue. Tell doctor at next visit.

WARNINGS & PRECAUTIONS

Don't take if:
- You are allergic to any progestin hormone.
- You may be pregnant.
- You have liver or gallbladder disease.
- You have had thrombophlebitis, embolism or stroke.
- You have unexplained vaginal bleeding.
- You have had breast or uterine cancer.

Before you start, consult your doctor:
- If you have heart or kidney disease.
- If you have diabetes.
- If you have a seizure disorder.
- If you suffer migraines.
- If you are easily depressed.

Over age 60:
Not recommended.

Pregnancy:
May harm child. Discontinue at first sign of pregnancy.

Breast-feeding:
Drug passes into milk. Avoid drug or discontinue nursing until you finish medicine. Consult doctor for advice on maintaining milk supply.

Infants & children:
Use only for female children under medical supervision.

Prolonged use:
No problems expected.

Skin & sunlight:
No problems expected.

Driving, piloting or hazardous work:
No problems expected.

Airplane passengers:
No problems expected.

Discontinuing:
Consult doctor. This medicine stays in the body and causes fetal abnormalities. Wait at least 3 months before becoming pregnant.

Others:
- Patients with diabetes must be monitored closely.
- Symptoms of blood clot in leg, brain or lung are: chest, groin, leg pain; sudden, severe headache; loss of coordination; vision change; shortness of breath; slurred speech.

INTERACTION WITH OTHER DRUGS

GENERIC NAME OR DRUG CLASS	COMBINED EFFECT
Antihistamines	Decreased norgestrel effect.
Oxyphenbutazone	Decreased norgestrel effect.
Phenobarbital	Decreased norgestrel effect.
Phenothiazines	Increased phenothiazine effect.
Phenylbutazone	Decreased norgestrel effect.

INTERACTION WITH OTHER SUBSTANCES

INTERACTS WITH	COMBINED EFFECT
Alcohol:	None expected.
Beverages:	None expected.
Cocaine:	Decreased norgestrel effect.
Foods: Salt	Fluid retention.
Marijuana:	Possible menstrual irregularities or bleeding between periods.
Tobacco:	Possible blood clots in lung, brain, legs. Avoid.

NORTRIPTYLINE

BRAND NAMES

Aventyl
Pamelor

GENERAL INFORMATION

Habit forming? No
Prescription needed? Yes
Available as generic? Yes
Drug class: Antidepressant (tricyclic)

USES

Gradually relieves, but doesn't cure, symptoms of depression.

DOSAGE & USAGE INFORMATION

How to take:
- Capsule—Swallow with liquid.
- Liquid—Use measuring spoon.

When to take:
At the same time each day, usually bedtime.

If you forget a dose:
Bedtime dose—If you forget your once-a-day bedtime dose, don't take it more than 3 hours late. If more than 3 hours, wait for next scheduled dose. Don't double this dose.

What drug does:
Probably affects part of brain that controls messages between nerve cells.

Time lapse before drug works:
Begins in 1 to 2 weeks. May require 4 to 6 weeks for maximum benefit.

Don't take with:
- Non-prescription drugs without consulting doctor.
- See Interaction column and consult doctor.

OVERDOSE

Symptoms:
Hallucinations, convulsions, coma.

What to do:
- Dial 0 (operator) or 911 (emergency) for an ambulance or medical help. Then give first aid immediately.
- If patient is unconscious and not breathing, give mouth-to-mouth breathing. If there is no heartbeat, use cardiac massage and mouth-to-mouth breathing (CPR). Don't try to make patient vomit. If you can't get help quickly, take patient to nearest emergency facility.
- Additional emergency information on page 886.

POSSIBLE ADVERSE REACTIONS OR SIDE EFFECTS

SYMPTOMS	FREQUENCY	WHAT TO DO
Brain & nervous system:		
● Hallucinations, shakiness, dizziness, fainting.	Infrequent	3
● Headache	Common	4
● Seizures	Rare	1
● Insomnia	Common	5
Skin:		
Rash, itch.	Rare	3
Eyes:		
Blurred vision, pain.	Infrequent	3
Ears, nose, throat:		
● Sore throat.	Rare	3
● Dry mouth or unpleasant taste.	Common	4
Digestive:		
● Constipation or diarrhea, nausea, indigestion.	Common	4
● Vomiting	Infrequent	3
● "Sweet tooth"	Common	5
Heart & lungs:		
Irregular heartbeat or slow pulse.	Infrequent	3
Blood vessels, muscles, bones, joints, kidneys, allergic, blood:	None expected.	
Genital, urinary:		
Difficulty urinating.	Infrequent	4
Liver:		
Jaundice (yellow skin and eyes).	Rare	3
Others:		
● Fever	Rare	3
● Fatigue, weakness.	Common	4

1 - Life-threatening. Seek emergency treatment immediately.
2 - Discontinue. Seek emergency treatment.
3 - Discontinue. Call doctor right away.
4 - Continue. Call doctor when convenient.
5 - Continue. Tell doctor at next visit.

NORTRIPTYLINE

 WARNINGS & PRECAUTIONS

Don't take if:
- You are allergic to any tricyclic antidepressant.
- You drink alcohol.
- You have had a heart attack within 6 weeks.
- You have glaucoma.
- You have taken MAO inhibitors within 2 weeks.
- Patient is younger than 12.

Before you start, consult your doctor:
- If you will have surgery within 2 months, including dental surgery, requiring general or spinal anesthesia.
- If you have an enlarged prostate.
- If you have heart disease or high blood pressure.
- If you have stomach or intestinal problems.
- If you have an overactive thyroid.
- If you have asthma.
- If you have liver disease.

Over age 60:
More likely to develop urination difficulty and side effects under *Brain & nervous system*, opposite.

Pregnancy:
Studies inconclusive on harm to unborn child. Animal studies show fetal abnormalities. Decide with your doctor whether drug benefits justify risk to unborn child.

Breast-feeding:
Drug passes into milk. Avoid drug or discontinue nursing until you finish medicine. Consult doctor for advice on maintaining milk supply.

Infants & children:
Don't give to children younger than 12.

Prolonged use:
No problems expected.

Skin & sunlight:
May cause rash or intensify sunburn in areas exposed to sun or sunlamp.

Driving, piloting or hazardous work:
Don't drive or pilot aircraft until you learn how medicine affects you. Don't work around dangerous machinery. Don't climb ladders or work in high places. Danger increases if you drink alcohol or take medicine affecting alertness and reflexes.

Airplane passengers:
No problems expected.

Discontinuing:
Don't discontinue without consulting doctor. Dose may require gradual reduction if you have taken drug for a long time. Doses of other drugs may also require adjustment.

 INTERACTION WITH OTHER DRUGS

GENERIC NAME OR DRUG CLASS	COMBINED EFFECT
Anticoagulants (oral)	Increased anticoagulant effect.
Anticholinergics	Increased sedation.
Antihistamines	Increased antihistamine effect.
Barbiturates	Decreased antidepressant effect.
Clonidine	Decreased clonidine effect.
Diuretics (thiazide)	Increased nortriptyline effect.
Ethchlorvynol	Delirium
Guanethidine	Decreased guanethidine effect.
MAO inhibitors	Fever, delirium, convulsions.
Methyldopa	Decreased methyldopa effect.
Narcotics	Dangerous oversedation.
Phenytoin	Decreased phenytoin effect.
Quinidine	Irregular heartbeat.
Sedatives	Dangerous oversedation.
Sympathomimetics	Increased sympathomimetic effect.
Thyroid hormones	Irregular heartbeat.

 INTERACTION WITH OTHER SUBSTANCES

INTERACTS WITH	COMBINED EFFECT
Alcohol: Beverages or medicines with alcohol.	Excessive intoxication. Avoid.
Beverages:	None expected.
Cocaine:	Excessive intoxication. Avoid.
Foods:	None expected.
Marijuana:	Excessive drowsiness. Avoid.
Tobacco:	None expected.

NYLIDRIN

BRAND NAMES

Arlidin   Pervadil
Arlidin Forte Rolidrin
Circlidrin

GENERAL INFORMATION

Habit forming? No
Prescription needed? Yes
Available as generic? Yes
Drug class: Vasodilator

USES

- Improves poor circulation in extremities.
- Reduces dizziness caused by poor circulation in inner ear.

DOSAGE & USAGE INFORMATION

How to take:
Tablet—Swallow with liquid or food to lessen stomach irritation. If you can't swallow whole, crumble tablet and take with liquid or food.

When to take:
At the same times each day.

If you forget a dose:
Take as soon as you remember up to 2 hours late. If more than 2 hours, wait for next scheduled dose (don't double this dose).

What drug does:
Stimulates nerves that dilate blood vessels, increasing oxygen and nutrients.

Time lapse before drug works:
10 to 30 minutes.

Don't take with:
See Interaction column and consult doctor.

OVERDOSE

Symptoms:
Blood-pressure drop; nausea, vomiting; rapid, irregular heartbeat, chest pain; blurred vision; metallic taste.

What to do:
- Dial 0 (operator) or 911 (emergency) for an ambulance or medical help. Then give first aid immediately.
- If patient is unconscious and not breathing, give mouth-to-mouth breathing. If there is no heartbeat, use cardiac massage and mouth-to-mouth breathing (CPR). Don't try to make patient vomit. If you can't get help quickly, take patient to nearest emergency facility.
- Additional emergency information on page 886.

POSSIBLE ADVERSE REACTIONS OR SIDE EFFECTS

SYMPTOMS	FREQUENCY	WHAT TO DO
Brain & nervous system:		
● Dizziness	Infrequent	4
● Headache, nervousness.	Rare	4
● Trembling	Rare	3
Skin:		
Flushed face.	Rare	4
Eyes:		
Blurred vision.	Common	4
Ears, nose, throat:		
Metallic taste.	Common	5
Digestive:		
Nausea, vomiting.	Rare	4
Heart & lungs:		
● Chest pain.	Common	3
● Rapid or irregular heartbeat.	Infrequent	3
Blood vessels:		
● Fever	Common	4
● Chills	Rare	3
● Low blood pressure on standing.	Common	4
Muscles, bones, joints:	None expected.	
Genital, urinary:		
Decreased or difficult urination.	Common	4
Kidneys:	None expected.	
Liver:	None expected.	
Allergic:	None expected.	
Blood:	None expected.	
Others:		
Weakness, tiredness.	Infrequent	4

1- Life-threatening. Seek emergency treatment immediately.
2- Discontinue. Seek emergency treatment.
3- Discontinue. Call doctor right away.
4- Continue. Call doctor when convenient.
5- Continue. Tell doctor at next visit.
6- No action necessary.

WARNINGS & PRECAUTIONS

Don't take if:
- You are allergic to any vasodilator drugs.
- You have had a heart attack or stroke within 4 weeks.
- You have an active peptic ulcer.

Before you start, consult your doctor:
- If you have had heart disease, heart-rhythm disorders (especially rapid heartbeat), a stroke or poor circulation to the brain.
- If you have glaucoma.
- If you have an overactive thyroid gland.
- If you plan to become pregnant within medication period.
- If you use tobacco.

Over age 60:
Adverse reactions and side effects may be more frequent and severe than in younger persons.

Pregnancy:
No proven harm to unborn child. Avoid if possible.

Breast-feeding:
No proven problems. Consult doctor.

Infants & children:
Not recommended.

Prolonged use:
No problems expected.

Skin & sunlight:
No problems expected.

Driving, piloting or hazardous work:
Don't drive or pilot aircraft until you learn how medicine affects you. Don't work around dangerous machinery. Don't climb ladders or work in high places. Danger increases if you drink alcohol or take medicine affecting alertness and reflexes, such as antihistamines, tranquilizers, sedatives, pain medicine, narcotics and mind-altering drugs.

Airplane passengers:
No problems expected.

Discontinuing:
Don't discontinue without consulting doctor. If your condition worsens, contact your doctor immediately. Dose may require gradual reduction if you have taken drug for a long time. Doses of other drugs may also require adjustment.

Others:
No problems expected.

INTERACTION WITH OTHER DRUGS

GENERIC NAME OR DRUG CLASS	COMBINED EFFECT
Beta-adrenergic blockers	Decreased effect of nylidrin.
Phenothiazines	Increased blood level of phenothiazines.

INTERACTION WITH OTHER SUBSTANCES

INTERACTS WITH	COMBINED EFFECT
Alcohol:	Possible increased stomach-acid secretion. Use with caution.
Beverages:	None expected.
Cocaine:	Increased adverse effects of nylidrin.
Foods:	None expected.
Marijuana:	None expected.
Tobacco:	Decreased nylidrin effect. Worsens circulation. Avoid.

NYSTATIN

BRAND NAMES

Achrostatin V (M)
Declostatin (M)
Korostatin
Mycolog (M)
Mycostatin
Nadostine

Nilstat
O-V statin
Terrastatin (M)

GENERAL INFORMATION

Habit forming? No
Prescription needed? Yes
Available as generic? Yes
Drug class: Antifungal

 USES

Treatment of fungus infections susceptible to nystatin.

 DOSAGE & USAGE INFORMATION

How to take:
- Tablet or capsule—Swallow with liquid. If you can't swallow whole, crumble tablet or open capsule and take with liquid or food.
- Suppositories—Remove wrapper and moisten suppository with water. Gently insert larger end into vagina. Push well into vagina with finger.
- Ointment, cream or lotion—Use as directed by doctor and label.
- Liquid—Take as directed. Instruction varies by preparation.

When to take:
At the same time each day.

If you forget a dose:
Take as soon as you remember up to 2 hours late. If more than 2 hours, wait for next scheduled dose (don't double this dose).

What drug does:
Prevents growth and reproduction of fungus.

Time lapse before drug works:
Begins immediately. May require 3 weeks for maximum benefit, depending on location and severity of infection.

Don't take with:
See Interaction column and consult doctor.

 OVERDOSE

Symptoms:
Mild overdose may cause nausea, vomiting, diarrhea.

What to do:
Overdose unlikely to threaten life. If person takes much larger amount than prescribed, call doctor, poison-control center or hospital emergency room for instructions.

 POSSIBLE ADVERSE REACTIONS OR SIDE EFFECTS

SYMPTOMS	FREQUENCY	WHAT TO DO
Brain & nervous system:	None expected.	
Skin: Mild irritation, itch at application site.	Infrequent	3
Eyes:	None expected.	
Ears, nose, throat:	None expected.	
Digestive: Nausea, stomach pain, vomiting, diarrhea.	Common (at high doses)	3
Heart & lungs:	None expected.	
Blood vessels:	None expected.	
Muscles, bones, joints:	None expected.	
Genital, urinary:	None expected.	
Kidneys:	None expected.	
Liver:	None expected.	
Allergic:	None expected.	
Blood:	None expected.	
Others:	None expected.	

1- Life-threatening. Seek emergency treatment immediately.
2- Discontinue. Seek emergency treatment.
3- Discontinue. Call doctor right away.
4- Continue. Call doctor when convenient.
5- Continue. Tell doctor at next visit.
6- No action necessary.

WARNINGS & PRECAUTIONS

Don't take if:
You are allergic to nystatin.

Before you start, consult your doctor:
If you plan to become pregnant within medication period.

Over age 60:
No problems expected.

Pregnancy:
No proven harm to unborn child. Avoid if possible.

Breast-feeding:
No proven problems. Consult doctor.

Infants & children:
No problems expected.

Prolonged use:
No problems expected.

Skin & sunlight:
No problems expected.

Driving, piloting or hazardous work:
No problems expected.

Airplane passengers:
No problems expected.

Discontinuing:
Don't discontinue without doctor's advice until you complete prescribed dose, even though symptoms diminish or disappear.

Others:
No problems expected.

 INTERACTION WITH OTHER DRUGS

GENERIC NAME OR DRUG CLASS	COMBINED EFFECT
None	

 INTERACTION WITH OTHER SUBSTANCES

INTERACTS WITH	COMBINED EFFECT
Alcohol:	None expected.
Beverages:	None expected.
Cocaine:	None expected.
Foods:	None expected.
Marijuana:	None expected.
Tobacco:	None expected.

OPIUM

BRAND NAMES

Pantopon

GENERAL INFORMATION

Habit forming? Yes
Prescription needed? Yes
Available as generic? Yes
Drug class: Narcotic

 USES

Relieves pain.

 DOSAGE & USAGE INFORMATION

How to take:
- Tablet or capsule—Swallow with liquid. If you can't swallow whole, crumble tablet or open capsule and take with liquid or food.
- Drops or liquid—Dilute dose in beverage before swallowing.

When to take:
When needed. No more often than every 4 hours.

If you forget a dose:
Take as soon as you remember. Wait 4 hours for next dose.

What drug does:
Blocks pain messages to brain and spinal cord.

Time lapse before drug works:
30 minutes.

Don't take with:
See Interaction column and consult doctor.

 OVERDOSE

Symptoms:
Deep sleep; slow breathing; slow pulse; flushed, warm skin; constricted pupils.

What to do:
- Dial 0 (operator) or 911 (emergency) for an ambulance or medical help. Then give first aid immediately.
- If patient is unconscious and not breathing, give mouth-to-mouth breathing. If there is no heartbeat, use cardiac massage and mouth-to-mouth breathing (CPR). Don't try to make patient vomit. If you can't get help quickly, take patient to nearest emergency facility.
- Additional emergency information on page 886.

POSSIBLE ADVERSE REACTIONS OR SIDE EFFECTS

SYMPTOMS	FREQUENCY	WHAT TO DO
Brain & nervous system: Depression, confusion, hallucinations.	Infrequent	4
Skin: • Hives, rash, itch, face swelling.	Rare	3
• Flushed face.	Common	4
Eyes: Blurred vision.	Rare	4
Ears, nose, throat:	None expected.	
Digestive: Severe constipation, abdominal pain, vomiting.	Infrequent	3
Heart & lungs: Slow heartbeat, irregular breathing.	Rare	3
Blood vessels:	None expected.	
Muscles, bones, joints:	None expected.	
Genital, urinary: Difficult urination.	Common	4
Kidneys: Less urine.	Common	4
Liver:	None expected.	
Allergic:	None expected.	
Blood:	None expected.	
Others: Unusual tiredness.	Common	4

1- Life-threatening. Seek emergency treatment immediately.
2- Discontinue. Seek emergency treatment.
3- Discontinue. Call doctor right away.
4- Continue. Call doctor when convenient.
5- Continue. Tell doctor at next visit.
6- No action necessary.

WARNINGS & PRECAUTIONS

Don't take if:
You are allergic to any narcotic.

Before you start, consult your doctor:
If you have impaired liver or kidney function.

Over age 60:
More likely to be drowsy, dizzy, unsteady or constipated. Avoid prolonged use.

Pregnancy:
Studies inconclusive on harm to unborn child. Animal studies show fetal abnormalities. Decide with your doctor whether drug benefits justify risk to unborn child. Abuse by pregnant woman will result in addicted newborn. Withdrawal can be life-threatening.

Breast-feeding:
Drug filters into milk. May depress infant. Avoid.

Infants & children:
Not recommended

Prolonged use:
Causes psychological and physical dependence.

Skin & sunlight:
No problems expected.

Driving, piloting or hazardous work:
Don't drive or pilot aircraft until you learn how medicine affects you. Don't work around dangerous machinery. Don't climb ladders or work in high places. Danger increases if you drink alcohol or take medicine affecting alertness and reflexes, such as antihistamines, tranquilizers, sedatives, pain medicine, other narcotics and mind-altering drugs.

Airplane passengers:
No proven problems.

Discontinuing:
May be unnecessary to finish medicine. Follow doctor's instructions.

Others:
No problems expected.

INTERACTION WITH OTHER DRUGS

GENERIC NAME OR DRUG CLASS	COMBINED EFFECT
Analgesics	Increased analgesic effect.
Antidepressants	Increased sedative effect.
Antihistamines	Increased sedative effect.
Mind-altering drugs	Increased sedative effect.
Narcotics (other)	Increased narcotic effect.
Phenothiazines	Increased phenothiazine effect.
Sedatives	Increased sedative effect.
Sleep inducers	Increased sedative effect.
Tranquilizers	Increased sedative effect.

INTERACTION WITH OTHER SUBSTANCES

INTERACTS WITH	COMBINED EFFECT
Alcohol:	Increases alcohol's intoxicating effect. Avoid.
Beverages:	None expected.
Cocaine:	Increased cocaine effect.
Foods:	None expected.
Marijuana:	Impaired physical and mental performance.
Tobacco:	None expected.

ORPHENADRINE

BRAND NAMES

Disipal	Norflex
Flexoject	Norgesic (M)
Flexon	Norgesic Forte (M)
Marflex	Ro-Orphena
Myolin	Tega-Flex
Neocyten	X-Otag

GENERAL INFORMATION

Habit forming? No
Prescription needed? U.S.: Yes
Canada: No
Available as generic? Yes
Drug class: Muscle relaxant, anticholinergic, antihistamine, antiparkinsonism

USES

- Reduces muscle-strain discomfort.
- Relieves symptoms of Parkinson's disease.

DOSAGE & USAGE INFORMATION

How to take:
Tablet—Swallow with liquid. If you can't swallow whole, crumble tablet and take with liquid or food.

When to take:
At the same times each day.

If you forget a dose:
Take as soon as you remember up to 6 hours late. If more than 6 hours, wait for next scheduled dose (don't double this dose).

What drug does:
Sedative and analgesic effects reduce spasm and pain in skeletal muscles.

Time lapse before drug works:
1 to 2 hours.

Don't take with:
See Interaction column and consult doctor.

OVERDOSE

Symptoms:
Fainting, confusion, widely dilated pupils, rapid pulse, convulsions, coma.

What to do:
- Dial 0 (operator) or 911 (emergency) for an ambulance or medical help. Then give first aid immediately.
- Additional emergency information on page 886.

POSSIBLE ADVERSE REACTIONS OR SIDE EFFECTS

SYMPTOMS	FREQUENCY	WHAT TO DO
Brain & nervous system: Weakness, headache, dizziness, drowsiness, agitation, tremor, confusion.	Infrequent	3
Skin: Rash or itch.	Rare	3
Eyes: Blurred vision, dilated pupils.	Rare	3
Ears, nose, throat: Dry mouth.	Infrequent	4
Digestive: Nausea, vomiting, constipation.	Infrequent	4
Heart & lungs: Rapid or pounding heartbeat.	Infrequent	3
Blood vessels:	None expected.	
Muscles, bones, joints:	None expected.	
Genital, urinary: Urinary hesitancy or retention.	Infrequent	4
Kidneys:	None expected.	
Liver:	None expected.	
Allergic:	None expected.	
Blood:	None expected.	
Others:	None expected.	

1- Life-threatening. Seek emergency treatment immediately.
2- Discontinue. Seek emergency treatment.
3- Discontinue. Call doctor right away.
4- Continue. Call doctor when convenient.
5- Continue. Tell doctor at next visit.
6- No action necessary.

ORPHENADRINE

WARNINGS & PRECAUTIONS

Don't take if:
You are allergic to orphenadrine.

Before you start, consult your doctor:
- If you have glaucoma.
- If you have myasthenia gravis.
- If you have difficulty emptying bladder.
- If you have had heart disease or heart-rhythm disturbance.
- If you have had a peptic ulcer.

Over age 60:
Adverse reactions and side effects may be more frequent and severe than in younger persons.

Pregnancy:
No proven harm to unborn child. Avoid if possible.

Breast-feeding:
No proven problems. Consult doctor.

Infants & children:
Not recommended for children younger than 12.

Prolonged use:
Increased internal-eye pressure.

Skin & sunlight:
No problems expected.

Driving, piloting or hazardous work:
Don't drive or pilot aircraft until you learn how medicine affects you. Don't work around dangerous machinery. Don't climb ladders or work in high places. Danger increases if you drink alcohol or take medicine affecting alertness and reflexes, such as antihistamines, tranquilizers, sedatives, pain medicine, narcotics and mind-altering drugs.

Airplane passengers:
No problems expected.

Discontinuing:
May be unnecessary to finish medicine. Follow doctor's instructions.

Others:
No problems expected.

INTERACTION WITH OTHER DRUGS

GENERIC NAME OR DRUG CLASS	COMBINED EFFECT
Anticholinergics	Increased anticholinergic effect.
Chlorpromazine	Hypoglycemia (low blood sugar).
Griseofulvin	Decreased griseofulvin effect.
Levodopa	Increased effect of levodopa. (Improves effectiveness in treating Parkinson's disease.)
Phenylbutazone	Decreased phenylbutazone effect.
Propoxyphene	Possible confusion, nervousness, tremors.

INTERACTION WITH OTHER SUBSTANCES

INTERACTS WITH	COMBINED EFFECT
Alcohol:	Increased drowsiness. Avoid.
Beverages:	None expected.
Cocaine:	Decreased orphenadrine effect. Avoid.
Foods:	None expected.
Marijuana:	Increased drowsiness, mouth dryness, muscle weakness, fainting.
Tobacco:	None expected.

OXACILLIN

BRAND NAMES

Bactocill
Prostaphlin

GENERAL INFORMATION

Habit forming? No
Prescription needed? Yes
Available as generic? Yes
Drug class: Antibiotic (penicillin)

USES

Treatment of bacterial infections that are susceptible to oxacillin.

DOSAGE & USAGE INFORMATION

How to take:
- Tablets or capsules—Swallow with liquid on an empty stomach 1 hour before or 2 hours after eating.
- Liquid—Take with cold beverage. Liquid form is perishable and effective for only 7 days at room temperature. Effective for 14 days if stored in refrigerator. Don't freeze.

When to take:
Follow instructions on prescription label or side of package. Doses should be evenly spaced. For example, 4 times a day means every 6 hours.

If you forget a dose:
Take as soon as you remember. Continue regular schedule.

What drug does:
Destroys susceptible bacteria. Does not kill viruses.

Time lapse before drug works:
May be several days before medicine affects infection.

Don't take with:
See Interaction column and consult doctor.

OVERDOSE

Symptoms:
Severe diarrhea, nausea or vomiting.

What to do:
Overdose unlikely to threaten life. If person takes much larger amount than prescribed, call doctor, poison-control center or hospital emergency room for instructions.

POSSIBLE ADVERSE REACTIONS OR SIDE EFFECTS

SYMPTOMS	FREQUENCY	WHAT TO DO
Brain & nervous system:	None expected.	
Skin: Hives, rash, intense itch soon after a dose.	Rare	1
Eyes:	None expected.	
Ears, nose, throat: Dark or discolored tongue.	Common	5
Digestive: Mild nausea, vomiting, diarrhea.	Infrequent	4
Heart & lungs:	None expected.	
Blood vessels: Unexplained bleeding.	Rare	3
Muscles, bones, joints:	None expected.	
Genital, urinary:	None expected.	
Kidneys:	None expected.	
Liver:	None expected.	
Allergic: Life-threatening anaphylaxis may occur!	Rare	1 See page 888.
Blood:	None expected.	
Others:	None expected.	

1- Life-threatening. Seek emergency treatment immediately.
2- Discontinue. Seek emergency treatment.
3- Discontinue. Call doctor right away.
4- Continue. Call doctor when convenient.
5- Continue. Tell doctor at next visit.
6- No action necessary.

OXACILLIN

WARNINGS & PRECAUTIONS

Don't take if:
You are allergic to oxacillin, cephalosporin antibiotics, other penicillins or penicillamine. Life-threatening reaction may occur.

Before you start, consult your doctor:
If you are allergic to any substance or drug.

Over age 60:
You may have skin reactions, particularly around genitals and anus.

Pregnancy:
Studies inconclusive on harm to unborn child. Animal studies show fetal abnormalities. Decide with your doctor whether drug benefits justify risk to unborn child.

Breast-feeding:
Drug passes into milk. Child may become sensitive to penicillins and have allergic reactions to penicillin drugs. Avoid oxacillin or discontinue nursing until you finish medicine. Consult doctor for advice on maintaining milk supply.

Infants & children:
No problems expected.

Prolonged use:
You may become more susceptible to infections caused by germs not responsive to oxacillin.

Skin & sunlight:
No problems expected.

Driving, piloting or hazardous work:
Usually not dangerous. Most hazardous reactions likely to occur a few minutes after taking oxacillin.

Airplane passengers:
No problems expected.

Discontinuing:
Don't discontinue without doctor's advice until you complete prescribed dose, even though symptoms diminish or disappear.

Others:
No problems expected.

INTERACTION WITH OTHER DRUGS

GENERIC NAME OR DRUG CLASS	COMBINED EFFECT
Chloramphenicol	Decreased effect of both drugs.
Erythromycins	Decreased effect of both drugs.
Paromomycin	Decreased effect of both drugs.
Tetracyclines	Decreased effect of both drugs.
Troleandomycin	Decreased effect of both drugs.

INTERACTION WITH OTHER SUBSTANCES

INTERACTS WITH	COMBINED EFFECT
Alcohol:	Occasional stomach irritation.
Beverages:	None expected.
Cocaine:	No proven problems.
Foods:	None expected.
Marijuana:	No proven problems.
Tobacco:	None expected.

OXANDROLONE

BRAND NAMES

Anavar

Habit forming? No
Prescription needed? Yes

GENERAL INFORMATION

Available as generic? Yes
Drug class: Androgen (male sex hormone)

USES

- Corrects male hormone deficiency.
- Reduces "male menopause" symptoms (loss of sex drive, depression, anxiety).
- Decreases calcium loss of osteoporosis (softened bones).
- Blocks growth of breast-cancer cells in females.
- Corrects undescended testicles in male children.
- Reduces breast pain and fullness following childbirth.
- Augments treatment of aplastic anemia.
- Stimulates weight gain after illness, injury or for chronically underweight persons.
- Stimulates growth in treatment of dwarfism.

DOSAGE & USAGE INFORMATION

How to take:
- Tablets—With food to lessen stomach irritation.
- Injection—Once or twice a month.

When to take:
At the same time each day.

If you forget a dose:
Take as soon as you remember up to 2 hours late. If more than 2 hours, wait for next scheduled dose (don't double this dose).

What drug does:
- Stimulates cells that produce male sex characteristics.
- Replaces hormone deficiencies.
- Stimulates red-blood-cell production.
- Suppresses production of estrogen (female sex hormone).

Time lapse before drug works:
Varies with problems treated. May require 2 or 3 months of regular use for desired effects.

Don't take with:
See Interaction column and consult doctor.

OVERDOSE

Overdose unlikely to threaten life. If person takes much larger amount than prescribed, call doctor, poison-control center or hospital emergency room for instructions.

POSSIBLE ADVERSE REACTIONS OR SIDE EFFECTS

SYMPTOMS	FREQUENCY	WHAT TO DO
Brain & nervous system:		
Depression or confusion.	Infrequent	3
Skin:		
● Flushed face.	Infrequent	3
● Rash or itch.	Infrequent	3
● Hives	Rare	2
● Acne or oily skin in females.	Common	4
Eyes, heart & lungs, blood vessels, kidneys, blood:	None expected.	
Ears, nose, throat:		
● Deep voice.	Common	4
● Sore mouth.	Common	5
● Sore throat, fever.	Rare	3
Digestive:		
● Nausea, vomiting, diarrhea.	Infrequent	3
● Abdominal pain.	Rare	3
● Black stool.	Rare	2
Muscles, bones, joints:		
Swollen feet or legs.	Infrequent	3
Genital, urinary:		
● Enlarged clitoris or frequent erections.	Common	4
● Vaginal bleeding.	Infrequent	3
Liver:		
Jaundice (yellow skin and eyes).	Infrequent	2
Allergic:		
Intense itching, weakness, loss of consciousness.	Rare	1
Others:		
● Higher sex drive.	Common	5
● Swollen breasts in men.	Common	4

1- Life-threatening. Seek emergency treatment immediately.
2- Discontinue. Seek emergency treatment.
3- Discontinue. Call doctor right away.
4- Continue. Call doctor when convenient.
5- Continue. Tell doctor at next visit.

OXANDROLONE

WARNINGS & PRECAUTIONS

Don't take if:
You are allergic to any male hormone.

Before you start, consult your doctor:
- If you might be pregnant.
- If you have cancer of prostate.
- If you have heart disease or arteriosclerosis.
- If you have kidney or liver disease.
- If you have breast cancer (males).
- If you have high blood pressure.
- If you have migraine attacks.
- If you have high level of blood calcium.
- If you have epilepsy.

Over age 60:
- May stimulate sexual activity.
- Can make high blood pressure or heart disease worse.
- Can enlarge prostate and cause urinary retention.

Pregnancy:
Risk to unborn child outweighs drug benefits. Don't use.

Breast-feeding:
Drug passes into milk. Avoid drug or discontinue nursing until you finish medicine. Consult doctor for advice on maintaining milk supply.

Infants & children:
Don't give to children younger than 2. Use with older children only under medical supervision.

Prolonged use:
- Reduces sperm count and volume of semen.
- Possible kidney stones.
- Unnatural hair growth and deep voice in women.

Skin & sunlight:
No problems expected.

Driving, piloting or hazardous work:
No problems expected.

Airplane passengers:
No problems expected.

Discontinuing:
No problems expected.

Others:
- May cause atrophy of testicles.
- Will not increase strength in athletes.

INTERACTION WITH OTHER DRUGS

GENERIC NAME OR DRUG CLASS	COMBINED EFFECT
Anticoagulants	Increased anticoagulant effect.
Antidiabetics (oral)	Increased antidiabetic effect.
Chlorzoxazone	Decreases oxandrolone effect.
Oxyphenbutazone	Decreased oxandrolone effect.
Phenobarbital	Decreased oxandrolone effect.
Phenylbutazone	Decreased oxandrolone effect.

INTERACTION WITH OTHER SUBSTANCES

INTERACTS WITH	COMBINED EFFECT
Alcohol:	None expected.
Beverages:	None expected.
Cocaine:	No proven problems.
Foods: Salt	Excessive fluid retention (edema). Decrease salt intake while taking male hormones.
Marijuana:	Decreased blood levels of oxandrolone.
Tobacco:	No proven problems.

OXAZEPAM

BRAND NAMES

Apo-Oxazepam
Ox-Pam
Serax

GENERAL INFORMATION

Habit forming? Yes
Prescription needed? Yes
Available as generic? No
Drug class: Tranquilizer (benzodiazepine)

 USES

Treatment for nervousness or tension.

 DOSAGE & USAGE INFORMATION

How to take:
Tablet or capsule—Swallow with liquid. If you can't swallow whole, crumble tablet or open capsule and take with liquid or food.

When to take:
At the same time each day, according to instructions on prescription label.

If you forget a dose:
Take as soon as you remember up to 2 hours late. If more than 2 hours, wait for next scheduled dose (don't double this dose).

What drug does:
Affects limbic system of brain—part that controls emotions.

Time lapse before drug works:
2 hours. May take 6 weeks for full benefit.

Don't take with:
See Interaction column and consult doctor.

 OVERDOSE

Symptoms:
Drowsiness, weakness, tremor, stupor, coma.

What to do:
- Dial 0 (operator) or 911 (emergency) for an ambulance or medical help. Then give first aid immediately.
- If patient is unconscious and not breathing, give mouth-to-mouth breathing. If there is no heartbeat, use cardiac massage and mouth-to-mouth breathing (CPR). Don't try to make patient vomit. If you can't get help quickly, take patient to nearest emergency facility.
- Additional emergency information on page 886.

POSSIBLE ADVERSE REACTIONS OR SIDE EFFECTS

SYMPTOMS	FREQUENCY	WHAT TO DO
Brain & nervous system:		
● Clumsiness, drowsiness, dizziness.	Common	4
● Hallucinations, confusion, depression, irritability.	Infrequent	3
Skin:		
Rash, itch.	Infrequent	3
Eyes:		
Vision changes.	Infrequent	3
Ears, nose, throat:		
Mouth, throat ulcers.	Rare	3
Digestive:		
Constipation or diarrhea, nausea, vomiting.	Infrequent	4
Heart & lungs:		
Slow heartbeat, breathing difficulty.	Rare	2
Blood vessels:	None expected.	
Muscles, bones, joints:	None expected.	
Genital, urinary:		
Urination difficulty.	Infrequent	4
Kidneys:	None expected.	
Liver:		
Jaundice (yellow eyes and skin).	Rare	3
Allergic:	None expected.	
Blood:	None expected.	
Others:	None expected.	

1- Life-threatening. Seek emergency treatment immediately.
2- Discontinue. Seek emergency treatment.
3- Discontinue. Call doctor right away.
4- Continue. Call doctor when convenient.
5- Continue. Tell doctor at next visit.
6- No action necessary.

WARNINGS & PRECAUTIONS

Don't take if:
- You are allergic to any benzodiazepine.
- You have myasthenia gravis.
- You have glaucoma.
- You are active or recovering alcoholic.
- Patient is younger than 6 months.

Before you start, consult your doctor:
- If you have liver, kidney or lung disease.
- If you have diabetes, epilepsy or porphyria.

Over age 60:
Adverse reactions and side effects may be more frequent and severe than in younger persons. You need smaller doses for shorter periods of time. May develop agitation, rage or "hangover effect."

Pregnancy:
Risk to unborn child outweighs drug benefits. Don't use.

Breast-feeding:
Drug passes into milk. Avoid drug or discontinue nursing until you finish medicine. Consult doctor for advice on maintaining milk supply.

Infants & children:
Use only under medical supervision for children older than 6 months.

Prolonged use:
May impair liver function.

Skin & sunlight:
No problems expected.

Driving, piloting or hazardous work:
Don't drive or pilot aircraft until you learn how medicine affects you. Don't work around dangerous machinery. Don't climb ladders or work in high places. Danger increases if you drink alcohol or take medicine affecting alertness and reflexes.

Airplane passengers:
No problems expected.

Discontinuing:
Don't discontinue without consulting doctor. Dose may require gradual reduction if you have taken drug for a long time. Doses of other drugs may also require adjustment.

Others:
- Hot weather, heavy exercise and profuse sweat may reduce excretion and cause overdose.
- Blood sugar may rise in diabetics, requiring insulin adjustment.

INTERACTION WITH OTHER DRUGS

GENERIC NAME OR DRUG CLASS	COMBINED EFFECT
Anticonvulsants	Change in seizure frequency or severity.
Antidepressants	Increased sedative effect of both drugs.
Antihistamines	Increased sedative effect of both drugs.
Antihypertensives	Excessively low blood pressure.
Cimetidine	Excess sedation.
Disulfiram	Increased oxazepam effect.
MAO inhibitors	Convulsions, deep sedation, rage.
Narcotics	Increased sedative effect of both drugs.
Sedatives	Increased sedative effect of both drugs.
Sleep inducers	Increased sedative effect of both drugs.
Tranquilizers	Increased sedative effect of both drugs.

INTERACTION WITH OTHER SUBSTANCES

INTERACTS WITH	COMBINED EFFECT
Alcohol:	Heavy sedation. Avoid.
Beverages:	None expected.
Cocaine:	Decreased oxazepam effect.
Foods:	None expected.
Marijuana:	Heavy sedation. Avoid.
Tobacco:	Decreased oxazepam effect.

OXTRIPHYLLINE

BRAND NAMES

Choledyl

GENERAL INFORMATION

Habit forming? No
Prescription needed? Canada—No
U.S: High strength—Yes
Low strength—No
Available as generic? Yes
Drug class: Bronchodilator (xanthine)

 ## USES

Treatment for bronchial asthma symptoms.

 ## DOSAGE & USAGE INFORMATION

How to take:
- Tablet or capsule—Swallow with liquid.
- Extended-release tablets or capsules—Swallow each dose whole. If you take regular tablets, you may chew or crush them.
- Suppositories—Remove wrapper and moisten suppository with water. Gently insert larger end into rectum. Push well into rectum with finger.
- Syrup—Take as directed on bottle.
- Enema—Use as directed on label.

When to take:
Most effective taken on empty stomach 1 hour before or 2 hours after eating. However, may take with food to lessen stomach upset.

If you forget a dose:
Take as soon as you remember up to 2 hours late. If more than 2 hours, wait for next scheduled dose (don't double this dose).

What drug does:
Relaxes and expands bronchial tubes.

Time lapse before drug works:
15 to 30 minutes.

Don't take with:
See Interaction column and consult doctor.

 ## OVERDOSE

Symptoms:
Restlessness, irritability, confusion, delirium, convulsions, rapid pulse, coma.

What to do:
- Dial 0 (operator) or 911 (emergency) for an ambulance or medical help. Then give first aid immediately.
- Additional emergency information on page 886.

 ## POSSIBLE ADVERSE REACTIONS OR SIDE EFFECTS

SYMPTOMS	FREQUENCY	WHAT TO DO
Brain & nervous system:		
● Headache, irritability, nervousness, restlessness, insomnia.	Common	4
● Dizziness or lightheadedness.	Infrequent	4
Skin:		
● Rash or hives.	Infrequent	3
● Flushed face.	Infrequent	4
Eyes:	None expected.	
Ears, nose, throat:	None expected.	
Digestive:		
● Nausea, vomiting, stomach pain.	Common	4
● Diarrhea, appetite loss.	Infrequent	3
Heart & lungs:		
● Rapid breathing.	Infrequent	3
● Irregular heartbeat.	Infrequent	3
Blood vessels:	None expected.	
Muscles, bones, joints:	None expected.	
Genital, urinary:	None expected.	
Kidneys:	None expected.	
Liver:	None expected.	
Allergic:	None expected.	
Blood:	None expected.	
Others:	None expected.	

1 - Life-threatening. Seek emergency treatment immediately.
2 - Discontinue. Seek emergency treatment.
3 - Discontinue. Call doctor right away.
4 - Continue. Call doctor when convenient.
5 - Continue. Tell doctor at next visit.
6 - No action necessary.

WARNINGS & PRECAUTIONS

Don't take if:
- You are allergic to any bronchodilator.
- You have an active peptic ulcer.

Before you start, consult your doctor:
- If you have had impaired kidney or liver function.
- If you have gastritis.
- If you have a peptic ulcer.
- If you have high blood pressure or heart disease.
- If you take medication for gout.

Over age 60:
Adverse reactions and side effects may be more frequent and severe than in younger persons.

Pregnancy:
Risk to unborn child outweighs drug benefits. Don't use.

Breast-feeding:
Drug passes into milk. Avoid drug or discontinue nursing until you finish medicine. Consult doctor for advice on maintaining milk supply.

Infants & children:
Use only under medical supervision.

Prolonged use:
Stomach irritation.

Skin & sunlight:
No problems expected.

Driving, piloting or hazardous work:
Avoid if lightheaded or dizzy. Otherwise, no problems expected.

Airplane passengers:
No problems expected.

Discontinuing:
May be unnecessary to finish medicine. Follow doctor's instructions.

Others:
No problems expected.

INTERACTION WITH OTHER DRUGS

GENERIC NAME OR DRUG CLASS	COMBINED EFFECT
Allopurinol	Decreased allopurinol effect.
Ephedrine	Increased effect of both drugs.
Epinephrine	Increased effect of both drugs.
Erythromycin	Increased oxtriphylline effect.
Furosemide	Increased furosemide effect.
Lincomycins	Increased oxtriphylline effect.
Lithium	Decreased lithium effect.
Probenecid	Decreased effect of both drugs.
Propranolol	Decreased oxtriphylline effect.
Rauwolfia alkaloids	Rapid heartbeat.
Sulfinpyrazone	Decreased sulfinpyrazone effect.
Troleandomycin	Increased oxtriphylline effect.

INTERACTION WITH OTHER SUBSTANCES

INTERACTS WITH	COMBINED EFFECT
Alcohol:	None expected.
Beverages: Caffeine drinks	Nervousness and insomnia.
Cocaine:	Excess stimulation. Avoid.
Foods:	None expected.
Marijuana:	Slightly increased antiasthmatic effect of oxtriphylline.
Tobacco:	Decreased oxtriphylline effect.

OXYCODONE

BRAND NAMES

Percodan (M)

GENERAL INFORMATION

Habit forming? Yes
Prescription needed? Yes
Available as generic? Yes
Drug class: Narcotic

USES

- Relieves pain.
- Suppresses cough.

DOSAGE & USAGE INFORMATION

How to take:

- Tablet or capsule—Swallow with liquid. If you can't swallow tablet or capsule whole, crumble or open and take with liquid or food.
- Drops or liquid—Dilute dose in beverage before swallowing.

When to take:

When needed. No more often than every 4 hours.

If you forget a dose:

Take as soon as you remember. Wait 4 hours for next dose.

What drug does:

- Reduces sensitivity of brain's cough-control center.
- Blocks pain messages to brain and spinal cord.

Time lapse before drug works:

30 minutes.

Don't take with:

See Interaction column and consult doctor.

OVERDOSE

Symptoms:

Deep sleep; slow breathing; slow pulse; flushed, warm skin; constricted pupils.

What to do:

- Dial 0 (operator) or 911 (emergency) for an ambulance or medical help. Then give first aid immediately.
- Additional emergency information on page 886.

POSSIBLE ADVERSE REACTIONS OR SIDE EFFECTS

SYMPTOMS	FREQUENCY	WHAT TO DO
Brain & nervous system: Depression, confusion, hallucinations.	Infrequent	4
Skin:		
● Hives, rash, itch, face swelling.	Rare	3
● Flushed face.	Common	4
Eyes: Blurred vision.	Rare	4
Ears, nose, throat:	None expected.	
Digestive: Severe constipation, abdominal pain, vomiting.	Infrequent	3
Heart & lungs: Slow heartbeat, irregular breathing.	Rare	3
Blood vessels:	None expected.	
Muscles, bones, joints:	None expected.	
Genital, urinary: Difficult urination.	Common	4
Kidneys: Less urine.	Common	4
Liver:	None expected.	
Allergic:	None expected.	
Blood:	None expected.	
Others: Unusual tiredness.	Common	4

1- Life-threatening. Seek emergency treatment immediately.
2- Discontinue. Seek emergency treatment.
3- Discontinue. Call doctor right away.
4- Continue. Call doctor when convenient.
5- Continue. Tell doctor at next visit.
6- No action necessary.

OXYCODONE

WARNINGS & PRECAUTIONS

Don't take if:
You are allergic to any narcotic.

Before you start, consult your doctor:
If you have impaired liver or kidney function.

Over age 60:
More likely to be drowsy, dizzy, unsteady or constipated. Avoid prolonged use.

Pregnancy:
Studies inconclusive on harm to unborn child. Animal studies show fetal abnormalities. Decide with your doctor whether drug benefits justify risk to unborn child. Abuse by pregnant woman will result in addicted newborn. Withdrawal can be life-threatening.

Breast-feeding:
Drug filters into milk. May depress infant. Avoid.

Infants & children:
Not recommended.

Prolonged use:
Causes psychological and physical dependence.

Skin & sunlight:
No problems expected.

Driving, piloting or hazardous work:
Don't drive or pilot aircraft until you learn how medicine affects you. Don't work around dangerous machinery. Don't climb ladders or work in high places. Danger increases if you drink alcohol or take medicine affecting alertness and reflexes, such as antihistamines, tranquilizers, sedatives, pain medicine, other narcotics and mind-altering drugs.

Airplane passengers:
No proven problems.

Discontinuing:
May be unnecessary to finish medicine. Follow doctor's instructions.

Others:
No problems expected.

INTERACTION WITH OTHER DRUGS

GENERIC NAME OR DRUG CLASS	COMBINED EFFECT
Analgesics	Increased analgesic effect.
Antidepressants	Increased sedative effect.
Antihistamines	Increased sedative effect.
Mind-altering drugs	Increased sedative effect.
Narcotics (other)	Increased narcotic effect.
Phenothiazines	Increased phenothiazine effect.
Sedatives	Increased sedative effect.
Sleep inducers	Increased sedative effect.
Tranquilizers	Increased sedative effect.

INTERACTION WITH OTHER SUBSTANCES

INTERACTS WITH	COMBINED EFFECT
Alcohol:	Increases alcohol's intoxicating effect. Avoid.
Beverages:	None expected.
Cocaine:	Increased cocaine effect.
Foods:	None expected.
Marijuana:	Impairs physical and mental peformance.
Tobacco:	None expected.

OXYMETAZOLINE

BRAND NAMES

Afrin
Duration
Nafrine
Otrivin
St. Joseph Decongestant for Children

GENERAL INFORMATION

Habit forming? No
Prescription needed? No
Available as generic? No
Drug class: Sympathomimetic

 ## USES

Relieves congestion of nose, sinuses and throat from allergies and infections.

 ## DOSAGE & USAGE INFORMATION

How to take:
Nasal solution, nasal spray—Use as directed on label. Avoid contamination. Don't use same container for more than 1 person.

When to take:
When needed, no more often than every 4 hours.

If you forget a dose:
Take as soon as you remember. Wait 4 hours for next dose.

What drug does:
Constricts walls of small arteries in nose, sinuses and eustachian tubes.

Time lapse before drug works:
5 to 30 minutes.

Don't take with:
- Non-prescription drugs for allergy, cough or cold without consulting doctor.
- See Interaction column and consult doctor.

 ## OVERDOSE

Symptoms:
Headache, sweating, anxiety, agitation, rapid and irregular heartbeat.

What to do:
- Dial 0 (operator) or 911 (emergency) for an ambulance or medical help. Then give first aid immediately.
- If patient is unconscious and not breathing, give mouth-to-mouth breathing. If there is no heartbeat, use cardiac massage and mouth-to-mouth breathing (CPR). If you can't get help quickly, take patient to nearest emergency facility.
- Additional emergency information on page 886.

 ## POSSIBLE ADVERSE REACTIONS OR SIDE EFFECTS

SYMPTOMS	FREQUENCY	WHAT TO DO
Brain & nervous system: Headache or lightheadedness, insomnia, nervousness.	Infrequent	4
Skin:	None expected.	
Eyes:	None expected.	
Ears, nose, throat: Runny, stuffy, burning, dry or stinging nose, sneezing.	Common	4
Digestive:	None expected.	
Heart & lungs: Fast, irregular or pounding heartbeat.	Common	4
Blood vessels:	None expected.	
Muscles, bones, joints:	None expected.	
Genital, urinary:	None expected.	
Kidneys:	None expected.	
Liver:	None expected.	
Allergic:	None expected.	
Blood:	None expected.	
Others:	None expected.	

1 - Life-threatening. Seek emergency treatment immediately.
2 - Discontinue. Seek emergency treatment.
3 - Discontinue. Call doctor right away.
4 - Continue. Call doctor when convenient.
5 - Continue. Tell doctor at next visit.
6 - No action necessary.

WARNINGS & PRECAUTIONS

Don't take if:
You are allergic to any sympathomimetic nasal spray.

Before you start, consult your doctor:
- If you have heart disease or high blood pressure.
- If you have diabetes.
- If you have overactive thyroid.
- If you have taken MAO inhibitors in past 2 weeks.

Over age 60:
Adverse reactions and side effects may be more frequent and severe than in younger persons.

Pregnancy:
No proven harm to unborn child. Avoid if possible.

Breast-feeding:
No proven problems. Consult doctor.

Infants & children:
Don't give to children younger than 2.

Prolonged use:
Drug may lose effectiveness, cause increased congestion ("rebound effect," see page 851) and irritate nasal membranes.

Skin & sunlight:
No problems expected.

Driving, piloting or hazardous work:
No problems expected.

Airplane passengers:
No problems expected.

Discontinuing:
May be unnecessary to finish medicine. Follow doctor's instructions.

Others:
No problems expected.

INTERACTION WITH OTHER DRUGS

GENERIC NAME OR DRUG CLASS	COMBINED EFFECT
MAO inhibitors	Dangerous blood-pressure rise.
Sympathomimetics	Increased effect of both drugs, especially harmful side effects.

INTERACTION WITH OTHER SUBSTANCES

INTERACTS WITH	COMBINED EFFECT
Alcohol:	None expected.
Beverages: Caffeine drinks	Nervousness or insomnia.
Cocaine:	Overstimulation. Avoid.
Foods:	None expected.
Marijuana:	Overstimulation. Avoid.
Tobacco:	None expected.

OXYMETHOLONE

BRAND NAMES

Adroyd
Anadrol-50
Anapolon 50

Habit forming? No
Prescription needed? Yes

GENERAL INFORMATION

Available as generic? Yes
Drug class: Androgen (male sex hormone)

USES

- Corrects male hormone deficiency.
- Reduces "male menopause" symptoms (loss of sex drive, depression, anxiety).
- Decreases calcium loss of osteoporosis (softened bones).
- Blocks growth of breast-cancer cells in females.
- Corrects undescended testicles in male children.
- Reduces breast pain and fullness following childbirth.
- Augments treatment of aplastic anemia.
- Stimulates weight gain after illness, injury or for chronically underweight persons.
- Stimulates growth in treatment of dwarfism.

DOSAGE & USAGE INFORMATION

How to take:
- Tablets—With food to lessen stomach irritation.
- Injection—Once or twice a month.

When to take:
At the same time each day.

If you forget a dose:
Take as soon as you remember up to 2 hours late. If more than 2 hours, wait for next scheduled dose (don't double this dose).

What drug does:
- Stimulates cells that produce male sex characteristics.
- Replaces hormone deficiencies.
- Stimulates red-blood-cell production.
- Suppresses production of estrogen (female sex hormone).

Time lapse before drug works:
Varies with problems treated. May require 2 or 3 months of regular use for desired effects.

Don't take with:
See Interaction column and consult doctor.

OVERDOSE

Overdose unlikely to threaten life. If person takes much larger amount than prescribed, call doctor, poison-control center or hospital emergency room for instructions.

POSSIBLE ADVERSE REACTIONS OR SIDE EFFECTS

SYMPTOMS	FREQUENCY	WHAT TO DO
Brain & nervous system:		
Depression or confusion.	Infrequent	3
Skin:		
• Flushed face.	Infrequent	3
• Rash or itch.	Infrequent	3
• Hives	Rare	2
• Acne or oily skin in females.	Common	4
Eyes, heart & lungs, blood vessels, kidneys, blood:	None expected.	
Ears, nose, throat:		
• Deep voice.	Common	4
• Sore mouth.	Common	5
• Sore throat, fever.	Rare	3
Digestive:		
• Nausea, vomiting, diarrhea.	Infrequent	3
• Abdominal pain.	Rare	3
• Black stool.	Rare	2
Muscles, bones, joints:		
Swollen feet or legs.	Infrequent	3
Genital, urinary:		
• Enlarged clitoris or frequent erections.	Common	4
• Vaginal bleeding.	Infrequent	3
Liver:		
Jaundice (yellow skin and eyes).	Infrequent	2
Allergic:		
Intense itching, weakness, loss of consciousness.	Rare	1
Others:		
• Higher sex drive.	Common	5
• Swollen breasts in men.	Common	4

1-Life-threatening. Seek emergency treatment immediately.
2-Discontinue. Seek emergency treatment.
3-Discontinue. Call doctor right away.
4-Continue. Call doctor when convenient.
5-Continue. Tell doctor at next visit.

OXYMETHOLONE

WARNINGS & PRECAUTIONS

Don't take if:
You are allergic to any male hormone.

Before you start, consult your doctor:
- If you might be pregnant.
- If you have cancer of prostate.
- If you have heart disease or arteriosclerosis.
- If you have kidney or liver disease.
- If you have breast cancer (males).
- If you have high blood pressure.
- If you have migraine attacks.
- If you have high level of blood calcium.
- If you have epilepsy.

Over age 60:
- May stimulate sexual activity.
- Can make high blood pressure or heart disease worse.
- Can enlarge prostate and cause urinary retention.

Pregnancy:
Risk to unborn child outweighs drug benefits. Don't use.

Breast-feeding:
Drug passes into milk. Avoid drug or discontinue nursing until you finish medicine. Consult doctor for advice on maintaining milk supply.

Infants & children:
Don't give to children younger than 2. Use with older children only under medical supervision.

Prolonged use:
- Reduces sperm count and volume of semen.
- Possible kidney stones.
- Unnatural hair growth and deep voice in women.

Skin & sunlight:
No problems expected.

Driving, piloting or hazardous work:
No problems expected.

Airplane passengers:
No problems expected.

Discontinuing:
No problems expected.

Others:
- May cause atrophy of testicles.
- Will not increase strength in athletes.

INTERACTION WITH OTHER DRUGS

GENERIC NAME OR DRUG CLASS	COMBINED EFFECT
Anticoagulants	Increased anticoagulant effect.
Antidiabetics (oral)	Increased antidiabetic effect.
Chlorzoxazone	Decreased oxymetholone effect.
Oxyphenbutazone	Decreased oxymetholone effect.
Phenobarbital	Decreased oxymetholone effect.
Phenylbutazone	Decreased oxymetholone effect.

INTERACTION WITH OTHER SUBSTANCES

INTERACTS WITH	COMBINED EFFECT
Alcohol:	None expected.
Beverages:	None expected.
Cocaine:	No proven problems.
Foods: Salt	Excessive fluid retention (edema). Decrease salt intake while taking male hormones.
Marijuana:	Decreased blood levels of oxymetholone.
Tobacco:	No proven problems.

OXYMORPHONE

BRAND NAMES

Numorphan

GENERAL INFORMATION

Habit forming? Yes
Prescription needed? Yes
Available as generic? Yes
Drug class: Narcotic

 ## USES

Relieves pain.

 ## DOSAGE & USAGE INFORMATION

How to take:
- Tablet or capsule—Swallow with liquid. If you can't swallow whole, crumble tablet or open capsule and take with liquid or food.
- Drops or liquid—Dilute dose in beverage before swallowing.

When to take:
When needed. No more often than every 4 hours.

If you forget a dose:
Take as soon as you remember. Wait 4 hours for next dose.

What drug does:
Blocks pain messages to brain and spinal cord.

Time lapse before drug works:
30 minutes.

Don't take with:
See Interaction column and consult doctor.

 ## OVERDOSE

Symptoms:
Deep sleep; slow breathing; slow pulse; flushed, warm skin; constricted pupils.

What to do:
- Dial 0 (operator) or 911 (emergency) for an ambulance or medical help. Then give first aid immediately.
- If patient is unconscious and not breathing, give mouth-to-mouth breathing. If there is no heartbeat, use cardiac massage and mouth-to-mouth breathing (CPR). Don't try to make patient vomit. If you can't get help quickly, take patient to nearest emergency facility.
- Additional emergency information on page 886.

 ## POSSIBLE ADVERSE REACTIONS OR SIDE EFFECTS

SYMPTOMS	FREQUENCY	WHAT TO DO
Brain & nervous system: Depression, confusion, hallucinations.	Infrequent	4
Skin:		
• Hives, rash, itch, face swelling.	Rare	3
• Flushed face.	Common	4
Eyes: Blurred vision	Rare	4
Ears, nose, throat:	None expected.	
Digestive: Severe constipation, abdominal pain, vomiting.	Infrequent	3
Heart & lungs: Slow heartbeat, irregular breathing.	Rare	3
Blood vessels:	None expected.	
Muscles, bones, joints:	None expected.	
Genital, urinary: Difficult urination.	Common	4
Kidneys: Less urine.	Common	4
Liver:	None expected.	
Allergic:	None expected.	
Blood:	None expected.	
Others: Unusual tiredness.	Common	4

1 - Life-threatening. Seek emergency treatment immediately.
2 - Discontinue. Seek emergency treatment.
3 - Discontinue. Call doctor right away.
4 - Continue. Call doctor when convenient.
5 - Continue. Tell doctor at next visit.
6 - No action necessary.

OXYMORPHONE

 ## WARNINGS & PRECAUTIONS

Don't take if:
You are allergic to any narcotic.

Before you start, consult your doctor:
If you have impaired liver or kidney function.

Over age 60:
More likely to be drowsy, dizzy, unsteady or constipated. Avoid prolonged use.

Pregnancy:
Studies inconclusive on harm to unborn child. Animal studies show fetal abnormalities. Decide with your doctor whether drug benefits justify risk to unborn child. Abuse by pregnant woman will result in addicted newborn. Withdrawal can be life-threatening.

Breast-feeding:
Drug filters into milk. May depress infant. Avoid.

Infants & children:
Not recommended.

Prolonged use:
Causes psychological and physical dependence.

Skin & sunlight:
No problems expected.

Driving, piloting or hazardous work:
Don't drive or pilot aircraft until you learn how medicine affects you. Don't work around dangerous machinery. Don't climb ladders or work in high places. Danger increases if you drink alcohol or take medicine affecting alertness and reflexes, such as antihistamines, tranquilizers, sedatives, pain medicine, other narcotics and mind-altering drugs.

Airplane passengers:
No proven problems.

Discontinuing:
May be unnecessary to finish medicine. Follow doctor's instructions.

Others:
No problems expected.

 ## INTERACTION WITH OTHER DRUGS

GENERIC NAME OR DRUG CLASS	COMBINED EFFECT
Analgesics	Increased analgesic effect.
Antidepressants	Increased sedative effect.
Antihistamines	Increased sedative effect.
Mind-altering drugs	Increased sedative effect.
Narcotics (other)	Increased narcotic effect.
Phenothiazines	Increased phenothiazine effect.
Sedatives	Increased sedative effect.
Sleep inducers	Increased sedative effect.
Tranquilizers	Increased sedative effect.

 ## INTERACTION WITH OTHER SUBSTANCES

INTERACTS WITH	COMBINED EFFECT
Alcohol:	Increases alcohol's intoxicating effect. Avoid.
Beverages:	None expected.
Cocaine:	Increased cocaine effect.
Foods:	None expected.
Marijuana:	Impairs physical and mental performance.
Tobacco:	None expected.

OXYPHENBUTAZONE

BRAND NAMES

Oxalid
Oxybutazone
Tandearil

Habit forming? No
Prescription needed? Yes

GENERAL INFORMATION

Available as generic? Yes
Drug class: Antiinflammatory (non-steroid)

USES

- Treatment for joint pain, stiffness, inflammation and swelling of arthritis and gout.
- Pain reliever.
- Treatment for dysmenorrhea (painful or difficult menstruation).

DOSAGE & USAGE INFORMATION

How to take:
Tablet or capsule—Swallow with liquid or food to lessen stomach irritation. If you can't swallow whole, crumble tablet or open capsule and take with liquid or food.

When to take:
At the same times each day.

If you forget a dose:
Take as soon as you remember up to 2 hours late. If more than 2 hours, wait for next scheduled dose (don't double this dose).

What drug does:
Reduces tissue concentration of prostaglandins (hormones which produce inflammation and pain).

Time lapse before drug works:
Begins in 4 to 24 hours. May require 3 weeks regular use for maximum benefit.

Don't take with:
See Interaction column and consult doctor.

OVERDOSE

Symptoms:
Confusion, agitation, incoherence, convulsions, possible hemorrhage from stomach or intestine, coma.

What to do:
- Dial 0 (operator) or 911 (emergency) for an ambulance or medical help. Then give first aid immediately.
- Additional emergency information on page 886.

POSSIBLE ADVERSE REACTIONS OR SIDE EFFECTS

SYMPTOMS	FREQUENCY	WHAT TO DO
Brain & nervous system:		
• Depression, drowsiness.	Infrequent	4
• Convulsions, confusion.	Rare	3
• Dizziness	Common	4
• Headache	Common	5
Skin:		
Rash, hives or itch.	Rare	3
Eyes:		
Blurred vision.	Rare	3
Ears, nose, throat:		
• Ringing in ears.	Infrequent	4
• Sore throat, fever, mouth ulcers.	Rare	3
Digestive:		
• Black stools, vomiting blood.	Rare	3
• Stomach upset.	Common	4
• Constipation or diarrhea, vomiting.	Infrequent	4
Heart & lungs:		
Breathing difficulty, tightness in chest.	Rare	3
Blood vessels:		
Unusual bleeding or bruising.	Rare	3
Muscles, bones, joints:		
Swollen feet, legs.	Infrequent	4
Genital, urinary:		
• Bloody urine.	Rare	3
• Difficult, painful or frequent urination.	Rare	4
Kidneys, allergic, blood, liver:	None expected.	
Others:		
• Fatigue, weakness.	Rare	4
• Weight gain.	Rare	4

1- Life-threatening. Seek emergency treatment immediately.
2- Discontinue. Seek emergency treatment.
3- Discontinue. Call doctor right away.
4- Continue. Call doctor when convenient.
5- Continue. Tell doctor at next visit.

OXYPHENBUTAZONE

WARNINGS & PRECAUTIONS

Don't take if:
- You are allergic to aspirin or any non-steroid, antiinflammatory drug.
- You have gastritis, peptic ulcer, enteritis, ileitis, ulcerative colitis.
- Patient is younger than 15.

Before you start, consult your doctor:
- If you have epilepsy.
- If you have Parkinson's disease.
- If you have been mentally ill.
- If you have had kidney disease or impaired kidney function, asthma, high blood pressure, heart failure, temporal arthritis, or polymyalgia rheumatica.

Over age 60:
Adverse reactions and side effects may be more frequent and severe than in younger persons.

Pregnancy:
Studies inconclusive on harm to unborn child. Animal studies show fetal abnormalities. Decide with your doctor whether drug benefits justify risk to unborn child.

Breast-feeding:
Drug filters into milk. May harm child. Avoid.

Infants & children:
Not recommended for those younger than 15. Use only under medical supervision.

Prolonged use:
- Eye damage.
- May cause rare bone-marrow damage, jaundice (yellow skin and eyes), reduced hearing.
- Periodic blood counts recommended if you use a long time.

Skin & sunlight:
No problems expected.

Driving, piloting or hazardous work:
Don't drive or pilot aircraft until you learn how medicine affects you. Don't work around dangerous machinery. Don't climb ladders or work in high places. Danger increases if you drink alcohol or take medicine affecting alertness and reflexes, such as antihistamines, tranquilizers, sedatives, pain medicine, narcotics and mind-altering drugs.

Airplane passengers:
No problems expected.

Discontinuing:
Don't discontinue without consulting doctor. Dose may require gradual reduction if you have taken drug for a long time. Doses of other drugs may also require adjustment.

INTERACTION WITH OTHER DRUGS

GENERIC NAME OR DRUG CLASS	COMBINED EFFECT
Anticoagulants (oral)	Increased anticoagulant effect.
Aspirin	Possible stomach ulcer.
Antidiabetics (oral)	Increased antidiabetic effect.
Chloroquine	Possible skin toxicity.
Digitoxin	Decreased digitoxin effect.
Gold compounds	Increased toxicity to skin and bone marrow.
Hydroxychloroquine	Possible skin toxicity.
Methotrexate	Increased toxicity of both drugs to bone marrow.
Penicillamine	Possible toxicity.
Phenytoin	Possible toxic phenytoin effect.
Trimethoprim	Possible bone-marrow toxicity.

INTERACTION WITH OTHER SUBSTANCES

INTERACTS WITH	COMBINED EFFECT
Alcohol:	Possible stomach ulcer or bleeding.
Beverages:	None expected.
Cocaine:	None expected.
Foods:	None expected.
Marijuana:	Increased pain relief from oxyphenbutazone.
Tobacco:	None expected.

OXYTETRACYCLINE

BRAND NAMES

Oxlopar
Oxy-Kesso-Tetra
Terramycin
Tetramine
Urobiotic (M)

GENERAL INFORMATION

Habit forming? No
Prescription needed? Yes
Available as generic? Yes
Drug class: Antibiotic (tetracycline)

 ## USES

- Treatment for infections susceptible to oxytetracycline. Will not cure virus infections such as colds or flu.
- Treatment for acne.

 ## DOSAGE & USAGE INFORMATION

How to take:
- Tablet, capsule or syrup—Take on empty stomach 1 hour before or 2 hours after eating. If you can't swallow whole, crumble tablet or open capsule and take with liquid or food.
- Liquid—Shake well. Take with measuring spoon.

When to take:
At the same times each day, evenly spaced.

If you forget a dose:
Take as soon as you remember up to 2 hours late. If more than 2 hours, wait for next scheduled dose (don't double this dose).

What drug does:
Prevents germ growth and reproduction.

Time lapse before drug works:
- Infections—May require 5 days to affect infection.
- Acne—May require 4 weeks to affect acne.

Don't take with:
- Non-prescription drugs without consulting doctor.
- See Interaction column and consult doctor.

 ## OVERDOSE

Symptoms:
Severe nausea, vomiting, diarrhea.

What to do:
Overdose unlikely to threaten life. If person takes much larger amount than prescribed, call doctor, poison-control center or hospital emergency room for instructions.

POSSIBLE ADVERSE REACTIONS OR SIDE EFFECTS

SYMPTOMS	FREQUENCY	WHAT TO DO
Brain & nervous system: Headache	Infrequent	3
Skin: • Itching around rectum and genitals.	Common	3
• Rash	Infrequent	3
Eyes: Blurred vision.	Rare	3
Ears, nose, throat: • Dark tongue.	Common	5
• Sore mouth or tongue.	Common	2
• Excessive thirst.	Infrequent	4
Digestive: Nausea, vomiting, diarrhea, abdominal burning.	Common	2
Heart & lungs:	None expected.	
Blood vessels:	None expected.	
Muscles, bones, joints:	None expected.	
Genital, urinary: Increased urination.	Infrequent	4
Kidneys:	None expected.	
Liver: Jaundice (yellow eyes and skin) in pregnant women.	Rare	3
Allergic:	None expected.	
Blood:	None expected.	
Others:	None expected.	

1- Life-threatening. Seek emergency treatment immediately.
2- Discontinue. Seek emergency treatment.
3- Discontinue. Call doctor right away.
4- Continue. Call doctor when convenient.
5- Continue. Tell doctor at next visit.
6- No action necessary.

WARNINGS & PRECAUTIONS

Don't take if:
You are allergic to any tetracycline antibiotic.

Before you start, consult your doctor:
• If you have kidney or liver disease.
• If you have lupus.
• If you have myasthenia gravis.

Over age 60:
Dosage usually less than in younger adults. More likely to cause itching around rectum. Ask you doctor how to prevent it.

Pregnancy:
Risk to unborn child outweighs drug benefits. Don't use.

Breast-feeding:
Drug passes into milk. Avoid drug or discontinue nursing until you finish medicine. Consult doctor for advice on maintaining milk supply.

Infants & children:
May cause permanent teeth malformation or discoloration in children less than 8 years old. Don't use.

Prolonged use:
• You may become more susceptible to infections caused by germs not responsive to oxytetracycline.
• May cause rare problems in liver, kidney or bone marrow. Periodic laboratory blood studies, liver- and kidney-function tests recommended if you use drug a long time.

Skin & sunlight:
May cause rash or intensify sunburn in areas exposed to sun or sunlamp.

Driving, piloting or hazardous work:
No problems expected.

Airplane passengers:
No problems expected.

Discontinuing:
Don't discontinue without doctor's advice until you complete prescribed dose, even though symptoms diminish or disappear.

Others:
No problems expected.

INTERACTION WITH OTHER DRUGS

GENERIC NAME OR DRUG CLASS	COMBINED EFFECT
Antacids	Decreased oxytetracycline effect.
Anticoagulants (oral)	Increased anticoagulant effect.
Contraceptives (oral)	Decreased contraceptive effect.
Digitalis preparations	Increased digitalis effect.
Mineral supplements (iron, calcium, magnesium, zinc)	Decreased oxytetracycline absorption. Separate doses by 1 to 2 hours.
Lithium	Increased lithium effect.
Penicillins	Decreased penicillin effect.
Sodium bicarbonate	Decreased oxytetracycline effect.

INTERACTION WITH OTHER SUBSTANCES

INTERACTS WITH	COMBINED EFFECT
Alcohol:	Possible liver damage. Avoid.
Beverages: Milk	Decreased oxytetracycline absorption. Take dose 2 hours after or 1 hour before drinking.
Cocaine:	No proven problems.
Foods: Dairy products	Decreased oxytetracycline absorption. Take dose 2 hours after or 1 hour before eating.
Marijuana:	No interactions expected, but marijuana may slow body's recovery. Avoid.
Tobacco:	None expected.

PAPAVERINE

BRAND NAMES

Cerebid	Kavrin	Pavacap	Pavatran
Cerespan	Myobid	Pavadon	Paverolan
Copavin (M)	Octapav	Pavakey	Ro-Papan
Dipav	P-200	Pavased	Sustaverine
Dylate	P-A-V	Pavasule	Vasospan
Hyobid	Pavabid	Pavatest	

GENERAL INFORMATION

Habit forming? No
Prescription needed? Yes
Available as generic? Yes
Drug class: Vasodilator

USES

Improves poor circulation in the extremities or brain.

DOSAGE & USAGE INFORMATION

How to take:
- Tablet or capsule—Swallow with liquid or food to lessen stomach irritation. If you can't swallow whole, crumble tablet or open capsule and take with liquid or food.
- Extended-release tablets or capsules—Swallow whole with liquid.
- Liquid—Follow label instructions.

When to take:
At the same times each day.

If you forget a dose:
Take as soon as you remember up to 2 hours late. If more than 2 hours, wait for next scheduled dose (don't double this dose).

What drug does:
Relaxes and expands blood-vessel walls, allowing better distribution of oxygen and nutrients.

Time lapse before drug works:
30 to 60 minutes.

Don't take with:
- Non-prescription drugs without consulting doctor.
- See Interaction column and consult doctor.

OVERDOSE

Symptoms:
Weakness, fainting, flush, sweating, stupor, irregular heartbeat.

What to do:
- Dial 0 (operator) or 911 (emergency) for an ambulance or medical help. Then give first aid immediately.
- Additional emergency information on page 886.

POSSIBLE ADVERSE REACTIONS OR SIDE EFFECTS

SYMPTOMS	FREQUENCY	WHAT TO DO
Brain & nervous system: Drowsiness, dizziness, headache.	Common	4
Skin: • Flushed face.	Common	4
• Rash, itch.	Infrequent	3
Eyes: Blurred or double vision.	Infrequent	3
Ears, nose, throat: Dry mouth, throat.	Common	5
Digestive: Stomach irritation, indigestion, nausea, mild constipation.	Common	4
Heart & lungs: Deep breathing, rapid heartbeat.	Infrequent	4
Blood vessels: Low blood pressure, causing lethargy or dizziness (especially on change of position).	Common	4
Muscles, bones, joints, genital, urinary, kidneys, allergic, blood:	None expected.	
Liver: Jaundice (yellow skin and eyes).	Rare	3
Others: Weakness	Infrequent	3

1- Life-threatening. Seek emergency treatment immediately.
2- Discontinue. Seek emergency treatment.
3- Discontinue. Call doctor right away.
4- Continue. Call doctor when convenient.
5- Continue. Tell doctor at next visit.

WARNINGS & PRECAUTIONS

Don't take if:
You are allergic to any narcotic.

Before you start, consult your doctor:
- If you plan to become pregnant within medication period.
- If you have had a heart attack, heart disease, angina or stroke.
- If you have Parkinson's disease.

Over age 60:
Adverse reactions and side effects may be more frequent and severe than in younger persons.

Pregnancy:
No proven harm to unborn child. Avoid if possible.

Breast-feeding:
Drug filters into milk. May harm child. Avoid.

Infants & children:
Not recommended.

Prolonged use:
No problems expected.

Skin & sunlight:
No problems expected.

Driving, piloting or hazardous work:
Don't drive or pilot aircraft until you learn how medicine affects you. Don't work around dangerous machinery. Don't climb ladders or work in high places. Danger increases if you drink alcohol or take medicine affecting alertness and reflexes, such as antihistamines, tranquilizers, sedatives, pain medicine, narcotics and mind-altering drugs.

Airplane passengers:
No problems expected.

Discontinuing:
May be unnecessary to finish medicine. If drug does not help in 1 to 2 weeks, consult doctor about discontinuing.

Others:
- Periodic liver-function tests recommended.
- Internal eye-pressure measurements recommended if you have glaucoma.

INTERACTION WITH OTHER DRUGS

GENERIC NAME OR DRUG CLASS	COMBINED EFFECT
Levodopa	Decreased levodopa effect.
Narcotics	Increased papaverine effect.
Pain relievers	Increased papaverine effect.
Sedatives	Increased papaverine effect.
Tranquilizers	Increased papaverine effect.

INTERACTION WITH OTHER SUBSTANCES

INTERACTS WITH	COMBINED EFFECT
Alcohol:	None expected.
Beverages:	None expected.
Cocaine:	Decreased papaverine effect.
Foods:	None expected.
Marijuana:	None expected.
Tobacco:	Decrease in papaverine's dilation of blood vessels.

PARA-AMINOSALICYLIC ACID (PAS)

BRAND NAMES

Nemasol	P.A.S. Acid
Parasal	Pasna
P.A.S.	Teebacin

GENERAL INFORMATION

Habit forming? No
Prescription needed? Yes
Available as generic? Yes
Drug class: Antitubercular

 ## USES

Treatment for tuberculosis.

 ## DOSAGE & USAGE INFORMATION

How to take:
- Tablet—Swallow with liquid or food to lessen stomach irritation.
- Powder—Dissolve dose in water. Stir well and drink all liquid.

When to take:
At the same times each day.

If you forget a dose:
Take as soon as you remember up to 2 hours late. If more than 2 hours, wait for next scheduled dose (don't double this dose).

What drug does:
- Prevents growth of TB germs.
- Makes TB germs more susceptible to other antituberculosis drugs.

Time lapse before drug works:
6 months.

Don't take with:
See Interaction column and consult doctor.

 ## OVERDOSE

Symptoms:
Nausea, vomiting, diarrhea; rapid breathing; convulsions.

What to do:
- Dial 0 (operator) or 911 (emergency) for an ambulance or medical help. Then give first aid immediately.
- Additional emergency information on page 886.

POSSIBLE ADVERSE REACTIONS OR SIDE EFFECTS

SYMPTOMS	FREQUENCY	WHAT TO DO
Brain & nervous system:		
• Headache	Infrequent	4
• Confusion	Infrequent	3
Skin:		
Itching, dry, puffy skin.	Infrequent	4
Eyes:		
Light sensitivity.	Infrequent	4
Ears, nose, throat:		
Sore throat, fever.	Infrequent	4
Digestive:		
• Constipation or vomiting.	Infrequent	4
• Diarrhea or stomach pain.	Common	4
Heart & lungs, blood vessels, muscles, bones, joints, allergic, blood:	None expected.	
Genital, urinary:		
• Painful urination.	Common	3
• Bloody urine.	Infrequent	3
Kidneys:		
Low back pain.	Common	3
Liver:		
Jaundice (yellow skin and eyes).	Rare	3
Others:		
• Chills	Common	3
• Swelling in front of neck.	Infrequent	4
• Changed menstrual pattern. Decreased sex drive in men.	Infrequent	5
• Fatigue, weakness.	Infrequent	4

1- Life-threatening. Seek emergency treatment immediately.
2- Discontinue. Seek emergency treatment.
3- Discontinue. Call doctor right away.
4- Continue. Call doctor when convenient.
5- Continue. Tell doctor at next visit.

PARA-AMINOSALICYLIC ACID (PAS)

 ## WARNINGS & PRECAUTIONS

Don't take if:
- You are allergic to PAS, aspirin or other salicylates.
- Tablets have turned brownish or purplish.

Before you start, consult your doctor:
- If you have ulcers in stomach or duodenum.
- If you have liver or kidney disease.
- If you have epilepsy.
- If you have adrenal insufficiency.
- If you have heart disease or congestive heart failure.
- If you have cancer.
- If you have overactive thyroid.

Over age 60:
Adverse reactions and side effects may be more frequent and severe than in younger persons.

Pregnancy:
Risk to unborn child outweighs drug benefits. Don't use.

Breast-feeding:
No proven problems. Consult doctor.

Infants & children:
Use only under medical supervision.

Prolonged use:
Enlarged thyroid gland and decreased function.

Skin & sunlight:
No problems expected.

Driving, piloting or hazardous work:
No problems expected.

Airplane passengers:
No problems expected.

Discontinuing:
No problems expected.

Others:
- Treatment may need to continue for several years or indefinitely.
- Periodic blood tests and liver- and kidney-function studies recommended.

 ## INTERACTION WITH OTHER DRUGS

GENERIC NAME OR DRUG CLASS	COMBINED EFFECT
Aminobenzoic acid (PABA)	Decreased effect of PAS.
Anticoagulants (oral)	Increased anticoagulant effect.
Anticonvulsants (hydantoin)	Increased anticonvulsant effect.
Aspirin	Stomach irritation.
Barbiturates	Oversedation.
Folic acid	Decreased effect of folic acid.
Probenecid	Increased PAS effect. Possible toxicity.
Rifampin	Decreased rifampin effect.
Sulfa drugs	Decreased effect of sulfa drugs.
Sulfinpyrazone	Increased PAS effect. Possible toxicity.
Tetracyclines	Reduced absorption of PAS. Space doses 3 hours apart.

 ## INTERACTION WITH OTHER SUBSTANCES

INTERACTS WITH	COMBINED EFFECT
Alcohol:	Possible liver disease.
Beverages:	None expected
Cocaine:	None expected.
Foods:	None expected.
Marijuana:	None expected.
Tobacco:	None expected, but tobacco smoking may slow recovery. Avoid.

PARAMETHASONE

BRAND NAMES

Haldrone

GENERAL INFORMATION

Habit forming? No
Prescription needed? Yes
Available as generic? No
Drug class: Cortisone drug (adrenal corticosteroid)

USES

- Reduces inflammation caused by many different medical problems.
- Treatment for some allergic diseases, blood disorders, kidney diseases, asthma and emphysema.
- Replaces corticosteroid deficiencies.

DOSAGE & USAGE INFORMATION

How to take:
Tablet—Swallow with liquid or food to lessen stomach irritation. If you can't swallow whole, crumble tablet and take with liquid or food.

When to take:
At the same times each day. Take once-a-day or once-every-other-day doses in mornings.

If you forget a dose:
- Several-doses-per-day prescription—Take as soon as you remember up to 2 hours late. If more than 2 hours, wait for next scheduled dose (don't double this dose).
- Once-a-day dose or less—Wait for next dose. Double this dose.

What drug does:
Decreases inflammatory responses.

Time lapse before drug works:
2 to 4 days.

Don't take with:
See Interaction column and consult doctor.

OVERDOSE

Symptoms:
Headache, convulsions, heart failure.

What to do:
- Dial 0 (operator) or 911 (emergency) for an ambulance or medical help. Then give first aid immediately.
- Additional emergency information on page 886.

POSSIBLE ADVERSE REACTIONS OR SIDE EFFECTS

SYMPTOMS	FREQUENCY	WHAT TO DO
Brain & nervous system:		
Mood changes, insomnia, restlessness.	Infrequent	4
Skin:		
• Acne	Common	4
• Rash	Rare	3
• Poor wound healing.	Common	4
Eyes:		
Blurred vision, halos around lights.	Infrequent	3
Ears, nose, throat:		
• Sore throat, fever.	Infrequent	3
• Thirst	Common	4
Digestive:		
• Indigestion, nausea, vomiting.	Common	4
• Bloody or black, tarry stool.	Infrequent	2
Heart & lungs:		
Irregular heartbeat.	Rare	2
Blood vessels, kidneys, liver, allergic, blood:	None expected.	
Muscles, bones, joints:		
Muscle cramps, swollen legs, feet.	Infrequent	3
Genital, urinary:		
Frequent urination.	Infrequent	4
Others:		
• Weight gain, round face.	Infrequent	4
• Fatigue, weakness.	Infrequent	4
• TB recurrence.	Infrequent	4
• Irregular menstrual periods.	Infrequent	4

1-Life-threatening. Seek emergency treatment immediately.
2-Discontinue. Seek emergency treatment.
3-Discontinue. Call doctor right away.
4-Continue. Call doctor when convenient.

WARNINGS & PRECAUTIONS

Don't take if:
- You are allergic to any cortisone drug.
- You have tuberculosis or fungus infection.
- You have herpes infection of eyes, lips or genitals.

Before you start, consult your doctor:
- If you have had tuberculosis.
- If you have congestive heart failure.
- If you have diabetes.
- If you have peptic ulcer.
- If you have glaucoma.
- If you have underactive thyroid.
- If you have high blood pressure.
- If you have myasthenia gravis.
- If you have blood clots in legs or lungs.

Over age 60:
Adverse reactions and side effects may be more frequent and severe than in younger persons. Likely to aggravate edema, diabetes or ulcers. Likely to cause cataracts and osteoporosis (softening of the bones).

Pregnancy:
Risk to unborn child outweighs drug benefits. Don't use.

Breast-feeding:
Drug passes into milk. Avoid drug or discontinue nursing until you finish medicine. Consult doctor for advice on maintaining milk supply.

Infants & children:
Use only under medical supervision.

Prolonged use:
- Retards growth in children.
- Possible glaucoma, cataracts, diabetes, fragile bones and thin skin.
- Functional dependence.

Skin & sunlight:
No problems expected.

Driving, piloting or hazardous work:
No problems expected.

Airplane passengers:
No problems expected.

Discontinuing:
- Don't discontinue without doctor's advice until you complete prescribed dose, even though symptoms diminish or disappear.
- Drug affects your response to surgery, illness, injury or stress for 2 years after discontinuing. Tell about drug to anyone who takes medical care of you within 2 years.

Others:
Avoid immunizations if possible.

INTERACTION WITH OTHER DRUGS

GENERIC NAME OR DRUG CLASS	COMBINED EFFECT
Amphoterecin B	Potassium depletion.
Anticholinergics	Possible glaucoma.
Anticoagulants (oral)	Decreased anticoagulant effect.
Anticonvulsants (hydantoin)	Decreased paramethasone effect.
Antidiabetics (oral)	Decreased antidiabetic effect.
Antihistamines	Decreased paramethasone effect.
Aspirin	Increased paramethasone effect.
Barbiturates	Decreased paramethasone effect. Oversedation.
Beta-adrenergic blockers	Decreased paramethasone effect.
Chloral hydrate	Decreased paramethasone effect.
Chlorthalidone	Potassium depletion.
Cholinergics	Decreased cholinergic effect.
Contraceptives (oral)	Increased paramethasone effect.
Digitalis preparations	Dangerous potassium depletion. Possible digitalis toxicity.

Additional interactions on page 840.

INTERACTION WITH OTHER SUBSTANCES

INTERACTS WITH	COMBINED EFFECT
Alcohol:	Risk of stomach ulcers.
Beverages:	No proven problems.
Cocaine:	Overstimulation. Avoid.
Foods:	No proven problems.
Marijuana:	Decreased immunity.
Tobacco:	Increased paramethasone effect. Possible toxicity.

PAREGORIC

BRAND NAMES

Brown Mixture (M)
CM with Paregoric (M)
Diban (M)
Donnagel-PG (M)
Kaoparin (M)

Opium Tincture
Parepectolin (M)
Pomalin

GENERAL INFORMATION

Habit forming? Yes
Prescription needed? Yes
Available as generic? Yes
Drug class: Narcotic, antidiarrheal

USES

Reduces intestinal cramps and diarrhea.

DOSAGE & USAGE INFORMATION

How to take:
Drops or liquid—Dilute dose in beverage before swallowing.

When to take:
As needed for diarrhea, no more often than every 4 hours.

If you forget a dose:
Take as soon as you remember. Wait 4 hours for next dose.

What drug does:
Anesthetizes surface membranes of intestines and blocks nerve impulses.

Time lapse before drug works:
2 to 6 hours.

Don't take with:
See Interaction column and consult doctor.

OVERDOSE

Symptoms:
Deep sleep; slow breathing; slow pulse; flushed, warm skin; constricted pupils.

What to do:
- Dial 0 (operator) or 911 (emergency) for an ambulance or medical help. Then give first aid immediately.
- If patient is unconscious and not breathing, give mouth-to-mouth breathing. If there is no heartbeat, use cardiac massage and mouth-to-mouth breathing (CPR). Don't try to make patient vomit. If you can't get help quickly, take patient to nearest emergency facility.
- Additional emergency information on page 886.

POSSIBLE ADVERSE REACTIONS OR SIDE EFFECTS

SYMPTOMS	FREQUENCY	WHAT TO DO
Brain & nervous system:		
● Depression	Rare	4
● Dizziness	Common	4
Skin:		
● Hives, itch, rash.	Rare	3
● Flushed face.	Common	4
Eyes:	None expected.	
Ears, nose, throat:	None expected.	
Digestive: Severe constipation, abdominal pain, vomiting.	Infrequent	3
Heart & lungs: Slow heartbeat, irregular breathing.	Rare	3
Blood vessels:	None expected.	
Muscles, bones, joints:	None expected.	
Genital, urinary: Difficult urination.	Common	4
Kidneys:	None expected.	
Liver:	None expected.	
Allergic:	None expected.	
Blood:	None expected.	
Others: Unusual tiredness.	Common	4

1- Life-threatening. Seek emergency treatment immediately.
2- Discontinue. Seek emergency treatment.
3- Discontinue. Call doctor right away.
4- Continue. Call doctor when convenient.
5- Continue. Tell doctor at next visit.
6- No action necessary.

PAREGORIC

 WARNINGS & PRECAUTIONS

Don't take if:
You are allergic to any narcotic.

Before you start, consult your doctor:
If you have impaired liver or kidney function.

Over age 60:
More likely to be drowsy, dizzy, unsteady or constipated.

Pregnancy:
No proven harm to unborn child. Avoid if possible.

Breast-feeding:
Drug filters into milk. May depress infant. Avoid.

Infants & children:
Use only under medical supervision.

Prolonged use:
Causes psychological and physical dependence.

Skin & sunlight:
No problems expected.

Driving, piloting or hazardous work:
Don't drive or pilot aircraft until you learn how medicine affects you. Don't work around dangerous machinery. Don't climb ladders or work in high places. Danger increases if you drink alcohol or take medicine affecting alertness and reflexes, such as antihistamines, tranquilizers, sedatives, pain medicine, narcotics and mind-altering drugs.

Airplane passengers:
No problems expected.

Discontinuing:
May be unnecessary to finish medicine. Follow doctor's instructions.

Others:
No problems expected.

 INTERACTION WITH OTHER DRUGS

GENERIC NAME OR DRUG CLASS	COMBINED EFFECT
Analgesics	Increased analgesic effect.
Antidepressants	Increased sedative effect.
Antihistamines	Increased sedative effect.
Mind-altering drugs	Increased sedative effect.
Narcotics (other)	Increased narcotic effect.
Phenothiazines	Increased sedative effect of paregoric.
Sedatives	Excessive sedation.
Sleep inducers	Increased effect of sleep inducers.
Tranquilizers	Increased tranquilizer effect.

 INTERACTION WITH OTHER SUBSTANCES

INTERACTS WITH	COMBINED EFFECT
Alcohol:	Increases alcohol's intoxicating effect. Avoid.
Beverages:	None expected.
Cocaine:	None expected.
Foods:	None expected.
Marijuana:	Impairs physical and mental performance.
Tobacco:	None expected.

PARGYLINE

BRAND NAMES

Eutonyl

Habit forming? No
Prescription needed? Yes
Available as generic? Yes

GENERAL INFORMATION

Drug class: MAO inhibitor
(monamine oxidase inhibitor),
antidepressant

 USES

Treatment for high blood pressure.

 DOSAGE & USAGE INFORMATION

How to take:
Tablet—Swallow with liquid. If you can't swallow whole, crumble tablet and take with liquid or food.

When to take:
At the same times each day.

If you forget a dose:
Take as soon as you remember up to 2 hours late. If more than 2 hours, wait for next scheduled dose (don't double this dose).

What drug does:
Inhibits nerve transmissions in brain.

Time lapse before drug works:
4 to 6 weeks for maximum effect.

Don't take with:
- Non-prescription diet pills, nose drops, medicine for asthma, cough, cold or allergy, or medicine containing caffeine or alcohol.
- See Interaction column and consult doctor.

 OVERDOSE

Symptoms:
Restlessness, agitation, fever, convulsions, coma.

What to do:
- Dial 0 (operator) or 911 (emergency) for an ambulance or medical help. Then give first aid immediately.
- Additional emergency information on page 886.

 POSSIBLE ADVERSE REACTIONS OR SIDE EFFECTS

SYMPTOMS	FREQUENCY	WHAT TO DO
Brain & nervous system:		
● Fainting	Infrequent	2
● Severe headache.	Infrequent	3
● Dizziness when changing position.	Common	5
● Hallucinations, insomnia, nightmares.	Infrequent	4
Skin:		
Rash	Rare	3
Eyes, blood vessels, kidneys, allergic, blood:	None expected.	
Ears, nose, throat:		
Dry mouth.	Common	5
Digestive:		
● Diarrhea	Infrequent	4
● Constipation	Common	5
● Nausea, vomiting.	Rare	3
Heart & lungs:		
● Rapid or pounding heartbeat.	Infrequent	4
● Chest pain.	Infrequent	3
Muscles, bones, joints:		
Stiff neck.	Rare	3
Genital, urinary:		
Difficult urination.	Common	5
Liver:		
Jaundice (yellow skin and eyes).	Rare	3
Others:		
● Swollen feet, legs.	Infrequent	4
● Fever	Rare	3
● Lower sex drive.	Infrequent	5
● Fatigue, weakness.	Common	4

1- Life-threatening. Seek emergency treatment immediately.
2- Discontinue. Seek emergency treatment.
3- Discontinue. Call doctor right away.
4- Continue. Call doctor when convenient.
5- Continue. Tell doctor at next visit.

PARGYLINE

WARNINGS & PRECAUTIONS

Don't take if:
- You are allergic to any MAO inhibitor.
- You have heart disease, congestive heart failure, heart-rhythm irregularities or high blood pressure.
- You have liver or kidney disease.

Before you start, consult your doctor:
- If you are alcoholic.
- If you have asthma.
- If you have had a stroke.
- If you have diabetes or epilepsy.
- If you have overactive thyroid.
- If you have schizophrenia.
- If you have Parkinson's disease.
- If you have adrenal-gland tumor.
- If you will have surgery within 2 months, including dental surgery, requiring general or spinal anesthesia.

Over age 60:
Not recommended.

Pregnancy:
No proven harm to unborn child. Avoid if possible.

Breast-feeding:
Safety not established. Consult doctor.

Infants & children:
Not recommended.

Prolonged use:
May be toxic to liver.

Skin & sunlight:
May cause rash or intensify sunburn in areas exposed to sun or sunlamp.

Driving, piloting or hazardous work:
Don't drive or pilot aircraft until you learn how medicine affects you. Don't work around dangerous machinery. Don't climb ladders or work in high places. Danger increases if you drink alcohol or take medicine affecting alertness and reflexes.

Airplane passengers:
No problems expected.

Discontinuing:
- Don't discontinue without doctor's advice until you complete prescribed dose, even though symptoms diminish or disappear.
- Follow precautions regarding foods, drinks and other medicines for 2 weeks after discontinuing.

Others:
- May affect blood-sugar levels in patients with diabetes.
- Fever may indicate that MAO inhibitor dose requires adjustment.

INTERACTION WITH OTHER DRUGS

GENERIC NAME OR DRUG CLASS	COMBINED EFFECT
Amphetamines	Blood-pressure rise to life-threatening level.
Anticonvulsants	Changed seizure pattern.
Antidepressants (tricyclic)	Blood-pressure rise to life-threatening level.
Antidiabetics (oral and insulin)	Excessively low blood sugar.
Antihypertensives	Excessively low blood pressure.
Caffeine	Irregular heartbeat or high blood pressure.
Carbamazepine	Fever, seizures. Avoid.
Cyclobenzaprine	Fever, seizures. Avoid.
Diuretics	Excessively low blood pressure.
Guanethidine	Blood-pressure rise to life-threatening level.
Levodopa	Sudden, severe blood-pressure rise.
MAO inhibitors (other)	High fever, convulsions, death.

Additional interactions on page 840.

INTERACTION WITH OTHER SUBSTANCES

INTERACTS WITH	COMBINED EFFECT
Alcohol:	Increased sedation to dangerous level.
Beverages: Caffeine drinks	Irregular heartbeat or high blood pressure.
Drinks containing tyramine (see page 851).	Blood-pressure rise to life-threatening level.
Cocaine:	Overstimulation. Possibly fatal.
Foods: Foods containing tyramine (see page 851).	Blood-pressure rise to life-threatening level.
Marijuana:	Overstimulation. Avoid.
Tobacco:	No proven problems.

PENICILLAMINE

BRAND NAMES

Cuprimine
Depen

GENERAL INFORMATION

Habit forming? No
Prescription needed? Yes
Available as generic? Yes
Drug class: Chelating agent, antirheumatic,
antidote (heavy-metal)

USES

- Treatment for rheumatoid arthritis.
- Prevention of kidney stones.
- Treatment for heavy-metal poisoning.

DOSAGE & USAGE INFORMATION

How to take:
Tablets or capsules—With liquid on an empty stomach 1 hour before or 2 hours after eating.

When to take:
At the same times each day.

If you forget a dose:
- 1 dose a day—Take as soon as you remember up to 12 hours late. If more than 12 hours, wait for next scheduled dose (don't double this dose).
- More than 1 dose a day—Take as soon as you remember up to 2 hours late. If more than 2 hours, wait for next scheduled dose (don't double this dose).

What drug does:
- Combines with heavy metals so kidney can excrete them.
- Combines with cysteine (amino acid found in many foods) to prevent cysteine kidney stones.
- May improve protective function of some white-blood cells against rheumatoid arthritis.

Time lapse before drug works:
2 to 3 months.

Don't take with:
See Interaction column and consult doctor.

OVERDOSE

Symptoms:
Ulcers, sores, convulsions, coughing up blood, coma.

What to do:
- Dial 0 (operator) or 911 (emergency) for an ambulance or medical help. Then give first aid immediately.
- Additional emergency information on page 886.

POSSIBLE ADVERSE REACTIONS OR SIDE EFFECTS

SYMPTOMS	FREQUENCY	WHAT TO DO
Brain & nervous system:	None expected.	
Skin: Rash, itch.	Common	3
Eyes: Double or blurred vision, pain.	Rare	3
Ears, nose, throat:		
● Sore throat, fever.	Infrequent	3
● Ringing in ears.	Rare	3
● Ulcer, sores, white spots in mouth.	Rare	3
Digestive: Appetite loss, nausea, diarrhea, vomiting.	Infrequent	4
Heart & lungs: Breathing difficulty, coughing up blood.	Rare	3
Blood vessels: Unusual bruising.	Infrequent	3
Muscles, bones, joints:		
● Joint pain.	Common	3
● Swollen feet, legs.	Infrequent	3
Genital, urinary: Bloody or cloudy urine.	Infrequent	3
Kidneys, allergic, blood:	None expected.	
Liver: Jaundice (yellow skin and eyes).	Rare	3
Others:		
● Fever, swollen lymph glands.	Common	3
● Weight gain.	Infrequent	3
● Fatigue, weakness.	Infrequent	3

1- Life-threatening. Seek emergency treatment immediately.
2- Discontinue. Seek emergency treatment.
3- Discontinue. Call doctor right away.
4- Continue. Call doctor when convenient.

PENICILLAMINE

WARNINGS & PRECAUTIONS

Don't take if:
- You are allergic to penicillamine.
- You have severe anemia.

Before you start, consult your doctor:
- If you have kidney disease.
- If you are allergic to any penicillin antibiotic.

Over age 60:
More likely to damage blood cells and kidneys.

Pregnancy:
Risk to unborn child outweighs drug benefits. Don't use.

Breast-feeding:
Drug filters into milk. May harm child. Avoid.

Infants & children:
Use only under medical supervision.

Prolonged use:
May damage blood cells, kidney, liver.

Skin & sunlight:
No problems expected.

Driving, piloting or hazardous work:
No problems expected.

Airplane passengers:
No problems expected.

Discontinuing:
No problems expected.

Others:
Request laboratory studies on blood and urine every 2 weeks. Kidney- and liver-function studies recommended every 6 months.

INTERACTION WITH OTHER DRUGS

GENERIC NAME OR DRUG CLASS	COMBINED EFFECT
Gold compounds	Damage to blood cells and kidney.
Immunosuppressants	Damage to blood cells and kidney.
Iron supplements	Decreased effect of penicillamine. Wait 2 hours between doses.
Oxyphenbutazone	Damage to blood cells and kidney.
Phenylbutazone	Damage to blood cells and kidney.
Quinine	Damage to blood cells and kidney.

INTERACTION WITH OTHER SUBSTANCES

INTERACTS WITH	COMBINED EFFECT
Alcohol:	Increased side effects of penicillamine.
Beverages:	None expected.
Cocaine:	Increased side effects of penicillamine.
Foods:	None expected.
Marijuana:	Increased side effects of penicillamine.
Tobacco:	None expected.

PENICILLIN G

BRAND NAMES

Bicillin	Penioral
Crystapen	Pentids
Crysticillin	Permapen
Duracillin	Pfizerpen G
Megacillin	Wycillin

GENERAL INFORMATION

Habit forming? No
Prescription needed? Yes
Available as generic? Yes
Drug class: Antibiotic (penicillin)

 USES

Treatment of bacterial infections that are susceptible to penicillin G.

 DOSAGE & USAGE INFORMATION

How to take:
- Tablets or capsules—Swallow with liquid on an empty stomach 1 hour before or 2 hours after eating.
- Liquid—Take with cold beverage. Liquid form is perishable and effective for only 7 days at room temperature. Effective for 14 days if stored in refrigerator. Don't freeze.

When to take:
Follow instructions on prescription label or side of package. Doses should be evenly spaced. For example, 4 times a day means every 6 hours.

If you forget a dose:
Take as soon as you remember. Continue regular schedule.

What drug does:
Destroys susceptible bacteria. Does not kill viruses.

Time lapse before drug works:
May be several days before medicine affects infection.

Don't take with:
See Interaction column and consult doctor.

 OVERDOSE

Symptoms:
Severe diarrhea, nausea or vomiting.

What to do:
Overdose unlikely to threaten life. If person takes much larger amount than prescribed, call doctor, poison-control center or hospital emergency room for instructions.

 POSSIBLE ADVERSE REACTIONS OR SIDE EFFECTS

SYMPTOMS	FREQUENCY	WHAT TO DO
Brain & nervous system:	None expected.	
Skin: Hives, rash, intense itch soon after a dose.	Rare	1
Eyes:	None expected.	
Ears, nose, throat: Dark or discolored tongue.	Common	5
Digestive: Mild nausea, vomiting, diarrhea.	Infrequent	4
Heart & lungs:	None expected.	
Blood vessels: Unexplained bleeding.	Rare	3
Muscles, bones, joints:	None expected.	
Genital, urinary:	None expected.	
Kidneys:	None expected.	
Liver:	None expected.	
Allergic: Life-threatening anaphylaxis may occur!	Rare	1 See page 888.
Blood:	None expected.	
Others:	None expected.	

1- Life-threatening. Seek emergency treatment immediately.
2- Discontinue. Seek emergency treatment.
3- Discontinue. Call doctor right away.
4- Continue. Call doctor when convenient.
5- Continue. Tell doctor at next visit.
6- No action necessary.

WARNINGS & PRECAUTIONS

Don't take if:
You are allergic to penicillin G, cephalosporin antibiotics, other penicillins or penicillamine. Life-threatening reaction may occur.

Before you start, consult your doctor:
If you are allergic to any substance or drug.

Over age 60:
You may have skin reactions, particularly around genitals and anus.

Pregnancy:
Studies inconclusive on harm to unborn child. Animal studies show fetal abnormalities. Decide with your doctor whether drug benefits justify risk to unborn child.

Breast-feeding:
Drug passes into milk. Child may become sensitive to penicillins and have allergic reactions to penicillin drugs. Avoid penicillin G or discontinue nursing until you finish medicine. Consult doctor for advice on maintaining milk supply.

Infants & children:
No problems expected.

Prolonged use:
You may become more susceptible to infections caused by germs not responsive to penicillin G.

Skin & sunlight:
No problems expected.

Driving, piloting or hazardous work:
Usually not dangerous. Most hazardous reactions likely to occur a few minutes after taking penicillin G.

Airplane passengers:
No problems expected.

Discontinuing:
Don't discontinue without doctor's advice until you complete prescribed dose, even though symptoms diminish or disappear.

Others:
Urine sugar test for diabetes may show false positive result.

INTERACTION WITH OTHER DRUGS

GENERIC NAME OR DRUG CLASS	COMBINED EFFECT
Chloramphenicol	Decreased effect of both drugs.
Erythromycins	Decreased effect of both drugs.
Paromomycin	Decreased effect of both drugs.
Tetracyclines	Decreased effect of both drugs.
Troleandomycin	Decreased effect of both drugs.

INTERACTION WITH OTHER SUBSTANCES

INTERACTS WITH	COMBINED EFFECT
Alcohol:	Occasional stomach irritation.
Beverages:	None expected.
Cocaine:	No proven problems.
Foods:	Decreased effect of penicillin G.
Marijuana:	No proven problems.
Tobacco:	None expected.

PENICILLIN V

BRAND NAMES

Betapen-VK	Pfizerpen VK
Compocillin VK	Robicillin VK
Ledercillin VK	Uticillin VK
Novapen V	V-Cillin
Pen-Vee K	Veetids
Penapar VK	

GENERAL INFORMATION

Habit forming? No
Prescription needed? Yes
Available as generic? Yes
Drug class: Antibiotic (penicillin)

 USES

- Treatment of bacterial infections that are susceptible to penicillin V.
- Prevention of streptococcal infections in susceptible persons such as those with heart valves damaged by rheumatic fever.

 DOSAGE & USAGE INFORMATION

How to take:
- Tablets or capsules—Swallow with liquid on an empty stomach 1 hour before meals or 2 hours after eating.
- Liquid—Take with cold beverage. Liquid form is perishable and effective for only 7 days at room temperature. Effective for 14 days if stored in refrigerator. Don't freeze.

When to take:
Follow instructions on prescription label or side of package. Doses should be evenly spaced. For example, 4 times a day means every 6 hours.

If you forget a dose:
Take as soon as you remember. Continue regular schedule.

What drug does:
Destroys susceptible bacteria. Does not kill viruses.

Time lapse before drug works:
May be several days before penicillin V affects infection.

Don't take with:
See Interaction column and consult doctor.

 OVERDOSE

Symptoms:
Severe diarrhea, nausea or vomiting.

What to do:
Overdose unlikely to threaten life. If person takes much larger amount than prescribed, call doctor, poison-control center or hospital emergency room for instructions.

 POSSIBLE ADVERSE REACTIONS OR SIDE EFFECTS

SYMPTOMS	FREQUENCY	WHAT TO DO
Brain & nervous system:	None expected.	
Skin: Hives, rash, intense itch soon after a dose.	Rare	1
Eyes:	None expected.	
Ears, nose, throat: Dark or discolored tongue.	Common	5
Digestive: Mild nausea, vomiting, diarrhea.	Infrequent	4
Heart & lungs:	None expected.	
Blood vessels: Unexplained bleeding.	Rare	3
Muscles, bones, joints:	None expected.	
Genital, urinary:	None expected.	
Kidneys:	None expected.	
Liver:	None expected.	
Allergic: Life-threatening anaphylaxis may occur!	Rare	1 See page 888.
Blood:	None expected.	
Others:	None expected.	

1- Life-threatening. Seek emergency treatment immediately.
2- Discontinue. Seek emergency treatment.
3- Discontinue. Call doctor right away.
4- Continue. Call doctor when convenient.
5- Continue. Tell doctor at next visit.
6- No action necessary.

WARNINGS & PRECAUTIONS

Don't take if:
You are allergic to penicillin V, cephalosporin antibiotics, other penicillins or penicillamine. Life-threatening reaction may occur.

Before you start, consult your doctor:
If you are allergic to any substance or drug.

Over age 60:
You may have skin reactions, particularly around genitals and anus.

Pregnancy:
Studies inconclusive on danger to unborn child. Decide with your doctor whether drug benefits justify risk to unborn child.

Breast-feeding:
Drug passes into milk. Child may become sensitive to penicillin. Child more likely to have future allergic reactions to penicillin. Avoid penicillin V or discontinue nursing until you finish medicine. Consult doctor for advice on maintaining milk supply.

Infants & children:
No problems expected.

Prolonged use:
You may become more susceptible to infections caused by germs not responsive to penicillin V.

Skin & sunlight:
No problems expected.

Driving, piloting or hazardous work:
Usually not dangerous. Most hazardous reactions likely to occur a few minutes after taking penicillin V.

Airplane passengers:
No problems expected.

Discontinuing:
Don't discontinue without doctor's advice until you have finished prescribed dose, even if symptoms diminish or disappear.

Others:
No problems expected.

INTERACTION WITH OTHER DRUGS

GENERIC NAME OR DRUG CLASS	COMBINED EFFECT
Chloramphenicol	Decreased effect of both drugs.
Erythromycins	Decreased effect of both drugs.
Paromomycin	Decreased effect of both drugs.
Tetracyclines	Decreased effect of both drugs.
Troleandomycin	Decreased effect of both drugs.

INTERACTION WITH OTHER SUBSTANCES

INTERACTS WITH	COMBINED EFFECT
Alcohol:	Occasional stomach irritation.
Beverages:	None expected.
Cocaine:	No proven problems.
Foods:	Decreased effect of penicillin V.
Marijuana:	No proven problems.
Tobacco:	None expected.

PENTAERYTHRITOL TETRANITRATE

BRAND NAMES

Duotrate Peritrate
Kaytrate P.E.T.N.
Naptrate
Pentestan
Pentraspan
Pentritol

GENERAL INFORMATION

Habit forming? No
Prescription needed? Yes
Available as generic? Yes
Drug class: Antianginal (nitrate)

 ## USES

Reduces frequency and severity of angina attacks.

 ## DOSAGE & USAGE INFORMATION

How to take:
- Regular tablet—Swallow with liquid. You may chew or crush it.
- Extended-release tablets or capsules—Swallow each dose whole with liquid.

When to take:
Take at the same times each day, 1 or 2 hours after meals.

If you forget a dose:
Take as soon as you remember up to 2 hours late. If more than 2 hours, wait for next scheduled dose (don't double this dose).

What drug does:
Relaxes blood vessels, increasing blood flow to heart muscle.

Time lapse before drug works:
30 minutes.

Don't take with:
See Interaction column and consult doctor.

 ## OVERDOSE

Symptoms:
Vomiting, sweating, shortness of breath, loss of consciousness.

What to do:
- Dial 0 (operator) or 911 (emergency) for an ambulance or medical help. Then give first aid immediately.
- Additional emergency information on page 886.

 ## POSSIBLE ADVERSE REACTIONS OR SIDE EFFECTS

SYMPTOMS	FREQUENCY	WHAT TO DO
Brain & nervous system:		
● Headache	Common	5
● Fainting	Infrequent	3
Skin:		
● Rash	Rare	3
● Flushed face and neck.	Common	5
Eyes:	None expected.	
Ears, nose, throat:	None expected.	
Digestive: Nausea, vomiting.	Common	5
Heart & lungs: Rapid heartbeat.	Common	5
Blood vessels:	None expected.	
Muscles, bones, joints:	None expected.	
Genital, urinary:	None expected.	
Kidneys:	None expected.	
Liver:	None expected.	
Allergic:	None expected.	
Blood:	None expected.	
Others:	None expected.	

1- Life-threatening. Seek emergency treatment immediately.
2- Discontinue. Seek emergency treatment.
3- Discontinue. Call doctor right away.
4- Continue. Call doctor when convenient.
5- Continue. Tell doctor at next visit.
6- No action necessary.

PENTAERYTHRITOL TETRANITRATE

 WARNINGS & PRECAUTIONS

Don't take if:
You are allergic to nitrates, including nitroglycerin.

Before you start, consult your doctor:
If you have glaucoma.

Over age 60:
Adverse reactions and side effects may be more frequent and severe than in younger persons.

Pregnancy:
No proven harm to unborn child. Avoid if possible.

Breast-feeding:
No proven problems. Consult your doctor.

Infants & children:
Not recommended.

Prolonged use:
Drug may become less effective and require higher doses.

Skin & sunlight:
No problems expected.

Driving, piloting or hazardous work:
Don't drive or pilot aircraft until you learn how medicine affects you. Don't work around dangerous machinery. Don't climb ladders or work in high places. Danger increases if you drink alcohol or take medicine affecting alertness and reflexes, such as antihistamines, tranquilizers, sedatives, pain medicine, narcotics and mind-altering drugs.

Airplane passengers:
No problems expected.

Discontinuing:
Don't discontinue without doctor's advice until you complete prescribed dose, even though symptoms diminish or disappear.

Others:
Periodic laboratory blood studies recommended if you take pentaerythritol tetranitrate.

 INTERACTION WITH OTHER DRUGS

GENERIC NAME OR DRUG CLASS	COMBINED EFFECT
Anticholinergics	Increased internal eye pressure.
Antidepressants (tricyclic)	Excessive blood-pressure drop.
Antihypertensives	Excessive blood-pressure drop.
Beta-adrenergic blockers	Excessive blood-pressure drop.
Cholinergics	Decreased cholinergic effect.
Ephedrine	Decreased effect of pentaerythritol tetranitrate.

 INTERACTION WITH OTHER SUBSTANCES

INTERACTS WITH	COMBINED EFFECT
Alcohol:	Excessive blood-pressure drop.
Beverages:	None expected.
Cocaine:	Flushed face and headache. Avoid
Foods:	None expected.
Marijuana:	Decreased effect of pentaerythritol tetranitrate.
Tobacco:	Decreased effect of pentaerythritol tetranitrate.

PENTAZOCINE

BRAND NAMES

Talwin

GENERAL INFORMATION

Habit forming? Yes
Prescription needed? Yes
Available as generic? Yes
Drug class: Narcotic

USES

Relieves pain.

DOSAGE & USAGE INFORMATION

How to take:
- Tablet or capsule—Swallow with liquid. If you can't swallow whole, crumble tablet or open capsule and take with liquid or food.
- Drops or liquid—Dilute dose in beverage before swallowing.

When to take:
When needed. No more often than every 4 hours.

If you forget a dose:
Take as soon as you remember. Wait 4 hours for next dose.

What drug does:
Blocks pain messages to brain and spinal cord.

Time lapse before drug works:
30 minutes.

Don't take with:
See Interaction column and consult doctor.

OVERDOSE

Symptoms:
Deep sleep; slow breathing; slow pulse; flushed, warm skin; constricted pupils.

What to do:
- Dial 0 (operator) or 911 (emergency) for an ambulance or medical help. Then give first aid immediately.
- If patient is unconscious and not breathing, give mouth-to-mouth breathing. If there is no heartbeat, use cardiac massage and mouth-to-mouth breathing (CPR). Don't try to make patient vomit. If you can't get help quickly, take patient to nearest emergency facility.
- Additional emergency information on page 886.

POSSIBLE ADVERSE REACTIONS OR SIDE EFFECTS

SYMPTOMS	FREQUENCY	WHAT TO DO
Brain & nervous system: Depression, confusion, hallucinations.	Infrequent	4
Skin: • Hives, rash, itch, face swelling.	Rare	3
• Flushed face.	Common	4
Eyes: Blurred vision.	Rare	4
Ears, nose, throat: Difficulty in swallowing.	Common	4
Digestive: Severe constipation, abdominal pain, vomiting.	Infrequent	3
Heart & lungs: Slow heartbeat, irregular breathing.	Rare	3
Blood vessels:	None expected.	
Muscles, bones, joints:	None expected.	
Genital, urinary: Difficult urination.	Common	4
Kidneys: Less urine.	Common	4
Liver:	None expected.	
Allergic:	None expected.	
Blood:	None expected.	
Others: Unusual tiredness.	Common	4

1- Life-threatening. Seek emergency treatment immediately.
2- Discontinue. Seek emergency treatment.
3- Discontinue. Call doctor right away.
4- Continue. Call doctor when convenient.
5- Continue. Tell doctor at next visit.
6- No action necessary.

WARNINGS & PRECAUTIONS

Don't take if:
You are allergic to any narcotic.

Before you start, consult your doctor:
If you have impaired heart, liver or kidney function.

Over age 60:
More likely to be drowsy, dizzy, unsteady or constipated. Avoid prolonged use.

Pregnancy:
Studies inconclusive on harm to unborn child. Animal studies show fetal abnormalities. Decide with your doctor whether drug benefits justify risk to unborn child. Abuse by pregnant woman will result in addicted newborn. Withdrawal can be life-threatening.

Breast-feeding:
Drug filters into milk. May depress infant. Avoid.

Infants & children:
Not recommended

Prolonged use:
Causes psychological and physical dependence.

Skin & sunlight:
No problems expected.

Driving, piloting or hazardous work:
Don't drive or pilot aircraft until you learn how medicine affects you. Don't work around dangerous machinery. Don't climb ladders or work in high places. Danger increases if you drink alcohol or take medicine affecting alertness and reflexes, such as antihistamines, tranquilizers, sedatives, pain medicine, other narcotics and mind-altering drugs.

Airplane passengers:
No proven problems.

Discontinuing:
May be unnecessary to finish medicine. Follow doctor's instructions.

Others:
No problems expected.

INTERACTION WITH OTHER DRUGS

GENERIC NAME OR DRUG CLASS	COMBINED EFFECT
Analgesics	Increased analgesic effect.
Antidepressants	Increased sedative effect.
Antihistamines	Increased sedative effect.
Mind-altering drugs	Increased sedative effect.
Narcotics (other)	Increased narcotic effect.
Phenothiazines	Increased phenothiazine effect.
Sedatives	Increased sedative effect.
Sleep inducers	Increased sedative effect.
Tranquilizers	Increased sedative effect.

INTERACTION WITH OTHER SUBSTANCES

INTERACTS WITH	COMBINED EFFECT
Alcohol:	Increases alcohol's intoxicating effect. Avoid.
Beverages:	None expected.
Cocaine:	Increased cocaine effect.
Foods:	None expected.
Marijuana:	Impairs physical and mental performance.
Tobacco:	None expected.

PENTOBARBITAL

BRAND NAMES

Carbrital (M)
Nembutal
Nova-Rectal
Pentogen
Quless

GENERAL INFORMATION

Habit forming? Yes
Prescription needed? Yes
Available as generic? Yes
Drug class: Sedative, hypnotic (barbiturate)

USES

- Reduces anxiety or nervous tension (low dose).
- Relieves insomnia (higher bedtime dose).

DOSAGE & USAGE INFORMATION

How to take:
- Tablet, capsule or liquid—Swallow with food or liquid to lessen stomach irritation. If you can't swallow whole, crumble tablet or open capsule and take with liquid or food.
- Suppositories—Remove wrapper and moisten suppository with water. Gently insert larger end into rectum. Push well into rectum with finger.

When to take:
At the same times each day.

If you forget a dose:
Take as soon as you remember up to 2 hours late. If more than 2 hours, wait for next scheduled dose (don't double this dose).

What drug does:
May partially block nerve impulses at nerve-cell connections.

Time lapse before drug works:
60 minutes.

Don't take with:
- Non-prescription drugs without consulting doctor.
- See Interaction column and consult doctor.

OVERDOSE

Symptoms:
Deep sleep, weak pulse, coma.

What to do:
- Dial 0 (operator) or 911 (emergency) for an ambulance or medical help. Then give first aid immediately.
- Additional emergency information on page 886.

POSSIBLE ADVERSE REACTIONS OR SIDE EFFECTS

SYMPTOMS	FREQUENCY	WHAT TO DO
Brain & nervous system:		
● Dizziness, drowsiness, "hangover effect."	Common	4
● Depression, confusion, slurred speech.	Infrequent	4
● Agitation	Rare	3
Skin:		
● Rash or hives.	Infrequent	3
● Face, lip swelling.	Infrequent	3
Eyes:		
Eyelid swelling.	Infrequent	3
Ears, nose, throat:		
Sore throat, fever.	Infrequent	3
Digestive:		
Diarrhea, nausea, vomiting.	Infrequent	4
Heart & lungs:		
● Slow heartbeat.	Rare	3
● Breathing difficulty.	Rare	3
Blood vessels:		
Unexplained bleeding or bruising.	Rare	4
Muscles, bones, joints:		
Joint or muscle pain.	Infrequent	4
Genital, urinary:	None expected.	
Kidneys:	None expected.	
Liver:		
Jaundice (yellow skin and eyes).	Rare	3
Allergic:	None expected.	
Blood:	None expected.	
Others:	None expected.	

1- Life-threatening. Seek emergency treatment immediately.
2- Discontinue. Seek emergency treatment.
3- Discontinue. Call doctor right away.
4- Continue. Call doctor when convenient.

WARNINGS & PRECAUTIONS

Don't take if:
- You are allergic to any barbiturate.
- You have porphyria.

Before you start, consult your doctor:
- If you have epilepsy.
- If you have kidney or liver damage.
- If you have asthma.
- If you have anemia.
- If you have chronic pain.
- If you will have surgery within 2 months, including dental surgery, requiring general or spinal anesthesia.

Over age 60:
Adverse reactions and side effects may be more frequent and severe than in younger persons. Use small doses.

Pregnancy:
Risk to unborn child outweighs drug benefits. Don't use.

Breast-feeding:
Drug passes into milk. Avoid drug or discontinue nursing until you finish medicine. Consult doctor for advice on maintaining milk supply.

Infants & children:
Use only under doctor's supervision.

Prolonged use:
- May cause addiction, anemia, chronic intoxication.
- May lower body temperature, making exposure to cold temperatures hazardous.

Skin & sunlight:
May cause rash or intensify sunburn in areas exposed to sun or sunlamp.

Driving, piloting or hazardous work:
Don't drive or pilot aircraft until you learn how medicine affects you. Don't work around dangerous machinery. Don't climb ladders or work in high places. Danger increases if you drink alcohol or take medicine affecting alertness and reflexes.

Airplane passengers:
No problems expected.

Discontinuing:
May be unnecessary to finish medicine. Follow doctor's instructions. If you develop withdrawal symptoms of hallucinations, agitation or sleeplessness after discontinuing, call doctor right away.

Others:
No problems expected.

INTERACTION WITH OTHER DRUGS

GENERIC NAME OR DRUG CLASS	COMBINED EFFECT
Anticoagulants (oral)	Decreased anticoagulant effect.
Anticonvulsants	Changed seizure patterns.
Antidepressants (tricyclic)	Decreased antidepressant effect.
Antidiabetics (oral)	Increased pentobarbital effect.
Antihistamines	Dangerous sedation. Avoid.
Antiinflammatory drugs (non-steroidal)	Decreased antiinflammatory effect.
Aspirin	Decreased aspirin effect.
Beta-adrenergic blockers	Decreased effect of beta-adrenergic blocker.
Contraceptives (oral)	Decreased contraceptive effect.
Cortisone drugs	Decreased cortisone effect.
Digitoxin	Decreased digitoxin effect.
Doxycycline	Decreased doxycycline effect.
Griseofulvin	Decreased griseofulvin effect.

Additional interactions on page 840.

INTERACTION WITH OTHER SUBSTANCES

INTERACTS WITH	COMBINED EFFECT
Alcohol:	Possible fatal oversedation. Avoid.
Beverages:	None expected.
Cocaine:	Decreased pentobarbital effect.
Foods:	None expected.
Marijuana:	Excessive sedation. Avoid.
Tobacco:	None expected.

PERPHENAZINE

BRAND NAMES

Etrafon (M)
Phenazine
Trilafon

GENERAL INFORMATION

Habit forming? No
Prescription needed? Yes
Available as generic? Yes
Drug class: Tranquilizer, antiemetic (phenothiazine)

 ## USES

- Stops nausea, vomiting.
- Reduces anxiety, agitation.

 ## DOSAGE & USAGE INFORMATION

How to take:

- Tablet or capsule—Swallow with liquid or food to lessen stomach irritation.
- Suppositories—Remove wrapper and moisten suppository with water. Gently insert into rectum, large end first.
- Drops or liquid—Dilute dose in beverage.

When to take:

- Nervous and mental disorders—Take at the same times each day.
- Nausea and vomiting—Take as needed, no more often than every 4 hours.

If you forget a dose:

- Nervous and mental disorders—Take up to 2 hours late. If more than 2 hours, wait for next scheduled dose (don't double this).
- Nausea and vomiting—Take as soon as you remember. Wait 4 hours for next dose.

What drug does:

- Suppresses brain's vomiting center.
- Suppresses brain centers that control abnormal emotions and behavior.

Time lapse before drug works:

- Nausea and vomiting—1 hour or less.
- Nervous and mental disorders—4-6 weeks.

Don't take with:

- Antacid or medicine for diarrhea.
- Non-prescription drug for cough, cold or allergy.
- See Interaction column and consult doctor.

 ## OVERDOSE

Symptoms:
Stupor, convulsions, coma.

What to do:

- Dial 0 (operator) or 911 (emergency) for an ambulance or medical help. Then give first aid immediately.
- Additional emergency information on page 886.

POSSIBLE ADVERSE REACTIONS OR SIDE EFFECTS

SYMPTOMS	FREQUENCY	WHAT TO DO
Brain & nervous system:		
• Restlessness, tremor.	Common	3
• Fainting	Infrequent	2
• Drowsiness	Common	3
Skin:		
• Rash	Infrequent	3
• Less perspiration.	Common	4
Eyes:		
Vision changes.	Rare	3
Ears, nose, throat:		
• Sore throat, fever.	Rare	3
• Dry mouth, nasal congestion.	Common	4
Digestive:		
Constipation	Common	4
Heart & lungs, blood vessels, kidneys, allergic, blood:	None expected.	
Muscles, bones, joints:		
Muscle spasms of face and neck, unsteady gait.	Common	2
Genital, urinary:		
Urination difficulty.	Infrequent	4
Liver:		
Jaundice (yellow eyes and skin).	Rare	3
Others:		
Less interest in sex, breast swelling, change in menstrual pattern.	Infrequent	4

1-Life-threatening. Seek emergency treatment immediately.
2-Discontinue. Seek emergency treatment.
3-Discontinue. Call doctor right away.
4-Continue. Call doctor when convenient.
5-Continue. Tell doctor at next visit.
6-No action necessary.

PERPHENAZINE

 ## WARNINGS & PRECAUTIONS

Don't take if:
- You are allergic to any phenothiazine.
- You have a blood or bone-marrow disease.

Before you start, consult your doctor:
- If you will have surgery within 2 months, including dental surgery, requiring general or spinal anesthesia.
- If you have asthma, emphysema or other lung disorder.
- If you take non-prescription ulcer medicine, asthma medicine or amphetamines.

Over age 60:
Adverse reactions and side effects may be more frequent and severe than in younger persons. More likely to develop involuntary movement of jaws, lips, tongue, chewing. Report this to your doctor immediately. Early treatment can help.

Pregnancy:
Risk to unborn child outweighs drug benefits. Don't use.

Breast-feeding:
Drug passes into milk. Avoid drug or discontinue nursing until you finish medicine. Consult doctor for advice on maintaining milk supply.

Infants & children:
Don't give to children younger than 2.

Prolonged use:
May lead to tardive dyskinesia (involuntary movement of jaws, lips, tongue, chewing).

Skin & sunlight:
May cause rash or intensify sunburn in areas exposed to sun or sunlamp. Skin may remain sensitive for 3 months after discontinuing.

Driving, piloting or hazardous work:
Don't drive or pilot aircraft until you learn how medicine affects you. Don't work around dangerous machinery. Don't climb ladders or work in high places. Danger increases if you drink alcohol or take medicine affecting alertness and reflexes.

Airplane passengers:
No problems expected.

Discontinuing:
- Nervous and mental disorders—Don't discontinue without doctor's advice until you complete prescribed dose, even though symptoms diminish or disappear.
- Nausea and vomiting—May be unnecessary to finish medicine. Follow doctor's instructions.

 ## INTERACTION WITH OTHER DRUGS

GENERIC NAME OR DRUG CLASS	COMBINED EFFECT
Anticholinergics	Increased anticholinergic effect.
Antidepressants (tricyclic)	Increased perphenazine effect.
Antihistamines	Increased antihistamine effect.
Appetite suppressants	Decreased suppressant effect.
Levodopa	Decreased levodopa effect.
Mind-altering drugs	Increased effect of mind-altering drugs.
Narcotics	Increased narcotic effect.
Phenytoin	Increased phenytoin effect.
Quinidine	Impaired heart function. Dangerous mixture.
Sedatives	Increased sedative effect.
Tranquilizers (other)	Increased tranquilizer effect.

 ## INTERACTION WITH OTHER SUBSTANCES

INTERACTS WITH	COMBINED EFFECT
Alcohol:	Dangerous oversedation.
Beverages:	None expected.
Cocaine:	Decreased perphenazine effect. Avoid.
Foods:	None expected.
Marijuana:	Drowsiness. May increase antinausea effect.
Tobacco:	None expected.

PHENACETIN

BRAND NAMES

A.P.C.-Demerol (M)
A.P.C. Tablets (M)
Aspirin Compound
 with Codeine (M)
Emprazil (M)
Fiorinal (M)

P.A.C. Compound (M)
Percodan (M)
Sinubid (M)
SK-65 Compound (M)
Soma Compound (M)
Synalgos (M)

GENERAL INFORMATION

Habit forming? No
Prescription needed? No
Available as generic? Yes
Drug class: Analgesic, fever reducer

 USES

- Relieves pain.
- Reduces fever.

 DOSAGE & USAGE INFORMATION

How to take:
- Tablet or capsule—Swallow with liquid or food to lessen stomach irritation. You may chew or crush tablets.
- Extended-release tablets or capsules—Swallow each dose whole with liquid.

When to take:
At the same times each day.

If you forget a dose:
Take as soon as you remember up to 2 hours late. If more than 2 hours, wait for next scheduled dose (don't double this dose).

What drug does:
Reduces level of prostaglandins, a chemical involved in producing inflammation, fever, pain.

Time lapse before drug works:
15 minutes.

Don't take with:
See Interaction column and consult doctor.

 OVERDOSE

Symptoms:
Sweating, bloody urine, convulsions, coma.

What to do:
- Dial 0 (operator) or 911 (emergency) for an ambulance or medical help. Then give first aid immediately.
- Additional emergency information on page 886.

POSSIBLE ADVERSE REACTIONS OR SIDE EFFECTS

SYMPTOMS	FREQUENCY	WHAT TO DO
Brain & nervous system: Confusion, drowsiness.	Infrequent	4
Skin: Rash, itch, hives.	Infrequent	3
Eyes:	None expected.	
Ears, nose, throat: Sore throat, fever, sores in mouth.	Infrequent	3
Digestive:		
• Nausea	Infrequent	4
• Black, tarry or bloody stools.	Rare	2
Heart & lungs:	None expected.	
Blood vessels: Easy bruising.	Rare	3
Muscles, bones, joints: Swollen feet, legs.	Rare	3
Genital, urinary: Bloody urine.	Rare	3
Kidneys:	None expected.	
Liver:	None expected.	
Allergic:	None expected.	
Blood: Anemia	Rare	3
Others:		
• Blue fingernails.	Rare	3
• Fatigue, weakness.	Rare	3

1-Life-threatening. Seek emergency treatment immediately.
2-Discontinue. Seek emergency treatment.
3-Discontinue. Call doctor right away.
4-Continue. Call doctor when convenient.
5-Continue. Tell doctor at next visit.
6-No action necessary.

PHENACETIN

WARNINGS & PRECAUTIONS

Don't take if:
You are allergic to phenacetin, aspirin or any of the many mixtures which contain either.

Before you start, consult your doctor:
● If you have kidney or liver disease.
● If you have G6PD deficiency.

Over age 60:
Adverse reactions and side effects may be more frequent and severe than in younger persons.

Pregnancy:
May cause anemia in newborn. Avoid if possible.

Breast-feeding:
Drug passes into milk. Avoid drug or discontinue nursing until you finish medicine. Consult doctor for advice on maintaining milk supply.

Infants & children:
Not recommended.

Prolonged use:
Kidney damage. Don't take regularly without medical advice.

Skin & sunlight:
No problems expected.

Driving, piloting or hazardous work:
No problems expected.

Airplane passengers:
No problems expected.

Discontinuing:
May be unnecessary to finish medicine. Follow doctor's instructions.

Others:
No problems expected.

INTERACTION WITH OTHER DRUGS

GENERIC NAME OR DRUG CLASS	COMBINED EFFECT
Phenobarbital	Decreased phenacetin effect.

INTERACTION WITH OTHER SUBSTANCES

INTERACTS WITH	COMBINED EFFECT
Alcohol:	None expected.
Beverages:	None expected.
Cocaine:	None expected.
Foods:	None expected.
Marijuana:	Increased pain relief.
Tobacco:	None expected.

PHENAZOPYRIDINE

BRAND NAMES

Azo-100
Azodine
Azo-Gantanol (M)
Azo-Gantrisin (M)
Azo-Mandelamine (M)
Azo-Standard

Azotrex
Di-Azo
Phen-Azo
Phenazodine
Pyridiate
Pyridium

Pyridium Plus (M)
Pyrodine
Thiosulfil-A (M)
Urobiotic (M)

GENERAL INFORMATION

Habit forming? No
Prescription needed? Yes
Available as generic? Yes
Drug class: Analgesic (urinary)

 ## USES

Relieves pain of lower urinary-tract irritation,
as in cystitis, urethritis or prostatitis.
Relieves symptoms only. Phenazopyridine
alone does not cure infections.

 ## DOSAGE & USAGE INFORMATION

How to take:
Tablet or capsule—Swallow with liquid or
food to lessen stomach irritation.

When to take:
At the same times each day.

If you forget a dose:
Take as soon as you remember up to 2 hours
late. If more than 2 hours, wait for next
scheduled dose (don't double this dose).

What drug does:
Anesthetizes lower urinary tract. Relieves
pain, burning, pressure and urgency to
urinate.

Time lapse before drug works:
1 to 2 hours.

Don't take with:
No restrictions.

 ## OVERDOSE

Symptoms:
Shortness of breath, weakness.

What to do:
Overdose unlikely to threaten life. If person
takes much larger amount than prescribed,
call doctor, poison-control center or hospital
emergency room for instructions.

 ## POSSIBLE ADVERSE REACTIONS OR SIDE EFFECTS

SYMPTOMS	FREQUENCY	WHAT TO DO
Brain & nervous system: Headache	Rare	4
Skin: Rash	Rare	3
Eyes:	None expected.	
Ears, nose, throat:	None expected.	
Digestive: Indigestion	Infrequent	4
Heart & lungs:	None expected.	
Blood vessels:	None expected.	
Muscles, bones, joints:	None expected.	
Genital, urinary: Red-orange urine.	Common	6
Kidneys:	None expected.	
Liver: Jaundice (yellow skin and eyes).	Rare	3
Allergic:	None expected.	
Blood: Anemia	Rare	4
Others: Fatigue, weakness.	Infrequent	4

1- Life-threatening. Seek emergency
   treatment immediately.
2- Discontinue. Seek emergency treatment.
3- Discontinue. Call doctor right away.
4- Continue. Call doctor when convenient.
5- Continue. Tell doctor at next visit.
6- No action necessary.

WARNINGS & PRECAUTIONS

Don't take if:
- You have hepatitis.
- You are allergic to any urinary analgesic.

Before you start, consult your doctor:
If you have kidney or liver disease.

Over age 60:
Adverse reactions and side effects may be more frequent and severe than in younger persons.

Pregnancy:
No proven harm to unborn child. Avoid if possible.

Breast-feeding:
No problems expected.

Infants & children:
Not recommended.

Prolonged use:
- Orange or yellow skin.
- Anemia. Occasional blood studies recommended.

Skin & sunlight:
No problems expected.

Driving, piloting or hazardous work:
No problems expected.

Airplane passengers:
No problems expected.

Discontinuing:
May be unnecessary to finish medicine. Follow doctor's instructions.

Others:
No problems expected.

INTERACTION WITH OTHER DRUGS

GENERIC NAME OR DRUG CLASS	COMBINED EFFECT
None	

INTERACTION WITH OTHER SUBSTANCES

INTERACTS WITH	COMBINED EFFECT
Alcohol:	None expected.
Beverages:	None expected.
Cocaine:	None expected.
Foods:	None expected.
Marijuana:	None expected.
Tobacco:	None expected.

PHENDIMETRAZINE

BRAND NAMES

Adphen	Di-Ap-Trol	Minus	Trimstat
Anorex	Ex-Obese	Obestrol	Trimtabs
Bacarate	Limit	Reducto	Weightrol

See complete brand names list, page 827.

GENERAL INFORMATION

Habit forming? Yes
Prescription needed? Yes
Available as generic? Yes
Drug class: Appetite suppressant

 USES

Suppresses appetite.

 DOSAGE & USAGE INFORMATION

How to take:
- Tablet or capsule—Swallow with liquid. You may chew or crush tablet.
- Extended-release tablets or capsules—Swallow each dose whole with liquid.

When to take:
- Long-acting forms—10 to 14 hours before bedtime.
- Short-acting forms—1 hour before meals. Last dose no later than 4 to 6 hours before bedtime.

If you forget a dose:
- Long-acting form—Take as soon as you remember up to 2 hours late. If more than 2 hours, wait for next scheduled dose (don't double this dose).
- Short-acting form—Wait for next scheduled dose. Don't double this dose.

What drug does:
Apparently stimulates brain's appetite-control center.

Time lapse before drug works:
Begins in about 1 hour. Short-acting form lasts 4 hours. Long-acting form lasts 14 hours.

Don't take with:
- Non-prescription drugs without consulting doctor.
- See Interaction column and consult doctor.

 OVERDOSE

Symptoms:
Irritability, overactivity, trembling, insomnia, mood changes, rapid heartbeat, confusion, disorientation, hallucinations, convulsions, coma.

What to do:
- Dial 0 (operator) or 911 (emergency) for an ambulance or medical help. Then give first aid immediately.
- Additional information on page 886.

POSSIBLE ADVERSE REACTIONS OR SIDE EFFECTS

SYMPTOMS	FREQUENCY	WHAT TO DO
Brain & nervous system:		
● Irritability, nervousness, insomnia.	Common	4
● Mood changes.	Rare	3
Skin:		
● Hair loss.	Rare	4
● Rash or hives.	Rare	3
Eyes:		
Blurred vision.	Infrequent	4
Ears, nose, throat:		
Unpleasant taste or dry mouth.	Infrequent	4
Digestive:		
Constipation or diarrhea, nausea, vomiting, cramps.	Infrequent	4
Heart & lungs:		
● Irregular or pounding heartbeat.	Infrequent	3
● Breathing difficulty.	Rare	3
Blood vessels, muscles, bones, joints, kidneys, liver, allergic, blood:	None expected.	
Genital, urinary:		
Urinary urgency and difficulty.	Infrequent	3
Others:		
● False sense of well-being.	Common	4
● Changes in sex drive.	Infrequent	4
● Sweat increase.	Infrequent	4

1—Life-threatening. Seek emergency treatment immediately.
2—Discontinue. Seek emergency treatment.
3—Discontinue. Call doctor right away.
4—Continue. Call doctor when convenient.

WARNINGS & PRECAUTIONS

Don't take if:
- You are allergic to any sympathomimetic or phenylpropanolamine.
- You have glaucoma.
- You have taken MAO inhibitors within 2 weeks.
- You plan to become pregnant within medication period.
- You have a history of drug abuse.

Before you start, consult your doctor:
- If you have high blood pressure or heart disease.
- If you have an overactive thyroid, nervous tension or "anxiety."
- If you have epilepsy.

Over age 60:
Adverse reactions and side effects may be more frequent and severe than in younger persons.

Pregnancy:
Safety not established. Avoid.

Breast-feeding:
No proven problems. Consult doctor.

Infants & children:
Don't give to children younger than 12.

Prolonged use:
Loses effectiveness. Avoid.

Skin & sunlight:
No problems expected.

Driving, piloting or hazardous work:
Don't drive or pilot aircraft until you learn how medicine affects you. Don't work around dangerous machinery. Don't climb ladders or work in high places. Danger increases if you drink alcohol or take medicine affecting alertness and reflexes, such as antihistamines, tranquilizers, sedatives, pain medicine, narcotics and mind-altering drugs.

Airplane passengers:
No problems expected.

Discontinuing:
Don't discontinue without consulting doctor. Dose may require gradual reduction if you have taken drug for a long time. Doses of other drugs may also require adjustment.

Others:
Don't increase dose.

INTERACTION WITH OTHER DRUGS

GENERIC NAME OR DRUG CLASS	COMBINED EFFECT
Appetite suppressants (other)	Dangerous overstimulation.
Caffeine	Increased stimulant effect of phendimetrazine.
Guanethidine	Decreased guanethidine effect.
Hydralazine	Decreased hydralazine effect.
MAO inhibitors	Dangerous blood-pressure rise.
Methyldopa	Decreased methyldopa effect.
Phenothiazines	Decreased phendimetrazine effect.
Rauwolfia alkaloids	Decreased effect of rauwolfia alkaloids.

INTERACTION WITH OTHER SUBSTANCES

INTERACTS WITH	COMBINED EFFECT
Alcohol: Beer, chianti wines, vermouth.	Dangerous blood-pressure rise.
Beverages: • Caffeine drinks • Drinks containing tyramine (see page 851).	Excessive stimulation. Blood-pressure rise.
Cocaine:	Excessive stimulation.
Foods: Foods containing tyramine (see page 851).	Blood-pressure rise.
Marijuana:	Frequent use—Irregular heartbeat.
Tobacco:	None expected.

PHENELZINE

BRAND NAMES

Nardil

Habit forming? No
Prescription needed? Yes
Available as generic? No

GENERAL INFORMATION

Drug class: MAO inhibitor
(monamine oxidase inhibitor),
antidepressant

 USES

Treatment for depression.

 DOSAGE & USAGE INFORMATION

How to take:
Tablet—Swallow with liquid. If you can't swallow whole, crumble tablet and take with liquid or food.

When to take:
At the same times each day.

If you forget a dose:
Take as soon as you remember up to 2 hours late. If more than 2 hours, wait for next scheduled dose (don't double this dose).

What drug does:
Inhibits nerve transmissions in brain that may cause depression.

Time lapse before drug works:
4 to 6 weeks for maximum effect.

Don't take with:
- Non-prescription diet pills, nose drops, medicine for asthma, cough, cold or allergy, or medicine containing caffeine or alcohol.
- See Interaction column and consult doctor.

 OVERDOSE

Symptoms:
Restlessness, agitation, fever, convulsions, coma.

What to do:
- Dial 0 (operator) or 911 (emergency) for an ambulance or medical help. Then give first aid immediately.
- Additional emergency information on page 886.

POSSIBLE ADVERSE REACTIONS OR SIDE EFFECTS

SYMPTOMS	FREQUENCY	WHAT TO DO
Brain & nervous system:		
• Fainting	Infrequent	2
• Severe headache.	Infrequent	3
• Dizziness when changing position.	Common	5
• Hallucinations, insomnia, nightmares.	Infrequent	4
Skin:		
Rash	Rare	3
Eyes, blood vessels, kidneys, allergic, blood:		
	None expected.	
Ears, nose, throat:		
Dry mouth.	Common	5
Digestive:		
• Diarrhea	Infrequent	4
• Constipation	Common	5
• Nausea, vomiting.	Rare	3
Heart & lungs:		
• Rapid or pounding heartbeat.	Infrequent	4
• Chest pain.	Infrequent	3
Muscles, bones, joints:		
Stiff neck.	Rare	3
Genital, urinary:		
Difficult urination.	Common	5
Liver:		
Jaundice (yellow skin and eyes).	Rare	3
Others:		
• Swollen feet, legs.	Infrequent	4
• Fever	Rare	3
• Lower sex drive.	Infrequent	5
• Fatigue, weakness.	Common	4

1- Life-threatening. Seek emergency treatment immediately.
2- Discontinue. Seek emergency treatment.
3- Discontinue. Call doctor right away.
4- Continue. Call doctor when convenient.
5- Continue. Tell doctor at next visit.

WARNINGS & PRECAUTIONS

Don't take if:
- You are allergic to any MAO inhibitor.
- You have heart disease, congestive heart failure, heart-rhythm irregularities or high blood pressure.
- You have liver or kidney disease.

Before you start, consult your doctor:
- If you are alcoholic.
- If you have asthma.
- If you have had a stroke.
- If you have diabetes or epilepsy.
- If you have overactive thyroid.
- If you have schizophrenia.
- If you have Parkinson's disease.
- If you have adrenal-gland tumor.
- If you will have surgery within 2 months, including dental surgery, requiring general or spinal anesthesia.

Over age 60:
Not recommended.

Pregnancy:
No proven harm to unborn child. Avoid if possible.

Breast-feeding:
Safety not established. Consult doctor.

Infants & children:
Not recommended.

Prolonged use:
May be toxic to liver.

Skin & sunlight:
May cause rash or intensify sunburn in areas exposed to sun or sunlamp.

Driving, piloting or hazardous work:
Don't drive or pilot aircraft until you learn how medicine affects you. Don't work around dangerous machinery. Don't climb ladders or work in high places. Danger increases if you drink alcohol or take medicine affecting alertness and reflexes.

Airplane passengers:
No problems expected.

Discontinuing:
- Don't discontinue without doctor's advice until you complete prescribed dose, even though symptoms diminish or disappear.
- Follow precautions regarding foods, drinks and other medicines for 2 weeks after discontinuing.

Others:
- May affect blood-sugar levels in patients with diabetes.
- Fever may indicate that MAO inhibitor dose requires adjustment.

INTERACTION WITH OTHER DRUGS

GENERIC NAME OR DRUG CLASS	COMBINED EFFECT
Amphetamines	Blood-pressure rise to life-threatening level.
Anticonvulsants	Changed seizure pattern.
Antidepressants (tricyclic)	Blood-pressure rise to life-threatening level.
Antidiabetics (oral and insulin)	Excessively low blood sugar.
Antihypertensives	Excessively low blood pressure.
Caffeine	Irregular heartbeat or high blood pressure.
Carbamazepine	Fever, seizures. Avoid.
Cyclobenzaprine	Fever, seizures. Avoid.
Diuretics	Excessively low blood pressure.
Guanethidine	Blood-pressure rise to life-threatening level.
Levodopa	Sudden, severe blood pressure rise.
MAO inhibitors (other)	High fever, convulsions, death.

Additional interactions on page 840.

INTERACTION WITH OTHER SUBSTANCES

INTERACTS WITH	COMBINED EFFECT
Alcohol:	Increased sedation to dangerous level.
Beverages: Caffeine drinks	Irregular heartbeat or high blood pressure.
Drinks containing tyramine (see page 851).	Blood-pressure rise to life-threatening level.
Cocaine:	Overstimulation. Possibly fatal.
Foods: Foods containing tyramine (see page 851).	Blood-pressure rise to life-threatening level.
Marijuana:	Overstimulation. Avoid.
Tobacco:	No proven problems.

PHENIRAMINE

BRAND NAMES

Citra Capsules (M)   Triaminicin (M)
Fiogesic (M)   Triaminicol (M)
Inhistor   Tussagesic (M)
Robitussin-AC (M)   Tussaminic (M)
Triaminic (M)

See complete brand names list, page 827.

 USES

Reduces allergic symptoms such as hay fever, hives, rash or itching.

 DOSAGE & USAGE INFORMATION

How to take:
- Tablet, syrup or capsule—Swallow with liquid or food to lessen stomach irritation.
- Extended-release tablets or capsules—Swallow each dose whole.

When to take:
Varies with form. Follow label directions.

If you forget a dose:
Take as soon as you remember up to 2 hours late. If more than 2 hours, wait for next scheduled dose (don't double this dose).

What drug does:
Blocks action of histamine after an allergic response triggers histamine release in sensitive cells.

Time lapse before drug works:
30 minutes.

Don't take with:
See Interaction column and consult doctor.

 OVERDOSE

Symptoms:
Convulsions, red face, hallucinations, coma.

What to do:
- Dial 0 (operator) or 911 (emergency) for an ambulance or medical help. Then give first aid immediately.
- Additional emergency information on page 886.

GENERAL INFORMATION

Habit forming? No
Prescription needed? High strength: Yes
Low strength: No
Available as generic? Yes
Drug class: Antihistamine

 POSSIBLE ADVERSE REACTIONS OR SIDE EFFECTS

SYMPTOMS	FREQUENCY	WHAT TO DO
Brain & nervous system:		
• Nightmares, agitation, irritability.	Rare	3
• Drowsiness, dizziness.	Common	5
Skin:	None expected.	
Eyes:		
• Vision changes.	Infrequent	3
• Less tolerance for contact lenses.	Infrequent	4
Ears, nose, throat:		
• Sore throat, fever.	Rare	3
• Dry mouth, nose, throat.	Common	5
Digestive:		
• Nausea	Common	5
• Appetite loss.	Infrequent	5
Heart & lungs:		
Rapid heartbeat.	Rare	3
Blood vessels:		
Unusual bleeding or bruising.	Rare	3
Muscles, bones, joints, kidneys, liver, allergic, blood:	None expected.	
Genital, urinary:		
Urination difficulty.	Infrequent	4
Others:		
Fatigue, weakness.	Rare	3

1- Life-threatening. Seek emergency treatment immediately.
2- Discontinue. Seek emergency treatment.
3- Discontinue. Call doctor right away.
4- Continue. Call doctor when convenient.
5- Continue. Tell doctor at next visit.
6- No action necessary.

PHENIRAMINE

WARNINGS & PRECAUTIONS

Don't take if:
You are allergic to any antihistamine.

Before you start, consult your doctor:
- If you have glaucoma.
- If you have enlarged prostate.
- If you have asthma.
- If you have kidney disease.
- If you have peptic ulcer.
- If you will have surgery within 2 months, including dental surgery, requiring general or spinal anesthesia.

Over age 60:
Don't exceed recommended dose. Adverse reactions and side effects may be more frequent and severe than in younger persons, especially urination difficulty, diminished alertness and other brain and nervous-system symptoms.

Pregnancy:
No proven harm to unborn child. Avoid if possible.

Breast-feeding:
Drug passes into milk. Avoid drug or discontinue nursing until you finish medicine. Consult doctor for advice on maintaining milk supply.

Infants & children:
Not recommended for premature or newborn infants. Otherwise, no problems expected.

Prolonged use:
Avoid. May damage bone-marrow and nerve cells.

Skin & sunlight:
May cause rash or intensify sunburn in areas exposed to sun or sunlamp.

Driving, piloting or hazardous work:
Don't drive or pilot aircraft until you learn how medicine affects you. Don't work around dangerous machinery. Don't climb ladders or work in high places. Danger increases if you drink alcohol or take medicine affecting alertness and reflexes, such as antihistamines, tranquilizers, sedatives, pain medicine, narcotics and mind-altering drugs.

Airplane passengers:
No problems expected.

Discontinuing:
No problems expected.

Others:
May mask symptoms of hearing damage from aspirin, other salicylates, cisplatin, paromomycin, vancomycin or anticonvulsants. Consult doctor if you use these.

INTERACTION WITH OTHER DRUGS

GENERIC NAME OR DRUG CLASS	COMBINED EFFECT
Anticholinergics	Increased anticholinergic effect.
Antidepressants	Excess sedation. Avoid.
Antihistamines (other)	Excess sedation. Avoid.
Hypnotics	Excess sedation. Avoid.
MAO inhibitors	Increased pheniramine effect.
Mind-altering drugs	Excess sedation. Avoid.
Narcotics	Excess sedation. Avoid.
Sedatives	Excess sedation. Avoid.
Sleep inducers	Excess sedation. Avoid.
Tranquilizers	Excess sedation. Avoid.

INTERACTION WITH OTHER SUBSTANCES

INTERACTS WITH	COMBINED EFFECT
Alcohol:	Excess sedation. Avoid.
Beverages: Caffeine drinks	Less pheniramine sedation.
Cocaine:	Decreased pheniramine effect. Avoid.
Foods:	None expected.
Marijuana:	Excess sedation. Avoid.
Tobacco:	None expected.

PHENMETRAZINE

BRAND NAMES

Preludin

GENERAL INFORMATION

Habit forming? Yes
Prescription needed? Yes
Available as generic? Yes
Drug class: Appetite suppressant

 ## USES

Suppresses appetite.

 ## DOSAGE & USAGE INFORMATION

How to take:
- Tablet—Swallow with liquid. You may chew or crush tablet.
- Extended-release tablets—Swallow each dose whole with liquid.

When to take:
- Long-acting forms—10 to 14 hours before bedtime.
- Short-acting forms—1 hour before meals. Last dose no later than 4 to 6 hours before bedtime.

If you forget a dose:
- Long-acting form—Take as soon as you remember up to 2 hours late. If more than 2 hours, wait for next scheduled dose (don't double this dose).
- Short-acting form—Wait for next scheduled dose. Don't double this dose.

What drug does:
Apparently stimulates brain's appetite-control center.

Time lapse before drug works:
Begins in 1 hour. Short-acting form lasts 4 hours. Long-acting form lasts 14 hours.

Don't take with:
- Non-prescription drugs without consulting doctor.
- See Interaction column and consult doctor.

 ## OVERDOSE

Symptoms:
Irritability, overactivity, trembling, insomnia, mood changes, rapid heartbeat, confusion, disorientation, hallucinations, convulsions, coma.

What to do:
- Dial 0 (operator) or 911 (emergency) for an ambulance or medical help. Then give first aid immediately.
- Additional emergency information on page 886.

POSSIBLE ADVERSE REACTIONS OR SIDE EFFECTS

SYMPTOMS	FREQUENCY	WHAT TO DO
Brain & nervous system:		
• Irritability, nervousness, insomnia.	Common	4
• Mood changes.	Rare	3
Skin:		
• Hair loss.	Rare	4
• Rash or hives.	Rare	3
Eyes:		
Blurred vision.	Infrequent	4
Ears, nose, throat:		
Unpleasant taste or dry mouth.	Infrequent	4
Digestive:		
Constipation or diarrhea, nausea, vomiting, cramps.	Infrequent	4
Heart & lungs:		
• Irregular or pounding heartbeat.	Infrequent	3
• Breathing difficulty.	Rare	3
Blood vessels, muscles, bones, joints, kidneys, liver, allergic, blood:	None expected.	
Genital, urinary:		
Urinary urgency and difficulty.	Infrequent	3
Others:		
• False sense of well-being.	Common	4
• Changes in sex drive.	Infrequent	4
• Sweat increase.	Infrequent	4

1- Life-threatening. Seek emergency treatment immediately.
2- Discontinue. Seek emergency treatment.
3- Discontinue. Call doctor right away.
4- Continue. Call doctor when convenient.

WARNINGS & PRECAUTIONS

Don't take if:
- You are allergic to any sympathomimetic or phenylpropanolamine.
- You have glaucoma.
- You have taken MAO inhibitors within 2 weeks.
- You plan to become pregnant within medication period.
- You have a history of drug abuse.

Before you start, consult your doctor:
- If you have high blood pressure or heart disease.
- If you have an overactive thyroid, nervous tension or "anxiety."
- If you have epilepsy.

Over age 60:
Adverse reactions and side effects may be more frequent and severe than in younger persons.

Pregnancy:
Safety not established. Avoid.

Breast-feeding:
No proven problems. Consult doctor.

Infants & children:
Don't give to children younger than 12.

Prolonged use:
Loses effectiveness. Avoid.

Skin & sunlight:
No problems expected.

Driving, piloting or hazardous work:
Don't drive or pilot aircraft until you learn how medicine affects you. Don't work around dangerous machinery. Don't climb ladders or work in high places. Danger increases if you drink alcohol or take medicine affecting alertness and reflexes, such as antihistamines, tranquilizers, sedatives, pain medicine, narcotics and mind-altering drugs.

Airplane passengers:
No problems expected.

Discontinuing:
Don't discontinue without consulting doctor. Dose may require gradual reduction if you have taken drug for a long time. Doses of other drugs may also require adjustment.

Others:
Don't increase dose.

 INTERACTION WITH OTHER DRUGS

GENERIC NAME OR DRUG CLASS	COMBINED EFFECT
Appetite suppressants (other)	Dangerous overstimulation.
Caffeine	Increased stimulant effect of phenmetrazine.
Guanethidine	Decreased guanethidine effect.
Hydralazine	Decreased hydralazine effect.
MAO inhibitors	Dangerous blood-pressure rise.
Methyldopa	Decreased methyldopa effect.
Phenothiazines	Decreased phenmetrazine effect.
Rauwolfia alkaloids	Decreased effect of rauwolfia alkaloids.

 INTERACTION WITH OTHER SUBSTANCES

INTERACTS WITH	COMBINED EFFECT
Alcohol: Beer, chianti wines, vermouth.	Dangerous blood-pressure rise.
Beverages: ● Caffeine drinks	Excessive stimulation.
● Drinks containing tyramine (see page 851).	Blood-pressure rise.
Cocaine:	Excessive stimulation.
Foods: Foods containing tyramine (see page 851).	Blood-pressure rise.
Marijuana:	Frequent use—Irregular heartbeat.
Tobacco:	None expected.

PHENOBARBITAL

BRAND NAMES

Anaspaz-PB (M)   Probital (M)
Eskabarb   Sedadrops
Gardenal   SK-Phenobarbital
Nova-Pheno   Solfoton
See complete brand names list, page 827.

GENERAL INFORMATION

Habit forming? Yes
Prescription needed? Yes
Available as generic? Yes
Drug class: Sedative,
hypnotic (barbiturate), anticonvulsant

USES

- Reduces anxiety or nervous tension (low dose).
- Relieves insomnia (higher bedtime dose).
- Prevents convulsions or seizures, such as epilepsy.

DOSAGE & USAGE INFORMATION

How to take:
- Tablet, liquid or capsule—Swallow with liquid or food to lessen stomach irritation. If you can't swallow whole, crumble tablet or open capsule and take with liquid or food.
- Extended-release tablets or capsules—Swallow each dose whole.
- Drops—Dilute dose in beverage before swallowing.

When to take:
At the same times each day.

If you forget a dose:
Take as soon as you remember up to 2 hours late. If more than 2 hours, wait for next scheduled dose (don't double this dose).

What drug does:
May partially block nerve impulses at nerve-cell connections.

Time lapse before drug works:
60 minutes.

Don't take with:
- Non-prescription drugs without consulting doctor.
- See Interaction column and consult doctor.

OVERDOSE

Symptoms:
Deep sleep, weak pulse, coma.

What to do:
- Dial 0 (operator) or 911 (emergency) for an ambulance or medical help. Then give first aid immediately.
- Additional emergency information on page 886.

POSSIBLE ADVERSE REACTIONS OR SIDE EFFECTS

SYMPTOMS	FREQUENCY	WHAT TO DO
Brain & nervous system:		
• Dizziness, drowsiness, "hangover effect."	Common	4
• Depression, confusion, slurred speech.	Infrequent	4
• Agitation	Rare	3
Skin:		
• Rash or hives.	Infrequent	3
• Face, lip swelling.	Infrequent	3
Eyes:		
Eyelid swelling.	Infrequent	3
Ears, nose, throat:		
Sore throat, fever.	Infrequent	3
Digestive:		
Diarrhea, nausea, vomiting.	Infrequent	4
Heart & lungs:		
• Slow heartbeat.	Rare	3
• Breathing difficulty.	Rare	3
Blood vessels:		
Unexplained bleeding or bruising.	Rare	4
Muscles, bones, joints:		
Joint or muscle pain.	Infrequent	4
Genital, urinary:	None expected.	
Kidneys:	None expected.	
Liver:		
Jaundice (yellow skin and eyes).	Rare	3
Allergic:	None expected.	
Blood:	None expected.	
Others:	None expected.	

1-Life-threatening. Seek emergency treatment immediately.
2-Discontinue. Seek emergency treatment.
3-Discontinue. Call doctor right away.
4-Continue. Call doctor when convenient.

PHENOBARBITAL

WARNINGS & PRECAUTIONS

Don't take if:
- You are allergic to any barbiturate.
- You have porphyria.

Before you start, consult your doctor:
- If you have epilepsy.
- If you have kidney or liver damage.
- If you have asthma.
- If you have anemia.
- If you have chronic pain.
- If you will have surgery within 2 months, including dental surgery, requiring general or spinal anesthesia.

Over age 60:
Adverse reactions and side effects may be more frequent and severe than in younger persons. Use small doses.

Pregnancy:
Risk to unborn child outweighs drug benefits. Don't use.

Breast-feeding:
Drug passes into milk. Avoid drug or discontinue nursing until you finish medicine. Consult doctor for advice on maintaining milk supply.

Infants & children:
Use only under doctor's supervision.

Prolonged use:
- May cause addiction, anemia, chronic intoxication.
- May lower body temperature, making exposure to cold temperatures hazardous.

Skin & sunlight:
May cause rash or intensify sunburn in areas exposed to sun or sunlamp.

Driving, piloting or hazardous work:
Don't drive or pilot aircraft until you learn how medicine affects you. Don't work around dangerous machinery. Don't climb ladders or work in high places. Danger increases if you drink alcohol or take medicine affecting alertness and reflexes.

Airplane passengers:
No problems expected.

Discontinuing:
May be unnecessary to finish medicine. Follow doctor's instructions. If you develop withdrawal symptoms of hallucinations, agitation or sleeplessness after discontinuing, call doctor right away.

Others:
No problems expected.

INTERACTION WITH OTHER DRUGS

GENERIC NAME OR DRUG CLASS	COMBINED EFFECT
Anticoagulants (oral)	Decreased anticoagulant effect.
Anticonvulsants	Changed seizure patterns.
Antidepressants (tricyclic)	Decreased antidepressant effect.
Antidiabetics (oral)	Increased phenobarbital effect.
Antihistamines	Dangerous sedation. Avoid.
Antiinflammatory drugs (non-steroidal)	Decreased antiinflammatory effect.
Aspirin	Decreased aspirin effect.
Beta-adrenergic blockers	Decreased effect of beta-adrenergic blocker.
Contraceptives (oral)	Decreased contraceptive effect.
Cortisone drugs	Decreased cortisone effect.
Digitoxin	Decreased digitoxin effect.
Doxycycline	Decreased doxycycline effect.
Griseofulvin	Decreased griseofulvin effect.

Additional interactions on page 840.

INTERACTION WITH OTHER SUBSTANCES

INTERACTS WITH	COMBINED EFFECT
Alcohol:	Possible fatal oversedation. Avoid.
Beverages:	None expected.
Cocaine:	Decreased phenobarbital effect.
Foods:	None expected.
Marijuana:	Excessive sedation. Avoid.
Tobacco:	None expected.

PHENOLPHTHALEIN

BRAND NAMES

Alophen	Feen-A-Mint
Correctol	Phenolax
Espotabs	Prulet
Evac-U-Gen	
Evac-U-Lax	
Ex-Lax	

GENERAL INFORMATION

Habit forming? No
Prescription needed? No
Available as generic? Yes
Drug class: Laxative (stimulant)

USES

Constipation relief.

DOSAGE & USAGE INFORMATION

How to take:
- Tablet or wafer—Swallow with liquid. If you can't swallow whole, chew or crumble and take with liquid or food.
- Liquid—Drink 6 to 8 glasses of water each day, in addition to one taken with each dose.
- Chewable tablets—Chew thoroughly before swallowing.

When to take:
Usually at bedtime with a snack, unless directed otherwise.

If you forget a dose:
Take as soon as you remember.

What drug does:
Acts on smooth muscles of intestine wall to cause vigorous bowel movement.

Time lapse before drug works:
6 to 10 hours.

Don't take with:
- See Interaction column and consult doctor.
- Don't take within 2 hours of taking another medicine. Laxative interferes with medicine absorption.

OVERDOSE

Symptoms:
Vomiting, electrolyte depletion.

What to do:
Overdose unlikely to threaten life. If person takes much larger amount than prescribed, call doctor, poison-control center or hospital emergency room for instructions.

POSSIBLE ADVERSE REACTIONS OR SIDE EFFECTS

SYMPTOMS	FREQUENCY	WHAT TO DO
Brain & nervous system: Irritability, confusion, headache.	Rare	3
Skin: Rash	Rare	3
Eyes:	None expected.	
Ears, nose, throat:	None expected.	
Digestive: Belching, cramps, nausea.	Infrequent	4
Heart & lungs: Breathing difficulty, irregular heartbeat.	Rare	3
Blood vessels:	None expected.	
Muscles, bones, joints: Muscle cramps.	Rare	3
Genital, urinary: Pink to orange urine.	Common	6
Kidneys: Burning on urination.	Rare	4
Liver:	None expected.	
Allergic:	None expected.	
Blood:	None expected.	
Others: • Rectal irritation.	Common	4
• Dangerous potassium loss.	Infrequent	3
• Unusual tiredness or weakness.	Rare	3

1- Life-threatening. Seek emergency treatment immediately.
2- Discontinue. Seek emergency treatment.
3- Discontinue. Call doctor right away.
4- Continue. Call doctor when convenient.
5- Continue. Tell doctor at next visit.
6- No action necessary.

PHENOLPHTHALEIN

WARNINGS & PRECAUTIONS

Don't take if:
- You have symptoms of appendicitis, inflamed bowel or intestinal blockage.
- You are allergic to a stimulant laxative.
- You have missed a bowel movement for only 1 or 2 days.

Before you start, consult your doctor:
- If you have a colostomy or ileostomy.
- If you have congestive heart disease.
- If you have diabetes.
- If you have high blood pressure.
- If you have a laxative habit.
- If you have rectal bleeding.
- If you take other laxatives.

Over age 60:
Adverse reactions and side effects may be more frequent and severe than in younger persons.

Pregnancy:
Risk to mother and unborn child outweighs drug benefits. Don't use.

Breast-feeding:
Drug passes into milk. Avoid drug or discontinue nursing until you finish medicine. Consult doctor for advice on maintaining milk supply.

Infants & children:
Use only under medical supervision.

Prolonged use:
Don't take for more than 1 week unless under a doctor's supervision. May cause laxative dependence.

Skin & sunlight:
No problems expected.

Driving, piloting or hazardous work:
No problems expected.

Airplane passengers:
No problems expected.

Discontinuing:
May be unnecessary to finish medicine. Follow doctor's instructions.

Others:
Don't take to "flush out" your system or as a "tonic."

INTERACTION WITH OTHER DRUGS

GENERIC NAME OR DRUG CLASS	COMBINED EFFECT
Antacids	Tablet coating may dissolve too rapidly, irritating stomach or bowel.
Antihypertensives	May cause dangerous low potassium level.
Diuretics	May cause dangerous low potassium level.

INTERACTION WITH OTHER SUBSTANCES

INTERACTS WITH	COMBINED EFFECT
Alcohol:	None expected.
Beverages: Milk	Tablet coating may dissolve too rapidly, irritating stomach or bowel.
Cocaine:	None expected.
Foods:	None expected.
Marijuana:	None expected.
Tobacco:	None expected.

PHENPROCOUMON

BRAND NAMES

Liquamar
Marcumar

GENERAL INFORMATION

Habit forming? No
Prescription needed? Yes
Available as generic? Yes
Drug class: Anticoagulant

 USES

Reduces blood clots. Used for abnormal clotting inside blood vessels.

 DOSAGE & USAGE INFORMATION

How to take:
Tablet—Swallow with liquid. If you can't swallow whole, crumble tablet and take with liquid or food.

When to take:
At the same time each day.

If you forget a dose:
Take as soon as you remember up to 12 hours late. If more than 12 hours, wait for next scheduled dose (don't double this dose). Inform your doctor of any missed doses.

What drug does:
Blocks action of vitamin K necessary for blood clotting.

Time lapse before drug works:
36 to 48 hours.

Don't take with:
See Interaction column and consult doctor.

 OVERDOSE

Symptoms:
Bloody vomit and bloody or black stools, red urine.

What to do:
- Dial 0 (operator) or 911 (emergency) for an ambulance or medical help. Then give first aid immediately.
- Additional emergency information on page 886.

 POSSIBLE ADVERSE REACTIONS OR SIDE EFFECTS

SYMPTOMS	FREQUENCY	WHAT TO DO
Brain & nervous system:		
Dizziness, headache.	Rare	3
Skin:		
Rash, hives, itch.	Infrequent	3
Eyes:		
Blurred vision.	Infrequent	3
Ears, nose, throat:		
• Sore throat.	Infrequent	3
• Mouth sores.	Rare	3
Digestive:		
• Black stools or bloody vomit.	Infrequent	2
• Diarrhea, cramps, nausea, vomiting.	Infrequent	4
• Bloating, gas.	Common	5
Heart & lungs:		
Coughing up blood.	Infrequent	2
Blood vessels:		
Easy bruising, bleeding.	Infrequent	3
Muscles, bones, joints:		
Swollen feet, legs.	Infrequent	4
Genital, urinary:		
Cloudy or red urine.	Infrequent	3
Kidneys:		
Back pain.	Infrequent	3
Liver:		
Jaundice (yellow skin and eyes).	Infrequent	3
Allergic, blood:	None expected.	
Others:		
• Fever, chills.	Infrequent	3
• Hair loss.	Infrequent	4
• Fatigue, weakness.	Infrequent	3

1-Life-threatening. Seek emergency treatment immediately.
2-Discontinue. Seek emergency treatment.
3-Discontinue. Call doctor right away.
4-Continue. Call doctor when convenient.
5-Continue. Tell doctor at next visit.

WARNINGS & PRECAUTIONS

Don't take if:
- You have been allergic to any oral anticoagulant.
- You have a bleeding disorder.
- You have an active peptic ulcer.
- You have ulcerative colitis.

Before you start, consult your doctor:
- If you take any other drugs, including non-prescription drugs.
- If you have high blood pressure.
- If you have heavy or prolonged menstrual periods.
- If you have diabetes.
- If you have a bladder catheter.
- If you have serious liver or kidney disease.
- If you will have surgery within 2 months, including dental surgery, requiring general or spinal anesthesia.

Over age 60:
Adverse reactions and side effects may be more frequent and severe than in younger persons.

Pregnancy:
Risk to unborn child outweighs drug benefits. Don't use.

Breast-feeding:
Drug filters into milk. May harm child. Avoid.

Infants & children:
Use only under doctor's supervision.

Prolonged use:
No problems expected.

Skin & sunlight:
No problems expected.

Driving, piloting or hazardous work:
- Avoid hazardous activities that could cause injury.
- Don't drive if you feel dizzy or have blurred vision.

Airplane passengers:
No problems expected.

Discontinuing:
Don't discontinue without consulting doctor. Dose may require gradual reduction if you have taken drug for a long time. Doses of other drugs may also require adjustment.

Others:
Carry identification to state you take anticoagulants.

INTERACTION WITH OTHER DRUGS

GENERIC NAME OR DRUG CLASS	COMBINED EFFECT
Acetaminophen	Increased phenprocoumon effect.
Allopurinol	Increased phenprocoumon effect.
Androgens	Increased phenprocoumon effect.
Antacids (large doses)	Decreased phenprocoumon effect.
Antibiotics	Increased phenprocoumon effect.
Anticonvulsants (hydantoin)	Increased effect of both drugs.
Antidepressants (tricyclic)	Increased phenprocoumon effect.
Antidiabetics (oral)	Increased phenprocoumon effect.
Antihistamines	Unpredictable increased or decreased anticoagulant effect.
Barbiturates	Decreased phenprocoumon effect.

Additional interactions on page 840.

INTERACTION WITH OTHER SUBSTANCES

INTERACTS WITH	COMBINED EFFECT
Alcohol:	Can increase or decrease effect of anticoagulant. Use with caution.
Beverages:	None expected.
Cocaine:	None expected.
Foods: High in vitamin K such as fish, liver, spinach, cabbage.	May decrease anticoagulant effect.
Marijuana:	None expected.
Tobacco:	None expected.

PHENSUXIMIDE

BRAND NAMES

Milontin

GENERAL INFORMATION

Habit forming? No
Prescription needed? Yes
Available as generic? No
Drug class: Anticonvulsant (succinimide)

USES

Controls seizures in treatment of epilepsy.

DOSAGE & USAGE INFORMATION

How to take:
Capsule or syrup—Swallow with liquid or food to lessen stomach irritation.

When to take:
Every day in regularly-spaced doses, according to prescription.

If you forget a dose:
Take as soon as you remember up to 2 hours late. If more than 2 hours, wait for next scheduled dose (don't double this dose).

What drug does:
Depresses nerve transmissions in part of brain that controls muscles.

Time lapse before drug works:
3 hours.

Don't take with:
See Interaction column and consult doctor.

OVERDOSE

Symptoms:
Coma

What to do:
- Dial 0 (operator) or 911 (emergency) for an ambulance or medical help. Then give first aid immediately.
- If patient is unconscious and not breathing, give mouth-to-mouth breathing. If there is no heartbeat, use cardiac massage and mouth-to-mouth breathing (CPR). Don't try to make patient vomit. If you can't get help quickly, take patient to nearest emergency facility.
- Additional emergency information on page 886.

POSSIBLE ADVERSE REACTIONS OR SIDE EFFECTS

SYMPTOMS	FREQUENCY	WHAT TO DO
Brain & nervous system: Dizziness, drowsiness, headache, irritability, mood changes.	Infrequent	4
Skin: Rash	Rare	3
Eyes:	None expected.	
Ears, nose, throat: Sore throat, fever.	Rare	3
Digestive: Nausea, vomiting, stomach cramps, appetite loss.	Common	4
Heart & lungs:	None expected.	
Blood vessels:	None expected.	
Muscles, bones, joints:	None expected.	
Genital, urinary:	None expected.	
Kidneys:	None expected.	
Liver:	None expected.	
Allergic:	None expected.	
Blood: Unusual bleeding or bruising.	Rare	3
Others: Swollen lymph glands.	Rare	4

1-Life-threatening. Seek emergency treatment immediately.
2-Discontinue. Seek emergency treatment.
3-Discontinue. Call doctor right away.
4-Continue. Call doctor when convenient.
5-Continue. Tell doctor at next visit.
6-No action necessary.

WARNINGS & PRECAUTIONS

Don't take if:
You are allergic to any succinimide anticonvulsant.

Before you start, consult your doctor:
- If you plan to become pregnant within medication period.
- If you take other anticonvulsants.
- If you have blood disease.
- If you have kidney or liver disease.

Over age 60:
Adverse reactions and side effects may be more frequent and severe than in younger persons.

Pregnancy:
Risk to unborn child outweighs drug benefits. Don't use.

Breast-feeding:
Drug passes into milk. Avoid drug or discontinue nursing.

Infants & children:
Use only under medical supervision.

Prolonged use:
No problems expected.

Skin & sunlight:
No problems expected.

Driving, piloting or hazardous work:
Don't drive or pilot aircraft until you learn how medicine affects you. Don't work around dangerous machinery. Don't climb ladders or work in high places. Danger increases if you drink alcohol or take medicine affecting alertness and reflexes, such as antihistamines, tranquilizers, sedatives, pain medicine, narcotics and mind-altering drugs.

Airplane passengers:
No problems expected.

Discontinuing:
Don't discontinue without doctor's advice until you complete prescribed dose, even though symptoms diminish or disappear.

Others:
- Your response to medicine should be checked regularly by your doctor. Dose and schedule may have to be altered frequently to fit individual needs.
- Periodic blood-cell counts, kidney- and liver-function studies recommended.

 INTERACTION WITH OTHER DRUGS

GENERIC NAME OR DRUG CLASS	COMBINED EFFECT
Anticonvulsants (other)	Increased effect of both drugs.
Antidepressants (tricyclic)	May provoke seizures.
Antipsychotics	May provoke seizures.

 INTERACTION WITH OTHER SUBSTANCES

INTERACTS WITH	COMBINED EFFECT
Alcohol:	May provoke seizures.
Beverages:	None expected.
Cocaine:	May provoke seizures.
Foods:	None expected.
Marijuana:	May provoke seizures.
Tobacco:	None expected.

PHENTERMINE

BRAND NAMES

Adipex-D	Obephen	Parmine
Fastin	Obermine	Phentrol
Ionamin	Obestrin-30	Wilpowr

GENERAL INFORMATION

Habit forming? Yes
Prescription needed? Yes
Available as generic? Yes
Drug class: Appetite suppressant

USES

Suppresses appetite.

DOSAGE & USAGE INFORMATION

How to take:
- Tablet or capsule—Swallow with liquid. You may chew or crush tablet.
- Extended-release tablets or capsules—Swallow each dose whole with liquid.

When to take:
- Long-acting forms—10 to 14 hours before bedtime.
- Short-acting forms—1 hour before meals. Last dose no later than 4 to 6 hours before bedtime.

If you forget a dose:
- Long-acting form—Take as soon as you remember up to 2 hours late. If more than 2 hours, wait for next scheduled dose (don't double this dose).
- Short-acting form—Wait for next scheduled dose. Don't double this dose.

What drug does:
Apparently stimulates brain's appetite-control center.

Time lapse before drug works:
Begins in 1 hour. Short-acting form lasts 4 hours. Long-acting form lasts 14 hours.

Don't take with:
- Non-prescription drugs without consulting doctor.
- See Interaction column and consult doctor.

OVERDOSE

Symptoms:
Irritability, overactivity, trembling, insomnia, mood changes, rapid heartbeat, confusion, disorientation, hallucinations, convulsions, coma.

What to do:
- Dial 0 (operator) or 911 (emergency) for an ambulance or medical help. Then give first aid immediately.
- Additional emergency information on page 886.

POSSIBLE ADVERSE REACTIONS OR SIDE EFFECTS

SYMPTOMS	FREQUENCY	WHAT TO DO
Brain & nervous system:		
• Irritability, nervousness, insomnia.	Common	4
• Mood changes.	Rare	3
Skin:		
• Hair loss.	Rare	4
• Rash or hives.	Rare	3
Eyes:		
Blurred vision.	Infrequent	4
Ears, nose, throat:		
Unpleasant taste or dry mouth.	Infrequent	4
Digestive:		
Constipation or diarrhea, nausea, vomiting, cramps.	Infrequent	4
Heart & lungs:		
• Irregular or pounding heartbeat.	Infrequent	3
• Breathing difficulty.	Rare	3
Blood vessels, muscles, bones, joints, kidneys, liver, allergic, blood:	None expected.	
Genital, urinary:		
Urinary urgency and difficulty.	Infrequent	3
Others:		
• False sense of well-being.	Common	4
• Changes in sex drive.	Infrequent	4
• Sweat increase.	Infrequent	4

1-Life-threatening. Seek emergency treatment immediately.
2-Discontinue. Seek emergency treatment.
3-Discontinue. Call doctor right away.
4-Continue. Call doctor when convenient.

WARNINGS & PRECAUTIONS

Don't take if:
- You are allergic to any sympathomimetic or phenylpropanolamine.
- You have glaucoma.
- You have taken MAO inhibitors within 2 weeks.
- You plan to become pregnant within medication period.
- You have a history of drug abuse.

Before you start, consult your doctor:
- If you have high blood pressure or heart disease.
- If you have an overactive thyroid, nervous tension or "anxiety."
- If you have epilepsy.

Over age 60:
Adverse reactions and side effects may be more frequent and severe than in younger persons.

Pregnancy:
Safety not established. Avoid.

Breast-feeding:
No proven problems. Consult doctor.

Infants & children:
Don't give to children younger than 12.

Prolonged use:
Loses effectiveness. Avoid.

Skin & sunlight:
No problems expected.

Driving, piloting or hazardous work:
Don't drive or pilot aircraft until you learn how medicine affects you. Don't work around dangerous machinery. Don't climb ladders or work in high places. Danger increases if you drink alcohol or take medicine affecting alertness and reflexes, such as antihistamines, tranquilizers, sedatives, pain medicine, narcotics and mind-altering drugs.

Airplane passengers:
No problems expected.

Discontinuing:
Don't discontinue without consulting doctor. Dose may require gradual reduction if you have taken drug for a long time. Doses of other drugs may also require adjustment.

Others:
Don't increase dose.

INTERACTION WITH OTHER DRUGS

GENERIC NAME OR DRUG CLASS	COMBINED EFFECT
Appetite suppressants (other)	Dangerous overstimulation.
Caffeine	Increased stimulant effect of phentermine.
Guanethidine	Decreased guanethidine effect.
Hydralazine	Decreased hydralazine effect.
MAO inhibitors	Dangerous blood-pressure rise.
Methyldopa	Decreased methyldopa effect.
Phenothiazines	Decreased phentermine effect.
Rauwolfia alkaloids	Decreased effect of rauwolfia alkaloids.

INTERACTION WITH OTHER SUBSTANCES

INTERACTS WITH	COMBINED EFFECT
Alcohol: Beer, chianti wines, vermouth.	Dangerous blood pressure rise.
Beverages: • Caffeine drinks • Drinks containing tyramine (see page 851).	Excessive stimulation. Blood-pressure rise.
Cocaine:	Excessive stimulation.
Foods: Foods containing tyramine (see page 851).	Blood-pressure rise.
Marijuana:	Frequent use—Irregular heartbeat.
Tobacco:	None expected.

PHENYLBUTAZONE

BRAND NAMES

Butagesic   Sterazolidin
Phenbutazone
See complete brand names list, page 828.

 USES

- Treatment for joint pain, stiffness, inflammation and swelling of arthritis and gout.
- Pain reliever.
- Treatment for dysmenorrhea (painful or difficult menstruation).

DOSAGE & USAGE INFORMATION

How to take:
Tablet or capsule—Swallow with liquid or food to lessen stomach irritation. If you can't swallow whole, crumble tablet or open capsule and take with liquid or food.

When to take:
At the same times each day.

If you forget a dose:
Take as soon as you remember up to 2 hours late. If more than 2 hours, wait for next scheduled dose (don't double this dose).

What drug does:
Reduces tissue concentration of prostaglandins (hormones which produce inflammation and pain).

Time lapse before drug works:
Begins in 4 to 24 hours. May require 3 weeks regular use for maximum benefit.

Don't take with:
See Interaction column and consult doctor.

 OVERDOSE

Symptoms:
Confusion, agitation, incoherence, convulsions, possible hemorrhage from stomach or intestine, coma.

What to do:
- Dial 0 (operator) or 911 (emergency) for an ambulance or medical help. Then give first aid immediately.
- Additional emergency information on page 886.

GENERAL INFORMATION

Habit forming? No
Prescription needed? Yes
Available as generic? Yes
Drug class: Antiinflammatory (non-steroid)

 POSSIBLE ADVERSE REACTIONS OR SIDE EFFECTS

SYMPTOMS	FREQUENCY	WHAT TO DO
Brain & nervous system:		
• Depression, drowsiness.	Infrequent	4
• Convulsions, confusion.	Rare	3
• Dizziness	Common	4
• Headache	Common	5
Skin:		
Rash, hives or itch.	Rare	3
Eyes:		
Blurred vision.	Rare	3
Ears, nose, throat:		
• Ringing in ears.	Infrequent	4
• Sore throat, fever, mouth ulcers.	Rare	3
Digestive:		
• Black stools, vomiting blood.	Rare	3
• Stomach upset.	Common	4
• Constipation or diarrhea, vomiting.	Infrequent	4
Heart & lungs:		
Breathing difficulty, tightness in chest.	Rare	3
Blood vessels:		
Unusual bleeding or bruising.	Rare	3
Muscles, bones, joints:		
Swollen feet, legs.	Infrequent	4
Genital, urinary:		
• Bloody urine.	Rare	3
• Difficult, painful or frequent urination.	Rare	4
Kidneys, allergic, blood, liver:	None expected.	
Others:		
• Fatigue, weakness.	Rare	4
• Weight gain.	Rare	4

1- Life-threatening. Seek emergency treatment immediately.
2- Discontinue. Seek emergency treatment.
3- Discontinue. Call doctor right away.
4- Continue. Call doctor when convenient.
5- Continue. Tell doctor at next visit.

WARNINGS & PRECAUTIONS

Don't take if:
- You are allergic to aspirin or any non-steroid, antiinflammatory drug.
- You have gastritis, peptic ulcer, enteritis, ileitis, ulcerative colitis.
- Patient is younger than 15.

Before you start, consult your doctor:
- If you have epilepsy.
- If you have Parkinson's disease.
- If you have been mentally ill.
- If you have had kidney disease or impaired kidney function, asthma, high blood pressure, heart failure, temporal arthritis, or polymyalgia rheumatica.

Over age 60:
Adverse reactions and side effects may be more frequent and severe than in younger persons.

Pregnancy:
Studies inconclusive on harm to unborn child. Animal studies show fetal abnormalities. Decide with your doctor whether drug benefits justify risk to unborn child.

Breast-feeding:
Drug filters into milk. May harm child. Avoid.

Infants & children:
Not recommended for those younger than 15. Use only under medical supervision.

Prolonged use:
- Eye damage.
- May cause rare bone-marrow damage, jaundice (yellow skin and eyes), reduced hearing.
- Periodic blood counts recommended if you use a long time.

Skin & sunlight:
No problems expected.

Driving, piloting or hazardous work:
Don't drive or pilot aircraft until you learn how medicine affects you. Don't work around dangerous machinery. Don't climb ladders or work in high places. Danger increases if you drink alcohol or take medicine affecting alertness and reflexes, such as antihistamines, tranquilizers, sedatives, pain medicine, narcotics and mind-altering drugs.

Airplane passengers:
No problems expected.

Discontinuing:
Don't discontinue without consulting doctor. Dose may require gradual reduction if you have taken drug for a long time. Doses of other drugs may also require adjustment.

 ## INTERACTION WITH OTHER DRUGS

GENERIC NAME OR DRUG CLASS	COMBINED EFFECT
Anticoagulants (oral)	Increased anticoagulant effect.
Aspirin	Possible stomach ulcer.
Antidiabetics (oral)	Increased antidiabetic effect.
Chloroquine	Possible skin toxicity.
Digitoxin	Decreased digitoxin effect.
Gold compounds	Increased toxicity to skin and bone marrow.
Hydroxychloroquine	Possible skin toxicity.
Methotrexate	Increased toxicity of both drugs to bone marrow.
Penicillamine	Possible toxicity.
Phenytoin	Possible toxic phenytoin effect.
Trimethoprim	Possible bone-marrow toxicity.

 ## INTERACTION WITH OTHER SUBSTANCES

INTERACTS WITH	COMBINED EFFECT
Alcohol:	Possible stomach ulcer or bleeding.
Beverages:	None expected.
Cocaine:	None expected.
Foods:	None expected.
Marijuana:	Increased pain relief from phenylbutazone.
Tobacco:	None expected.

PHENYLEPHRINE

BRAND NAMES

4-Way Tablets (M)
4-Way Nasal Spray (M)
Chlor-Trimeton (M)
Contac (M)
Coricidin Mist
Co-Tylenol (M)

Duo-Medihaler (M)
Isophrin
Neo-Synephrine
Super Anahist

See complete brand names list, page 828.

GENERAL INFORMATION

Habit forming? No
Prescription needed? No
Available as generic? Yes
Drug class: Sympathomimetic

 ## USES

Temporary relief of congestion of nose, sinuses and throat caused by allergies, colds or sinusitis.

 ## DOSAGE & USAGE INFORMATION

How to take:
- Syrup, tablet or capsule—Swallow with liquid or food to lessen stomach irritation.
- Extended-release tablets or capsules—Swallow each dose whole.
- Nasal solution, nasal spray, nasal jelly—Take as directed on package.

When to take:
As needed, no more often than every 4 hours.

If you forget a dose:
Take when you remember. Wait 4 hours for next dose. Never double a dose.

What drug does:
Contracts blood-vessel walls of nose, sinus and throat tissues, enlarging airways.

Time lapse before drug works:
5 to 30 minutes.

Don't take with:
- Non-prescription drugs for asthma, cough, cold, allergy, appetite suppressants, sleeping pills or drugs containing caffeine without consulting doctor.
- See Interaction column and consult doctor.

 ## OVERDOSE

Symptoms:
Headache, heart palpitations, vomiting, blood-pressure rise, slow and forceful pulse.

What to do:
- Dial 0 (operator) or 911 (emergency) for an ambulance or medical help. Then give first aid immediately.
- Additional emergency information on page 886.

POSSIBLE ADVERSE REACTIONS OR SIDE EFFECTS

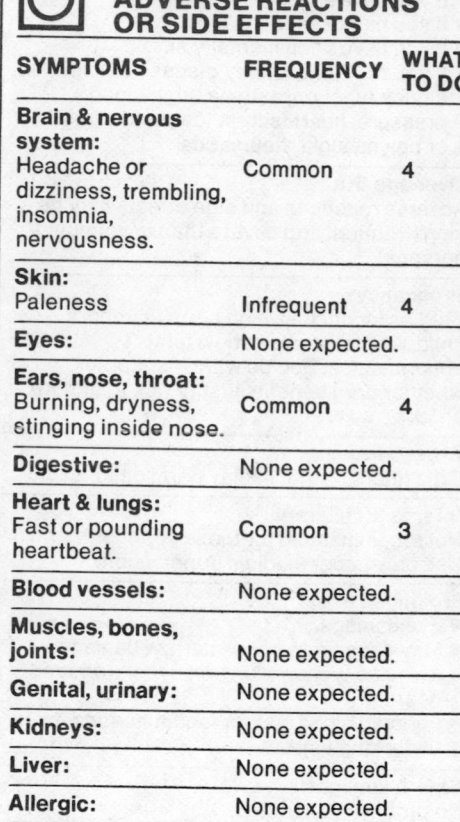

SYMPTOMS	FREQUENCY	WHAT TO DO
Brain & nervous system: Headache or dizziness, trembling, insomnia, nervousness.	Common	4
Skin: Paleness	Infrequent	4
Eyes: None expected.		
Ears, nose, throat: Burning, dryness, stinging inside nose.	Common	4
Digestive: None expected.		
Heart & lungs: Fast or pounding heartbeat.	Common	3
Blood vessels: None expected.		
Muscles, bones, joints: None expected.		
Genital, urinary: None expected.		
Kidneys: None expected.		
Liver: None expected.		
Allergic: None expected.		
Blood: None expected.		
Others: Unusual sweating.	Rare	3

1- Life-threatening. Seek emergency treatment immediately.
2- Discontinue. Seek emergency treatment.
3- Discontinue. Call doctor right away.
4- Continue. Call doctor when convenient.
5- Continue. Tell doctor at next visit.
6- No action necessary.

WARNINGS & PRECAUTIONS

Don't take if:
You are allergic to any sympathomimetic.

Before you start, consult your doctor:
- If you have high blood pressure.
- If you have heart disease.
- If you have diabetes.
- If you have overactive thyroid.
- If you have taken MAO inhibitors in past 2 weeks.

Over age 60:
Adverse reactions and side effects may be more frequent and severe than in younger persons.

Pregnancy:
Risk to unborn child outweighs drug benefits. Don't use.

Breast-feeding:
Drug passes into milk. Avoid drug or discontinue nursing until you finish medicine. Consult doctor for advice on maintaining milk supply.

Infants & children:
Use only under close supervision.

Prolonged use:
- "Rebound" congestion (see page 851) and chemical irritation of nasal membranes.
- May cause functional dependence.

Skin & sunlight:
No problems expected.

Driving, piloting or hazardous work:
No problems expected.

Airplane passengers:
No problems expected.

Discontinuing:
May be unnecessary to finish medicine. Follow doctor's instructions.

Others:
No problems expected.

INTERACTION WITH OTHER DRUGS

GENERIC NAME OR DRUG CLASS	COMBINED EFFECT
Amphetamines	Increased nervousness.
Antiasthmatics	Nervous stimulation.
Antihypertensives	Decreased antihypertensive effect.
MAO inhibitors	Dangerous blood-pressure rise.
Sedatives	Decreased sedative effect.
Tranquilizers	Decreased tranquilizer effect.

INTERACTION WITH OTHER SUBSTANCES

INTERACTS WITH	COMBINED EFFECT
Alcohol:	None expected.
Beverages: Caffeine drinks	Excess brain stimulation.
Cocaine:	Excess brain stimulation.
Foods:	None expected.
Marijuana:	None expected.
Tobacco:	None expected.

PHENYLPROPANOLAMINE

BRAND NAMES

Allerest (M)	Dimetapp (M)	Sinubid (M)
Caldecon (M)	4-Way Nasal	Sinutab (M)
Coffee-Break	Spray (M)	Triaminicin (M)
Contac (M)	Naldecon (M)	Triaminicol (M)
Control (M)	Sinarest	Tussagesic (M)
Dietac	Sine-Off (M)	

See complete brand names list, page 829.

GENERAL INFORMATION

Habit forming? No
Prescription needed? Low strength: No
High strength: Yes
Available as generic? Yes
Drug class: Sympathomimetic

USES

- Relieves bronchial asthma.
- Decreases congestion of breathing passages.
- Suppresses allergic reactions.
- Decreases appetite.

DOSAGE & USAGE INFORMATION

How to take:
- Tablet or capsule—Swallow with liquid. You may chew or crush tablet.
- Extended-release tablets or capsules—Swallow each dose whole.
- Syrup—Take as directed on bottle.

When to take:
As needed, no more often than every 4 hours.

If you forget a dose:
Take up to 2 hours late. If more than 2 hours, wait for next dose (don't double this dose).

What drug does:
- Prevents cells from releasing allergy-causing chemicals (histamines).
- Relaxes muscles of bronchial tubes.
- Decreases blood-vessel size and blood flow, thus causing decongestion.

Time lapse before drug works:
30 to 60 minutes.

Don't take with:
- Non-prescription drugs for cough, cold, allergy or asthma without consulting doctor.
- See Interaction column and consult doctor.

OVERDOSE

Symptoms:
Severe anxiety, confusion, delirium, muscle tremors, rapid and irregular pulse.

What to do:
- Dial 0 (operator) or 911 (emergency) for an ambulance or medical help. Then give first aid immediately.
- Additional emergency information on page 886.

POSSIBLE ADVERSE REACTIONS OR SIDE EFFECTS

SYMPTOMS	FREQUENCY	WHAT TO DO
Brain & nervous system:		
• Nervousness, headache.	Common	4
• Dizziness	Infrequent	4
Skin: Paleness	Common	4
Eyes:	None expected.	
Ears, nose, throat:	None expected.	
Digestive: Appetite loss, nausea, vomiting.	Infrequent	4
Heart & lungs:		
• Irregular heartbeat.	Infrequent	3
• Rapid heartbeat.	Common	3
• Tightness in chest.	Rare	3
Blood vessels:	None expected.	
Muscles, bones, joints:	None expected.	
Genital, urinary: Difficult urination.	Infrequent	4
Kidneys:	None expected.	
Liver:	None expected.	
Allergic:	None expected.	
Blood:	None expected.	
Others: Insomnia	Common	5

1- Life-threatening. Seek emergency treatment immediately.
2- Discontinue. Seek emergency treatment.
3- Discontinue. Call doctor right away.
4- Continue. Call doctor when convenient.
5- Continue. Tell doctor at next visit.
6- No action necessary.

PHENYLPROPANOLAMINE

 WARNINGS & PRECAUTIONS

Don't take if:
You are allergic to any sympathomimetic drug.

Before you start, consult your doctor:
- If you have high blood pressure.
- If you have diabetes.
- If you have overactive thyroid gland.
- If you have difficulty urinating.
- If you have taken any MAO inhibitors in past 2 weeks.
- If you have taken digitalis preparations in the last 7 days.
- If you will have surgery within 2 months, including dental surgery, requiring general or spinal anesthesia.

Over age 60:
More likely to develop high blood pressure, heart-rhythm disturbances, angina and to feel drug's stimulant effects.

Pregnancy:
No proven harm to unborn child. Avoid if possible.

Breast-feeding:
Drug passes into milk. Avoid drug or discontinue nursing until you finish medicine. Consult doctor for advice on maintaining milk supply.

Infants & children:
No special problems expected.

Prolonged use:
- Excessive doses—Rare toxic psychosis.
- Men with enlarged prostate gland may have more urination difficulty.

Skin & sunlight:
No known problems.

Driving, piloting or hazardous work:
No restrictions unless you feel dizzy.

Airplane passengers:
No problems expected.

Discontinuing:
May be unnecessary to finish medicine. Follow doctor's instructions.

Others:
No problems expected.

 INTERACTION WITH OTHER DRUGS

GENERIC NAME OR DRUG CLASS	COMBINED EFFECT
Anesthetics (general)	Increased phenylpropanolamine effect.
Antidepressants (tricyclic)	Increased effect of phenylpropanolamine. Excessive stimulation of heart and blood pressure.
Antihypertensives	Decreased antihypertensive effect.
Digitalis preparations	Serious heart-rhythm disturbances.
Epinephrine	Increased epinephrine effect.
Ergot preparations	Serious blood-pressure rise.
Guanethidine	Decreased effect of both drugs.
MAO inhibitors	Increased phenylpropanolamine effect. Dangerous blood-pressure rise.

 INTERACTION WITH OTHER SUBSTANCES

INTERACTS WITH	COMBINED EFFECT
Alcohol:	None expected.
Beverages: Caffeine drinks	Nervousness or insomnia.
Cocaine:	Rapid heartbeat. Avoid.
Foods:	None expected.
Marijuana:	Rapid heartbeat, possible heart-rhythm disturbance. Avoid.
Tobacco:	None expected.

PHENYLTOLOXAMINE

BRAND NAMES

Amaril D (M) Sinubid (M)
Naldecol (M) Sinutab (M)
Naldecon (M) Tussionex (M)
Percogesic (M)

GENERAL INFORMATION

Habit forming? No
Prescription needed? No
Available as generic? No
Drug class: Antihistamine

 USES

Relieves symptoms of hay fever, allergic reactions and infections of nose and throat.

 DOSAGE & USAGE INFORMATION

How to take:
- Extended-release tablets or capsules—Swallow each dose whole with liquid.
- Syrup—Take as directed on label.
- Pediatric drops—Dilute dose in beverage before swallowing.

When to take:
As needed, no more often than every 3 hours.

If you forget a dose:
Take as soon as you remember. Wait 3 hours for next dose (don't double this dose).

What drug does:
Blocks histamine action in sensitized tissues.

Time lapse before drug works:
30 minutes.

Don't take with:
- Non-prescription drugs containing alcohol without consulting doctor.
- See Interaction column and consult doctor.

 OVERDOSE

Symptoms:
- Adults—Drowsiness, confusion, incoordination, unsteadiness, muscle tremors, stupor, coma.
- Children—Excitement, hallucinations, overactivity, convulsions.

What to do:
- Dial 0 (operator) or 911 (emergency) for an ambulance or medical help. Then give first aid immediately.
- Additional emergency information on page 886.

POSSIBLE ADVERSE REACTIONS OR SIDE EFFECTS

SYMPTOMS	FREQUENCY	WHAT TO DO
Brain & nervous system:		
• Nightmares agitation, irritability, (especially children).	Rare	3
• Drowsiness	Common	5
• Confusion	Infrequent	4
Skin:	None expected.	
Eyes:		
Vision changes.	Rare	3
Ears, nose, throat:		
• Sore throat, fever.	Rare	3
• Dry mouth, nose, throat, ringing or buzzing in ears.	Infrequent	4
Digestive:		
• Appetite loss.	Infrequent	4
• Stomach upset or pain.	Infrequent	3
Heart & lungs:		
• Thick bronchial secretions.	Common	5
• Rapid heartbeat.	Infrequent	3
Blood vessels:		
Unusual bleeding or bruising.	Rare	3
Muscles, bones, joints, kidneys, liver, allergic, blood:	None expected.	
Genital, urinary:		
Difficult or painful urination.	Infrequent	4
Others:		
• Unusual sweating.	Rare	4
• Fatigue, weakness.	Rare	3

1- Life-threatening. Seek emergency treatment immediately.
2- Discontinue. Seek emergency treatment.
3- Discontinue. Call doctor right away.
4- Continue. Call doctor when convenient.
5- Continue. Tell doctor at next visit.

WARNINGS & PRECAUTIONS

Don't take if:
- You are allergic to any antihistamine.
- You have asthma attacks.
- You have glaucoma.
- You have urination difficulty.

Before you start, consult your doctor:
- If you have reacted badly to any antihistamine.
- If you have had peptic ulcer disease.
- If you will have surgery within 2 months, including dental surgery, requiring general or spinal anesthesia.

Over age 60:
Likely to be drowsy, dizzy or lethargic and have impaired thinking, judgment and memory. Increases urination problems from enlarged prostate gland.

Pregnancy:
No proven problems. Consult doctor.

Breast-feeding:
Drug passes into milk. Avoid drug or discontinue nursing until you finish medicine. Consult doctor for advice on maintaining milk supply.

Infants & children:
Use only under medical supervision.

Prolonged use:
No problems expected.

Skin & sunlight:
May cause rash or intensify sunburn in areas exposed to sun or sunlamp.

Driving, piloting or hazardous work:
Don't drive or pilot aircraft until you learn how medicine affects you. Don't work around dangerous machinery. Don't climb ladders or work in high places. Danger increases if you drink alcohol or take medicine affecting alertness and reflexes.

Airplane passengers:
Take 30 to 60 minutes before departure.

Discontinuing:
May be unnecessary to finish medicine. Follow doctor's instructions.

Others:
No problems expected.

INTERACTION WITH OTHER DRUGS

GENERIC NAME OR DRUG CLASS	COMBINED EFFECT
Amphetamines	Decreased effect of phenyltoloxamine, especially drowsiness.
Anticholinergics	Increased anticholinergic effect.
Anticonvulsants (hydantoin)	Changed pattern of epileptic seizures.
Antidepressants	Increased antidepressant effect.
Narcotics	Increased sedation.
Pain relievers	Increased sedation.
Sedatives	Increased sedation.
Sleep inducers	Increased sedation.
Tranquilizers	Increased sedation.

INTERACTION WITH OTHER SUBSTANCES

INTERACTS WITH	COMBINED EFFECT
Alcohol:	Rapid, excessive sedation. Use caution.
Beverages:	None expected.
Cocaine:	Decreased phenyltoloxamine effect.
Foods:	None expected.
Marijuana:	Excessive sedation.
Tobacco:	None expected.

PHENYTOIN

BRAND NAMES

Dantoin   Diphenylan
Dilantin   Diphenylhydantoin
Di-Phen

GENERAL INFORMATION

Habit forming? No
Prescription needed? Yes
Available as generic? Yes
Drug class: Anticonvulsant (hydantoin)

 ## USES

- Prevents epileptic seizures.
- Stabilizes irregular heartbeat.

 ## DOSAGE & USAGE INFORMATION

How to take:
- Tablet or capsule—Swallow with liquid.
- Extended-release tablets or capsules—Swallow each dose whole. If you take regular tablets, you may chew or crush them.

When to take:
At the same time each day.

If you forget a dose:
- If drug taken 1 time per day—Take as soon as you remember up to 12 hours late. If more than 12 hours, wait for next scheduled dose (don't double this dose).
- If taken several times per day—Take as soon as possible, then return to regular schedule.

What drug does:
Promotes sodium loss from nerve fibers. This lessens excitability and inhibits spread of nerve impulses.

Time lapse before drug works:
7 to 10 days continual use.

Don't take with:
See Interaction column and consult doctor.

 ## OVERDOSE

Symptoms:
Jerky eye movements; stagger; slurred speech; imbalance; drowsiness; blood-pressure drop; slow, shallow breathing; coma.

What to do:
- Dial 0 (operator) or 911 (emergency) for an ambulance or medical help. Then give first aid immediately.
- Additional emergency information on page 886.

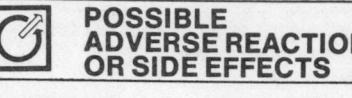 ## POSSIBLE ADVERSE REACTIONS OR SIDE EFFECTS

SYMPTOMS	FREQUENCY	WHAT TO DO
Brain & nervous system:		
• Mild dizziness, drowsiness.	Common	4
• Headache, sleeplessness.	Infrequent	4
• Hallucinations, confusion, slurred speech, stagger.	Infrequent	3
Skin:		
Rash	Infrequent	3
Eyes:		
Vision changes.	Infrequent	3
Ears, nose, throat:		
Sore throat, fever.	Rare	3
Digestive:		
• Stomach pain.	Rare	3
• Constipation, nausea, vomiting.	Common	4
• Diarrhea	Infrequent	4
Heart & lungs, genital, urinary, kidneys, allergic blood:	None expected.	
Blood vessels:		
Unusual bleeding or bruising.	Rare	3
Muscles, bones, joints:		
Muscle twitching.	Infrequent	4
Liver:		
Jaundice (yellow skin and eyes).	Rare	3
Others:		
Increased body and facial hair.	Infrequent	5

1- Life-threatening. Seek emergency treatment immediately.
2- Discontinue. Seek emergency treatment.
3- Discontinue. Call doctor right away.
4- Continue. Call doctor when convenient.
5- Continue. Tell doctor at next visit.

WARNINGS & PRECAUTIONS

Don't take if:
You are allergic to any hydantoin anticonvulsant.

Before you start, consult your doctor:
- If you have had impaired liver function or disease.
- If you will have surgery within 2 months, including dental surgery, requiring general or spinal anesthesia.

Over age 60:
Adverse reactions and side effects may be more frequent and severe than in younger persons.

Pregnancy:
Risk to unborn child outweighs drug benefits. Don't use.

Breast-feeding:
Drug passes into milk. Avoid drug or discontinue nursing until you finish medicine. Consult doctor for advice on maintaining milk supply.

Infants & children:
Use only under medical supervision.

Prolonged use:
- Weakened bones.
- Lymph gland enlargement.
- Possible liver damage.
- Numbness and tingling of hands and feet.
- Continual back-and-forth eye movements.
- Bleeding, swollen or tender gums.

Skin & sunlight:
May cause rash or intensify sunburn in areas exposed to sun or sunlamp.

Driving, piloting or hazardous work:
Don't drive or pilot aircraft until you learn how medicine affects you. Don't work around dangerous machinery. Don't climb ladders or work in high places. Danger increases if you drink alcohol or take medicine affecting alertness and reflexes.

Airplane passengers:
No problems expected.

Discontinuing:
Don't discontinue without consulting doctor. Dose may require gradual reduction if you have taken drug for a long time. Doses of other drugs may also require adjustment.

INTERACTION WITH OTHER DRUGS

GENERIC NAME OR DRUG CLASS	COMBINED EFFECT
Anticoagulants	Increased effect of both drugs.
Antidepressants (tricyclic)	Need to adjust phenytoin dose.
Antihypertensives	Increased effect of antihypertensive.
Aspirin	Increased phenytoin effect.
Barbiturates	Changed seizure pattern.
Carbonic anhydrase inhibitors	Increased chance of bone disease.
Chloramphenicol	Increased phenytoin effect.
Contraceptives (oral)	Increased seizures.
Cortisone drugs	Decreased cortisone effect.
Digitalis preparations	Decreased digitalis effect.
Disulfiram	Increased phenytoin effect.
Estrogens	Increased phenytoin effect.
Furosemide	Decreased furosemide effect.
Glutethimide	Decreased phenytoin effect.

See additional Interactions, page 842.

INTERACTION WITH OTHER SUBSTANCES

INTERACTS WITH	COMBINED EFFECT
Alcohol:	Possible decreased anticonvulsant effect. Use with caution.
Beverages:	None expected.
Cocaine:	Possible seizures.
Foods:	None expected.
Marijuana:	Drowsiness, unsteadiness, decreased anticonvulsant effect.
Tobacco:	None expected.

PILOCARPINE

BRAND NAMES

Adsorbocarpine	Ocusert Pilo-40
Almocarpine	Pilocar
Isopto Carpine	Pilocel
Miocarpine	Pilomiotin
Nova-Carpine	P.V. Carpine
Ocusert Pilo-20	

GENERAL INFORMATION

Habit forming? No
Prescription needed? U.S.: Yes; Canada: No
Available as generic? Yes
Drug class: Antiglaucoma

 ## USES

Treatment for glaucoma.

 ## DOSAGE & USAGE INFORMATION

How to take:
- Drops—Apply to eyes. Close eyes for 1 or 2 minutes to absorb medicine.
- Eye system—Follow label directions.

When to take:
As directed on label.

If you forget a dose:
Apply as soon as possible and return to prescribed schedule. Don't double dose.

What drug does:
Reduces internal eye pressure.

Time lapse before drug works:
15 to 30 minutes.

Don't take with:
See Interaction column and consult doctor.

 ## OVERDOSE

Symptoms:
If swallowed—Nausea, vomiting, diarrhea, forceful urination, profuse sweating, rapid pulse, breathing difficulty, loss of consciousness.

What to do:
- Dial O (operator) or 911 (emergency) for an ambulance or medical help. Then give first aid immediately.
- If patient is unconscious and not breathing, give mouth-to-mouth breathing. If there is no heartbeat, use cardiac massage and mouth-to-mouth breathing (CPR). Don't try to make patient vomit. If you can't get help quickly, take patient to nearest emergency facility.
- Additional emergency information on page 886.

POSSIBLE ADVERSE REACTIONS OR SIDE EFFECTS

SYMPTOMS	FREQUENCY	WHAT TO DO
Brain & nervous system:		
Headache	Infrequent	3
Skin:		
Profuse sweating.	Infrequent	4
Eyes:		
• Pain, blurred or altered vision.	Common	4
• Eye irritation or twitching.	Infrequent	3
Ears, nose, throat:		
Unusual saliva flow.	Infrequent	4
Digestive:		
Nausea, vomiting, diarrhea.	Infrequent	3
Heart & lungs:		
Breathing difficulty.	Infrequent	3
Blood vessels:	None expected.	
Muscles, bones, joints:		
Muscle tremors.	Infrequent	3
Genital, urinary:	None expected.	
Kidneys:	None expected.	
Liver:	None expected.	
Allergic:	None expected.	
Blood:	None expected.	
Others:	None expected.	

1- Life-threatening. Seek emergency treatment immediately.
2- Discontinue. Seek emergency treatment.
3- Discontinue. Call doctor right away.
4- Continue. Call doctor when convenient.
5- Continue. Tell doctor at next visit.
6- No action necessary.

WARNINGS & PRECAUTIONS

Don't take if:
You are allergic to pilocarpine.

Before you start, consult your doctor:
- If you take sedatives, sleeping pills, tranquilizers, antidepressants, antihistamines, narcotics or mind-altering drugs.
- If you have asthma.
- If you have conjunctivitis (pink eye).

Over age 60:
Adverse reactions and side effects may be more frequent and severe than in younger persons.

Pregnancy:
No proven harm to unborn child. Avoid if possible.

Breast-feeding:
No proven problems. Consult doctor.

Infants & children:
Not recommended.

Prolonged use:
You may develop tolerance for drug, making it ineffective.

Skin & sunlight:
No problems expected.

Driving, piloting or hazardous work:
Don't drive or pilot aircraft until you learn how medicine affects you. Don't work around dangerous machinery. Don't climb ladders or work in high places. Danger increases if you drink alcohol or take medicine affecting alertness and reflexes, such as antihistamines, tranquilizers, sedatives, pain medicine, narcotics and mind-altering drugs.

Airplane passengers:
No problems expected.

Discontinuing:
Doctor may discontinue and substitute another drug to keep treatment effective.

Others:
- Can provoke asthma attack in susceptible individuals.
- Drops may impair vision for 2 to 3 hours.

INTERACTION WITH OTHER DRUGS

GENERIC NAME OR DRUG CLASS	COMBINED EFFECT
Amphetamines	Decreased pilocarpine effect.
Anticholinergics	Decreased pilocarpine effect.
Appetite suppressants	Decreased pilocarpine effect.
Cortisone drugs	Decreased pilocarpine effect.
Phenothiazines	Decreased pilocarpine effect.

INTERACTION WITH OTHER SUBSTANCES

INTERACTS WITH	COMBINED EFFECT
Alcohol:	May prolong alcohol's effect on brain.
Beverages:	None expected.
Cocaine:	Decreased pilocarpine effect. Avoid.
Foods:	None expected.
Marijuana:	Used once or twice weekly—May help lower internal eye pressure.
Tobacco:	None expected.

PIPERACETAZINE

BRAND NAMES

Quide

GENERAL INFORMATION

Habit forming? No
Prescription needed? Yes
Available as generic? Yes
Drug class: Tranquilizer, antiemetic (phenothiazine)

USES

- Stops nausea, vomiting.
- Reduces anxiety, agitation.

DOSAGE & USAGE INFORMATION

How to take:
- Tablet or capsule—Swallow with liquid or food to lessen stomach irritation.
- Suppositories—Remove wrapper and moisten suppository with water. Gently insert into rectum, large end first.
- Drops or liquid—Dilute dose in beverage.

When to take:
- Nervous and mental disorders—Take at the same times each day.
- Nausea and vomiting—Take as needed, no more often than every 4 hours.

If you forget a dose:
- Nervous and mental disorders—Take up to 2 hours late. If more than 2 hours, wait for next scheduled dose (don't double this).
- Nausea and vomiting—Take as soon as you remember. Wait 4 hours for next dose.

What drug does:
- Suppresses brain's vomiting center.
- Suppresses brain centers that control abnormal emotions and behavior.

Time lapse before drug works:
- Nausea and vomiting—1 hour or less.
- Nervous and mental disorders—4-6 weeks.

Don't take with:
- Antacid or medicine for diarrhea.
- Non-prescription drug for cough, cold or allergy.
- See Interaction column and consult doctor.

OVERDOSE

Symptoms:
Stupor, convulsions, coma.

What to do:
- Dial O (operator) or 911 (emergency) for an ambulance or medical help. Then give first aid immediately.
- Additional emergency information on page 886.

POSSIBLE ADVERSE REACTIONS OR SIDE EFFECTS

SYMPTOMS	FREQUENCY	WHAT TO DO
Brain & nervous system:		
• Restlessness, tremor.	Common	3
• Fainting	Infrequent	2
• Drowsiness	Common	3
Skin:		
• Rash	Infrequent	3
• Less perspiration.	Common	4
Eyes:		
Vision changes.	Rare	3
Ears, nose, throat:		
• Sore throat, fever.	Rare	3
• Dry mouth, nasal congestion.	Common	4
Digestive:		
Constipation	Common	4
Heart & lungs, blood vessels, kidneys, allergic, blood:	None expected.	
Muscles, bones, joints:		
Muscle spasms of face and neck, unsteady gait.	Common	2
Genital, urinary:		
Urination difficulty.	Infrequent	4
Liver:		
Jaundice (yellow eyes and skin).	Rare	3
Others:		
Less interest in sex, breast swelling, change in menstrual pattern.	Infrequent	4

1-Life-threatening. Seek emergency treatment immediately.
2-Discontinue. Seek emergency treatment.
3-Discontinue. Call doctor right away.
4-Continue. Call doctor when convenient.
5-Continue. Tell doctor at next visit.
6-No action necessary.

WARNINGS & PRECAUTIONS

Don't take if:
- You are allergic to any phenothiazine.
- You have a blood or bone-marrow disease.

Before you start, consult your doctor:
- If you will have surgery within 2 months, including dental surgery, requiring general or spinal anesthesia.
- If you have asthma, emphysema or other lung disorder.
- If you take non-prescription ulcer medicine, asthma medicine or amphetamines.

Over age 60:
Adverse reactions and side effects may be more frequent and severe than in younger persons. More likely to develop involuntary movement of jaws, lips, tongue, chewing. Report this to your doctor immediately. Early treatment can help.

Pregnancy:
Risk to unborn child outweighs drug benefits. Don't use.

Breast-feeding:
Drug passes into milk. Avoid drug or discontinue nursing until you finish medicine. Consult doctor for advice on maintaining milk supply.

Infants & children:
Don't give to children younger than 2.

Prolonged use:
May lead to tardive dyskinesia (involuntary movement of jaws, lips, tongue, chewing).

Skin & sunlight:
May cause rash or intensify sunburn in areas exposed to sun or sunlamp. Skin may remain sensitive for 3 months after discontinuing.

Driving, piloting or hazardous work:
Don't drive or pilot aircraft until you learn how medicine affects you. Don't work around dangerous machinery. Don't climb ladders or work in high places. Danger increases if you drink alcohol or take medicine affecting alertness and reflexes.

Airplane passengers:
No problems expected.

Discontinuing:
- Nervous and mental disorders—Don't discontinue without doctor's advice until you complete prescribed dose, even though symptoms diminish or disappear.
- Nausea and vomiting—May be unnecessary to finish medicine. Follow doctor's instructions.

INTERACTION WITH OTHER DRUGS

GENERIC NAME OR DRUG CLASS	COMBINED EFFECT
Anticholinergics	Increased anticholinergic effect.
Antidepressants (tricyclic)	Increased piperacetazine effect.
Antihistamines	Increased antihistamine effect.
Appetite suppressants	Decreased suppressant effect.
Levodopa	Decreased levodopa effect.
Mind-altering drugs	Increased effect of mind-altering drugs.
Narcotics	Increased narcotic effect.
Phenytoin	Increased phenytoin effect.
Quinidine	Impaired heart function. Dangerous mixture.
Sedatives	Increased sedative effect.
Tranquilizers (other)	Increased tranquilizer effect.

INTERACTION WITH OTHER SUBSTANCES

INTERACTS WITH	COMBINED EFFECT
Alcohol:	Dangerous oversedation.
Beverages:	None expected.
Cocaine:	Decreased piperacetazine effect. Avoid.
Foods:	None expected.
Marijuana:	Drowsiness. May increase antinausea effect.
Tobacco:	None expected.

POLOXAMER 188

BRAND NAMES

Alaxin

GENERAL INFORMATION

Habit forming? No
Prescription needed? No
Available as generic? Yes
Drug class: Laxative (emollient)

 ## USES

Constipation relief.

 ## DOSAGE & USAGE INFORMATION

How to take:
- Tablet or capsule—Swallow with liquid. Don't open capsules.
- Drops—Dilute dose in beverage before swallowing.
- Syrup—Take as directed on bottle.

When to take:
At the same time each day, preferably bedtime.

If you forget a dose:
Take as soon as you remember. Wait 12 hours for next dose. Return to regular schedule.

What drug does:
Makes stool hold fluid so it is easier to pass.

Time lapse before drug works:
2 to 3 days of continual use.

Don't take with:
- Other medicines at same time. Wait 2 hours.
- See Interaction column and consult doctor.

 ## OVERDOSE

Symptoms:
Appetite loss, nausea, vomiting, diarrhea.

What to do:
Overdose unlikely to threaten life. If person takes much larger amount than prescribed, call doctor, poison-control center or hospital emergency room for instructions.

 ## POSSIBLE ADVERSE REACTIONS OR SIDE EFFECTS

SYMPTOMS	FREQUENCY	WHAT TO DO
Brain & nervous system:	None expected.	
Skin: Rash	Rare	3
Eyes:	None expected.	
Ears, nose, throat: Throat irritation (liquid only).	Infrequent	4
Digestive: Intestinal and stomach cramps.	Infrequent	4
Heart & lungs:	None expected.	
Blood vessels:	None expected.	
Muscles, bones, joints:	None expected.	
Genital, urinary:	None expected.	
Kidneys:	None expected.	
Liver:	None expected.	
Allergic:	None expected.	
Blood:	None expected.	
Others:	None expected.	

1 - Life-threatening. Seek emergency treatment immediately.
2 - Discontinue. Seek emergency treatment.
3 - Discontinue. Call doctor right away.
4 - Continue. Call doctor when convenient.
5 - Continue. Tell doctor at next visit.
6 - No action necessary.

POLOXAMER 188

WARNINGS & PRECAUTIONS

Don't take if:
● You are allergic to any emollient laxative.
● You have abdominal pain and fever that might be appendicitis.

Before you start, consult your doctor:
● If you are taking other laxatives.
● To be sure constipation isn't a sign of a serious disorder.

Over age 60:
You must drink 6 to 8 glasses of fluid every 24 hours for drug to work.

Pregnancy:
No problems expected. Consult doctor.

Breast-feeding:
No problems expected.

Infants & children:
No problems expected.

Prolonged use:
Avoid. Overuse of laxatives may damage intestine lining.

Skin & sunlight:
No problems expected.

Driving, piloting or hazardous work:
No problems expected.

Airplane passengers:
No problems expected.

Discontinuing:
May be unnecessary to finish medicine. Follow doctor's instructions.

Others:
No problems expected.

INTERACTION WITH OTHER DRUGS

GENERIC NAME OR DRUG CLASS	COMBINED EFFECT
Danthron	Possible liver damage.
Digitalis preparations	Toxic absorption of digitalis.
Mineral oil	Increased mineral oil absorption into bloodstream. Avoid.
Phenolphthalein	Increased phenolphthalein absorption. Possible toxicity.

INTERACTION WITH OTHER SUBSTANCES

INTERACTS WITH	COMBINED EFFECT
Alcohol:	None expected.
Beverages:	None expected.
Cocaine:	None expected.
Foods:	None expected.
Marijuana:	None expected.
Tobacco:	None expected.

POLYCARBOPHIL CALCIUM

BRAND NAMES

Mitrolan

GENERAL INFORMATION

Habit forming? No
Prescription needed? No
Available as generic? No
Drug class: Laxative (bulk-forming), antidiarrheal

 ## USES

- Relieves constipation and prevents straining for bowel movement.
- Stops diarrhea.

 ## DOSAGE & USAGE INFORMATION

How to take:
- Tablets (laxative)—Swallow with 8 oz. cold liquid. Drink 6 to 8 glasses of water each day in addition to the one with each dose.
- Tablets (diarrhea)—Take without water at half-hour intervals.

When to take:
At the same times each day.

If you forget a dose:
Take as soon as you remember. Resume regular schedule.

What drug does:
Absorbs water, stimulating the bowel to form a soft, bulky stool and decreasing watery diarrhea.

Time lapse before drug works:
May require 2 or 3 days to begin, then works in 12 to 24 hours.

Don't take with:
- See Interaction column and consult doctor.
- Don't take within 2 hours of taking another medicine.

 ## OVERDOSE

Symptoms:
None expected.

What to do:
Overdose unlikely to threaten life. If person takes much larger amount than prescribed, call doctor, poison-control center or hospital emergency room for instructions.

 ## POSSIBLE ADVERSE REACTIONS OR SIDE EFFECTS

SYMPTOMS	FREQUENCY	WHAT TO DO
Brain & nervous system:	None expected.	
Skin: Itch, rash.	Rare	3
Eyes:	None expected.	
Ears, nose, throat: Swallowing difficulty, "lump in throat" sensation.	Infrequent	4
Digestive:		
• Intestinal blockage.	Rare	3
• Nausea, vomiting, diarrhea.	Infrequent	4
Heart & lungs: Asthma	Rare	3
Blood vessels:	None expected.	
Muscles, bones, joints:	None expected.	
Genital, urinary:	None expected.	
Kidneys:	None expected.	
Liver:	None expected.	
Allergic:	None expected.	
Blood:	None expected.	
Others:	None expected.	

1 - Life-threatening. Seek emergency treatment immediately.
2 - Discontinue. Seek emergency treatment.
3 - Discontinue. Call doctor right away.
4 - Continue. Call doctor when convenient.
5 - Continue. Tell doctor at next visit.
6 - No action necessary.

POLYCARBOPHIL CALCIUM

 WARNINGS & PRECAUTIONS

Don't take if:
- You are allergic to any bulk-forming laxative.
- You have symptoms of appendicitis, inflamed bowel or intestinal blockage.
- You have missed a bowel movement for only 1 or 2 days.

Before you start, consult your doctor:
- If you have diabetes.
- If you have a laxative habit.
- If you have rectal bleeding.
- If you have difficulty swallowing.
- If you take other laxatives.

Over age 60:
Adverse reactions and side effects may be more frequent and severe than in younger persons.

Pregnancy:
Most bulk-forming laxatives contain sodium or sugars which may cause fluid retention. Avoid if possible.

Breast-feeding:
No problems expected.

Infants & children:
Use only under medical supervision.

Prolonged use:
Don't take for more than 1 week unless under a doctor's supervision. May cause laxative dependence.

Skin & sunlight:
No problems expected.

Driving, piloting or hazardous work:
No problems expected.

Airplane passengers:
No problems expected.

Discontinuing:
May be unnecessary to finish medicine. Follow doctor's instructions.

Others:
Don't take to "flush out" your system or as a "tonic."

 INTERACTION WITH OTHER DRUGS

GENERIC NAME OR DRUG CLASS	COMBINED EFFECT
Antibiotics	Decreased antibiotic effect.
Anticoagulants	Decreased anticoagulant effect.
Digitalis preparations	Decreased digitalis effect.
Salicylates (including aspirin)	Decreased salicylate effect.

 INTERACTION WITH OTHER SUBSTANCES

INTERACTS WITH	COMBINED EFFECT
Alcohol:	None expected.
Beverages:	None expected.
Cocaine:	None expected.
Foods:	None expected.
Marijuana:	None expected.
Tobacco:	None expected.

POLYTHIAZIDE

BRAND NAMES

Renese

GENERAL INFORMATION

Habit forming? No
Prescription needed? Yes
Available as generic? Yes
Drug class: Antihypertensive,
diuretic (thiazide)

USES

- Controls, but doesn't cure, high blood pressure.
- Reduces fluid retention (edema) caused by conditions such as heart disorders and liver disease.

DOSAGE & USAGE INFORMATION

How to take:
Tablet or capsule—Swallow with 8 oz. of liquid. If you can't swallow whole, crumble tablet or open capsule and take with liquid or food. Don't exceed dose.

When to take:
At the same time each day.

If you forget a dose:
Take as soon as you remember up to 2 hours late. If more than 2 hours, wait for next scheduled dose (don't double this dose).

What drug does:
- Forces sodium and water excretion, reducing body fluid.
- Relaxes muscle cells of small arteries.
- Reduced body fluid and relaxed arteries lower blood pressure.

Time lapse before drug works:
4 to 6 hours. May require several weeks to lower blood pressure.

Don't take with:
- See Interaction column and consult doctor.
- Non-prescription drugs without consulting doctor.

OVERDOSE

Symptoms:
Cramps, weakness, drowsiness, weak pulse, coma.

What to do:
- Dial 0 (operator) or 911 (emergency) for an ambulance or medical help. Then give first aid immediately.
- Additional emergency information on page 886.

POSSIBLE ADVERSE REACTIONS OR SIDE EFFECTS

SYMPTOMS	FREQUENCY	WHAT TO DO
Brain & nervous system:		
• Dizziness	Infrequent	4
• Mood changes.	Infrequent	4
• Headaches	Infrequent	4
Skin:		
Rash or hives.	Rare	2
Eyes:		
Blurred vision.	Infrequent	3
Ears, nose, throat:		
• Sore throat, fever.	Rare	3
• Dry mouth, thirst.	Infrequent	5
Digestive:		
Severe abdominal pain, nausea, vomiting.	Infrequent	3
Heart & lungs:		
Irregular heartbeat, weak pulse.	Infrequent	3
Blood vessels:	None expected.	
Muscles, bones, joints:		
Weakness, tiredness.	Infrequent	4
Genital, urinary:	None expected.	
Kidneys:	None expected.	
Liver:		
Jaundice (yellow skin and eyes).	Rare	3
Allergic:	None expected.	
Blood:	None expected.	
Others:		
Weight changes.	Infrequent	4

1- Life-threatening. Seek emergency treatment immediately.
2- Discontinue. Seek emergency treatment.
3- Discontinue. Call doctor right away.
4- Continue. Call doctor when convenient.
5- Continue. Tell doctor at next visit.
6- No action necessary.

POLYTHIAZIDE

WARNINGS & PRECAUTIONS

Don't take if:
You are allergic to any thiazide diuretic drug.

Before you start, consult your doctor:
- If you are allergic to any sulfa drug.
- If you have gout.
- If you have liver, pancreas or kidney disorder.

Over age 60:
Adverse reactions and side effects may be more frequent and severe than in younger persons, especially dizziness and excessive potassium loss.

Pregnancy:
Risk to unborn child outweighs drug benefits. Don't use.

Breast-feeding:
Drug passes into milk. Avoid drug or discontinue nursing.

Infants & children:
No problems expected.

Prolonged use:
You may need medicine to treat high blood pressure for the rest of your life.

Skin & sunlight:
May cause rash or intensify sunburn in areas exposed to sun or sunlamp.

Driving, piloting or hazardous work:
Don't drive or pilot aircraft until you learn how medicine affects you. Don't work around dangerous machinery. Don't climb ladders or work in high places. Danger increases if you drink alcohol or take medicine affecting alertness and reflexes, such as antihistamines, tranquilizers, sedatives, pain medicine, narcotics and mind-altering drugs.

Airplane passengers:
No problems expected.

Discontinuing:
Don't discontinue without medical advice.

Others:
- Hot weather and fever may cause dehydration and drop in blood pressure. Dose may require temporary adjustment. Weigh daily and report any unexpected weight decreases to your doctor.
- May cause rise in uric acid, leading to gout.
- May cause blood-sugar rise in diabetics.

INTERACTION WITH OTHER DRUGS

GENERIC NAME OR DRUG CLASS	COMBINED EFFECT
Allopurinol	Decreased allopurinol effect.
Antidepressants (tricyclic)	Dangerous drop in blood pressure. Avoid combination unless under medical supervision.
Barbiturates	Increased polythiazide effect.
Cholestyramine	Decreased polythiazide effect.
Cortisone drugs	Excessive potassium loss that causes dangerous heart rhythms.
Digitalis preparations	Excessive potassium loss that causes dangerous heart rhythms.
Diuretics (thiazide)	Increased effect of other thiazide diuretics.
Lithium	Increased effect of lithium.
MAO inhibitors	Increased polythiazide effect.
Probenecid	Decreased probenecid effect.

INTERACTION WITH OTHER SUBSTANCES

INTERACTS WITH	COMBINED EFFECT
Alcohol:	Dangerous blood-pressure drop.
Beverages:	None expected.
Cocaine:	None expected.
Foods: Licorice	Excessive potassium loss that causes dangerous heart rhythms.
Marijuana:	May increase blood pressure.
Tobacco:	None expected.

POTASSIUM ACETATE, POTASSIUM BICARBONATE & POTASSIUM CITRATE

BRAND NAMES

Potassium Triplex
Tri-K
Trikates

GENERAL INFORMATION

Habit forming? No
Prescription needed? Yes
Available as generic? Yes
Drug class: Mineral supplement (potassium)

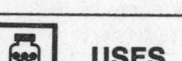 ## USES

Treatment for potassium deficiency from illness, diuretics, cortisone drugs or digitalis preparations.

 ## DOSAGE & USAGE INFORMATION

How to take:
- Tablet or capsule—Swallow with liquid or food to lessen stomach irritation. You may chew or crush tablet.
- Extended-release tablets or capsules—Swallow each dose whole with liquid.
- Effervescent tablets, granules, powder or liquid—Dilute dose in water.

When to take:
At the same times each day, preferably with food or immediately after meals.

If you forget a dose:
Take as soon as you remember. Don't double next dose.

What drug does:
Preserves or restores normal function of nerve cells, heart and skeletal-muscle cells, kidneys and stomach-juice secretion.

Time lapse before drug works:
12 to 24 hours.

Don't take with:
See Interaction column and consult doctor.

 ## OVERDOSE

Symptoms:
Paralysis of arms and legs, irregular heartbeat, blood-pressure drop, convulsions, coma, cardiac arrest.

What to do:
- Dial 0 (operator) or 911 (emergency) for an ambulance or medical help. Then give first aid immediately.
- Additional emergency information on page 886.

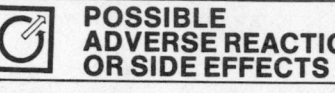 ## POSSIBLE ADVERSE REACTIONS OR SIDE EFFECTS

SYMPTOMS	FREQUENCY	WHAT TO DO
Brain & nervous system:		
● Numbness and tingling in hands and feet.	Rare	4
● Confusion	Rare	3
Skin:	None expected.	
Eyes:	None expected.	
Ears, nose, throat:	None expected.	
Digestive: Diarrhea, nausea, vomiting, stomach discomfort.	Infrequent	4
Heart & lungs: Irregular heartbeat, breathing difficulty.	Rare	3
Blood vessels:	None expected.	
Muscles, bones, joints: Unusual fatigue, weakness, heaviness of legs.	Rare	3
Genital, urinary:	None expected.	
Kidneys:	None expected.	
Liver:	None expected.	
Allergic:	None expected.	
Blood:	None expected.	
Others:	None expected.	

1- Life-threatening. Seek emergency treatment immediately.
2- Discontinue. Seek emergency treatment.
3- Discontinue. Call doctor right away.
4- Continue. Call doctor when convenient.
5- Continue. Tell doctor at next visit.
6- No action necessary.

POTASSIUM ACETATE, POTASSIUM BICARBONATE & POTASSIUM CITRATE

WARNINGS & PRECAUTIONS

Don't take if:
- You are allergic to any potassium supplement.
- You have kidney disease.

Before you start, consult your doctor:
- If you have Addison's disease.
- If you have heart disease.
- If you have intestinal blockage.
- If you have a stomach ulcer.
- If you use diuretics.
- If you use heart medicine.
- If you use laxatives or have chronic diarrhea.
- If you use salt substitutes or low-salt milk.

Over age 60:
Observe dose schedule strictly. Potassium balance is critical. Deviation above or below normal can have serious results.

Pregnancy:
No problems expected if you adhere strictly to prescribed dose.

Breast-feeding:
Studies inconclusive on harm to infant. Consult doctor.

Infants & children:
Use only under doctor's supervision.

Prolonged use:
Slows absorption of vitamin B-12. May cause anemia.

Skin & sunlight:
No problems expected.

Driving, piloting or hazardous work:
No problems expected.

Airplane passengers:
No problems expected.

Discontinuing:
Don't discontinue without consulting doctor. Dose may require gradual reduction if you have taken drug for a long time. Doses of other drugs may also require adjustment.

Others:
Overdose or underdose serious. Frequent laboratory blood studies recommended.

INTERACTION WITH OTHER DRUGS

GENERIC NAME OR DRUG CLASS	COMBINED EFFECT
Digitalis preparations	Possible irregular heartbeat.
Diuretics (thiazide)	Decreased potassium effect.
Spironolactone	Dangerous rise in blood potassium.
Triamterene	Dangerous rise in blood potassium.

INTERACTION WITH OTHER SUBSTANCES

INTERACTS WITH	COMBINED EFFECT
Alcohol:	None expected.
Beverages: Salty drinks such as tomato juice, commercial thirst quenchers.	Increased fluid retention.
Cocaine:	May cause irregular heartbeat.
Foods: Salty foods.	Increased fluid retention.
Marijuana:	May cause irregular heartbeat.
Tobacco:	None expected.

POTASSIUM BICARBONATE & CITRIC ACID

BRAND NAMES

K-Lyte

GENERAL INFORMATION

Habit forming? No
Prescription needed? Yes
Available as generic? Yes
Drug class: Mineral supplement (potassium)

USES

Treatment for potassium deficiency from illness, diuretics, cortisone drugs or digitalis preparations.

DOSAGE & USAGE INFORMATION

How to take:
- Tablet or capsule—Swallow with liquid or food to lessen stomach irritation. You may chew or crush tablet.
- Extended-release tablets or capsules— Swallow each dose whole with liquid.
- Effervescent tablets, granules, powder or liquid—Dilute dose in water.

When to take:
At the same times each day, preferably with food or immediately after meals.

If you forget a dose:
Take as soon as you remember. Don't double next dose.

What drug does:
Preserves or restores normal function of nerve cells, heart and skeletal-muscle cells, kidneys and stomach-juice secretion.

Time lapse before drug works:
12 to 24 hours.

Don't take with:
See Interaction column and consult doctor.

OVERDOSE

Symptoms:
Paralysis of arms and legs, irregular heartbeat, blood-pressure drop, convulsions, coma, cardiac arrest.

What to do:
- Dial 0 (operator) or 911 (emergency) for an ambulance or medical help. Then give first aid immediately.
- Additional emergency information on page 886.

POSSIBLE ADVERSE REACTIONS OR SIDE EFFECTS

SYMPTOMS	FREQUENCY	WHAT TO DO
Brain & nervous system:		
• Numbness and tingling in hands and feet.	Rare	4
• Confusion.	Rare	3
Skin:	None expected.	
Eyes:	None expected.	
Ears, nose, throat:	None expected.	
Digestive: Diarrhea, nausea, vomiting, stomach discomfort.	Infrequent	4
Heart & lungs: Irregular heartbeat, breathing difficulty.	Rare	3
Blood vessels:	None expected.	
Muscles, bones, joints: Unusual fatigue, weakness, heaviness of legs.	Rare	3
Genital, urinary:	None expected.	
Kidneys:	None expected.	
Liver:	None expected.	
Allergic:	None expected.	
Blood:	None expected.	
Others:	None expected.	

1- Life-threatening. Seek emergency treatment immediately.
2- Discontinue. Seek emergency treatment.
3- Discontinue. Call doctor right away.
4- Continue. Call doctor when convenient.
5- Continue. Tell doctor at next visit.
6- No action necessary.

POTASSIUM BICARBONATE & CITRIC ACID

WARNINGS & PRECAUTIONS

Don't take if:
- You are allergic to any potassium supplement.
- You have kidney disease.

Before you start, consult your doctor:
- If you have Addison's disease.
- If you have heart disease.
- If you have intestinal blockage.
- If you have a stomach ulcer.
- If you use diuretics.
- If you use heart medicine.
- If you use laxatives or have chronic diarrhea.
- If you use salt substitutes or low-salt milk.

Over age 60:
Observe dose schedule strictly. Potassium balance is critical. Deviation above or below normal can have serious results.

Pregnancy:
No problems expected if you adhere strictly to prescribed dose.

Breast-feeding:
Studies inconclusive on harm to infant. Consult doctor.

Infants & children:
Use only under doctor's supervision.

Prolonged use:
Slows absorption of vitamin B-12. May cause anemia.

Skin & sunlight:
No problems expected.

Driving, piloting or hazardous work:
No problems expected.

Airplane passengers:
No problems expected.

Discontinuing:
Don't discontinue without consulting doctor. Dose may require gradual reduction if you have taken drug for a long time. Doses of other drugs may also require adjustment.

Others:
Overdose or underdose serious. Frequent laboratory blood studies recommended.

INTERACTION WITH OTHER DRUGS

GENERIC NAME OR DRUG CLASS	COMBINED EFFECT
Digitalis preparations	Possible irregular heartbeat.
Diuretics (thiazide)	Decreased potassium effect.
Spironolactone	Dangerous rise in blood potassium.
Triamterene	Dangerous rise in blood potassium.

INTERACTION WITH OTHER SUBSTANCES

INTERACTS WITH	COMBINED EFFECT
Alcohol:	None expected.
Beverages: Salty drinks such as tomato juice, commercial thirst quenchers.	Increased fluid retention.
Cocaine:	May cause irregular heartbeat.
Foods: Salty foods.	Increased fluid retention.
Marijuana:	May cause irregular heartbeat.
Tobacco:	None expected.

POTASSIUM BICARBONATE, POTASSIUM CARBONATE & POTASSIUM CHLORIDE

BRAND NAMES

KEFF

GENERAL INFORMATION

Habit forming? No
Prescription needed? Yes
Available as generic? Yes
Drug class: Mineral supplement (potassium)

USES

Treatment for potassium deficiency from illness, diuretics, cortisone drugs or digitalis preparations.

DOSAGE & USAGE INFORMATION

How to take:
- Tablet or capsule—Swallow with liquid or food to lessen stomach irritation. You may chew or crush tablet.
- Extended-release tablets or capsules—Swallow each dose whole with liquid.
- Effervescent tablets, granules, powder or liquid—Dilute dose in water.

When to take:
At the same times each day, preferably with food or immediately after meals.

If you forget a dose:
Take as soon as you remember. Don't double next dose.

What drug does:
Preserves or restores normal function of nerve cells, heart and skeletal-muscle cells, kidneys and stomach-juice secretion.

Time lapse before drug works:
12 to 24 hours.

Don't take with:
See Interaction column and consult doctor.

OVERDOSE

Symptoms:
Paralysis of arms and legs, irregular heartbeat, blood-pressure drop, convulsions, coma, cardiac arrest.

What to do:
- Dial 0 (operator) or 911 (emergency) for an ambulance or medical help. Then give first aid immediately.
- Additional emergency information on page 886.

POSSIBLE ADVERSE REACTIONS OR SIDE EFFECTS

SYMPTOMS	FREQUENCY	WHAT TO DO
Brain & nervous system:		
• Numbness and tingling in hands and feet.	Rare	4
• Confusion	Rare	3
Skin:	None expected.	
Eyes:	None expected.	
Ears, nose, throat:	None expected.	
Digestive: Diarrhea, nausea, vomiting, stomach discomfort.	Infrequent	4
Heart & lungs: Irregular heartbeat, breathing difficulty.	Rare	3
Blood vessels:	None expected.	
Muscles, bones, joints: Unusual fatigue, weakness, heaviness of legs.	Rare	3
Genital, urinary:	None expected.	
Kidneys:	None expected.	
Liver:	None expected.	
Allergic:	None expected.	
Blood:	None expected.	
Others:	None expected.	

1- Life-threatening. Seek emergency treatment immediately.
2- Discontinue. Seek emergency treatment.
3- Discontinue. Call doctor right away.
4- Continue. Call doctor when convenient.
5- Continue. Tell doctor at next visit.
6- No action necessary.

POTASSIUM BICARBONATE, POTASSIUM CARBONATE & POTASSIUM CHLORIDE

WARNINGS & PRECAUTIONS

Don't take if:
- You are allergic to any potassium supplement.
- You have kidney disease.

Before you start, consult your doctor:
- If you have Addison's disease.
- If you have heart disease.
- If you have intestinal blockage.
- If you have a stomach ulcer.
- If you use diuretics.
- If you use heart medicine.
- If you use laxatives or have chronic diarrhea.
- If you use salt substitutes or low-salt milk.

Over age 60:
Observe dose schedule strictly. Potassium balance is critical. Deviation above or below normal can have serious results.

Pregnancy:
No problems expected if you adhere strictly to prescribed dose.

Breast-feeding:
Studies inconclusive on harm to infant. Consult doctor.

Infants & children:
Use only under doctor's supervision.

Prolonged use:
Slows absorption of vitamin B-12. May cause anemia.

Skin & sunlight:
No problems expected.

Driving, piloting or hazardous work:
No problems expected.

Airplane passengers:
No problems expected.

Discontinuing:
Don't discontinue without consulting doctor. Dose may require gradual reduction if you have taken drug for a long time. Doses of other drugs may also require adjustment.

Others:
Overdose or underdose serious. Frequent laboratory blood studies recommended.

INTERACTION WITH OTHER DRUGS

GENERIC NAME OR DRUG CLASS	COMBINED EFFECT
Digitalis preparations	Possible irregular heartbeat.
Diuretics (thiazide)	Decreased potassium effect.
Spironolactone	Dangerous rise in blood potassium.
Triamterene	Dangerous rise in blood potassium.

INTERACTION WITH OTHER SUBSTANCES

INTERACTS WITH	COMBINED EFFECT
Alcohol:	None expected.
Beverages: Salty drinks such as tomato juice, commercial thirst quenchers.	Increased fluid retention.
Cocaine:	May cause irregular heartbeat.
Foods: Salty foods.	Increased fluid retention.
Marijuana:	May cause irregular heartbeat.
Tobacco:	None expected.

POTASSIUM BICARBONATE & POTASSIUM CHLORIDE

BRAND NAMES

Klorvess

GENERAL INFORMATION

Habit forming? No
Prescription needed? Yes
Available as generic? Yes
Drug class: Mineral supplement (potassium)

 ## USES

Treatment for potassium deficiency from illness, diuretics, cortisone drugs or digitalis preparations.

 ## DOSAGE & USAGE INFORMATION

How to take:
- Tablet or capsule—Swallow with liquid or food to lessen stomach irritation. You may chew or crush tablet.
- Extended-release tablets or capsules— Swallow each dose whole with liquid.
- Effervescent tablets, granules, powder or liquid—Dilute dose in water.

When to take:
At the same times each day, preferably with food or immediately after meals.

If you forget a dose:
Take as soon as you remember. Don't double next dose.

What drug does:
Preserves or restores normal function of nerve cells, heart and skeletal-muscle cells, kidneys and stomach-juice secretion.

Time lapse before drug works:
12 to 24 hours.

Don't take with:
See Interaction column and consult doctor.

 ## OVERDOSE

Symptoms:
Paralysis of arms and legs, irregular heartbeat, blood-pressure drop, convulsions, coma, cardiac arrest.

What to do:
- Dial 0 (operator) or 911 (emergency) for an ambulance or medical help. Then give first aid immediately.
- Additional emergency information on page 886.

 ## POSSIBLE ADVERSE REACTIONS OR SIDE EFFECTS

SYMPTOMS	FREQUENCY	WHAT TO DO
Brain & nervous system:		
• Numbness and tingling in hands and feet.	Rare	4
• Confusion	Rare	3
Skin:	None expected.	
Eyes:	None expected.	
Ears, nose, throat:	None expected.	
Digestive: Diarrhea, nausea, vomiting, stomach discomfort.	Infrequent	4
Heart & lungs: Irregular heartbeat, breathing difficulty.	Rare	3
Blood vessels:	None expected.	
Muscles, bones, joints: Unusual fatigue, weakness, heaviness of legs.	Rare	3
Genital, urinary:	None expected.	
Kidneys:	None expected.	
Liver:	None expected.	
Allergic:	None expected.	
Blood:	None expected.	
Others:	None expected.	

1- Life-threatening. Seek emergency treatment immediately.
2- Discontinue. Seek emergency treatment.
3- Discontinue. Call doctor right away.
4- Continue. Call doctor when convenient.
5- Continue. Tell doctor at next visit.
6- No action necessary.

POTASSIUM BICARBONATE & POTASSIUM CHLORIDE

WARNINGS & PRECAUTIONS

Don't take if:
- You are allergic to any potassium supplement.
- You have kidney disease.

Before you start, consult your doctor:
- If you have Addison's disease.
- If you have heart disease.
- If you have intestinal blockage.
- If you have a stomach ulcer.
- If you use diuretics.
- If you use heart medicine.
- If you use laxatives or have chronic diarrhea.
- If you use salt substitutes or low-salt milk.

Over age 60:
Observe dose schedule strictly. Potassium balance is critical. Deviation above or below normal can have serious results.

Pregnancy:
No problems expected if you adhere strictly to prescribed dose.

Breast-feeding:
Studies inconclusive on harm to infant. Consult doctor.

Infants & children:
Use only under doctor's supervision.

Prolonged use:
Slows absorption of vitamin B-12. May cause anemia.

Skin & sunlight:
No problems expected.

Driving, piloting or hazardous work:
No problems expected.

Airplane passengers:
No problems expected.

Discontinuing:
Don't discontinue without consulting doctor. Dose may require gradual reduction if you have taken drug for a long time. Doses of other drugs may also require adjustment.

Others:
Overdose or underdose serious. Frequent laboratory blood studies recommended.

INTERACTION WITH OTHER DRUGS

GENERIC NAME OR DRUG CLASS	COMBINED EFFECT
Digitalis preparations	Possible irregular heartbeat.
Diuretics (thiazide)	Decreased potassium effect.
Spironolactone	Dangerous rise in blood potassium.
Triamterene	Dangerous rise in blood potassium.

INTERACTION WITH OTHER SUBSTANCES

INTERACTS WITH	COMBINED EFFECT
Alcohol:	None expected.
Beverages: Salty drinks such as tomato juice, commercial thirst quenchers.	Increased fluid retention.
Cocaine:	May cause irregular heartbeat.
Foods: Salty foods.	Increased fluid retention.
Marijuana:	May cause irregular heartbeat.
Tobacco:	None expected.

POTASSIUM BICARBONATE, POTASSIUM CHLORIDE & CITRIC ACID

BRAND NAMES

K-Lyte/Cl

GENERAL INFORMATION

Habit forming? No
Prescription needed? Yes
Available as generic? Yes
Drug class: Mineral supplement (potassium)

USES

Treatment for potassium deficiency from illness, diuretics, cortisone drugs or digitalis preparations.

DOSAGE & USAGE INFORMATION

How to take:
- Tablet or capsule—Swallow with liquid or food to lessen stomach irritation. You may chew or crush tablet.
- Extended-release tablets or capsules—Swallow each dose whole with liquid.
- Effervescent tablets, granules, powder or liquid—Dilute dose in water.

When to take:
At the same times each day, preferably with food or immediately after meals.

If you forget a dose:
Take as soon as you remember. Don't double next dose.

What drug does:
Preserves or restores normal function of nerve cells, heart and skeletal-muscle cells, kidneys and stomach-juice secretion.

Time lapse before drug works:
12 to 24 hours.

Don't take with:
See Interaction column and consult doctor.

OVERDOSE

Symptoms:
Paralysis of arms and legs, irregular heartbeat, blood-pressure drop, convulsions, coma, cardiac arrest.

What to do:
- Dial 0 (operator) or 911 (emergency) for an ambulance or medical help. Then give first aid immediately.
- Additional emergency information on page 886.

POSSIBLE ADVERSE REACTIONS OR SIDE EFFECTS

SYMPTOMS	FREQUENCY	WHAT TO DO
Brain & nervous system:		
● Numbness and tingling in hands and feet.	Rare	4
● Confusion	Rare	3
Skin:	None expected.	
Eyes:	None expected.	
Ears, nose, throat:	None expected.	
Digestive: Diarrhea, nausea, vomiting, stomach discomfort.	Infrequent	4
Heart & lungs: Irregular heartbeat, breathing difficulty.	Rare	3
Blood vessels:	None expected.	
Muscles, bones, joints: Unusual fatigue, weakness, heaviness of legs.	Rare	3
Genital, urinary:	None expected.	
Kidneys:	None expected.	
Liver:	None expected.	
Allergic:	None expected.	
Blood:	None expected.	
Others:	None expected.	

1- Life-threatening. Seek emergency treatment immediately.
2- Discontinue. Seek emergency treatment.
3- Discontinue. Call doctor right away.
4- Continue. Call doctor when convenient.
5- Continue. Tell doctor at next visit.
6- No action necessary.

POTASSIUM BICARBONATE, POTASSIUM CHLORIDE & CITRIC ACID

 ## WARNINGS & PRECAUTIONS

Don't take if:
- You are allergic to any potassium supplement.
- You have kidney disease.

Before you start, consult your doctor:
- If you have Addison's disease.
- If you have heart disease.
- If you have intestinal blockage.
- If you have a stomach ulcer.
- If you use diuretics.
- If you use heart medicine.
- If you use laxatives or have chronic diarrhea.
- If you use salt substitutes or low-salt milk.

Over age 60:
Observe dose schedule strictly. Potassium balance is critical. Deviation above or below normal can have serious results.

Pregnancy:
No problems expected if you adhere strictly to prescribed dose.

Breast-feeding:
Studies inconclusive on harm to infant. Consult doctor.

Infants & children:
Use only under doctor's supervision.

Prolonged use:
Slows absorption of vitamin B-12. May cause anemia.

Skin & sunlight:
No problems expected.

Driving, piloting or hazardous work:
No problems expected.

Airplane passengers:
No problems expected.

Discontinuing:
Don't discontinue without consulting doctor. Dose may require gradual reduction if you have taken drug for a long time. Doses of other drugs may also require adjustment.

Others:
Overdose or underdose serious. Frequent laboratory blood studies recommended.

 ## INTERACTION WITH OTHER DRUGS

GENERIC NAME OR DRUG CLASS	COMBINED EFFECT
Digitalis preparations	Possible irregular heartbeat.
Diuretics (thiazide)	Decreased potassium effect.
Spironolactone	Dangerous rise in blood potassium.
Triamterene	Dangerous rise in blood potassium.

 ## INTERACTION WITH OTHER SUBSTANCES

INTERACTS WITH	COMBINED EFFECT
Alcohol:	None expected.
Beverages: Salty drinks such as tomato juice, commercial thirst quenchers.	Increased fluid retention.
Cocaine:	May cause irregular heartbeat.
Foods: Salty foods.	Increased fluid retention.
Marijuana:	May cause irregular heartbeat.
Tobacco:	None expected.

POTASSIUM BICARBONATE, POTASSIUM CHLORIDE & POTASSIUM CITRATE

BRAND NAMES

Kaochlor-Eff

GENERAL INFORMATION

Habit forming? No
Prescription needed? Yes
Available as generic? Yes
Drug class: Mineral supplement (potassium)

USES

Treatment for potassium deficiency from illness, diuretics, cortisone drugs or digitalis preparations.

DOSAGE & USAGE INFORMATION

How to take:
- Tablet or capsule—Swallow with liquid or food to lessen stomach irritation. You may chew or crush tablet.
- Extended-release tablets or capsules—Swallow each dose whole with liquid.
- Effervescent tablets, granules, powder or liquid—Dilute dose in water.

When to take:
At the same times each day, preferably with food or immediately after meals.

If you forget a dose:
Take as soon as you remember. Don't double next dose.

What drug does:
Preserves or restores normal function of nerve cells, heart and skeletal-muscle cells, kidneys and stomach-juice secretion.

Time lapse before drug works:
12 to 24 hours.

Don't take with:
See Interaction column and consult doctor.

OVERDOSE

Symptoms:
Paralysis of arms and legs, irregular heartbeat, blood-pressure drop, convulsions, coma, cardiac arrest.

What to do:
- Dial 0 (operator) or 911 (emergency) for an ambulance or medical help. Then give first aid immediately.
- Additional emergency information on page 886.

POSSIBLE ADVERSE REACTIONS OR SIDE EFFECTS

SYMPTOMS	FREQUENCY	WHAT TO DO
Brain & nervous system:		
• Numbness and tingling in hands and feet.	Rare	4
• Confusion	Rare	3
Skin:	None expected.	
Eyes:	None expected.	
Ears, nose, throat:	None expected.	
Digestive: Diarrhea, nausea, vomiting, stomach discomfort.	Infrequent	4
Heart & lungs: Irregular heartbeat, breathing difficulty.	Rare	3
Blood vessels:	None expected.	
Muscles, bones, joints: Unusual fatigue, weakness, heaviness of legs.	Rare	3
Genital, urinary:	None expected.	
Kidneys:	None expected.	
Liver:	None expected.	
Allergic:	None expected.	
Blood:	None expected.	
Others:	None expected.	

1- Life-threatening. Seek emergency treatment immediately.
2- Discontinue. Seek emergency treatment.
3- Discontinue. Call doctor right away.
4- Continue. Call doctor when convenient.
5- Continue. Tell doctor at next visit.
6- No action necessary.

POTASSIUM BICARBONATE, POTASSIUM CHLORIDE & POTASSIUM CITRATE

 ## WARNINGS & PRECAUTIONS

Don't take if:
- You are allergic to any potassium supplement.
- You have kidney disease.

Before you start, consult your doctor:
- If you have Addison's disease.
- If you have heart disease.
- If you have intestinal blockage.
- If you have a stomach ulcer.
- If you use diuretics.
- If you use heart medicine.
- If you use laxatives or have chronic diarrhea.
- If you use salt substitutes or low-salt milk.

Over age 60:
Observe dose schedule strictly. Potassium balance is critical. Deviation above or below normal can have serious results.

Pregnancy:
No problems expected if you adhere strictly to prescribed dose.

Breast-feeding:
Studies inconclusive on harm to infant. Consult doctor.

Infants & children:
Use only under doctor's supervision.

Prolonged use:
Slows absorption of vitamin B-12. May cause anemia.

Skin & sunlight:
No problems expected.

Driving, piloting or hazardous work:
No problems expected.

Airplane passengers:
No problems expected.

Discontinuing:
Don't discontinue without consulting doctor. Dose may require gradual reduction if you have taken drug for a long time. Doses of other drugs may also require adjustment.

Others:
Overdose or underdose serious. Frequent laboratory blood studies recommended.

 ## INTERACTION WITH OTHER DRUGS

GENERIC NAME OR DRUG CLASS	COMBINED EFFECT
Digitalis preparations	Possible irregular heartbeat.
Diuretics (thiazide)	Decreased potassium effect.
Spironolactone	Dangerous rise in blood potassium.
Triamterene	Dangerous rise in blood potassium.

 ## INTERACTION WITH OTHER SUBSTANCES

INTERACTS WITH	COMBINED EFFECT
Alcohol:	None expected.
Beverages: Salty drinks such as tomato juice, commercial thirst quenchers.	Increased fluid retention.
Cocaine:	May cause irregular heartbeat.
Foods: Salty foods.	Increased fluid retention.
Marijuana:	May cause irregular heartbeat.
Tobacco:	None expected.

POTASSIUM CHLORIDE

BRAND NAMES

Kaochlor	KLOR-10%
Kaon-Cl	KLOR-CON
Kato	Klotrix
Kay-Ciel	Potassium chloride solution USP
K-Lor	Slow-K

GENERAL INFORMATION

Habit forming? No
Prescription needed? Yes
Available as generic? Yes
Drug class: Mineral supplement
(potassium)

 USES

Treatment for potassium deficiency from illness, diuretics, cortisone drugs or digitalis preparations.

 DOSAGE & USAGE INFORMATION

How to take:
- Tablet or capsule—Swallow with liquid or food to lessen stomach irritation. You may chew or crush tablet.
- Extended-release tablets or capsules— Swallow each dose whole with liquid.
- Effervescent tablets, granules, powder or liquid—Dilute dose in water.

When to take:
At the same times each day, preferably with food or immediately after meals.

If you forget a dose:
Take as soon as you remember. Don't double next dose.

What drug does:
Preserves or restores normal function of nerve cells, heart and skeletal-muscle cells, kidneys and stomach-juice secretion.

Time lapse before drug works:
12 to 24 hours.

Don't take with:
See Interaction column and consult doctor.

 OVERDOSE

Symptoms:
Paralysis of arms and legs, irregular heartbeat, blood-pressure drop, convulsions, coma, cardiac arrest.

What to do:
- Dial 0 (operator) or 911 (emergency) for an ambulance or medical help. Then give first aid immediately.
- Additional emergency information on page 886.

POSSIBLE ADVERSE REACTIONS OR SIDE EFFECTS

SYMPTOMS	FREQUENCY	WHAT TO DO
Brain & nervous system:		
• Numbness and tingling in hands and feet.	Rare	4
• Confusion	Rare	3
Skin:	None expected.	
Eyes:	None expected.	
Ears, nose, throat:	None expected.	
Digestive: Diarrhea, nausea, vomiting, stomach discomfort.	Infrequent	4
Heart & lungs: Irregular heartbeat, breathing difficulty.	Rare	3
Blood vessels:	None expected.	
Muscles, bones, joints: Unusual fatigue, weakness, heaviness of legs.	Rare	3
Genital, urinary:	None expected.	
Kidneys:	None expected.	
Liver:	None expected.	
Allergic:	None expected.	
Blood:	None expected.	
Others:	None expected.	

1- Life-threatening. Seek emergency treatment immediately.
2- Discontinue. Seek emergency treatment.
3- Discontinue. Call doctor right away.
4- Continue. Call doctor when convenient.
5- Continue. Tell doctor at next visit.
6- No action necessary.

POTASSIUM CHLORIDE

 ## WARNINGS & PRECAUTIONS

Don't take if:
- You are allergic to any potassium supplement.
- You have kidney disease.

Before you start, consult your doctor:
- If you have Addison's disease.
- If you have heart disease.
- If you have intestinal blockage.
- If you have a stomach ulcer.
- If you use diuretics.
- If you use heart medicine.
- If you use laxatives or have chronic diarrhea.
- If you use salt substitutes or low-salt milk.

Over age 60:
Observe dose schedule strictly. Potassium balance is critical. Deviation above or below normal can have serious results.

Pregnancy:
No problems expected if you adhere strictly to prescribed dose.

Breast-feeding:
Studies inconclusive on harm to infant. Consult doctor.

Infants & children:
Use only under doctor's supervision.

Prolonged use:
Slows absorption of vitamin B-12. May cause anemia.

Skin & sunlight:
No problems expected.

Driving, piloting or hazardous work:
No problems expected.

Airplane passengers:
No problems expected.

Discontinuing:
Don't discontinue without consulting doctor. Dose may require gradual reduction if you have taken drug for a long time. Doses of other drugs may also require adjustment.

Others:
Overdose or underdose serious. Frequent laboratory blood studies recommended.

 ## INTERACTION WITH OTHER DRUGS

GENERIC NAME OR DRUG CLASS	COMBINED EFFECT
Digitalis preparations	Possible irregular heartbeat.
Diuretics (thiazide)	Decreased potassium effect.
Spironolactone	Dangerous rise in blood potassium.
Triamterene	Dangerous rise in blood potassium.

 ## INTERACTION WITH OTHER SUBSTANCES

INTERACTS WITH	COMBINED EFFECT
Alcohol:	None expected.
Beverages: Salty drinks such as tomato juice, commercial thirst quenchers.	Increased fluid retention.
Cocaine:	May cause irregular heartbeat.
Foods: Salty foods.	Increased fluid retention.
Marijuana:	May cause irregular heartbeat.
Tobacco:	None expected.

POTASSIUM CHLORIDE & POTASSIUM GLUCONATE

BRAND NAMES

Kolyum

GENERAL INFORMATION

Habit forming? No
Prescription needed? Yes
Available as generic? Yes
Drug class: Mineral supplement (potassium)

USES

Treatment for potassium deficiency from illness, diuretics, cortisone drugs or digitalis preparations.

DOSAGE & USAGE INFORMATION

How to take:
- Tablet or capsule—Swallow with liquid or food to lessen stomach irritation. You may chew or crush tablet.
- Extended-release tablets or capsules— Swallow each dose whole with liquid.
- Effervescent tablets, granules, powder or liquid—Dilute dose in water.

When to take:
At the same times each day, preferably with food or immediately after meals.

If you forget a dose:
Take as soon as you remember. Don't double next dose.

What drug does:
Preserves or restores normal function of nerve cells, heart and skeletal-muscle cells, kidneys and stomach-juice secretion.

Time lapse before drug works:
12 to 24 hours.

Don't take with:
See Interaction column and consult doctor.

OVERDOSE

Symptoms:
Paralysis of arms and legs, irregular heartbeat, blood-pressure drop, convulsions, coma, cardiac arrest.

What to do:
- Dial 0 (operator) or 911 (emergency) for an ambulance or medical help. Then give first aid immediately.
- Additional emergency information on page 886.

POSSIBLE ADVERSE REACTIONS OR SIDE EFFECTS

SYMPTOMS	FREQUENCY	WHAT TO DO
Brain & nervous system:		
• Numbness and tingling in hands and feet.	Rare	4
• Confusion	Rare	3
Skin:	None expected.	
Eyes:	None expected.	
Ears, nose, throat:	None expected.	
Digestive: Diarrhea, nausea, vomiting, stomach discomfort.	Infrequent	4
Heart & lungs: Irregular heartbeat, breathing difficulty.	Rare	3
Blood vessels:	None expected.	
Muscles, bones, joints: Unusual fatigue, weakness, heaviness of legs.	Rare	3
Genital, urinary:	None expected.	
Kidneys:	None expected.	
Liver:	None expected.	
Allergic:	None expected.	
Blood:	None expected.	
Others:	None expected.	

1- Life-threatening. Seek emergency treatment immediately.
2- Discontinue. Seek emergency treatment.
3- Discontinue. Call doctor right away.
4- Continue. Call doctor when convenient.
5- Continue. Tell doctor at next visit.
6- No action necessary.

POTASSIUM CHLORIDE & POTASSIUM GLUCONATE

WARNINGS & PRECAUTIONS

Don't take if:
- You are allergic to any potassium supplement.
- You have kidney disease.

Before you start, consult your doctor:
- If you have Addison's disease.
- If you have heart disease.
- If you have intestinal blockage.
- If you have a stomach ulcer.
- If you use diuretics.
- If you use heart medicine.
- If you use laxatives or have chronic diarrhea.
- If you use salt substitutes or low-salt milk.

Over age 60:
Observe dose schedule strictly. Potassium balance is critical. Deviation above or below normal can have serious results.

Pregnancy:
No problems expected if you adhere strictly to prescribed dose.

Breast-feeding:
Studies inconclusive on harm to infant. Consult doctor.

Infants & children:
Use only under doctor's supervision.

Prolonged use:
Slows absorption of vitamin B-12. May cause anemia.

Skin & sunlight:
No problems expected.

Driving, piloting or hazardous work:
No problems expected.

Airplane passengers:
No problems expected.

Discontinuing:
Don't discontinue without consulting doctor. Dose may require gradual reduction if you have taken drug for a long time. Doses of other drugs may also require adjustment.

Others:
Overdose or underdose serious. Frequent laboratory blood studies recommended.

INTERACTION WITH OTHER DRUGS

GENERIC NAME OR DRUG CLASS	COMBINED EFFECT
Digitalis preparations	Possible irregular heartbeat.
Diuretics (thiazide)	Decreased potassium effect.
Spironolactone	Dangerous rise in blood potassium.
Triamterene	Dangerous rise in blood potassium.

INTERACTION WITH OTHER SUBSTANCES

INTERACTS WITH	COMBINED EFFECT
Alcohol:	None expected.
Beverages: Salty drinks such as tomato juice, commercial thirst quenchers.	Increased fluid retention.
Cocaine:	May cause irregular heartbeat.
Foods: Salty foods.	Increased fluid retention.
Marijuana:	May cause irregular heartbeat.
Tobacco:	None expected.

POTASSIUM CITRATE & POTASSIUM GLUCONATE

BRAND NAMES

Twin-K

GENERAL INFORMATION

Habit forming? No
Prescription needed? Yes
Available as generic? Yes
Drug class: Mineral supplement (potassium)

 USES

Treatment for potassium deficiency from illness, diuretics, cortisone drugs or digitalis preparations.

 DOSAGE & USAGE INFORMATION

How to take:
- Tablet or capsule—Swallow with liquid or food to lessen stomach irritation. You may chew or crush tablet.
- Extended-release tablets or capsules—Swallow each dose whole with liquid.
- Effervescent tablets, granules, powder or liquid—Dilute dose in water.

When to take:
At the same times each day, preferably with food or immediately after meals.

If you forget a dose:
Take as soon as you remember. Don't double next dose.

What drug does:
Preserves or restores normal function of nerve cells, heart and skeletal-muscle cells, kidneys and stomach-juice secretion.

Time lapse before drug works:
12 to 24 hours.

Don't take with:
See Interaction column and consult doctor.

 OVERDOSE

Symptoms:
Paralysis of arms and legs, irregular heartbeat, blood-pressure drop, convulsions, coma, cardiac arrest.

What to do:
- Dial 0 (operator) or 911 (emergency) for an ambulance or medical help. Then give first aid immediately.
- Additional emergency information on page 886.

 POSSIBLE ADVERSE REACTIONS OR SIDE EFFECTS

SYMPTOMS	FREQUENCY	WHAT TO DO
Brain & nervous system:		
• Numbness and tingling in hands and feet.	Rare	4
• Confusion	Rare	3
Skin:	None expected.	
Eyes:	None expected.	
Ears, nose, throat:	None expected.	
Digestive: Diarrhea, nausea, vomiting, stomach discomfort.	Infrequent	4
Heart & lungs: Irregular heartbeat, breathing difficulty.	Rare	3
Blood vessels:	None expected.	
Muscles, bones, joints: Unusual fatigue, weakness, heaviness of legs.	Rare	3
Genital, urinary:	None expected.	
Kidneys:	None expected.	
Liver:	None expected.	
Allergic:	None expected.	
Blood:	None expected.	
Others:	None expected.	

1- Life-threatening. Seek emergency treatment immediately.
2- Discontinue. Seek emergency treatment.
3- Discontinue. Call doctor right away.
4- Continue. Call doctor when convenient.
5- Continue. Tell doctor at next visit.
6- No action necessary.

POTASSIUM CITRATE & POTASSIUM GLUCONATE

WARNINGS & PRECAUTIONS

Don't take if:
- You are allergic to any potassium supplement.
- You have kidney disease.

Before you start, consult your doctor:
- If you have Addison's disease.
- If you have heart disease.
- If you have intestinal blockage.
- If you have a stomach ulcer.
- If you use diuretics.
- If you use heart medicine.
- If you use laxatives or have chronic diarrhea.
- If you use salt substitutes or low-salt milk.

Over age 60:
Observe dose schedule strictly. Potassium balance is critical. Deviation above or below normal can have serious results.

Pregnancy:
No problems expected if you adhere strictly to prescribed dose.

Breast-feeding:
Studies inconclusive on harm to infant. Consult doctor.

Infants & children:
Use only under doctor's supervision.

Prolonged use:
Slows absorption of vitamin B-12. May cause anemia.

Skin & sunlight:
No problems expected.

Driving, piloting or hazardous work:
No problems expected.

Airplane passengers:
No problems expected.

Discontinuing:
Don't discontinue without consulting doctor. Dose may require gradual reduction if you have taken drug for a long time. Doses of other drugs may also require adjustment.

Others:
Overdose or underdose serious. Frequent laboratory blood studies recommended.

INTERACTION WITH OTHER DRUGS

GENERIC NAME OR DRUG CLASS	COMBINED EFFECT
Digitalis preparations	Possible irregular heartbeat.
Diuretics (thiazide)	Decreased potassium effect.
Spironolactone	Dangerous rise in blood potassium.
Triamterene	Dangerous rise in blood potassium.

INTERACTION WITH OTHER SUBSTANCES

INTERACTS WITH	COMBINED EFFECT
Alcohol:	None expected.
Beverages: Salty drinks such as tomato juice, commercial thirst quenchers.	Increased fluid retention.
Cocaine:	May cause irregular heartbeat.
Foods: Salty foods.	Increased fluid retention.
Marijuana:	May cause irregular heartbeat.
Tobacco:	None expected.

POTASSIUM GLUCONATE

BRAND NAMES

Kaon
K-10

GENERAL INFORMATION

Habit forming? No
Prescription needed? Yes
Available as generic? Yes
Drug class: Mineral supplement (potassium)

 USES

Treatment for potassium deficiency from illness, diuretics, cortisone drugs or digitalis preparations.

 DOSAGE & USAGE INFORMATION

How to take:
- Tablet or capsule—Swallow with liquid or food to lessen stomach irritation. You may chew or crush tablet.
- Extended-release tablets or capsules—Swallow each dose whole with liquid.
- Effervescent tablets, granules, powder or liquid—Dilute dose in water.

When to take:
At the same times each day, preferably with food or immediately after meals.

If you forget a dose:
Take as soon as you remember. Don't double next dose.

What drug does:
Preserves or restores normal function of nerve cells, heart and skeletal-muscle cells, kidneys and stomach-juice secretion.

Time lapse before drug works:
12 to 24 hours.

Don't take with:
See Interaction column and consult doctor.

 OVERDOSE

Symptoms:
Paralysis of arms and legs, irregular heartbeat, blood-pressure drop, convulsions, coma, cardiac arrest.

What to do:
- Dial 0 (operator) or 911 (emergency) for an ambulance or medical help. Then give first aid immediately.
- Additional emergency information on page 886.

POSSIBLE ADVERSE REACTIONS OR SIDE EFFECTS

SYMPTOMS	FREQUENCY	WHAT TO DO
Brain & nervous system:		
• Numbness and tingling in hands and feet.	Rare	4
• Confusion	Rare	3
Skin:	None expected.	
Eyes:	None expected.	
Ears, nose, throat:	None expected.	
Digestive: Diarrhea, nausea, vomiting, stomach discomfort.	Infrequent	4
Heart & lungs: Irregular heartbeat, breathing difficulty.	Rare	3
Blood vessels:	None expected.	
Muscles, bones, joints: Unusual fatigue, weakness, heaviness of legs.	Rare	3
Genital, urinary:	None expected.	
Kidneys:	None expected.	
Liver:	None expected.	
Allergic:	None expected.	
Blood:	None expected.	
Others:	None expected.	

1- Life-threatening. Seek emergency treatment immediately.
2- Discontinue. Seek emergency treatment.
3- Discontinue. Call doctor right away.
4- Continue. Call doctor when convenient.
5- Continue. Tell doctor at next visit.
6- No action necessary.

POTASSIUM GLUCONATE

 ## WARNINGS & PRECAUTIONS

Don't take if:
- You are allergic to any potassium supplement.
- You have kidney disease.

Before you start, consult your doctor:
- If you have Addison's disease.
- If you have heart disease.
- If you have intestinal blockage.
- If you have a stomach ulcer.
- If you use diuretics.
- If you use heart medicine.
- If you use laxatives or have chronic diarrhea.
- If you use salt substitutes or low-salt milk.

Over age 60:
Observe dose schedule strictly. Potassium balance is critical. Deviation above or below normal can have serious results.

Pregnancy:
No problems expected if you adhere strictly to prescribed dose.

Breast-feeding:
Studies inconclusive on harm to infant. Consult doctor.

Infants & children:
Use only under doctor's supervision.

Prolonged use:
Slows absorption of vitamin B-12. May cause anemia.

Skin & sunlight:
No problems expected.

Driving, piloting or hazardous work:
No problems expected.

Airplane passengers:
No problems expected.

Discontinuing:
Don't discontinue without consulting doctor. Dose may require gradual reduction if you have taken drug for a long time. Doses of other drugs may also require adjustment.

Others:
Overdose or underdose serious. Frequent laboratory blood studies recommended.

 ## INTERACTION WITH OTHER DRUGS

GENERIC NAME OR DRUG CLASS	COMBINED EFFECT
Digitalis preparations	Possible irregular heartbeat.
Diuretics (thiazide)	Decreased potassium effect.
Spironolactone	Dangerous rise in blood potassium.
Triamterene	Dangerous rise in blood potassium.

 ## INTERACTION WITH OTHER SUBSTANCES

INTERACTS WITH	COMBINED EFFECT
Alcohol:	None expected.
Beverages: Salty drinks such as tomato juice, commercial thirst quenchers.	Increased fluid retention.
Cocaine:	May cause irregular heartbeat.
Foods: Salty foods.	Increased fluid retention.
Marijuana:	May cause irregular heartbeat.
Tobacco:	None expected.

PRAZEPAM

BRAND NAMES

Centrax

GENERAL INFORMATION

Habit forming? Yes
Prescription needed? Yes
Available as generic? No
Drug class: Tranquilizer (benzodiazepine)

USES

Treatment for nervousness or tension.

DOSAGE & USAGE INFORMATION

How to take:
Tablet or capsule—Swallow with liquid. If you can't swallow whole, crumble tablet or open capsule and take with liquid or food.

When to take:
At the same time each day, according to instructions on prescription label.

If you forget a dose:
Take as soon as you remember up to 2 hours late. If more than 2 hours, wait for next scheduled dose (don't double this dose).

What drug does:
Affects limbic system of brain—part that controls emotions.

Time lapse before drug works:
2 hours. May take 6 weeks for full benefit.

Don't take with:
See Interaction column and consult doctor.

OVERDOSE

Symptoms:
Drowsiness, weakness, tremor, stupor, coma.

What to do:
- Dial 0 (operator) or 911 (emergency) for an ambulance or medical help. Then give first aid immediately.
- If patient is unconscious and not breathing, give mouth-to-mouth breathing. If there is no heartbeat, use cardiac massage and mouth-to-mouth breathing (CPR). Don't try to make patient vomit. If you can't get help quickly, take patient to nearest emergency facility.
- Additional emergency information on page 886.

POSSIBLE ADVERSE REACTIONS OR SIDE EFFECTS

SYMPTOMS	FREQUENCY	WHAT TO DO
Brain & nervous system:		
• Clumsiness, drowsiness, dizziness.	Common	4
• Hallucinations, confusion, depression, irritability.	Infrequent	3
Skin:		
Rash, itch.	Infrequent	3
Eyes:		
Vision changes.	Infrequent	3
Ears, nose, throat:		
Mouth, throat ulcers.	Rare	3
Digestive:		
Constipation or diarrhea, nausea, vomiting.	Infrequent	4
Heart & lungs:		
Slow heartbeat, breathing difficulty.	Rare	2
Blood vessels:	None expected.	
Muscles, bones, joints:	None expected.	
Genital, urinary:		
Urination difficulty.	Infrequent	4
Kidneys:	None expected.	
Liver:		
Jaundice (yellow eyes and skin).	Rare	3
Allergic:	None expected.	
Blood:	None expected.	
Others:	None expected.	

1- Life-threatening. Seek emergency treatment immediately.
2- Discontinue. Seek emergency treatment.
3- Discontinue. Call doctor right away.
4- Continue. Call doctor when convenient.
5- Continue. Tell doctor at next visit.
6- No action necessary.

WARNINGS & PRECAUTIONS

Don't take if:
- You are allergic to any benzodiazepine.
- You have myasthenia gravis.
- You have glaucoma.
- You are active or recovering alcoholic.
- Patient is younger than 6 months.

Before you start, consult your doctor:
- If you have liver, kidney or lung disease.
- If you have diabetes, epilepsy or porphyria.

Over age 60:
Adverse reactions and side effects may be more frequent and severe than in younger persons. You need smaller doses for shorter periods of time. May develop agitation, rage or "hangover effect."

Pregnancy:
Risk to unborn child outweighs drug benefits. Don't use.

Breast-feeding:
Drug passes into milk. Avoid drug or discontinue nursing until you finish medicine. Consult doctor for advice on maintaining milk supply.

Infants & children:
Use only under medical supervision for children older than 6 months.

Prolonged use:
May impair liver function.

Skin & sunlight:
No problems expected.

Driving, piloting or hazardous work:
Don't drive or pilot aircraft until you learn how medicine affects you. Don't work around dangerous machinery. Don't climb ladders or work in high places. Danger increases if you drink alcohol or take medicine affecting alertness and reflexes.

Airplane passengers:
No problems expected.

Discontinuing:
Don't discontinue without consulting doctor. Dose may require gradual reduction if you have taken drug for a long time. Doses of other drugs may also require adjustment.

Others:
- Hot weather, heavy exercise and profuse sweat may reduce excretion and cause overdose.
- Blood sugar may rise in diabetics, requiring insulin adjustment.

INTERACTION WITH OTHER DRUGS

GENERIC NAME OR DRUG CLASS	COMBINED EFFECT
Anticonvulsants	Change in seizure frequency or severity.
Antidepressants	Increased sedative effect of both drugs.
Antihistamines	Increased sedative effect of both drugs.
Antihypertensives	Excessively low blood pressure.
Cimetidine	Excess sedation.
Disulfiram	Increased prazepam effect.
MAO inhibitors	Convulsions, deep sedation, rage.
Narcotics	Increased sedative effect of both drugs.
Sedatives	Increased sedative effect of both drugs.
Sleep inducers	Increased sedative effect of both drugs.
Tranquilizers	Increased sedative effect of both drugs.

INTERACTION WITH OTHER SUBSTANCES

INTERACTS WITH	COMBINED EFFECT
Alcohol:	Heavy sedation. Avoid.
Beverages:	None expected.
Cocaine:	Decreased prazepam effect.
Foods:	None expected.
Marijuana:	Heavy sedation. Avoid.
Tobacco:	Decreased prazepam effect.

PRAZOSIN

BRAND NAMES

Minipress
Minizide (M)

GENERAL INFORMATION

Habit forming? No
Prescription needed? Yes
Available as generic? No
Drug class: Antihypertensive

USES

- Treatment for high blood pressure.
- Improves congestive heart failure.

DOSAGE & USAGE INFORMATION

How to take:
Tablet or capsule—Swallow with liquid. If you can't swallow whole, crumble tablet or open capsule and take with liquid or food.

When to take:
At the same times each day.

If you forget a dose:
Take as soon as you remember up to 2 hours late. If more than 2 hours, wait for next scheduled dose (don't double this dose).

What drug does:
Expands and relaxes blood-vessel walls to lower blood pressure.

Time lapse before drug works:
30 minutes.

Don't take with:
See Interaction column and consult doctor.

OVERDOSE

Symptoms:
Extreme weakness; loss of consciousness; cold, sweaty skin; weak, rapid pulse; coma.

What to do:
- Dial 0 (operator) or 911 (emergency) for an ambulance or medical help. Then give first aid immediately.
- If patient is unconscious and not breathing, give mouth-to-mouth breathing. If there is no heartbeat, use cardiac massage and mouth-to-mouth breathing (CPR). Don't try to make patient vomit. If you can't get help quickly, take patient to nearest emergency facility.
- Additional emergency information on page 886.

POSSIBLE ADVERSE REACTIONS OR SIDE EFFECTS

SYMPTOMS	FREQUENCY	WHAT TO DO
Brain & nervous system:		
● Vivid dreams, drowsiness, dizziness.	Common	4
● Headache, irritability, depression.	Infrequent	5
Skin:		
Rash or itch.	Infrequent	3
Eyes:		
Blurred vision.	Infrequent	3
Ears, nose, throat:		
Dry mouth, stuffy nose.	Infrequent	5
Digestive:		
Appetite loss, constipation or diarrhea, stomach pain, nausea, vomiting.	Infrequent	4
Heart & lungs:		
● Rapid heartbeat.	Common	3
● Shortness of breath, chest pain.	Infrequent	3
Blood vessels, kidneys, liver, allergic, blood:	None expected.	
Muscles, bones, joints:		
● Fluid retention.	Infrequent	4
● Joint, muscle aches.	Infrequent	4
Genital, urinary:		
● More urination.	Infrequent	5
● Decreased sexual function.	Rare	4

1-Life-threatening. Seek emergency treatment immediately.
2-Discontinue. Seek emergency treatment.
3-Discontinue. Call doctor right away.
4-Continue. Call doctor when convenient.
5-Continue. Tell doctor at next visit.

WARNINGS & PRECAUTIONS

Don't take if:
- You are allergic to prazosin.
- You are depressed.
- You will have surgery within 2 months, including dental surgery, requiring general or spinal anesthesia.

Before you start, consult your doctor:
- If you experience lightheadedness or fainting with other antihypertensive drugs.
- If you are easily depressed.
- If you have impaired brain circulation or have had a stroke.
- If you have coronary heart disease (with or without angina).
- If you have kidney disease or impaired liver function.

Over age 60:
Begin with no more than 1 mg. per day for first 3 days. Increases should be gradual and supervised by your doctor. Don't stand while taking. Sudden changes in position may cause falls. Sit or lie down promptly if you feel dizzy. If you have impaired brain circulation or coronary heart disease, excessive lowering of blood pressure should be avoided. Report problems to your doctor immediately.

Pregnancy:
Studies inconclusive on harm to unborn child. Animal studies show fetal abnormalities. Decide with your doctor whether drug benefits justify risk to child.

Breast-feeding:
No proven problems. Consult doctor.

Infants & children:
Not recommended.

Prolonged use:
No problems expected.

Skin & sunlight:
No problems expected.

Driving, piloting or hazardous work:
Don't drive or pilot aircraft until you learn how medicine affects you. Don't work around dangerous machinery. Don't climb ladders or work in high places.

Airplane passengers:
No problems expected.

Discontinuing:
Don't discontinue without doctor's advice until you complete prescribed dose, even though symptoms diminish or disappear.

Others:
First dose likely to cause fainting. Take it at night and get out of bed slowly next morning.

INTERACTION WITH OTHER DRUGS

GENERIC NAME OR DRUG CLASS	COMBINED EFFECT
Amitriptyline	Acute agitation.
Amphetamines	Decreased prazosin effect.
Antihypertensives (other)	Increased effect of other drugs.
Chlorpromazine	Acute agitation.
MAO inhibitors	Blood-pressure drop.
Nitroglycerin	Prolonged effect of prazosin.

INTERACTION WITH OTHER SUBSTANCES

INTERACTS WITH	COMBINED EFFECT
Alcohol:	Excessive blood-pressure drop.
Beverages:	None expected.
Cocaine:	Decreased prazosin effect. Avoid.
Foods:	None expected.
Marijuana:	Possible fainting. Avoid.
Tobacco:	Possible spasm of coronary arteries. Avoid.

PREDNISOLONE

BRAND NAMES

Cortalone	Meticortelone
Delta-Cortef	Nor-Pred-TBA
Fernisolone-P	Pred Cor-TBA
Hydeltrasol	Savacort 50 & 100
Hydeltra-TBA	Sterane
Metalone-TBA	

GENERAL INFORMATION

Habit forming? No
Prescription needed? Yes
Available as generic? Yes
Drug class: Cortisone drug (adrenal corticosteroid)

 ## USES

- Reduces inflammation caused by many different medical problems.
- Treatment for some allergic diseases, blood disorders, kidney diseases, asthma and emphysema.
- Replaces corticosteroid deficiencies.

 ## DOSAGE & USAGE INFORMATION

How to take:
Tablet—Swallow with liquid or food to lessen stomach irritation. If you can't swallow whole, crumble tablet and take with liquid or food.

When to take:
At the same times each day. Take once-a-day or once-every-other-day doses in mornings.

If you forget a dose:
- Several-doses-per-day prescription—Take as soon as you remember up to 2 hours late. If more than 2 hours, wait for next scheduled dose (don't double this dose).
- Once-a-day dose or less—Wait for next dose. Double this dose.

What drug does:
Decreases inflammatory responses.

Time lapse before drug works:
2 to 4 days.

Don't take with:
See Interaction column and consult doctor.

 ## OVERDOSE

Symptoms:
Headache, convulsions, heart failure.

What to do:
- Dial 0 (operator) or 911 (emergency) for an ambulance or medical help. Then give first aid immediately.
- Additional emergency information on page 886.

 ## POSSIBLE ADVERSE REACTIONS OR SIDE EFFECTS

SYMPTOMS	FREQUENCY	WHAT TO DO
Brain & nervous system:		
Mood changes, insomnia, restlessness.	Infrequent	4
Skin:		
● Acne	Common	4
● Rash	Rare	3
● Poor wound healing.	Common	4
Eyes:		
Blurred vision, halos around lights.	Infrequent	3
Ears, nose, throat:		
● Sore throat, fever.	Infrequent	3
● Thirst	Common	4
Digestive:		
● Indigestion, nausea, vomiting.	Common	4
● Bloody or black, tarry stool.	Infrequent	2
Heart & lungs:		
Irregular heartbeat.	Rare	2
Blood vessels, kidneys, liver, allergic, blood:	None expected.	
Muscles, bones, joints:		
Muscle cramps, swollen legs, feet.	Infrequent	3
Genital, urinary:		
Frequent urination.	Infrequent	4
Others:		
● Weight gain, round face.	Infrequent	4
● Fatigue, weakness.	Infrequent	4
● TB recurrence.	Infrequent	4
● Irregular menstrual periods.	Infrequent	4

1- Life-threatening. Seek emergency treatment immediately.
2- Discontinue. Seek emergency treatment.
3- Discontinue. Call doctor right away.
4- Continue. Call doctor when convenient.

PREDNISOLONE

WARNINGS & PRECAUTIONS

Don't take if:
- You are allergic to any cortisone drug.
- You have tuberculosis or fungus infection.
- You have herpes infection of eyes, lips or genitals.

Before you start, consult your doctor:
- If you have had tuberculosis.
- If you have congestive heart failure.
- If you have diabetes.
- If you have peptic ulcer.
- If you have glaucoma.
- If you have underactive thyroid.
- If you have high blood pressure.
- If you have myasthenia gravis.
- If you have blood clots in legs or lungs.

Over age 60:
Adverse reactions and side effects may be more frequent and severe than in younger persons. Likely to aggravate edema, diabetes or ulcers. Likely to cause cataracts and osteoporosis (softening of the bones).

Pregnancy:
Risk to unborn child outweighs drug benefits. Don't use.

Breast-feeding:
Drug passes into milk. Avoid drug or discontinue nursing until you finish medicine. Consult doctor for advice on maintaining milk supply.

Infants & children:
Use only under medical supervision.

Prolonged use:
- Retards growth in children.
- Possible glaucoma, cataracts, diabetes, fragile bones and thin skin.
- Functional dependence.

Skin & sunlight:
No problems expected.

Driving, piloting or hazardous work:
No problems expected.

Airplane passengers:
No problems expected.

Discontinuing:
- Don't discontinue without doctor's advice until you complete prescribed dose, even though symptoms diminish or disappear.
- Drug affects your response to surgery, illness, injury or stress for 2 years after discontinuing. Tell about drug to anyone who takes medical care of you within 2 years.

Others:
Avoid immunizations if possible.

INTERACTION WITH OTHER DRUGS

GENERIC NAME OR DRUG CLASS	COMBINED EFFECT
Amphotericin B	Potassium depletion.
Anticholinergics	Possible glaucoma.
Anticoagulants (oral)	Decreased anticoagulant effect.
Anticonvulsants (hydantoin)	Decreased prednisolone effect.
Antidiabetics (oral)	Decreased antidiabetic effect.
Antihistamines	Decreased prednisolone effect.
Aspirin	Increased prednisolone effect.
Barbiturates	Decreased prednisolone effect. Oversedation.
Beta-adrenergic blockers	Decreased prednisolone effect.
Chloral hydrate	Decreased prednisolone effect.
Chlorthalidone	Potassium depletion.
Cholinergics	Decreased cholinergic effect.
Contraceptives (oral)	Increased prednisolone effect.
Digitalis preparations	Dangerous potassium depletion. Possible digitalis toxicity.
Diuretics (thiazide)	Potassium depletion.

Additional interactions on page 842.

INTERACTION WITH OTHER SUBSTANCES

INTERACTS WITH	COMBINED EFFECT
Alcohol:	Risk of stomach ulcers.
Beverages:	No proven problems.
Cocaine:	Overstimulation. Avoid.
Foods:	No proven problems.
Marijuana:	Decreased immunity.
Tobacco:	Increased prednisolone effect. Possible toxicity.

PREDNISONE

BRAND NAMES

Colisone	Meticorten	Sterapred
Cortan	Orasone	Sterazolidin (M)
Deltasone	Paracort	Winpred
Liquid-Pred	SK-Prednisone	

GENERAL INFORMATION

Habit forming? No
Prescription needed? Yes
Available as generic? Yes
Drug class: Cortisone drug (adrenal corticosteroid)

USES

- Reduces inflammation caused by many different medical problems.
- Treatment for some allergic diseases, blood disorders, kidney diseases, asthma and emphysema.
- Replaces corticosteroid deficiencies.

DOSAGE & USAGE INFORMATION

How to take:
Tablet or syrup—Swallow with liquid or food to lessen stomach irritation. If you can't swallow whole, crumble tablet.

When to take:
At the same times each day. Take once-a-day or once-every-other-day doses in mornings.

If you forget a dose:
- Several-doses-per-day prescription—Take as soon as you remember up to 2 hours late. If more than 2 hours, wait for next scheduled dose (don't double this dose).
- Once-a-day dose or less—Wait for next dose. Double this dose.

What drug does:
Decreases inflammatory responses.

Time lapse before drug works:
2 to 4 days.

Don't take with:
See Interaction column and consult doctor.

OVERDOSE

Symptoms:
Headache, convulsions, heart failure.

What to do:
- Dial 0 (operator) or 911 (emergency) for an ambulance or medical help. Then give first aid immediately.
- Additional emergency information on page 886.

POSSIBLE ADVERSE REACTIONS OR SIDE EFFECTS

SYMPTOMS	FREQUENCY	WHAT TO DO
Brain & nervous system:		
Mood changes, insomnia, restlessness.	Infrequent	4
Skin:		
• Acne	Common	4
• Rash	Rare	3
• Poor wound healing.	Common	4
Eyes:		
Blurred vision, halos around lights.	Infrequent	3
Ears, nose, throat:		
• Sore throat, fever.	Infrequent	3
• Thirst	Common	4
Digestive:		
• Indigestion, nausea, vomiting.	Common	4
• Bloody or black, tarry stool.	Infrequent	2
Heart & lungs:		
Irregular heartbeat.	Rare	2
Blood vessels, kidneys, liver, allergic, blood:	None expected.	
Muscles, bones, joints:		
Muscle cramps, swollen legs, feet.	Infrequent	3
Genital, urinary:		
Frequent urination.	Infrequent	4
Others:		
• Weight gain, round face.	Infrequent	4
• Fatigue, weakness.	Infrequent	4
• TB recurrence.	Infrequent	4
• Irregular menstrual periods.	Infrequent	4

1- Life-threatening. Seek emergency treatment immediately.
2- Discontinue. Seek emergency treatment.
3- Discontinue. Call doctor right away.
4- Continue. Call doctor when convenient.

PREDNISONE

WARNINGS & PRECAUTIONS

Don't take if:
- You are allergic to any cortisone drug.
- You have tuberculosis or fungus infection.
- You have herpes infection of eyes, lips or genitals.

Before you start, consult your doctor:
- If you have had tuberculosis.
- If you have congestive heart failure.
- If you have diabetes.
- If you have peptic ulcer.
- If you have glaucoma.
- If you have underactive thyroid.
- If you have high blood pressure.
- If you have myasthenia gravis.
- If you have blood clots in legs or lungs.

Over age 60:
Adverse reactions and side effects may be more frequent and severe than in younger persons. Likely to aggravate edema, diabetes or ulcers. Likely to cause cataracts and osteoporosis (softening of the bones).

Pregnancy:
Risk to unborn child outweighs drug benefits. Don't use.

Breast-feeding:
Drug passes into milk. Avoid drug or discontinue nursing until you finish medicine. Consult doctor for advice on maintaining milk supply.

Infants & children:
Use only under medical supervision.

Prolonged use:
- Retards growth in children.
- Possible glaucoma, cataracts, diabetes, fragile bones and thin skin.
- Functional dependence.

Skin & sunlight:
No problems expected.

Driving, piloting or hazardous work:
No problems expected.

Airplane passengers:
No problems expected.

Discontinuing:
- Don't discontinue without doctor's advice until you complete prescribed dose, even though symptoms diminish or disappear.
- Drug affects your response to surgery, illness, injury or stress for 2 years after discontinuing. Tell about drug to anyone who takes medical care of you within 2 years.

Others:
Avoid immunizations if possible.

INTERACTION WITH OTHER DRUGS

GENERIC NAME OR DRUG CLASS	COMBINED EFFECT
Amphoterecin B	Potassium depletion.
Anticholinergics	Possible glaucoma.
Anticoagulants (oral)	Decreased anticoagulant effect.
Anticonvulsants (hydantoin)	Decreased prednisone effect.
Antidiabetics (oral)	Decreased antidiabetic effect.
Antihistamines	Decreased prednisone effect.
Aspirin	Increased prednisone effect.
Barbiturates	Decreased prednisone effect. Oversedation.
Beta-adrenergic blockers	Decreased prednisone effect.
Chloral hydrate	Decreased prednisone effect.
Chlorthalidone	Potassium depletion.
Cholinergics	Decreased cholinergic effect.
Contraceptives (oral)	Increased prednisone effect.
Digitalis preparations	Dangerous potassium depletion. Possible digitalis toxicity.
Diuretics (thiazide)	Potassium depletion.

Additional interactions on page 842.

INTERACTION WITH OTHER SUBSTANCES

INTERACTS WITH	COMBINED EFFECT
Alcohol:	Risk of stomach ulcers.
Beverages:	No proven problems.
Cocaine:	Overstimulation. Avoid.
Foods:	No proven problems.
Marijuana:	Decreased immunity.
Tobacco:	Increased prednisone effect. Possible toxicity.

PRIMIDONE

BRAND NAMES

Mysoline
Sertan

GENERAL INFORMATION

Habit forming? No
Prescription needed? Yes
Available as generic? Yes
Drug class: Anticonvulsant

USES

Prevents epileptic seizures.

DOSAGE & USAGE INFORMATION

How to take:
- Tablet or capsule—Swallow with liquid. If you can't swallow whole, crumble tablet or open capsule and take with liquid or food.
- Liquid—If desired, dilute dose in beverage before swallowing.

When to take:
Daily in regularly spaced doses, according to doctor's prescription.

If you forget a dose:
Take as soon as you remember up to 2 hours late. If more than 2 hours, wait for next scheduled dose (don't double this dose).

What drug does:
Probably inhibits repetitious spread of impulses along nerve pathways.

Time lapse before drug works:
2 to 3 weeks.

Don't take with:
See Interaction column and consult doctor.

OVERDOSE

Symptoms:
Slow, shallow breathing; weak, rapid pulse; confusion, deep sleep, coma.

What to do:
- Dial 0 (operator) or 911 (emergency) for an ambulance or medical help. Then give first aid immediately.
- If patient is unconscious and not breathing, give mouth-to-mouth breathing. If there is no heartbeat, use cardiac massage and mouth-to-mouth breathing (CPR). Don't try to make patient vomit. If you can't get help quickly, take patient to nearest emergency facility.
- Additional emergency information on page 886.

POSSIBLE ADVERSE REACTIONS OR SIDE EFFECTS

SYMPTOMS	FREQUENCY	WHAT TO DO
Brain & nervous system:		
• Confusion	Common	4
• Clumsiness, dizziness, drowsiness.	Common	5
• Headache	Infrequent	4
Skin:		
Rash or hives.	Rare	3
Eyes:		
• Vision change.	Common	4
• Eyelid swelling.	Rare	4
Ears, nose, throat:	None expected.	
Digestive:		
Nausea, vomiting, appetite loss.	Infrequent	4
Heart & lungs:		
Breathing difficulty.	Common	3
Blood vessels:	None expected.	
Muscles, bones, joints:	None expected.	
Genital, urinary:		
Decreased sexual ability.	Rare	5
Kidneys:	None expected.	
Liver:	None expected.	
Allergic:	None expected.	
Blood:	None expected.	
Others:		
• Unusual excitement, particularly in children.	Infrequent	3
• Fatigue, weakness.	Rare	3

1 - Life-threatening. Seek emergency treatment immediately.
2 - Discontinue. Seek emergency treatment.
3 - Discontinue. Call doctor right away.
4 - Continue. Call doctor when convenient.
5 - Continue. Tell doctor at next visit.
6 - No action necessary.

PRIMIDONE

WARNINGS & PRECAUTIONS

Don't take if:
- You are allergic to any barbiturate.
- You have had porphyria.

Before you start, consult your doctor:
- If you have had liver, kidney or lung disease or asthma.
- If you have lupus.

Over age 60:
Adverse reactions and side effects may be more frequent and severe than in younger persons.

Pregnancy:
Studies inconclusive on harm to unborn child. Animal studies show fetal abnormalities. Decide with your doctor whether drug benefits justify risk to unborn child.

Breast-feeding:
Drug filters into milk. May harm child. Avoid.

Infants & children:
Use only under medical supervision.

Prolonged use:
- Enlarged lymph and thyroid glands.
- Anemia
- Rickets in children and osteomalacia (insufficient calcium to bones) in adults.

Skin & sunlight:
None expected.

Driving, piloting or hazardous work:
Don't drive or pilot aircraft until you learn how medicine affects you. Don't work around dangerous machinery. Don't climb ladders or work in high places. Danger increases if you drink alcohol or take medicine affecting alertness and reflexes.

Airplane passengers:
No problems expected.

Discontinuing:
Don't discontinue abruptly or without doctor's advice until you complete prescribed dose, even though symptoms diminish or disappear.

Others:
- Tell doctor if you become ill or injured and must interrupt dose schedule.
- Periodic laboratory blood tests of drug level recommended.

INTERACTION WITH OTHER DRUGS

GENERIC NAME OR DRUG CLASS	COMBINED EFFECT
Anticoagulants (oral)	Decreased primidone effect.
Anticonvulsants (other)	Changed seizure pattern.
Antidepressants	Increased antidepressant effect.
Antidiabetics	Increased effect of primidone sedation.
Antihistamines	Increased effect of primidone sedation.
Aspirin	Decreased aspirin effect.
Contraceptives (oral)	Decreased contraceptive effect.
Cortisone drugs	Decreased cortisone effect.
Digitalis preparations	Decreased digitalis effect.
Griseofulvin	Decreased griseofulvin effect.
Isoniazid	Increased isoniazid effect.
MAO inhibitors	Increased effect of primidone sedation.
Mind-altering drugs	Increased effect of mind-altering drugs.

Additional interactions on page 842.

INTERACTION WITH OTHER SUBSTANCES

INTERACTS WITH	COMBINED EFFECT
Alcohol:	Dangerous sedative effect. Avoid.
Beverages:	None expected.
Cocaine:	Decreased primidone effect.
Foods:	Possible need for more vitamin D.
Marijuana:	Decreased anticonvulsant effect of primidone. Drowsiness, unsteadiness.
Tobacco:	None expected.

PROBENECID

BRAND NAMES

Benacen
Benemid
Benuryl
ColBENEMID (M)
Probalan
SK-Probenecid

GENERAL INFORMATION

Habit forming? No
Prescription needed? Yes
Available as generic? Yes
Drug class: Antigout (uricosuric)

USES

- Treatment for chronic gout.
- Increases blood levels of penicillins and cephalosporins.

DOSAGE & USAGE INFORMATION

How to take:
Tablet or capsule—Swallow with liquid or food to lessen stomach irritation. If you can't swallow whole, crumble tablet or open capsule and take with liquid or food.

When to take:
At the same time each day.

If you forget a dose:
Take as soon as you remember up to 12 hours late. If more than 12 hours, wait for next scheduled dose (don't double this dose).

What drug does:
- Forces kidneys to excrete uric acid.
- Reduces amount of penicillin excreted in urine.

Time lapse before drug works:
May require several months of regular use to prevent acute gout.

Don't take with:
- Non-prescription drugs containing aspirin or caffeine.
- See Interaction column and consult doctor.

OVERDOSE

Symptoms:
Breathing difficulty, severe nervous agitation, convulsions, delirium, coma.

What to do:
- Dial 0 (operator) or 911 (emergency) for an ambulance or medical help. Then give first aid immediately.
- Additional emergency information on page 886.

POSSIBLE ADVERSE REACTIONS OR SIDE EFFECTS

SYMPTOMS	FREQUENCY	WHAT TO DO
Brain & nervous system:		
• Headache	Common	4
• Dizziness	Infrequent	4
Skin:		
Flushed face, itching.	Infrequent	4
Eyes:	None expected.	
Ears, nose, throat:		
Sore throat.	Rare	3
Digestive:		
Appetite loss, nausea, vomiting.	Common	4
Heart & lungs:		
Breathing difficulty.	Rare	3
Blood vessels:		
Unusual bleeding or bruising.	Rare	3
Muscles, bones, joints:		
Red, painful joint.	Rare	3
Genital, urinary:		
• Bloody urine.	Infrequent	3
• Painful or frequent urination.	Infrequent	5
Kidneys:		
Low back pain.	Infrequent	3
Liver:		
Jaundice (yellow skin and eyes).	Rare	3
Allergic:	None expected.	
Blood:	None expected.	
Others:		
Fever	Rare	3

1- Life-threatening. Seek emergency treatment immediately.
2- Discontinue. Seek emergency treatment.
3- Discontinue. Call doctor right away.
4- Continue. Call doctor when convenient.
5- Continue. Tell doctor at next visit.

PROBENECID

WARNINGS & PRECAUTIONS

Don't take if:
- You are allergic to any uricosuric.
- You have acute gout.
- Patient is younger than 2.

Before you start, consult your doctor:
- If you have had kidney stones or kidney disease.
- If you have a peptic ulcer.
- If you have bone-marrow or blood-cell disease.

Over age 60:
Adverse reactions and side effects may be more frequent and severe than in younger persons.

Pregnancy:
Studies inconclusive on harm to unborn child. Animal studies show fetal abnormalities. Decide with your doctor whether drug benefits justify risk to unborn child.

Breast-feeding:
No proven problems.

Infants & children:
Not recommended.

Prolonged use:
Possible kidney damage.

Skin & sunlight:
No problems expected.

Driving, piloting or hazardous work:
Avoid if you feel dizzy. Otherwise, no problems expected.

Airplane passengers:
No problems expected.

Discontinuing:
Don't discontinue without consulting doctor. Dose may require gradual reduction if you have taken drug for a long time. Doses of other drugs may also require adjustment.

Others:
If signs of gout attack develop while taking medicine, consult doctor.

INTERACTION WITH OTHER DRUGS

GENERIC NAME OR DRUG CLASS	COMBINED EFFECT
Acetohexamide	Increased acetohexamide effect.
Anticoagulants (oral)	Increased anticoagulant effect.
Aspirin	Decreased probenecid effect.
Cephalosporins	Increased cephalosporin effect.
Dapsone	Increased dapsone effect. Increased toxicity.
Diuretics (thiazide)	Decreased probenecid effect.
Indomethacin	Increased adverse effects of indomethacin.
Methotrexate	Increased methotrexate toxicity.
Nitrofurantoin	Increased effect of nitrofurantoin.
Para-aminosalicylic acid (PAS)	Increased effect of para-aminosalicylic acid.
Penicillins	Enhanced penicillin effect.
Pyrazinamide	Decreased probenecid effect.

Additional interactions on page 842.

INTERACTION WITH OTHER SUBSTANCES

INTERACTS WITH	COMBINED EFFECT
Alcohol:	Decreased probenecid effect.
Beverages: Caffeine drinks	Loss of probenecid effectiveness.
Cocaine:	None expected.
Foods:	None expected.
Marijuana:	Daily use—Decreased probenecid effect.
Tobacco:	None expected.

PROCAINAMIDE

BRAND NAMES

Procan
Procan SR
Procamide
Procapan
Pronestyl
Sub-Quin

GENERAL INFORMATION

Habit forming? No
Prescription needed? Yes
Available as generic? Yes
Drug class: Antiarrhythmic

 USES

Stabilizes irregular heartbeat.

 DOSAGE & USAGE INFORMATION

How to take:
- Tablet or capsule—Swallow with liquid.
- Extended-release tablets or capsules—Swallow each dose whole. If you take regular tablets, you may chew or crush them.

When to take:
Best taken on empty stomach, 1 hour before or 2 hours after meals. If necessary, may be taken with food or milk to lessen stomach upset.

If you forget a dose:
Take as soon as you remember up to 2 hours late. If more than 2 hours, wait for next scheduled dose (don't double this dose).

What drug does:
Slows activity of pacemaker (rhythm-control center of heart) and delays transmission of electrical impulses.

Time lapse before drug works:
30 to 60 minutes.

Don't take with:
See Interaction column and consult doctor.

 OVERDOSE

Symptoms:
Fast and irregular heartbeat, stupor, fainting, cardiac arrest.

What to do:
- Dial 0 (operator) or 911 (emergency) for an ambulance or medical help. Then give first aid immediately.
- Additional emergency information on page 886.

 POSSIBLE ADVERSE REACTIONS OR SIDE EFFECTS

SYMPTOMS	FREQUENCY	WHAT TO DO
Brain & nervous system:		
● Hallucinations, confusion, depression.	Rare	3
● Dizziness	Infrequent	4
Skin: Itch, rash.	Rare	3
Eyes:	None expected.	
Ears, nose, throat: Sore throat, fever.	Rare	3
Digestive: Diarrhea, appetite loss, nausea, vomiting.	Common	4
Heart & lungs: Painful breathing.	Infrequent	3
Blood vessels:	None expected.	
Muscles, bones, joints: Joint pain.	Infrequent	3
Genital, urinary:	None expected.	
Kidneys:	None expected.	
Liver:	None expected.	
Allergic:	None expected.	
Blood:	None expected.	
Others:		
● Fever	Rare	3
● Fatigue	Rare	4

1- Life-threatening. Seek emergency treatment immediately.
2- Discontinue. Seek emergency treatment.
3- Discontinue. Call doctor right away.
4- Continue. Call doctor when convenient.
5- Continue. Tell doctor at next visit.
6- No action necessary.

WARNINGS & PRECAUTIONS

Don't take if:
- You are allergic to procainamide.
- You have myasthenia gravis.

Before you start, consult your doctor:
- If you are allergic to local anesthetics that end in "caine."
- If you have had liver or kidney disease or impaired kidney function.
- If you have had lupus.
- If you take digitalis preparations.
- If you will have surgery within 2 months, including dental surgery, requiring general or spinal anesthesia.

Over age 60:
Adverse reactions and side effects may be more frequent and severe than in younger persons.

Pregnancy:
No proven harm to unborn child. Avoid if possible.

Breast-feeding:
No proven problems. Consult doctor.

Infants & children:
Not recommended.

Prolonged use:
May cause lupus-like illness.

Skin & sunlight:
No problems expected.

Driving, piloting or hazardous work:
Use caution if you feel dizzy or weak. Otherwise, no problems expected.

Airplane passengers:
No problems expected.

Discontinuing:
Don't discontinue without doctor's advice until you complete prescribed dose, even though symptoms diminish or disappear.

Others:
No problems expected.

INTERACTION WITH OTHER DRUGS

GENERIC NAME OR DRUG CLASS	COMBINED EFFECT
Acetazolamide	Increased procainamide effect.
Ambenonium	Decreased ambenonium effect.
Antihypertensives	Increased antihypertensive effect.
Antimyasthenics	Decreased antimyasthenic effect.
Anticholinergics	Increased anticholinergic effect.
Kanamycin	Severe muscle weakness, impaired breathing.
Neomycin	Severe muscle weakness, impaired breathing.

INTERACTION WITH OTHER SUBSTANCES

INTERACTS WITH	COMBINED EFFECT
Alcohol:	None expected.
Beverages: Caffeine drinks, iced drinks.	Irregular heartbeat.
Cocaine:	Decreased procainamide effect.
Foods:	None expected.
Marijuana:	None expected.
Tobacco:	Decreased procainamide effect.

PROCHLORPERAZINE

BRAND NAMES

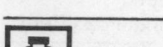

Combid (M)
Compazine
Eskatrol (M)
Stemetil

GENERAL INFORMATION

Habit forming? No
Prescription needed? Yes
Available as generic? Yes
Drug class: Tranquilizer, antiemetic (phenothiazine)

USES

- Stops nausea, vomiting.
- Reduces anxiety, agitation.

DOSAGE & USAGE INFORMATION

How to take:
- Tablet or capsule—Swallow with liquid or food to lessen stomach irritation.
- Suppositories—Remove wrapper and moisten suppository with water. Gently insert into rectum, large end first.
- Drops or liquid—Dilute dose in beverage.

When to take:
- Nervous and mental disorders—Take at the same times each day.
- Nausea and vomiting—Take as needed, no more often than every 4 hours.

If you forget a dose:
- Nervous and mental disorders—Take up to 2 hours late. If more than 2 hours, wait for next scheduled dose (don't double this).
- Nausea and vomiting—Take as soon as you remember. Wait 4 hours for next dose.

What drug does:
- Suppresses brain's vomiting center.
- Suppresses brain centers that control abnormal emotions and behavior.

Time lapse before drug works:
- Nausea and vomiting—1 hour or less.
- Nervous and mental disorders—4-6 weeks.

Don't take with:
- Antacid or medicine for diarrhea.
- Non-prescription drug for cough, cold or allergy.
- See Interaction column and consult doctor.

OVERDOSE

Symptoms:
Stupor, convulsions, coma.

What to do:
- Dial 0 (operator) or 911 (emergency) for an ambulance or medical help. Then give first aid immediately.
- Additional emergency information on page 886.

POSSIBLE ADVERSE REACTIONS OR SIDE EFFECTS

SYMPTOMS	FREQUENCY	WHAT TO DO
Brain & nervous system:		
• Restlessness, tremor.	Common	3
• Fainting	Infrequent	2
• Drowsiness	Common	3
Skin:		
• Rash	Infrequent	3
• Less perspiration.	Common	4
Eyes:		
Vision changes.	Rare	3
Ears, nose, throat:		
• Sore throat, fever.	Rare	3
• Dry mouth, nasal congestion.	Common	4
Digestive:		
Constipation	Common	4
Heart & lungs, blood vessels, kidneys, allergic, blood:	None expected.	
Muscles, bones, joints:		
Muscle spasms of face and neck, unsteady gait.	Common	2
Genital, urinary:		
Urination difficulty.	Infrequent	4
Liver:		
Jaundice (yellow eyes and skin).	Rare	3
Others:		
Less interest in sex, breast swelling, change in menstrual pattern.	Infrequent	4

1- Life-threatening. Seek emergency treatment immediately.
2- Discontinue. Seek emergency treatment.
3- Discontinue. Call doctor right away.
4- Continue. Call doctor when convenient.
5- Continue. Tell doctor at next visit.
6- No action necessary.

WARNINGS & PRECAUTIONS

Don't take if:
- You are allergic to any phenothiazine.
- You have a blood or bone-marrow disease.

Before you start, consult your doctor:
- If you will have surgery within 2 months, including dental surgery, requiring general or spinal anesthesia.
- If you have asthma, emphysema or other lung disorder.
- If you take non-prescription ulcer medicine, asthma medicine or amphetamines.

Over age 60:
Adverse reactions and side effects may be more frequent and severe than in younger persons. More likely to develop involuntary movement of jaws, lips, tongue, chewing. Report this to your doctor immediately. Early treatment can help.

Pregnancy:
Risk to unborn child outweighs drug benefits. Don't use.

Breast-feeding:
Drug passes into milk. Avoid drug or discontinue nursing until you finish medicine. Consult doctor for advice on maintaining milk supply.

Infants & children:
Don't give to children younger than 2.

Prolonged use:
May lead to tardive dyskinesia (involuntary movement of jaws, lips, tongue, chewing).

Skin & sunlight:
May cause rash or intensify sunburn in areas exposed to sun or sunlamp. Skin may remain sensitive for 3 months after discontinuing.

Driving, piloting or hazardous work:
Don't drive or pilot aircraft until you learn how medicine affects you. Don't work around dangerous machinery. Don't climb ladders or work in high places. Danger increases if you drink alcohol or take medicine affecting alertness and reflexes.

Airplane passengers:
No problems expected.

Discontinuing:
- Nervous and mental disorders—Don't discontinue without doctor's advice until you complete prescribed dose, even though symptoms diminish or disappear.
- Nausea and vomiting—May be unnecessary to finish medicine. Follow doctor's instructions.

INTERACTION WITH OTHER DRUGS

GENERIC NAME OR DRUG CLASS	COMBINED EFFECT
Anticholinergics	Increased anticholinergic effect.
Antidepressants (tricyclic)	Increased prochlorperazine effect.
Antihistamines	Increased antihistamine effect.
Appetite suppressants	Decreased suppressant effect.
Levodopa	Decreased levodopa effect.
Mind-altering drugs	Increased effect of mind-altering drugs.
Narcotics	Increased narcotic effect.
Phenytoin	Increased phenytoin effect.
Quinidine	Impaired heart function. Dangerous mixture.
Sedatives	Increased sedative effect.
Tranquilizers (other)	Increased tranquilizer effect.

INTERACTION WITH OTHER SUBSTANCES

INTERACTS WITH	COMBINED EFFECT
Alcohol:	Dangerous oversedation.
Beverages:	None expected.
Cocaine:	Decreased prochlorperazine effect. Avoid.
Foods:	None expected.
Marijuana:	Drowsiness. May increase antinausea effect.
Tobacco:	None expected.

PROCYCLIDINE

BRAND NAMES

Kemadrin

GENERAL INFORMATION

Habit forming? No
Prescription needed? Yes
Available as generic? No
Drug class: Antidyskinetic, antiparkinsonism

 USES

- Treatment of Parkinson's disease.
- Treatment of adverse effects of phenothiazines.

 DOSAGE & USAGE INFORMATION

How to take:
Tablets or capsules—Take with food to lessen stomach irritation.

When to take:
At the same times each day.

If you forget a dose:
Take as soon as you remember up to 2 hours late. If more than 2 hours, wait for next scheduled dose (don't double this dose).

What drug does:
- Balances chemical reactions necessary to send nerve impulses within base of brain.
- Improves muscle control and reduces stiffness.

Time lapse before drug works:
1 to 2 hours.

Don't take with:
- Non-prescription drugs for colds, cough or allergy.
- See Interaction column and consult doctor.

 OVERDOSE

Symptoms:
Agitation, dilated pupils, hallucinations, dry mouth, rapid heartbeat, sleepiness.

What to do:
- Dial 0 (operator) or 911 (emergency) for an ambulance or medical help. Then give first aid immediately.
- If patient is unconscious and not breathing, give mouth-to-mouth breathing. If there is no heartbeat, use cardiac massage and mouth-to-mouth breathing (CPR). Don't try to make patient vomit. If you can't get help quickly, take patient to nearest emergency facility.
- Additional emergency information on page 886.

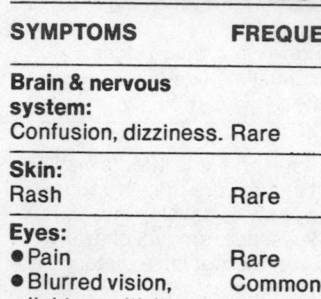 **POSSIBLE ADVERSE REACTIONS OR SIDE EFFECTS**

SYMPTOMS	FREQUENCY	WHAT TO DO
Brain & nervous system: Confusion, dizziness.	Rare	4
Skin: Rash	Rare	3
Eyes:		
• Pain	Rare	3
• Blurred vision, light sensitivity.	Common	4
Ears, nose, throat: Sore mouth or tongue.	Rare	4
Digestive:		
• Constipation	Common	4
• Nausea, vomiting.	Common	4
Heart & lungs:	None expected.	
Blood vessels:	None expected.	
Muscles, bones, joints:		
• Muscle cramps.	Rare	4
• Numbness, weakness in hands or feet.	Rare	4
Genital, urinary: Difficult or painful urination.	Common	5
Kidneys:	None expected.	
Liver:	None expected.	
Allergic:	None expected.	
Blood:	None expected.	
Others:	None expected.	

1- Life-threatening. Seek emergency treatment immediately.
2- Discontinue. Seek emergency treatment.
3- Discontinue. Call doctor right away.
4- Continue. Call doctor when convenient.
5- Continue. Tell doctor at next visit.
6- No action necessary.

WARNINGS & PRECAUTIONS

Don't take if:
You are allergic to any antidyskinetic.

Before you start, consult your doctor:
- If you have had glaucoma.
- If you have had high blood pressure or heart disease.
- If you have had impaired liver function.
- If you have had kidney disease or urination difficulty.

Over age 60:
More sensitive to drug. Aggravates symptoms of enlarged prostate. Causes impaired thinking, hallucinations, nightmares. Consult doctor about any of these.

Pregnancy:
Studies inconclusive on harm to unborn child. Animal studies show fetal abnormalities. Decide with your doctor whether drug benefits justify risk to unborn child.

Breast-feeding:
No problems expected.

Infants & children:
Not recommended for children 3 and younger. Use for older children only under doctor's supervision.

Prolonged use:
Possible glaucoma.

Skin & sunlight:
No problems expected.

Driving, piloting or hazardous work:
Don't drive or pilot aircraft until you learn how medicine affects you. Don't work around dangerous machinery. Don't climb ladders or work in high places. Danger increases if you drink alcohol or take medicine affecting alertness and reflexes, such as antihistamines, tranquilizers, sedatives, pain medicine, narcotics and mind-altering drugs.

Airplane passengers:
No problems expected.

Discontinuing:
Don't discontinue without consulting doctor. Dose may require gradual reduction if you have taken drug for a long time. Doses of other drugs may also require adjustment.

Others:
- Internal eye pressure should be measured regularly.
- Avoid becoming overheated.

INTERACTION WITH OTHER DRUGS

GENERIC NAME OR DRUG CLASS	COMBINED EFFECT
Amantadine	Increased amantadine effect.
Antidepressants (tricyclic)	Increased procyclidine effect. May cause glaucoma.
Antihistamines	Increased procyclidine effect.
Levodopa	Increased levodopa effect. Improved results in treating Parkinson's disease.
Meperidine	Increased procyclidine effect.
MAO inhibitors	Increased procyclidine effect.
Orphenadrine	Increased procyclidine effect.
Phenothiazines	Behavior changes.
Primidone	Excessive sedation.
Procainamide	Increased procainamide effect.
Quinidine	Increased procyclidine effect.
Tranquilizers	Excessive sedation.

INTERACTION WITH OTHER SUBSTANCES

INTERACTS WITH	COMBINED EFFECT
Alcohol:	None expected.
Beverages:	None expected.
Cocaine:	Decreased procyclidine effect. Avoid.
Foods:	None expected.
Marijuana:	None expected.
Tobacco:	None expected.

PROMAZINE

BRAND NAMES

Norzine
Promanyl
Sparine

GENERAL INFORMATION

Habit forming? No
Prescription needed? Yes
Available as generic? Yes
Drug class: Tranquilizer, antiemetic (phenothiazine)

USES

- Stops nausea, vomiting.
- Reduces anxiety, agitation.

DOSAGE & USAGE INFORMATION

How to take:
- Tablet or capsule—Swallow with liquid or food to lessen stomach irritation.
- Suppositories—Remove wrapper and moisten suppository with water. Gently insert into rectum, large end first.
- Drops or liquid—Dilute dose in beverage.

When to take:
- Nervous and mental disorders—Take at the same times each day.
- Nausea and vomiting—Take as needed, no more often than every 4 hours.

If you forget a dose:
- Nervous and mental disorders—Take up to 2 hours late. If more than 2 hours, wait for next scheduled dose (don't double this).
- Nausea and vomiting—Take as soon as you remember. Wait 4 hours for next dose.

What drug does:
- Suppresses brain's vomiting center.
- Suppresses brain centers that control abnormal emotions and behavior.

Time lapse before drug works:
- Nausea and vomiting—1 hour or less.
- Nervous and mental disorders—4-6 weeks.

Don't take with:
- Antacid or medicine for diarrhea.
- Non-prescription drug for cough, cold or allergy.
- See Interaction column and consult doctor.

OVERDOSE

Symptoms:
Stupor, convulsions, coma.

What to do:
- Dial 0 (operator) or 911 (emergency) for an ambulance or medical help. Then give first aid immediately.
- Additional emergency information on page 886.

POSSIBLE ADVERSE REACTIONS OR SIDE EFFECTS

SYMPTOMS	FREQUENCY	WHAT TO DO
Brain & nervous system:		
• Restlessness, tremor.	Common	3
• Fainting	Infrequent	2
• Drowsiness	Common	3
Skin:		
• Rash	Infrequent	3
• Less perspiration.	Common	4
Eyes:		
Vision changes.	Rare	3
Ears, nose, throat:		
• Sore throat, fever.	Rare	3
• Dry mouth, nasal congestion.	Common	4
Digestive:		
Constipation	Common	4
Heart & lungs, blood vessels, kidneys, allergic, blood:	None expected.	
Muscles, bones, joints:		
Muscle spasms of face and neck, unsteady gait.	Common	2
Genital, urinary:		
Urination difficulty.	Infrequent	4
Liver:		
Jaundice (yellow eyes and skin).	Rare	3
Others:		
Less interest in sex, breast swelling, change in menstrual pattern.	Infrequent	4

1- Life-threatening. Seek emergency treatment immediately.
2- Discontinue. Seek emergency treatment.
3- Discontinue. Call doctor right away.
4- Continue. Call doctor when convenient.
5- Continue. Tell doctor at next visit.
6- No action necessary.

WARNINGS & PRECAUTIONS

Don't take if:
- You are allergic to any phenothiazine.
- You have a blood or bone-marrow disease.

Before you start, consult your doctor:
- If you will have surgery within 2 months, including dental surgery, requiring general or spinal anesthesia.
- If you have asthma, emphysema or other lung disorder.
- If you take non-prescription ulcer medicine, asthma medicine or amphetamines.

Over age 60:
Adverse reactions and side effects may be more frequent and severe than in younger persons. More likely to develop involuntary movement of jaws, lips, tongue, chewing. Report this to your doctor immediately. Early treatment can help.

Pregnancy:
Risk to unborn child outweighs drug benefits. Don't use.

Breast-feeding:
Drug passes into milk. Avoid drug or discontinue nursing until you finish medicine. Consult doctor for advice on maintaining milk supply.

Infants & children:
Don't give to children younger than 2.

Prolonged use:
May lead to tardive dyskinesia (involuntary movement of jaws, lips, tongue, chewing).

Skin & sunlight:
May cause rash or intensify sunburn in areas exposed to sun or sunlamp. Skin may remain sensitive for 3 months after discontinuing.

Driving, piloting or hazardous work:
Don't drive or pilot aircraft until you learn how medicine affects you. Don't work around dangerous machinery. Don't climb ladders or work in high places. Danger increases if you drink alcohol or take medicine affecting alertness and reflexes.

Airplane passengers:
No problems expected.

Discontinuing:
- Nervous and mental disorders—Don't discontinue without doctor's advice until you complete prescribed dose, even though symptoms diminish or disappear.
- Nausea and vomiting—May be unnecessary to finish medicine. Follow doctor's instructions.

INTERACTION WITH OTHER DRUGS

GENERIC NAME OR DRUG CLASS	COMBINED EFFECT
Anticholinergics	Increased anticholinergic effect.
Antidepressants (tricyclic)	Increased promazine effect.
Antihistamines	Increased antihistamine effect.
Appetite suppressants	Decreased suppressant effect.
Levodopa	Decreased levodopa effect.
Mind-altering drugs	Increased effect of mind-altering drugs.
Narcotics	Increased narcotic effect.
Phenytoin	Increased phenytoin effect.
Quinidine	Impaired heart function. Dangerous mixture.
Sedatives	Increased sedative effect.
Tranquilizers (other)	Increased tranquilizer effect.

INTERACTION WITH OTHER SUBSTANCES

INTERACTS WITH	COMBINED EFFECT
Alcohol:	Dangerous oversedation.
Beverages:	None expected.
Cocaine:	Decreased promazine effect. Avoid.
Foods:	None expected.
Marijuana:	Drowsiness. May increase antinausea effect.
Tobacco:	None expected.

PROMETHAZINE

BRAND NAMES

Baymethazine	Mepergan Fortis (M)	Prosedin
Fellozine	Pentazine	Provigan
Ganphen	Phenergan	Remsed
Histanil	Phenerhist	Synalgos (M)
K-Phen	Prorex	ZiPan

GENERAL INFORMATION

Habit forming? No
Prescription needed? Yes
Available as generic? Yes
Drug class: Antihistamine,
tranquilizer (phenothiazine)

USES

- Stops nausea, vomiting and dizziness of motion sickness.
- Produces mild sedation and light sleep.
- Reduces allergic symptoms of hay fever and hives.

DOSAGE & USAGE INFORMATION

How to take:
- Tablets or liquid—Swallow with water.
- Suppositories—Remove wrapper and moisten suppository with water. Gently insert larger end into rectum. Push well into rectum with finger.

When to take:
Take as needed, no more often than every 12 hours.

If you forget a dose:
Take as soon as you remember. Wait 12 hours for next dose.

What drug does:
- Blocks stimulation of brain's vomiting center.
- Suppresses brain centers that control abnormal emotions and behavior.
- Blocks histamine action in sensitized cells.

Time lapse before drug works:
1 to 2 hours.

Don't take with:
- Antacid or medicine for diarrhea.
- Non-prescription drug for cough, cold or allergy.
- See Interaction column and consult doctor.

OVERDOSE

Symptoms:
Stupor, convulsions, coma.

What to do:
- Dial 0 (operator) or 911 (emergency) for an ambulance or medical help. Then give first aid immediately.
- Additional emergency information on page 886.

POSSIBLE ADVERSE REACTIONS OR SIDE EFFECTS

SYMPTOMS	FREQUENCY	WHAT TO DO
Brain & nervous system:		
• Restlessness, tremor, drowsiness.	Common	3
• Fainting	Infrequent	2
Skin:		
• Rash	Infrequent	3
• Less perspiration.	Common	4
Eyes:		
Vision changes.	Rare	3
Ears, nose, throat:		
• Sore throat, fever.	Rare	3
• Dry mouth, nasal congestion.	Common	4
Digestive:		
Constipation	Common	4
Heart & lungs:	None expected.	
Blood vessels:	None expected.	
Muscles, bones, joints:		
Muscle spasms of face and neck, unsteady gait.	Infrequent	3
Genital, urinary:		
Urination difficulty.	Infrequent	4
Kidneys:	None expected.	
Liver:		
Jaundice (yellow eyes and skin).	Rare	3
Allergic:	None expected.	
Blood:	None expected.	
Others:		
Less interest in sex, breast swelling, menstrual changes.	Infrequent	4

1 - Life-threatening. Seek emergency treatment immediately.
2 - Discontinue. Seek emergency treatment.
3 - Discontinue. Call doctor right away.
4 - Continue. Call doctor when convenient.

WARNINGS & PRECAUTIONS

Don't take if:
- You are allergic to any phenothiazine.
- You have a blood or bone-marrow disease.

Before you start, consult your doctor:
- If you will have surgery within 2 months, including dental surgery, requiring general or spinal anesthesia.
- If you have asthma, emphysema or other lung disorder.
- If you take non-prescription ulcer medicine, asthma medicine or amphetamines.

Over age 60:
Adverse reactions and side effects may be more frequent and severe than in younger persons. More likely to develop tardive dyskinesia (involuntary movement of jaws, lips, tongue, chewing). Report this to your doctor immediately. Early treatment can help.

Pregnancy:
Risk to unborn child outweighs drug benefits. Don't use.

Breast-feeding:
Drug passes into milk. Avoid drug or discontinue nursing until you finish medicine. Consult doctor for advice on maintaining milk supply.

Infants & children:
Don't give to children younger than 2.

Prolonged use:
May lead to tardive dyskinesia (involuntary movement of jaws, lips, tongue, chewing).

Skin & sunlight:
May cause rash or intensify sunburn in areas exposed to sun or sunlamp. Skin may remain sensitive for 3 months after discontinuing.

Driving, piloting or hazardous work:
Don't drive or pilot aircraft until you learn how medicine affects you. Don't work around dangerous machinery. Don't climb ladders or work in high places. Danger increases if you drink alcohol or take medicine affecting alertness and reflexes.

Airplane passengers:
No problems expected.

Discontinuing:
- Nervous and mental disorders—Don't discontinue without doctor's advice until you complete prescribed dose, even though symptoms diminish or disappear.
- Nausea, vomiting or allergy—May be unnecessary to finish medicine. Follow doctor's instructions.

INTERACTION WITH OTHER DRUGS

GENERIC NAME OR DRUG CLASS	COMBINED EFFECT
Antacids	Decreased promethazine effect.
Anticholinergics	Increased anticholinergic effect.
Anticonvulsants (hydantoin)	Increased anticonvulsant effect.
Antidepressants (tricyclic)	Increased promethazine effect.
Antihistamines (other)	Increased antihistamine effect.
Appetite suppressants	Decreased suppressant effect.
Barbiturates	Oversedation.
Guanethidine	Decreased guanethidine effect.
Levodopa	Decreased levodopa effect.
MAO inhibitors	Increased promethazine effect.
Mind-altering drugs	Increased effect of mind-altering drugs.
Narcotics	Increased narcotic effect.
Sedatives	Increased sedative effect.
Tranquilizers (other)	Increased tranquilizer effect.

INTERACTION WITH OTHER SUBSTANCES

INTERACTS WITH	COMBINED EFFECT
Alcohol:	Dangerous oversedation.
Beverages:	None expected.
Cocaine:	Decreased promethazine effect. Avoid.
Foods:	None expected.
Marijuana:	Drowsiness. May increase antinausea effect.
Tobacco:	None expected.

PROPANTHELINE

BRAND NAMES

Banlin
Norpanth
Novopropanthil
Pro-Banthine
Pro-Banthine with
 Phenobarbital (M)

Propanthel
Ropanth
SK-Propantheline

GENERAL INFORMATION

Habit forming? No
Prescription needed? Low strength: No
High strength: Yes
Available as generic? Yes
Drug class: Antispasmodic, anticholinergic

 ## USES

Reduces spasms of digestive system, bladder and urethra.

 ## DOSAGE & USAGE INFORMATION

How to take:
Tablet—Swallow with liquid or food to lessen stomach irritation.

When to take:
30 minutes before meals (unless directed otherwise by doctor).

If you forget a dose:
Take as soon as you remember up to 2 hours late. If more than 2 hours, wait for next scheduled dose (don't double this dose).

What drug does:
Blocks nerve impulses at parasympathetic nerve endings, preventing muscle contractions and gland secretions of organs involved.

Time lapse before drug works:
15 to 30 minutes.

Don't take with:
See Interaction column and consult doctor.

 ## OVERDOSE

Symptoms:
Dilated pupils; rapid pulse and breathing; dizziness; fever; hallucinations; confusion; slurred speech; agitation; flushed face; convulsions; coma.

What to do:
- Dial 0 (operator) or 911 (emergency) for an ambulance or medical help. Then give first aid immediately.
- Additional emergency information on page 886.

POSSIBLE ADVERSE REACTIONS OR SIDE EFFECTS

SYMPTOMS	FREQUENCY	WHAT TO DO
Brain & nervous system:		
• Headache	Infrequent	4
• Confusion, delirium.	Common	3
Skin:		
Rash or hives.	Rare	3
Eyes:		
Pain, blurred vision.	Rare	3
Ears, nose, throat:		
Dryness	Common	6
Digestive:		
• Constipation	Common	5
• Nausea, vomiting.	Common	4
Heart & lungs:		
Rapid heartbeat.	Common	3
Blood vessels:	None expected.	
Muscles, bones, joints:	None expected.	
Genital, urinary:		
Difficult urination.	Infrequent	4
Kidneys:	None expected.	
Liver:	None expected.	
Allergic:	None expected.	
Blood:	None expected.	
Others:		
Less perspiration.	Common	4

1- Life-threatening. Seek emergency treatment immediately.
2- Discontinue. Seek emergency treatment.
3- Discontinue. Call doctor right away.
4- Continue. Call doctor when convenient.
5- Continue. Tell doctor at next visit.
6- No action necessary.

PROPANTHELINE

WARNINGS & PRECAUTIONS

Don't take if:
- You are allergic to any anticholinergic.
- You have trouble with stomach bloating.
- You have difficulty emptying your bladder completely.
- You have narrow-angle glaucoma.
- You have severe ulcerative colitis.

Before you start, consult your doctor:
- If you have open-angle glaucoma.
- If you have angina.
- If you have chronic bronchitis or asthma.
- If you have hiatal hernia.
- If you have liver disease.
- If you have enlarged prostate.
- If you have myasthenia gravis.
- If you have peptic ulcer.
- If you will have surgery within 2 months, including dental surgery, requiring general or spinal anesthesia.

Over age 60:
Adverse reactions and side effects may be more frequent and severe than in younger persons.

Pregnancy:
Studies inconclusive on harm to unborn child. Animal studies show fetal abnormalities. Decide with your doctor whether drug benefits justify risk to unborn child.

Breast-feeding:
Drug passes into milk and decreases milk flow. Avoid drug or discontinue nursing until you finish medicine. Consult doctor for advice on maintaining milk supply.

Infants & children:
Use only under medical supervision.

Prolonged use:
Chronic constipation, possible fecal impaction. Consult doctor immediately.

Skin & sunlight:
No problems expected.

Driving, piloting or hazardous work:
Use disqualifies you for piloting aircraft. Otherwise, no problems expected.

Airplane passengers:
No problems expected.

Discontinuing:
May be unnecessary to finish medicine. Follow doctor's instructions.

Others:
No problems expected.

INTERACTION WITH OTHER DRUGS

GENERIC NAME OR DRUG CLASS	COMBINED EFFECT
Amantadine	Increased propantheline effect.
Anticholinergics (other)	Increased propantheline effect.
Antidepressants (tricyclic)	Increased propantheline effect.
Antihistamines	Increased propantheline effect.
Cortisone drugs	Increased internal eye pressure.
Haloperidol	Increased internal eye pressure.
MAO inhibitors	Increased propantheline effect.
Meperidine	Increased propantheline effect.
Methylphenidate	Increased propantheline effect.
Orphenadrine	Increased propantheline effect.
Phenothiazines	Increased propantheline effect.
Pilocarpine	Loss of pilocarpine effect in glaucoma treatment.
Vitamin C	Decreased propantheline effect. Avoid large doses of vitamin C.

INTERACTION WITH OTHER SUBSTANCES

INTERACTS WITH	COMBINED EFFECT
Alcohol:	None expected.
Beverages:	None expected.
Cocaine:	Excessively rapid heartbeat. Avoid.
Foods:	None expected.
Marijuana:	Drowsiness and dry mouth.
Tobacco:	None expected.

PROPOXYPHENE

BRAND NAMES

Algodex	Pargesic 65	642
Darvon	Pro-65	
Depronal-SA	Proxagesic	
Dolene	Proxene	
Novoproproxyn	SK-65	

GENERAL INFORMATION

Habit forming? Yes
Prescription needed? Yes
Available as generic? Yes
Drug class: Narcotic

 USES

Relieves pain.

 DOSAGE & USAGE INFORMATION

How to take:
- Tablet or capsule—Swallow with liquid. If you can't swallow whole, crumble tablet or open capsule and take with liquid or food.
- Drops or liquid—Dilute dose in beverage before swallowing.

When to take:
When needed. No more often than every 4 hours.

If you forget a dose:
Take as soon as you remember. Wait 4 hours for next dose.

What drug does:
Blocks pain message to brain and spinal cord.

Time lapse before drug works:
30 minutes.

Don't take with:
See Interaction column and consult doctor.

 OVERDOSE

Symptoms:
Deep sleep; slow breathing; slow pulse; flushed, warm skin; constricted pupils.

What to do:
- Dial 0 (operator) or 911 (emergency) for an ambulance or medical help. Then give first aid immediately.
- If patient is unconscious and not breathing, give mouth-to-mouth breathing. If there is no heartbeat, use cardiac massage and mouth-to-mouth breathing (CPR). Don't try to make patient vomit. If you can't get help quickly, take patient to nearest emergency facility.
- Additional emergency information on page 886.

POSSIBLE ADVERSE REACTIONS OR SIDE EFFECTS

SYMPTOMS	FREQUENCY	WHAT TO DO
Brain & nervous system: Depression, confusion, hallucinations.	Infrequent	4
Skin:		
• Hives, rash, itch, face swelling.	Rare	3
• Flushed face.	Common	4
Eyes: Blurred vision.	Rare	4
Ears, nose, throat:	None expected.	
Digestive: Severe constipation, abdominal pain, vomiting.	Infrequent	3
Heart & lungs: Slow heartbeat, irregular breathing.	Rare	3
Blood vessels:	None expected.	
Muscles, bones, joints:	None expected.	
Genital, urinary: Difficult urination.	Common	4
Kidneys: Less urine.	Common	4
Liver:	None expected.	
Allergic:	None expected.	
Blood:	None expected.	
Others: Unusual tiredness.	Common	4

1- Life-threatening. Seek emergency treatment immediately.
2- Discontinue. Seek emergency treatment.
3- Discontinue. Call doctor right away.
4- Continue. Call doctor when convenient.
5- Continue. Tell doctor at next visit.
6- No action necessary.

WARNINGS & PRECAUTIONS

Don't take if:
You are allergic to any narcotic.

Before you start, consult your doctor:
If you have impaired liver or kidney function.

Over age 60:
More likely to be drowsy, dizzy, unsteady or constipated. Avoid prolonged use.

Pregnancy:
Studies inconclusive on harm to unborn child. Animal studies show fetal abnormalities. Decide with your doctor whether drug benefits justify risk to unborn child. Abuse by pregnant woman will result in addicted newborn. Withdrawal can be life-threatening.

Breast-feeding:
Drug filters into milk. May depress infant. Avoid.

Infants & children:
Not recommended.

Prolonged use:
Causes psychological and physical dependence.

Skin & sunlight:
No problems expected.

Driving, piloting or hazardous work:
Don't drive or pilot aircraft until you learn how medicine affects you. Don't work around dangerous machinery. Don't climb ladders or work in high places. Danger increases if you drink alcohol or take medicine affecting alertness and reflexes, such as antihistamines, tranquilizers, sedatives, pain medicine, other narcotics and mind-altering drugs.

Airplane passengers:
No proven problems.

Discontinuing:
May be unnecessary to finish medicine. Follow doctor's instructions.

Others:
No problems expected.

INTERACTION WITH OTHER DRUGS

GENERIC NAME OR DRUG CLASS	COMBINED EFFECT
Analgesics	Increased analgesic effect.
Antidepressants	Increased sedative effect.
Antihistamines	Increased sedative effect.
Mind-altering drugs	Increased sedative effect.
Narcotics (other)	Increased narcotic effect.
Phenothiazines	Increased phenothiazine effect.
Sedatives	Increased sedative effect.
Sleep inducers	Increased sedative effect.
Tranquilizers	Increased sedative effect.

INTERACTION WITH OTHER SUBSTANCES

INTERACTS WITH	COMBINED EFFECT
Alcohol:	Increases alcohol's intoxicating effect. Avoid.
Beverages:	None expected.
Cocaine:	Increased cocaine effect.
Foods:	None expected.
Marijuana:	Impairs physical and mental performance.
Tobacco:	None expected.

PROPRANOLOL

BRAND NAMES

Inderal
Inderide (M)

GENERAL INFORMATION

Habit forming? No
Prescription needed? Yes
Available as generic? No
Drug class: Beta-adrenergic blocker

USES

- Reduces angina attacks.
- Stabilizes irregular heartbeat.
- Lowers blood pressure.
- Reduces frequency of migraine headaches. (Does not relieve headache pain.)
- Other uses prescribed by your doctor.

DOSAGE & USAGE INFORMATION

How to take:
Tablet or capsule—Swallow with liquid. If you can't swallow whole, crumble tablet or open capsule and take with liquid or food.

When to take:
With meals or immediately after.

If you forget a dose:
Take as soon as you remember. Return to regular schedule, but allow 3 hours between doses.

What drug does:
- Blocks certain actions of sympathetic nervous system.
- Lowers heart's oxygen requirements.
- Slows nerve impulses through heart.
- Reduces blood vessel contraction in heart, scalp and other body parts.

Time lapse before drug works:
1 to 4 hours.

Don't take with:
Non-prescription drugs or drugs in Interaction column without consulting doctor.

OVERDOSE

Symptoms:
Weakness, slow or weak pulse, blood pressure drop, fainting, convulsions, cold and sweaty skin.

What to do:
- Dial O (operator) or 911 (emergency) for an ambulance or medical help. Then give first aid immediately.
- Additional emergency information on page 886.

POSSIBLE ADVERSE REACTIONS OR SIDE EFFECTS

SYMPTOMS	FREQUENCY	WHAT TO DO
Brain & nervous system:		
● Hallucinations, nightmares, insomnia, headache.	Infrequent	3
● Confusion, depression, reduced alertness.	Infrequent	4
● Drowsiness, numbness or tingling of fingers or toes, dizziness.	Common	4
Skin:		
Rash	Rare	3
Eyes:	None expected.	
Ears, nose, throat:		
Sore throat, fever.	Rare	3
Digestive:		
● Diarrhea, nausea.	Common	4
● Constipation	Infrequent	5
Heart & lungs:		
● Pulse slower than 50 beats per minute.	Common	3
● Breathing difficulty.	Infrequent	3
Blood vessels:		
Cold hands, feet.	Common	5
Muscles, bones, joints, genital, urinary, kidneys, liver, allergic:	None expected.	
Blood:		
Unusual bleeding and bruising.	Rare	4
Others:		
● Fatigue, weakness.	Common	4
● Dry mouth, eyes, skin.	Common	5

1 - Life-threatening. Seek emergency treatment immediately.
2 - Discontinue. Seek emergency treatment.
3 - Discontinue. Call doctor right away.
4 - Continue. Call doctor when convenient.
5 - Continue. Tell doctor at next visit.

WARNINGS & PRECAUTIONS

Don't take if:
- You are allergic to any beta-adrenergic blocker.
- You have asthma.
- You have hay fever symptoms.
- You have taken MAO inhibitors in past 2 weeks.

Before you start, consult your doctor:
- If you have heart disease or poor circulation to the extremities.
- If you have hay fever, asthma, chronic bronchitis, emphysema.
- If you have overactive thyroid function.
- If you have impaired liver or kidney function.
- If you will have surgery within 2 months, including dental surgery, requiring general or spinal anesthesia.
- If you have diabetes or hypoglycemia.

Over age 60:
Adverse reactions and side effects may be more frequent and severe than in younger persons.

Pregnancy:
Risk to unborn child outweighs drug benefits. Don't use.

Breast-feeding:
Drug passes into milk. Avoid drug or discontinue nursing until you finish medicine. Consult doctor for advice on maintaining milk supply.

Infants & children:
Not recommended.

Prolonged use:
Weakens heart muscle contractions.

Skin & sunlight:
No problems expected.

Driving, piloting or hazardous work:
Don't drive or pilot aircraft until you learn how medicine affects you. Don't work around dangerous machinery. Don't climb ladders or work in high places. Danger increases if you drink alcohol or take medicine affecting alertness and reflexes.

Airplane passengers:
No problems expected.

Discontinuing:
Don't discontinue without consulting doctor. Dose may require gradual reduction if you have taken drug for a long time. Doses of other drugs may also require adjustment.

Others:
May mask hypoglycemia.

INTERACTION WITH OTHER DRUGS

GENERIC NAME OR DRUG CLASS	COMBINED EFFECT
Antidiabetics	Increased antidiabetic effect.
Antihistamines	Decreased antihistamine effect.
Antihypertensives	Increased antihypertensive effect.
Antiinflammatory drugs	Decreased antiinflammatory effect.
Barbiturates	Increased barbiturate effect. Dangerous sedation.
Digitalis preparations	Can either increase or decrease heart rate. Improves irregular heartbeat.
Narcotics	Increased narcotic effect. Dangerous sedation.
Phenytoin	Increased propranolol effect.
Quinidine	Slows heart excessively.
Reserpine	Increased reserpine effect. Excessive sedation and depression.

INTERACTION WITH OTHER SUBSTANCES

INTERACTS WITH	COMBINED EFFECT
Alcohol:	Excessive blood-pressure drop. Avoid.
Beverages:	None expected.
Cocaine:	Irregular heartbeat. Avoid.
Foods:	None expected.
Marijuana:	Daily use—Impaired circulation to hands and feet.
Tobacco:	Possible irregular heartbeat.

PROTRIPTYLINE

BRAND NAMES

Vivactil

GENERAL INFORMATION

Habit forming? No
Prescription needed? Yes
Available as generic? No
Drug class: Antidepressant (tricyclic)

USES

Gradually relieves, but doesn't cure, symptoms of depression.

DOSAGE & USAGE INFORMATION

How to take:
Tablet—Swallow with liquid.

When to take:
At the same time each day, usually bedtime.

If you forget a dose:
Bedtime dose—If you forget your once-a-day bedtime dose, don't take it more than 3 hours late. If more than 3 hours, wait for next scheduled dose. Don't double this dose.

What drug does:
Probably affects part of brain that controls messages between nerve cells.

Time lapse before drug works:
Begins in 1 to 2 weeks. May require 4 to 6 weeks for maximum benefit.

Don't take with:
- Non-prescription drugs without consulting doctor.
- See Interaction column and consult doctor.

OVERDOSE

Symptoms:
Hallucinations, convulsions, coma.

What to do:
- Dial 0 (operator) or 911 (emergency) for an ambulance or medical help. Then give first aid immediately.
- If patient is unconscious and not breathing, give mouth-to-mouth breathing. If there is no heartbeat, use cardiac massage and mouth-to-mouth breathing (CPR). Don't try to make patient vomit. If you can't get help quickly, take patient to nearest emergency facility.
- Additional emergency information on page 886.

POSSIBLE ADVERSE REACTIONS OR SIDE EFFECTS

SYMPTOMS	FREQUENCY	WHAT TO DO
Brain & nervous system:		
• Hallucinations, shakiness, dizziness, fainting.	Infrequent	3
• Headache	Common	4
• Seizures	Rare	1
• Insomnia	Common	5
Skin:		
Rash, itch.	Rare	3
Eyes:		
Blurred vision, pain.	Infrequent	3
Ears, nose, throat:		
• Sore throat.	Rare	3
• Dry mouth or unpleasant taste.	Common	4
Digestive:		
• Constipation or diarrhea, nausea, indigestion.	Common	4
• Vomiting	Infrequent	3
• "Sweet tooth"	Common	5
Heart & lungs:		
Irregular heartbeat or slow pulse.	Infrequent	3
Blood vessels, muscles, bones, joints, kidneys, allergic, blood:	None expected.	
Genital, urinary:		
Difficulty urinating.	Infrequent	4
Liver:		
Jaundice (yellow skin and eyes).	Rare	3
Others:		
• Fever	Rare	3
• Fatigue, weakness.	Common	4

1 - Life-threatening. Seek emergency treatment immediately.
2 - Discontinue. Seek emergency treatment.
3 - Discontinue. Call doctor right away.
4 - Continue. Call doctor when convenient.
5 - Continue. Tell doctor at next visit.

PROTRIPTYLINE

WARNINGS & PRECAUTIONS

Don't take if:
- You are allergic to any tricyclic antidepressant.
- You drink alcohol.
- You have had a heart attack within 6 weeks.
- You have glaucoma.
- You have taken MAO inhibitors within 2 weeks.
- Patient is younger than 12.

Before you start, consult your doctor:
- If you will have surgery within 2 months, including dental surgery, requiring general or spinal anesthesia.
- If you have an enlarged prostate.
- If you have heart disease or high blood pressure.
- If you have stomach or intestinal problems.
- If you have an overactive thyroid.
- If you have asthma.
- If you have liver disease.

Over age 60:
More likely to develop urination difficulty and side effects under Brain & nervous system.

Pregnancy:
Studies inconclusive on harm to unborn child. Animal studies show fetal abnormalities. Decide with your doctor whether drug benefits justify risk to unborn child.

Breast-feeding:
Drug passes into milk. Avoid drug or discontinue nursing until you finish medicine. Consult doctor for advice on maintaining milk supply.

Infants & children:
Don't give to children younger than 12.

Prolonged use:
No problems expected.

Skin & sunlight:
May cause rash or intensify sunburn in areas exposed to sun or sunlamp.

Driving, piloting or hazardous work:
Don't drive or pilot aircraft until you learn how medicine affects you. Don't work around dangerous machinery. Don't climb ladders or work in high places. Danger increases if you drink alcohol or take medicine affecting alertness and reflexes.

Airplane passengers:
No problems expected.

Discontinuing:
Don't discontinue without consulting doctor. Dose may require gradual reduction if you have taken drug for a long time. Doses of other drugs may also require adjustment.

INTERACTION WITH OTHER DRUGS

GENERIC NAME OR DRUG CLASS	COMBINED EFFECT
Anticoagulants (oral)	Increased anticoagulant effect.
Anticholinergics	Increased sedation.
Antihistamines	Increased antihistamine effect.
Barbiturates	Decreased antidepressant effect.
Clonidine	Decreased clonidine effect.
Diuretics (thiazide)	Increased protriptyline effect.
Ethchlorvynol	Delirium
Guanethidine	Decreased guanethidine effect.
MAO inhibitors	Fever, delirium, convulsions.
Methyldopa	Decreased methyldopa effect.
Narcotics	Dangerous oversedation.
Phenytoin	Decreased phenytoin effect.
Quinidine	Irregular heartbeat.
Sedatives	Dangerous oversedation.
Sympathomimetics	Increased sympathomimetic effect.
Thyroid hormones	Irregular heartbeat.

INTERACTION WITH OTHER SUBSTANCES

INTERACTS WITH	COMBINED EFFECT
Alcohol: Beverages or medicines with alcohol.	Excessive intoxication. Avoid.
Beverages:	None expected.
Cocaine:	Excessive intoxication. Avoid.
Foods:	None expected.
Marijuana:	Excessive drowsiness. Avoid.
Tobacco:	None expected.

PSEUDOEPHEDRINE

BRAND NAMES

Actifed (M)	Dimacol (M)	Fedahist (M)
Afrinol	Disophrol (M)	Fedrazil (M)
Cenafed	Drixoral (M)	Neobid
D-Feda	Eltor	Novafed (M)
Deconamine (M)	Emprazil (M)	Sudafed

See complete brand names list, page 829.

See complete brand names list, page 829.

GENERAL INFORMATION

Habit forming? No
Prescription needed?
U.S.: Low strength—No
High strength—Yes
Canada: No
Available as generic? Yes
Drug class: Sympathomimetic

USES

Reduces congestion of nose, sinuses and throat from allergies and infections.

DOSAGE & USAGE INFORMATION

How to take:
- Tablet or capsule—Swallow with liquid. You may chew or crush tablet.
- Extended-release tablets or capsules—Swallow each dose whole.
- Syrup—Take as directed on label.

When to take:
- At the same times each day.
- To prevent insomnia, take last dose of day a few hours before bedtime.

If you forget a dose:
Take up to 2 hours late. If more than 2 hours, wait for next dose (don't double this).

What drug does:
Decreases blood volume in nasal tissues, shrinking tissues and enlarging airways.

Time lapse before drug works:
15 to 20 minutes.

Don't take with:
- See Interaction column and consult doctor.
- Non-prescription drugs with caffeine without consulting doctor.

OVERDOSE

Symptoms:
Nervousness, restlessness, headache, rapid or irregular heartbeat, sweating, nausea, vomiting, anxiety, confusion, delirium, muscle tremors.

What to do:
- Dial 0 (operator) or 911 (emergency) for an ambulance or medical help. Then give first aid immediately.
- Additional emergency information on page 886.

POSSIBLE ADVERSE REACTIONS OR SIDE EFFECTS

SYMPTOMS	FREQUENCY	WHAT TO DO
Brain & nervous system:		
• Hallucinations, seizures.	Rare	2
• Agitation, insomnia.	Common	5
• Dizziness, headache, trembling, weakness.	Infrequent	4
Skin, eyes, ears, nose, throat, blood vessels, muscles, bones, joints, kidneys, liver, allergic, blood:	None expected.	
Digestive: Nausea or vomiting.	Infrequent	3
Heart & lungs: Irregular or slow heartbeat, breathing difficulty, unusually fast or pounding heartbeat.	Infrequent	3
Genital, urinary: Difficult or painful urination.	Infrequent	3
Others:		
• Increased sweating.	Infrequent	3
• Paleness	Infrequent	5

1- Life-threatening. Seek emergency treatment immediately.
2- Discontinue. Seek emergency treatment.
3- Discontinue. Call doctor right away.
4- Continue. Call doctor when convenient.
5- Continue. Tell doctor at next visit.

PSEUDOEPHEDRINE

WARNINGS & PRECAUTIONS

Don't take if:
You are allergic to any sympathomimetic drug.

Before you start, consult your doctor:
- If you have overactive thyroid or diabetes.
- If you have taken any MAO inhibitors in past 2 weeks.
- If you take digitalis preparations or have high blood pressure or heart disease.
- If you will have surgery within 2 months, including dental surgery, requiring general or spinal anesthesia.
- If you have urination difficulty.

Over age 60:
Adverse reactions and side effects may be more frequent and severe than in younger persons.

Pregnancy:
No proven harm to unborn child. Avoid if possible.

Breast-feeding:
Drug passes into milk. Avoid drug or discontinue nursing until you finish medicine. Consult doctor for advice on maintaining milk supply.

Infants & children:
Keep dose low or avoid.

Prolonged use:
No proven problems.

Skin & sunlight:
No problems expected.

Driving, piloting or hazardous work:
Avoid if you feel dizzy. Otherwise, no problems expected..

Airplane passengers:
Use 30 minutes before departure. Repeat every 4 hours.

Discontinuing:
May be unnecessary to finish medicine. Follow doctor's instructions.

Others:
No problems expected.

INTERACTION WITH OTHER DRUGS

GENERIC NAME OR DRUG CLASS	COMBINED EFFECT
Antidepressants (tricyclic)	Increased pseudoephedrine effect.
Antihypertensives	Decreased antihypertensive effect.
Beta-adrenergic blockers	Decreased effect of beta-adrenergic blockers.
Digitalis preparations	Irregular heartbeat.
Epinephrine	Increased epinephrine effect. Excessive heart stimulation and blood-pressure increase.
Ergot preparations	Serious blood-pressure rise.
Guanethidine	Decreased effect of both drugs.
MAO inhibitors	Increased pseudoephedrine effect.

INTERACTION WITH OTHER SUBSTANCES

INTERACTS WITH	COMBINED EFFECT
Alcohol:	None expected.
Beverages: Caffeine drinks	Nervousness or insomnia.
Cocaine:	Dangerous stimulation. Avoid.
Foods:	None expected.
Marijuana:	Rapid heartbeat.
Tobacco:	None expected.

PSYLLIUM

BRAND NAMES

Effersyllium	Mucilose	Syllact
Hydrocil	Plova	V-Lax
Konsyl	Senokot with Psyllium (M)	
L.A. Formula	Siblin	
Metamucil	Sof-Cil (M)	
Modane Bulk		

GENERAL INFORMATION

Habit forming? No
Prescription needed? No
Available as generic? Yes
Drug class: Laxative (bulk-forming)

 ## USES

Relieves constipation and prevents straining for bowel movement.

 ## DOSAGE & USAGE INFORMATION

How to take:
Powder, flakes or granules—Dilute dose in 8 oz. cold water or fruit juice.

When to take:
At the same time each day, preferably morning.

If you forget a dose:
Take as soon as you remember. Resume regular schedule.

What drug does:
Absorbs water, stimulating the bowel to form a soft, bulky stool.

Time lapse before drug works:
May require 2 or 3 days to begin, then works in 12 to 24 hours.

Don't take with:
- See Interaction column and consult doctor.
- Don't take within 2 hours of taking another medicine.

 ## OVERDOSE

Symptoms:
None expected.

What to do:
Overdose unlikely to threaten life. If person takes much larger amount than prescribed, call doctor, poison-control center or hospital emergency room for instructions.

POSSIBLE ADVERSE REACTIONS OR SIDE EFFECTS

SYMPTOMS	FREQUENCY	WHAT TO DO
Brain & nervous system:	None expected.	
Skin: Itch, rash.	Rare	3
Eyes:	None expected.	
Ears, nose, throat: Swallowing difficulty, "lump in throat" sensation.	Infrequent	4
Digestive: Intestinal blockage.	Rare	3
Heart & lungs: Asthma	Rare	3
Blood vessels:	None expected.	
Muscles, bones, joints:	None expected.	
Genital, urinary:	None expected.	
Kidneys:	None expected.	
Liver:	None expected.	
Allergic:	None expected.	
Blood:	None expected.	
Others:	None expected.	

1- Life-threatening. Seek emergency treatment immediately.
2- Discontinue. Seek emergency treatment.
3- Discontinue. Call doctor right away.
4- Continue. Call doctor when convenient.
5- Continue. Tell doctor at next visit.
6- No action necessary.

WARNINGS & PRECAUTIONS

Don't take if:
- You are allergic to any bulk-forming laxative.
- You have symptoms of appendicitis, inflamed bowel or intestinal blockage.
- You have missed a bowel movement for only 1 or 2 days.

Before you start, consult your doctor:
- If you have diabetes.
- If you have kidney disease.
- If you have a laxative habit.
- If you have rectal bleeding.
- If you have difficulty swallowing.
- If you take other laxatives.

Over age 60:
Adverse reactions and side effects may be more frequent and severe than in younger persons.

Pregnancy:
Most bulk-forming laxatives contain sodium or sugars which may cause fluid retention. Avoid if possible.

Breast-feeding:
No problems expected.

Infants & children:
Use only under medical supervision.

Prolonged use:
Don't take for more than 1 week unless under a doctor's supervision. May cause laxative dependence.

Skin & sunlight:
No problems expected.

Driving, piloting or hazardous work:
No problems expected.

Airplane passengers:
No problems expected.

Discontinuing:
May be unnecessary to finish medicine. Follow doctor's instructions.

Others:
Don't take to "flush out" your system, or as a "tonic."

INTERACTION WITH OTHER DRUGS

GENERIC NAME OR DRUG CLASS	COMBINED EFFECT
Antibiotics	Decreased antibiotic effect.
Anticoagulants	Decreased anticoagulant effect.
Digitalis preparations	Decreased digitalis effect.
Salicylates (including aspirin)	Decreased salicylate effect.

INTERACTION WITH OTHER SUBSTANCES

INTERACTS WITH	COMBINED EFFECT
Alcohol:	None expected.
Beverages:	None expected.
Cocaine:	None expected.
Foods:	None expected.
Marijuana:	None expected.
Tobacco:	None expected.

PYRIDOSTIGMINE

BRAND NAMES

Mestinon
Regonol

GENERAL INFORMATION

Habit forming? No
Prescription needed? Yes
Available as generic? Yes
Drug class: Cholinergic (anticholinesterase)

USES

- Treatment of myasthenia gravis.
- Treatment of urinary retention and abdominal distention.
- Antidote to adverse effects of muscle relaxants used in surgery.

DOSAGE & USAGE INFORMATION

How to take:
- Tablet or syrup—Swallow with liquid or food to lessen stomach irritation.
- Extended-release tablets or capsules—Swallow each dose whole. If you take regular tablets, you may chew or crush them.

When to take:
As directed, usually 3 or 4 times a day.

If you forget a dose:
Take as soon as you remember up to 2 hours late. If more than 2 hours, wait for next scheduled dose (don't double this dose).

What drug does:
Inhibits the chemical activity of an enzyme (cholinesterase) so nerve impulses can cross the junction of nerves and muscles.

Time lapse before drug works:
3 hours.

Don't take with:
See Interaction column and consult doctor.

OVERDOSE

Symptoms:
Muscle weakness, cramps, twitching or clumsiness; severe diarrhea, nausea, vomiting, stomach cramps or pain; breathing difficulty; confusion, irritability, nervousness, restlessness, fear; unusually slow heartbeat; seizures.

What to do:
- Dial 0 (operator) or 911 (emergency) for an ambulance or medical help. Then give first aid immediately.
- Additional emergency information on page 886.

POSSIBLE ADVERSE REACTIONS OR SIDE EFFECTS

SYMPTOMS	FREQUENCY	WHAT TO DO
Brain & nervous system: Confusion, irritability.	Infrequent	2
Skin:	None expected.	
Eyes: Constricted pupils, watery eyes.	Infrequent	4
Ears, nose, throat: Excess saliva.	Common	4
Digestive: Mild diarrhea, nausea, vomiting, stomach cramps or pain.	Common	3
Heart & lungs: Lung congestion.	Infrequent	4
Blood vessels:	None expected.	
Muscles, bones, joints:	None expected.	
Genital, urinary: Frequent urge to urinate.	Infrequent	4
Kidneys:	None expected.	
Liver:	None expected.	
Allergic:	None expected.	
Blood:	None expected.	
Others: Unusual sweating.	Common	4

1-Life-threatening. Seek emergency treatment immediately.
2-Discontinue. Seek emergency treatment.
3-Discontinue. Call doctor right away.
4-Continue. Call doctor when convenient.
5-Continue. Tell doctor at next visit.
6-No action necessary.

PYRIDOSTIGMINE

WARNINGS & PRECAUTIONS

Don't take if:
- You are allergic to any cholinergic or bromide.
- You take mecamylamine.

Before you start, consult your doctor:
- If you plan to become pregnant within medication period.
- If you have bronchial asthma.
- If you have heartbeat irregularities.
- If you have urinary obstruction or urinary-tract infection.

Over age 60:
Adverse reactions and side effects may be more frequent and severe than in younger persons.

Pregnancy:
No proven harm to unborn child. Avoid if possible. May increase uterus contractions close to delivery.

Breast-feeding:
No problems expected, but consult doctor.

Infants & children:
Not recommended.

Prolonged use:
Medication may lose effectiveness. Discontinuing for a few days may restore effect.

Skin & sunlight:
No problems expected.

Driving, piloting or hazardous work:
Don't drive or pilot aircraft until you learn how medicine affects you. Don't work around dangerous machinery. Don't climb ladders or work in high places. Danger increases if you drink alcohol or take medicine affecting alertness and reflexes, such as antihistamines, tranquilizers, sedatives, pain medicine, narcotics and mind-altering drugs.

Airplane passengers:
No problems expected.

Discontinuing:
Don't discontinue without doctor's advice until you complete prescribed dose, even though symptoms diminish or disappear.

Others:
No problems expected.

INTERACTION WITH OTHER DRUGS

GENERIC NAME OR DRUG CLASS	COMBINED EFFECT
Anesthetics (local or general)	Decreased pyridostigmine effect.
Antiarrhythmics	Decreased pyridostigmine effect.
Antibiotics	Decreased pyridostigmine effect.
Anticholinergics	Decreased pyridostigmine effect. May mask severe side effects.
Cholinergics (other)	Reduced intestinal-tract function. Possible brain and nervous-system toxicity.
Mecamylamine	Decreased pyridostigmine effect.
Quinidine	Decreased pyridostigmine effect.

INTERACTION WITH OTHER SUBSTANCES

INTERACTS WITH	COMBINED EFFECT
Alcohol:	No proven problems with small doses.
Beverages:	None expected.
Cocaine:	Decreased pyridostigmine effect. Avoid.
Foods:	None expected.
Marijuana:	No proven problems.
Tobacco:	No proven problems.

PYRIDOXINE (VITAMIN B-6)

BRAND NAMES

Beesix
Bendectin (M)
Hexa-Betalin
Hexacrest

Hexavibex
Pyroxine
Tex Six T.R.

GENERAL INFORMATION

Habit forming? No
Prescription needed? High strength: Yes
Low strength: No
Available as generic? Yes
Drug class: Vitamin supplement

USES

- Prevention and treatment of pyridoxine deficiency.
- Treatment of some forms of anemia.

DOSAGE & USAGE INFORMATION

How to take:
- Tablets—Swallow with liquid.
- Extended-release tablets—Swallow each dose whole with liquid.

When to take:
At the same times each day.

If you forget a dose:
Take as soon as you remember, then resume regular schedule.

What drug does:
Acts as co-enzyme in carbohydrate, protein and fat metabolism.

Time lapse before drug works:
15 to 20 minutes.

Don't take with:
- Levodopa—Small amounts of pyridoxine will nullify levodopa effect. Carbidopa-levodopa combination not affected by this interaction.
- See Interaction column and consult doctor.

OVERDOSE

Symptoms:
None expected.

What to do:
Overdose unlikely to threaten life.

POSSIBLE ADVERSE REACTIONS OR SIDE EFFECTS

SYMPTOMS	FREQUENCY	WHAT TO DO
Brain & nervous system:	None expected.	
Skin:	None expected.	
Eyes:	None expected.	
Ears, nose, throat:	None expected.	
Digestive:	None expected.	
Heart & lungs:	None expected.	
Blood vessels:	None expected.	
Muscles, bones, joints:	None expected.	
Genital, urinary:	None expected.	
Kidneys:	None expected.	
Liver:	None expected.	
Allergic:	None expected.	
Blood:	None expected.	
Others:	None expected.	

1- Life-threatening. Seek emergency treatment immediately.
2- Discontinue. Seek emergency treatment.
3- Discontinue. Call doctor right away.
4- Continue. Call doctor when convenient.
5- Continue. Tell doctor at next visit.
6- No action necessary.

PYRIDOXINE (VITAMIN B-6)

 WARNINGS & PRECAUTIONS

Don't take if:
You are allergic to pyridoxine.

Before you start, consult your doctor:
If you are pregnant or breast-feeding.

Over age 60:
No problems expected.

Pregnancy:
Don't exceed recommended dose.

Breast-feeding:
Don't exceed recommended dose.

Infants & children:
Don't exceed recommended dose.

Prolonged use:
Large doses for more than 1 month may cause toxicity.

Skin & sunlight:
No problems expected.

Driving, piloting or hazardous work:
No problems expected.

Airplane passengers:
No problems expected.

Discontinuing:
No problems expected.

Others:
Regular pyridoxine supplements recommended if you take chloramphenicol, cycloserine, ethionamide, hydralazine, immunosuppressants, isoniazid or penicillamine. These decrease pyridoxine absorption and can cause anemia or tingling and numbness in hands and feet.

 INTERACTION WITH OTHER DRUGS

GENERIC NAME OR DRUG CLASS	COMBINED EFFECT
Chloramphenicol	Decreased pyridoxine effect.
Contraceptives (oral)	Decreased pyridoxine effect.
Cycloserine	Decreased pyridoxine effect.
Ethionamide	Decreased pyridoxine effect.
Hydralazine	Decreased pyridoxine effect.
Immunosuppressants	Decreased pyridoxine effect.
Isoniazid	Decreased pyridoxine effect.
Penicillamine	Decreased pyridoxine effect.
Levodopa	Decreased levodopa effect.

 INTERACTION WITH OTHER SUBSTANCES

INTERACTS WITH	COMBINED EFFECT
Alcohol:	None expected.
Beverages:	None expected.
Cocaine:	None expected.
Foods:	None expected.
Marijuana:	None expected.
Tobacco:	May decrease pyridoxine absorption. Decreased pyridoxine effect.

PYRILAMINE

BRAND NAMES

Allertoc
Dormarex
Somnicaps

GENERAL INFORMATION

Habit forming? No
Prescription needed? No
Available as generic? Yes
Drug class: Antihistamine

USES

- Reduces allergic symptoms such as hay fever, hives, rash or itching.
- Prevents motion sickness, nausea, vomiting.
- Induces sleep.

DOSAGE & USAGE INFORMATION

How to take:
Tablet or capsule—Swallow with liquid or food to lessen stomach irritation.

When to take:
Varies with form. Follow label directions.

If you forget a dose:
Take as soon as you remember up to 2 hours late. If more than 2 hours, wait for next scheduled dose (don't double this dose).

What drug does:
Blocks action of histamine after an allergic response triggers histamine release in sensitive cells.

Time lapse before drug works:
30 minutes.

Don't take with:
See Interaction column and consult doctor.

OVERDOSE

Symptoms:
Convulsions, red face, hallucinations, coma.

What to do:
- Dial 0 (operator) or 911 (emergency) for an ambulance or medical help. Then give first aid immediately.
- If patient is unconscious and not breathing, give mouth-to-mouth breathing. If there is no heartbeat, use cardiac massage and mouth-to-mouth breathing (CPR). Don't try to make patient vomit. If you can't get help quickly, take patient to nearest emergency facility.
- Additional emergency information on page 886.

POSSIBLE ADVERSE REACTIONS OR SIDE EFFECTS

SYMPTOMS	FREQUENCY	WHAT TO DO
Brain & nervous system:		
• Nightmares, agitation, irritability.	Rare	3
• Drowsiness, dizziness.	Common	5
Skin:	None expected.	
Eyes:		
• Vision changes.	Infrequent	3
• Less tolerance for contact lenses.	Infrequent	4
Ears, nose, throat:		
• Sore throat, fever.	Rare	3
• Dry mouth, nose, throat.	Common	5
Digestive:		
• Nausea	Common	5
• Appetite loss.	Infrequent	5
Heart & lungs:		
Rapid heartbeat.	Rare	3
Blood vessels:		
Unusual bleeding or bruising.	Rare	3
Muscles, bones, joints, kidneys, liver, allergic, blood:	None expected.	
Genital, urinary:		
Urination difficulty.	Infrequent	4
Others:		
Fatigue, weakness.	Rare	3

1- Life-threatening. Seek emergency treatment immediately.
2- Discontinue. Seek emergency treatment.
3- Discontinue. Call doctor right away.
4- Continue. Call doctor when convenient.
5- Continue. Tell doctor at next visit.
6- No action necessary.

WARNINGS & PRECAUTIONS

Don't take if:
You are allergic to any antihistamine.

Before you start, consult your doctor:
- If you have glaucoma.
- If you have enlarged prostate.
- If you have asthma.
- If you have kidney disease.
- If you have peptic ulcer.
- If you will have surgery within 2 months, including dental surgery, requiring general or spinal anesthesia.

Over age 60:
Don't exceed recommended dose. Adverse reactions and side effects may be more frequent and severe than in younger persons, especially urination difficulty, diminished alertness and other brain and nervous-system symptoms.

Pregnancy:
No proven harm to unborn child. Avoid if possible.

Breast-feeding:
Drug passes into milk. Avoid drug or discontinue nursing until you finish medicine. Consult doctor for advice on maintaining milk supply.

Infants & children:
Not recommended for premature or newborn infants. Otherwise, no problems expected.

Prolonged use:
Avoid. May damage bone marrow and nerve cells.

Skin & sunlight:
May cause rash or intensify sunburn in areas exposed to sun or sunlamp.

Driving, piloting or hazardous work:
Don't drive or pilot aircraft until you learn how medicine affects you. Don't work around dangerous machinery. Don't climb ladders or work in high places. Danger increases if you drink alcohol or take medicine affecting alertness and reflexes, such as antihistamines, tranquilizers, sedatives, pain medicine, narcotics and mind-altering drugs.

Airplane passengers:
No problems expected.

Discontinuing:
No problems expected.

Others:
May mask symptoms of hearing damage from aspirin, other salicylates, cisplatin, paromomycin, vancomycin or anticonvulsants. Consult doctor if you use these.

INTERACTION WITH OTHER DRUGS

GENERIC NAME OR DRUG CLASS	COMBINED EFFECT
Anticholinergics	Increased anticholinergic effect.
Antidepressants	Excess sedation. Avoid.
Antihistamines (other)	Excess sedation. Avoid.
Hypnotics	Excess sedation. Avoid.
MAO inhibitors	Increased pyrilamine effect.
Mind-altering drugs	Excess sedation. Avoid.
Narcotics	Excess sedation. Avoid.
Sedatives	Excess sedation. Avoid.
Sleep inducers	Excess sedation. Avoid.
Tranquilizers	Excess sedation. Avoid.

INTERACTION WITH OTHER SUBSTANCES

INTERACTS WITH	COMBINED EFFECT
Alcohol:	Excess sedation. Avoid.
Beverages: Caffeine drinks	Less pyrilamine sedation.
Cocaine:	Decreased pyrilamine effect. Avoid.
Foods:	None expected.
Marijuana:	Excess sedation. Avoid.
Tobacco:	None expected.

PYRVINIUM

BRAND NAMES

Povan

GENERAL INFORMATION

Habit forming? No
Prescription needed? Yes
Available as generic? No
Drug class: Antihelminthic (antiworm medication)

 USES

Treatment for pinworm infestation.

 DOSAGE & USAGE INFORMATION

How to take:
- Tablet—Swallow whole with food or liquid. Don't crush or chew tablet.
- Liquid—Take with food or liquid.

When to take:
According to label instructions. Usually a single dose, which may be repeated in 2 or 3 weeks.

If you forget a dose:
Take when remembered.

What drug does:
Interferes with a metabolic process in the infecting parasite and kills it.

Time lapse before drug works:
12 hours.

Don't take with:
Non-prescription drugs for pinworms.

 OVERDOSE

Symptoms:
Increased severity of adverse reactions and side effects.

What to do:
Overdose unlikely to threaten life. If person takes much larger amount than prescribed, call doctor, poison-control center or hospital emergency room for instructions.

 POSSIBLE ADVERSE REACTIONS OR SIDE EFFECTS

SYMPTOMS	FREQUENCY	WHAT TO DO
Brain & nervous system: Dizziness	Rare	4
Skin: Rash	Rare	3
Eyes:	None expected.	
Ears, nose, throat:	None expected.	
Digestive: Stomach cramps, nausea, vomiting.	Rare	4
Heart & lungs:	None expected.	
Blood vessels:	None expected.	
Muscles, bones, joints:	None expected.	
Genital, urinary:	None expected.	
Kidneys:	None expected.	
Liver:	None expected.	
Allergic:	None expected.	
Blood:	None expected.	
Others:	None expected.	

1- Life-threatening. Seek emergency treatment immediately.
2- Discontinue. Seek emergency treatment.
3- Discontinue. Call doctor right away.
4- Continue. Call doctor when convenient.
5- Continue. Tell doctor at next visit.
6- No action necessary.

WARNINGS & PRECAUTIONS

Don't take if:
You are allergic to any antihelminthic drug.

Before you start, consult your doctor:
- If you have kidney or liver disease.
- If you have a bowel disease or inflammation.

Over age 60:
Adverse reactions and side effects may be more frequent and severe than in younger persons.

Pregnancy:
No proven harm to unborn child. Avoid if possible.

Breast-feeding:
No problems expected, but consult doctor.

Infants & children:
No problems expected.

Prolonged use:
Not recommended.

Skin & sunlight:
May cause rash or intensify sunburn in areas exposed to sun or sunlamp.

Driving, piloting or hazardous work:
Avoid if you feel dizzy. Otherwise, no problems expected.

Airplane passengers:
No problems expected.

Discontinuing:
Don't discontinue without doctor's advice until you complete prescribed dose, even though symptoms diminish or disappear.

Others:
- This medicine is a dye that permanently stains most materials. Teeth will be stained a few days. Stool and vomit may be red.
- Pinworm infestations are highly contagious. All family members should be treated at the same time.

INTERACTION WITH OTHER DRUGS

GENERIC NAME OR DRUG CLASS	COMBINED EFFECT
None	

INTERACTION WITH OTHER SUBSTANCES

INTERACTS WITH	COMBINED EFFECT
Alcohol:	None expected.
Beverages:	None expected.
Cocaine:	None expected.
Foods:	None expected.
Marijuana:	None expected.
Tobacco:	None expected.

QUINESTROL

BRAND NAMES

Estrovis

GENERAL INFORMATION

Habit forming? No
Prescription needed? Yes
Available as generic? Yes
Drug class: Female sex hormone (estrogen)

 USES

- Treatment for symptoms of menopause and menstrual-cycle irregularity.
- Replacement for female hormone deficiency.

 DOSAGE & USAGE INFORMATION

How to take:
Tablet—Swallow with liquid. If you can't swallow whole, crumble tablet and take with liquid or food.

When to take:
At the same time each day.

If you forget a dose:
Take as soon as you remember up to 12 hours late. If more than 12 hours, wait for next scheduled dose (don't double this dose).

What drug does:
Restores normal estrogen level in tissues.

Time lapse before drug works:
10 to 20 days.

Don't take with:
See Interaction column and consult doctor.

 OVERDOSE

Symptoms:
Nausea, vomiting, fluid retention, breast enlargement and discomfort, abnormal vaginal bleeding.

What to do:
Overdose unlikely to threaten life. If person takes much larger amount than prescribed, call doctor, poison-control center or hospital emergency room for instructions.

 POSSIBLE ADVERSE REACTIONS OR SIDE EFFECTS

SYMPTOMS	FREQUENCY	WHAT TO DO
Brain & nervous system: Depression, dizziness, irritability.	Infrequent	4
Skin:		
• Rash	Infrequent	3
• Brown blotches.	Infrequent	5
• Hair loss.	Infrequent	5
Eyes, ears, nose, throat, heart & lungs, muscles, bones, joints, kidneys, allergic, blood:	None expected.	
Digestive:		
• Stomach or side pain.	Infrequent	3
• Stomach cramps.	Common	3
• Appetite loss.	Common	4
• Nausea, diarrhea.	Common	5
• Vomiting	Infrequent	4
Blood vessels: Swollen ankles, feet.	Common	5
Genital, urinary: Vaginal discharge or bleeding.	Infrequent	5
Liver: Jaundice (yellow skin and eyes).	Rare	3
Others:		
• Breast lumps.	Infrequent	4
• Swollen, tender breasts.	Common	5
• Changes in sex drive.	Infrequent	5

1- Life-threatening. Seek emergency treatment immediately.
2- Discontinue. Seek emergency treatment.
3- Discontinue. Call doctor right away.
4- Continue. Call doctor when convenient.
5- Continue. Tell doctor at next visit.

WARNINGS & PRECAUTIONS

Don't take if:
- You are allergic to any estrogen-containing drugs.
- You have impaired liver function.
- You have had blood clots, stroke or heart attack.
- You have unexplained vaginal bleeding.

Before you start, consult your doctor:
- If you have had cancer of breast or reproductive organs, fibrocystic breast disease, fibroid tumors of the uterus or endometriosis.
- If you have had migraine headaches, epilepsy or porphyria.
- If you have diabetes, high blood pressure, asthma, congestive heart failure, kidney disease or gallstones.
- If you plan to become pregnant within 3 months.

Over age 60:
Controversial. You and your doctor must decide if drug risks outweigh benefits.

Pregnancy:
Risk to unborn child outweighs drug benefits. Don't use.

Breast-feeding:
Drug filters into milk. May harm child. Avoid.

Infants & children:
Not recommended.

Prolonged use:
Increased growth of fibroid tumors of uterus. Possible association with cancer of uterus.

Skin & sunlight:
May cause rash or intensify sunburn in areas exposed to sun or sunlamp.

Driving, piloting or hazardous work:
No problems expected.

Airplane passengers:
No problems expected.

Discontinuing:
You may need to discontinue quinestrol periodically. Consult your doctor.

Others:
In rare instances, may cause blood clot in lung, brain or leg. Symptoms are *sudden* severe headache, coordination loss, vision change, chest pain, breathing difficulty, slurred speech, pain in legs or groin. Seek emergency treatment immediately.

INTERACTION WITH OTHER DRUGS

GENERIC NAME OR DRUG CLASS	COMBINED EFFECT
Anticoagulants (oral)	Decreased anticoagulant effect.
Anticonvulsants (hydantoin)	Increased seizures.
Antidiabetics (oral)	Unpredictable increase or decrease in blood sugar.
Clofibrate	Decreased clofibrate effect.
Carbamazepine	Increased seizures.
Meprobamate	Increased quinestrol effect.
Phenobarbital	Decreased quinestrol effect.
Primidone	Decreased quinestrol effect.
Rifampin	Decreased quinestrol effect.
Thyroid hormones	Decreased thyroid effect.

INTERACTION WITH OTHER SUBSTANCES

INTERACTS WITH	COMBINED EFFECT
Alcohol:	None expected.
Beverages:	None expected.
Cocaine:	No proven problems.
Foods:	None expected.
Marijuana:	Possible menstrual irregularities and bleeding between periods.
Tobacco:	Increased risk of blood clots leading to stroke or heart attack.

QUINETHAZONE

BRAND NAMES

Hydromox

GENERAL INFORMATION

Habit forming? No
Prescription needed? Yes
Available as generic? Yes
Drug class: Antihypertensive,
diuretic (thiazide)

USES

- Controls, but doesn't cure, high blood pressure.
- Reduces fluid retention (edema) caused by conditions such as heart disorders and liver disease.

DOSAGE & USAGE INFORMATION

How to take:
Tablet or capsule—Swallow with liquid. If you can't swallow whole, crumble tablet or open capsule and take with liquid or food. Don't exceed dose.

When to take:
At the same time each day.

If you forget a dose:
Take as soon as you remember up to 2 hours late. If more than 2 hours, wait for next scheduled dose (don't double this dose).

What drug does:
- Forces sodium and water excretion, reducing body fluid.
- Relaxes muscle cells of small arteries.
- Reduced body fluid and relaxed arteries lower blood pressure.

Time lapse before drug works:
4 to 6 hours. May require several weeks to lower blood pressure.

Don't take with:
- See Interaction column and consult doctor.
- Non-prescription drugs without consulting doctor.

OVERDOSE

Symptoms:
Cramps, weakness, drowsiness, weak pulse, coma.

What to do:
- Dial 0 (operator) or 911 (emergency) for an ambulance or medical help. Then give first aid immediately.
- Additional emergency information on page 886.

POSSIBLE ADVERSE REACTIONS OR SIDE EFFECTS

SYMPTOMS	FREQUENCY	WHAT TO DO
Brain & nervous system:		
● Dizziness	Infrequent	4
● Mood changes.	Infrequent	4
● Headaches	Infrequent	4
Skin:		
Rash or hives.	Rare	2
Eyes:		
Blurred vision.	Infrequent	3
Ears, nose, throat:		
● Sore throat, fever.	Rare	3
● Dry mouth, thirst.	Infrequent	5
Digestive:		
Severe abdominal pain, nausea, vomiting.	Infrequent	3
Heart & lungs:		
Irregular heartbeat, weak pulse.	Infrequent	3
Blood vessels:	None expected.	
Muscles, bones, joints:		
Weakness, tiredness.	Infrequent	4
Genital, urinary:	None expected.	
Kidneys:	None expected.	
Liver:		
Jaundice (yellow skin and eyes).	Rare	3
Allergic:	None expected.	
Blood:	None expected.	
Others:		
Weight changes.	Infrequent	4

1- Life-threatening. Seek emergency treatment immediately.
2- Discontinue. Seek emergency treatment.
3- Discontinue. Call doctor right away.
4- Continue. Call doctor when convenient.
5- Continue. Tell doctor at next visit.
6- No action necessary.

QUINETHAZONE

WARNINGS & PRECAUTIONS

Don't take if:
You are allergic to any thiazide diuretic drug.

Before you start, consult your doctor:
• If you are allergic to any sulfa drug.
• If you have gout.
• If you have liver, pancreas or liver disorder.

Over age 60:
Adverse reactions and side effects may be more frequent and severe than in younger persons, especially dizziness and excessive potassium loss.

Pregnancy:
Risk to unborn child outweighs drug benefits. Don't use.

Breast-feeding:
Drug passes into milk. Avoid drug or discontinue nursing.

Infants & children:
No problems expected.

Prolonged use:
You may need medicine to treat high blood pressure for the rest of your life.

Skin & sunlight:
May cause rash or intensify sunburn in areas exposed to sun or sunlamp.

Driving, piloting or hazardous work:
Don't drive or pilot aircraft until you learn how medicine affects you. Don't work around dangerous machinery. Don't climb ladders or work in high places. Danger increases if you drink alcohol or take medicine affecting alertness and reflexes, such as antihistamines, tranquilizers, sedatives, pain medicine, narcotics and mind-altering drugs.

Airplane passengers:
No problems expected.

Discontinuing:
Don't discontinue without medical advice.

Others:
• Hot weather and fever may cause dehydration and drop in blood pressure. Dose may require temporary adjustment. Weigh daily and report any unexpected weight decreases to your doctor.
• May cause rise in uric acid, leading to gout.
• May cause blood-sugar rise in diabetics.

INTERACTION WITH OTHER DRUGS

GENERIC NAME OR DRUG CLASS	COMBINED EFFECT
Allopurinol	Decreased allopurinol effect.
Antidepressants (tricyclic)	Dangerous drop in blood pressure. Avoid combination unless under medical supervision.
Barbiturates	Increased quinethazone effect.
Cholestyramine	Decreased quinethazone effect.
Cortisone drugs	Excessive potassium loss that causes dangerous heart rhythms.
Digitalis preparations	Excessive potassium loss that causes dangerous heart rhythms.
Diuretics (thiazide)	Increased effect of other thiazide diuretics.
Lithium	Increased effect of lithium.
MAO Inhibitors	Increased quinethazone effect.
Probenecid	Decreased probenecid effect.

INTERACTION WITH OTHER SUBSTANCES

INTERACTS WITH	COMBINED EFFECT
Alcohol:	Dangerous blood-pressure drop.
Beverages:	None expected.
Cocaine:	None expected.
Foods: Licorice	Excessive potassium loss that causes dangerous heart rhythms.
Marijuana:	May increase blood pressure.
Tobacco:	None expected.

QUINIDINE

BRAND NAMES

Biquin Durules Quinidex Extentabs
Cardioquin Quinobarb (M)
Cin-Quin Quinora
Duraquin
Quinaglute Dura-Tabs
Quinate

Habit forming? No
Prescription needed? U.S.: Yes, Canada: No
Available as generic? Yes
Drug class: Antiarrhythmic

 ## USES

Corrects heart-rhythm disorders.

 ## DOSAGE & USAGE INFORMATION

How to take:
- Tablet or capsule—Swallow liquid or with food to lessen stomach irritation.
- Extended-release tablets or capsules— Swallow each dose whole. If you take regular tablets, you may chew or crush them.

When to take:
At the same times each day.

If you forget a dose:
Take as soon as you remember up to 2 hours late. If more than 2 hours, wait for next scheduled dose (don't double this dose).

What drug does:
Delays nerve impulses to the heart to regulate heartbeat.

Time lapse before drug works:
2 to 4 hours.

Don't take with:
See Interaction column and consult doctor.

 ## OVERDOSE

Symptoms:
Confusion, severe blood-pressure drop, breathing difficulty, fainting.

What to do:
- Dial 0 (operator) or 911 (emergency) for an ambulance or medical help. Then give first aid immediately.
- If patient is unconscious and not breathing, give mouth-to-mouth breathing. If there is no heartbeat, use cardiac massage and mouth-to-mouth breathing (CPR). Don't try to make patient vomit. If you can't get help quickly, take patient to nearest emergency facility.
- Additional emergency information on page 886.

 ## POSSIBLE ADVERSE REACTIONS OR SIDE EFFECTS

SYMPTOMS	FREQUENCY	WHAT TO DO
Brain & nervous system: Dizziness, lightheadedness, fainting, headache, confusion.	Infrequent	3
Skin: Rash	Infrequent	3
Eyes: Vision changes.	Infrequent	3
Ears, nose, throat: Ringing in ears.	Infrequent	4
Digestive: Bitter taste, diarrhea, nausea, vomiting.	Common	3
Heart & lungs: Breathing difficulty, rapid heartbeat.	Infrequent	3
Blood vessels: Unusual bleeding or bruising.	Rare	3
Muscles, bones, joints:	None expected.	
Genital, urinary:	None expected.	
Kidneys:	None expected.	
Liver:	None expected.	
Allergic:	None expected.	
Blood:	None expected.	
Others: Weakness	Rare	4

1- Life-threatening. Seek emergency treatment immediately.
2- Discontinue. Seek emergency treatment.
3- Discontinue. Call doctor right away.
4- Continue. Call doctor when convenient.
5- Continue. Tell doctor at next visit.
6- No action necessary.

WARNINGS & PRECAUTIONS

Don't take if:
- You are allergic to quinidine.
- You have an active infection.

Before you start, consult your doctor:
About any drug you take, including non-prescription drugs.

Over age 60:
Adverse reactions and side effects may be more frequent and severe than in younger persons.

Pregnancy:
Risk to unborn child outweighs drug benefits. Don't use.

Breast-feeding:
Drug filters into milk. May harm child. Avoid.

Infants & children:
No problems expected.

Prolonged use:
No problems expected.

Skin & sunlight:
No problems expected.

Driving, piloting or hazardous work:
Don't drive or pilot aircraft until you learn how medicine affects you. Don't work around dangerous machinery. Don't climb ladders or work in high places. Danger increases if you drink alcohol or take medicine affecting alertness and reflexes, such as antihistamines, tranquilizers, sedatives, pain medicine, narcotics and mind-altering drugs.

Airplane passengers:
No problems expected.

Discontinuing:
Don't discontinue without doctor's advice until you complete prescribed dose, even though symptoms diminish or disappear.

Others:
No problems expected.

INTERACTION WITH OTHER DRUGS

GENERIC NAME OR DRUG CLASS	COMBINED EFFECT
Anticholinergics	Increased anticholinergic effect.
Anticoagulants	Increased anticoagulant effect.
Antihypertensives	Increased antihypertensive effect.
Cholinergics	Decreased cholinergic effect.
Digitalis preparations	Slows heartbeat excessively.
Phenytoin	Increased quinidine effect.
Propranolol	Slows heartbeat excessively.
Pyrimethamine	Increased quinidine effect.
Rauwolfia alkaloids	Seriously disturbs heart rhythms.

INTERACTION WITH OTHER SUBSTANCES

INTERACTS WITH	COMBINED EFFECT
Alcohol:	None expected.
Beverages: Caffeine drinks	Causes rapid heartbeat. Use sparingly.
Cocaine:	Irregular heartbeat. Avoid.
Foods:	None expected.
Marijuana:	Can cause fainting.
Tobacco:	Irregular heartbeat. Avoid.

QUININE

BRAND NAMES

Coco-Quinine
Quinamm (M)
Quine

GENERAL INFORMATION

Habit forming? No
Prescription needed? Yes
Available as generic? Yes
Drug class: Antiprotozoal

USES

Treatment or prevention of malaria.

DOSAGE & USAGE INFORMATION

How to take:
Liquid, tablet or capsule—Swallow with liquid or food to lessen stomach irritation.

When to take:
- Prevention—At the same time each day, usually at bedtime.
- Treatment—At the same times each day in evenly spaced doses.

If you forget a dose:
- Prevention—Take as soon as you remember up to 12 hours late. If more than 12 hours, wait for next scheduled dose (don't double this dose).
- Treatment—Take as soon as you remember up to 2 hours late. If more than 2 hours, wait for next scheduled dose (don't double this dose).

What drug does:
- Reduces contractions of skeletal muscles.
- Increases blood flow.
- Interferes with genes in malaria microorganisms.

Time lapse before drug works:
May require several days or weeks for maximum effect.

Don't take with:
See Interaction column and consult doctor.

OVERDOSE

Symptoms:
Severe impairment of vision and hearing; severe nausea, vomiting, diarrhea; shallow breathing, fast heartbeat; apprehension, confusion, delirium.

What to do:
- Dial 0 (operator) or 911 (emergency) for an ambulance or medical help. Then give first aid immediately.
- Additional emergency information on page 886.

POSSIBLE ADVERSE REACTIONS OR SIDE EFFECTS

SYMPTOMS	FREQUENCY	WHAT TO DO
Brain & nervous system: Dizziness, headache.	Common	4
Skin: Rash, hives, itch.	Infrequent	3
Eyes: Blurred or changed vision.	Common	3
Ears, nose, throat:		
• Ringing or buzzing in ears, impaired hearing.	Common	5
• Sore throat, fever.	Rare	3
Digestive: Stomach discomfort, mild nausea, vomiting, diarrhea.	Common	4
Heart & lungs: Breathing difficulty.	Infrequent	3
Blood vessels: Unusual bleeding or bruising.	Rare	3
Muscles, bones, joints: Unusual tiredness or weakness.	Rare	3
Genital, urinary:	None expected.	
Kidneys:	None expected.	
Liver:	None expected.	
Allergic:	None expected.	
Blood:	None expected.	
Others:	None expected.	

1- Life-threatening. Seek emergency treatment immediately.
2- Discontinue. Seek emergency treatment.
3- Discontinue. Call doctor right away.
4- Continue. Call doctor when convenient.
5- Continue. Tell doctor at next visit.
6- No action necessary.

WARNINGS & PRECAUTIONS

Don't take if:
You are allergic to quinine or quinidine.

Before you start, consult your doctor:
- If you plan to become pregnant within medication period.
- If you have asthma.
- If you have eye disease, hearing problems or ringing in the ears.
- If you have heart disease.
- If you have myasthenia gravis.

Over age 60:
Adverse reactions and side effects may be more frequent and severe than in younger persons.

Pregnancy:
Risk to unborn child outweighs drug benefits. Don't use.

Breast-feeding:
Drug filters into milk. May harm child. Avoid.

Infants & children:
Use only under medical supervision.

Prolonged use:
May develop headache, blurred vision, nausea, temporary hearing loss, but seldom need to discontinue because of these symptoms.

Skin & sunlight:
No problems expected.

Driving, piloting or hazardous work:
Avoid if you feel dizzy or have blurred vision Otherwise, no problems expected.

Airplane passengers:
No problems expected.

Discontinuing:
Don't discontinue without doctor's advice until you complete prescribed dose, even though symptoms diminish or disappear.

Others:
Don't confuse with quinidine, a medicine for heart-rhythm problems.

INTERACTION WITH OTHER DRUGS

GENERIC NAME OR DRUG CLASS	COMBINED EFFECT
Antacids (with aluminum hydroxide)	Decreased quinine effect.
Anticoagulants	Increased anticoagulant effect.
Quinidine	Possible toxic effects of quinine.
Sodium bicarbonate	Possible toxic effects of quinine.

INTERACTION WITH OTHER SUBSTANCES

INTERACTS WITH	COMBINED EFFECT
Alcohol:	No proven problems.
Beverages:	None expected.
Cocaine:	No proven problems.
Foods:	None expected.
Marijuana:	No proven problems.
Tobacco:	None expected.

RANITIDINE

BRAND NAMES

Zantac

GENERAL INFORMATION

Habit forming? No
Prescription needed? Yes
Available as generic? No
Drug class: Histamine H2 antagonist

 USES

- Treatment for duodenal ulcer.
- Decreases acid in stomach.

 DOSAGE & USAGE INFORMATION

How to take:
Tablets—Swallow with liquid.

When to take:
At same times each day.

If you forget a dose:
Take as soon as you remember up to 2 hours late. If more than 2 hours, wait for next scheduled dose (don't double this dose).

What drug does:
Decreases stomach-acid production.

Time lapse before drug works:
2 to 3 hours.

Don't take with:
- Alcohol
- See Interaction column and consult doctor.

 OVERDOSE

Symptoms:
Muscular tremors, vomiting, rapid breathing, coma.

What to do:
- Dial 0 (operator) or 911 (emergency) for an ambulance or medical help. Then give first aid immediately.
- If patient is unconscious and not breathing, give mouth-to-mouth breathing. If there is no heartbeat, use cardiac massage and mouth-to-mouth breathing (CPR). Don't try to make patient vomit. If you can't get help quickly, take patient to nearest emergency facility.
- Additional emergency information on page 886.

 POSSIBLE ADVERSE REACTIONS OR SIDE EFFECTS

SYMPTOMS	FREQUENCY	WHAT TO DO
Brain & nervous system: Headache, dizziness.	Infrequent	4
Skin: Rash	Infrequent	3
Eyes:	None expected.	
Ears, nose, throat:	None expected.	
Digestive: Constipation, abdominal pain, nausea.	Infrequent	4
Heart & lungs:	None expected.	
Blood vessels:	None expected.	
Muscles, bones, joints:	None expected.	
Genital, urinary:	None expected.	
Kidneys:	None expected.	
Liver: Jaundice (yellow skin and eyes).	Rare	3
Allergic:	None expected.	
Blood:	None expected.	
Others:	None expected.	

1- Life-threatening. Seek emergency treatment immediately.
2- Discontinue. Seek emergency treatment.
3- Discontinue. Call doctor right away.
4- Continue. Call doctor when convenient.
5- Continue. Tell doctor at next visit.
6- No action necessary.

WARNINGS & PRECAUTIONS

Don't take if:
You are allergic to any histamine H2 antagonist.

Before you start, consult your doctor:
If you have kidney disease.

Over age 60:
Adverse reactions and side effects may be more frequent and severe than in younger persons.

Pregnancy:
No proven harm to unborn child. Avoid if possible.

Breast-feeding:
Drug passes into milk. Avoid drug or discontinue nursing until you finish medicine. Consult doctor for advice on maintaining milk supply.

Infants & children:
Not recommended.

Prolonged use:
Not recommended. Use for short term only.

Skin & sunlight:
No problems expected.

Driving, piloting or hazardous work:
Avoid if you feel dizzy. Otherwise, no problems expected.

Airplane passengers:
No problems expected

Discontinuing:
Don't discontinue without consulting doctor until you finish prescribed dose, even though symptoms diminish or disappear.

Others:
No problems expected.

INTERACTION WITH OTHER DRUGS

GENERIC NAME OR DRUG CLASS	COMBINED EFFECT
None	

INTERACTION WITH OTHER SUBSTANCES

INTERACTS WITH	COMBINED EFFECT
Alcohol:	Decreased ranitidine effect.
Beverages:	None expected.
Cocaine:	No proven problems.
Foods:	None expected.
Marijuana:	No proven problems.
Tobacco:	Decreased ranitidine effect.

RAUWOLFIA SERPENTINA

BRAND NAMES

Raudixin
Raulfia
Raupoid
Rauserpa

GENERAL INFORMATION

Habit forming? No
Prescription needed? Yes
Available as generic? Yes
Drug class: Antihypertensive, tranquilizer
(rauwolfia alkaloid)

USES

- Treatment for high blood pressure.
- Tranquilizer for mental and emotional disturbances.

DOSAGE & USAGE INFORMATION

How to take:
Tablet—Swallow with liquid or food to lessen stomach irritation. If you can't swallow whole, crumble tablet and take with liquid or food.

When to take:
At the same times each day.

If you forget a dose:
Take as soon as you remember up to 2 hours late. If more than 2 hours, wait for next scheduled dose (don't double this dose).

What drug does:
- Interferes with nerve impulses and relaxes blood-vessel muscles, reducing blood pressure.
- Suppresses brain centers that control emotions.

Time lapse before drug works:
3 weeks continual use required to determine effectiveness.

Don't take with:
See Interaction column and consult doctor.

OVERDOSE

Symptoms:
Drowsiness; slow, weak pulse; slow, shallow breathing; diarrhea; coma; flush; low body temperature.

What to do:
- Dial 0 (operator) or 911 (emergency) for an ambulance or medical help. Then give first aid immediately.
- Additional emergency information on page 886.

POSSIBLE ADVERSE REACTIONS OR SIDE EFFECTS

SYMPTOMS	FREQUENCY	WHAT TO DO
Brain & nervous system:		
● Trembling hands.	Infrequent	4
● Headache, drowsiness or faintness, lethargy.	Common	5
● Depression	Common	4
Skin:		
Rash or itch.	Rare	3
Eyes:		
Redness	Common	5
Ears, nose, throat:		
● Sore throat, fever.	Rare	3
● Stuffy nose.	Common	5
Digestive:		
● Stomach pain, nausea, vomiting.	Rare	3
● Black stool, bloody vomit.	Infrequent	3
Heart & lungs:		
Chest pain, shortness of breath, irregular or slow heartbeat.	Infrequent	3
Blood vessels:		
Unusual bleeding or bruising.	Rare	3
Muscles, bones, joints:		
Stiffness	Infrequent	3
Genital, urinary:		
● Painful urination.	Rare	4
● Impotence, lower sex drive.	Common	5
Kidneys, allergic, blood, others:	None expected.	
Liver:		
Jaundice (yellow skin and eyes).	Rare	3

1 - Life-threatening. Seek emergency treatment immediately.
2 - Discontinue. Seek emergency treatment.
3 - Discontinue. Call doctor right away.
4 - Continue. Call doctor when convenient.
5 - Continue. Tell doctor at next visit.

RAUWOLFIA SERPENTINA

WARNINGS & PRECAUTIONS

Don't take if:
- You are allergic to any rauwolfia alkaloid.
- You are depressed.
- You have active peptic ulcer.
- You have ulcerative colitis.

Before you start, consult your doctor:
- If you have been depressed.
- If you have had peptic ulcer, ulcerative colitis or gallstones.
- If you have epilepsy.
- If you will have surgery within 2 months, including dental surgery, requiring general or spinal anesthesia.

Over age 60:
Adverse reactions and side effects may be more frequent and severe than in younger persons.

Pregnancy:
Studies inconclusive on harm to unborn child. Animal studies show fetal abnormalities. Decide with your doctor whether drug benefits justify risk to unborn child.

Breast-feeding:
Drug passes into milk. Avoid drug or discontinue nursing until you finish medicine. Consult doctor for advice on maintaining milk supply.

Infants & children:
Not recommended.

Prolonged use:
Causes cancer in laboratory animals. Consult your doctor if you have family or personal history of cancer.

Skin & sunlight:
No problems expected.

Driving, piloting or hazardous work:
Avoid if you feel drowsy, dizzy or faint. Otherwise, no problems expected.

Airplane passengers:
No problems expected.

Discontinuing:
Don't discontinue without consulting doctor. Dose may require gradual reduction if you have taken drug for a long time. Doses of other drugs may also require adjustment.

Others:
Consult your doctor if you do isometric exercises. These raise blood pressure. Drug may intensify blood-pressure rise.

INTERACTION WITH OTHER DRUGS

GENERIC NAME OR DRUG CLASS	COMBINED EFFECT
Anticoagulants (oral)	Unpredictable increased or decreased effect of anticoagulant.
Anticonvulsants	Serious change in seizure pattern.
Antidepressants	Increased antidepressant effect.
Antihistamines	Increased antihistamine effect.
Aspirin	Decreased aspirin effect.
Beta-adrenergic blockers	Increased effect of rauwolfia serpentina. Excessive sedation.
Digitalis preparations	Irregular heartbeat.
Levodopa	Decreased levodopa effect.
MAO inhibitors	Severe depression.
Mind-altering drugs	Excessive sedation.
Narcotics	Increased narcotic effect.

Additional interactions on page 843.

INTERACTION WITH OTHER SUBSTANCES

INTERACTS WITH	COMBINED EFFECT
Alcohol:	Increased intoxication. Use with extreme caution.
Beverages: Carbonated drinks	Decreased rauwolfia serpentina effect.
Cocaine:	Decreased rauwolfia serpentina effect.
Foods: Spicy foods	Possible digestive upset.
Marijuana:	Occasional use—Mild drowsiness. Daily use—Moderate drowsiness, low blood pressure, depression.
Tobacco:	No problems expected.

RESERPINE

BRAND NAMES

Alkarau	Metatensin (M)	Reserpoid
Broserpine	Naquival (M)	Sandril
Dralserp	Oreticyl (M)	Serpasil
Harmonyl-D (M)	Rau-Sed	

See complete brand names list, page 830.

GENERAL INFORMATION

Habit forming? No
Prescription needed? Yes
Available as generic? Yes
Drug class: Antihypertensive, tranquilizer
(rauwolfia alkaloid)

USES

- Treatment for high blood pressure.
- Tranquilizer for mental and emotional disturbances.

DOSAGE & USAGE INFORMATION

How to take:
Tablet—Swallow with liquid or food to lessen stomach irritation. If you can't swallow whole, crumble tablet and take with liquid or food.

When to take:
At the same times each day.

If you forget a dose:
Take as soon as you remember up to 2 hours late. If more than 2 hours, wait for next scheduled dose (don't double this dose).

What drug does:
- Interferes with nerve impulses and relaxes blood-vessel muscles, reducing blood pressure.
- Suppresses brain centers that control emotions.

Time lapse before drug works:
3 weeks continual use required to determine effectiveness.

Don't take with:
See Interaction column and consult doctor.

OVERDOSE

Symptoms:
Drowsiness; slow, weak pulse; slow, shallow breathing; diarrhea; coma; flush; low body temperature.

What to do:
- Dial 0 (operator) or 911 (emergency) for an ambulance or medical help. Then give first aid immediately.
- Additional emergency information on page 886.

POSSIBLE ADVERSE REACTIONS OR SIDE EFFECTS

SYMPTOMS	FREQUENCY	WHAT TO DO
Brain & nervous system:		
• Trembling hands.	Infrequent	4
• Headache, drowsiness or faintness, lethargy.	Common	5
• Depression	Common	4
Skin:		
Rash or itch.	Rare	3
Eyes:		
Redness	Common	5
Ears, nose, throat:		
• Sore throat, fever.	Rare	3
• Stuffy nose.	Common	5
Digestive:		
• Stomach pain, nausea, vomiting.	Rare	3
• Black stool, bloody vomit.	Infrequent	3
Heart & lungs:		
Chest pain, shortness of breath, irregular or slow heartbeat.	Infrequent	3
Blood vessels:		
Unusual bleeding or bruising.	Rare	3
Muscles, bones, joints:		
Stiffness	Infrequent	3
Genital, urinary:		
• Painful urination.	Rare	4
• Impotence, lower sex drive.	Common	5
Kidneys, allergic, blood, others:	None expected.	
Liver:		
Jaundice (yellow skin and eyes).	Rare	3

1- Life-threatening. Seek emergency treatment immediately.
2- Discontinue. Seek emergency treatment.
3- Discontinue. Call doctor right away.
4- Continue. Call doctor when convenient.
5- Continue. Tell doctor at next visit.

WARNINGS & PRECAUTIONS

Don't take if:
- You are allergic to any rauwolfia alkaloid.
- You are depressed.
- You have active peptic ulcer.
- You have ulcerative colitis.

Before you start, consult your doctor:
- If you have been depressed.
- If you have had peptic ulcer, ulcerative colitis or gallstones.
- If you have epilepsy.
- If you will have surgery within 2 months, including dental surgery, requiring general or spinal anesthesia.

Over age 60:
Adverse reactions and side effects may be more frequent and severe than in younger persons.

Pregnancy:
Studies inconclusive on harm to unborn child. Animal studies show fetal abnormalities. Decide with your doctor whether drug benefits justify risk to unborn child.

Breast-feeding:
Drug passes into milk. Avoid drug or discontinue nursing until you finish medicine. Consult doctor for advice on maintaining milk supply.

Infants & children:
Not recommended.

Prolonged use:
Causes cancer in laboratory animals. Consult your doctor if you have family or personal history of cancer.

Skin & sunlight:
No problems expected.

Driving, piloting or hazardous work:
Avoid if you feel drowsy, dizzy or faint. Otherwise, no problems expected.

Airplane passengers:
No problems expected.

Discontinuing:
Don't discontinue without consulting doctor. Dose may require gradual reduction if you have taken drug for a long time. Doses of other drugs may also require adjustment.

Others:
Consult your doctor if you do isometric exercises. These raise blood pressure. Drug may intensify blood-pressure rise.

INTERACTION WITH OTHER DRUGS

GENERIC NAME OR DRUG CLASS	COMBINED EFFECT
Anticoagulants (oral)	Unpredictable increased or decreased effect of anticoagulant.
Anticonvulsants	Serious change in seizure pattern.
Antidepressants	Increased antidepressant effect.
Antihistamines	Increased antihistamine effect.
Aspirin	Decreased aspirin effect.
Beta-adrenergic blockers	Increased effect of reserpine. Excessive sedation.
Digitalis preparations	Irregular heartbeat.
Levodopa	Decreased levodopa effect.
MAO inhibitors	Severe depression.
Mind-altering drugs	Excessive sedation.
Narcotics	Increased narcotic effect.

Additional interactions on page 843.

INTERACTION WITH OTHER SUBSTANCES

INTERACTS WITH	COMBINED EFFECT
Alcohol:	Increased intoxication. Use with extreme caution.
Beverages: Carbonated drinks	Decreased reserpine effect.
Cocaine:	Decreased reserpine effect.
Foods: Spicy foods	Possible digestive upset.
Marijuana:	Occasional use—Mild drowsiness. Daily use—Moderate drowsiness, low blood pressure, depression.
Tobacco:	No problems expected.

RIFAMPIN

BRAND NAMES

Rifadin
Rifomycin
Rifamate (M)
Rimactane
Rofact

GENERAL INFORMATION

Habit forming? No
Prescription needed? Yes
Available as generic? No
Drug class: Antibiotic (rifamycin)

 USES

Treatment for tuberculosis and other infections. Requires daily use for 1 to 2 years.

DOSAGE & USAGE INFORMATION

How to take:
Capsule—Swallow with liquid. If you can't swallow whole, open capsule and take with liquid or small amount of food. For child, mix with small amount of applesauce or jelly.

When to take:
1 hour before or 2 hours after a meal.

If you forget a dose:
Take as soon as you remember up to 2 hours late. If more than 2 hours, wait for next scheduled dose (don't double this dose).

What drug does:
Prevents multiplication of tuberculosis germs.

Time lapse before drug works:
Usually 2 weeks. May require 1 to 2 years without missed doses for maximum benefit.

Don't take with:
See Interaction column and consult doctor.

 OVERDOSE

Symptoms:
Slow, shallow breathing; weak, rapid pulse; cold, sweaty skin; coma.

What to do:
- Dial 0 (operator) or 911 (emergency) for an ambulance or medical help. Then give first aid immediately.
- If patient is unconscious and not breathing, give mouth-to-mouth breathing. If there is no heartbeat, use cardiac massage and mouth-to-mouth breathing (CPR). Don't try to make patient vomit. If you can't get help quickly, take patient to nearest emergency facility.
- Additional emergency information on page 886.

 POSSIBLE ADVERSE REACTIONS OR SIDE EFFECTS

SYMPTOMS	FREQUENCY	WHAT TO DO
Brain & nervous system:		
● Headache	Infrequent	5
● Dizziness, unsteady gait, confusion.	Infrequent	4
Skin:		
Rash, itch.	Infrequent	3
Eyes:		
Blurred vision.	Infrequent	3
Ears, nose, throat:		
Sore throat, mouth or tongue.	Rare	3
Digestive:		
● Diarrhea	Common	4
● Appetite loss, vomiting.	Rare	4
Heart & lungs:		
Breathing difficulty.	Infrequent	3
Blood vessels:	None expected.	
Muscles, bones, joints:		
Muscle, bone pain.	Infrequent	4
Genital, urinary:		
Less urination.	Rare	4
Kidneys:	None expected.	
Liver:		
Jaundice (yellow skin and eyes).	Rare	3
Allergic:	None expected.	
Blood:	None expected.	
Others:		
Reddish urine, stool, saliva, sweat and tears.	Common	4

1-Life-threatening. Seek emergency treatment immediately.
2-Discontinue. Seek emergency treatment.
3-Discontinue. Call doctor right away.
4-Continue. Call doctor when convenient.
5-Continue. Tell doctor at next visit.
6-No action necessary.

WARNINGS & PRECAUTIONS

Don't take if:
- You are allergic to rifampin.
- You wear soft contact lenses.

Before you start, consult your doctor:
If you are alcoholic or have liver disease.

Over age 60:
Adverse reactions and side effects may be more frequent and severe than in younger persons.

Pregnancy:
Studies inconclusive on harm to unborn child. Animal studies show fetal abnormalities. Decide with your doctor whether drug benefits justify risk to unborn child.

Breast-feeding:
No proven problems. Consult doctor.

Infants & children:
Use only under medical supervision.

Prolonged use:
You may become more susceptible to infections caused by germs not responsive to rifampin.

Skin & sunlight:
No problems expected.

Driving, piloting or hazardous work:
Don't drive or pilot aircraft until you learn how medicine affects you. Don't work around dangerous machinery. Don't climb ladders or work in high places. Danger increases if you drink alcohol or take medicine affecting alertness and reflexes, such as antihistamines, tranquilizers, sedatives, pain medicine, narcotics and mind-altering drugs.

Airplane passengers:
No problems expected.

Discontinuing:
Don't discontinue without doctor's advice until you complete prescribed dose, even though symptoms diminish or disappear.

Others:
No problems expected.

INTERACTION WITH OTHER DRUGS

GENERIC NAME OR DRUG CLASS	COMBINED EFFECT
Anticoagulants (oral)	Decreased anticoagulant effect.
Barbiturates	Decreased barbiturate effect.
Contraceptives (oral)	Decreased contraceptive effect.
Cortisone drugs	Decreased effect of cortisone drugs.
Dapsone	Decreased dapsone effect.
Digitoxin	Decreased digitoxin effect.
Isoniazid	Possible toxicity to liver.
Methadone	Decreased methadone effect.
Para-aminosalicylic acid (PAS)	Decreased rifampin effect.
Probenecid	Possible toxicity to liver.
Tolbutamide	Decreased tolbutamide effect.
Trimethoprim	Decreased trimethoprim effect.

INTERACTION WITH OTHER SUBSTANCES

INTERACTS WITH	COMBINED EFFECT
Alcohol:	Possible toxicity to liver.
Beverages:	None expected.
Cocaine:	No proven problems.
Foods:	None expected.
Marijuana:	No proven problems.
Tobacco:	None expected.

SCOPOLAMINE (HYOSCINE)

BRAND NAMES

Barbidonna (M)   Levamine (M)
Donnatal (M)   Omnibel (M)
Kinesed (M)

See complete brand names list, page 830.

See complete brand names list, page 830.

GENERAL INFORMATION

Habit forming? No
Prescription needed? Low strength: No
High strength: Yes
Available as generic? Yes
Drug class: Antispasmodic, anticholinergic

USES

- Reduces spasms of digestive system, bladder and urethra.
- Relieves painful menstruation.
- Prevents motion sickness.

DOSAGE & USAGE INFORMATION

How to take:
- Tablet or capsule—Swallow with liquid or food to lessen stomach irritation.
- Extended-release tablets or capsules—Swallow each dose whole.
- Drops—Dilute dose in beverage.
- Skin discs—Clean application site. Change application sites with each dose.

When to take:
- Motion sickness—Apply disc 30 minutes before departure.
- Other uses—Take 30 minutes before meals (unless directed otherwise by doctor).

If you forget a dose:
Take up to 2 hours late. If more than 2 hours, wait for next dose (don't double this).

What drug does:
Blocks nerve impulses at parasympathetic nerve endings, preventing muscle contractions and gland secretions of organs involved.

Time lapse before drug works:
15 to 30 minutes.

Don't take with:
See Interaction column and consult doctor.

OVERDOSE

Symptoms:
Dilated pupils; rapid pulse and breathing; dizziness; fever; hallucinations; confusion; slurred speech; agitation; flushed face; convulsions; coma.

What to do:
- Dial 0 (operator) or 911 (emergency) for an ambulance or medical help. Then give first aid immediately.
- Additional emergency information on page 886.

POSSIBLE ADVERSE REACTIONS OR SIDE EFFECTS

SYMPTOMS	FREQUENCY	WHAT TO DO
Brain & nervous system:		
• Headache	Infrequent	4
• Confusion, delirium.	Common	3
Skin:		
Rash or hives.	Rare	3
Eyes:		
Pain, blurred vision.	Rare	3
Ears, nose, throat:		
Dryness	Common	6
Digestive:		
• Constipation	Common	5
• Nausea, vomiting.	Common	4
Heart & lungs:		
Rapid heartbeat.	Common	3
Blood vessels:	None expected.	
Muscles, bones, joints:	None expected.	
Genital, urinary:		
Difficult urination.	Infrequent	4
Kidneys:	None expected.	
Liver:	None expected.	
Allergic:	None expected.	
Blood:	None expected.	
Others:		
Less perspiration.	Common	4

1- Life-threatening. Seek emergency treatment immediately.
2- Discontinue. Seek emergency treatment.
3- Discontinue. Call doctor right away.
4- Continue. Call doctor when convenient.
5- Continue. Tell doctor at next visit.
6- No action necessary.

SCOPOLAMINE (HYOSCINE)

WARNINGS & PRECAUTIONS

Don't take if:
- You are allergic to any anticholinergic.
- You have trouble with stomach bloating.
- You have difficulty emptying your bladder completely.
- You have narrow-angle glaucoma.
- You have severe ulcerative colitis.

Before you start, consult your doctor:
- If you have open-angle glaucoma.
- If you have angina.
- If you have chronic bronchitis or asthma.
- If you have hiatal hernia.
- If you have liver disease.
- If you have enlarged prostate.
- If you have myasthenia gravis.
- If you have peptic ulcer.
- If you will have surgery within 2 months, including dental surgery, requiring general or spinal anesthesia.

Over age 60:
Adverse reactions and side effects may be more frequent and severe than in younger persons.

Pregnancy:
Studies inconclusive on harm to unborn child. Animal studies show fetal abnormalities. Decide with your doctor whether drug benefits justify risk to unborn child.

Breast-feeding:
Drug passes into milk and decreases milk flow. Avoid drug or discontinue nursing until you finish medicine. Consult doctor for advice on maintaining milk supply.

Infants & children:
Use only under medical supervision.

Prolonged use:
Chronic constipation, possible fecal impaction. Consult doctor immediately.

Skin & sunlight:
No problems expected.

Driving, piloting or hazardous work:
Use disqualifies you for piloting aircraft. Otherwise, no problems expected.

Airplane passengers:
No problems expected.

Discontinuing:
May be unnecessary to finish medicine. Follow doctor's instructions.

Others:
No problems expected.

INTERACTION WITH OTHER DRUGS

GENERIC NAME OR DRUG CLASS	COMBINED EFFECT
Amantadine	Increased scopolamine effect.
Anticholinergics (other)	Increased scopolamine effect.
Antidepressants (tricyclic)	Increased scopolamine effect.
Antihistamines	Increased scopolamine effect.
Cortisone drugs	Increased internal-eye pressure.
Haloperidol	Increased internal-eye pressure.
MAO inhibitors	Increased scopolamine effect.
Meperidine	Increased scopolamine effect.
Methylphenidate	Increased scopolamine effect.
Orphenadrine	Increased scopolamine effect.
Phenothiazines	Increased scopolamine effect.
Pilocarpine	Loss of pilocarpine effect in glaucoma treatment.
Vitamin C	Decreased scopolamine effect. Avoid large doses of vitamin C.

INTERACTION WITH OTHER SUBSTANCES

INTERACTS WITH	COMBINED EFFECT
Alcohol:	None expected.
Beverages:	None expected.
Cocaine:	Excessively rapid heartbeat. Avoid.
Foods:	None expected.
Marijuana:	Drowsiness and dry mouth.
Tobacco:	None expected.

SECOBARBITAL

BRAND NAMES

Secogen
Seconal
Seral
Tuinal (M)

GENERAL INFORMATION

Habit forming? Yes
Prescription needed? Yes
Available as generic? Yes
Drug class: Sedative, hypnotic (barbiturate)

 ## USES

- Reduces anxiety or nervous tension (low dose).
- Relieves insomnia (higher bedtime dose).

 ## DOSAGE & USAGE INFORMATION

How to take:
- Tablet, capsule or liquid—Swallow with food or liquid to lessen stomach irritation. If you can't swallow whole, crumble tablet or open capsule and take with liquid or food.
- Suppositories—Remove wrapper and moisten suppository with water. Gently insert larger end into rectum. Push well into rectum with finger.

When to take:
At the same times each day.

If you forget a dose:
Take as soon as you remember up to 2 hours late. If more than 2 hours, wait for next scheduled dose (don't double this dose).

What drug does:
May partially block nerve impulses at nerve-cell connections.

Time lapse before drug works:
60 minutes.

Don't take with:
- Non-prescription drugs without consulting doctor.
- See Interaction column and consult doctor.

 ## OVERDOSE

Symptoms:
Deep sleep, weak pulse, coma.

What to do:
- Dial O (operator) or 911 (emergency) for an ambulance or medical help. Then give first aid immediately.
- Additional emergency information on page 886.

POSSIBLE ADVERSE REACTIONS OR SIDE EFFECTS

SYMPTOMS	FREQUENCY	WHAT TO DO
Brain & nervous system:		
• Dizziness, drowsiness, "hangover effect."	Common	4
• Depression, confusion, slurred speech.	Infrequent	4
• Agitation	Rare	3
Skin:		
• Rash or hives.	Infrequent	3
• Face, lip swelling.	Infrequent	3
Eyes:		
Eyelid swelling.	Infrequent	3
Ears, nose, throat:		
Sore throat, fever.	Infrequent	3
Digestive:		
Diarrhea, nausea, vomiting.	Infrequent	4
Heart & lungs:		
• Slow heartbeat.	Rare	3
• Breathing difficulty.	Rare	3
Blood vessels:		
Unexplained bleeding or bruising.	Rare	4
Muscles, bones, joints:		
Joint or muscle pain.	Infrequent	4
Genital, urinary:	None expected.	
Kidneys:	None expected.	
Liver:		
Jaundice (yellow skin and eyes).	Rare	3
Allergic:	None expected.	
Blood:	None expected.	
Others:	None expected.	

1 - Life-threatening. Seek emergency treatment immediately.
2 - Discontinue. Seek emergency treatment.
3 - Discontinue. Call doctor right away.
4 - Continue. Call doctor when convenient.

WARNINGS & PRECAUTIONS

Don't take if:
- You are allergic to any barbiturate.
- You have porphyria.

Before you start, consult your doctor:
- If you have epilepsy.
- If you have kidney or liver damage.
- If you have asthma.
- If you have anemia.
- If you have chronic pain.
- If you will have surgery within 2 months, including dental surgery, requiring general or spinal anesthesia.

Over age 60:
Adverse reactions and side effects may be more frequent and severe than in younger persons. Use small doses.

Pregnancy:
Risk to unborn child outweighs drug benefits. Don't use.

Breast-feeding:
Drug passes into milk. Avoid drug or discontinue nursing until you finish medicine. Consult doctor for advice on maintaining milk supply.

Infants & children:
Use only under doctor's supervision.

Prolonged use:
- May cause addiction, anemia, chronic intoxication.
- May lower body temperature, making exposure to cold temperatures hazardous.

Skin & sunlight:
May cause rash or intensify sunburn in areas exposed to sun or sunlamp.

Driving, piloting or hazardous work:
Don't drive or pilot aircraft until you learn how medicine affects you. Don't work around dangerous machinery. Don't climb ladders or work in high places. Danger increases if you drink alcohol or take medicine affecting alertness and reflexes.

Airplane passengers:
No problems expected.

Discontinuing:
May be unnecessary to finish medicine. Follow doctor's instructions. If you develop withdrawal symptoms of hallucinations, agitation or sleeplessness after discontinuing, call doctor right away.

Others:
No problems expected.

INTERACTION WITH OTHER DRUGS

GENERIC NAME OR DRUG CLASS	COMBINED EFFECT
Anticoagulants (oral)	Decreased anticoagulant effect.
Anticonvulsants	Changed seizure patterns.
Antidepressants (tricyclic)	Decreased antidepressant effect.
Antidiabetics (oral)	Increased secobarbital effect.
Antihistamines	Dangerous sedation. Avoid.
Antiinflammatory drugs (non-steroidal)	Decreased antiinflammatory effect.
Aspirin	Decreased aspirin effect.
Beta-adrenergic blockers	Decreased effect of beta-adrenergic blocker.
Contraceptives (oral)	Decreased contraceptive effect.
Cortisone drugs	Decreased cortisone effect.
Digitoxin	Decreased digitoxin effect.
Doxycycline	Decreased doxycycline effect.
Griseofulvin	Decreased griseofulvin effect.

Additional interactions on page 843.

INTERACTION WITH OTHER SUBSTANCES

INTERACTS WITH	COMBINED EFFECT
Alcohol:	Possible fatal oversedation. Avoid.
Beverages:	None expected.
Cocaine:	Decreased secobarbital effect.
Foods:	None expected.
Marijuana:	Excessive sedation. Avoid.
Tobacco:	None expected.

SENNA

BRAND NAMES

Black Draught
Casa-Fru
Dr. Caldwell's Senna Laxative
Fletcher's Castoria
Senexon
Senokot

Swiss Kriss
X-Prep

GENERAL INFORMATION

Habit forming? No
Prescription needed? No
Available as generic? Yes
Drug class: Laxative (stimulant)

 ## USES

Constipation relief.

 ## DOSAGE & USAGE INFORMATION

How to take:
- Tablet—Swallow with liquid. If you can't swallow whole, chew or crumble tablet and take with liquid or food.
- Liquid, granules—Drink 6 to 8 glasses of water each day, in addition to one taken with each dose.

When to take:
Usually at bedtime with a snack, unless directed otherwise.

If you forget a dose:
Take as soon as you remember.

What drug does:
Acts on smooth muscles of intestine wall to cause vigorous bowel movement.

Time lapse before drug works:
6 to 10 hours.

Don't take with:
- See Interaction column and consult doctor.
- Don't take within 2 hours of taking another medicine. Laxative interferes with medicine absorption.

 ## OVERDOSE

Symptoms:
Vomiting, electrolyte depletion.

What to do:
Overdose unlikely to threaten life. If person takes much larger amount than prescribed, call doctor, poison-control center or hospital emergency room for instructions.

 ## POSSIBLE ADVERSE REACTIONS OR SIDE EFFECTS

SYMPTOMS	FREQUENCY	WHAT TO DO
Brain & nervous system: Irritability, confusion, headache.	Rare	3
Skin: Rash	Rare	3
Eyes:	None expected.	
Ears, nose, throat:	None expected.	
Digestive: Belching, cramps, nausea.	Infrequent	4
Heart & lungs: Breathing difficulty, irregular heartbeat.	Rare	3
Blood vessels:	None expected.	
Muscles, bones, joints: Muscle cramps.	Rare	3
Genital, urinary: Yellow-brown or red-violet urine.	Common	6
Kidneys: Burning on urination.	Rare	4
Liver:	None expected.	
Allergic:	None expected.	
Blood:	None expected.	
Others: • Rectal irritation.	Common	4
• Dangerous potassium loss.	Infrequent	3
• Unusual tiredness or weakness.	Rare	3

1- Life-threatening. Seek emergency treatment immediately.
2- Discontinue. Seek emergency treatment.
3- Discontinue. Call doctor right away.
4- Continue. Call doctor when convenient.
5- Continue. Tell doctor at next visit.
6- No action necessary.

WARNINGS & PRECAUTIONS

Don't take if:
- You have symptoms of appendicitis, inflamed bowel or intestinal blockage.
- You are allergic to a stimulant laxative.
- You have missed a bowel movement for only 1 or 2 days.

Before you start, consult your doctor:
- If you have a colostomy or ileostomy.
- If you have congestive heart disease.
- If you have diabetes.
- If you have high blood pressure.
- If you have a laxative habit.
- If you have rectal bleeding.
- If you take other laxatives.

Over age 60:
Adverse reactions and side effects may be more frequent and severe than in younger persons.

Pregnancy:
Risk to mother and unborn child outweighs drug benefits. Don't use.

Breast-feeding:
Drug passes into milk. Avoid drug or discontinue nursing until you finish medicine. Consult doctor for advice on maintaining milk supply.

Infants & children:
Use only under medical supervision.

Prolonged use:
Don't take for more than 1 week unless under a doctor's supervision. May cause laxative dependence.

Skin & sunlight:
No problems expected.

Driving, piloting or hazardous work:
No problems expected.

Airplane passengers:
No problems expected.

Discontinuing:
May be unnecessary to finish medicine. Follow doctor's instructions.

Others:
Don't take to "flush out" your system or as a "tonic."

INTERACTION WITH OTHER DRUGS

GENERIC NAME OR DRUG CLASS	COMBINED EFFECT
Antihypertensives	May cause dangerous low potassium level.
Diuretics	May cause dangerous low potassium level.

INTERACTION WITH OTHER SUBSTANCES

INTERACTS WITH	COMBINED EFFECT
Alcohol:	None expected.
Beverages:	None expected.
Cocaine:	None expected.
Foods:	None expected.
Marijuana:	None expected.
Tobacco:	None expected.

SENNOSIDES A & B

BRAND NAMES

Glysennid

GENERAL INFORMATION

Habit forming? No
Prescription needed? No
Available as generic? Yes
Drug class: Laxative (stimulant)

 ## USES

Constipation relief.

 ## DOSAGE & USAGE INFORMATION

How to take:
- Tablet—Swallow with liquid. If you can't swallow whole, chew or crumble tablet and take with liquid or food.
- Liquid, granules—Drink 6 to 8 glasses of water each day, in addition to one taken with each dose.

When to take:
Usually at bedtime with a snack, unless directed otherwise.

If you forget a dose:
Take as soon as you remember.

What drug does:
Acts on smooth muscles of intestine wall to cause vigorous bowel movement.

Time lapse before drug works:
6 to 10 hours.

Don't take with:
- See Interaction column and consult doctor.
- Don't take within 2 hours of taking another medicine. Laxative interferes with medicine absorption.

 ## OVERDOSE

Symptoms:
Vomiting, electrolyte depletion.

What to do:
Overdose unlikely to threaten life. If person takes much larger amount than prescribed, call doctor, poison-control center or hospital emergency room for instructions.

POSSIBLE ADVERSE REACTIONS OR SIDE EFFECTS

SYMPTOMS	FREQUENCY	WHAT TO DO
Brain & nervous system: Irritability, confusion, headache.	Rare	3
Skin: Rash	Rare	3
Eyes:	None expected.	
Ears, nose, throat:	None expected.	
Digestive: Belching, cramps, nausea.	Infrequent	4
Heart & lungs: Breathing difficulty, irregular heartbeat.	Rare	3
Blood vessels:	None expected.	
Muscles, bones, joints: Muscle cramps.	Rare	3
Genital, urinary: Yellow-brown or red-violet urine.	Common	6
Kidneys: Burning on urination.	Rare	4
Liver:	None expected.	
Allergic:	None expected.	
Blood:	None expected.	
Others: • Rectal irritation.	Common	4
• Dangerous potassium loss.	Infrequent	3
• Unusual tiredness or weakness.	Rare	3

1- Life-threatening. Seek emergency treatment immediately.
2- Discontinue. Seek emergency treatment.
3- Discontinue. Call doctor right away.
4- Continue. Call doctor when convenient.
5- Continue. Tell doctor at next visit.
6- No action necessary.

WARNINGS & PRECAUTIONS

Don't take if:
- You have symptoms of appendicitis, inflamed bowel or intestinal blockage.
- You are allergic to a stimulant laxative.
- You have missed a bowel movement for only 1 or 2 days.

Before you start, consult your doctor:
- If you have a colostomy or ileostomy.
- If you have congestive heart disease.
- If you have diabetes.
- If you have high blood pressure.
- If you have a laxative habit.
- If you have rectal bleeding.
- If you take other laxatives.

Over age 60:
Adverse reactions and side effects may be more frequent and severe than in younger persons.

Pregnancy:
Risk to mother and unborn child outweighs drug benefits. Don't use.

Breast-feeding:
Drug passes into milk. Avoid drug or discontinue nursing until you finish medicine. Consult doctor for advice on maintaining milk supply.

Infants & children:
Use only under medical supervision.

Prolonged use:
Don't take for more than 1 week unless under a doctor's supervision. May cause laxative dependence.

Skin & sunlight:
No problems expected.

Driving, piloting or hazardous work:
No problems expected.

Airplane passengers:
No problems expected.

Discontinuing:
May be unnecessary to finish medicine. Follow doctor's instructions.

Others:
Don't take to "flush out" your system or as a "tonic."

 INTERACTION WITH OTHER DRUGS

GENERIC NAME OR DRUG CLASS	COMBINED EFFECT
Antihypertensives	May cause dangerous low potassium level.
Diuretics	May cause dangerous low potassium level.

 INTERACTION WITH OTHER SUBSTANCES

INTERACTS WITH	COMBINED EFFECT
Alcohol:	None expected.
Beverages:	None expected.
Cocaine:	None expected.
Foods:	None expected.
Marijuana:	None expected.
Tobacco:	None expected.

SIMETHICONE

BRAND NAMES

Di-Gel (M)
Gas-X
Mylicon
Ovol
Silain

GENERAL INFORMATION

Habit forming? No
Prescription needed? No
Available as generic? Yes
Drug class: Antiflatulent

USES

- Treatment for retention of abdominal gas.
- Used prior to x-ray of abdomen to reduce gas shadows.

DOSAGE & USAGE INFORMATION

How to take:
- Tablet—Swallow with liquid.
- Liquid—Dissolve in water. Drink complete dose.
- Chewable tablets—Chew completely. Don't swallow whole.

When to take:
After meals and at bedtime.

If you forget a dose:
Take when remembered if needed.

What drug does:
Reduces surface tension of gas bubbles in stomach.

Time lapse before drug works:
10 minutes.

Don't take with:
No restrictions.

OVERDOSE

Symptoms:
None expected.

What to do:
Overdose unlikely to threaten life.

POSSIBLE ADVERSE REACTIONS OR SIDE EFFECTS

SYMPTOMS	FREQUENCY	WHAT TO DO
Brain & nervous system:	None expected.	
Skin:	None expected.	
Eyes:	None expected.	
Ears, nose, throat:	None expected.	
Digestive:	None expected.	
Heart & lungs:	None expected.	
Blood vessels:	None expected.	
Muscles, bones, joints:	None expected.	
Genital, urinary:	None expected.	
Kidneys:	None expected.	
Liver:	None expected.	
Allergic:	None expected.	
Blood:	None expected.	
Others:	None expected.	

1- Life-threatening. Seek emergency treatment immediately.
2- Discontinue. Seek emergency treatment.
3- Discontinue. Call doctor right away.
4- Continue. Call doctor when convenient.
5- Continue. Tell doctor at next visit.
6- No action necessary.

SIMETHICONE

WARNINGS & PRECAUTIONS

Don't take if:
You are allergic to simethicone.

Before you start, consult your doctor:
No problems expected.

Over age 60:
No problems expected.

Pregnancy:
No proven harm to unborn child. Avoid if possible.

Breast-feeding:
No problems expected.

Infants & children:
Not recommended.

Prolonged use:
No problems expected.

Skin & sunlight:
No problems expected.

Driving, piloting or hazardous work:
No problems expected.

Airplane passengers:
No problems expected.

Discontinuing:
May be unnecessary to finish medicine. Discontinue when symptoms disappear.

Others:
No problems expected.

INTERACTION WITH OTHER DRUGS

GENERIC NAME OR DRUG CLASS	COMBINED EFFECT
None	

INTERACTION WITH OTHER SUBSTANCES

INTERACTS WITH	COMBINED EFFECT
Alcohol:	None expected.
Beverages:	None expected.
Cocaine:	None expected.
Foods:	None expected.
Marijuana:	None expected.
Tobacco:	None expected.

SODIUM BICARBONATE

BRAND NAMES

Alka-Seltzer Antacid
Alka-Citrate Compound
Bell/ans
Bisodol Powder
Brioschi
Bromo Seltzer

Chembicarb
Eno
Fizrin
Seidlitz Powder
Soda Mint

GENERAL INFORMATION

Habit forming? No
Prescription needed? No
Available as generic? Yes
Drug class: Antacid

 ## USES

Treatment for hyperacidity in upper gastrointestinal tract, including stomach and esophagus. Symptoms may be heartburn or acid indigestion. Diseases include peptic ulcer, gastritis, esophagitis, hiatal hernia.

 ## DOSAGE & USAGE INFORMATION

How to take:
• Tablet—Swallow with liquid.
• Chewable tablets or wafers—Chew well before swallowing.
• Powder—Dilute dose in beverage before swallowing.

When to take:
1 to 3 hours after meals unless directed otherwise by your doctor.

If you forget a dose:
Take as soon as you remember.

What drug does:
• Neutralizes some of the hydrochloric acid in the stomach.
• Reduces action of pepsin, a digestive enzyme.

Time lapse before drug works:
15 minutes.

Don't take with:
Other medicines at the same time. Decreases absorption of other drugs.

 ## OVERDOSE

Symptoms:
Weakness, fatigue, dizziness.

What to do:
Overdose unlikely to threaten life. If person takes much larger amount than prescribed, call doctor, poison-control center or hospital emergency room for instructions.

 ## POSSIBLE ADVERSE REACTIONS OR SIDE EFFECTS

SYMPTOMS	FREQUENCY	WHAT TO DO
Brain & nervous system: Mood changes.	Infrequent	4
Skin:	None expected.	
Eyes:	None expected.	
Ears, nose, throat:	None expected.	
Digestive:		
• Constipation, appetite loss.	Common	4
• Nausea, vomiting.	Infrequent	4
• Lower abdominal pain and swelling.	Infrequent	3
• Belching	Common	5
Heart & lungs:	None expected.	
Blood vessels:	None expected.	
Muscles, bones, joints: Bone pain, muscle weakness.	Infrequent	3
Genital, urinary:	None expected.	
Kidneys:	None expected.	
Liver:	None expected.	
Allergic:	None expected.	
Blood:	None expected.	
Others:		
• Swelling of wrists or ankles.	Infrequent	3
• Weight loss.	Infrequent	4
• Weight gain.	Common	4

1- Life-threatening. Seek emergency treatment immediately.
2- Discontinue. Seek emergency treatment.
3- Discontinue. Call doctor right away.
4- Continue. Call doctor when convenient.
5- Continue. Tell doctor at next visit.
6- No action necessary.

SODIUM BICARBONATE

WARNINGS & PRECAUTIONS

Don't take if:
You are allergic to any antacid.

Before you start, consult your doctor:
- If you have kidney disease, liver disease, high blood pressure or congestive heart failure.
- If you have chronic constipation or diarrhea.
- If you have symptoms of appendicitis.
- If you have stomach or intestinal bleeding.

Over age 60:
Adverse reactions and side effects may be more frequent and severe than in younger persons. Diarrhea or constipation particularly likely.

Pregnancy:
Risk to unborn child outweighs drug benefits. Don't use.

Breast-feeding:
Drug passes into milk. Avoid drug or discontinue nursing until you finish medicine. Consult doctor for advice on maintaining milk supply.

Infants & children:
Use only under medical supervision.

Prolonged use:
Prolonged use with calcium supplements or milk leads to too much calcium in blood.

Skin & sunlight:
No problems expected.

Driving, piloting or hazardous work:
No problems expected.

Airplane passengers:
No problems expected.

Discontinuing:
May be unnecessary to finish medicine. Follow doctor's instructions.

Others:
Don't take longer than 2 weeks unless under medical supervision.

INTERACTION WITH OTHER DRUGS

GENERIC NAME OR DRUG CLASS	COMBINED EFFECT
Amphetamine	Increased amphetamine effect.
Anticoagulants	Decreased anticoagulant effect.
Iron supplements	Decreased iron effect.
Meperidine	Increased meperidine effect.
Nalidixic acid	Decreased effect of nalidixic acid.
Oxyphenbutazone	Decreased oxyphenbutazone effect.
Para-aminosalicylic acid (PAS)	Decreased PAS effect.
Penicillins	Decreased penicillin effect.
Pentobarbital	Decreased pentobarbital effect.
Phenylbutazone	Decreased phenylbutazone effect.
Pseudoephedrine	Increased pseudoephedrine effect.
Quinidine	Increased quinidine effect.
Salicylates	Decreased salicylate effect.
Sulfa drugs	Decreased sulfa effect.
Tetracyclines	Decreased tetracycline effect.

INTERACTION WITH OTHER SUBSTANCES

INTERACTS WITH	COMBINED EFFECT
Alcohol:	Decreased antacid effect.
Beverages:	No proven problems.
Cocaine:	No proven problems.
Foods:	Decreased antacid effect. Wait 1 hour after eating.
Marijuana:	No proven problems.
Tobacco:	Decreased antacid effect.

SODIUM CARBONATE

BRAND NAMES

Rolaids (M)

GENERAL INFORMATION

Habit forming? No
Prescription needed? No
Available as generic? Yes
Drug class: Antacid

USES

Treatment for hyperacidity in upper gastrointestinal tract, including stomach and esophagus. Symptoms may be heartburn or acid indigestion. Diseases include peptic ulcer, gastritis, esophagitis, hiatal hernia.

DOSAGE & USAGE INFORMATION

How to take:
Chewable tablets or wafers—Chew well before swallowing.

When to take:
1 to 3 hours after meals unless directed otherwise by your doctor.

If you forget a dose:
Take as soon as you remember.

What drug does:
- Neutralizes some of the hydrochloric acid in the stomach.
- Reduces action of pepsin, a digestive enzyme.

Time lapse before drug works:
15 minutes.

Don't take with:
Other medicines at the same time. Decreases absorption of other drugs.

OVERDOSE

Symptoms:
Weakness, fatigue, dizziness.

What to do:
Overdose unlikely to threaten life. If person takes much larger amount than prescribed, call doctor, poison-control center or hospital emergency room for instructions.

POSSIBLE ADVERSE REACTIONS OR SIDE EFFECTS

SYMPTOMS	FREQUENCY	WHAT TO DO
Brain & nervous system: Mood changes.	Infrequent	4
Skin:	None expected.	
Eyes:	None expected.	
Ears, nose, throat:	None expected.	
Digestive:		
• Constipation, appetite loss.	Common	4
• Nausea, vomiting.	Infrequent	4
• Lower abdominal pain and swelling.	Infrequent	3
Heart & lungs:	None expected.	
Blood vessels:	None expected.	
Muscles, bones, joints: Bone pain, muscle weakness.	Infrequent	3
Genital, urinary:	None expected.	
Kidneys:	None expected.	
Liver:	None expected.	
Allergic:	None expected.	
Blood:	None expected.	
Others:		
• Swelling of wrists or ankles.	Infrequent	3
• Weight loss.	Infrequent	4

1- Life-threatening. Seek emergency treatment immediately.
2- Discontinue. Seek emergency treatment.
3- Discontinue. Call doctor right away.
4- Continue. Call doctor when convenient.
5- Continue. Tell doctor at next visit.
6- No action necessary.

SODIUM CARBONATE

WARNINGS & PRECAUTIONS

Don't take if:
You are allergic to any antacid.

Before you start, consult your doctor:
- If you have kidney disease, liver disease, high blood pressure or congestive heart failure.
- If you have chronic constipation or diarrhea.
- If you have symptoms of appendicitis.
- If you have stomach or intestinal bleeding.

Over age 60:
Adverse reactions and side effects may be more frequent and severe than in younger persons. Diarrhea or constipation particularly likely.

Pregnancy:
Risk to unborn child outweighs drug benefits. Don't use.

Breast-feeding:
Drug passes into milk. Avoid drug or discontinue nursing until you finish medicine. Consult doctor for advice on maintaining milk supply.

Infants & children:
Use only under medical supervision.

Prolonged use:
Fluid retention.

Skin & sunlight:
No problems expected.

Driving, piloting or hazardous work:
No problems expected.

Airplane passengers:
No problems expected.

Discontinuing:
May be unnecessary to finish medicine. Follow doctor's instructions.

Others:
Don't take longer than 2 weeks unless under medical supervision.

INTERACTION WITH OTHER DRUGS

GENERIC NAME OR DRUG CLASS	COMBINED EFFECT
Anticoagulants	Decreased anticoagulant effect.
Chlorpromazine	Decreased chlorpromazine effect.
Digitalis preparations	Decreased digitalis effect.
Iron supplements	Decreased iron effect.
Meperidine	Increased meperidine effect.
Nalidixic acid	Decreased effect of nalidixic acid.
Oxyphenbutazone	Decreased oxyphenbutazone effect.
Para-aminosalicylic acid (PAS)	Decreased PAS effect.
Penicillins	Decreased penicillin effect.
Pentobarbital	Decreased pentobarbital effect.
Phenylbutazone	Decreased phenylbutazone effect.
Pseudoephedrine	Increased pseudoephedrine effect.
Sulfa drugs	Decreased sulfa effect.
Tetracyclines	Decreased tetracycline effect.
Vitamins A and C	Decreased vitamin effect.

INTERACTION WITH OTHER SUBSTANCES

INTERACTS WITH	COMBINED EFFECT
Alcohol:	Decreased antacid effect.
Beverages:	No proven problems.
Cocaine:	No proven problems.
Foods:	Decreased antacid effect. Wait 1 hour after eating.
Marijuana:	No proven problems.
Tobacco:	Decreased antacid effect.

SODIUM FLUORIDE

BRAND NAMES

Denta-Fl
Flo-Tab
Fluorident
Fluoritab
Fluorodex

Flura
Karidium
Luride
Nafeen
Pediaflor

Pedi-Dent
Stay-Flo
Studaflor

Numerous other multiple vitamin-mineral supplements.

GENERAL INFORMATION

Habit forming? No
Prescription needed? Yes
Available as generic? Yes
Drug class: Mineral supplement
(fluoride)

 ## USES

Reduces tooth cavities.

 ## DOSAGE & USAGE INFORMATION

How to take:
- Tablet—Swallow with liquid or crumble tablet and take with liquid (*not* milk) or food.
- Liquid—Measure with dropper and take directly or with liquid.
- Chewable tablets—Chew slowly and thoroughly before swallowing.

When to take:
Usually at bedtime after teeth are thoroughly brushed.

If you forget a dose:
Take as soon as you remember. Don't double a forgotten dose. Return to schedule.

What drug does:
Provides supplemental fluoride to combat tooth decay.

Time lapse before drug works:
8 weeks to provide maximum effect.

Don't take with:
- Other medicine simultaneously.
- See Interaction column.

 ## OVERDOSE

Symptoms:
Stomach cramps or pain, nausea, faintness, vomiting (possibly bloody), diarrhea, black stools, shallow breathing.

What to do:
- Dial 0 (operator) or 911 (emergency) for an ambulance or medical help. Then give first aid immediately.
- Additional emergency information on page 886.

 ## POSSIBLE ADVERSE REACTIONS OR SIDE EFFECTS

SYMPTOMS	FREQUENCY	WHAT TO DO
Brain & nervous system:	None expected.	
Skin: Rash	Infrequent	3
Eyes:	None expected.	
Ears, nose, throat: Sores in mouth and lips.	Rare	3
Digestive: Severe upsets only with overdose.	Rare	2
Heart & lungs:	None expected.	
Blood vessels:	None expected.	
Muscles, bones, joints:	None expected.	
Genital, urinary:	None expected.	
Kidneys:	None expected.	
Liver:	None expected.	
Allergic:	None expected.	
Blood:	None expected.	
Others:	None expected.	

1- Life-threatening. Seek emergency treatment immediately.
2- Discontinue. Seek emergency treatment.
3- Discontinue. Call doctor right away.
4- Continue. Call doctor when convenient.
5- Continue. Tell doctor at next visit.
6- No action necessary.

WARNINGS & PRECAUTIONS

Don't take if:
- Your water supply contains 0.7 parts fluoride per million. Too much fluoride stains teeth permanently.
- You are allergic to any fluoride-containing product.
- You have underactive thyroid.

Before you start, consult your doctor:
Not necessary.

Over age 60:
No problems expected.

Pregnancy:
No problems expected.

Breast-feeding:
No problems expected.

Infants & children:
No problems expected except accidental overdose. Keep vitamin-mineral supplements out of children's reach.

Prolonged use:
Excess may cause discolored teeth and decreased calcium in blood.

Skin & sunlight:
No problems expected.

Driving, piloting or hazardous work:
No problems expected.

Airplane passengers:
No problems expected.

Discontinuing:
No problems expected.

Others:
Store in original plastic container. Fluoride decomposes glass.

INTERACTION WITH OTHER DRUGS

GENERIC NAME OR DRUG CLASS	COMBINED EFFECT
None	

INTERACTION WITH OTHER SUBSTANCES

INTERACTS WITH	COMBINED EFFECT
Alcohol:	None expected.
Beverages: Milk	Prevents absorption of fluoride. Space dose 2 hours before or after milk.
Cocaine:	None expected.
Foods:	None expected.
Marijuana:	None expected.
Tobacco:	None expected.

SODIUM PHOSPHATE

BRAND NAMES

Phospho-Soda
Sal Hepatica

GENERAL INFORMATION

Habit forming? No
Prescription needed? No
Available as generic? Yes
Drug class: Laxative (hyperosmotic)

 USES

Constipation relief.

 DOSAGE & USAGE INFORMATION

How to take:
Liquid, effervescent tablet or powder—Dilute dose in beverage before swallowing.

When to take:
Usually once a day, preferably in the morning.

If you forget a dose:
Take as soon as you remember up to 8 hours before bedtime. If later, wait for next scheduled dose (don't double this dose). Don't take at bedtime.

What drug does:
Draws water into bowel from other body tissues. Causes distention through fluid accumulation, which promotes soft stool and accelerates bowel motion.

Time lapse before drug works:
30 minutes to 3 hours.

Don't take with:
See Interaction column and consult doctor.

 OVERDOSE

Symptoms:
Fluid depletion, weakness, vomiting, fainting.

What to do:
Overdose unlikely to threaten life. If person takes much larger amount than prescribed, call doctor, poison-control center or hospital emergency room for instructions.

POSSIBLE ADVERSE REACTIONS OR SIDE EFFECTS

SYMPTOMS	FREQUENCY	WHAT TO DO
Brain & nervous system: Dizziness, confusion.	Rare	4
Skin:	None expected.	
Eyes:	None expected.	
Ears, nose, throat: Increased thirst.	Infrequent	5
Digestive: Cramps, nausea, diarrhea, gas.	Infrequent	5
Heart & lungs: Irregular heartbeat.	Infrequent	3
Blood vessels:	None expected.	
Muscles, bones, joints:	None expected.	
Genital, urinary:	None expected.	
Kidneys:	None expected.	
Liver:	None expected.	
Allergic:	None expected.	
Blood:	None expected.	
Others: Tiredness or weakness.	Rare	4

1 - Life-threatening. Seek emergency treatment immediately.
2 - Discontinue. Seek emergency treatment.
3 - Discontinue. Call doctor right away.
4 - Continue. Call doctor when convenient.
5 - Continue. Tell doctor at next visit.
6 - No action necessary.

SODIUM PHOSPHATE

WARNINGS & PRECAUTIONS

Don't take if:
- You are allergic to any hyperosmotic laxative.
- You have symptoms of appendicitis, inflamed bowel or intestinal blockage.
- You have missed a bowel movement for only 1 or 2 days.

Before you start, consult your doctor:
- If you have congestive heart disease.
- If you have diabetes.
- If you have high blood pressure.
- If you have a colostomy or ileostomy.
- If you have kidney disease.
- If you have a laxative habit.
- If you have rectal bleeding.
- If you take another laxative.

Over age 60:
Adverse reactions and side effects may be more frequent and severe than in younger persons.

Pregnancy:
Salt content may cause fluid retention and swelling. Avoid if possible.

Breast-feeding:
No problems expected.

Infants & children:
Use only under medical supervision.

Prolonged use:
Don't take for more than 1 week unless under a doctor's supervision. May cause laxative dependence.

Skin & sunlight:
No problems expected.

Driving, piloting or hazardous work:
No problems expected.

Airplane passengers:
No problems expected.

Discontinuing:
May be unnecessary to finish medicine. Follow doctor's instructions.

Others:
- Don't take to "flush out" your system or as a "tonic."
- Don't take within 2 hours of taking another medicine.

INTERACTION WITH OTHER DRUGS

GENERIC NAME OR DRUG CLASS	COMBINED EFFECT
Chlordiazepoxide	Decreased chlordiazepoxide effect.
Chlorpromazine	Decreased chlorpromazine effect.
Dicumarol	Decreased dicumarol effect.
Digoxin	Decreased digoxin effect.
Isoniazid	Decreased isoniazid effect.
Tetracyclines	Possible intestinal blockage.

INTERACTION WITH OTHER SUBSTANCES

INTERACTS WITH	COMBINED EFFECT
Alcohol:	None expected.
Beverages:	None expected.
Cocaine:	None expected.
Foods:	None expected.
Marijuana:	None expected.
Tobacco:	None expected.

SPIRONOLACTONE

BRAND NAMES

Aldactazide (M)
Aldactone

GENERAL INFORMATION

Habit forming? No
Prescription needed? Yes
Available as generic? No
Drug class: Antihypertensive, diuretic

 USES

- Reduces high blood pressure.
- Prevents fluid retention.

 DOSAGE & USAGE INFORMATION

How to take:
Tablet—Swallow with liquid or food to lessen stomach irritation. If you can't swallow whole, crumble tablet and take with liquid or food.

When to take:
- 1 dose a day—Take after breakfast.
- More than 1 dose a day—Take last dose no later than 6 p.m.

If you forget a dose:
- 1 dose a day—Take as soon as you remember up to 12 hours late. If more than 12 hours, wait for next scheduled dose (don't double this dose).
- More than 1 dose a day—Take as soon as you remember. Wait 6 hours for next dose.

What drug does:
- Increases sodium and water excretion through increased urine production, decreasing body fluid and blood pressure.
- Retains potassium.

Time lapse before drug works:
3 to 5 days.

Don't take with:
See Interaction column and consult doctor.

 OVERDOSE

Symptoms:
Thirst, drowsiness, confusion, fatigue, weakness, nausea, vomiting, irregular heartbeat, excessive blood-pressure drop.

What to do:
- Dial 0 (operator) or 911 (emergency) for an ambulance or medical help. Then give first aid immediately.
- Additional emergency information on page 886.

POSSIBLE ADVERSE REACTIONS OR SIDE EFFECTS

SYMPTOMS	FREQUENCY	WHAT TO DO
Brain & nervous system: Drowsiness or headache.	Common	4
Skin:		
• Rash or itch.	Rare	3
• Confusion	Infrequent	3
Eyes:	None expected.	
Ears, nose, throat:		
• Deep voice in women.	Rare	5
• Thirst	Common	4
Digestive: Nausea, vomiting, diarrhea.	Common	4
Heart & lungs: Irregular heartbeat, shortness of breath.	Infrequent	3
Blood vessels:	None expected.	
Muscles, bones, joints: Numbness, tingling in hands or feet.	Infrequent	4
Genital, urinary:	None expected.	
Kidneys:	None expected.	
Liver:	None expected.	
Allergic:	None expected.	
Blood:	None expected.	
Others:		
• Irregular menstruation, breast tenderness, change in sex drive.	Infrequent	4
• Unusual sweating.	Infrequent	3

1 - Life-threatening. Seek emergency treatment immediately.
2 - Discontinue. Seek emergency treatment.
3 - Discontinue. Call doctor right away.
4 - Continue. Call doctor when convenient.
5 - Continue. Tell doctor at next visit.
6 - No action necessary.

SPIRONOLACTONE

WARNINGS & PRECAUTIONS

Don't take if:
- You are allergic to spironolactone.
- You have impaired kidney function.
- Your serum potassium level is high.

Before you start, consult your doctor:
- If you have had kidney or liver disease.
- If you will have surgery within 2 months, including dental surgery, requiring general or spinal anesthesia.

Over age 60:
- Limit use to 2 to 3 weeks if possible.
- Adverse reactions and side effects may be more frequent and severe than in younger persons.
- Heat or fever can reduce blood pressure. May require dose adjustment.
- Overdose and extended use may cause blood clots.

Pregnancy:
No proven harm to unborn child. Avoid if possible.

Breast-feeding:
No proven problems. Consult doctor.

Infants & children:
Use only under medical supervision.

Prolonged use:
Potassium retention with irregular heartbeat, unusual weakness and confusion.

Skin & sunlight:
No problems expected.

Driving, piloting or hazardous work:
Avoid if you feel drowsy. Otherwise, no problems expected.

Airplane passengers:
No problems expected.

Discontinuing:
Consult doctor about adjusting doses of other drugs.

Others:
No problems expected.

INTERACTION WITH OTHER DRUGS

GENERIC NAME OR DRUG CLASS	COMBINED EFFECT
Anticoagulants (oral)	Decreased anticoagulant effect.
Antihypertensives (other)	Increased antihypertensive effect.
Aspirin	Decreased spironolactone effect.
Digitalis preparations	Decreased digitalis effect.
Diuretics (other)	Increased effect of both drugs. Beneficial if needed and dose correct.
Laxatives	Reduced potassium levels.
Lithium	Likely lithium toxicity.
Potassium supplements	Dangerous potassium retention.
Sodium bicarbonate	Reduces high potassium levels.
Triamterene	Dangerous potassium retention.

INTERACTION WITH OTHER SUBSTANCES

INTERACTS WITH	COMBINED EFFECT
Alcohol:	None expected.
Beverages: Low-salt milk	Possible potassium toxicity.
Cocaine:	Decreased spironolactone effect.
Foods: Salt	Don't restrict unless directed by doctor.
Salt substitutes	Possible potassium toxicity.
Marijuana:	Increased thirst, fainting.
Tobacco:	None expected.

STANOZOLOL

BRAND NAMES

Winstrol

Habit forming? No
Prescription needed? Yes

GENERAL INFORMATION

Available as generic? Yes
Drug class: Androgen (male sex hormone)

 USES

- Corrects male hormone deficiency.
- Reduces "male menopause" symptoms (loss of sex drive, depression, anxiety).
- Decreases calcium loss of osteoporosis (softened bones).
- Blocks growth of breast-cancer cells in females.
- Corrects undescended testicles in male children.
- Reduces breast pain and fullness following childbirth.
- Augments treatment of aplastic anemia.
- Stimulates weight gain after illness, injury or for chronically underweight persons.
- Stimulates growth in treatment of dwarfism.

 DOSAGE & USAGE INFORMATION

How to take:
- Tablets—With food to lessen stomach irritation.
- Injection—Once or twice a month.

When to take:
At the same time each day.

If you forget a dose:
Take as soon as you remember up to 2 hours late. If more than 2 hours, wait for next scheduled dose (don't double this dose).

What drug does:
- Stimulates cells that produce male sex characteristics.
- Replaces hormone deficiencies.
- Stimulates red-blood-cell production.
- Suppresses production of estrogen (female sex hormone).

Time lapse before drug works:
Varies with problems treated. May require 2 or 3 months of regular use for desired effects.

Don't take with:
See Interaction column and consult doctor.

 OVERDOSE

Overdose unlikely to threaten life. If person takes much larger amount than prescribed, call doctor, poison-control center or hospital emergency room for instructions.

POSSIBLE ADVERSE REACTIONS OR SIDE EFFECTS

SYMPTOMS	FREQUENCY	WHAT TO DO
Brain & nervous system:		
Depression or confusion.	Infrequent	3
Skin:		
• Flushed face.	Infrequent	3
• Rash or itch.	Infrequent	3
• Hives	Rare	2
• Acne or oily skin in females.	Common	4
Eyes, heart & lungs, blood vessels, kidneys, blood:	None expected.	
Ears, nose, throat:		
• Deep voice.	Common	4
• Sore mouth.	Common	5
• Sore throat, fever.	Rare	3
Digestive:		
• Nausea, vomiting, diarrhea.	Infrequent	3
• Abdominal pain.	Rare	3
• Black stool.	Rare	2
Muscles, bones, joints:		
Swollen feet or legs.	Infrequent	3
Genital, urinary:		
• Enlarged clitoris or frequent erections.	Common	4
• Vaginal bleeding.	Infrequent	3
Liver:		
Jaundice (yellow skin and eyes).	Infrequent	2
Allergic:		
Intense itching, weakness, loss of consciousness.	Rare	1
Others:		
• Higher sex drive.	Common	5
• Swollen breasts in men.	Common	4

1- Life-threatening. Seek emergency treatment immediately.
2- Discontinue. Seek emergency treatment.
3- Discontinue. Call doctor right away.
4- Continue. Call doctor when convenient.
5- Continue. Tell doctor at next visit.

STANOZOLOL

WARNINGS & PRECAUTIONS

Don't take if:
You are allergic to any male hormone.

Before you start, consult your doctor:
- If you might be pregnant.
- If you have cancer of prostate.
- If you have heart disease or arteriosclerosis.
- If you have kidney or liver disease.
- If you have breast cancer (males).
- If you have high blood pressure.
- If you have migraine attacks.
- If you have high level of blood calcium.
- If you have epilepsy.

Over age 60:
- May stimulate sexual activity.
- Can make high blood pressure or heart disease worse.
- Can enlarge prostate and cause urinary retention.

Pregnancy:
Risk to unborn child outweighs drug benefits. Don't use.

Breast-feeding:
Drug passes into milk. Avoid drug or discontinue nursing until you finish medicine. Consult doctor for advice on maintaining milk supply.

Infants & children:
Don't give to children younger than 2. Use with older children only under medical supervision.

Prolonged use:
- Reduces sperm count and volume of semen.
- Possible kidney stones.
- Unnatural hair growth and deep voice in women.

Skin & sunlight:
No problems expected.

Driving, piloting or hazardous work:
No problems expected.

Airplane passengers:
No problems expected.

Discontinuing:
No problems expected.

Others:
- May cause atrophy of testicles.
- Will not increase strength in athletes.

INTERACTION WITH OTHER DRUGS

GENERIC NAME OR DRUG CLASS	COMBINED EFFECT
Anticoagulants	Increased anticoagulant effect.
Antidiabetics (oral)	Increased antidiabetic effect.
Chlorzoxazone	Decreased stanozolol effect.
Oxyphenbutazone	Decreased stanozolol effect.
Phenobarbital	Decreased stanozolol effect.
Phenylbutazone	Decreased stanozolol effect.

INTERACTION WITH OTHER SUBSTANCES

INTERACTS WITH	COMBINED EFFECT
Alcohol:	None expected.
Beverages:	None expected.
Cocaine:	No proven problems.
Foods: Salt	Excessive fluid retention (edema). Decrease salt intake while taking male hormones.
Marijuana:	Decreased blood levels of stanozolol.
Tobacco:	No proven problems.

SULFACYTINE

BRAND NAMES

Renoquid

GENERAL INFORMATION

Habit forming? No
Prescription needed? Yes
Available as generic? Yes
Drug class: Sulfa (sulfonamide)

USES

Treatment for infections responsive to this drug.

DOSAGE & USAGE INFORMATION

How to take:
Tablet—Swallow with liquid. Instructions to take on empty stomach mean 1 hour before or 2 hours after eating.

When to take:
At the same times each day, evenly spaced.

If you forget a dose:
Take as soon as you remember up to 2 hours late. If more than 2 hours, wait for next scheduled dose (don't double this dose).

What drug does:
Interferes with a nutrient (folic acid) necessary for growth and reproduction of bacteria. Will not attack viruses.

Time lapse before drug works:
2 to 5 days to affect infection.

Don't take with:
See Interaction column and consult doctor.

OVERDOSE

Symptoms:
Less urine; bloody urine; coma.

What to do:
- Dial O (operator) or 911 (emergency) for an ambulance or medical help. Then give first aid immediately.
- Additional emergency information on page 886.

POSSIBLE ADVERSE REACTIONS OR SIDE EFFECTS

SYMPTOMS	FREQUENCY	WHAT TO DO
Brain & nervous system: Headache, dizziness.	Common	4
Skin:		
• Itch, rash.	Common	3
• Redness, peeling, blistering.	Infrequent	3
Eyes:	None expected.	
Ears, nose, throat: Sore throat, fever.	Infrequent	3
Digestive:		
• Swallowing difficulty.	Infrequent	3
• Appetite loss, nausea, vomiting, diarrhea.	Common	4
Heart & lungs:	None expected.	
Blood vessels: Unusual bruising.	Infrequent	3
Muscles, bones, joints: Aching joints, muscles.	Infrequent	3
Genital, urinary: Painful urination.	Rare	3
Kidneys: Low back pain.	Rare	3
Liver: Jaundice (yellow skin and eyes).	Infrequent	3
Allergic:	None expected.	
Blood:	None expected.	
Others:	None expected.	

1-Life-threatening. Seek emergency treatment immediately.
2-Discontinue. Seek emergency treatment.
3-Discontinue. Call doctor right away.
4-Continue. Call doctor when convenient.

WARNINGS & PRECAUTIONS

Don't take if:
You are allergic to any sulfa drug.

Before you start, consult your doctor:
- If you are allergic to carbonic anhydrase inhibitors, oral antidiabetics or thiazide diuretics.
- If you are allergic by nature.
- If you have liver or kidney disease.
- If you have porphyria.
- If you have developed anemia from use of any drug.

Over age 60:
Adverse reactions and side effects may be more frequent and severe than in younger persons.

Pregnancy:
Risk to unborn child outweighs drug benefits. Don't use.

Breast-feeding:
Drug passes into milk. Avoid drug or discontinue nursing until you finish medicine. Consult doctor for advice on maintaining milk supply.

Infants & children:
Don't give to infants younger than 1 month.

Prolonged use:
- May enlarge thyroid gland.
- You may become more susceptible to infections caused by germs not responsive to this drug.
- Request frequent blood counts, liver- and kidney-function studies.

Skin & sunlight:
May cause rash or intensify sunburn in areas exposed to sun or sunlamp.

Driving, piloting or hazardous work:
Avoid if you feel dizzy. Otherwise, no problems expected.

Airplane passengers:
No problems expected.

Discontinuing:
Don't discontinue without doctor's advice until you complete prescribed dose, even though symptoms diminish or disappear.

Others:
- Drink 2 quarts of liquid each day to prevent adverse reactions.
- If you require surgery, tell anesthetist you take sulfa. Pentothal anesthesia should not be used.

INTERACTION WITH OTHER DRUGS

GENERIC NAME OR DRUG CLASS	COMBINED EFFECT
Anticoagulants (oral)	Increased anticoagulant effect.
Anticonvulsants (hydantoin)	Toxic effect on brain.
Aspirin	Increased sulfa effect.
Isoniazid	Possible anemia.
Methenamine	Possible kidney blockage.
Methotrexate	Increased methotrexate effect.
Oxyphenbutazone	Increased sulfa effect.
Para-aminosalicylic acid (PAS)	Decreased sulfa effect.
Penicillins	Decreased penicillin effect.
Phenylbutazone	Increased sulfa effect.
Probenecid	Increased sulfa effect.
Sulfinpyrazone	Increased sulfa effect.
Trimethoprim	Increased sulfa effect.
Vitamin C	Possible kidney damage. Avoid large doses of vitamin C.

INTERACTION WITH OTHER SUBSTANCES

INTERACTS WITH	COMBINED EFFECT
Alcohol:	Increased alcohol effect.
Beverages: Less than 2 quarts of fluid daily.	Kidney damage.
Cocaine:	None expected.
Foods:	None expected.
Marijuana:	None expected.
Tobacco:	None expected.

SULFAMETHOXAZOLE

BRAND NAMES

Azo Gantanol (M)   Septra (M)
Bactrim (M)   SMZ-TMP
Cetamide
Gantanol
Gantrisin

GENERAL INFORMATION

Habit forming? No
Prescription needed? Yes
Available as generic? Yes
Drug class: Sulfa (sulfonamide)

 ## USES

Treatment for infections responsive to this drug.

 ## DOSAGE & USAGE INFORMATION

How to take:
- Tablet—Swallow with liquid. Instructions to take on empty stomach mean 1 hour before or 2 hours after eating.
- Liquid—Shake carefully before measuring.

When to take:
At the same times each day, evenly spaced.

If you forget a dose:
Take as soon as you remember up to 2 hours late. If more than 2 hours, wait for next scheduled dose (don't double this dose).

What drug does:
Interferes with a nutrient (folic acid) necessary for growth and reproduction of bacteria. Will not attack viruses.

Time lapse before drug works:
2 to 5 days to affect infection.

Don't take with:
See Interaction column and consult doctor.

 ## OVERDOSE

Symptoms:
Less urine; bloody urine; coma.

What to do:
- Dial O (operator) or 911 (emergency) for an ambulance or medical help. Then give first aid immediately.
- Additional emergency information on page 886.

 ## POSSIBLE ADVERSE REACTIONS OR SIDE EFFECTS

SYMPTOMS	FREQUENCY	WHAT TO DO
Brain & nervous system: Headache, dizziness.	Common	4
Skin:		
• Itch, rash.	Common	3
• Redness, peeling, blistering.	Infrequent	3
Eyes:	None expected.	
Ears, nose, throat: Sore throat, fever.	Infrequent	3
Digestive:		
• Swallowing difficulty.	Infrequent	3
• Appetite loss, nausea, vomiting, diarrhea.	Common	4
Heart & lungs:	None expected.	
Blood vessels: Unusual bruising.	Infrequent	3
Muscles, bones, joints: Aching joints, muscles.	Infrequent	3
Genital, urinary: Painful urination.	Rare	3
Kidneys: Low back pain.	Rare	3
Liver: Jaundice (yellow skin and eyes).	Infrequent	3
Allergic:	None expected.	
Blood:	None expected.	
Others:	None expected.	

1- Life-threatening. Seek emergency treatment immediately.
2- Discontinue. Seek emergency treatment.
3- Discontinue. Call doctor right away.
4- Continue. Call doctor when convenient.

SULFAMETHOXAZOLE

WARNINGS & PRECAUTIONS

Don't take if:
You are allergic to any sulfa drug.

Before you start, consult your doctor:
- If you are allergic to carbonic anhydrase inhibitors, oral antidiabetics or thiazide diuretics.
- If you are allergic by nature.
- If you have liver or kidney disease.
- If you have porphyria.
- If you have developed anemia from use of any drug.

Over age 60:
Adverse reactions and side effects may be more frequent and severe than in younger persons.

Pregnancy:
Risk to unborn child outweighs drug benefits. Don't use.

Breast-feeding:
Drug passes into milk. Avoid drug or discontinue nursing until you finish medicine. Consult doctor for advice on maintaining milk supply.

Infants & children:
Don't give to infants younger than 1 month.

Prolonged use:
- May enlarge thyroid gland.
- You may become more susceptible to infections caused by germs not responsive to this drug.
- Request frequent blood counts, liver- and kidney-function studies.

Skin & sunlight:
May cause rash or intensify sunburn in areas exposed to sun or sunlamp.

Driving, piloting or hazardous work:
Avoid if you feel dizzy. Otherwise, no problems expected.

Airplane passengers:
No problems expected.

Discontinuing:
Don't discontinue without doctor's advice until you complete prescribed dose, even though symptoms diminish or disappear.

Others:
- Drink 2 quarts of liquid each day to prevent adverse reactions.
- If you require surgery, tell anesthetist you take sulfa. Pentothal anesthesia should not be used.

INTERACTION WITH OTHER DRUGS

GENERIC NAME OR DRUG CLASS	COMBINED EFFECT
Anticoagulants (oral)	Increased anticoagulant effect.
Anticonvulsants (hydantoin)	Toxic effect on brain.
Aspirin	Increased sulfa effect.
Isoniazid	Possible anemia.
Methenamine	Possible kidney blockage.
Methotrexate	Increased methotrexate effect.
Oxyphenbutazone	Increased sulfa effect.
Para-aminosalicylic acid (PAS)	Decreased sulfa effect.
Penicillins	Decreased penicillin effect.
Phenylbutazone	Increased sulfa effect.
Probenecid	Increased sulfa effect.
Sulfinpyrazone	Increased sulfa effect.
Trimethoprim	Increased sulfa effect.
Vitamin C	Possible kidney damage. Avoid large doses of vitamin C.

INTERACTION WITH OTHER SUBSTANCES

INTERACTS WITH	COMBINED EFFECT
Alcohol:	Increased alcohol effect.
Beverages: Less than 2 quarts of fluid daily.	Kidney damage.
Cocaine:	None expected.
Foods:	None expected.
Marijuana:	None expected.
Tobacco:	None expected.

SULFASALAZINE

BRAND NAMES

Azulfidine
Salazopyrin
SAS-500

GENERAL INFORMATION

Habit forming? No
Prescription needed? Yes
Available as generic? Yes
Drug class: Sulfa (sulfonamide)

 ## USES

Treatment for ulceration and bleeding during active phase of ulcerative colitis.

 ## DOSAGE & USAGE INFORMATION

How to take:
- Tablet—Swallow with liquid. Instructions to take on empty stomach mean 1 hour before or 2 hours after eating.
- Liquid—Shake carefully before measuring.

When to take:
At the same times each day, evenly spaced.

If you forget a dose:
Take as soon as you remember up to 2 hours late. If more than 2 hours, wait for next scheduled dose (don't double this dose).

What drug does:
Antiinflammatory action reduces tissue destruction in colon.

Time lapse before drug works:
2 to 5 days.

Don't take with:
See Interaction column and consult doctor.

 ## OVERDOSE

Symptoms:
Less urine; bloody urine; coma.

What to do:
- Dial O (operator) or 911 (emergency) for an ambulance or medical help. Then give first aid immediately.
- Additional emergency information on page 886.

 ## POSSIBLE ADVERSE REACTIONS OR SIDE EFFECTS

SYMPTOMS	FREQUENCY	WHAT TO DO
Brain & nervous system: Headache, dizziness.	Common	4
Skin:		
• Itch, rash.	Common	3
• Redness, peeling, blistering.	Infrequent	3
Eyes:	None expected.	
Ears, nose, throat: Sore throat, fever.	Infrequent	3
Digestive:		
• Swallowing difficulty.	Infrequent	3
• Appetite loss, nausea, vomiting, diarrhea.	Common	4
Heart & lungs:	None expected.	
Blood vessels: Unusual bruising.	Infrequent	3
Muscles, bones, joints: Aching joints, muscles.	Infrequent	3
Genital, urinary:		
• Painful urination.	Rare	3
• Orange urine.	Common	5
Kidneys: Low back pain.	Rare	3
Liver: Jaundice (yellow skin and eyes).	Infrequent	3
Allergic:	None expected.	
Blood:	None expected.	
Others:	None expected.	

1- Life-threatening. Seek emergency treatment immediately.
2- Discontinue. Seek emergency treatment.
3- Discontinue. Call doctor right away.
4- Continue. Call doctor when convenient.
5- Continue. Tell doctor at next visit.

SULFASALAZINE

WARNINGS & PRECAUTIONS

Don't take if:
You are allergic to any sulfa drug.

Before you start, consult your doctor:
- If you are allergic to carbonic anhydrase inhibitors, oral antidiabetics or thiazide diuretics.
- If you are allergic by nature.
- If you have liver or kidney disease.
- If you have porphyria.
- If you have developed anemia from use of any drug.

Over age 60:
Adverse reactions and side effects may be more frequent and severe than in younger persons.

Pregnancy:
Risk to unborn child outweighs drug benefits. Don't use.

Breast-feeding:
Drug passes into milk. Avoid drug or discontinue nursing until you finish medicine. Consult doctor for advice on maintaining milk supply.

Infants & children:
Don't give to infants younger than 1 month.

Prolonged use:
- May enlarge thyroid gland.
- You may become more susceptible to infections caused by germs not responsive to this drug.
- Request frequent blood counts, liver- and kidney-function studies.

Skin & sunlight:
May cause rash or intensify sunburn in areas exposed to sun or sunlamp.

Driving, piloting or hazardous work:
Avoid if you feel dizzy. Otherwise, no problems expected.

Airplane passengers:
No problems expected.

Discontinuing:
Don't discontinue without doctor's advice until you complete prescribed dose, even though symptoms diminish or disappear.

Others:
- Drink 2 quarts of liquid each day to prevent adverse reactions.
- If you require surgery, tell anesthetist you take sulfa. Pentothal anesthesia should not be used.

INTERACTION WITH OTHER DRUGS

GENERIC NAME OR DRUG CLASS	COMBINED EFFECT
Antibiotics	Decreased sulfasalazine effect.
Anticoagulants (oral)	Increased anticoagulant effect.
Anticonvulsants (hydantoin)	Toxic effect on brain.
Aspirin	Increased sulfa effect.
Digoxin	Decreased digoxin effect.
Iron supplements	Decreased sulfa effect.
Isoniazid	Possible anemia.
Methenamine	Possible kidney blockage.
Methotrexate	Increased methotrexate effect.
Oxyphenbutazone	Increased sulfa effect.
Para-aminosalicylic acid (PAS)	Decreased sulfa effect.
Penicillins	Decreased penicillin effect.
Phenylbutazone	Increased sulfa effect.
Probenecid	Increased sulfa effect.
Sulfinpyrazone	Increased sulfa effect.
Trimethoprim	Increased sulfa effect.
Vitamin C	Possible kidney damage. Avoid large doses of vitamin C.

INTERACTION WITH OTHER SUBSTANCES

INTERACTS WITH	COMBINED EFFECT
Alcohol:	Increased alcohol effect.
Beverages: Less than 2 quarts of fluid daily.	Kidney damage.
Cocaine:	None expected.
Foods:	None expected.
Marijuana:	None expected.
Tobacco:	None expected.

SULFINPYRAZONE

BRAND NAMES

Anturan
Anturane
Zynol

GENERAL INFORMATION

Habit forming? No
Prescription needed? Yes
Available as generic? No
Drug class: Antigout (uricosuric)

 USES

- Treatment for chronic gout.
- Reduces severity of recurrent heart attack. (This use is experimental and not yet approved by F.D.A.)

 DOSAGE & USAGE INFORMATION

How to take:
Tablet or capsule—Swallow with liquid or food to lessen stomach irritation. If you can't swallow whole, crumble tablet or open capsule and take with liquid or food.

When to take:
At the same times each day.

If you forget a dose:
Take as soon as you remember up to 2 hours late. If more than 2 hours, wait for next scheduled dose (don't double this dose).

What drug does:
Reduces uric-acid level in blood and tissues by increasing amount of uric acid secreted in urine by kidneys.

Time lapse before drug works:
May require 6 months to prevent gout attacks.

Don't take with:
See Interaction column and consult doctor.

 OVERDOSE

Symptoms:
Breathing difficulty, imbalance, convulsions, coma.

What to do:
- Dial 0 (operator) or 911 (emergency) for an ambulance or medical help. Then give first aid immediately.
- If patient is unconscious and not breathing, give mouth-to-mouth breathing. If there is no heartbeat, use cardiac massage and mouth-to-mouth breathing (CPR). Don't try to make patient vomit. If you can't get help quickly, take patient to nearest emergency facility.
- Additional emergency information on page 886.

POSSIBLE ADVERSE REACTIONS OR SIDE EFFECTS

SYMPTOMS	FREQUENCY	WHAT TO DO
Brain & nervous system:	None expected.	
Skin: Rash	Infrequent	4
Eyes:	None expected.	
Ears, nose, throat: Sore throat, fever.	Rare	3
Digestive:		
• Bloody or black, tarry stools.	Rare	2
• Nausea, vomiting, stomach pain.	Infrequent	4
Heart & lungs:	None expected.	
Blood vessels: Unusual bleeding or bruising.	Rare	3
Muscles, bones, joints: Red, painful joint.	Rare	3
Genital, urinary:		
• Bloody urine.	Rare	3
• Difficult or painful urination.	Infrequent	3
Kidneys: Low back pain.	Infrequent	4
Liver:	None expected.	
Allergic:	None expected.	
Blood:	None expected.	
Others: Fatigue or weakness.	Rare	3

1 - Life-threatening. Seek emergency treatment immediately.
2 - Discontinue. Seek emergency treatment.
3 - Discontinue. Call doctor right away.
4 - Continue. Call doctor when convenient.
5 - Continue. Tell doctor at next visit.
6 - No action necessary.

SULFINPYRAZONE

WARNINGS & PRECAUTIONS

Don't take if:
- You are allergic to any uricosuric.
- You have acute gout.
- You have active ulcers (stomach or duodenal), enteritis or ulcerative colitis.
- You have blood-cell disorders.
- You are allergic to oxyphenbutazone or phenylbutazone.

Before you start, consult your doctor:
If you have kidney or blood disease.

Over age 60:
Adverse reactions and side effects may be more frequent and severe than in younger persons. You require lower dose because of decreased kidney function.

Pregnancy:
Studies inconclusive on harm to unborn child. Animal studies show fetal abnormalities. Decide with your doctor whether drug benefits justify risk to unborn child.

Breast-feeding:
No proven problems. Consult doctor.

Infants & children:
Not recommended.

Prolonged use:
Possible kidney damage.

Skin & sunlight:
No problems expected.

Driving, piloting or hazardous work:
No problems expected.

Airplane passengers:
No problems expected.

Discontinuing:
Don't discontinue without consulting doctor. Dose may require gradual reduction if you have taken drug for a long time. Doses of other drugs may also require adjustment.

Others:
- Drink 10 to 12 glasses of water each day you take this medicine.
- Periodic blood and urine laboratory tests recommended.

INTERACTION WITH OTHER DRUGS

GENERIC NAME OR DRUG CLASS	COMBINED EFFECT
Anticoagulants (oral)	Increased anticoagulant effect.
Antidiabetics (oral)	Increased antidiabetic effect.
Aspirin	Bleeding tendency. Decreased sulfinpyrazone effect.
Cephalexin	Increased effect of cephalexin.
Cephradine	Increased effect of cephradine.
Contraceptives (oral)	Increased bleeding between menstrual periods.
Diuretics	Decreased sulfinpyrazone effect.
Insulin	Increased insulin effect.
Penicillins	Increased penicillin effect.
Probenecid	Possible increased sulfinpyrazone effect.
Salicylates	Bleeding tendency. Decreased sulfinpyrazone effect.
Sulfa drugs	Increased effect of sulfa drugs.

INTERACTION WITH OTHER SUBSTANCES

INTERACTS WITH	COMBINED EFFECT
Alcohol:	Decreased sulfinpyrazone effect.
Beverages: Caffeine drinks	Decreased sulfinpyrazone effect.
Cocaine:	None expected.
Foods:	None expected.
Marijuana:	Occasional use—None expected. Daily use—May increase blood level of uric acid.
Tobacco:	None expected.

SULFISOXAZOLE

BRAND NAMES

Azo-Gantrisin (M)	Lipo Gantrisin	Sulfagen
Azo-Soxazole (M)	Novosoxazole	Sulfizin
Barazole	Rosoxol	Sulfizole
Chemovag	SK-Soxazole	Urisoxin
Gantrisin	Sosol	
G-Sox	Soxa	

GENERAL INFORMATION

Habit forming? No
Prescription needed? Yes
Available as generic? Yes
Drug class: Sulfa (sulfonamide)

 ## USES

Treatment for infections responsive to this drug.

 ## DOSAGE & USAGE INFORMATION

How to take:
- Tablet—Swallow with liquid. Instructions to take on empty stomach mean 1 hour before or 2 hours after eating.
- Liquid—Shake carefully before measuring.

When to take:
At the same times each day, evenly spaced.

If you forget a dose:
Take as soon as you remember up to 2 hours late. If more than 2 hours, wait for next scheduled dose (don't double this dose).

What drug does:
Interferes with a nutrient (folic acid) necessary for growth and reproduction of bacteria. Will not attack viruses.

Time lapse before drug works:
2 to 5 days to affect infection.

Don't take with:
See Interaction column and consult doctor.

 ## OVERDOSE

Symptoms:
Less urine; bloody urine; coma.

What to do:
- Dial O (operator) or 911 (emergency) for an ambulance or medical help. Then give first aid immediately.
- Additional emergency information on page 886.

POSSIBLE ADVERSE REACTIONS OR SIDE EFFECTS

SYMPTOMS	FREQUENCY	WHAT TO DO
Brain & nervous system: Headache, dizziness.	Common	4
Skin:		
• Itch, rash.	Common	3
• Redness, peeling, blistering.	Infrequent	3
Eyes:	None expected.	
Ears, nose, throat: Sore throat, fever.	Infrequent	3
Digestive:		
• Swallowing difficulty.	Infrequent	3
• Appetite loss, nausea, vomiting, diarrhea.	Common	4
Heart & lungs:	None expected.	
Blood vessels: Unusual bruising.	Infrequent	3
Muscles, bones, joints: Aching joints, muscles.	Infrequent	3
Genital, urinary: Painful urination.	Rare	3
Kidneys: Low back pain.	Rare	3
Liver: Jaundice (yellow skin and eyes).	Infrequent	3
Allergic:	None expected.	
Blood:	None expected.	
Others:	None expected.	

1- Life-threatening. Seek emergency treatment immediately.
2- Discontinue. Seek emergency treatment.
3- Discontinue. Call doctor right away.
4- Continue. Call doctor when convenient.

SULFISOXAZOLE

WARNINGS & PRECAUTIONS

Don't take if:
You are allergic to any sulfa drug.

Before you start, consult your doctor:
- If you are allergic to carbonic anhydrase inhibitors, oral antidiabetics or thiazide diuretics.
- If you are allergic by nature.
- If you have liver or kidney disease.
- If you have porphyria.
- If you have developed anemia from use of any drug.

Over age 60:
Adverse reactions and side effects may be more frequent and severe than in younger persons.

Pregnancy:
Risk to unborn child outweighs drug benefits. Don't use.

Breast-feeding:
Drug passes into milk. Avoid drug or discontinue nursing until you finish medicine. Consult doctor for advice on maintaining milk supply.

Infants & children:
Don't give to infants younger than 1 month.

Prolonged use:
- May enlarge thyroid gland.
- You may become more susceptible to infections caused by germs not responsive to this drug.
- Request frequent blood counts, liver- and kidney-function studies.

Skin & sunlight:
May cause rash or intensify sunburn in areas exposed to sun or sunlamp.

Driving, piloting or hazardous work:
Avoid if you feel dizzy. Otherwise, no problems expected.

Airplane passengers:
No problems expected.

Discontinuing:
Don't discontinue without doctor's advice until you complete prescribed dose, even though symptoms diminish or disappear.

Others:
- Drink 2 quarts of liquid each day to prevent adverse reactions.
- If you require surgery, tell anesthetist you take sulfa. Pentothal anesthesia should not be used.

INTERACTION WITH OTHER DRUGS

GENERIC NAME OR DRUG CLASS	COMBINED EFFECT
Anticoagulants (oral)	Increased anticoagulant effect.
Anticonvulsants (hydantoin)	Toxic effect on brain.
Aspirin	Increased sulfa effect.
Isoniazid	Possible anemia.
Methenamine	Possible kidney blockage.
Methotrexate	Increased methotrexate effect.
Oxyphenbutazone	Increased sulfa effect.
Para-aminosalicylic acid (PAS)	Decreased sulfa effect.
Penicillins	Decreased penicillin effect.
Phenylbutazone	Increased sulfa effect.
Probenecid	Increased sulfa effect.
Sulfinpyrazone	Increased sulfa effect.
Trimethoprim	Increased sulfa effect.
Vitamin C	Possible kidney damage. Avoid large doses of vitamin C.

INTERACTION WITH OTHER SUBSTANCES

INTERACTS WITH	COMBINED EFFECT
Alcohol:	Increased alcohol effect.
Beverages: Less than 2 quarts of fluid daily.	Kidney damage.
Cocaine:	None expected.
Foods:	None expected.
Marijuana:	None expected.
Tobacco:	None expected.

SULINDAC

BRAND NAMES

Clinoril

Habit forming? No
Prescription needed? Yes

GENERAL INFORMATION

Available as generic? Yes
Drug class: Antiinflammatory (non-steroid)

 USES

- Treatment for joint pain, stiffness, inflammation and swelling of arthritis and gout.
- Pain reliever.

 DOSAGE & USAGE INFORMATION

How to take:
Tablet—Swallow with liquid or food to lessen stomach irritation. If you can't swallow whole, crumble tablet and take with liquid or food.

When to take:
At the same times each day.

If you forget a dose:
Take as soon as you remember up to 2 hours late. If more than 2 hours, wait for next scheduled dose (don't double this dose).

What drug does:
Reduces tissue concentration of prostaglandins (hormones which produce inflammation and pain).

Time lapse before drug works:
Begins in 4 to 24 hours. May require 3 weeks regular use for maximum benefit.

Don't take with:
See Interaction column and consult doctor.

 OVERDOSE

Symptoms:
Confusion, agitation, incoherence, convulsions, possible hemorrhage from stomach or intestine, coma.

What to do:
- Dial 0 (operator) or 911 (emergency) for an ambulance or medical help. Then give first aid immediately.
- Additional emergency information on page 886.

 POSSIBLE ADVERSE REACTIONS OR SIDE EFFECTS

SYMPTOMS	FREQUENCY	WHAT TO DO
Brain & nervous system:		
• Depression, drowsiness.	Infrequent	4
• Convulsions, confusion.	Rare	3
• Dizziness	Common	4
• Headache	Common	5
Skin:		
Rash, hives or itch.	Rare	3
Eyes:		
Blurred vision.	Rare	3
Ears, nose, throat:		
Ringing in ears.	Infrequent	4
Digestive:		
• Bloody or black, tarry stools.	Rare	3
• Nausea, pain.	Common	4
• Constipation or diarrhea, vomiting.	Infrequent	4
Heart & lungs:		
Breathing difficulty, tightness in chest, rapid heartbeat.	Rare	3
Blood vessels:		
Unusual bleeding or bruising.	Rare	3
Muscles, bones, joints:		
Swollen feet, legs.	Infrequent	4
Genital, urinary:		
• Bloody urine.	Rare	3
• Difficult, painful or frequent urination.	Rare	4
Kidneys, allergic, blood:	None expected.	
Liver:		
Jaundice (yellow skin and eyes).	Rare	3
Others:		
Fatigue, weakness.	Rare	4

1 - Life-threatening. Seek emergency treatment immediately.
2 - Discontinue. Seek emergency treatment.
3 - Discontinue. Call doctor right away.
4 - Continue. Call doctor when convenient.
5 - Continue. Tell doctor at next visit.

SULINDAC

WARNINGS & PRECAUTIONS

Don't take if:
- You are allergic to aspirin or any non-steroid, antiinflammatory drug.
- You have gastritis, peptic ulcer, enteritis, ileitis, ulcerative colitis, asthma, heart failure, high blood pressure or bleeding problems.
- You have had recent rectal bleeding and suppository form has been prescribed.
- Patient is younger than 15.

Before you start, consult your doctor:
- If you have epilepsy.
- If you have Parkinson's disease.
- If you have been mentally ill.
- If you have had kidney disease or impaired kidney function.

Over age 60:
Adverse reactions and side effects may be more frequent and severe than in younger persons.

Pregnancy:
Studies inconclusive on harm to unborn child. Decide with your doctor whether drug benefits justify risk to unborn child.

Breast-feeding:
May harm child. Avoid.

Infants & children:
Not recommended for those younger than 15. Use only under medical supervision.

Prolonged use:
- Eye damage.
- Reduced hearing.
- Sore throat, fever.
- Weight gain.

Skin & sunlight:
No problems expected.

Driving, piloting or hazardous work:
Don't drive or pilot aircraft until you learn how medicine affects you. Don't work around dangerous machinery. Don't climb ladders or work in high places. Danger increases if you drink alcohol or take medicine affecting alertness and reflexes, such as antihistamines, tranquilizers, sedatives, pain medicine, narcotics and mind-altering drugs.

Airplane passengers:
No problems expected.

Discontinuing:
Don't discontinue without consulting doctor. Dose may require gradual reduction if you have taken drug for a long time. Doses of other drugs may also require adjustment.

Others:
No problems expected.

INTERACTION WITH OTHER DRUGS

GENERIC NAME OR DRUG CLASS	COMBINED EFFECT
Anticoagulants (oral)	Increased risk of bleeding.
Aspirin	Increased risk of stomach ulcer.
Cortisone drugs	Increased risk of stomach ulcer.
Furosemide	Decreased diuretic effect of furosemide.
Oxyphenbutazone	Possible stomach ulcer.
Phenylbutazone	Possible stomach ulcer.
Probenecid	Increased sulindac effect.
Thyroid hormones	Rapid heartbeat, blood-pressure rise.

INTERACTION WITH OTHER SUBSTANCES

INTERACTS WITH	COMBINED EFFECT
Alcohol:	Possible stomach ulcer or bleeding.
Beverages:	None expected.
Cocaine:	None expected.
Foods:	None expected.
Marijuana:	Increased pain relief from sulindac.
Tobacco:	None expected.

TALBUTAL (BUTALBITAL)

BRAND NAMES

Fiorinal (M)
Lotusate
Plexonal (M)
Sandoptal

GENERAL INFORMATION

Habit forming? Yes
Prescription needed? Yes
Available as generic? Yes
Drug class: Sedative, hypnotic (barbiturate)

 ## USES

- Reduces anxiety or nervous tension (low dose).
- Relieves insomnia (higher bedtime dose).

 ## DOSAGE & USAGE INFORMATION

How to take:
Tablet or capsule—Swallow with liquid or food to lessen stomach irritation. If you can't swallow whole, crumble tablet or open capsule and take with liquid or food.

When to take:
At the same times each day.

If you forget a dose:
Take as soon as you remember up to 2 hours late. If more than 2 hours, wait for next scheduled dose (don't double this dose).

What drug does:
May partially block nerve impulses at nerve-cell connections.

Time lapse before drug works:
60 minutes.

Don't take with:
- Non-prescription drugs without consulting doctor.
- See Interaction column and consult doctor.

 ## OVERDOSE

Symptoms:
Deep sleep, weak pulse, coma.

What to do:
- Dial 0 (operator) or 911 (emergency) for an ambulance or medical help. Then give first aid immediately.
- Additional emergency information on page 886.

POSSIBLE ADVERSE REACTIONS OR SIDE EFFECTS

SYMPTOMS	FREQUENCY	WHAT TO DO
Brain & nervous system:		
• Dizziness, drowsiness, "hangover effect."	Common	4
• Depression, confusion, slurred speech.	Infrequent	4
• Agitation	Rare	3
Skin:		
• Rash or hives.	Infrequent	3
• Face, lip swelling.	Infrequent	3
Eyes:		
Eyelid swelling.	Infrequent	3
Ears, nose, throat:		
Sore throat, fever.	Infrequent	3
Digestive:		
Diarrhea, nausea, vomiting.	Infrequent	4
Heart & lungs:		
• Slow heartbeat.	Rare	3
• Breathing difficulty.	Rare	3
Blood vessels:		
Unexplained bleeding or bruising.	Rare	4
Muscles, bones, joints:		
Joint or muscle pain.	Infrequent	4
Genital, urinary:	None expected.	
Kidneys:	None expected.	
Liver:		
Jaundice (yellow skin and eyes).	Rare	3
Allergic:	None expected.	
Blood:	None expected.	
Others:	None expected.	

1- Life-threatening. Seek emergency treatment immediately.
2- Discontinue. Seek emergency treatment.
3- Discontinue. Call doctor right away.
4- Continue. Call doctor when convenient.

TALBUTAL (BUTALBITAL)

WARNINGS & PRECAUTIONS

Don't take if:
- You are allergic to any barbiturate.
- You have porphyria.

Before you start, consult your doctor:
- If you have epilepsy.
- If you have kidney or liver damage.
- If you have asthma.
- If you have anemia.
- If you have chronic pain.
- If you will have surgery within 2 months, including dental surgery, requiring general or spinal anesthesia.

Over age 60:
Adverse reactions and side effects may be more frequent and severe than in younger persons. Use small doses.

Pregnancy:
Risk to unborn child outweighs drug benefits. Don't use.

Breast-feeding:
Drug passes into milk. Avoid drug or discontinue nursing until you finish medicine. Consult doctor for advice on maintaining milk supply.

Infants & children:
Use only under doctor's supervision.

Prolonged use:
- May cause addiction, anemia, chronic intoxication.
- May lower body temperature, making exposure to cold temperatures hazardous.

Skin & sunlight:
May cause rash or intensify sunburn in areas exposed to sun or sunlamp.

Driving, piloting or hazardous work:
Don't drive or pilot aircraft until you learn how medicine affects you. Don't work around dangerous machinery. Don't climb ladders or work in high places. Danger increases if you drink alcohol or take medicine affecting alertness and reflexes.

Airplane passengers:
No problems expected.

Discontinuing:
May be unnecessary to finish medicine. Follow doctor's instructions. If you develop withdrawal symptoms of hallucinations, agitation or sleeplessness after discontinuing, call doctor right away.

Others:
No problems expected.

INTERACTION WITH OTHER DRUGS

GENERIC NAME OR DRUG CLASS	COMBINED EFFECT
Anticoagulants (oral)	Decreased anticoagulant effect.
Anticonvulsants	Changed seizure patterns.
Antidepressants (tricyclic)	Decreased antidepressant effect.
Antidiabetics (oral)	Increased talbutal (butalbital) effect.
Antihistamines	Dangerous sedation. Avoid.
Antiinflammatory drugs (non-steroidal)	Decreased antiinflammatory effect.
Aspirin	Decreased aspirin effect.
Beta-adrenergic blockers	Decreased effect of beta-adrenergic blocker.
Contraceptives (oral)	Decreased contraceptive effect.
Cortisone drugs	Decreased cortisone effect.
Digitoxin	Decreased digitoxin effect.
Doxycycline	Decreased doxycycline effect.
Griseofulvin	Decreased griseofulvin effect.

Additional interactions on page 843.

INTERACTION WITH OTHER SUBSTANCES

INTERACTS WITH	COMBINED EFFECT
Alcohol:	Possible fatal oversedation. Avoid.
Beverages:	None expected.
Cocaine:	Decreased talbutal (butalbital) effect.
Foods:	None expected.
Marijuana:	Excessive sedation. Avoid.
Tobacco:	None expected.

TEMAZEPAM

BRAND NAMES

Restoril

GENERAL INFORMATION

Habit forming? Yes
Prescription needed? Yes
Available as generic? No
Drug class: Tranquilizer (benzodiazepine)

USES

Treatment for insomnia.

DOSAGE & USAGE INFORMATION

How to take:
Tablet or capsule—Swallow with liquid. If you can't swallow whole, crumble tablet or open capsule and take with liquid or food.

When to take:
At the same time each day, according to instructions on prescription label.

If you forget a dose:
Take as soon as you remember up to 2 hours late. If more than 2 hours, wait for next scheduled dose (don't double this dose).

What drug does:
Affects limbic system of brain—part that controls emotions. Induces near-normal sleep pattern.

Time lapse before drug works:
30 minutes.

Don't take with:
See Interaction column and consult doctor.

OVERDOSE

Symptoms:
Drowsiness, weakness, tremor, stupor, coma.

What to do:
- Dial 0 (operator) or 911 (emergency) for an ambulance or medical help. Then give first aid immediately.
- If patient is unconscious and not breathing, give mouth-to-mouth breathing. If there is no heartbeat, use cardiac massage and mouth-to-mouth breathing (CPR). Don't try to make patient vomit. If you can't get help quickly, take patient to nearest emergency facility.
- Additional emergency information on page 886.

POSSIBLE ADVERSE REACTIONS OR SIDE EFFECTS

SYMPTOMS	FREQUENCY	WHAT TO DO
Brain & nervous system:		
● Clumsiness, drowsiness, dizziness.	Common	4
● Hallucinations, confusion, depression, irritability.	Infrequent	3
Skin:		
Rash, itch.	Infrequent	3
Eyes:		
Vision changes.	Infrequent	3
Ears, nose, throat:		
Mouth, throat ulcers.	Rare	3
Digestive:		
Constipation or diarrhea, nausea, vomiting.	Infrequent	4
Heart & lungs:		
Slow heartbeat, breathing difficulty.	Rare	2
Blood vessels:	None expected.	
Muscles, bones, joints:	None expected.	
Genital, urinary:		
Urination difficulty.	Infrequent	4
Kidneys:	None expected.	
Liver:		
Jaundice (yellow eyes and skin).	Rare	3
Allergic:	None expected.	
Blood:	None expected.	
Others:	None expected.	

1- Life-threatening. Seek emergency treatment immediately.
2- Discontinue. Seek emergency treatment.
3- Discontinue. Call doctor right away.
4- Continue. Call doctor when convenient.
5- Continue. Tell doctor at next visit.
6- No action necessary.

WARNINGS & PRECAUTIONS

Don't take if:
- You are allergic to any benzodiazepine.
- You have myasthenia gravis.
- You have glaucoma.
- You are active or recovering alcoholic.
- Patient is younger than 6 months.

Before you start, consult your doctor:
- If you have liver, kidney or lung disease.
- If you have diabetes, epilepsy or porphyria.

Over age 60:
Adverse reactions and side effects may be more frequent and severe than in younger persons. May develop agitation, rage or "hangover effect."

Pregnancy:
Risk to unborn child outweighs drug benefits. Don't use.

Breast-feeding:
Drug passes into milk. Avoid drug or discontinue nursing until you finish medicine. Consult doctor for advice on maintaining milk supply.

Infants & children:
Use only under medical supervision for children older than 6 months.

Prolonged use:
May impair liver function.

Skin & sunlight:
No problems expected.

Driving, piloting or hazardous work:
Don't drive or pilot aircraft until you learn how medicine affects you. Don't work around dangerous machinery. Don't climb ladders or work in high places. Danger increases if you drink alcohol or take medicine affecting alertness and reflexes.

Airplane passengers:
No problems expected.

Discontinuing:
Don't discontinue without doctor's advice until you complete prescribed dose, even though symptoms diminish or disappear.

Others:
- Hot weather, heavy exercise and profuse sweat may reduce excretion and cause overdose.
- Blood sugar may rise in diabetics, requiring insulin adjustment.

INTERACTION WITH OTHER DRUGS

GENERIC NAME OR DRUG CLASS	COMBINED EFFECT
Anticonvulsants	Change in seizure frequency or severity.
Antidepressants	Increased sedative effect of both drugs.
Antihistamines	Increased sedative effect of both drugs.
Antihypertensives	Excessively low blood pressure.
Cimetidine	Excess sedation.
Disulfiram	Increased temazepam effect.
MAO inhibitors	Convulsions, deep sedation, rage.
Narcotics	Increased sedative effect of both drugs.
Sedatives	Increased sedative effect of both drugs.
Tranquilizers	Increased sedative effect of both drugs.

INTERACTION WITH OTHER SUBSTANCES

INTERACTS WITH	COMBINED EFFECT
Alcohol:	Heavy sedation. Avoid.
Beverages:	None expected.
Cocaine:	Decreased temazepam effect.
Foods:	None expected.
Marijuana:	Heavy sedation. Avoid.
Tobacco:	Decreased temazepam effect.

TERBUTALINE

BRAND NAMES

Brethine
Bricanyl

GENERAL INFORMATION

Habit forming? No
Prescription needed? Yes
Available as generic? No
Drug class: Sympathomimetic

USES

Treatment of bronchial asthma, bronchitis
and emphysema.

DOSAGE & USAGE INFORMATION

How to take:
Tablet or capsule—Swallow with liquid or
food to lessen stomach irritation.

When to take:
At the same times each day.

If you forget a dose:
Take as soon as you remember up to 2 hours
late. If more than 2 hours, wait for next
scheduled dose (don't double this dose).

What drug does:
Dilates constricted bronchial tubes.

Time lapse before drug works:
30 minutes.

Don't take with:
See Interaction column and consult doctor.

OVERDOSE

Symptoms:
Rapid heartbeat, chest pain, tremors.

What to do:
- Dial 0 (operator) or 911 (emergency) for an
  ambulance or medical help. Then give first
  aid immediately.
- If patient is unconscious and not breathing,
  give mouth-to-mouth breathing. If there is
  no heartbeat, use cardiac massage and
  mouth-to-mouth breathing (CPR). Don't try
  to make patient vomit. If you can't get help
  quickly, take patient to nearest emergency
  facility.
- Additional emergency information on page
  886.

POSSIBLE ADVERSE REACTIONS OR SIDE EFFECTS

SYMPTOMS	FREQUENCY	WHAT TO DO
Brain & nervous system:		
• Headache, nervousness, restlessness, trembling.	Common	4
• Drowsiness	Infrequent	3
Skin:	None expected.	
Eyes:	None expected.	
Ears, nose, throat:	None expected.	
Digestive: Nausea, vomiting.	Infrequent	3
Heart & lungs: Fast or pounding heartbeat.	Infrequent	3
Blood vessels:	None expected.	
Muscles, bones, joints: Cramps, weakness.	Infrequent	3
Genital, urinary:	None expected.	
Kidneys:	None expected.	
Liver:	None expected.	
Allergic:	None expected.	
Blood:	None expected.	
Others: Unusual sweating.	Infrequent	4

1- Life-threatening. Seek emergency
   treatment immediately.
2- Discontinue. Seek emergency treatment.
3- Discontinue. Call doctor right away.
4- Continue. Call doctor when convenient.
5- Continue. Tell doctor at next visit.
6- No action necessary.

WARNINGS & PRECAUTIONS

Don't take if:
You are allergic to any sympathomimetic.

Before you start, consult your doctor:
- If you have diabetes.
- If you have heart disease or high blood pressure.
- If you have overactive thyroid.
- If you have had seizures.
- If you take non-prescription amphetamines or other asthma medicines.

Over age 60:
Adverse reactions and side effects may be more frequent and severe than in younger persons.

Pregnancy:
No proven harm to unborn child. Avoid if possible. May prolong labor and delivery.

Breast-feeding:
No proven problems. Avoid if possible.

Infants & children:
Use only under medical supervision.

Prolonged use:
No problems expected.

Skin & sunlight:
No problems expected.

Driving, piloting or hazardous work:
Avoid if you feel drowsy. Otherwise, no problems expected.

Airplane passengers:
No problems expected.

Discontinuing:
May be unnecessary to finish medicine. Follow doctor's instructions.

Others:
If troubled breathing does not improve or worsens after using medicine, don't increase dose. Consult doctor.

INTERACTION WITH OTHER DRUGS

GENERIC NAME OR DRUG CLASS	COMBINED EFFECT
Beta-adrenergic blockers	Decreased terbutaline effect.
Ephedrine	Increased terbutaline effect. Excess heart stimulation.
Epinephrine	Increased terbutaline effect. Excess heart stimulation.
MAO inhibitors	Increased terbutaline effect. Dangerous. Avoid.
Sympathomimetics	Increased terbutaline effect.

INTERACTION WITH OTHER SUBSTANCES

INTERACTS WITH	COMBINED EFFECT
Alcohol:	None expected.
Beverages:	None expected.
Cocaine:	Overstimulation.
Foods:	None expected.
Marijuana:	Possible increased therapeutic effect of terbutaline. May cause lung disorders to worsen.
Tobacco:	No interactions expected, but smoking may slow body's recovery. Avoid.

TERPIN HYDRATE

BRAND NAMES

Cotussis (M)
Prunicodeine (M)
Terpin Hydrate and
  Codeine Syrup (M)
Terpin Hydrate Elixir

GENERAL INFORMATION

Habit forming? Yes
Prescription needed? No
Available as generic? Yes
Drug class: Expectorant

USES

Decreases cough due to simple bronchial irritation.

DOSAGE & USAGE INFORMATION

How to take:
Follow each dose with 8 oz. water. Works better in combination with a cool-air vaporizer.

When to take:
3 to 4 times each day, spaced at least 4 hours apart.

If you forget a dose:
Take as soon as you remember. Wait 4 hours for next dose.

What drug does:
Loosens mucus in bronchial tubes to make mucus easier to cough up.

Time lapse before drug works:
10 to 15 minutes.

Don't take with:
See Interaction column and consult doctor.

OVERDOSE

Symptoms:
Nausea, drowsiness.

What to do:
Overdose unlikely to threaten life. If person takes much larger amount than prescribed, call doctor, poison-control center or hospital emergency room for instructions.

POSSIBLE ADVERSE REACTIONS OR SIDE EFFECTS

SYMPTOMS	FREQUENCY	WHAT TO DO
Brain & nervous system: Symptoms of alcohol intoxication, especially in children.	Rare	3
Skin:	None expected.	
Eyes:	None expected.	
Ears, nose, throat:	None expected.	
Digestive: Nausea, vomiting, stomach pain.	Infrequent	4
Heart & lungs:	None expected.	
Blood vessels:	None expected.	
Muscles, bones, joints:	None expected.	
Genital, urinary:	None expected.	
Kidneys:	None expected.	
Liver:	None expected.	
Allergic:	None expected.	
Blood:	None expected.	
Others:	None expected.	

1 - Life-threatening. Seek emergency treatment immediately.
2 - Discontinue. Seek emergency treatment.
3 - Discontinue. Call doctor right away.
4 - Continue. Call doctor when convenient.
5 - Continue. Tell doctor at next visit.
6 - No action necessary.

WARNINGS & PRECAUTIONS

Don't take if:
- You are allergic to terpin hydrate.
- You are a recovering or active alcoholic.

Before you start, consult your doctor:
If you plan to become pregnant within medication period.

Over age 60:
No problems expected.

Pregnancy:
Risk to unborn child outweighs drug benefits. Don't use.

Breast-feeding:
Drug filters into milk. May harm child. Avoid.

Infants & children:
Use only under medical supervision.

Prolonged use:
Habit forming.

Skin & sunlight:
No problems expected.

Driving, piloting or hazardous work:
Don't drive or pilot aircraft until you learn how medicine affects you. Don't work around dangerous machinery. Don't climb ladders or work in high places. Danger increases if you drink alcohol or take medicine affecting alertness and reflexes, such as antihistamines, tranquilizers, sedatives, pain medicine, narcotics and mind-altering drugs.

Airplane passengers:
No problems expected.

Discontinuing:
May be unnecessary to finish medicine. Follow doctor's instructions.

Others:
- Exceeding recommended doses may cause intoxication; drug is 42.5% alcohol.
- Frequently combined with codeine, which increases hazards.

INTERACTION WITH OTHER DRUGS

GENERIC NAME OR DRUG CLASS	COMBINED EFFECT
Antidepressants	Increased effect of terpin hydrate.
Antihistamines	Increased effect of terpin hydrate.
Muscle relaxants	Increased effect of terpin hydrate.
Narcotics	Increased effect of terpin hydrate.
Sedatives	Increased effect of terpin hydrate.
Sleep inducers	Increased effect of terpin hydrate.
Tranquilizers	Increased effect of terpin hydrate.

INTERACTION WITH OTHER SUBSTANCES

INTERACTS WITH	COMBINED EFFECT
Alcohol:	Increased sedative effect of both drugs. Avoid.
Beverages:	None expected.
Cocaine:	Unpredictable effect on nervous system. Avoid.
Foods:	None expected.
Marijuana:	Unpredictable effect on nervous system. Avoid.
Tobacco:	None expected.

TESTOSTERONE

BRAND NAMES

Delatestryl
Depo-Testosterone
Oreton

Habit forming? No
Prescription needed? Yes

GENERAL INFORMATION

Available as generic? Yes
Drug class: Androgen (male sex hormone)

USES

- Corrects male hormone deficiency.
- Reduces "male menopause" symptoms (loss of sex drive, depression, anxiety).
- Decreases calcium loss of osteoporosis (softened bones).
- Blocks growth of breast-cancer cells in females.
- Corrects undescended testicles in male children.
- Reduces breast pain and fullness following childbirth.
- Augments treatment of aplastic anemia.
- Stimulates weight gain after illness, injury or for chronically underweight persons.
- Stimulates growth in treatment of dwarfism.

DOSAGE & USAGE INFORMATION

How to take:
- Tablets—With food to lessen stomach irritation.
- Injection—Once or twice a month.

When to take:
At the same time each day.

If you forget a dose:
Take as soon as you remember up to 2 hours late. If more than 2 hours, wait for next scheduled dose (don't double this dose).

What drug does:
- Stimulates cells that produce male sex characteristics.
- Replaces hormone deficiencies.
- Stimulates red-blood-cell production.
- Suppresses production of estrogen (female sex hormone).

Time lapse before drug works:
Varies with problems treated. May require 2 or 3 months of regular use for desired effects.

Don't take with:
See Interaction column and consult doctor.

OVERDOSE

Overdose unlikely to threaten life. If person takes much larger amount than prescribed, call doctor, poison-control center or hospital emergency room for instructions.

POSSIBLE ADVERSE REACTIONS OR SIDE EFFECTS

SYMPTOMS	FREQUENCY	WHAT TO DO
Brain & nervous system:		
Depression or confusion.	Infrequent	3
Skin:		
• Flushed face.	Infrequent	3
• Rash or itch.	Infrequent	3
• Hives	Rare	2
• Acne or oily skin in females.	Common	4
Eyes, heart & lungs, blood vessels, kidneys, blood:	None expected.	
Ears, nose, throat:		
• Deep voice.	Common	4
• Sore mouth.	Common	5
• Sore throat, fever.	Rare	3
Digestive:		
• Nausea, vomiting, diarrhea.	Infrequent	3
• Abdominal pain.	Rare	3
• Black stool.	Rare	2
Muscles, bones, joints:		
Swollen feet or legs.	Infrequent	3
Genital, urinary:		
• Enlarged clitoris or frequent erections.	Common	4
• Vaginal bleeding.	Infrequent	3
Liver:		
Jaundice (yellow skin and eyes).	Infrequent	2
Allergic:		
Intense itching, weakness, loss of consciousness.	Rare	1
Others:		
• Higher sex drive.	Common	5
• Swollen breasts in men.	Common	4

1- Life-threatening. Seek emergency treatment immediately.
2- Discontinue. Seek emergency treatment.
3- Discontinue. Call doctor right away.
4- Continue. Call doctor when convenient.
5- Continue. Tell doctor at next visit.

WARNINGS & PRECAUTIONS

Don't take if:
You are allergic to any male hormone.

Before you start, consult your doctor:
- If you might be pregnant.
- If you have cancer of prostate.
- If you have heart disease or arteriosclerosis.
- If you have kidney or liver disease.
- If you have breast cancer (males).
- If you have high blood pressure.
- If you have migraine attacks.
- If you have high level of blood calcium.
- If you have epilepsy.

Over age 60:
- May stimulate sexual activity.
- Can make high blood pressure or heart disease worse.
- Can enlarge prostate and cause urinary retention.

Pregnancy:
Risk to unborn child outweighs drug benefits. Don't use.

Breast-feeding:
Drug passes into milk. Avoid drug or discontinue nursing until you finish medicine. Consult doctor for advice on maintaining milk supply.

Infants & children:
Don't give to children younger than 2. Use with older children only under medical supervision.

Prolonged use:
- Reduces sperm count and volume of semen.
- Possible kidney stones.
- Unnatural hair growth and deep voice in women.

Skin & sunlight:
No problems expected.

Driving, piloting or hazardous work:
No problems expected.

Airplane passengers:
No problems expected.

Discontinuing:
No problems expected.

Others:
- May cause atrophy of testicles.
- Will not increase strength in athletes.

INTERACTION WITH OTHER DRUGS

GENERIC NAME OR DRUG CLASS	COMBINED EFFECT
Anticoagulants	Increased anticoagulant effect.
Antidiabetics (oral)	Increased antidiabetic effect.
Chlorzoxazone	Decreased testosterone effect.
Oxyphenbutazone	Decreased testosterone effect.
Phenobarbital	Decreased testosterone effect.
Phenylbutazone	Decreased testosterone effect.

INTERACTION WITH OTHER SUBSTANCES

INTERACTS WITH	COMBINED EFFECT
Alcohol:	None expected.
Beverages:	None expected.
Cocaine:	No proven problems.
Foods: Salt	Excessive fluid retention (edema). Decrease salt intake while taking male hormones.
Marijuana:	Decreased blood levels of testosterone.
Tobacco:	No proven problems.

TETRACYCLINE

BRAND NAMES

Achromycin	Neo-Tetrine	SK-Tetracycline
Achrostatin V (M)	Nor-tet	Tetrachel
Bio-Tetra	Novotetra	Tetracyn
Bristacycline	Panmycin	Tetracyrine
Cyclopar	Retet	Tetrastatin (M)
Medicycline	Robitet	Tetrex

See complete brand names list, page 831.

GENERAL INFORMATION

Habit forming? No
Prescription needed? Yes
Available as generic? Yes
Drug class: Antibiotic (tetracycline)

USES

- Treatment for infections susceptible to tetracycline. Will not cure virus infections such as colds or flu.
- Treatment for acne.

DOSAGE & USAGE INFORMATION

How to take:
- Tablet or capsule—Take on empty stomach 1 hour before or 2 hours after eating. If you can't swallow whole, crumble tablet or open capsule and take with liquid or food.
- Liquid—Shake well. Take with measuring spoon.

When to take:
At the same times each day, evenly spaced.

If you forget a dose:
Take as soon as you remember up to 2 hours late. If more than 2 hours, wait for next scheduled dose (don't double this dose).

What drug does:
Prevents germ growth and reproduction.

Time lapse before drug works:
- Infections—May require 5 days to affect infection.
- Acne—May require 4 weeks to affect acne.

Don't take with:
- Non-prescription drugs without consulting doctor.
- See Interaction column and consult doctor.

OVERDOSE

Symptoms:
Severe nausea, vomiting, diarrhea.

What to do:
Overdose unlikely to threaten life. If person takes much larger amount than prescribed, call doctor, poison-control center or hospital emergency room for instructions.

POSSIBLE ADVERSE REACTIONS OR SIDE EFFECTS

SYMPTOMS	FREQUENCY	WHAT TO DO
Brain & nervous system: Headache	Infrequent	3
Skin:		
• Itching around rectum and genitals.	Common	3
• Rash	Infrequent	3
Eyes: Blurred vision.	Rare	3
Ears, nose, throat:		
• Dark tongue.	Common	5
• Sore mouth or tongue.	Common	2
• Excessive thirst.	Infrequent	4
Digestive: Nausea, vomiting, diarrhea, abdominal burning.	Common	2
Heart & lungs:	None expected.	
Blood vessels:	None expected.	
Muscles, bones, joints:	None expected.	
Genital, urinary: Increased urination.	Infrequent	4
Kidneys:	None expected.	
Liver: Jaundice (yellow eyes and skin) in pregnant women.	Rare	3
Allergic:	None expected.	
Blood:	None expected.	
Others:	None expected.	

1- Life-threatening. Seek emergency treatment immediately.
2- Discontinue. Seek emergency treatment.
3- Discontinue. Call doctor right away.
4- Continue. Call doctor when convenient.
5- Continue. Tell doctor at next visit.
6- No action necessary.

TETRACYCLINE

WARNINGS & PRECAUTIONS

Don't take if:
You are allergic to any tetracycline antibiotic.

Before you start, consult your doctor:
- If you have kidney or liver disease.
- If you have lupus.
- If you have myasthenia gravis.

Over age 60:
Dosage usually less than in younger adults. More likely to cause itching around rectum. Ask you doctor how to prevent it.

Pregnancy:
Risk to unborn child outweighs drug benefits. Don't use.

Breast-feeding:
Drug passes into milk. Avoid drug or discontinue nursing until you finish medicine. Consult doctor for advice on maintaining milk supply.

Infants & children:
May cause permanent teeth malformation or discoloration in children less than 8 years old. Don't use.

Prolonged use:
- You may become more susceptible to infections caused by germs not responsive to tetracycline.
- May cause rare problems in liver, kidney or bone marrow. Periodic laboratory blood studies, liver- and kidney-function tests recommended if you use drug a long time.

Skin & sunlight:
May cause rash or intensify sunburn in areas exposed to sun or sunlamp.

Driving, piloting or hazardous work:
No problems expected.

Airplane passengers:
No problems expected.

Discontinuing:
Don't discontinue without doctor's advice until you complete prescribed dose, even though symptoms diminish or disappear.

Others:
No problems expected.

INTERACTION WITH OTHER DRUGS

GENERIC NAME OR DRUG CLASS	COMBINED EFFECT
Antacids	Decreased tetracycline effect.
Anticoagulants (oral)	Increased anticoagulant effect.
Contraceptives (oral)	Decreased contraceptive effect.
Digitalis preparations	Increased digitalis effect.
Mineral supplements (iron, calcium, magnesium, zinc)	Decreased tetracycline absorption. Separate doses by 1 to 2 hours.
Lithium	Increased lithium effect.
Penicillins	Decreased penicillin effect.
Sodium bicarbonate	Decreased tetracycline effect.

INTERACTION WITH OTHER SUBSTANCES

INTERACTS WITH	COMBINED EFFECT
Alcohol:	Possible liver damage. Avoid.
Beverages: Milk	Decreased tetracycline absorption. Take dose 2 hours after or 1 hour before drinking.
Cocaine:	No proven problems.
Foods: Dairy products	Decreased tetracycline absorption. Take dose 2 hours after or 1 hour before eating.
Marijuana:	No interactions expected, but marijuana may slow body's recovery. Avoid.
Tobacco:	None expected.

THEOPHYLLINE

BRAND NAMES

Accurbron	Elixophyllin	Theoclear
Aerolate	Physpan	Theo-Dur
Asthmophylline	Slophyllin	Theolair
Bronkodyl	Somophyllin-T	Theolixir
Elixicon	Theobid	Theophyl

See complete brand names list, page 831.

GENERAL INFORMATION

Habit forming? No
Prescription needed? Canada—No
U.S: High strength—Yes
Low strength—No
Available as generic? Yes
Drug class: Bronchodilator (xanthine)

 ## USES

Treatment for bronchial asthma symptoms.

 ## DOSAGE & USAGE INFORMATION

How to take:
- Tablet or capsule—Swallow with liquid.
- Extended-release tablets or capsules—Swallow each dose whole. If you take regular tablets, you may chew or crush them.
- Suppositories—Remove wrapper and moisten suppository with water. Gently insert larger end into rectum. Push well into rectum with finger.
- Syrup—Take as directed on bottle.
- Enema—Use as directed on label.

When to take:
Most effective taken on empty stomach 1 hour before or 2 hours after eating. However, may take with food to lessen stomach upset.

If you forget a dose:
Take as soon as you remember up to 2 hours late. If more than 2 hours, wait for next scheduled dose (don't double this dose).

What drug does:
Relaxes and expands bronchial tubes.

Time lapse before drug works:
15 to 30 minutes.

Don't take with:
See Interaction column and consult doctor.

 ## OVERDOSE

Symptoms:
Restlessness, irritability, confusion, delirium, convulsions, rapid pulse, coma.

What to do:
- Dial 0 (operator) or 911 (emergency) for an ambulance or medical help. Then give first aid immediately.
- Additional emergency information on page 886.

 ## POSSIBLE ADVERSE REACTIONS OR SIDE EFFECTS

SYMPTOMS	FREQUENCY	WHAT TO DO
Brain & nervous system:		
● Headache, irritability, nervousness, restlessness, insomnia.	Common	4
● Dizziness or lightheadedness.	Infrequent	4
Skin:		
● Rash or hives.	Infrequent	3
● Flushed face.	Infrequent	4
Eyes:	None expected.	
Ears, nose, throat:	None expected.	
Digestive:		
● Nausea, vomiting, stomach pain.	Common	4
● Diarrhea, appetite loss.	Infrequent	3
Heart & lungs:		
● Rapid breathing.	Infrequent	3
● Irregular heartbeat.	Infrequent	3
Blood vessels:	None expected.	
Muscles, bones, joints:	None expected.	
Genital, urinary:	None expected.	
Kidneys:	None expected.	
Liver:	None expected.	
Allergic:	None expected.	
Blood:	None expected.	
Others:	None expected.	

1-Life-threatening. Seek emergency treatment immediately.
2-Discontinue. Seek emergency treatment.
3-Discontinue. Call doctor right away.
4-Continue. Call doctor when convenient.
5-Continue. Tell doctor at next visit.
6-No action necessary.

THEOPHYLLINE

WARNINGS & PRECAUTIONS

Don't take if:
- You are allergic to any bronchodilator.
- You have an active peptic ulcer.

Before you start, consult your doctor:
- If you have had impaired kidney or liver function.
- If you have gastritis.
- If you have a peptic ulcer.
- If you have high blood pressure or heart disease.
- If you take medication for gout.

Over age 60:
Adverse reactions and side effects may be more frequent and severe than in younger persons.

Pregnancy:
Risk to unborn child outweighs drug benefits. Don't use.

Breast-feeding:
Drug passes into milk. Avoid drug or discontinue nursing until you finish medicine. Consult doctor for advice on maintaining milk supply.

Infants & children:
Use only under medical supervision.

Prolonged use:
Stomach irritation.

Skin & sunlight:
No problems expected.

Driving, piloting or hazardous work:
Avoid if lightheaded or dizzy. Otherwise, no problems expected.

Airplane passengers:
No problems expected.

Discontinuing:
May be unnecessary to finish medicine. Follow doctor's instructions.

Others:
No problems expected.

INTERACTION WITH OTHER DRUGS

GENERIC NAME OR DRUG CLASS	COMBINED EFFECT
Allopurinol	Decreased allopurinol effect.
Ephedrine	Increased effect of both drugs.
Epinephrine	Increased effect of both drugs.
Erythromycin	Increased theophylline effect.
Furosemide	Increased furosemide effect.
Lincomycins	Increased theophylline effect.
Lithium	Decreased lithium effect.
Probenecid	Decreased effect of both drugs.
Propranolol	Decreased theophylline effect.
Rauwolfia alkaloids	Rapid heartbeat.
Sulfinpyrazone	Decreased sulfinpyrazone effect.
Troleandomycin	Increased theophylline effect.

INTERACTION WITH OTHER SUBSTANCES

INTERACTS WITH	COMBINED EFFECT
Alcohol:	None expected.
Beverages: Caffeine drinks	Nervousness and insomnia.
Cocaine:	Excess stimulation. Avoid.
Foods:	None expected.
Marijuana:	Slightly increased antiasthmatic effect of theophylline.
Tobacco:	Decreased theophylline effect.

THIAMINE (VITAMIN B-1)

BRAND NAMES

Betalin S
Betaxin
Bewon
Pan-B-1
Numerous other multiple vitamin-mineral supplements.

GENERAL INFORMATION

Habit forming? No
Prescription needed? No
Available as generic? Yes
Drug class: Vitamin supplement

 ## USES

- Dietary supplement to promote normal growth, development and health.
- Treatment for beri-beri (a thiamine-deficiency disease).
- Dietary supplement for alcoholism, cirrhosis, overactive thyroid, infection, breast-feeding, absorption diseases, pregnancy, prolonged diarrhea, burns.

 ## DOSAGE & USAGE INFORMATION

How to take:
Tablet or liquid—Swallow with beverage or food to lessen stomach irritation.

When to take:
At the same time each day.

If you forget a dose:
Take when remembered. Return to regular schedule.

What drug does:
- Promotes normal growth and development.
- Combines with an enzyme to metabolize carbohydrates.

Time lapse before drug works:
15 minutes.

Don't take with:
See Interaction column and consult doctor.

 ## OVERDOSE

Symptoms:
Increased severity of adverse reactions and side effects.

What to do:
Overdose unlikely to threaten life. If person takes much larger amount than prescribed, call doctor, poison-control center or hospital emergency room for instructions.

 ## POSSIBLE ADVERSE REACTIONS OR SIDE EFFECTS

SYMPTOMS	FREQUENCY	WHAT TO DO
Brain & nervous system:	None expected.	
Skin: Rash or itch.	Rare	3
Eyes:	None expected.	
Ears, nose, throat:	None expected.	
Digestive:	None expected.	
Heart & lungs: Wheezing	Rare	2
Blood vessels:	None expected.	
Muscles, bones, joints:	None expected.	
Genital, urinary:	None expected.	
Kidneys:	None expected.	
Liver:	None expected.	
Allergic: Life-threatening anaphylaxis may occur when given intravenously.	Rare	1 See Page 888.
Blood:	None expected.	
Others:	None expected.	

1- Life-threatening. Seek emergency treatment immediately.
2- Discontinue. Seek emergency treatment.
3- Discontinue. Call doctor right away.
4- Continue. Call doctor when convenient.
5- Continue. Tell doctor at next visit.
6- No action necessary.

THIAMINE (VITAMIN B-1)

 ## WARNINGS & PRECAUTIONS

Don't take if:
You are allergic to any B vitamin.

Before you start, consult your doctor:
If you have liver or kidney disease.

Over age 60:
No problems expected.

Pregnancy:
No problems expected.

Breast-feeding:
No problems expected.

Infants & children:
No problems expected.

Prolonged use:
No problems expected.

Skin & sunlight:
No problems expected.

Driving, piloting or hazardous work:
No problems expected.

Airplane passengers:
No problems expected.

Discontinuing:
No problems expected.

Others:
A balanced diet should provide enough thiamine for healthy people to make supplement unnecessary. Best dietary sources of thiamine are whole-grain cereals and meats.

 ## INTERACTION WITH OTHER DRUGS

GENERIC NAME OR DRUG CLASS	COMBINED EFFECT
Barbiturates	Decreased thiamine effect.

 ## INTERACTION WITH OTHER SUBSTANCES

INTERACTS WITH	COMBINED EFFECT
Alcohol:	None expected.
Beverages: Carbonates, citrates (additives listed on many beverage labels).	Decreased thiamine effect.
Cocaine:	None expected.
Foods: Carbonates, citrates (additives listed on many food labels).	Decreased thiamine effect.
Marijuana:	None expected.
Tobacco:	None expected.

THIORIDAZINE

BRAND NAMES

Mellaril
Novoridazine
Thioril

GENERAL INFORMATION

Habit forming? No
Prescription needed? Yes
Available as generic? Yes
Drug class: Tranquilizer, antiemetic (phenothiazine)

USES

- Stops nausea, vomiting.
- Reduces anxiety, agitation.

DOSAGE & USAGE INFORMATION

How to take:
- Tablet or capsule—Swallow with liquid or food to lessen stomach irritation.
- Suppositories—Remove wrapper and moisten suppository with water. Gently insert into rectum, large end first.
- Drops or liquid—Dilute dose in beverage.

When to take:
- Nervous and mental disorders—Take at the same times each day.
- Nausea and vomiting—Take as needed, no more often than every 4 hours.

If you forget a dose:
- Nervous and mental disorders—Take up to 2 hours late. If more than 2 hours, wait for next scheduled dose (don't double this).
- Nausea and vomiting—Take as soon as you remember. Wait 4 hours for next dose.

What drug does:
- Suppresses brain's vomiting center.
- Suppresses brain centers that control abnormal emotions and behavior.

Time lapse before drug works:
- Nausea and vomiting—1 hour or less.
- Nervous and mental disorders—4-6 weeks.

Don't take with:
- Antacid or medicine for diarrhea.
- Non-prescription drug for cough, cold or allergy.
- See Interaction column and consult doctor.

OVERDOSE

Symptoms:
Stupor, convulsions, coma.

What to do:
- Dial 0 (operator) or 911 (emergency) for an ambulance or medical help. Then give first aid immediately.
- Additional emergency information on page 886.

POSSIBLE ADVERSE REACTIONS OR SIDE EFFECTS

SYMPTOMS	FREQUENCY	WHAT TO DO
Brain & nervous system:		
• Restlessness, tremor.	Common	3
• Fainting	Infrequent	2
• Drowsiness	Common	3
Skin:		
• Rash	Infrequent	3
• Less perspiration.	Common	4
Eyes:		
Vision changes.	Rare	3
Ears, nose, throat:		
• Sore throat, fever.	Rare	3
• Dry mouth, nasal congestion.	Common	4
Digestive:		
Constipation	Common	4
Heart & lungs, blood vessels, kidneys, allergic, blood:		
	None expected.	
Muscles, bones, joints:		
Muscle spasms of face and neck, unsteady gait.	Common	2
Genital, urinary:		
Urination difficulty.	Infrequent	4
Liver:		
Jaundice (yellow eyes and skin).	Rare	3
Others:		
Less interest in sex, breast swelling, change in menstrual pattern.	Infrequent	4

1-Life-threatening. Seek emergency treatment immediately.
2-Discontinue. Seek emergency treatment.
3-Discontinue. Call doctor right away.
4-Continue. Call doctor when convenient.
5-Continue. Tell doctor at next visit.
6-No action necessary.

THIORIDAZINE

WARNINGS & PRECAUTIONS

Don't take if:
- You are allergic to any phenothiazine.
- You have a blood or bone-marrow disease.

Before you start, consult your doctor:
- If you will have surgery within 2 months, including dental surgery, requiring general or spinal anesthesia.
- If you have asthma, emphysema or other lung disorder.
- If you take non-prescription ulcer medicine, asthma medicine or amphetamines.

Over age 60:
Adverse reactions and side effects may be more frequent and severe than in younger persons. More likely to develop involuntary movement of jaws, lips, tongue, chewing. Report this to your doctor immediately. Early treatment can help.

Pregnancy:
Risk to unborn child outweighs drug benefits. Don't use.

Breast-feeding:
Drug passes into milk. Avoid drug or discontinue nursing until you finish medicine. Consult doctor for advice on maintaining milk supply.

Infants & children:
Don't give to children younger than 2.

Prolonged use:
May lead to tardive dyskinesia (involuntary movement of jaws, lips, tongue, chewing).

Skin & sunlight:
May cause rash or intensify sunburn in areas exposed to sun or sunlamp. Skin may remain sensitive for 3 months after discontinuing.

Driving, piloting or hazardous work:
Don't drive or pilot aircraft until you learn how medicine affects you. Don't work around dangerous machinery. Don't climb ladders or work in high places. Danger increases if you drink alcohol or take medicine affecting alertness and reflexes.

Airplane passengers:
No problems expected.

Discontinuing:
- Nervous and mental disorders—Don't discontinue without doctor's advice until you complete prescribed dose, even though symptoms diminish or disappear.
- Nausea and vomiting—May be unnecessary to finish medicine. Follow doctor's instructions.

INTERACTION WITH OTHER DRUGS

GENERIC NAME OR DRUG CLASS	COMBINED EFFECT
Anticholinergics	Increased anticholinergic effect.
Antidepressants (tricyclic)	Increased thioridazine effect.
Antihistamines	Increased antihistamine effect.
Appetite suppressants	Decreased suppressant effect.
Levodopa	Decreased levodopa effect.
Mind-altering drugs	Increased effect of mind-altering drugs.
Narcotics	Increased narcotic effect.
Phenytoin	Increased phenytoin effect.
Quinidine	Impaired heart function. Dangerous mixture.
Sedatives	Increased sedative effect.
Tranquilizers (other)	Increased tranquilizer effect.

INTERACTION WITH OTHER SUBSTANCES

INTERACTS WITH	COMBINED EFFECT
Alcohol:	Dangerous oversedation.
Beverages:	None expected.
Cocaine:	Decreased thioridazine effect. Avoid.
Foods:	None expected.
Marijuana:	Drowsiness. May increase antinausea effect.
Tobacco:	None expected.

THIOTHIXENE

BRAND NAMES

Navane

GENERAL INFORMATION

Habit forming? No
Prescription needed? Yes
Available as generic? No

Drug class: Tranquilizer
(thioxanthine), antiemetic

USES

- Reduces anxiety, agitation, psychosis.
- Stops vomiting.

DOSAGE & USAGE INFORMATION

How to take:
- Capsule—Swallow with liquid. If you can't swallow whole, open capsule and take with liquid or food.
- Syrup—Dilute dose in beverage before swallowing.

When to take:
At the same time each day.

If you forget a dose:
Take as soon as you remember up to 2 hours late. If more than 2 hours, wait for next scheduled dose (don't double this dose).

What drug does:
Corrects imbalance of nerve impulses.

Time lapse before drug works:
3 weeks.

Don't take with:
See Interaction column and consult doctor.

OVERDOSE

Symptoms:
Drowsiness, dizziness, weakness, muscle rigidity, twitching, tremors, confusion, dry mouth, blurred vision, rapid pulse, shallow breathing, low blood pressure, convulsions, coma.

What to do:
- Dial 0 (operator) or 911 (emergency) for an ambulance or medical help. Then give first aid immediately.
- If patient is unconscious and not breathing, give mouth-to-mouth breathing. If there is no heartbeat, use cardiac massage and mouth-to-mouth breathing (CPR). Don't try to make patient vomit. If you can't get help quickly, take patient to nearest emergency facility.
- Additional emergency information on page 886.

POSSIBLE ADVERSE REACTIONS OR SIDE EFFECTS

SYMPTOMS	FREQUENCY	WHAT TO DO
Brain & nervous system:		
• Fainting; restlessness; jerky, involuntary movements.	Common	3
• Dizziness, drowsiness.	Common	4
Skin:		
Rash	Infrequent	3
Eyes:		
Blurred vision.	Common	3
Ears, nose, throat:		
• Sore throat, fever.	Rare	3
• Dry mouth, nasal congestion.	Common	5
Digestive:		
Constipation	Common	4
Heart & lungs:		
Rapid heartbeat.	Common	3
Blood vessels, kidneys, allergic, blood:	None expected.	
Muscles, bones, joints:		
• Muscle spasms.	Common	4
• Shuffling walk.	Common	4
Genital, urinary:		
• Less sexual ability.	Infrequent	4
• Difficult urination.	Infrequent	4
Liver:		
Jaundice (yellow skin and eyes).	Rare	3
Others:		
• Less perspiration.	Common	4
• Menstrual changes.	Infrequent	5
• Breast swelling.	Infrequent	5

1- Life-threatening. Seek emergency treatment immediately.
2- Discontinue. Seek emergency treatment.
3- Discontinue. Call doctor right away.
4- Continue. Call doctor when convenient.
5- Continue. Tell doctor at next visit.

WARNINGS & PRECAUTIONS

Don't take if:
- You are allergic to any thioxanthine or phenothiazine tranquilizer.
- You have serious blood disorder.
- You have Parkinson's disease.
- Patient is younger than 12.

Before you start, consult your doctor:
- If you have had liver or kidney disease.
- If you have epilepsy or glaucoma.
- If you have high blood pressure or heart disease (especially angina).
- If you use alcohol daily.
- If you will have surgery within 2 months, including dental surgery, requiring general or spinal anesthesia.

Over age 60:
Adverse reactions and side effects may be more frequent and severe than in younger persons.

Pregnancy:
No proven harm to unborn child. Avoid if possible.

Breast-feeding:
Studies inconclusive. Consult your doctor.

Infants & children:
Not recommended.

Prolonged use:
- Pigment deposits in lens and retina of eye.
- Involuntary movements of jaws, lips, tongue (tardive dyskinesia).

Skin & sunlight:
May cause rash or intensify sunburn in areas exposed to sun or sunlamp.

Driving, piloting or hazardous work:
Don't drive or pilot aircraft until you learn how medicine affects you. Don't work around dangerous machinery. Don't climb ladders or work in high places. Danger increases if you drink alcohol or take medicine affecting alertness and reflexes.

Airplane passengers:
No problems expected.

Discontinuing:
Don't discontinue without consulting doctor. Dose may require gradual reduction if you have taken drug for a long time. Doses of other drugs may also require adjustment.

Others:
Hot temperatures increase chance of heat stroke.

INTERACTION WITH OTHER DRUGS

GENERIC NAME OR DRUG CLASS	COMBINED EFFECT
Anticholinergics	Increased anticholinergic effect.
Anticonvulsants	Change in seizure pattern.
Antidepressants (tricyclic)	Increased thiothixene effect. Excessive sedation.
Antihistamines	Increased thiothixene effect. Excessive sedation.
Antihypertensives	Excessively low blood pressure.
Barbiturates	Increased thiothixene effect. Excessive sedation.
Bethanechol	Decreased bethanechol effect.
Guanethidine	Decreased guanethidine effect.
Levodopa	Decreased levodopa effect.
MAO inhibitors	Excessive sedation.
Mind-altering drugs	Increased thiothixene effect. Excessive sedation.
Narcotics	Increased thiothixene effect. Excessive sedation.

Additional interactions on page 843.

INTERACTION WITH OTHER SUBSTANCES

INTERACTS WITH	COMBINED EFFECT
Alcohol:	Excessive brain depression. Avoid.
Beverages:	None expected.
Cocaine:	Decreased thiothixene effect. Avoid.
Foods:	None expected.
Marijuana:	Daily use—Fainting likely, possible psychosis.
Tobacco:	None expected.

THYROGLOBULIN

BRAND NAMES

Proloid

GENERAL INFORMATION

Habit forming? No
Prescription needed? Yes
Available as generic? Yes
Drug class: Thyroid hormone

USES

Replacement for thyroid hormone deficiency.

DOSAGE & USAGE INFORMATION

How to take:
- Tablet or capsule—Swallow with liquid.
- Extended-release tablets or capsules—Swallow each dose whole. If you take regular tablets, you may chew or crush them.

When to take:
At the same time each day before a meal or on awakening.

If you forget a dose:
Take as soon as you remember up to 12 hours late. If more than 12 hours, wait for next scheduled dose (don't double this dose).

What drug does:
Increases cell metabolism rate.

Time lapse before drug works:
48 hours.

Don't take with:
See Interaction column and consult doctor.

OVERDOSE

Symptoms:
"Hot" feeling, heart palpitations, nervousness, sweating, hand tremors, insomnia, rapid and irregular pulse, headache, irritability, diarrhea, weight loss, muscle cramps.

What to do:
Overdose unlikely to threaten life. If person takes much larger amount than prescribed, call doctor, poison-control center or hospital emergency room for instructions.

POSSIBLE ADVERSE REACTIONS OR SIDE EFFECTS

SYMPTOMS	FREQUENCY	WHAT TO DO
Brain & nervous system: Tremor, headache, irritability, insomnia.	Common	3
Skin: Hives, rash.	Infrequent	3
Eyes:	None expected.	
Ears, nose, throat:	None expected.	
Digestive:		
• Appetite change.	Common	4
• Diarrhea	Common	4
• Vomiting	Infrequent	3
Heart & lungs: Chest pain, rapid and irregular heartbeat, shortness of breath.	Infrequent	3
Blood vessels:	None expected.	
Muscles, bones, joints: Leg cramps.	Common	4
Genital, urinary:	None expected.	
Kidneys:	None expected.	
Liver:	None expected.	
Allergic:	None expected.	
Blood:	None expected.	
Others:		
• Change in menstrual periods.	Common	4
• Fever, heat sensitivity, unusual sweating.	Common	4
• Weight loss.	Common	4

1 - Life-threatening. Seek emergency treatment immediately.
2 - Discontinue. Seek emergency treatment.
3 - Discontinue. Call doctor right away.
4 - Continue. Call doctor when convenient.
5 - Continue. Tell doctor at next visit.
6 - No action necessary.

WARNINGS & PRECAUTIONS

Don't take if:
- You have had a heart attack within 6 weeks.
- You have no thyroid deficiency, but use this to lose weight.

Before you start, consult your doctor:
- If you have heart disease or high blood pressure.
- If you have diabetes.
- If you have Addison's disease, have had adrenal gland deficiency or use epinephrine, ephedrine or isoproterenol for asthma.

Over age 60:
More sensitive to thyroid hormone. May need smaller doses.

Pregnancy:
Considered safe if for thyroid deficiency only.

Breast-feeding:
Present in milk. Considered safe if dose is correct.

Infants & children:
Use only under medical supervision.

Prolonged use:
No problems expected, if dose is correct.

Skin & sunlight:
No problems expected.

Driving, piloting or hazardous work:
No problems expected.

Airplane passengers:
No problems expected.

Discontinuing:
Don't discontinue without consulting doctor. Dose may require gradual reduction if you have taken drug for a long time. Doses of other drugs may also require adjustment.

Others:
Digestive upsets, tremors, cramps, nervousness, insomnia or diarrhea may indicate need for dose adjustment.

INTERACTION WITH OTHER DRUGS

GENERIC NAME OR DRUG CLASS	COMBINED EFFECT
Amphetamines	Increased amphetamine effect.
Anticoagulants (oral)	Increased anticoagulant effect.
Antidepressants (tricyclic)	Increased antidepressant effect.
Antidiabetics	Antidiabetic may require adjustment.
Aspirin (large doses, continuous use)	Increased thyroglobulin effect.
Barbiturates	Decreased barbiturate effect.
Cholestyramine	Decreased thyroglobulin effect.
Contraceptives (oral)	Decreased thyroglobulin effect.
Cortisone drugs	Requires dose adjustment to prevent cortisone deficiency.
Digitalis preparations	Increased digitalis effect.
Ephedrine	Increased ephedrine effect.
Epinephrine	Increased epinephrine effect.
Methylphenidate	Increased methylphenidate effect.
Phenytoin	Increased thyroglobulin effect.

INTERACTION WITH OTHER SUBSTANCES

INTERACTS WITH	COMBINED EFFECT
Alcohol:	None expected.
Beverages:	None expected.
Cocaine:	Excess stimulation. Avoid.
Foods: Soybeans	Heavy consumption interferes with thyroid function.
Marijuana:	None expected.
Tobacco:	None expected.

THYROID

BRAND NAMES

S-P-T
Thyrar
Thyrocrine

GENERAL INFORMATION

Habit forming? No
Prescription needed? Yes
Available as generic? Yes
Drug class: Thyroid hormone

 USES

Replacement for thyroid hormone deficiency.

 DOSAGE & USAGE INFORMATION

How to take:
- Tablet or capsule—Swallow with liquid.
- Extended-release tablets or capsules—Swallow each dose whole. If you take regular tablets, you may chew or crush them.

When to take:
At the same time each day before a meal or on awakening.

If you forget a dose:
Take as soon as you remember up to 12 hours late. If more than 12 hours, wait for next scheduled dose (don't double this dose).

What drug does:
Increases cell metabolism rate.

Time lapse before drug works:
48 hours.

Don't take with:
See Interaction column and consult doctor.

 OVERDOSE

Symptoms:
"Hot" feeling, heart palpitations, nervousness, sweating, hand tremors, insomnia, rapid and irregular pulse, headache, irritability, diarrhea, weight loss, muscle cramps.

What to do:
Overdose unlikely to threaten life. If person takes much larger amount than prescribed, call doctor, poison-control center or hospital emergency room for instructions.

POSSIBLE ADVERSE REACTIONS OR SIDE EFFECTS

SYMPTOMS	FREQUENCY	WHAT TO DO
Brain & nervous system: Tremor, headache, irritability, insomnia.	Common	3
Skin: Hives, rash.	Infrequent	3
Eyes:	None expected.	
Ears, nose, throat:	None expected.	
Digestive:		
• Appetite change.	Common	4
• Diarrhea	Common	4
• Vomiting	Infrequent	3
Heart & lungs: Chest pain, rapid and irregular heartbeat, shortness of breath.	Infrequent	3
Blood vessels:	None expected.	
Muscles, bones, joints: Leg cramps.	Common	4
Genital, urinary:	None expected.	
Kidneys:	None expected.	
Liver:	None expected.	
Allergic:	None expected.	
Blood:	None expected.	
Others:		
• Change in menstrual periods.	Common	4
• Fever, heat sensitivity, unusual sweating.	Common	4
• Weight loss.	Common	4

1- Life-threatening. Seek emergency treatment immediately.
2- Discontinue. Seek emergency treatment.
3- Discontinue. Call doctor right away.
4- Continue. Call doctor when convenient.
5- Continue. Tell doctor at next visit.
6- No action necessary.

THYROID

WARNINGS & PRECAUTIONS

Don't take if:
- You have had a heart attack within 6 weeks.
- You have no thyroid deficiency, but use this to lose weight.

Before you start, consult your doctor:
- If you have heart disease or high blood pressure.
- If you have diabetes.
- If you have Addison's disease, have had adrenal gland deficiency or use epinephrine, ephedrine or isoproterenol for asthma.

Over age 60:
More sensitive to thyroid hormone. May need smaller doses.

Pregnancy:
Considered safe if for thyroid deficiency only.

Breast-feeding:
Present in milk. Considered safe if dose is correct.

Infants & children:
Use only under medical supervision.

Prolonged use:
No problems expected, if dose is correct.

Skin & sunlight:
No problems expected.

Driving, piloting or hazardous work:
No problems expected.

Airplane passengers:
No problems expected.

Discontinuing:
Don't discontinue without consulting doctor. Dose may require gradual reduction if you have taken drug for a long time. Doses of other drugs may also require adjustment.

Others:
Digestive upsets, tremors, cramps, nervousness, insomnia or diarrhea may indicate need for dose adjustment.

INTERACTION WITH OTHER DRUGS

GENERIC NAME OR DRUG CLASS	COMBINED EFFECT
Amphetamines	Increased amphetamine effect.
Anticoagulants (oral)	Increased anticoagulant effect.
Antidepressants (tricyclic)	Increased antidepressant effect.
Antidiabetics	Antidiabetic may require adjustment.
Aspirin (large doses, continuous use)	Increased thyroid effect.
Barbiturates	Decreased barbiturate effect.
Cholestyramine	Decreased thyroid effect.
Contraceptives (oral)	Decreased thyroid effect.
Cortisone drugs	Requires dose adjustment to prevent cortisone deficiency.
Digitalis preparations	Increased digitalis effect.
Ephedrine	Increased ephedrine effect.
Epinephrine	Increased epinephrine effect.
Methylphenidate	Increased methylphenidate effect.
Phenytoin	Increased thyroid effect.

INTERACTION WITH OTHER SUBSTANCES

INTERACTS WITH	COMBINED EFFECT
Alcohol:	None expected.
Beverages:	None expected.
Cocaine:	Excess stimulation. Avoid.
Foods: Soybeans	Heavy consumption interferes with thyroid function.
Marijuana:	None expected.
Tobacco:	None expected.

THYROXINE (T-4, LEVOTHYROXINE)

BRAND NAMES

Cytolen	Levothroid	Thyrolar (M)
Elthroxin	L-T-S	
Euthroid (M)	Noroxine	
Letter	Ro-Thyroxine	
Levoid	Synthroid	

GENERAL INFORMATION

Habit forming? No
Prescription needed? Yes
Available as generic? Yes
Drug class: Thyroid hormone

 ## USES

Replacement for thyroid hormone deficiency.

 ## DOSAGE & USAGE INFORMATION

How to take:
- Tablet or capsule—Swallow with liquid.
- Extended-release tablets or capsules—Swallow each dose whole. If you take regular tablets, you may chew or crush them.

When to take:
At the same time each day before a meal or on awakening.

If you forget a dose:
Take as soon as you remember up to 12 hours late. If more than 12 hours, wait for next scheduled dose (don't double this dose).

What drug does:
Increases cell metabolism rate.

Time lapse before drug works:
48 hours.

Don't take with:
See Interaction column and consult doctor.

 ## OVERDOSE

Symptoms:
"Hot" feeling, heart palpitations, nervousness, sweating, hand tremors, insomnia, rapid and irregular pulse, headache, irritability, diarrhea, weight loss, muscle cramps.

What to do:
Overdose unlikely to threaten life. If person takes much larger amount than prescribed, call doctor, poison-control center or hospital emergency room for instructions.

 ## POSSIBLE ADVERSE REACTIONS OR SIDE EFFECTS

SYMPTOMS	FREQUENCY	WHAT TO DO
Brain & nervous system: Tremor, headache, irritability, insomnia.	Common	3
Skin: Hives, rash.	Infrequent	3
Eyes:	None expected.	
Ears, nose, throat:	None expected.	
Digestive:		
• Appetite change.	Common	4
• Diarrhea	Common	4
• Vomiting	Infrequent	3
Heart & lungs: Chest pain, rapid and irregular heartbeat, shortness of breath.	Infrequent	3
Blood vessels:	None expected.	
Muscles, bones, joints: Leg cramps.	Common	4
Genital, urinary:	None expected.	
Kidneys:	None expected.	
Liver:	None expected.	
Allergic:	None expected.	
Blood:	None expected.	
Others:		
• Change in menstrual periods.	Common	4
• Fever, heat sensitivity, unusual sweating.	Common	4
• Weight loss.	Common	4

1-Life-threatening. Seek emergency treatment immediately.
2-Discontinue. Seek emergency treatment.
3-Discontinue. Call doctor right away.
4-Continue. Call doctor when convenient.
5-Continue. Tell doctor at next visit.
6-No action necessary.

THYROXINE (T-4, LEVOTHYROXINE)

WARNINGS & PRECAUTIONS

Don't take if:
- You have had a heart attack within 6 weeks.
- You have no thyroid deficiency, but use this to lose weight.

Before you start, consult your doctor:
- If you have heart disease or high blood pressure.
- If you have diabetes.
- If you have Addison's disease, have had adrenal gland deficiency or use epinephrine, ephedrine or isoproterenol for asthma.

Over age 60:
More sensitive to thyroid hormone. May need smaller doses.

Pregnancy:
Considered safe if for thyroid deficiency only.

Breast-feeding:
Present in milk. Considered safe if dose is correct.

Infants & children:
Use only under medical supervision.

Prolonged use:
No problems expected, if dose is correct.

Skin & sunlight:
No problems expected.

Driving, piloting or hazardous work:
No problems expected.

Airplane passengers:
No problems expected.

Discontinuing:
Don't discontinue without consulting doctor. Dose may require gradual reduction if you have taken drug for a long time. Doses of other drugs may also require adjustment.

Others:
Digestive upsets, tremors, cramps, nervousness, insomnia or diarrhea may indicate need for dose adjustment.

INTERACTION WITH OTHER DRUGS

GENERIC NAME OR DRUG CLASS	COMBINED EFFECT
Amphetamines	Increased amphetamine effect.
Anticoagulants (oral)	Increased anticoagulant effect.
Antidepressants (tricyclic)	Increased antidepressant effect.
Antidiabetics	Antidiabetic may require adjustment.
Aspirin (large doses, continuous use)	Increased thyroxine effect.
Barbiturates	Decreased barbiturate effect.
Cholestyramine	Decreased thyroxine effect.
Contraceptives (oral)	Decreased thyroxine effect.
Cortisone drugs	Requires dose adjustment to prevent cortisone deficiency.
Digitalis preparations	Increased digitalis effect.
Ephedrine	Increased ephedrine effect.
Epinephrine	Increased epinephrine effect.
Methylphenidate	Increased methylphenidate effect.
Phenytoin	Increased thyroxine effect.

INTERACTION WITH OTHER SUBSTANCES

INTERACTS WITH	COMBINED EFFECT
Alcohol:	None expected.
Beverages:	None expected.
Cocaine:	Excess stimulation. Avoid.
Foods: Soybeans	Heavy consumption interferes with thyroid function.
Marijuana:	None expected.
Tobacco:	None expected.

TICARCILLIN

BRAND NAMES

Ticar

GENERAL INFORMATION

Habit forming? No
Prescription needed? Yes
Available as generic? Yes
Drug class: Antibiotic (penicillin)

USES

Treatment of bacterial infections that are susceptible to ticarcillin.

DOSAGE & USAGE INFORMATION

How to take:
By injection only.

When to take:
Follow doctor's instructions.

If you forget a dose:
Consult doctor.

What drug does:
Destroys susceptible bacteria. Does not kill viruses.

Time lapse before drug works:
May be several days before medicine affects infection.

Don't take with:
See Interaction column and consult doctor.

OVERDOSE

Symptoms:
Severe diarrhea, nausea, edema or vomiting.

What to do:
Overdose unlikely to threaten life. If person takes much larger amount than prescribed, call doctor, poison-control center or hospital emergency room for instructions.

POSSIBLE ADVERSE REACTIONS OR SIDE EFFECTS

SYMPTOMS	FREQUENCY	WHAT TO DO
Brain & nervous system:	None expected.	
Skin: Hives, rash, intense itch soon after a dose.	Rare	1
Eyes:	None expected.	
Ears, nose, throat: Dark or discolored tongue.	Common	5
Digestive: Mild nausea, vomiting, diarrhea.	Infrequent	4
Heart & lungs:	None expected.	
Blood vessels: Unexplained bleeding.	Rare	3
Muscles, bones, joints:	None expected.	
Genital, urinary:	None expected.	
Kidneys:	None expected.	
Liver:	None expected.	
Allergic: Life-threatening anaphylaxis may occur!	Rare	1 See page 888.
Blood:	None expected.	
Others:	None expected.	

1- Life-threatening. Seek emergency treatment immediately.
2- Discontinue. Seek emergency treatment.
3- Discontinue. Call doctor right away.
4- Continue. Call doctor when convenient.
5- Continue. Tell doctor at next visit.
6- No action necessary.

WARNINGS & PRECAUTIONS

Don't take if:
You are allergic to ticarcillin, cephalosporin antibiotics, other penicillins or penicillamine. Life-threatening reaction may occur.

Before you start, consult your doctor:
If you are allergic to any substance or drug.

Over age 60:
You may have skin reactions, particularly around genitals and anus.

Pregnancy:
Studies inconclusive on harm to unborn child. Animal studies show fetal abnormalities. Decide with your doctor whether drug benefits justify risk to unborn child.

Breast-feeding:
Drug passes into milk. Child may become sensitive to penicillins and have allergic reactions to penicillin drugs. Avoid ticarcillin or discontinue nursing until you finish medicine. Consult doctor for advice on maintaining milk supply.

Infants & children:
No problems expected.

Prolonged use:
You may become more susceptible to infections caused by germs not responsive to ticarcillin.

Skin & sunlight:
No problems expected.

Driving, piloting or hazardous work:
Usually not dangerous. Most hazardous reactions likely to occur a few minutes after taking ticarcillin.

Airplane passengers:
No problems expected.

Discontinuing:
Don't discontinue without doctor's advice until you complete prescribed dose, even though symptoms diminish or disappear.

Others:
No problems expected.

INTERACTION WITH OTHER DRUGS

GENERIC NAME OR DRUG CLASS	COMBINED EFFECT
Chloramphenicol	Decreased effect of both drugs.
Erythromycins	Decreased effect of both drugs.
Paromomycin	Decreased effect of both drugs.
Tetracyclines	Decreased effect of both drugs.
Troleandomycin	Decreased effect of both drugs.

INTERACTION WITH OTHER SUBSTANCES

INTERACTS WITH	COMBINED EFFECT
Alcohol:	Occasional stomach irritation.
Beverages:	None expected.
Cocaine:	No proven problems.
Foods:	None expected.
Marijuana:	No proven problems.
Tobacco:	None expected.

TIMOLOL

BRAND NAMES

Blocadren

GENERAL INFORMATION

Habit forming? No
Prescription needed? Yes
Available as generic? No
Drug class: Beta-adrenergic blocker

USES

- Reduces angina attacks.
- Stabilizes irregular heartbeat.
- Lowers blood pressure.
- Reduces frequency of migraine headaches. (Does not relieve headache pain.)
- Other uses prescribed by your doctor.

DOSAGE & USAGE INFORMATION

How to take:
Tablet or capsule—Swallow with liquid. If you can't swallow whole, crumble tablet or open capsule and take with liquid or food.

When to take:
With meals or immediately after.

If you forget a dose:
Take as soon as you remember. Return to regular schedule, but allow 3 hours between doses.

What drug does:
- Blocks certain actions of sympathetic nervous system.
- Lowers heart's oxygen requirements.
- Slows nerve impulses through heart.
- Reduces blood vessel contraction in heart, scalp and other body parts.

Time lapse before drug works:
1 to 4 hours.

Don't take with:
Non-prescription drugs or drugs in Interaction column without consulting doctor.

OVERDOSE

Symptoms:
Weakness, slow or weak pulse, blood-pressure drop, fainting, convulsions, cold and sweaty skin.

What to do:
- Dial O (operator) or 911 (emergency) for an ambulance or medical help. Then give first aid immediately.
- Additional emergency information on page 886.

POSSIBLE ADVERSE REACTIONS OR SIDE EFFECTS

SYMPTOMS	FREQUENCY	WHAT TO DO
Brain & nervous system:		
• Hallucinations, nightmares, insomnia, headache.	Infrequent	3
• Confusion, depression, reduced alertness.	Infrequent	4
• Drowsiness, numbness or tingling of fingers or toes, dizziness.	Common	4
Skin: Rash	Rare	3
Eyes:	None expected.	
Ears, nose, throat: Sore throat, fever.	Rare	3
Digestive:		
• Diarrhea, nausea.	Common	4
• Constipation	Infrequent	5
Heart & lungs:		
• Pulse slower than 50 beats per minute.	Common	3
• Breathing difficulty.	Infrequent	3
Blood vessels: Cold hands, feet.	Common	5
Muscles, bones, joints, genital, urinary, kidneys, liver, allergic:	None expected.	
Blood: Unusual bleeding and bruising.	Rare	4
Others:		
• Fatigue, weakness.	Common	4
• Dry mouth, eyes, skin.	Common	5

1 - Life-threatening. Seek emergency treatment immediately.
2 - Discontinue. Seek emergency treatment.
3 - Discontinue. Call doctor right away.
4 - Continue. Call doctor when convenient.
5 - Continue. Tell doctor at next visit.

TIMOLOL

WARNINGS & PRECAUTIONS

Don't take if:
- You are allergic to any beta-adrenergic blocker.
- You have asthma.
- You have hay fever symptoms.
- You have taken MAO inhibitors in past 2 weeks.

Before you start, consult your doctor:
- If you have heart disease or poor circulation to the extremities.
- If you have hay fever, asthma, chronic bronchitis, emphysema.
- If you have overactive thyroid function.
- If you have impaired liver or kidney function.
- If you will have surgery within 2 months, including dental surgery, requiring general or spinal anesthesia.
- If you have diabetes or hypoglycemia.

Over age 60:
Adverse reactions and side effects may be more frequent and severe than in younger persons.

Pregnancy:
Risk to unborn child outweighs drug benefits. Don't use.

Breast-feeding:
Drug passes into milk. Avoid drug or discontinue nursing until you finish medicine. Consult doctor for advice on maintaining milk supply.

Infants & children:
Not recommended.

Prolonged use:
Weakens heart muscle contractions.

Skin & sunlight:
No problems expected.

Driving, piloting or hazardous work:
Don't drive or pilot aircraft until you learn how medicine affects you. Don't work around dangerous machinery. Don't climb ladders or work in high places. Danger increases if you drink alcohol or take medicine affecting alertness and reflexes.

Airplane passengers:
No problems expected.

Discontinuing:
Don't discontinue without consulting doctor. Dose may require gradual reduction if you have taken drug for a long time. Doses of other drugs may also require adjustment.

Others:
May mask hypoglycemia.

INTERACTION WITH OTHER DRUGS

GENERIC NAME OR DRUG CLASS	COMBINED EFFECT
Antidiabetics	Increased antidiabetic effect.
Antihistamines	Decreased antihistamine effect.
Antihypertensives	Increased antihypertensive effect.
Antiinflammatory drugs	Decreased antiinflammatory effect.
Barbiturates	Increased barbiturate effect. Dangerous sedation.
Digitalis preparations	Can either increase or decrease heart rate. Improves irregular heartbeat.
Narcotics	Increased narcotic effect. Dangerous sedation.
Phenytoin	Increased timolol effect.
Quinidine	Slows heart excessively.
Reserpine	Increased reserpine effect. Excessive sedation and depression.

INTERACTION WITH OTHER SUBSTANCES

INTERACTS WITH	COMBINED EFFECT
Alcohol:	Excessive blood-pressure drop. Avoid.
Beverages:	None expected.
Cocaine:	Irregular heartbeat. Avoid.
Foods:	None expected.
Marijuana:	Daily use—Impaired circulation to hands and feet.
Tobacco:	Possible irregular heartbeat.

TOLAZAMIDE

BRAND NAMES

Tolinase

GENERAL INFORMATION

Habit forming? No
Prescription needed? Yes
Available as generic? No
Drug class: Antidiabetic (oral), sulfonurea

USES

Treatment for diabetes in adults who can't control blood sugar by diet, weight loss and exercise.

DOSAGE & USAGE INFORMATION

How to take:
Tablet—Swallow with liquid or food to lessen stomach irritation. If you can't swallow whole, crumble tablet and take with liquid or food.

When to take:
At the same times each day.

If you forget a dose:
Take as soon as you remember up to 2 hours late. If more than 2 hours, wait for next scheduled dose (don't double this dose).

What drug does:
Stimulates pancreas to produce more insulin. Insulin in blood forces cells to use sugar in blood.

Time lapse before drug works:
3 to 4 hours. May require 2 weeks for maximum benefit.

Don't take with:
See Interaction column and consult doctor.

OVERDOSE

Symptoms:
Excessive hunger, nausea, anxiety, cool skin, cold sweats, drowsiness, rapid heartbeat, weakness, unconsciousness, coma.

What to do:
- Dial 0 (operator) or 911 (emergency) for an ambulance or medical help. Then give first aid immediately.
- Additional emergency information on page 886.

POSSIBLE ADVERSE REACTIONS OR SIDE EFFECTS

SYMPTOMS	FREQUENCY	WHAT TO DO
Brain & nervous system:		
● Dizziness	Common	3
● Fatigue	Rare	3
Skin:		
Itching or rash.	Rare	3
Eyes:	None expected.	
Ears, nose, throat:		
● Sore throat, fever.	Rare	3
● Ringing in ears.	Rare	3
Digestive:		
Diarrhea, loss of appetite, nausea, stomach pain, heartburn.	Common	4
Heart & lungs, muscles, bones, joints, genital, urinary, kidneys, allergic, blood:	None expected.	
Blood vessels:		
Unusual bleeding or bruising.	Rare	3
Liver:		
Jaundice (yellow skin and eyes).	Rare	3
Others:		
Low blood sugar (ravenous hunger, nausea, anxiety, cold sweats, cool skin, chills, drowsiness, nervousness, headache, rapid heartbeat, weakness).	Infrequent	2

1- Life-threatening. Seek emergency treatment immediately.
2- Discontinue. Seek emergency treatment.
3- Discontinue. Call doctor right away.
4- Continue. Call doctor when convenient.

TOLAZAMIDE

WARNINGS & PRECAUTIONS

Don't take if:
- You are allergic to any sulfonurea.
- You have impaired kidney or liver function.

Before you start, consult your doctor:
- If you have a severe infection.
- If you have thyroid disease.
- If you take insulin.
- If you have heart disease.

Over age 60:
Dose usually smaller than for younger adults. Avoid "low-blood-sugar" episodes because repeated ones can damage brain permanently.

Pregnancy:
No proven harm to unborn child. Avoid if possible.

Breast-feeding:
Drug filters into milk. May lower baby's blood sugar. Avoid.

Infants & children:
Don't give to infants or children.

Prolonged use:
None expected.

Skin & sunlight:
May cause rash or intensify sunburn in areas exposed to sun or sunlamp.

Driving, piloting or hazardous work:
No problems expected unless you develop hypoglycemia (low blood sugar). If so, avoid driving or hazardous activity.

Airplane passengers:
No problems expected.

Discontinuing:
Don't discontinue without consulting doctor. Dose may require gradual reduction if you have taken drug for a long time. Doses of other drugs may also require adjustment.

Others:
- Don't exceed 1500 mg. in 1 day.
- Hypoglycemia (low blood sugar) may occur, even with proper dose schedule. You must balance medicine, diet and exercise.

INTERACTION WITH OTHER DRUGS

GENERIC NAME OR DRUG CLASS	COMBINED EFFECT
Androgens	Increased tolazamide effect.
Anticoagulants (oral)	Unpredictable prothrombin times (see page 850).
Anticonvulsants (hydantoin)	Decreased tolazamide effect.
Antiinflammatory drugs (non-steroidal)	Increased tolazamide effect.
Aspirin	Increased tolazamide effect.
Beta-adrenergic blockers	Increased tolazamide effect.
Chloramphenicol	Increased tolazamide effect.
Clofibrate	Increased tolazamide effect.
Contraceptives (oral)	Decreased tolazamide effect.
Cortisone drugs	Decreased tolazamide effect.
Diuretics (thiazide)	Decreased tolazamide effect.
Epinephrine	Decreased tolazamide effect.
Estrogens	Increased tolazamide effect.
Guanethidine	Unpredictable tolazamide effect.

Additional interactions on page 843.

INTERACTION WITH OTHER SUBSTANCES

INTERACTS WITH	COMBINED EFFECT
Alcohol:	Disulfiram reaction (see page 848). Avoid.
Beverages:	None expected.
Cocaine:	No proven problems.
Foods:	None expected.
Marijuana:	Decreased tolazamide effect. Avoid.
Tobacco:	None expected.

TOLBUTAMIDE

BRAND NAMES

Mobenol
Neo-Dibetic
Novobutamide
Oramide

Orinase
SK-Tolbutamide
Tolbutone

GENERAL INFORMATION

Habit forming? No
Prescription needed? Yes
Available as generic? No
Drug class: Antidiabetic (oral), sulfonurea

 ## USES

Treatment for diabetes in adults who can't control blood sugar by diet, weight loss and exercise.

 ## DOSAGE & USAGE INFORMATION

How to take:
Tablet—Swallow with liquid or food to lessen stomach irritation. If you can't swallow whole, crumble tablet and take with liquid or food.

When to take:
At the same times each day.

If you forget a dose:
Take as soon as you remember up to 2 hours late. If more than 2 hours, wait for next scheduled dose (don't double this dose).

What drug does:
Stimulates pancreas to produce more insulin. Insulin in blood forces cells to use sugar in blood.

Time lapse before drug works:
3 to 4 hours. May require 2 weeks for maximum benefit.

Don't take with:
See Interaction column and consult doctor.

 ## OVERDOSE

Symptoms:
Excessive hunger, nausea, anxiety, cool skin, cold sweats, drowsiness, rapid heartbeat, weakness, unconsciousness, coma.

What to do:
- Dial 0 (operator) or 911 (emergency) for an ambulance or medical help. Then give first aid immediately.
- Additional emergency information on page 886.

POSSIBLE ADVERSE REACTIONS OR SIDE EFFECTS

SYMPTOMS	FREQUENCY	WHAT TO DO
Brain & nervous system:		
• Dizziness	Common	3
• Fatigue	Rare	3
Skin:		
Itching or rash.	Rare	3
Eyes:	None expected.	
Ears, nose, throat:		
• Sore throat, fever.	Rare	3
• Ringing in ears.	Rare	3
Digestive:		
Diarrhea, loss of appetite, nausea, stomach pain, heartburn.	Common	4
Heart & lungs, muscles, bones, joints, genital, urinary, kidneys, allergic, blood:	None expected.	
Blood vessels:		
Unusual bleeding or bruising.	Rare	3
Liver:		
Jaundice (yellow skin and eyes).	Rare	3
Others:		
Low blood sugar (ravenous hunger, nausea, anxiety, cold sweats, cool skin, chills, drowsiness, nervousness, headache, rapid heartbeat, weakness).	Infrequent	2

1 - Life-threatening. Seek emergency treatment immediately.
2 - Discontinue. Seek emergency treatment.
3 - Discontinue. Call doctor right away.
4 - Continue. Call doctor when convenient.

WARNINGS & PRECAUTIONS

Don't take if:
- You are allergic to any sulfonurea.
- You have impaired kidney or liver function.

Before you start, consult your doctor:
- If you have a severe infection.
- If you have thyroid disease.
- If you take insulin.
- If you have heart disease.

Over age 60:
Dose usually smaller than for younger adults. Avoid "low-blood-sugar" episodes because repeated ones can damage brain permanently.

Pregnancy:
No proven harm to unborn child. Avoid if possible.

Breast-feeding:
Drug filters into milk. May lower baby's blood sugar. Avoid.

Infants & children:
Don't give to infants or children.

Prolonged use:
None expected.

Skin & sunlight:
May cause rash or intensify sunburn in areas exposed to sun or sunlamp.

Driving, piloting or hazardous work:
No problems expected unless you develop hypoglycemia (low blood sugar). If so, avoid driving or hazardous activity.

Airplane passengers:
No problems expected.

Discontinuing:
Don't discontinue without consulting doctor. Dose may require gradual reduction if you have taken drug for a long time. Doses of other drugs may also require adjustment.

Others:
- Don't exceed 1500 mg. in 1 day.
- Hypoglycemia (low blood sugar) may occur, even with proper dose schedule. You must balance medicine, diet and exercise.

 ## INTERACTION WITH OTHER DRUGS

GENERIC NAME OR DRUG CLASS	COMBINED EFFECT
Androgens	Increased tolbutamide effect.
Anticoagulants (oral)	Unpredictable prothrombin times (see page 850).
Anticonvulsants (hydantoin)	Decreased tolbutamide effect.
Antiinflammatory drugs (non-steroidal)	Increased tolbutamide effect.
Aspirin	Increased tolbutamide effect.
Beta-adrenergic blockers	Increased tolbutamide effect.
Chloramphenicol	Increased tolbutamide effect.
Clofibrate	Increased tolbutamide effect.
Contraceptives (oral)	Decreased tolbutamide effect.
Cortisone drugs	Decreased tolbutamide effect.
Diuretics (thiazide)	Decreased tolbutamide effect.
Epinephrine	Decreased tolbutamide effect.
Estrogens	Increased tolbutamide effect.
Guanethidine	Unpredictable tolbutamide effect.

Additional interactions on page 844.

 ## INTERACTION WITH OTHER SUBSTANCES

INTERACTS WITH	COMBINED EFFECT
Alcohol:	Disulfiram reaction (see page 848). Avoid.
Beverages:	None expected.
Cocaine:	No proven problems.
Foods:	None expected.
Marijuana:	Decreased tolbutamide effect. Avoid.
Tobacco:	None expected.

TOLMETIN

BRAND NAMES

Tolectin
Tolectin DS

Habit forming? No
Prescription needed? Yes

USES

- Treatment for joint pain, stiffness, inflammation and swelling of arthritis and gout.
- Pain reliever.

DOSAGE & USAGE INFORMATION

How to take:
Tablet or capsule—Swallow with liquid or food to lessen stomach irritation. If you can't swallow whole, crumble tablet or open capsule and take with liquid or food.

When to take:
At the same times each day.

If you forget a dose:
Take as soon as you remember up to 2 hours late. If more than 2 hours, wait for next scheduled dose (don't double this dose).

What drug does:
Reduces tissue concentration of prostaglandins (hormones which produce inflammation and pain).

Time lapse before drug works:
Begins in 4 to 24 hours. May require 3 weeks regular use for maximum benefit.

Don't take with:
See Interaction column and consult doctor.

OVERDOSE

Symptoms:
Confusion, agitation, incoherence, convulsions, possible hemorrhage from stomach or intestine, coma.

What to do:
- Dial 0 (operator) or 911 (emergency) for an ambulance or medical help. Then give first aid immediately.
- Additional emergency information on page 886.

GENERAL INFORMATION

Available as generic? No
Drug class: Antiinflammatory (non-steroid)

POSSIBLE ADVERSE REACTIONS OR SIDE EFFECTS

SYMPTOMS	FREQUENCY	WHAT TO DO
Brain & nervous system:		
• Depression, drowsiness.	Infrequent	4
• Convulsions, confusion.	Rare	3
• Dizziness	Common	4
• Headache	Common	5
Skin:		
Rash, hives or itch.	Rare	3
Eyes:		
Blurred vision.	Rare	3
Ears, nose, throat:		
Ringing in ears.	Infrequent	4
Digestive:		
• Bloody or black, tarry stools.	Rare	3
• Nausea, pain.	Common	4
• Constipation or diarrhea, vomiting.	Infrequent	4
Heart & lungs:		
Breathing difficulty, tightness in chest, rapid heartbeat.	Rare	3
Blood vessels:		
Unusual bleeding or bruising.	Rare	3
Muscles, bones, joints:		
Swollen feet, legs.	Infrequent	4
Genital, urinary:		
• Bloody urine.	Rare	3
• Difficult, painful or frequent urination.	Rare	4
Kidneys, allergic, blood:		
	None expected.	
Liver:		
Jaundice (yellow skin and eyes).	Rare	3
Others:		
Fatigue, weakness.	Rare	4

1- Life-threatening. Seek emergency treatment immediately.
2- Discontinue. Seek emergency treatment.
3- Discontinue. Call doctor right away.
4- Continue. Call doctor when convenient.
5- Continue. Tell doctor at next visit.

WARNINGS & PRECAUTIONS

Don't take if:
- You are allergic to aspirin or any non-steroid, antiinflammatory drug.
- You have gastritis, peptic ulcer, enteritis, ileitis, ulcerative colitis, asthma, heart failure, high blood pressure or bleeding problems.
- Patient is younger than 15.

Before you start, consult your doctor:
- If you have epilepsy.
- If you have Parkinson's disease.
- If you have been mentally ill.
- If you have had kidney disease or impaired kidney function.

Over age 60:
Adverse reactions and side effects may be more frequent and severe than in younger persons.

Pregnancy:
Studies inconclusive on harm to unborn child. Decide with your doctor whether drug benefits justify risk to unborn child.

Breast-feeding:
May harm child. Avoid.

Infants & children:
Not recommended for anyone younger than 15. Use only under medical supervision.

Prolonged use:
- Eye damage.
- Reduced hearing.
- Sore throat, fever.
- Weight gain.

Skin & sunlight:
No problems expected.

Driving, piloting or hazardous work:
Don't drive or pilot aircraft until you learn how medicine affects you. Don't work around dangerous machinery. Don't climb ladders or work in high places. Danger increases if you drink alcohol or take medicine affecting alertness and reflexes, such as antihistamines, tranquilizers, sedatives, pain medicine, narcotics and mind-altering drugs.

Airplane passengers:
No problems expected.

Discontinuing:
Don't discontinue without consulting doctor. Dose may require gradual reduction if you have taken drug for a long time. Doses of other drugs may also require adjustment.

Others:
No problems expected.

INTERACTION WITH OTHER DRUGS

GENERIC NAME OR DRUG CLASS	COMBINED EFFECT
Anticoagulants (oral)	Increased risk of bleeding.
Aspirin	Increased risk of stomach ulcer.
Cortisone drugs	Increased risk of stomach ulcer.
Furosemide	Decreased diuretic effect of furosemide.
Oxyphenbutazone	Possible stomach ulcer.
Phenylbutazone	Possible stomach ulcer.
Probenecid	Increased tolmetin effect.
Thyroid hormones	Rapid heartbeat, blood-pressure rise.

INTERACTION WITH OTHER SUBSTANCES

INTERACTS WITH	COMBINED EFFECT
Alcohol:	Possible stomach ulcer or bleeding.
Beverages:	None expected.
Cocaine:	None expected.
Foods:	None expected.
Marijuana:	Increased pain relief from tolmetin.
Tobacco:	None expected.

TRANYLCYPROMINE

BRAND NAMES

Parnate

GENERAL INFORMATION

Habit forming? No
Prescription needed? Yes
Available as generic? No

Drug class: MAO inhibitor
(monamine oxidase inhibitor),
antidepressant

 ## USES

Treatment for depression.

 ## DOSAGE & USAGE INFORMATION

How to take:
Tablet—Swallow with liquid. If you can't swallow whole, crumble tablet and take with liquid or food.

When to take:
At the same times each day.

If you forget a dose:
Take as soon as you remember up to 2 hours late. If more than 2 hours, wait for next scheduled dose (don't double this dose).

What drug does:
Inhibits nerve transmissions in brain that may cause depression.

Time lapse before drug works:
4 to 6 weeks for maximum effect.

Don't take with:
- Non-prescription diet pills, nose drops, medicine for asthma, cough, cold or allergy, or medicine containing caffeine or alcohol.
- See Interaction column and consult doctor.

 ## OVERDOSE

Symptoms:
Restlessness, agitation, fever, convulsions, coma.

What to do:
- Dial 0 (operator) or 911 (emergency) for an ambulance or medical help. Then give first aid immediately.
- Additional emergency information on page 886.

 ## POSSIBLE ADVERSE REACTIONS OR SIDE EFFECTS

SYMPTOMS	FREQUENCY	WHAT TO DO
Brain & nervous system:		
• Fainting	Infrequent	2
• Severe headache.	Infrequent	3
• Dizziness when changing position.	Common	5
• Hallucinations, insomnia, nightmares.	Infrequent	4
Skin:		
Rash	Rare	3
Eyes, blood vessels, kidneys, allergic, blood:	None expected.	
Ears, nose, throat:		
Dry mouth.	Common	5
Digestive:		
• Diarrhea	Infrequent	4
• Constipation	Common	5
• Nausea, vomiting.	Rare	3
Heart & lungs:		
• Rapid or pounding heartbeat.	Infrequent	4
• Chest pain.	Infrequent	3
Muscles, bones, joints:		
Stiff neck.	Rare	3
Genital, urinary:		
Difficult urination.	Common	5
Liver:		
Jaundice (yellow skin and eyes).	Rare	3
Others:		
• Swollen feet, legs.	Infrequent	4
• Fever	Rare	3
• Lower sex drive.	Infrequent	5
• Fatigue, weakness.	Common	4

1- Life-threatening. Seek emergency treatment immediately.
2- Discontinue. Seek emergency treatment.
3- Discontinue. Call doctor right away.
4- Continue. Call doctor when convenient.
5- Continue. Tell doctor at next visit.

TRANYLCYPROMINE

WARNINGS & PRECAUTIONS

Don't take if:
- You are allergic to any MAO inhibitor.
- You have heart disease, congestive heart failure, heart-rhythm irregularities or high blood pressure.
- You have liver or kidney disease.

Before you start, consult your doctor:
- If you are alcoholic.
- If you have asthma.
- If you have had a stroke.
- If you have diabetes or epilepsy.
- If you have overactive thyroid.
- If you have schizophrenia.
- If you have Parkinson's disease.
- If you have adrenal-gland tumor.
- If you will have surgery within 2 months, including dental surgery, requiring general or spinal anesthesia.

Over age 60:
Not recommended.

Pregnancy:
No proven harm to unborn child. Avoid if possible.

Breast-feeding:
Safety not established. Consult doctor.

Infants & children:
Not recommended.

Prolonged use:
May be toxic to liver.

Skin & sunlight:
May cause rash or intensify sunburn in areas exposed to sun or sunlamp.

Driving, piloting or hazardous work:
Don't drive or pilot aircraft until you learn how medicine affects you. Don't work around dangerous machinery. Don't climb ladders or work in high places. Danger increases if you drink alcohol or take medicine affecting alertness and reflexes.

Airplane passengers:
No problems expected.

Discontinuing:
- Don't discontinue without doctor's advice until you complete prescribed dose, even though symptoms diminish or disappear.
- Follow precautions regarding foods, drinks and other medicines for 2 weeks after discontinuing.

Others:
- May affect blood-sugar levels in patients with diabetes.
- Fever may indicate that MAO inhibitor dose requires adjustment.

INTERACTION WITH OTHER DRUGS

GENERIC NAME OR DRUG CLASS	COMBINED EFFECT
Amphetamines	Blood-pressure rise to life-threatening level.
Anticonvulsants	Changed seizure pattern.
Antidepressants (tricyclic)	Blood-pressure rise to life-threatening level.
Antidiabetics (oral and insulin)	Excessively low blood sugar.
Antihypertensives	Excessively low blood pressure.
Caffeine	Irregular heartbeat or high blood pressure.
Carbamazepine	Fever, seizures. Avoid.
Cyclobenzaprine	Fever, seizures. Avoid.
Diuretics	Excessively low blood pressure.
Guanethidine	Blood-pressure rise to life-threatening level.
Levodopa	Sudden, severe blood-pressure rise.
MAO inhibitors (other)	High fever, convulsions, death.

Additional interactions on page 844.

INTERACTION WITH OTHER SUBSTANCES

INTERACTS WITH	COMBINED EFFECT
Alcohol:	Increased sedation to dangerous level.
Beverages: Caffeine drinks	Irregular heartbeat or high blood pressure.
Drinks containing tyramine (see page 851).	Blood-pressure rise to life-threatening level.
Cocaine:	Overstimulation. Possibly fatal.
Foods: Foods containing tyramine (see page 851).	Blood-pressure rise to life-threatening level.
Marijuana:	Overstimulation. Avoid.
Tobacco:	No proven problems.

TRETINOIN

BRAND NAMES

Retin-A
StieVAA

GENERAL INFORMATION

Habit forming? No
Prescription needed? Yes
Available as generic? No
Drug class: Antiacne (topical)

 USES

Treatment for acne, psoriasis, ichthyosis, keratosis, folliculitis, flat warts.

 DOSAGE & USAGE INFORMATION

How to use:
Wash skin with non-medicated soap, pat dry, wait 20 minutes before applying.
- Cream or gel—Apply to affected areas with fingertips and rub in gently.
- Solution—Apply to affected areas with gauze pad or cotton swab. Avoid getting too wet so medicine doesn't drip into eyes, mouth, lips or inside nose.

When to use:
At the same time each day.

If you forget an application:
Take as soon as you remember.

What drug does:
Increases skin-cell turnover so skin layer peels off more easily.

Time lapse before drug works:
2 to 3 weeks. May require 6 weeks for maximum improvement.

Don't use with:
- Benzoyl peroxide. Apply 12 hours apart.
- See Interaction column and consult doctor.

 OVERDOSE

Symptoms:
None expected.

What to do:
If person swallows drug, call doctor, poison-control center or hospital emergency room for instructions.

 POSSIBLE ADVERSE REACTIONS OR SIDE EFFECTS

SYMPTOMS	FREQUENCY	WHAT TO DO
Brain & nervous system:	None expected.	
Skin:		
• Blistering, crusting, severe burning, swelling.	Infrequent	3
• Pigment change in treated area, warmth or stinging, peeling.	Common	5
Eyes:	None expected.	
Ears, nose, throat:	None expected.	
Digestive:	None expected.	
Heart & lungs:	None expected.	
Blood vessels:	None expected.	
Muscles, bones, joints:	None expected.	
Genital, urinary:	None expected.	
Kidneys:	None expected.	
Liver:	None expected.	
Allergic:	None expected.	
Blood:	None expected.	
Others: Sensitivity to wind or cold.	Common	6

1- Life-threatening. Seek emergency treatment immediately.
2- Discontinue. Seek emergency treatment.
3- Discontinue. Call doctor right away.
4- Continue. Call doctor when convenient.
5- Continue. Tell doctor at next visit.
6- No action necessary.

WARNINGS & PRECAUTIONS

Don't take if:
- You are allergic to tretinoin.
- You are sunburned, windburned or have an open skin wound.

Before you start, consult your doctor:
If you have eczema.

Over age 60:
Not recommended.

Pregnancy:
No proven harm to unborn child. Avoid if possible.

Breast-feeding:
No problems expected.

Infants & children:
Not recommended.

Prolonged use:
No problems expected.

Skin & sunlight:
- May cause rash or intensify sunburn in areas exposed to sun or sunlamp.
- In some animal studies, tretinoin caused skin tumors to develop faster when treated area was exposed to ultraviolet light (sunlight or sunlamp). No proven similar effects in humans.

Driving, piloting or hazardous work:
No problems expected.

Airplane passengers:
No problems expected.

Discontinuing:
Don't discontinue without doctor's advice until you complete prescribed dose, even though symptoms diminish or disappear.

Others:
Acne may get worse before improvement starts in 2 or 3 weeks. Don't wash face more than 2 or 3 times daily.

INTERACTION WITH OTHER DRUGS

GENERIC NAME OR DRUG CLASS	COMBINED EFFECT
Antiacne topical preparations (other)	Severe skin irritation.
Cosmetics (medicated)	Severe skin irritation.
Skin preparations with alcohol	Severe skin irritation.
Soaps or cleansers (abrasive)	Severe skin irritation.

INTERACTION WITH OTHER SUBSTANCES

INTERACTS WITH	COMBINED EFFECT
Alcohol:	None expected.
Beverages:	None expected.
Cocaine:	None expected.
Foods:	None expected.
Marijuana:	None expected.
Tobacco:	None expected.

TRIAMCINOLONE

BRAND NAMES

Amcort
Aristocort
Aristospan
Cenocort Forte
Cino-40

Kenacort
Kenalog
Tramacort
Triacort

GENERAL INFORMATION

Habit forming? No
Prescription needed? Yes
Available as generic? Yes
Drug class: Cortisone drug (adrenal corticosteroid)

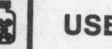

USES

- Reduces inflammation caused by many different medical problems.
- Treatment for some allergic diseases, blood disorders, kidney diseases, asthma and emphysema.
- Replaces corticosteroid deficiencies.

DOSAGE & USAGE INFORMATION

How to take:
Tablet or syrup—Swallow with liquid or food to lessen stomach irritation. If you can't swallow whole, crumble tablet.

When to take:
At the same times each day. Take once-a-day or once-every-other-day doses in mornings.

If you forget a dose:
- Several-doses-per-day prescription—Take as soon as you remember up to 2 hours late. If more than 2 hours, wait for next scheduled dose (don't double this dose).
- Once-a-day dose or less—Wait for next dose. Double this dose.

What drug does:
Decreases inflammatory responses.

Time lapse before drug works:
2 to 4 days.

Don't take with:
See Interaction column and consult doctor.

OVERDOSE

Symptoms:
Headache, convulsions, heart failure.

What to do:
- Dial 0 (operator) or 911 (emergency) for an ambulance or medical help. Then give first aid immediately.
- Additional emergency information on page 886.

POSSIBLE ADVERSE REACTIONS OR SIDE EFFECTS

SYMPTOMS	FREQUENCY	WHAT TO DO
Brain & nervous system:		
Mood changes, insomnia, restlessness.	Infrequent	4
Skin:		
• Acne	Common	4
• Rash	Rare	3
• Poor wound healing.	Common	4
Eyes:		
Blurred vision, halos around lights.	Infrequent	3
Ears, nose, throat:		
• Sore throat, fever.	Infrequent	3
• Thirst	Common	4
Digestive:		
• Indigestion, nausea, vomiting.	Common	4
• Bloody or black, tarry stool.	Infrequent	2
Heart & lungs:		
Irregular heartbeat.	Rare	2
Blood vessels, kidneys, liver, allergic, blood:	None expected.	
Muscles, bones, joints:		
Muscle cramps, swollen legs, feet.	Infrequent	3
Genital, urinary:		
Frequent urination.	Infrequent	4
Others:		
• Weight gain, round face.	Infrequent	4
• Fatigue, weakness.	Infrequent	4
• TB recurrence.	Infrequent	4
• Irregular menstrual periods.	Infrequent	4

1- Life-threatening. Seek emergency treatment immediately.
2- Discontinue. Seek emergency treatment.
3- Discontinue. Call doctor right away.
4- Continue. Call doctor when convenient.

WARNINGS & PRECAUTIONS

Don't take if:
- You are allergic to any cortisone drug.
- You have tuberculosis or fungus infection.
- You have herpes infection of eyes, lips or genitals.

Before you start, consult your doctor:
- If you have had tuberculosis.
- If you have congestive heart failure.
- If you have diabetes.
- If you have peptic ulcer.
- If you have glaucoma.
- If you have underactive thyroid.
- If you have high blood pressure.
- If you have myasthenia gravis.
- If you have blood clots in legs or lungs.

Over age 60:
Adverse reactions and side effects may be more frequent and severe than in younger persons. Likely to aggravate edema, diabetes or ulcers. Likely to cause cataracts and osteoporosis (softening of the bones).

Pregnancy:
Risk to unborn child outweighs drug benefits. Don't use.

Breast-feeding:
Drug passes into milk. Avoid drug or discontinue nursing until you finish medicine. Consult doctor for advice on maintaining milk supply.

Infants & children:
Use only under medical supervision.

Prolonged use:
- Retards growth in children.
- Possible glaucoma, cataracts, diabetes, fragile bones and thin skin.
- Functional dependence.

Skin & sunlight:
No problems expected.

Driving, piloting or hazardous work:
No problems expected.

Airplane passengers:
No problems expected.

Discontinuing:
- Don't discontinue without doctor's advice until you complete prescribed dose, even though symptoms diminish or disappear.
- Drug affects your response to surgery, illness, injury or stress for 2 years after discontinuing. Tell about drug to anyone who takes medical care of you within 2 years.

Others:
Avoid immunizations if possible.

INTERACTION WITH OTHER DRUGS

GENERIC NAME OR DRUG CLASS	COMBINED EFFECT
Amphoterecin B	Potassium depletion.
Anticholinergics	Possible glaucoma.
Anticoagulants (oral)	Decreased anticoagulant effect.
Anticonvulsants (hydantoin)	Decreased triamcinolone effect.
Antidiabetics (oral)	Decreased antidiabetic effect.
Antihistamines	Decreased triamcinolone effect.
Aspirin	Increased triamcinolone effect.
Barbiturates	Decreased triamcinolone effect. Oversedation.
Beta-adrenergic blockers	Decreased triamcinolone effect.
Chloral hydrate	Decreased triamcinolone effect.
Chlorthalidone	Potassium depletion.
Cholinergics	Decreased cholinergic effect.
Contraceptives (oral)	Increased triamcinolone effect.
Digitalis preparations	Dangerous potassium depletion. Possible digitalis toxicity.
Diuretics (thiazide)	Potassium depletion.

Additional interactions on page 844.

INTERACTION WITH OTHER SUBSTANCES

INTERACTS WITH	COMBINED EFFECT
Alcohol:	Risk of stomach ulcers.
Beverages:	No proven problems.
Cocaine:	Overstimulation. Avoid.
Foods:	No proven problems.
Marijuana:	Decreased immunity.
Tobacco:	Increased triamcinolone effect. Possible toxicity.

TRIAMTERENE

BRAND NAMES

Dyazide (M)
Dyrenium

GENERAL INFORMATION

Habit forming? No
Prescription needed? Yes
Available as generic? No
Drug class: Antihypertensive, diuretic

USES

- Reduces fluid retention (edema).
- Reduces potassium loss.

DOSAGE & USAGE INFORMATION

How to take:
Tablet or capsule—Swallow with liquid or food to lessen stomach irritation. If you can't swallow whole, crumble tablet or open capsule and take with liquid or food.

When to take:
- 1 dose per day—Take after breakfast.
- More than 1 dose per day—Take last dose no later than 6 p.m.

If you forget a dose:
Take as soon as you remember up to 6 hours late. If more than 6 hours, wait for next scheduled dose (don't double this dose).

What drug does:
Increases urine production to eliminate sodium and water from body while conserving potassium.

Time lapse before drug works:
2 hours. May require 2 to 3 days for maximum benefit.

Don't take with:
See Interaction column and consult doctor.

OVERDOSE

Symptoms:
Lethargy, irregular heartbeat, coma.

What to do:
- Dial 0 (operator) or 911 (emergency) for an ambulance or medical help. Then give first aid immediately.
- If patient is unconscious and not breathing, give mouth-to-mouth breathing. If there is no heartbeat, use cardiac massage and mouth-to-mouth breathing (CPR). Don't try to make patient vomit. If you can't get help quickly, take patient to nearest emergency facility.
- Additional emergency information on page 886.

POSSIBLE ADVERSE REACTIONS OR SIDE EFFECTS

SYMPTOMS	FREQUENCY	WHAT TO DO
Brain & nervous system:		
● Anxiety	Infrequent	5
● Drowsiness	Infrequent	3
● Headache	Rare	5
● Confusion	Infrequent	3
Skin:		
Rash	Rare	3
Eyes:	None expected.	
Ears, nose, throat:		
● Sore throat, fever.	Rare	3
● Dry mouth, thirst.	Infrequent	3
● Red, inflamed tongue.	Rare	3
Digestive:		
Diarrhea	Infrequent	4
Heart & lungs:		
Irregular heartbeat, shortness of breath.	Infrequent	3
Blood vessels:		
Unusual bleeding or bruising.	Rare	3
Muscles, bones, joints:	None expected.	
Genital, urinary:	None expected.	
Kidneys:	None expected.	
Liver:	None expected.	
Allergic:	None expected.	
Blood:	None expected.	
Others:		
Unusual tiredness, weakness.	Infrequent	3

1- Life-threatening. Seek emergency treatment immediately.
2- Discontinue. Seek emergency treatment.
3- Discontinue. Call doctor right away.
4- Continue. Call doctor when convenient.
5- Continue. Tell doctor at next visit.
6- No action necessary.

WARNINGS & PRECAUTIONS

Don't take if:
- You are allergic to triamterene.
- You have had severe liver or kidney disease.

Before you start, consult your doctor:
- If you have gout.
- If you have diabetes.
- If you will have surgery within 2 months, including dental surgery, requiring general or spinal anesthesia.

Over age 60:
- Warm weather or fever can decrease blood pressure. Dose may require adjustment.
- Extended use can increase blood clots.

Pregnancy:
No proven harm to unborn child. Avoid if possible.

Breast-feeding:
Present in milk. Avoid.

Infants & children:
Used infrequently. Use only under medical supervision.

Prolonged use:
Potassium retention which may lead to heart-rhythm problems.

Skin & sunlight:
May cause rash or intensify sunburn in areas exposed to sun or sunlamp.

Driving, piloting or hazardous work:
Avoid if you feel drowsy or confused. Otherwise, no problems expected.

Airplane passengers:
No problems expected.

Discontinuing:
Don't discontinue without consulting doctor. Dose may require gradual reduction if you have taken drug for a long time. Doses of other drugs may also require adjustment.

Others:
No problems expected.

INTERACTION WITH OTHER DRUGS

GENERIC NAME OR DRUG CLASS	COMBINED EFFECT
Antidiabetics (oral)	Decreased antidiabetic effect.
Antihypertensives (other)	Increased effect of other antihypertensives.
Digitalis preparations	Decreased digitalis effect.
Lithium	Increased lithium effect.
Spironolactone	Dangerous retention of potassium.

INTERACTION WITH OTHER SUBSTANCES

INTERACTS WITH	COMBINED EFFECT
Alcohol:	None expected.
Beverages:	None expected.
Cocaine:	Decreased triamterene effect.
Foods: Salt	Don't restrict unless directed by doctor.
Marijuana:	Daily use—Fainting likely.
Tobacco:	None expected.

TRICHLORMETHIAZIDE

BRAND NAMES

Metahydrin
Naqua

GENERAL INFORMATION

Habit forming? No
Prescription needed? Yes
Available as generic? Yes
Drug class: Antihypertensive,
diuretic (thiazide)

USES

- Controls, but doesn't cure, high blood pressure.
- Reduces fluid retention (edema) caused by conditions such as heart disorders and liver disease.

DOSAGE & USAGE INFORMATION

How to take:
Tablet or capsule—Swallow with liquid. If you can't swallow whole, crumble tablet or open capsule and take with liquid or food. Don't exceed dose.

When to take:
At the same time each day.

If you forget a dose:
Take as soon as you remember up to 2 hours late. If more than 2 hours, wait for next scheduled dose (don't double this dose).

What drug does:
- Forces sodium and water excretion, reducing body fluid.
- Relaxes muscle cells of small arteries.
- Reduced body fluid and relaxed arteries lower blood pressure.

Time lapse before drug works:
4 to 6 hours. May require several weeks to lower blood pressure.

Don't take with:
- See Interaction column and consult doctor.
- Non-prescription drugs without consulting doctor.

OVERDOSE

Symptoms:
Cramps, weakness, drowsiness, weak pulse, coma.

What to do:
- Dial O (operator) or 911 (emergency) for an ambulance or medical help. Then give first aid immediately.
- Additional emergency information on page 886.

POSSIBLE ADVERSE REACTIONS OR SIDE EFFECTS

SYMPTOMS	FREQUENCY	WHAT TO DO
Brain & nervous system:		
• Dizziness	Infrequent	4
• Mood changes.	Infrequent	4
• Headache	Infrequent	4
Skin:		
Rash or hives.	Rare	2
Eyes:		
Blurred vision.	Infrequent	3
Ears, nose, throat:		
• Sore throat, fever.	Rare	3
• Dry mouth, thirst.	Infrequent	5
Digestive:		
Severe abdominal pain, nausea, vomiting.	Infrequent	3
Heart & lungs:		
Irregular heartbeat, weak pulse.	Infrequent	3
Blood vessels:	None expected.	
Muscles, bones, joints:		
Weakness, tiredness.	Infrequent	4
Genital, urinary:	None expected.	
Kidneys:	None expected.	
Liver:		
Jaundice (yellow skin and eyes).	Rare	3
Allergic:	None expected.	
Blood:	None expected.	
Others:		
Weight changes.	Infrequent	4

1 - Life-threatening. Seek emergency treatment immediately.
2 - Discontinue. Seek emergency treatment.
3 - Discontinue. Call doctor right away.
4 - Continue. Call doctor when convenient.
5 - Continue. Tell doctor at next visit.
6 - No action necessary.

TRICHLORMETHIAZIDE

WARNINGS & PRECAUTIONS

Don't take if:
You are allergic to any thiazide diuretic drug.

Before you start, consult your doctor:
- If you are allergic to any sulfa drug.
- If you have gout.
- If you have liver, pancreas or kidney disorder.

Over age 60:
Adverse reactions and side effects may be more frequent and severe than in younger persons, especially dizziness and excessive potassium loss.

Pregnancy:
Risk to unborn child outweighs drug benefits. Don't use.

Breast-feeding:
Drug passes into milk. Avoid drug or discontinue nursing.

Infants & children:
No problems expected.

Prolonged use:
You may need medicine to treat high blood pressure for the rest of your life.

Skin & sunlight:
May cause rash or intensify sunburn in areas exposed to sun or sunlamp.

Driving, piloting or hazardous work:
Don't drive or pilot aircraft until you learn how medicine affects you. Don't work around dangerous machinery. Don't climb ladders or work in high places. Danger increases if you drink alcohol or take medicine affecting alertness and reflexes, such as antihistamines, tranquilizers, sedatives, pain medicine, narcotics and mind-altering drugs.

Airplane passengers:
No problems expected.

Discontinuing:
Don't discontinue without medical advice.

Others:
- Hot weather and fever may cause dehydration and drop in blood pressure. Dose may require temporary adjustment. Weigh daily and report any unexpected weight decreases to your doctor.
- May cause rise in uric acid, leading to gout.
- May cause blood-sugar rise in diabetics.

INTERACTION WITH OTHER DRUGS

GENERIC NAME OR DRUG CLASS	COMBINED EFFECT
Allopurinol	Decreased allopurinol effect.
Antidepressants (tricyclic)	Dangerous drop in blood pressure. Avoid combination unless under medical supervision.
Barbiturates	Increased trichlormethiazide effect.
Cholestyramine	Decreased trichlormethiazide effect.
Cortisone drugs	Excessive potassium loss that causes dangerous heart rhythms.
Digitalis preparations	Excessive potassium loss that causes dangerous heart rhythms.
Diuretics (thiazide)	Increased effect of other thiazide diuretics.
Lithium	Increased effect of lithium.
MAO inhibitors	Increased trichlormethiazide effect.
Probenecid	Decreased probenecid effect.

INTERACTION WITH OTHER SUBSTANCES

INTERACTS WITH	COMBINED EFFECT
Alcohol:	Dangerous blood-pressure drop.
Beverages:	None expected.
Cocaine:	None expected.
Foods: Licorice	Excessive potassium loss that causes dangerous heart rhythms.
Marijuana:	May increase blood pressure.
Tobacco:	None expected.

TRIDIHEXETHYL

BRAND NAMES

Milpath (M)
Pathibamate (M)
Pathilon

GENERAL INFORMATION

Habit forming? No
Prescription needed? Low strength: No
High strength: Yes
Available as generic? Yes
Drug class: Antispasmodic, anticholinergic

 ## USES

Reduces spasms of digestive system, bladder and urethra.

 ## DOSAGE & USAGE INFORMATION

How to take:
Tablet—Swallow with liquid or food to lessen stomach irritation.

When to take:
30 minutes before meals (unless directed otherwise by doctor).

If you forget a dose:
Take as soon as you remember up to 2 hours late. If more than 2 hours, wait for next scheduled dose (don't double this dose).

What drug does:
Blocks nerve impulses at parasympathetic nerve endings, preventing muscle contractions and gland secretions of organs involved.

Time lapse before drug works:
15 to 30 minutes.

Don't take with:
See Interaction column and consult doctor.

 ## OVERDOSE

Symptoms:
Dilated pupils; rapid pulse and breathing; dizziness; fever; hallucinations; confusion; slurred speech; agitation; flushed face; convulsions; coma.

What to do:
- Dial 0 (operator) or 911 (emergency) for an ambulance or medical help. Then give first aid immediately.
- Additional emergency information on page 886.

 ## POSSIBLE ADVERSE REACTIONS OR SIDE EFFECTS

SYMPTOMS	FREQUENCY	WHAT TO DO
Brain & nervous system:		
● Headache	Infrequent	4
● Confusion, delirium.	Common	3
Skin:		
Rash or hives.	Rare	3
Eyes:		
Pain, blurred vision.	Rare	3
Ears, nose, throat:		
Dryness	Common	6
Digestive:		
● Constipation	Common	5
● Nausea, vomiting.	Common	4
Heart & lungs:		
Rapid heartbeat.	Common	3
Blood vessels:	None expected.	
Muscles, bones, joints:	None expected.	
Genital, urinary:		
Difficult urination.	Infrequent	4
Kidneys:	None expected.	
Liver:	None expected.	
Allergic:	None expected.	
Blood:	None expected.	
Others:		
Less perspiration.	Common	4

1 - Life-threatening. Seek emergency treatment immediately.
2 - Discontinue. Seek emergency treatment.
3 - Discontinue. Call doctor right away.
4 - Continue. Call doctor when convenient.
5 - Continue. Tell doctor at next visit.
6 - No action necessary.

WARNINGS & PRECAUTIONS

Don't take if:
- You are allergic to any anticholinergic.
- You have trouble with stomach bloating.
- You have difficulty emptying your bladder completely.
- You have narrow-angle glaucoma.
- You have severe ulcerative colitis.

Before you start, consult your doctor:
- If you have open-angle glaucoma.
- If you have angina.
- If you have chronic bronchitis or asthma.
- If you have hiatal hernia.
- If you have liver disease.
- If you have enlarged prostate.
- If you have myasthenia gravis.
- If you have peptic ulcer.
- If you will have surgery within 2 months, including dental surgery, requiring general or spinal anesthesia.

Over age 60:
Adverse reactions and side effects may be more frequent and severe than in younger persons.

Pregnancy:
Studies inconclusive on harm to unborn child. Animal studies show fetal abnormalities. Decide with your doctor whether drug benefits justify risk to unborn child.

Breast-feeding:
Drug passes into milk and decreases milk flow. Avoid drug or discontinue nursing until you finish medicine. Consult doctor for advice on maintaining milk supply.

Infants & children:
Use only under medical supervision.

Prolonged use:
Chronic constipation, possible fecal impaction. Consult doctor immediately.

Skin & sunlight:
No problems expected.

Driving, piloting or hazardous work:
Use disqualifies you for piloting aircraft. Otherwise, no problems expected.

Airplane passengers:
No problems expected.

Discontinuing:
May be unnecessary to finish medicine. Follow doctor's instructions.

Others:
No problems expected.

INTERACTION WITH OTHER DRUGS

GENERIC NAME OR DRUG CLASS	COMBINED EFFECT
Amantadine	Increased tridihexethyl effect.
Anticholinergics (other)	Increased tridihexethyl effect.
Antidepressants (tricyclic)	Increased tridihexethyl effect.
Antihistamines	Increased tridihexethyl effect.
Cortisone drugs	Increased internal-eye pressure.
Haloperidol	Increased internal-eye pressure.
MAO inhibitors	Increased tridihexethyl effect.
Meperidine	Increased tridihexethyl effect.
Methylphenidate	Increased tridihexethyl effect.
Orphenadrine	Increased tridihexethyl effect.
Phenothiazines	Increased tridihexethyl effect.
Pilocarpine	Loss of pilocarpine effect in glaucoma treatment.
Vitamin C	Decreased tridihexethyl effect. Avoid large doses of vitamin C.

INTERACTION WITH OTHER SUBSTANCES

INTERACTS WITH	COMBINED EFFECT
Alcohol:	None expected.
Beverages:	None expected.
Cocaine:	Excessively rapid heartbeat. Avoid.
Foods:	None expected.
Marijuana:	Drowsiness and dry mouth.
Tobacco:	None expected.

TRIFLUOPERAZINE

BRAND NAMES

Clinazine
Novofluorazine
Pentazine
Solazine

Stelazine
Terfluzine
Triflurin
Tripazine

GENERAL INFORMATION

Habit forming? No
Prescription needed? Yes
Available as generic? Yes
Drug class: Tranquilizer, antiemetic (phenothiazine)

USES

- Stops nausea, vomiting.
- Reduces anxiety, agitation.

DOSAGE & USAGE INFORMATION

How to take:
- Tablet or capsule—Swallow with liquid or food to lessen stomach irritation.
- Suppositories—Remove wrapper and moisten suppository with water. Gently insert into rectum, large end first.
- Drops or liquid—Dilute dose in beverage.

When to take:
- Nervous and mental disorders—Take at the same times each day.
- Nausea and vomiting—Take as needed, no more often than every 4 hours.

If you forget a dose:
- Nervous and mental disorders—Take up to 2 hours late. If more than 2 hours, wait for next scheduled dose (don't double this).
- Nausea and vomiting—Take as soon as you remember. Wait 4 hours for next dose.

What drug does:
- Suppresses brain's vomiting center.
- Suppresses brain centers that control abnormal emotions and behavior.

Time lapse before drug works:
- Nausea and vomiting—1 hour or less.
- Nervous and mental disorders—4-6 weeks.

Don't take with:
- Antacid or medicine for diarrhea.
- Non-prescription drug for cough, cold or allergy.
- See Interaction column and consult doctor.

OVERDOSE

Symptoms:
Stupor, convulsions, coma.

What to do:
- Dial 0 (operator) or 911 (emergency) for an ambulance or medical help. Then give first aid immediately.
- Additional emergency information on page 886.

POSSIBLE ADVERSE REACTIONS OR SIDE EFFECTS

SYMPTOMS	FREQUENCY	WHAT TO DO
Brain & nervous system:		
● Restlessness, tremor.	Common	3
● Fainting	Infrequent	2
● Drowsiness	Common	3
Skin:		
● Rash	Infrequent	3
● Less perspiration.	Common	4
Eyes:		
Vision changes.	Rare	3
Ears, nose, throat:		
● Sore throat, fever.	Rare	3
● Dry mouth, nasal congestion.	Common	4
Digestive:		
Constipation	Common	4
Heart & lungs, blood vessels, kidneys, allergic, blood:	None expected.	
Muscles, bones, joints:		
Muscle spasms of face and neck, unsteady gait.	Common	2
Genital, urinary:		
Urination difficulty.	Infrequent	4
Liver:		
Jaundice (yellow eyes and skin).	Rare	3
Others:		
Less interest in sex, breast swelling, change in menstrual pattern.	Infrequent	4

1-Life-threatening. Seek emergency treatment immediately.
2-Discontinue. Seek emergency treatment.
3-Discontinue. Call doctor right away.
4-Continue. Call doctor when convenient.
5-Continue. Tell doctor at next visit.
6-No action necessary.

TRIFLUOPERAZINE

WARNINGS & PRECAUTIONS

Don't take if:
- You are allergic to any phenothiazine.
- You have a blood or bone-marrow disease.

Before you start, consult your doctor:
- If you will have surgery within 2 months, including dental surgery, requiring general or spinal anesthesia.
- If you have asthma, emphysema or other lung disorder.
- If you take non-prescription ulcer medicine, asthma medicine or amphetamines.

Over age 60:
Adverse reactions and side effects may be more frequent and severe than in younger persons. More likely to develop involuntary movement of jaws, lips, tongue, chewing. Report this to your doctor immediately. Early treatment can help.

Pregnancy:
Risk to unborn child outweighs drug benefits. Don't use.

Breast-feeding:
Drug passes into milk. Avoid drug or discontinue nursing until you finish medicine. Consult doctor for advice on maintaining milk supply.

Infants & children:
Don't give to children younger than 2.

Prolonged use:
May lead to tardive dyskinesia (involuntary movement of jaws, lips, tongue, chewing).

Skin & sunlight:
May cause rash or intensify sunburn in areas exposed to sun or sunlamp. Skin may remain sensitive for 3 months after discontinuing.

Driving, piloting or hazardous work:
Don't drive or pilot aircraft until you learn how medicine affects you. Don't work around dangerous machinery. Don't climb ladders or work in high places. Danger increases if you drink alcohol or take medicine affecting alertness and reflexes.

Airplane passengers:
No problems expected.

Discontinuing:
- Nervous and mental disorders—Don't discontinue without doctor's advice until you complete prescribed dose, even though symptoms diminish or disappear.
- Nausea and vomiting—May be unnecessary to finish medicine. Follow doctor's instructions.

INTERACTION WITH OTHER DRUGS

GENERIC NAME OR DRUG CLASS	COMBINED EFFECT
Anticholinergics	Increased anticholinergic effect.
Antidepressants (tricyclic)	Increased trifluoperazine effect.
Antihistamines	Increased antihistamine effect.
Appetite suppressants	Decreased suppressant effect.
Levodopa	Decreased levodopa effect.
Mind-altering drugs	Increased effect of mind-altering drugs.
Narcotics	Increased narcotic effect.
Phenytoin	Increased phenytoin effect.
Quinidine	Impaired heart function. Dangerous mixture.
Sedatives	Increased sedative effect.
Tranquilizers (other)	Increased tranquilizer effect.

INTERACTION WITH OTHER SUBSTANCES

INTERACTS WITH	COMBINED EFFECT
Alcohol:	Dangerous oversedation.
Beverages:	None expected.
Cocaine:	Decreased trifluoperazine effect. Avoid.
Foods:	None expected.
Marijuana:	Drowsiness. May increase antinausea effect.
Tobacco:	None expected.

TRIFLUPROMAZINE

BRAND NAMES

Psyquil
Vesprin

GENERAL INFORMATION

Habit forming? No
Prescription needed? Yes
Available as generic? Yes
Drug class: Tranquilizer, antiemetic (phenothiazine)

USES

- Stops nausea, vomiting.
- Reduces anxiety, agitation.

DOSAGE & USAGE INFORMATION

How to take:
- Tablet or capsule—Swallow with liquid or food to lessen stomach irritation.
- Suppositories—Remove wrapper and moisten suppository with water. Gently insert into rectum, large end first.
- Drops or liquid—Dilute dose in beverage.

When to take:
- Nervous and mental disorders—Take at the same times each day.
- Nausea and vomiting—Take as needed, no more often than every 4 hours.

If you forget a dose:
- Nervous and mental disorders—Take up to 2 hours late. If more than 2 hours, wait for next scheduled dose (don't double this).
- Nausea and vomiting—Take as soon as you remember. Wait 4 hours for next dose.

What drug does:
- Suppresses brain's vomiting center.
- Suppresses brain centers that control abnormal emotions and behavior.

Time lapse before drug works:
- Nausea and vomiting—1 hour or less.
- Nervous and mental disorders—4-6 weeks.

Don't take with:
- Antacid or medicine for diarrhea.
- Non-prescription drug for cough, cold or allergy.
- See Interaction column and consult doctor.

OVERDOSE

Symptoms:
Stupor, convulsions, coma.

What to do:
- Dial 0 (operator) or 911 (emergency) for an ambulance or medical help. Then give first aid immediately.
- Additional emergency information on page 886.

POSSIBLE ADVERSE REACTIONS OR SIDE EFFECTS

SYMPTOMS	FREQUENCY	WHAT TO DO
Brain & nervous system:		
● Restlessness, tremor.	Common	3
● Fainting	Infrequent	2
● Drowsiness	Common	3
Skin:		
● Rash	Infrequent	3
● Less perspiration.	Common	4
Eyes:		
Vision changes.	Rare	3
Ears, nose, throat:		
● Sore throat, fever.	Rare	3
● Dry mouth, nasal congestion.	Common	4
Digestive:		
Constipation	Common	4
Heart & lungs, blood vessels, kidneys, allergic, blood:	None expected.	
Muscles, bones, joints:		
Muscle spasms of face and neck, unsteady gait.	Common	2
Genital, urinary:		
Urination difficulty.	Infrequent	4
Liver:		
Jaundice (yellow eyes and skin).	Rare	3
Others:		
Less interest in sex, breast swelling, change in menstrual pattern.	Infrequent	4

1- Life-threatening. Seek emergency treatment immediately.
2- Discontinue. Seek emergency treatment.
3- Discontinue. Call doctor right away.
4- Continue. Call doctor when convenient.
5- Continue. Tell doctor at next visit.
6- No action necessary.

TRIFLUPROMAZINE

WARNINGS & PRECAUTIONS

Don't take if:
- You are allergic to any phenothiazine.
- You have a blood or bone-marrow disease.

Before you start, consult your doctor:
- If you will have surgery within 2 months, including dental surgery, requiring general or spinal anesthesia.
- If you have asthma, emphysema or other lung disorder.
- If you take non-prescription ulcer medicine, asthma medicine or amphetamines.

Over age 60:
Adverse reactions and side effects may be more frequent and severe than in younger persons. More likely to develop involuntary movement of jaws, lips, tongue, chewing. Report this to your doctor immediately. Early treatment can help.

Pregnancy:
Risk to unborn child outweighs drug benefits. Don't use.

Breast-feeding:
Drug passes into milk. Avoid drug or discontinue nursing until you finish medicine. Consult doctor for advice on maintaining milk supply.

Infants & children:
Don't give to children younger than 2.

Prolonged use:
May lead to tardive dyskinesia (involuntary movement of jaws, lips, tongue, chewing).

Skin & sunlight:
May cause rash or intensify sunburn in areas exposed to sun or sunlamp. Skin may remain sensitive for 3 months after discontinuing.

Driving, piloting or hazardous work:
Don't drive or pilot aircraft until you learn how medicine affects you. Don't work around dangerous machinery. Don't climb ladders or work in high places. Danger increases if you drink alcohol or take medicine affecting alertness and reflexes.

Airplane passengers:
No problems expected.

Discontinuing:
- Nervous and mental disorders—Don't discontinue without doctor's advice until you complete prescribed dose, even though symptoms diminish or disappear.
- Nausea and vomiting—May be unnecessary to finish medicine. Follow doctor's instructions.

INTERACTION WITH OTHER DRUGS

GENERIC NAME OR DRUG CLASS	COMBINED EFFECT
Anticholinergics	Increased anticholinergic effect.
Antidepressants (tricyclic)	Increased triflupromazine effect.
Antihistamines	Increased antihistamine effect.
Appetite suppressants	Decreased suppressant effect.
Levodopa	Decreased levodopa effect.
Mind-altering drugs	Increased effect of mind-altering drugs.
Narcotics	Increased narcotic effect.
Phenytoin	Increased phenytoin effect.
Quinidine	Impaired heart function. Dangerous mixture.
Sedatives	Increased sedative effect.
Tranquilizers (other)	Increased tranquilizer effect.

INTERACTION WITH OTHER SUBSTANCES

INTERACTS WITH	COMBINED EFFECT
Alcohol:	Dangerous oversedation.
Beverages:	None expected.
Cocaine:	Decreased triflupromazine effect. Avoid.
Foods:	None expected.
Marijuana:	Drowsiness. May increase antinausea effect.
Tobacco:	None expected.

TRIHEXYPHENIDYL

BRAND NAMES

Aparkane
Artane
Tremin

GENERAL INFORMATION

Habit forming? No
Prescription needed? Yes
Available as generic? No
Drug class: Antidyskinetic, antiparkinsonism

USES

- Treatment of Parkinson's disease.
- Treatment of adverse effects of phenothiazines.

DOSAGE & USAGE INFORMATION

How to take:
Tablets or capsules—Take with food to lessen stomach irritation.

When to take:
At the same times each day.

If you forget a dose:
Take as soon as you remember up to 2 hours late. If more than 2 hours, wait for next scheduled dose (don't double this dose).

What drug does:
- Balances chemical reactions necessary to send nerve impulses within base of brain.
- Improves muscle control and reduces stiffness.

Time lapse before drug works:
1 to 2 hours.

Don't take with:
- Non-prescription drugs for colds, cough or allergy.
- See Interaction column and consult doctor.

OVERDOSE

Symptoms:
Agitation, dilated pupils, hallucinations, dry mouth, rapid heartbeat, sleepiness.

What to do:
- Dial 0 (operator) or 911 (emergency) for an ambulance or medical help. Then give first aid immediately.
- If patient is unconscious and not breathing, give mouth-to-mouth breathing. If there is no heartbeat, use cardiac massage and mouth-to-mouth breathing (CPR). Don't try to make patient vomit. If you can't get help quickly, take patient to nearest emergency facility.
- Additional emergency information on page 886.

POSSIBLE ADVERSE REACTIONS OR SIDE EFFECTS

SYMPTOMS	FREQUENCY	WHAT TO DO
Brain & nervous system:		
Confusion, dizziness.	Rare	4
Skin:		
Rash	Rare	3
Eyes:		
• Pain	Rare	3
• Blurred vision, light sensitivity.	Common	4
Ears, nose, throat:		
Sore mouth or tongue.	Rare	4
Digestive:		
• Constipation	Common	4
• Nausea, vomiting.	Common	4
Heart & lungs:	None expected.	
Blood vessels:	None expected.	
Muscles, bones, joints:		
• Muscle cramps.	Rare	4
• Numbness, weakness in hands or feet.	Rare	4
Genital, urinary:		
Difficult or painful urination.	Common	5
Kidneys:	None expected.	
Liver:	None expected.	
Allergic:	None expected.	
Blood:	None expected.	
Others:	None expected.	

1- Life-threatening. Seek emergency treatment immediately.
2- Discontinue. Seek emergency treatment.
3- Discontinue. Call doctor right away.
4- Continue. Call doctor when convenient.
5- Continue. Tell doctor at next visit.
6- No action necessary.

TRIHEXYPHENIDYL

WARNINGS & PRECAUTIONS

Don't take if:
You are allergic to any antidyskinetic.

Before you start, consult your doctor:
- If you have had glaucoma.
- If you have had high blood pressure or heart disease.
- If you have had impaired liver function.
- If you have had kidney disease or urination difficulty.

Over age 60:
More sensitive to drug. Aggravates symptoms of enlarged prostate. Causes impaired thinking, hallucinations, nightmares. Consult doctor about any of these.

Pregnancy:
Studies inconclusive on harm to unborn child. Animal studies show fetal abnormalities. Decide with your doctor whether drug benefits justify risk to unborn child.

Breast-feeding:
No problems expected.

Infants & children:
Not recommended for children 3 and younger. Use for older children only under doctor's supervision.

Prolonged use:
Possible glaucoma.

Skin & sunlight:
No problems expected.

Driving, piloting or hazardous work:
Don't drive or pilot aircraft until you learn how medicine affects you. Don't work around dangerous machinery. Don't climb ladders or work in high places. Danger increases if you drink alcohol or take medicine affecting alertness and reflexes, such as antihistamines, tranquilizers, sedatives, pain medicine, narcotics and mind-altering drugs.

Airplane passengers:
No problems expected.

Discontinuing:
Don't discontinue without consulting doctor. Dose may require gradual reduction if you have taken drug for a long time. Doses of other drugs may also require adjustment.

Others:
- Internal eye pressure should be measured regularly.
- Avoid becoming overheated.

INTERACTION WITH OTHER DRUGS

GENERIC NAME OR DRUG CLASS	COMBINED EFFECT
Amantadine	Increased amantadine effect.
Antidepressants (tricyclic)	Increased trihexyphenidyl effect. May cause glaucoma.
Antihistamines	Increased trihexyphenidyl effect.
Levodopa	Increased levodopa effect. Improved results in treating Parkinson's disease.
Meperidine	Increased trihexyphenidyl effect.
MAO inhibitors	Increased trihexyphenidyl effect.
Orphenadrine	Increased trihexyphenidyl effect.
Phenothiazines	Behavior changes.
Primidone	Excessive sedation.
Procainamide	Increased procainamide effect.
Quinidine	Increased trihexyphenidyl effect.
Tranquilizers	Excessive sedation.

INTERACTION WITH OTHER SUBSTANCES

INTERACTS WITH	COMBINED EFFECT
Alcohol:	None expected.
Beverages:	None expected.
Cocaine:	Decreased trihexyphenidyl effect. Avoid.
Foods:	None expected.
Marijuana:	None expected.
Tobacco:	None expected.

TRIMEPRAZINE

BRAND NAMES

Panectyl
Temaril

GENERAL INFORMATION

Habit forming? No
Prescription needed? Yes
Available as generic? Yes
Drug class: Tranquilizer (phenothiazine), antihistamine

USES

Relieves itching of hives, skin allergies, chickenpox.

DOSAGE & USAGE INFORMATION

How to take:
- Tablet or syrup—Swallow with liquid or food to lessen stomach irritation.
- Extended-release capsules—Swallow each dose whole. If you take regular tablets, you may chew or crush them.

When to take:
At the same times each day.

If you forget a dose:
Take as soon as you remember up to 2 hours late. If more than 2 hours, wait for next scheduled dose (don't double this dose).

What drug does:
Blocks histamine action in skin.

Time lapse before drug works:
1 to 2 hours.

Don't take with:
- Antacid or medicine for diarrhea.
- Non-prescription drug for cough, cold or allergy.
- See Interaction column and consult doctor.

OVERDOSE

Symptoms:
Stupor, convulsions, coma.

What to do:
- Dial 0 (operator) or 911 (emergency) for an ambulance or medical help. Then give first aid immediately.
- Additional emergency information on page 886.

POSSIBLE ADVERSE REACTIONS OR SIDE EFFECTS

SYMPTOMS	FREQUENCY	WHAT TO DO
Brain & nervous system:		
• Restlessness, tremor, drowsiness.	Common	3
• Fainting	Infrequent	2
Skin:		
• Rash	Infrequent	3
• Less perspiration.	Common	4
Eyes:		
Vision changes.	Rare	3
Ears, nose, throat:		
• Sore throat, fever.	Rare	3
• Dry mouth, nasal congestion.	Common	4
Digestive:		
Constipation	Common	4
Heart & lungs:	None expected.	
Blood vessels:	None expected.	
Muscles, bones, joints:		
Muscle spasms of face and neck, unsteady gait.	Infrequent	3
Genital, urinary:		
Urination difficulty.	Infrequent	4
Kidneys:	None expected.	
Liver:		
Jaundice (yellow skin and eyes).	Rare	3
Allergic:	None expected.	
Blood:	None expected.	
Others:		
Less interest in sex, breast swelling, menstrual changes.	Infrequent	4

1- Life-threatening. Seek emergency treatment immediately.
2- Discontinue. Seek emergency treatment.
3- Discontinue. Call doctor right away.
4- Continue. Call doctor when convenient.

WARNINGS & PRECAUTIONS

Don't take if:
- You are allergic to any phenothiazine.
- You have a blood or bone-marrow disease.

Before you start, consult your doctor:
- If you will have surgery within 2 months, including dental surgery, requiring general or spinal anesthesia.
- If you have asthma, emphysema or other lung disorder.
- If you take non-prescription ulcer medicine, asthma medicine or amphetamines.

Over age 60:
Adverse reactions and side effects may be more frequent and severe than in younger persons. More likely to develop tardive dyskinesia (involuntary movement of jaws, lips, tongue, chewing). Report this to your doctor immediately. Early treatment can help.

Pregnancy:
Risk to unborn child outweighs drug benefits. Don't use.

Breast-feeding:
Drug passes into milk. Avoid drug or discontinue nursing until you finish medicine. Consult doctor for advice on maintaining milk supply.

Infants & children:
Don't give to children younger than 2.

Prolonged use:
May lead to tardive dyskinesia (involuntary movement of jaws, lips, tongue, chewing).

Skin & sunlight:
May cause rash or intensify sunburn in areas exposed to sun or sunlamp. Skin may remain sensitive for 3 months after discontinuing.

Driving, piloting or hazardous work:
Don't drive or pilot aircraft until you learn how medicine affects you. Don't work around dangerous machinery. Don't climb ladders or work in high places. Danger increases if you drink alcohol or take medicine affecting alertness and reflexes.

Airplane passengers:
No problems expected.

Discontinuing:
May be unnecessary to finish medicine. Follow doctor's instructions.

INTERACTION WITH OTHER DRUGS

GENERIC NAME OR DRUG CLASS	COMBINED EFFECT
Antacids	Decreased trimeprazine effect.
Anticholinergics	Increased anticholinergic effect.
Anticonvulsants (hydantoin)	Increased anticonvulsant effect.
Antidepressants (tricyclic)	Increased trimeprazine effect.
Antihistamines (other)	Increased antihistamine effect.
Appetite suppressants	Decreased suppressant effect.
Barbiturates	Oversedation.
Guanethidine	Decreased guanethidine effect.
Levodopa	Decreased levodopa effect.
MAO inhibitors	Increased trimeprazine effect.
Mind-altering drugs	Increased effect of mind-altering drugs.
Narcotics	Increased narcotic effect.
Sedatives	Increased sedative effect.
Tranquilizers	Increased tranquilizer effect. Avoid.

INTERACTION WITH OTHER SUBSTANCES

INTERACTS WITH	COMBINED EFFECT
Alcohol:	Dangerous oversedation.
Beverages:	None expected.
Cocaine:	Decreased effect of trimeprazine. Avoid.
Foods:	None expected.
Marijuana:	Drowsiness.
Tobacco:	None expected.

TRIMETHOBENZAMIDE

BRAND NAMES

Tigan
Tegamide

GENERAL INFORMATION

Habit forming? No
Prescription needed? Yes
Available as generic? Yes
Drug class: Antiemetic

USES

Reduces nausea and vomiting.

DOSAGE & USAGE INFORMATION

How to take:
- Capsule—Swallow with liquid. If you can't swallow whole, open capsule and take with liquid or food.
- Suppositories—Remove wrapper and moisten suppository with water. Gently insert larger end into rectum. Push well into rectum with finger.

When to take:
When needed, no more often than label directs.

If you forget a dose:
Take when you remember. Wait as long as label directs for next dose.

What drug does:
Possibly blocks nerve impulses to brain's vomiting centers.

Time lapse before drug works:
20 to 40 minutes.

Don't take with:
Non-prescription drugs or drugs in Interaction column without consulting doctor.

OVERDOSE

Symptoms:
Confusion, convulsions, coma.

What to do:
- Dial 0 (operator) or 911 (emergency) for an ambulance or medical help. Then give first aid immediately.
- If patient is unconscious and not breathing, give mouth-to-mouth breathing. If there is no heartbeat, use cardiac massage and mouth-to-mouth breathing (CPR). Don't try to make patient vomit. If you can't get help quickly, take patient to nearest emergency facility.
- Additional emergency information on page 886.

POSSIBLE ADVERSE REACTIONS OR SIDE EFFECTS

SYMPTOMS	FREQUENCY	WHAT TO DO
Brain & nervous system:		
• Dizziness, drowsiness, headache.	Infrequent	4
• Seizures, tremors, depression.	Rare	3
Skin:		
Rash	Infrequent	3
Eyes:		
Blurred vision.	Infrequent	3
Ears, nose, throat:		
Sore throat, fever.	Rare	3
Digestive:		
• Diarrhea	Infrequent	4
• Repeated vomiting.	Rare	3
Heart & lungs:	None expected.	
Blood vessels:		
Low blood pressure.	Infrequent	3
Muscles, bones, joints:		
• Muscle cramps.	Infrequent	4
• Back pain.	Rare	3
Genital, urinary:	None expected.	
Kidneys:	None expected.	
Liver:		
Jaundice (yellow skin and eyes).	Rare	3
Allergic:	None expected.	
Blood:	None expected.	
Others:		
Unusual tiredness.	Infrequent	4

1- Life-threatening. Seek emergency treatment immediately.
2- Discontinue. Seek emergency treatment.
3- Discontinue. Call doctor right away.
4- Continue. Call doctor when convenient.
5- Continue. Tell doctor at next visit.
6- No action necessary.

WARNINGS & PRECAUTIONS

Don't take if:
- You are allergic to trimethobenzamide.
- You are allergic to local anesthetics and have suppository form.

Before you start, consult your doctor:
If you have reacted badly to antihistamines.

Over age 60:
More susceptible to low blood pressure and sedative effects of this drug.

Pregnancy:
No proven harm to unborn child. Avoid if possible.

Breast-feeding:
No proven problems. Avoid if possible.

Infants & children:
- Injectable form not recommended.
- Avoid during viral infections. Drug may contribute to Reyes' syndrome.

Prolonged use:
- Damages blood-cell production of bone marrow.
- Causes Parkinson-like symptoms of tremors, rigidity.

Skin & sunlight:
Possible sun sensitivity. Use caution.

Driving, piloting or hazardous work:
- Use disqualifies you for piloting aircraft.
- Don't drive until you learn how medicine affects you. Don't work around dangerous machinery. Don't climb ladders or work in high places. Danger increases if you drink alcohol or take medicine affecting alertness and reflexes, such as antihistamines, tranquilizers, sedatives, pain medicine, narcotics and mind-altering drugs.

Airplane passengers:
No problems expected.

Discontinuing:
May be unnecessary to finish medicine. Follow doctor's instructions.

Others:
No problems expected.

INTERACTION WITH OTHER DRUGS

GENERIC NAME OR DRUG CLASS	COMBINED EFFECT
Antidepressants	Increased sedative effect.
Antihistamines	Increased sedative effect.
Barbiturates	Increased effect of both drugs.
Belladonna	Increased effect of both drugs.
Cholinergics	Increased effect of both drugs.
Mind-altering drugs	Increased effect of mind-altering drug.
Narcotics	Increased sedative effect.
Phenothiazines	Increased effect of both drugs.
Sedatives	Increased sedative effect.
Sleep inducers	Increased effect of sleep inducer.
Tranquilizers	Increased sedative effect.

INTERACTION WITH OTHER SUBSTANCES

INTERACTS WITH	COMBINED EFFECT
Alcohol:	Oversedation. Avoid.
Beverages:	None expected.
Cocaine:	None expected.
Foods:	None expected.
Marijuana:	Increased antinausea effect.
Tobacco:	None expected.

TRIMETHOPRIM

BRAND NAMES

Bactrim (M)
Proloprim
SMZ-TMP (M)
Septra (M)
Syraprim
Trimpex

GENERAL INFORMATION

Habit forming? No
Prescription needed? Yes
Available as generic? No
Drug class: Antimicrobial

 ## USES

- Treatment for urinary-tract infections susceptible to trimethoprim.
- Helps prevent recurrent urinary-tract infections if taken once a day.

 ## DOSAGE & USAGE INFORMATION

How to take:
- Tablet or capsule—Swallow with liquid or food to lessen stomach irritation.
- Drops—Dilute dose in beverage before swallowing.

When to take:
Space doses evenly in 24 hours to keep constant amount in urine.

If you forget a dose:
Take as soon as possible. Wait 5 to 6 hours before next dose. Then return to regular schedule.

What drug does:
Stops harmful bacterial germs from multiplying. Will not kill viruses.

Time lapse before drug works:
2 to 5 days.

Don't take with:
See Interaction column and consult doctor.

 ## OVERDOSE

Symptoms:
Nausea, vomiting, diarrhea.

What to do:
Overdose unlikely to threaten life. If person takes much larger amount than prescribed, call doctor, poison-control center or hospital emergency room for instructions.

 ## POSSIBLE ADVERSE REACTIONS OR SIDE EFFECTS

SYMPTOMS	FREQUENCY	WHAT TO DO
Brain & nervous system:		
Headache	Infrequent	4
Skin:		
• Blue fingernails, lips, skin.	Rare	2
• Rash, itch.	Common	3
Eyes:	None expected.	
Ears, nose, throat:		
Sore throat, fever.	Rare	3
Digestive:		
Diarrhea, nausea, vomiting, abdominal pain.	Infrequent	3
Heart & lungs:		
Breathing difficulty.	Rare	2
Blood vessels:	None expected.	
Muscles, bones, joints:	None expected.	
Genital, urinary:	None expected.	
Kidneys:	None expected.	
Liver:	None expected.	
Allergic:	None expected.	
Blood:	None expected.	
Others:	None expected.	

1- Life-threatening. Seek emergency treatment immediately.
2- Discontinue. Seek emergency treatment.
3- Discontinue. Call doctor right away.
4- Continue. Call doctor when convenient.
5- Continue. Tell doctor at next visit.
6- No action necessary.

WARNINGS & PRECAUTIONS

Don't take if:
You are allergic to trimethoprim or any sulfa drug.

Before you start, consult your doctor:
If you have had liver or kidney disease.

Over age 60:
- Reduced liver and kidney function may require reduced dose.
- More likely to have severe anal and genital itch.
- Increased susceptibility to anemia.

Pregnancy:
Studies inconclusive on harm to unborn child. Animal studies show fetal abnormalities. Decide with your doctor whether drug benefits justify risk to unborn child.

Breast-feeding:
No proven harm to unborn child. Avoid if possible.

Infants & children:
Use under medical supervision only.

Prolonged use:
Anemia

Skin & sunlight:
May cause rash or intensify sunburn in areas exposed to sun or sunlamp.

Driving, piloting or hazardous work:
No problems expected.

Airplane passengers:
No problems expected.

Discontinuing:
Don't discontinue without doctor's advice until you complete prescribed dose, even though symptoms diminish or disappear.

Others:
No problems expected.

INTERACTION WITH OTHER DRUGS

GENERIC NAME OR DRUG CLASS	COMBINED EFFECT
Diuretics (thiazide)	Unusual bleeding or bruising.
Sulfamethoxazole	Beneficial increase of sulfamethoxazole effect.

INTERACTION WITH OTHER SUBSTANCES

INTERACTS WITH	COMBINED EFFECT
Alcohol:	Increased alcohol effect with Bactrim or Septra.
Beverages:	None expected.
Cocaine:	No proven problems.
Foods:	None expected.
Marijuana:	None expected.
Tobacco:	None expected.

TRIMIPRAMINE

BRAND NAMES

Surmontil

GENERAL INFORMATION

Habit forming? No
Prescription needed? Yes
Available as generic? No
Drug class: Antidepressant (tricyclic)

 USES

Gradually relieves, but doesn't cure, symptoms of depression.

 DOSAGE & USAGE INFORMATION

How to take:
Capsule—Swallow with liquid.

When to take:
At the same time each day, usually bedtime.

If you forget a dose:
Bedtime dose—If you forget your once-a-day bedtime dose, don't take it more than 3 hours late. If more than 3 hours, wait for next scheduled dose. Don't double this dose.

What drug does:
Probably affects part of brain that controls messages between nerve cells.

Time lapse before drug works:
Begins in 1 to 2 weeks. May require 4 to 6 weeks for maximum benefit.

Don't take with:
- Non-prescription drugs without consulting doctor.
- See Interaction column and consult doctor.

 OVERDOSE

Symptoms:
Hallucinations, convulsions, coma.

What to do:
- Dial 0 (operator) or 911 (emergency) for an ambulance or medical help. Then give first aid immediately.
- If patient is unconscious and not breathing, give mouth-to-mouth breathing. If there is no heartbeat, use cardiac massage and mouth-to-mouth breathing (CPR). Don't try to make patient vomit. If you can't get help quickly, take patient to nearest emergency facility.
- Additional emergency information on page 886.

POSSIBLE ADVERSE REACTIONS OR SIDE EFFECTS

SYMPTOMS	FREQUENCY	WHAT TO DO
Brain & nervous system:		
• Hallucinations, shakiness, dizziness, fainting.	Infrequent	3
• Headache	Common	4
• Seizures	Rare	1
• Insomnia	Common	5
Skin:		
Rash, itch.	Rare	3
Eyes:		
Blurred vision, pain.	Infrequent	3
Ears, nose, throat:		
• Sore throat.	Rare	3
• Dry mouth or unpleasant taste.	Common	4
Digestive:		
• Constipation or diarrhea, nausea, indigestion.	Common	4
• Vomiting	Infrequent	3
• "Sweet tooth"	Common	5
Heart & lungs:		
Irregular heartbeat or slow pulse.	Infrequent	3
Blood vessels, muscles, bones, joints, kidneys, allergic, blood:	None expected.	
Genital, urinary:		
Difficulty urinating.	Infrequent	4
Liver:		
Jaundice (yellow skin and eyes).	Rare	3
Others:		
• Fever	Rare	3
• Fatigue, weakness.	Common	4

1 - Life-threatening. Seek emergency treatment immediately.
2 - Discontinue. Seek emergency treatment.
3 - Discontinue. Call doctor right away.
4 - Continue. Call doctor when convenient.
5 - Continue. Tell doctor at next visit.

TRIMIPRAMINE

WARNINGS & PRECAUTIONS

Don't take if:
- You are allergic to any tricyclic antidepressant.
- You drink alcohol.
- You have had a heart attack within 6 weeks.
- You have glaucoma.
- You have taken MAO inhibitors within 2 weeks.
- Patient is younger than 12.

Before you start, consult your doctor:
- If you will have surgery within 2 months, including dental surgery, requiring general or spinal anesthesia.
- If you have an enlarged prostate.
- If you have heart disease or high blood pressure.
- If you have stomach or intestinal problems.
- If you have an overactive thyroid.
- If you have asthma.
- If you have liver disease.

Over age 60:
More likely to develop urination difficulty and side effects under *Brain & nervous system*, opposite.

Pregnancy:
Studies inconclusive on harm to unborn child. Animal studies show fetal abnormalities. Decide with your doctor whether drug benefits justify risk to unborn child.

Breast-feeding:
Drug passes into milk. Avoid drug or discontinue nursing until you finish medicine. Consult doctor on maintaining milk supply.

Infants & children:
Don't give to children younger than 12.

Prolonged use:
No problems expected.

Skin & sunlight:
May cause rash or intensify sunburn in areas exposed to sun or sunlamp.

Driving, piloting or hazardous work:
Don't drive or pilot aircraft until you learn how medicine affects you. Don't work around dangerous machinery. Don't climb ladders or work in high places. Danger increases if you drink alcohol or take medicine affecting alertness and reflexes.

Airplane passengers:
No problems expected.

Discontinuing:
Don't discontinue without consulting doctor. Dose may require gradual reduction if you have taken drug for a long time. Doses of other drugs may also require adjustment.

INTERACTION WITH OTHER DRUGS

GENERIC NAME OR DRUG CLASS	COMBINED EFFECT
Anticoagulants (oral)	Increased anticoagulant effect.
Anticholinergics	Increased sedation.
Antihistamines	Increased antihistamine effect.
Barbiturates	Decreased antidepressant effect.
Clonidine	Decreased clonidine effect.
Diuretics (thiazide)	Increased trimipramine effect.
Ethchlorvynol	Delirium
Guanethidine	Decreased guanethidine effect.
MAO inhibitors	Fever, delirium, convulsions.
Methyldopa	Decreased methyldopa effect.
Narcotics	Dangerous oversedation.
Phenytoin	Decreased phenytoin effect.
Quinidine	Irregular heartbeat.
Sedatives	Dangerous oversedation.
Sympathomimetics	Increased sympathomimetic effect.
Thyroid hormones	Irregular heartbeat.

INTERACTION WITH OTHER SUBSTANCES

INTERACTS WITH	COMBINED EFFECT
Alcohol: Beverages or medicines with alcohol.	Excessive intoxication. Avoid.
Beverages:	None expected.
Cocaine:	Excessive intoxication. Avoid.
Foods:	None expected.
Marijuana:	Excessive drowsiness. Avoid.
Tobacco:	None expected.

TRIPELENNAMINE

BRAND NAMES

PBZ
PBZ-Lontabs
PBZ-SR
Pyribenzamine
Ro-Hist

GENERAL INFORMATION

Habit forming? No
Prescription needed? High strength: Yes
Low strength: No
Available as generic? Yes
Drug class: Antihistamine

USES

- Reduces allergic symptoms such as hay fever, hives, rash or itching.
- Induces sleep.

DOSAGE & USAGE INFORMATION

How to take:
- Tablet or liquid—Swallow with liquid or food to lessen stomach irritation.
- Extended-release tablets—Swallow each dose whole.

When to take:
Varies with form. Follow label directions.

If you forget a dose:
Take as soon as you remember up to 2 hours late. If more than 2 hours, wait for next scheduled dose (don't double this dose).

What drug does:
Blocks action of histamine after an allergic response triggers histamine release in sensitive cells.

Time lapse before drug works:
30 minutes.

Don't take with:
See Interaction column and consult doctor.

OVERDOSE

Symptoms:
Convulsions, red face, hallucinations, coma.

What to do:
- Dial 0 (operator) or 911 (emergency) for an ambulance or medical help. Then give first aid immediately.
- If patient is unconscious and not breathing, give mouth-to-mouth breathing. If there is no heartbeat, use cardiac massage and mouth-to-mouth breathing (CPR). Don't try to make patient vomit. If you can't get help quickly, take patient to nearest emergency facility.
- Additional emergency information on page 886.

POSSIBLE ADVERSE REACTIONS OR SIDE EFFECTS

SYMPTOMS	FREQUENCY	WHAT TO DO
Brain & nervous system:		
● Nightmares, agitation, irritability.	Rare	3
● Drowsiness, dizziness.	Common	5
Skin:	None expected.	
Eyes:		
● Vision changes.	Infrequent	3
● Less tolerance for contact lenses.	Infrequent	4
Ears, nose, throat:		
● Sore throat, fever.	Rare	3
● Dry mouth, nose, throat.	Common	5
Digestive:		
● Nausea	Common	5
● Appetite loss.	Infrequent	5
Heart & lungs:		
Rapid heartbeat.	Rare	3
Blood vessels:		
Unusual bleeding or bruising.	Rare	3
Muscles, bones, joints, kidneys, liver, allergic, blood:	None expected.	
Genital, urinary:		
Urination difficulty.	Infrequent	4
Others:		
Fatigue, weakness.	Rare	3

1- Life-threatening. Seek emergency treatment immediately.
2- Discontinue. Seek emergency treatment.
3- Discontinue. Call doctor right away.
4- Continue. Call doctor when convenient.
5- Continue. Tell doctor at next visit.
6- No action necessary.

WARNINGS & PRECAUTIONS

Don't take if:
You are allergic to any antihistamine.

Before you start, consult your doctor:
- If you have glaucoma.
- If you have enlarged prostate.
- If you have asthma.
- If you have kidney disease.
- If you have peptic ulcer.
- If you will have surgery within 2 months, including dental surgery, requiring general or spinal anesthesia.

Over age 60:
Don't exceed recommended dose. Adverse reactions and side effects may be more frequent and severe than in younger persons, especially urination difficulty, diminished alertness and other brain and nervous-system symptoms.

Pregnancy:
No proven harm to unborn child. Avoid if possible.

Breast-feeding:
Drug passes into milk. Avoid drug or discontinue nursing until you finish medicine. Consult doctor for advice on maintaining milk supply.

Infants & children:
Not recommended for premature or newborn infants. Otherwise, no problems expected.

Prolonged use:
Avoid. May damage bone marrow and nerve cells.

Skin & sunlight:
May cause rash or intensify sunburn in areas exposed to sun or sunlamp.

Driving, piloting or hazardous work:
Don't drive or pilot aircraft until you learn how medicine affects you. Don't work around dangerous machinery. Don't climb ladders or work in high places. Danger increases if you drink alcohol or take medicine affecting alertness and reflexes, such as antihistamines, tranquilizers, sedatives, pain medicine, narcotics and mind-altering drugs.

Airplane passengers:
No problems expected.

Discontinuing:
No problems expected.

Others:
May mask symptoms of hearing damage from aspirin, other salicylates, cisplatin, paromomycin, vancomycin or anticonvulsants. Consult doctor if you use these.

INTERACTION WITH OTHER DRUGS

GENERIC NAME OR DRUG CLASS	COMBINED EFFECT
Anticholinergics	Increased anticholinergic effect.
Antidepressants	Excess sedation. Avoid.
Antihistamines (other)	Excess sedation. Avoid.
Hypnotics	Excess sedation. Avoid.
MAO inhibitors	Increased tripelennamine effect.
Mind-altering drugs	Excess sedation. Avoid.
Narcotics	Excess sedation. Avoid.
Sedatives	Excess sedation. Avoid.
Sleep inducers	Excess sedation. Avoid.
Tranquilizers	Excess sedation. Avoid.

INTERACTION WITH OTHER SUBSTANCES

INTERACTS WITH	COMBINED EFFECT
Alcohol:	Excess sedation. Avoid.
Beverages: Caffeine drinks	Less tripelennamine sedation.
Cocaine:	Decreased tripelennamine effect. Avoid.
Foods:	None expected.
Marijuana:	Excess sedation. Avoid.
Tobacco:	None expected.

TRIPROLIDINE

BRAND NAMES

Actidil
Actifed (M)
Eldafed (M)

GENERAL INFORMATION

Habit forming? No
Prescription needed? Yes
Available as generic? Yes
Drug class: Antihistamine

 ## USES

- Reduces allergic symptoms such as hay fever, hives, rash or itching.
- Induces sleep.

 ## DOSAGE & USAGE INFORMATION

How to take:
Tablet or syrup—Swallow with liquid or food to lessen stomach irritation.

When to take:
Varies with form. Follow label directions.

If you forget a dose:
Take as soon as you remember up to 2 hours late. If more than 2 hours, wait for next scheduled dose (don't double this dose).

What drug does:
Blocks action of histamine after an allergic response triggers histamine release in sensitive cells.

Time lapse before drug works:
30 minutes.

Don't take with:
See Interaction column and consult doctor.

 ## OVERDOSE

Symptoms:
Convulsions, red face, hallucinations, coma.

What to do:
- Dial 0 (operator) or 911 (emergency) for an ambulance or medical help. Then give first aid immediately.
- If patient is unconscious and not breathing, give mouth-to-mouth breathing. If there is no heartbeat, use cardiac massage and mouth-to-mouth breathing (CPR). Don't try to make patient vomit. If you can't get help quickly, take patient to nearest emergency facility.
- Additional emergency information on page 886.

POSSIBLE ADVERSE REACTIONS OR SIDE EFFECTS

SYMPTOMS	FREQUENCY	WHAT TO DO
Brain & nervous system:		
• Nightmares, agitation, irritability.	Rare	3
• Drowsiness, dizziness.	Common	5
Skin:	None expected.	
Eyes:		
• Vision changes.	Infrequent	3
• Less tolerance for contact lenses.	Infrequent	4
Ears, nose, throat:		
• Sore throat, fever.	Rare	3
• Dry mouth, nose, throat.	Common	5
Digestive:		
• Nausea	Common	5
• Appetite loss.	Infrequent	5
Heart & lungs:		
Rapid heartbeat.	Rare	3
Blood vessels:		
Unusual bleeding or bruising.	Rare	3
Muscles, bones, joints, kidneys, liver, allergic, blood:	None expected.	
Genital, urinary:		
Urination difficulty.	Infrequent	4
Others:		
Fatigue, weakness.	Rare	3

1- Life-threatening. Seek emergency treatment immediately.
2- Discontinue. Seek emergency treatment.
3- Discontinue. Call doctor right away.
4- Continue. Call doctor when convenient.
5- Continue. Tell doctor at next visit.
6- No action necessary.

WARNINGS & PRECAUTIONS

Don't take if:
You are allergic to any antihistamine.

Before you start, consult your doctor:
- If you have glaucoma.
- If you have enlarged prostate.
- If you have asthma.
- If you have kidney disease.
- If you have peptic ulcer.
- If you will have surgery within 2 months, including dental surgery, requiring general or spinal anesthesia.

Over age 60:
Don't exceed recommended dose. Adverse reactions and side effects may be more frequent and severe than in younger persons, especially urination difficulty, diminished alertness and other brain and nervous-system symptoms.

Pregnancy:
No proven harm to unborn child. Avoid if possible.

Breast-feeding:
Drug passes into milk. Avoid drug or discontinue nursing until you finish medicine. Consult doctor for advice on maintaining milk supply.

Infants & children:
Not recommended for premature or newborn infants. Otherwise, no problems expected.

Prolonged use:
Avoid. May damage bone marrow and nerve cells.

Skin & sunlight:
May cause rash or intensify sunburn in areas exposed to sun or sunlamp.

Driving, piloting or hazardous work:
Don't drive or pilot aircraft until you learn how medicine affects you. Don't work around dangerous machinery. Don't climb ladders or work in high places. Danger increases if you drink alcohol or take medicine affecting alertness and reflexes, such as antihistamines, tranquilizers, sedatives, pain medicine, narcotics and mind-altering drugs.

Airplane passengers:
No problems expected.

Discontinuing:
No problems expected.

Others:
May mask symptoms of hearing damage from aspirin, other salicylates, cisplatin, paromomycin, vancomycin or anticonvulsants. Consult doctor if you use these.

INTERACTION WITH OTHER DRUGS

GENERIC NAME OR DRUG CLASS	COMBINED EFFECT
Anticholinergics	Increased anticholinergic effect.
Antidepressants	Excess sedation. Avoid.
Antihistamines (other)	Excess sedation. Avoid.
Hypnotics	Excess sedation. Avoid.
MAO inhibitors	Increased triprolidine effect.
Mind-altering drugs	Excess sedation. Avoid.
Narcotics	Excess sedation. Avoid.
Sedatives	Excess sedation. Avoid.
Sleep inducers	Excess sedation. Avoid.
Tranquilizers	Excess sedation. Avoid.

INTERACTION WITH OTHER SUBSTANCES

INTERACTS WITH	COMBINED EFFECT
Alcohol:	Excess sedation. Avoid.
Beverages: Caffeine drinks	Less triprolidine sedation.
Cocaine:	Decreased triprolidine effect. Avoid.
Foods:	None expected.
Marijuana:	Excess sedation. Avoid.
Tobacco:	None expected.

VERAPAMIL

BRAND NAMES

Calan
Isoptin

GENERAL INFORMATION

Habit forming? No
Prescription needed? Yes
Available as generic? No
Drug class: Calcium-channel blocker, antiarrhythmic,
antianginal

USES

- Prevents angina attacks.
- Stabilizes irregular heartbeat.

DOSAGE & USAGE INFORMATION

How to take:
Tablet—Swallow with liquid.

When to take:
At the same times each day 1 hour before or 2 hours after eating.

If you forget a dose:
Take as soon as you remember up to 2 hours late. If more than 2 hours, wait for next scheduled dose (don't double this dose).

What drug does:
- Reduces work that heart must perform.
- Reduces normal artery pressure.
- Increases oxygen to heart muscle.

Time lapse before drug works:
1 to 2 hours.

Don't take with:
See Interaction column and consult doctor.

OVERDOSE

Symptoms:
Unusually fast or unusually slow heartbeat, loss of consciousness, cardiac arrest.

What to do:
- Dial 0 (operator) or 911 (emergency) for an ambulance or medical help. Then give first aid immediately.
- If patient is unconscious and not breathing, give mouth-to-mouth breathing. If there is no heartbeat, use cardiac massage and mouth-to-mouth breathing (CPR). Don't try to make patient vomit. If you can't get help quickly, take patient to nearest emergency facility.
- Additional emergency information on page 886.

POSSIBLE ADVERSE REACTIONS OR SIDE EFFECTS

SYMPTOMS	FREQUENCY	WHAT TO DO
Brain & nervous system:		
● Dizziness	Infrequent	4
● Headache	Rare	5
● Fainting	Rare	3
Skin:	None expected.	
Eyes:	None expected.	
Ears, nose, throat:	None expected.	
Digestive: Nausea, constipation.	Infrequent	5
Heart & lungs:		
● Unusually fast or unusually slow heartbeat.	Infrequent	3
● Wheezing, cough, shortness of breath.	Infrequent	3
Blood vessels:	None expected.	
Muscles, bones, joints:		
● Numbness, tingling in hands and feet.	Infrequent	4
● Swelling of ankles, feet, legs.	Infrequent	4
Genital, urinary: Difficult urination.	Infrequent	4
Kidneys:	None expected.	
Liver:	None expected.	
Allergic:	None expected.	
Blood:	None expected.	
Others: Tiredness	Common	5

1- Life-threatening. Seek emergency treatment immediately.
2- Discontinue. Seek emergency treatment.
3- Discontinue. Call doctor right away.
4- Continue. Call doctor when convenient.
5- Continue. Tell doctor at next visit.
6- No action necessary.

WARNINGS & PRECAUTIONS

Don't take if:
- You are allergic to verapamil.
- You have very low blood pressure.

Before you start, consult your doctor:
- If you have kidney or liver disease.
- If you have high blood pressure.
- If you have heart disease other than coronary-artery disease.

Over age 60:
Adverse reactions and side effects may be more frequent and severe than in younger persons.

Pregnancy:
No proven harm to unborn child. Avoid if possible.

Breast-feeding:
Safety not established. Avoid if possible.

Infants & children:
Not recommended.

Prolonged use:
No problems expected.

Skin & sunlight:
No problems expected.

Driving, piloting or hazardous work:
Avoid if you feel dizzy. Otherwise, no problems expected.

Airplane passengers:
No problems expected.

Discontinuing:
Don't discontinue without doctor's advice until you complete prescribed dose, even though symptoms diminish or disappear.

Others:
Learn to check your own pulse rate. If it drops to 50 beats per minute or lower, don't take verapamil until your consult your doctor.

INTERACTION WITH OTHER DRUGS

GENERIC NAME OR DRUG CLASS	COMBINED EFFECT
Anticoagulants (oral)	Increased anticoagulant effect.
Anticonvulsants (hydantoin)	Increased anticonvulsant effect.
Antihypertensives	Dangerous blood-pressure drop.
Beta-adrenergic blockers	Possible irregular heartbeat.
Calcium (large doses)	Decreased verapamil effect.
Diuretics	Dangerous blood-pressure drop.
Digitalis preparations	Increased digitalis effect. May need to reduce dose.
Disopyramide	May cause dangerously slow, fast or irregular heartbeat.
Nitrates	Reduced angina attacks.
Quinidine	Increased quinidine effect.
Vitamin D (large doses)	Decreased verapamil effect.

INTERACTION WITH OTHER SUBSTANCES

INTERACTS WITH	COMBINED EFFECT
Alcohol:	Dangerously low blood pressure. Avoid.
Beverages:	None expected.
Cocaine:	Possible irregular heartbeat. Avoid.
Foods:	None expected.
Marijuana:	Possible irregular heartbeat. Avoid.
Tobacco:	Possible rapid heartbeat. Avoid.

VITAMIN A

BRAND NAMES

Acon
Afaxin
Alphalin
Aquasol A

Dispatabs
Sust-A

Numerous multiple vitamin-mineral supplements.

GENERAL INFORMATION

Habit forming? No
Prescription needed? No
Available as generic? Yes
Drug class: Vitamin supplement

USES

Dietary supplement to ensure normal growth and health, especially eyes and skin.

DOSAGE & USAGE INFORMATION

How to take:
Tablet or capsule—Swallow with liquid. If you can't swallow whole, crumble tablet or open capsule and take with liquid or food.

When to take:
At the same time each day.

If you forget a dose:
Take as soon as you remember. Resume regular schedule.

What drug does:
- Prevents night blindness.
- Promotes normal growth and health.

Time lapse before drug works:
Requires continual intake.

Don't take with:
See Interaction column and consult doctor.

OVERDOSE

Symptoms:
Increased adverse reactions and side effects. Jaundice (yellow eyes and skin) rare, but may occur with large doses.

What to do:
Overdose unlikely to threaten life. If person takes much larger amount than prescribed, call doctor, poison-control center or hospital emergency room for instructions.

POSSIBLE ADVERSE REACTIONS OR SIDE EFFECTS

SYMPTOMS	FREQUENCY	WHAT TO DO
Brain & nervous system:		
• Bulging soft spot on baby's head.	Rare	3
• Confusion, dizziness, drowsiness, headache, irritability.	Infrequent	4
Skin: Dry lips, peeling skin, hair loss.	Infrequent	4
Eyes: Double vision.	Rare	3
Ears, nose, throat:	None expected.	
Digestive: Diarrhea, appetite loss, nausea, vomiting.	Rare	4
Heart & lungs:	None expected.	
Blood vessels:	None expected.	
Muscles, bones, joints:	None expected.	
Genital, urinary:	None expected.	
Kidneys:	None expected.	
Liver:	None expected.	
Allergic:	None expected.	
Blood:	None expected.	
Others:	None expected.	

1- Life-threatening. Seek emergency treatment immediately.
2- Discontinue. Seek emergency treatment.
3- Discontinue. Call doctor right away.
4- Continue. Call doctor when convenient.
5- Continue. Tell doctor at next visit.
6- No action necessary.

WARNINGS & PRECAUTIONS

Don't take if:
You have chronic kidney failure.

Before you start, consult your doctor:
If you have any kidney disorder.

Over age 60:
No problems expected.

Pregnancy:
Don't take more than 6,000 units daily.

Breast-feeding:
No problems expected.

Infants & children:
- Avoid large doses.
- Keep vitamin-mineral supplements out of children's reach.

Prolonged use:
No problems expected.

Skin & sunlight:
No problems expected.

Driving, piloting or hazardous work:
No problems expected.

Airplane passengers:
No problems expected.

Discontinuing:
Don't discontinue without doctor's advice until you complete prescribed dose, even though symptoms diminish or disappear.

Others:
- Don't exceed dose. Too much over a long time may be harmful.
- A balanced diet should provide all the vitamin A a healthy person needs and prevent need for supplements. Best sources are liver, yellow-orange fruits and vegetables, dark-green, leafy vegetables, milk, butter and margarine.

INTERACTION WITH OTHER DRUGS

GENERIC NAME OR DRUG CLASS	COMBINED EFFECT
Cholestyramine	Decreased vitamin A absorption.
Mineral oil (long term)	Decreased vitamin A absorption.
Vitamin E (excess dose)	Vitamin A depletion.

INTERACTION WITH OTHER SUBSTANCES

INTERACTS WITH	COMBINED EFFECT
Alcohol:	None expected.
Beverages:	None expected.
Cocaine:	None expected.
Foods:	None expected.
Marijuana:	None expected.
Tobacco:	None expected.

VITAMIN B-12 (CYANOCOBALAMIN)

BRAND NAMES

Alphamin
Alpha Redisol
Anocobin
Betalin 12 Crystalline
Kaybovite
Neo-Betalin

Neo-Rubex
Redisol
Rubramin
Rubramin-PC
Sytobex

Numerous other multiple vitamin-mineral supplements.

GENERAL INFORMATION

Habit forming? No
Prescription needed? No
Available as generic? Yes
Drug class: Vitamin supplement

USES

- Dietary supplement for normal growth, development and health.
- Treatment for nerve damage.
- Treatment for pernicious anemia.
- Treatment and prevention of vitamin B-12 deficiencies in people who have had stomach or intestines surgically removed.
- Prevention of vitamin B-12 deficiency in strict vegetarians and persons with absorption diseases.

DOSAGE & USAGE INFORMATION

How to take:
- Tablets—Swallow with liquid.
- Injection—Follow doctor's directions.

When to take:
- Oral—At the same time each day.
- Injection—Follow doctor's directions.

If you forget a dose:
Take when remembered. Don't double next dose. Resume regular schedule.

What drug does:
Acts as enzyme to promote normal fat and carbohydrate metabolism and protein synthesis.

Time lapse before drug works:
15 minutes.

Don't take with:
See Interaction column and consult doctor.

OVERDOSE

Symptoms:
Increased adverse reactions and side effects.

What to do:
Overdose unlikely to threaten life. If person takes much larger amount than prescribed, call doctor, poison-control center or hospital emergency room for instructions.

POSSIBLE ADVERSE REACTIONS OR SIDE EFFECTS

SYMPTOMS	FREQUENCY	WHAT TO DO
Brain & nervous system:	None expected.	
Skin: Itching	Rare	3
Eyes:	None expected.	
Ears, nose, throat:	None expected.	
Digestive: Diarrhea	Rare	4
Heart & lungs: Wheezing	Rare	3
Blood vessels:	None expected.	
Muscles, bones, joints:	None expected.	
Genital, urinary:	None expected.	
Kidneys:	None expected.	
Liver:	None expected.	
Allergic: Life-threatening anaphylaxis may occur after injection.	Rare	1 See Page 888.
Blood:	None expected.	
Others:	None expected.	

1- Life-threatening. Seek emergency treatment immediately.
2- Discontinue. Seek emergency treatment.
3- Discontinue. Call doctor right away.
4- Continue. Call doctor when convenient.
5- Continue. Tell doctor at next visit.
6- No action necessary.

VITAMIN B-12 (CYANOCOBALAMIN)

WARNINGS & PRECAUTIONS

Don't take if:
You have Leber's disease (optic nerve atrophy).

Before you start, consult your doctor:
● If you have gout.
● If you have heart disease.

Over age 60:
No problems expected.

Pregnancy:
No problems expected.

Breast-feeding:
No problems expected.

Infants & children:
No problems expected.

Prolonged use:
No problems expected.

Skin & sunlight:
No problems expected.

Driving, piloting or hazardous work:
No problems expected.

Airplane passengers:
No problems expected.

Discontinuing:
Don't discontinue without doctor's advice until you complete prescribed dose, even though symptoms diminish or disappear.

Others:
● A balanced diet should provide all the vitamin B-12 a healthy person needs and make supplements unnecessary. Best sources are meat, fish, egg yolk and cheese.
● Tablets should be used only for diet supplements. All other uses of vitamin B-12 require injections.

INTERACTION WITH OTHER DRUGS

GENERIC NAME OR DRUG CLASS	COMBINED EFFECT
Anticonvulsants	Decreased absorption of vitamin B-12.
Aspirin	Decreased absorption of vitamin B-12.
Vitamin C (ascorbic acid)	Destroys vitamin B-12 if taken at same time. Take 2 hours apart.
Chloramphenicol	Decreased vitamin B-12 effect.
Colchicine	Decreased absorption of vitamin B-12.
Neomycin	Decreased absorption of vitamin B-12.
Potassium (extended-release forms)	Decreased absorption of vitamin B-12.

INTERACTION WITH OTHER SUBSTANCES

INTERACTS WITH	COMBINED EFFECT
Alcohol:	Decreased absorption of vitamin B-12.
Beverages:	None expected.
Cocaine:	None expected.
Foods:	None expected.
Marijuana:	None expected.
Tobacco:	None expected.

VITAMIN C (ASCORBIC ACID)

BRAND NAMES

Adenex	Ceri-Bid	Megascorb
Ascorbajen	Cevalin	Redoxon
Ascorbicap	Ce-Vi-Sol	
Ascoril	Cevita	
Cecon	C-Ject	
Cenolate	Liqui-Cee	

Numerous other multiple vitamin-mineral supplements.

GENERAL INFORMATION

Habit forming? No
Prescription needed? No
Available as generic? Yes
Drug class: Vitamin supplement

 ## USES

- Prevention and treatment of scurvy and other vitamin-C deficiencies.
- Treatment of anemia.
- Maintenance of acid urine.

 ## DOSAGE & USAGE INFORMATION

How to take:
- Tablets, capsules, liquid—Swallow with 8 oz. water.
- Extended-release tablets—Swallow whole.
- Drops—Squirt directly into mouth or mix with liquid or food.

When to take:
1, 2 or 3 times per day, as prescribed on label.

If you forget a dose:
Take as soon as you remember. Return to regular schedule.

What drug does:
- May help form collagen.
- Increases iron absorption from intestine.
- Contributes to hemoglobin and red-blood-cell production in bone marrow.

Time lapse before drug works:
1 week.

Don't take with:
See Interaction column and consult doctor.

 ## OVERDOSE

Symptoms:
Diarrhea, vomiting, dizziness.

What to do:
Overdose unlikely to threaten life. If person takes much larger amount than prescribed, call doctor, poison-control center or hospital emergency room for instructions.

 ## POSSIBLE ADVERSE REACTIONS OR SIDE EFFECTS

SYMPTOMS	FREQUENCY	WHAT TO DO
Brain & nervous system: Headache	Rare	5
Skin: Flushed face.	Infrequent	4
Eyes:	None expected.	
Ears, nose, throat:	None expected.	
Digestive: Mild diarrhea, nausea, vomiting.	Infrequent	3
Heart & lungs:	None expected.	
Blood vessels:	None expected.	
Muscles, bones, joints:	None expected.	
Genital, urinary:	None expected.	
Kidneys: Severe pain in lower abdomen (kidney stones).	Infrequent	3
Liver:	None expected.	
Allergic:	None expected.	
Blood: Anemia	Rare	3
Others:	None expected.	

1 - Life-threatening. Seek emergency treatment immediately.
2 - Discontinue. Seek emergency treatment.
3 - Discontinue. Call doctor right away.
4 - Continue. Call doctor when convenient.
5 - Continue. Tell doctor at next visit.
6 - No action necessary.

VITAMIN C (ASCORBIC ACID)

WARNINGS & PRECAUTIONS

Don't take if:
You are allergic to vitamin C.

Before you start, consult your doctor:
- If you have sickle-cell or other anemia.
- If you have had kidney stones.
- If you have gout.

Over age 60:
For daily doses of 1,000 mg. or more, drink at least 2 quarts of water daily.

Pregnancy:
No proven harm to unborn child. Avoid large doses.

Breast-feeding:
Avoid large doses.

Infants & children:
- Avoid large doses.
- Keep vitamin-mineral supplements out of children's reach.

Prolonged use:
Large doses for longer than 2 months may cause kidney stones.

Skin & sunlight:
No problems expected.

Driving, piloting or hazardous work:
No problems expected.

Airplane passengers:
No problems expected.

Discontinuing:
No problems expected.

Others:
- Store in cool, dry place.
- May cause inaccurate tests for sugar in urine or blood in stool.
- May cause crisis in patients with sickle-cell anemia.
- A balanced diet should provide all the vitamin C a healthy person needs and make supplements unnecessary. Best sources are citrus, strawberries, cantaloupe and raw peppers.

INTERACTION WITH OTHER DRUGS

GENERIC NAME OR DRUG CLASS	COMBINED EFFECT
Anticoagulants (oral)	Decreased anticoagulant effect.
Aspirin	Decreased vitamin C effect.
Anticholinergics	Decreased anticholinergic effect.
Barbiturates	Decreased vitamin C effect. Increased barbiturate effect.
Contraceptives (oral)	Decreased vitamin C effect.
Mineral oil	Decreased vitamin C effect.
Iron supplements	Increased iron effect.
Quinidine	Decreased quinidine effect.
Salicylates	Decreased vitamin C effect.
Sulfa drugs	Decreased vitamin C effect. Possible kidney stones.
Tetracyclines	Decreased vitamin C effect.

INTERACTION WITH OTHER SUBSTANCES

INTERACTS WITH	COMBINED EFFECT
Alcohol:	None expected.
Beverages:	None expected.
Cocaine:	None expected.
Foods:	None expected.
Marijuana:	None expected.
Tobacco:	Increased requirement for vitamin C.

VITAMIN D

BRAND NAMES

Calciferol
Calcifidiol
Calderol
Calcitriol
Deltalin
Dihydrotachysterol

Drisdol
Hykaterol
Ostoforte
Radiostol
Radiostol Forte
Rocaltrol

Numerous other multiple vitamin-mineral supplements.

GENERAL INFORMATION

Habit forming? No
Prescription needed? Low strength: No
High strength: Yes
Available as generic? Yes
Drug class: Vitamin supplement

 ## USES

- Dietary supplement.
- Prevention of rickets (bone disease).
- Treatment for hypocalcemia (low blood calcium) in kidney disease.
- Treatment for postoperative muscle contractions.

 ## DOSAGE & USAGE INFORMATION

How to take:
- Tablet or capsule—Swallow with liquid.
- Drops—Dilute dose in beverage.

When to take:
As directed, usually once a day at the same time each day.

If you forget a dose:
Take up to 12 hours late. If more than 12 hours, wait for next dose (don't double this).

What drug does:
Maintains growth and health. Prevents rickets. Essential so body can use calcium and phosphate.

Time lapse before drug works:
2 hours. May require 2 to 3 weeks of continual use for maximum effect.

Don't take with:
Non-prescription drugs or drugs in Interaction column without consulting doctor.

 ## OVERDOSE

Symptoms:
Severe stomach pain, nausea, vomiting, weight loss; bone and muscle pain; increased urination, cloudy urine; mood or mental changes (possible psychosis); high blood pressure, irregular heartbeat; eye irritation or light sensitivity; itchy skin.

What to do:
Overdose unlikely to threaten life. If person takes much larger amount than prescribed, call doctor, poison-control center or hospital emergency room for instructions.

POSSIBLE ADVERSE REACTIONS OR SIDE EFFECTS

SYMPTOMS	FREQUENCY	WHAT TO DO
Brain & nervous system: Headache	Infrequent	4
Skin:	None expected.	
Eyes:	None expected.	
Ears, nose, throat: Metallic taste in mouth, thirst, dry mouth.	Infrequent	4
Digestive: Constipation, appetite loss, nausea, vomiting.	Infrequent	4
Heart & lungs:	None expected.	
Blood vessels:	None expected.	
Muscles, bones, joints:	None expected.	
Genital, urinary:	None expected.	
Kidneys:	None expected.	
Liver:	None expected.	
Allergic:	None expected.	
Blood:	None expected.	
Others:	None expected.	

1- Life-threatening. Seek emergency treatment immediately.
2- Discontinue. Seek emergency treatment.
3- Discontinue. Call doctor right away.
4- Continue. Call doctor when convenient.
5- Continue. Tell doctor at next visit.
6- No action necessary.

WARNINGS & PRECAUTIONS

Don't take if:
You are allergic to medicine containing vitamin D.

Before you start, consult your doctor:
- If you plan to become pregnant while taking vitamin D.
- If you have epilepsy.
- If you have heart or blood-vessel disease.
- If you have kidney disease.

Over age 60:
Adverse reactions and side effects may be more frequent and severe than in younger persons.

Pregnancy:
Risk to unborn child outweighs drug benefits. Don't use.

Breast-feeding:
No problems expected, but consult doctor.

Infants & children:
- Avoid large doses.
- Keep vitamins out of children's reach.

Prolonged use:
No problems expected.

Skin & sunlight:
No problems expected.

Driving, piloting or hazardous work:
No problems expected.

Airplane passengers:
No problems expected.

Discontinuing:
Don't discontinue without doctor's advice until you complete prescribed dose, even though symptoms diminish or disappear.

Others:
- Don't exceed dose. Too much over a long time may be harmful.
- A balanced diet should provide all the vitamin D a healthy person needs and make supplements unnecessary. Best sources are fish and vitamin-D fortified milk and bread.

INTERACTION WITH OTHER DRUGS

GENERIC NAME OR DRUG CLASS	COMBINED EFFECT
Antacids (magnesium-containing)	Possible excess magnesium.
Anticonvulsants (hydantoin)	Decreased vitamin D effect.
Calcium (high doses)	Excess calcium in blood.
Calcium-channel blockers	Decreased effect of calcium-channel blockers.
Cholestyramine	Decreased vitamin D effect.
Digitalis preparations	Heartbeat irregularities.
Mineral oil	Decreased vitamin D effect.
Phenobarbital	Decreased vitamin D effect.
Phosphorous preparations	Accumulation of excess phosporous.
Vitamin D (other)	Possible toxicity.

INTERACTION WITH OTHER SUBSTANCES

INTERACTS WITH	COMBINED EFFECT
Alcohol:	None expected.
Beverages:	None expected.
Cocaine:	None expected.
Foods:	None expected.
Marijuana:	None expected.
Tobacco:	None expected.

VITAMIN E

BRAND NAMES

Aquasol E
Chew-E
Daltose
Eprolin
Pheryl-E
Numerous other multiple vitamin-mineral supplements.

GENERAL INFORMATION

Habit forming? No
Prescription needed? No
Available as generic? Yes
Drug class: Vitamin supplement

USES

- Dietary supplement to promote normal growth, development and health.
- Treatment and prevention of vitamin-E deficiency, especially in premature or low birth-weight infants.
- Treatment for fibrocystic disease of the breast.
- Treatment for circulatory problems to the lower extremities.
- Treatment for sickle-cell anemia.
- Treatment for lung toxicity from air pollution.

DOSAGE & USAGE INFORMATION

How to take:
- Tablet, capsule or chewable tablets—Swallow with liquid or food to lessen stomach irritation.
- Drops—Dilute dose in beverage before swallowing or squirt directly into mouth.

When to take:
At the same times each day.

If you forget a dose:
Take when you remember. Don't double next dose.

What drug does:
- Promotes normal growth and development.
- Prevents oxidation in body.

Time lapse before drug works:
Not determined.

Don't take with:
See Interaction column and consult doctor.

OVERDOSE

Symptoms:
Nausea, vomiting.

What to do:
Overdose unlikely to threaten life. If person takes much larger amount than prescribed, call doctor, poison-control center or hospital emergency room for instructions.

POSSIBLE ADVERSE REACTIONS OR SIDE EFFECTS

SYMPTOMS	FREQUENCY	WHAT TO DO
Brain & nervous system:	None expected.	
Skin:	None expected.	
Eyes:	None expected.	
Ears, nose, throat:	None expected.	
Digestive: Nausea, stomach pain.	Infrequent	4
Heart & lungs:	None expected.	
Blood vessels:	None expected.	
Muscles, bones, joints: Muscle aches, pain in lower legs.	Infrequent	4
Genital, urinary:	None expected.	
Kidneys:	None expected.	
Liver:	None expected.	
Allergic:	None expected.	
Blood:	None expected.	
Others: Fever, tiredness, weakness.	Infrequent	4

1- Life-threatening. Seek emergency treatment immediately.
2- Discontinue. Seek emergency treatment.
3- Discontinue. Call doctor right away.
4- Continue. Call doctor when convenient.
5- Continue. Tell doctor at next visit.
6- No action necessary.

VITAMIN E

WARNINGS & PRECAUTIONS

Don't take if:
You are allergic to vitamin E.

Before you start, consult your doctor:
- If you have had blood clots in leg veins (thrombophlebitis).
- If you have liver disease.

Over age 60:
No problems expected. Avoid excessive doses.

Pregnancy:
No problems expected with normal daily requirements. Don't exceed prescribed dose.

Breast-feeding:
No problems expected.

Infants & children:
Use only under medical supervision.

Prolonged use:
Toxic accumulation of vitamin E. Don't exceed recommended dose.

Skin & sunlight:
No problems expected.

Driving, piloting or hazardous work:
No problems expected.

Airplane passengers:
No problems expected.

Discontinuing:
No problems expected

Others:
A balanced diet should provide all the vitamin E a healthy person needs and make supplements unnecessary. Best sources are vegetable oils, whole-grain cereals, liver.

INTERACTION WITH OTHER DRUGS

GENERIC NAME OR DRUG CLASS	COMBINED EFFECT
Iron supplements	Decreased effect of iron supplement in patients with iron-deficiency anemia. Decreased vitamin E effect in healthy persons.
Vitamin A	Recommended dose of vitamin E— Increased benefit and decreased toxicity of vitamin A. Excess dose of vitamin E—Vitamin A depletion.

INTERACTION WITH OTHER SUBSTANCES

INTERACTS WITH	COMBINED EFFECT
Alcohol:	None expected.
Beverages:	None expected.
Cocaine:	None expected.
Foods:	None expected.
Marijuana:	None expected.
Tobacco:	None expected.

VITAMIN K

BRAND NAMES

AquaMEPHYTON   Phytonadione
Kappadione   Synkayvite
Konakion
Mephyton
Menadione
Menadiol

GENERAL INFORMATION

Habit forming? No
Prescription needed? No
Available as generic? Yes
Drug class: Vitamin supplement

USES

- Dietary supplement.
- Treatment for bleeding disorders and malabsorption diseases due to vitamin K deficiency.
- Treatment for hemorrhagic disease of the newborn.
- Treatment for bleeding due to overdose of oral anticoagulants.

DOSAGE & USAGE INFORMATION

How to take:
Tablet—Swallow with liquid. If you can't swallow whole, crumble tablet or open capsule and take with liquid or food.

When to take:
At the same time each day.

If you forget a dose:
Take as soon as you remember up to 12 hours late. If more than 12 hours, wait for next scheduled dose (don't double this dose).

What drug does:
- Promotes growth, development and good health.
- Supplies a necessary ingredient for blood clotting.

Time lapse before drug works:
15 to 30 minutes to support blood clotting.

Don't take with:
See Interaction column and consult doctor.

OVERDOSE

Symptoms:
Nausea, vomiting.

What to do:
Overdose unlikely to threaten life. If person takes much larger amount than prescribed, call doctor, poison-control center or hospital emergency room for instructions.

POSSIBLE ADVERSE REACTIONS OR SIDE EFFECTS

SYMPTOMS	FREQUENCY	WHAT TO DO
Brain & nervous system:	None expected.	
Skin:	None expected.	
Eyes:	None expected.	
Ears, nose, throat: Unusual taste.	Infrequent	4
Digestive:	None expected.	
Heart & lungs:	None expected.	
Blood vessels:	None expected.	
Muscles, bones, joints:	None expected.	
Genital, urinary:	None expected.	
Kidneys:	None expected.	
Liver:	None expected.	
Allergic:	None expected.	
Blood:	None expected.	
Others:	None expected.	

1-Life-threatening. Seek emergency treatment immediately.
2-Discontinue. Seek emergency treatment.
3-Discontinue. Call doctor right away.
4-Continue. Call doctor when convenient.
5-Continue. Tell doctor at next visit.
6-No action necessary.

VITAMIN K

WARNINGS & PRECAUTIONS

Don't take if:
- You are allergic to vitamin K.
- You have G6PD deficiency.
- You have liver disease.

Before you start, consult your doctor:
If you are pregnant.

Over age 60:
No problems expected.

Pregnancy:
Don't exceed dose.

Breast-feeding:
No problems expected.

Infants & children:
Phytonadione is the preferred form for hemorrhagic disease of the newborn.

Prolonged use:
No problems expected.

Skin & sunlight:
No problems expected.

Driving, piloting or hazardous work:
No problems expected.

Airplane passengers:
No problems expected.

Discontinuing:
No problems expected.

Others:
- Tell all doctors and dentists you consult that you take this medicine.
- Don't exceed dose. Too much over a long time may be harmful.
- A balanced diet should provide all the vitamin K a healthy person needs and make supplements unnecessary. Best sources are green, leafy vegetables, meat or dairy products.

INTERACTION WITH OTHER DRUGS

GENERIC NAME OR DRUG CLASS	COMBINED EFFECT
Anticoagulants (oral)	Decreased anticoagulant effect.
Cholestyramine	Decreased vitamin K effect.
Mineral oil (long term)	Vitamin K deficiency.
Sulfa drugs	Vitamin K deficiency.

INTERACTION WITH OTHER SUBSTANCES

INTERACTS WITH	COMBINED EFFECT
Alcohol:	None expected.
Beverages:	None expected.
Cocaine:	None expected.
Foods:	None expected.
Marijuana:	None expected.
Tobacco:	None expected.

WARFARIN POTASSIUM

BRAND NAMES

Athrombin-K

GENERAL INFORMATION

Habit forming? No
Prescription needed? Yes
Available as generic? Yes
Drug class: Anticoagulant

USES

Reduces blood clots. Used for abnormal clotting inside blood vessels.

DOSAGE & USAGE INFORMATION

How to take:
Tablet—Swallow with liquid. If you can't swallow whole, crumble tablet and take with liquid or food.

When to take:
At the same time each day.

If you forget a dose:
Take as soon as you remember up to 12 hours late. If more than 12 hours, wait for next scheduled dose (don't double this dose). Inform your doctor of any missed doses.

What drug does:
Blocks action of vitamin K necessary for blood clotting.

Time lapse before drug works:
36 to 48 hours.

Don't take with:
See Interaction column and consult doctor.

OVERDOSE

Symptoms:
Bloody vomit and bloody or black stools, red urine.

What to do:
- Dial 0 (operator) or 911 (emergency) for an ambulance or medical help. Then give first aid immediately.
- Additional emergency information on page 886.

POSSIBLE ADVERSE REACTIONS OR SIDE EFFECTS

SYMPTOMS	FREQUENCY	WHAT TO DO
Brain & nervous system: Dizziness, headache.	Rare	3
Skin: Rash, hives, itch.	Infrequent	3
Eyes: Blurred vision.	Infrequent	3
Ears, nose, throat:		
• Sore throat.	Infrequent	3
• Mouth sores.	Rare	3
Digestive:		
• Black stools or bloody vomit.	Infrequent	2
• Diarrhea, cramps, nausea, vomiting.	Infrequent	4
• Bloating, gas.	Common	5
Heart & lungs: Coughing up blood.	Infrequent	2
Blood vessels: Easy bruising, bleeding.	Infrequent	3
Muscles, bones, joints: Swollen feet, legs.	Infrequent	4
Genital, urinary: Cloudy or red urine.	Infrequent	3
Kidneys: Back pain.	Infrequent	3
Liver: Jaundice (yellow skin and eyes).	Infrequent	3
Allergic, blood:	None expected.	
Others:		
• Fever, chills.	Infrequent	3
• Hair loss.	Infrequent	4
• Fatigue, weakness.	Infrequent	3

1-Life-threatening. Seek emergency treatment immediately.
2-Discontinue. Seek emergency treatment.
3-Discontinue. Call doctor right away.
4-Continue. Call doctor when convenient.
5-Continue. Tell doctor at next visit.

WARFARIN POTASSIUM

WARNINGS & PRECAUTIONS

Don't take if:
- You have been allergic to any oral anticoagulant.
- You have a bleeding disorder.
- You have an active peptic ulcer.
- You have ulcerative colitis.

Before you start, consult your doctor:
- If you take any other drugs, including non-prescription drugs.
- If you have high blood pressure.
- If you have heavy or prolonged menstrual periods.
- If you have diabetes.
- If you have a bladder catheter.
- If you have serious liver or kidney disease.
- If you will have surgery within 2 months, including dental surgery, requiring general or spinal anesthesia.

Over age 60:
Adverse reactions and side effects may be more frequent and severe than in younger persons.

Pregnancy:
Risk to unborn child outweighs drug benefits. Don't use.

Breast-feeding:
Drug filters into milk. May harm child. Avoid.

Infants & children:
Use only under doctor's supervision.

Prolonged use:
No problems expected.

Skin & sunlight:
No problems expected.

Driving, piloting or hazardous work:
- Avoid hazardous activities that could cause injury.
- Don't drive if you feel dizzy or have blurred vision.

Airplane passengers:
No problems expected.

Discontinuing:
Don't discontinue without consulting doctor. Dose may require gradual reduction if you have taken drug for a long time. Doses of other drugs may also require adjustment.

Others:
Carry identification to state you take anticoagulants.

INTERACTION WITH OTHER DRUGS

GENERIC NAME OR DRUG CLASS	COMBINED EFFECT
Acetaminophen	Increased warfarin potassium effect.
Allopurinol	Increased warfarin potassium effect.
Androgens	Increased warfarin potassium effect.
Antacids (large doses)	Decreased warfarin potassium effect.
Antibiotics	Increased warfarin potassium effect.
Antidepressants (tricyclic)	Increased warfarin potassium effect.
Anticonvulsants (hydantoin)	Increased effect of both drugs.
Antidiabetics (oral)	Increased warfarin potassium effect.
Antihistamines	Unpredictable increased or decreased anticoagulant effect.
Barbiturates	Decreased warfarin potassium effect.
Benzodiazepines	Unpredictable increased or decreased anticoagulant effect.
Carbamazepine	Decreased warfarin potassium effect.

Additional interations on page 844.

Additional interations on page 844.

INTERACTION WITH OTHER SUBSTANCES

INTERACTS WITH	COMBINED EFFECT
Alcohol:	Can increase or decrease effect of anticoagulant. Use with caution.
Beverages:	None expected.
Cocaine:	None expected.
Foods: High in vitamin K such as fish, liver, spinach, cabbage.	May decrease anticoagulant effect.
Marijuana:	None expected.
Tobacco:	None expected.

WARFARIN SODIUM

BRAND NAMES

Coumadin
Panwarfin
Warfilone
Warnerin

Habit forming? No
Prescription needed? Yes
Available as generic? Yes
Drug class: Anticoagulant

 USES

Reduces blood clots. Used for abnormal clotting inside blood vessels.

 DOSAGE & USAGE INFORMATION

How to take:
Tablet—Swallow with liquid. If you can't swallow whole, crumble tablet and take with liquid or food.

When to take:
At the same time each day.

If you forget a dose:
Take as soon as you remember up to 12 hours late. If more than 12 hours, wait for next scheduled dose (don't double this dose). Inform your doctor of any missed doses.

What drug does:
Blocks action of vitamin K necessary for blood clotting.

Time lapse before drug works:
36 to 48 hours.

Don't take with:
See Interaction column and consult doctor.

 OVERDOSE

Symptoms:
Bloody vomit and bloody or black stools, red urine.

What to do:
- Dial 0 (operator) or 911 (emergency) for an ambulance or medical help. Then give first aid immediately.
- Additional emergency information on page 886.

POSSIBLE ADVERSE REACTIONS OR SIDE EFFECTS

SYMPTOMS	FREQUENCY	WHAT TO DO
Brain & nervous system:		
Dizziness, headache.	Rare	3
Skin:		
Rash, hives, itch.	Infrequent	3
Eyes:		
Blurred vision.	Infrequent	3
Ears, nose, throat:		
• Sore throat.	Infrequent	3
• Mouth sores.	Rare	3
Digestive:		
• Black stools or bloody vomit.	Infrequent	2
• Diarrhea, cramps, nausea, vomiting.	Infrequent	4
• Bloating, gas.	Common	5
Heart & lungs:		
Coughing up blood.	Infrequent	2
Blood vessels:		
Easy bruising, bleeding.	Infrequent	3
Muscles, bones, joints:		
Swollen feet, legs.	Infrequent	4
Genital, urinary:		
Cloudy or red urine.	Infrequent	3
Kidneys:		
Back pain.	Infrequent	3
Liver:		
Jaundice (yellow skin and eyes).	Infrequent	3
Allergic, blood:	None expected.	
Others:		
• Fever, chills.	Infrequent	3
• Hair loss.	Infrequent	4
• Fatigue, weakness.	Infrequent	3

1- Life-threatening. Seek emergency treatment immediately.
2- Discontinue. Seek emergency treatment.
3- Discontinue. Call doctor right away.
4- Continue. Call doctor when convenient.
5- Continue. Tell doctor at next visit.

WARNINGS & PRECAUTIONS

Don't take if:
- You have been allergic to any oral anticoagulant.
- You have a bleeding disorder.
- You have an active peptic ulcer.
- You have ulcerative colitis.

Before you start, consult your doctor:
- If you take any other drugs, including non-prescription drugs.
- If you have high blood pressure.
- If you have heavy or prolonged menstrual periods.
- If you have diabetes.
- If you have a bladder catheter.
- If you have serious liver or kidney disease.
- If you will have surgery within 2 months, including dental surgery, requiring general or spinal anesthesia.

Over age 60:
Adverse reactions and side effects may be more frequent and severe than in younger persons.

Pregnancy:
Risk to unborn child outweighs drug benefits. Don't use.

Breast-feeding:
Drug filters into milk. May harm child. Avoid.

Infants & children:
Use only under doctor's supervision.

Prolonged use:
No problems expected.

Skin & sunlight:
No problems expected.

Driving, piloting or hazardous work:
- Avoid hazardous activities that could cause injury.
- Don't drive if you feel dizzy or have blurred vision.

Airplane passengers:
No problems expected.

Discontinuing:
Don't discontinue without consulting doctor. Dose may require gradual reduction if you have taken drug for a long time. Doses of other drugs may also require adjustment.

Others:
Carry identification to state you take anticoagulants.

INTERACTION WITH OTHER DRUGS

GENERIC NAME OR DRUG CLASS	COMBINED EFFECT
Acetaminophen	Increased warfarin sodium effect.
Allopurinol	Increased warfarin sodium effect.
Androgens	Increased warfarin sodium effect.
Antacids (large doses)	Decreased warfarin sodium effect.
Antibiotics	Increased warfarin sodium effect.
Anticonvulsants (hydantoin)	Increased effect of both drugs.
Antidepressants (tricyclic)	Increased warfarin sodium effect.
Antidiabetics (oral)	Increased warfarin sodium effect.
Antihistamines	Unpredictable Increased or decreased anticoagulant effect.
Barbiturates	Decreased warfarin sodium effect.
Benzodiazepines	Unpredictable increased or decreased anticoagulant effect.
Carbamazepine	Decreased warfarin sodium effect.

Additional interactions on page 845.

INTERACTION WITH OTHER SUBSTANCES

INTERACTS WITH	COMBINED EFFECT
Alcohol:	Can increase or decrease effect of anticoagulant. Use with caution.
Beverages:	None expected.
Cocaine:	None expected.
Foods: High in vitamin K such as fish, liver, spinach, cabbage.	May decrease anticoagulant effect.
Marijuana:	None expected.
Tobacco:	None expected.

Additional Brand Names

The following drugs are alphabetized by generic name, shown in capital letters. The brand names that follow each generic name are a more complete list than appears on the drug charts. Brand names followed by an M in parentheses (M) are mixtures of more than one generic drug.

ACETAMINOPHEN

A-P-A-P Tablets
APAP
Aceta with Codeine Tablets (M)
Acetaminophen Elixir
Acetaminophen Suppositories
Acetaminophen with Codeine Tablets (M)
Anapap Tablets
Anaphen (M)
Anuphen Suppositories
Apamide Tablets
Arthralgen (M)
Arthralgen Tablets (M)
Axotal (M)
Bancap w/Codeine Capsules (M)
Banesin Forte Tablets (M)
Bromo-Seltzer (buffered acetaminophen)
Campain
Capital Tablets
Capital with Codeine Tablets (M)
Co-Tylenol (M)
Coastaldyne Tablets (M)
Coastalgesic (M)
Codap Tablets (M)
Colrex (M)
Covangesic (M)
D-Sinus Capsules (M)
Dapa Tablets
Dapase Tablets (M)
Darvocet-N (M)
Darvocet-N 100 (M)
Datril
Datril Elixir
Datril Tablets
Dialog (M)
Dolanex Elixir
Dolene AP-65 (M)
Dolor Tablets (M)
Duadacin (M)
Dularin (M)
Dularin Syrup
Dynosal Tablets (M)
Empracet with Codeine Tablets (M)

Endecon Tablets (M)
Esgic (M)
Excedrin (M)
Exdol
Febrogesic Capsules
Febrogesic Tablets
Fendol Tablets (M)
G-1 Tablets
G-2 (M)
Gaysal (M)
Guaiamine Capsules (M)
Hasacode Tablets (M)
Hi-Temp Tablets
Liquiprin
Liquiprin Drops
Liquix-C Capsules (M)
Lyteca Elixir
Lyteca Tablets
Medache (M)
Metrogesic Tablets (M)
Minotal (M)
NAPAP Capsules
Naldegesic Tablets (M)
Nebs Liquid
Nebs Tablets
Neopap Supprettes
Ornex Capsules (M)
Ossonate-Plus (M)
Parafon Forte (M)
Pavadon Elixir (M)
Percocet-5 (M)
Phenaphen
Phenaphen Tablets
Phenaphen with Codeine Capsules No. 4 (M)
Phenaphen with Codeine No. 3 Capsules (M)
Phendex Tablets
Phrenilin (M)
Presalin Tablets (M)
Prodolor (M)
Proval Drops
Proval Elixir
Provel Tablets
Rhinocaps Capsules (M)
Rhinspec Tablets (M)
Robigesic

Ronuvex
S-A-C Tablets (M)
SK-APAP
SK-APAP Elixir
SK-APAP Tablets
Salatin Capsules (M)
Saleto Tablets (M)
Saleto-D Capsules (M)
Salimeph Forte Tablets (M)
Salphenyl (M)
Sedapap (M)
Sinarest (M)
Sine-Off (M)
Sinutab (M)
Sinutab II (M)
Strascogesic Tablets (M)
Supac (M)
Sylapar Tablets (M)
T.P.I. (M)
Tapar
Tapar Elixir
Tapar Tablets
Temlo Syrup
Temlo Tablets
Tempra
Tempra Drops
Tempra Syrup
Tempra Tablets
Tenlap Elixir
Triaminicin (M)
Trigesic Tablets (M)
Trind Sryup
Tylenol
Tylenol Chewable Tablets
Tylenol Drops
Tylenol Elixir
Tylenol Extra Strength Capsules
Tylenol Tablets
Tylenol w/ Codeine Tablets (M)
Tylenol w/ Codeine Tablets No. 4 (M)
Valadol
Valadol Liquid
Valadol Tablets
Wygesic Tablets (M)

ANESTHETICS (TOPICAL)

Aero Caine Aerosol
Aero Caine-5 Aerosol
Americaine Aerosol
Americaine Ointment
Anbesol
Anestacon Solution
Benzocaine Topical
Benzocol Ointment

Burntame Aerosol
Butesin Picrate Ointment
Butyn Sulfate Solution
Caine Spray
Cal-Vi-Nol Ointment
Cetacaine Liquid
Cetacaine Ointment
Cetacaine Spray

Cetacine Gel
Chiggerex Ointment
Cyclaine Solution
Derma-Medicone Ointment
Dermo-Gen Dressing
Dibucaine Ointment
Diothane Ointment
Dyclone Solution

Foille Liquid
Foille Ointment
Hexathricin Aerospra
Hurricaine
Isotraine Cream
Lida-Mantle Cream
Lidocaine Ointment
Medicone Dressing
Morusan Ointment
Nupercainal Cream

Nupercainal Ointment
Nupercainal Spray
Panthocal A & D
Pontocaine Cream
Pontocaine Ointment
Quotane Lotion
Quotane Ointment
Rectal Medicone
Solarcaine Cream
Solarcaine Lotion

Solarcaine Spray
Surfacaine Cream
Surfacaine Ointment
Tega-Dyne Ointment
Tronolane
Tronothane Cream
Tronothane Jelly
Urolocaine Liquid
Xylocaine Ointment

ASPIRIN

A.P.C.-Demerol (M)
A.P.C w/Codeine 1/8 gr
    Tablets or Capsules (M)
A.P.C. Capsules (M)
A.P.C. w/Codeine 1 gr Tablets
    or Capsules (M)
A.P.C. w/Codeine 1/2 gr
    Tablets or Capsules (M)
A.P.C. w/Codeine 1/4 gr
    Tablets or Capsules (M)
A.S.A. & Codeine Compound
    Pulvules No. 2 (M)
A.S.A. & Codeine Compound
    Tablets No. 2 (M)
A.S.A. & Codeine Compound
    Pulvules No. 3 (M)
A.S.A. & Codeine Compound
    Tablets No. 3 (M)
A.S.A. & Codeine Compound
    Pulvules No. 4 (M)
A.S.A. Compound Pulvules (M)
A.S.A. Compound Tablets (M)
A.S.A. Enseals
A.S.A. Pulvules
A.S.A. Suppositories
A.S.A. Tablets
Acetophen (M)
Alka Seltzer Effervescent
    Tablets (M)
Aluminum ASA Tablets
    Chewable (M)
Amytal and Aspirin (M)
Anaphen (M)
Anexsia w/Codeine Tablets (M)
Ascodeen-30 Tablets (M)
Ascriptin A/D Tablets (M)
Ascriptin Tablets (M)
Ascriptin w/Codeine (M)
Ascriptin w/Codeine No. 2 (M)
Aspirin Compound with
    Codeine (M)
Aspirin Suppositories
Aspirin Suppositories
    Children's
Aspirin Tablets
Aspirin Tablets Children's
Aspirjen Jr.
Bancap w/Codeine Capsules
    (M)
Bayer Aspirin
Bayer Children's Aspirin
Bayer Timed-release Tablets
Bexophene Capsules (M)

Buff-A Comp. #3 (M)
Buff-A Tablets (M)
Buff-A-Comp (M)
Buffered ASA Tablets (M)
Calciphen Tablets (M)
Cama Inlay Tablets (M)
Causalin Tablets (M)
Cefinal (M)
Cirin (M)
Codalan #1 Tablets (M)
Codalan #2 Tablets (M)
Codalan #3 Tablets (M)
Codasa 1/2 gr Tablets (M)
Codasa 1/4 gr Tablets (M)
Codasa Forte Capsules (M)
Codasa-1 Capsules (M)
Codasa-II Capsules (M)
Coralsone (M)
Coricidin D (M)
Darvon Compound Pulvules (M)
Darvon Compound-65 Pulvules
    (M)
Dasicon Capsules (M)
Decagesic (M)
Dolene Compound-65
    Capsules (M)
Dolor Plus (M)
Dolor Tablets (M)
Duragesic Tablets (M)
Dynosal Tablets (M)
Ecotrin
Ecotrin Tablets, enteric coated
Elder 65 Compound Capsules
    (M)
Emagrin Forte Tablets
    (M)Emagrin Tablets (M)
Empirin Compound Tablets (M)
Empirin Compound w/Codeine
    No. 2 Tablets (M)
Empirin Compound w/Codeine
    No. 3 Tablets (M)
Empirin Compound w/Codeine
    No. 4 Tablets (M)
Empirin Compound w/Codeine
    No. 1 Tablets (M)
Emprazil Tablets (M)
Emprazil-C Tablets (M)
Entrophen
Equagesic (M)
Histadyl and ASA Compound
    (M)
ICN 65 Compound Capsules
    (M)
Kengesin (M)

Lanorinal (M)
Lemidyne w/Codeine 15 mg
    Tablets (M)
Lemidyne w/Codeine 30 mg
    Tablets (M)
Measurin Timed-release
    Tablets
Metrogesic #2 Tablets (M)
Metrogesic #3 Tablets (M)
Mobidin Tablets (M)
Nova-Phase
Novasen
P-A-C Compound Capsules (M)
P-A-C Compound Tablets (M)
P-A-C Compound w/Codeine
    1/4 gr Tablets (M)
P-A-C Compound w/Codeine
    1/2 gr Tablets (M)
P-A-C Compound w/Codeine
    1/2 gr Capsules (M)
Pabirin Buffered (M)
Pargesic Compound 65
    Capsules (M)
Percodan (M)
Persistin Tablets (M)
Phenodyne w/Codeine 1/2 gr
    Capsules (M)
Phenodyne w/Codeine 1/4 gr
    Capsules (M)
Poxy Compound-65 Capsules
    (M)
Presalin Tablets (M)
Progesic Compound-65
    Capsules (M)
Propoxychel Compound
    Capsules (M)
Propoxyphene HCl Compound
    Capsules (M)
Repro Compound 65 Capsules
    (M)
Rhinocaps Capsules (M)
SK-65 Compound Capsules
    (M)
Sal-Adult
Sal-Infant
Salatin Capsules (M)
Salatin w/Codeine 1/2 gr
    Tablets (M)
Salatin w/Codeine 1/4 gr
    Tablets (M)
Saleto Tablets (M)
Saleto for Children Tablets (M)
Salimeph Forte Tablets (M)

ADDITIONAL BRAND NAMES

ASPIRIN continued

Salocol Tablets (M)
Salsprin Tablets (M)
St. Joseph Aspirin
Stero-Darvon (M)

Supac (M)
Synalgos Capsules (M)
Talwin Compound Caplets
Triaminic Tablets (M)

Trigesic Tablets (M)
Zactirin Compound-100
  Tablets (M)
Zactirin Tablets (M)

ATROPINE

Almezyme (M)
Amocine (M)
Antrocol (M)
Arco-Lase (M)
Atrobarbital (M)
Atromal (M)
Atropine Bufopto
Atropisol
Atrosed (M)
Bar-Cy-A-Tab (M)
Bar-Cy-Amine (M)
Bar-Don (M)
Bar-Tropin (M)
Barbella (M)
Barbeloid (M)
Barbidonna-CR (M)
Belbutal (M)
Belkaloids (M)
Belladenal (M)
Bellergal (M)
Bellergal-S (M)
Bioxatphen (M)
Briabell (M)
Briaspaz (M)
Brobella (M)
Brobella-PB (M)
Buren (M)
Butibel (M)
Cerebel (M)
Chardonna (M)

Contac (M)
Copin (M)
Dallergy (M)
Donnacin (M)
Donnagel (M)
Donnamine (M)
Donnatal #2 (M)
Donnatal (M)
Donnatal Extentabs
Donnazyme (M)
Drinus (M)
Eldonal (M)
G.B.S. (M)
HASP (M)
Haponal (M)
Harvitrate (M)
Hyatal (M)
Hybephen (M)
Hycodan (M)
Hyonal (M)
Hyonatol (M)
Hytrona (M)
Isopto Atropine
Kalmedic
Kinesed (M)
Koryza (M)
Levamine (M)
Magnased (M)
Magnox (M)
Maso-Donna (M)
Neogel with sulfa (M)

Nilspasm (M)
P & A (M)
PAMA (M)
Palbar No. 2 (M)
Peece (M)
Prydon
Renalgin (M)
Ro Trim (M)
Sedamine (M)
Sedapar (M)
Sedatabs (M)
Sedralex (M)
Seds (M)
Spabelin
Spabelin (M)
Spasaid
Spasdel (M)
Spasidon (M)
Spasloids (M)
Spasmate
Spasmolin (M)
Spasquid (M)
Spastolate (M)
Spastosed (M)
Stannitol (M)
Thitrate
Unitral
Uriseptin (M)
Urogesic (M)
Zemarine (M)

BELLADONNA

Alised (M)
Amobel (M)
Atrocap (M)
Atrosed (M)
B & O Supprettes
B-Sed (M)
Barbidonna (M)
Bebetab (M)
Belap (M)
Belatol (M)
Belbarb (M)
Bellachar (M)
Belladenal (M)
Bellafedrol (M)
Bellergal (M)
Bellkatal (M)
Bello-phen (M)

Belphen (M)
Butabar Elixir
Butibel (M)
Butibel-Zyme (M)
Chardonna (M)
Coryztime (M)
Decobel (M)
Donabarb (M)
Donnafed Jr. (M)
Donnatal (M)
Donnazyme (M)
Fitacol (M)
Gastrolic
Gelcomul (M)
Hycoff Cold Caps
Hynaldyne (M)
Kamabel (M)
Kinesed (M)
Lanothal (M)
Mallenzyme (M)

Medi-Spas (M)
Nilspasm (M)
Phebe (M)
Phen-o-bel (M)
Phenobarbital and Belladonna
  (M)
Rectacort (M)
Sedapar (M)
Sedatromine
Spabelin (M)
Spasnil (M)
U-Tract
Ultabs (M)
Urilief
Urised (M)
Wigraine (M)
Woltac (M)
Wyanoids (M)

BROMPHENIRAMINE

Brocon Tablets (M)
Bromepaph Elixir (M)

Bromepath Elixir
Bromphen

Brompheniramine Tablets
Dimetane

BROMPHENIRAMINE continued

Dimetapp Elixir (M)
Dimetapp Extentabs
Dimetapp Extentabs (M)
Disophrol Chronotabs
Drixoral Tablets
Eldatapp Tablets
Eldatapp Tablets (M)
Histatapp Elixir
Histatapp Elixir (M)

Histatapp Tablets
Histatapp Tablets (M)
Poly-Histine Expectorant (M)
Poly-Histine-Dx
Poly-Histine-Dx Capsules (M)
Ralabromophen Decongestant
  Elixir
Rynatapp Elixir (M)
Symptom 3

Taltapp Duradisk Tablets (M)
Taltapp Duradisk Tablets
Taltapp Elixir
Taltapp Elixir (M)
Tapp Elixir
Tapp Elixir (M)
Tolabromophen Decongestant
  Elixir
Veltap Elixir

BUTABARBITAL

Butabell HMB Tablets (M)
Levamine Duracap
Broncholate Capsules (M)
Brondilate Tablets (M)
Butabell HMB Elixir
Butaserpazide-25 Tablets (M)
Butaserpazide-50 Tablets (M)
Butibel Elixir (M)

Butibel Tablets (M)
Buticaps
Butisol (M)
Butizide-25 Prestabs (M)
Butizide-50 Prestabs (M)
Cyclo-Bell Tablets
Cytospaz-SR Capsules
Levamine Duracap

Levamine Tablets
Numa-Dura-Tablets
Quibron Plus Capsules
Scolate Tablets
Sidonna Tablets
Sinate-M 1/2 Strength Tablets
Sinate-M Tablets
Tedral-25 Tablets

CAFFEINE

A.P.C. Capsules (M)
A.P.C.-Demerol (M)
A.P.C. w/Codeine Tablets (M)
A.S.A. & Codeine Compound
  Tablets (M)
A.S.A. Compound (M)
Anaphen (M)
Anexsia w/Codeine Tablets (M)
Asphac-G Tablets (M)
Aspirin Compound with
  Codeine (M)
Ban-Drow 2
Buxophene Capsules (M)
Buff-A-Comp (M)
Buff-A-Comp. #3 (M)
Buffadyne Tablets (M)
Butigetic (M)
Cafacetin (M)
Cafecon
Cafergot (M)
Cafermine (M)
Cafetrate
Cefinal (M)
Cenagesic (M)
Citrated Caffeine Tablets
Coastalgesic (M)
Codalan #3 Tablets (M)
Colrex (M)
Coriforte (M)
Coryban D (M)
Coryzaid (M)

Darvon Compound (M)
Darvon Compound-65 (M)
Dasicon Capsules (M)
Dolor Tablets (M)
Duadacin (M)
Dularin (M)
Dynosal Tablets (M)
Elder 65 Compound (M)
Emagrin Tablets (M)
Empirin Compound (M)
Empirin Compound w/Codeine
  Tablets (M)
Emprazil Tablets (M)
Emprazil-C Tablets (M)
Esgic (M)
Fendol Tablets (M)
Fiorinal (M)
Hista-Derfule (M)
Histadyl Compound (M)
ICN 65 Compound (M)
Kengesin (M)
Kirkaffeine Tablets
Lanorinal (M)
Lemidyne w/Codeine Tablets
  (M)
Medache (M)
Nodaca Timed-release
  Capsules
Nodoz
Nodoz Tablets
P-A-C Compound w/Codeine
  Tablets (M)

Pargesic Compound 65 (M)
Percodan (M)
Phenodyne Tablets (M)
Phenodyne w/Codeine
  Capsules (M)
Phensal Tablets (M)
Phrenilin (M)
Poxy Compound-65 (M)
Prodolor (M)
Progesic Compound-65 (M)
Propoxychel Compound-65 (M)
Propoxyphene Compound (M)
Pyrroxate Capsules (M)
Repro Compound 65 (M)
S-A-C Tablets (M)
SK-65 Compound (M)
Salatin Capsules (M)
Salatin w/Codeine Tablets (M)
Saleto Tablets (M)
Saleto-D Capsules
Salocol Tablets (M)
Sinarest (M)
Supac (M)
Synalgos (M)
Tirend
Triaminic Tablets (M)
Triaminicin Tablets (M)
Trigesic Tablets (M)
Vivarin
Zactirin (M)

CHLORPHENIRAMINE

AL-R
Acutuss Expectorant
  w/Codeine (M)
Alermine
Alka-Seltzer Plus Tablets (M)
Allerbid Tymcaps
Aller-chlor
Allerest Tablets (M)

Allerform Tablets
Allergesic Tablets (M)
Alumadrine Tablets
Anamine Syrup (M)
Anamine T.D. Capsules (M)
Anatuss Syrup
Antagonate
Cerose Compound Capsules
Children's Allerest (M)

Chloramate
Chlor-Histine Elixir (M)
Chlor-Span-8
Chlor-Span-12
Chlor-Trimeton
Chlor-Trimeton Decongestant
  Tablets (M)
Chlor-Trimeton Expectorant
  (M)

ADDITIONAL BRAND NAMES

CHLORPHENIRAMINE continued

Chlor-Trimeton Expectorant
w/Codeine (M)
Chlor-Trimeton Repetabs
Chlorafed Liquid (M)
Chloramate Unicelles
Chlormine
Chlorpheniramine Maleate
Tablets, Timed-release
Chlorpheniramine Maleate
Capsules, Sustained-release
Chlorpheniramine Maleate
Syrup
Chlorpheniramine Maleate
Tablets
Chlortab-4
Chlortab-8
Ciramine
Ciramine T.R.
Ciriforte Capsules
Co-Tylenol Liquid (M)
Co-Tylenol Tablets (M)
Codimal Capsules
Codimal Tablets
Codimal-L.A. Cenules (M)
Coldene Cough Formula
(Children)
Colrex Capsules (M)
Colrex Compound Capsules
(M)
Colrex Compound Elixir (M)
Colrex Decongestant Tablets
(M)
Colrex Syrup (M)
Conex Liquid (M)
Conex w/Codeine Liquid (M)
Conex-DA Tablets (M)
Cophene-X Capsules (M)
Cophene-XP Syrup (M)
Coricidin "D" Decongestant
Tablets
Coricidin Cough Formula Syrup
(M)
Coricidin Demilets (M)
Coricidin Tablets
Corilin Infant Liquid
Coryban-D Capsules (M)
Coryban-D Syrup (M)
Coryzaid Chewable Tablets
Cosea-8
Cosea-12
Cosea-D Capsules (M)
Cotrol-D Tablets (M)
Covanamine Liquid (M)
Covangesic Liquid (M)
Covangesic Tablets (M)
DM Plus Cough Syrup (M)
Dallergy Syrup (M)
Deconamine Capsules (M)
Deconamine Elixir (M)
Deconamine Tablets (M)
Dehist Capsules (M)
Demazin Repetabs (M)

Demazin Syrup (M)
Dextro-Tussin Syrup (M)
Dextromal Cough Syrup (M)
Donatussin Syrup (M)
Drinus Graduals (M)
Drinus Syrup (M)
Drize M Capsules (M)
Duadacin Capsules (M)
Duphrene Tablets (M)
Expectrosed Syrup (M)
Extendryl Capsules (M)
Fedahist Expectorant (M)
Fedahist Gyrocaps (M)
Fedahist Syrup (M)
Fedahist Tablets (M)
Fedahist-C Expectorant (M)
Fernhist Tablets (M)
Ginsopan Tablets (M)
Guaiahist TT Tablets (M)
Guaiamine Capsules (M)
Guistrey Fortis Tablets (M)
Hista-Vadrin Syrup (M)
Hista-Vadrin Tablets (M)
Histabid Duracaps (M)
Histalet DM Syrup (M)
Histalet Forte Tablets (M)
Histalet Syrup (M)
Histalon
Histamic Tablets (M)
Histapan-D Capsules (M)
Histaspan
Histaspan-Plus (M)
Histex
Historal Capsules (M)
Hycoff Cold Capsules (M)
Hycoff Cough Syrup (M)
Hycoff-A Cough Syrup
Hycoff-X Expectorant (M)
Hycomine Compound Tablets
(M)
Isoclor Expectorant (M)
Isoclor Liquid (M)
Isoclor Tablets (M)
Isoclor-Timesule (M)
Koryza Tablets (M)
Kronohist Kronocaps (M)
Lanatuss Expectorant (M)
Marhist Capsules (M)
Naldecon Pediatric Drops (M)
Naldecon Pediatric Syrup (M)
Naldecon Syrup (M)
Naldecon Tablets (M)
Naldetuss Syrup (M)
Napril Plateau Capsules (M)
Narine Gyrocaps (M)
Narspan Capsules (M)
Nasahist Capsules (M)
Neo-Codenyl-M Syrup (M)
Neotep Granucaps (M)
Nilcol Elixir (M)
Nilcol Tablets (M)
Nolamine Tablets (M)

Novafed A Liquid (M)
Novahistine Elixir (M)
Novahistine Expectorant (M)
Novahistine Fortis (M)
Novahistine LP Tablets (M)
Novahistine Melet (M)
Novahistine-DH Liquid (M)
Novopheniram
Omni-Tuss Suspension (M)
P.R. Syrup
Palohist Capsules (M)
Palohist Mild Capsules (M)
Partuss T.D. Tablets
Pediacof Cough Syrup (M)
Phenacol-DM Syrup (M)
Phenate Tablets (M)
Phenetron
Polaramine Expectorant (M)
Pseudo-Hist Liquid (M)
Pyma Timed Capsules (M)
Pyrroxate Capsules
Pyrroxate Tablets
Pyrroxate w/Codeine
Capsules (M)
Quelidrine Syrup (M)
Queltuss Liquid (M)
Rhinex DM (M)
Rhinex Tablets
Rhinex Ty-Med
Rynatan Pediatric Suspension
(M)
Rynatan Tablets (M)
Rynatuss Pediatric Suspension
(M)
Rynatuss Tablets (M)
Salphenyl Capsules (M)
Salphenyl Liquid (M)
Sinarest Tablets (M)
Singlet Tablets
Sinulin Tablets (M)
Sinovan Timed Capsules (M)
T.P.I. Tablets (M)
Tedral Anti-H Tablets (M)
Teldrin Spansules
Triaminicin Chewable Tablets
(M)
Tusquelin Syrup
Tuss-Ornade Liquid (M)
Tuss-Ornade Spansules (M)
Tussar SF Cough Syrup (M)
Tussar-2 Cough Syrup (M)
Tussi-Organidin (M)
Tussi-Organidin Expectorant
(M)
U.R.I. Capsules (M)
Wesmatic Forte Tablets (M)

CODEINE

A.P.C. w/Codeine Phosphate
Tablets (M)

Aceta with Codeine Tablets (M)
Acetaco Tablets (M)

Acetaminophen with Codeine
Tablets (M)

ADDITIONAL BRAND NAMES

CODEINE continued

Acetaminophen with Codeine Elixir (M)
Actifed-C Expectorant (M)
Adatuss Cough Syrup (M)
Ambenyl Expectorant (M)
Anaphen
Arthralgen Tablets (M)
Ascriptin with Codeine (M)
Aspirin Compound with Codeine (M)
Axotal (M)
Bancap with Codeine Capsules (M)
Banesin Forte Tablets (M)
Calcidrine Syrup (M)
Capital with Codeine Suspension (M)
Capital with Codeine Tablets (M)
Cetro Cirose Liquid (M)
Cheracol Syrup (M)
Co-Xan Elixir (M)
Co-Xan Syrup (M)
Coastaldyne Tablets (M)
Coastalgesic (M)
Codalan (M)
Codalex Cough Syrup (M)
Codap Tablets (M)
Codeine Sulfate Tablets
Codimal PH (M)
Coditrate Syrup (M)
Coditrate Tablets (M)
Colrex Compound Capsules (M)
Colrex Compound Elixir (M)
Copavin Pulvules (M)
Copavin Tablets (M)
Cotussis Cough Syrup (M)
Dapase Tablets (M)
Darvocet-N 100 (M)
Dialog (M)

Dimetane Expectorant-DC (M)
Dolene AP-65 (M)
Dolor Tablets (M)
Dularin (M)
Dynosal Tablets (M)
Empirin with Codeine (M)
Empracet with Codeine Phosphate Nos. 3 & 4 (M)
Empracet with Codeine Tablets (M)
Emprazil-C Tablets (M)
Ephedrol w/Codeine Liquid (M)
Esgic (M)
FL-Tussex Cough Syrup (M)
Florinal with Codeine (M)
G-2 (M)
G-3 Capsules (M)
Gaysal (M)
Hasacode Tablets (M)
Hycotuss Expectorant (M)
Isoclor Expectorant (M)
Liquix-C Capsules (M)
Lo-Tussin Syrup (M)
Maxigesic Capsules (M)
Metrogesic Tablets (M)
Minotal (M)
Novahistine DH (M)
Novahistine Expectorant (M)
Ossonate-Plus (M)
Pavadon Elixir (M)
Pediacof (M)
Phenaphen with Codeine Capsules No. 4 (M)
Phenaphen with Codeine Capsules (M)
Phenaphen with Codeine No. 3 Capsules (M)
Phenaphen-650 with Codeine Tablets (M)
Phenergan Expectorant with Codeine (M)

Phenergan VC Expectorant with Codeine (M)
Phrenilin (M)
Poly-Histine Expectorant with Codeine (M)
Presalin Tablets (M)
Prodolor (M)
Promethazine HCl Expectorant w/Codeine (M)
Prunicodeine Liquid (M)
Robitussin A-C (M)
Robitussin A-C Liquid (M)
Rotitussin-DAC (M)
S-A-C Tablets (M)
SK-APAP with Codeine Tablets (M)
Salatin Capsules (M)
Saleto Tablets (M)
Salimeph Forte Tablets (M)
Sedapap (M)
Soma Compound with Codeine (M)
Sorbase II Cough Syrup (M)
Strascogesic Tablets (M)
Supac (M)
Sylapar Tablets (M)
Terpin Hydrate w/Codeine Elixir (M)
Triaminic Expectorant with Codeine (M)
Trigesic Tablets (M)
Tussar SF (M)
Tussar-2 (M)
Tussend Expectorant (M)
Tussi-Organidin (M)
Tylenol w/ Codeine Tablets (M)
Tylenol w/ Codeine Tablets No. 4 (M)
Tylenol with Codeine Elixir (M)
Tylenol with Codeine Tablets (M)
Wygesic Tablets (M)

DEXTROMETHORPHAN

216 DM (M)
2/C-DM Liquid (M)
Anti-Tuss DM (M)
Balminil DM (M)
Benylin DM (M)
Cheracol D (M)
Cheracol D Cough Syrup (M)
Contratuss (M)
Cosanyl DM (M)
Cosanyl DM Cough Syrup (M)
Demo-Cincol
Dextro-Tussin GG (M)
Dormethan
Dristan Cough Formula (M)

Duad Koff Balls (M)
Endotussin-NN (M)
Formula 44-D (M)
Glycotuss-dM Syrup (M)
Glycotuss-dM Tablets (M)
Lixaminol AT Liquid (M)
Novahistine DMX Liquid (M)
Nyquil (M)
Ornacol Capsules (M)
Queltuss Tablets (M)
Robitussin-CF Liquid (M)
Robitussin-DM (M)
Robitussin-DM Cough Calmers (M)

Robitussin-DM Syrup (M)
Romilar (M)
Sedatuss
Silence is Golden Cough Syrup
Silexin (M)
Silexin Cough Syrup (M)
Sorbase Cough Syrup (M)
Sorbutuss Syrup (M)
St. Joseph Cough Syrup
Trind DM (M)
Trocal (M)
Tussagesic (M)
Tussaminic (M)
Unproco Capsules (M)
Vicks Cough Syrup (M)

EPHEDRINE

Acet-Am (M)
Aladrine Tablets (M)
Amesec (M)

Amesec Enseals (M)
Amesec Pulvules (M)
Amodrine Tablets (M)

Asminyl Tablets (M)
Benadryl w/Ephedrine Capsules (M)

ADDITIONAL BRAND NAMES

EPHEDRINE continued

Broncholate (M)
Brondilate Tablets (M)
Bronkolixir (M)
Bronkaid (M)
Bronkotabs (M)
Calcidrine (M)
Calcidrine Syrup (M)
Co-Xan Elixir (M)
Coryza Brengle Capsules (M)
Dainite Tablets (M)
Duovent (M)
Ectasule III Capsules (M)
Ectasule Minus
Ephed-Organidin (M)
Ephedrine and Amytal Pulvules (M)
Ephedrine and Nembutal-25 Capsules (M)

Ephedrine and Seconal Pulvules (M)
Ephedrol w/Codeine Liquid (M)
Epragen
Iso-Asminyl Tablets (M)
Isuprel
Luasmin Capsules (M)
Lufyllin-EPG Elixir (M)
Marax (M)
Mudrane GG Elixir (M)
Mudrane GG Tablets (M)
Mudrane Tablets (M)
Numa-Dura-Tablets (M)
Nyquil (M)
Phyldrox Tablets (M)
Pyribenazmine w/Ephedrine Tablets (M)
Pyribenzamine w/Ephedrine Capsules (M)
Quadrinal (M)

Quelidrine (M)
Quibron Plus (M)
Quibron Plus Elixir (M)
Slo-Fedrin A-60 Capsules (M)
Tedfern Tablets (M)
Tedral (M)
Tedral Anti-H Tablets (M)
Tedral Elixir (M)
Tedral S.A. Tablets (M)
Tedral Suspension (M)
Tedral Tablets (M)
Tedral-25 Tablets (M)
Thalfed Tablets (M)
Theotabs Tablets (M)
Verequad (M)
Verequad Suspension (M)
Verequad Tablets (M)
Wesmatic Capsules (M)

GUAIFENESIN

2/G-DM Liquid (M)
Actol Expectorant Syrup (M)
Actol Expectorant Tablets (M)
Ambenyl Expectorant (M)
Anti-Tuss (M)
Asbron Elixir (M)
Asbron G Elixir (M)
Asbron G Inlay-Tablets (M)
Asbron Inlay Tablets (M)
Asma Syrup (M)
Brexin Capsules (M)
Broncholate Capsules (M)
Broncholate Elixir (M)
Brondecon Elixir (M)
Brondecon Tablets (M)
Bronkolizir (M)
Bronkotabs (M)
Bronkotabs Hafs (M)
Cetro Cirose Liquid (M)
Cheracol Cough Syrup (M)
Cheracol D Cough Syrup (M)
Cheracol-D (M)
Chlor-Trimeton Expectorant (M)
Co-Xan Elixir (M)
Coditrate Syrup (M)
Coditrate Tablets (M)
Conar Expectorant (M)
Dilaudid Cough Syrup (M)

Dilor-G Tablets (M)
Dilor-G Elixir (M)
Dimetane Expectorant (M)
Dristan Cough Formula (M)
Duovent Tablets (M)
Emfaseen Capsules (M)
Emfaseen Liquid (M)
Formula 44-D (M)
Glycotuss (M)
Glycotuss-DM Syrup (M)
Glycotuss-DM Tablets (M)
Glytuss
Guaiahist Tablets (M)
Hycotuss Expectorant (M)
Hytuss
Luftodil Tablets (M)
Lufyllin-GG Elixir (M)
Lufyllin-EPG Tablets (M)
Lufyllin-GG Tablets (M)
Malotuss
Mudrane GG Elixir (M)
Mudrane GG Tablets (M)
Mudrane GG-2 Tablets (M)
Neospect Tablets (M)
Neothyllin-G Elixir (M)
Neothylline-G Tablets (M)
Novahistine (M)
Novahistine DMX Liquid (M)
Queltuss Tablets (M)

Quibron Capsules (M)
Quibron Elixir (M)
Quibron Plus (M)
Quibron Plus Capsules (M)
Robitussin (M)
Robitussin A-C Liquid (M)
Robitussin-DM Cough Calmers (M)
Robitussin-DM Syrup (M)
Silexin Cough Syrup (M)
Slo-Phyllin GG (M)
Slo-Phyllin GG Capsules (M)
Slo-Phyllin-GG Syrup (M)
Sorbase Cough Syrup (M)
Sorbase II Cough Syrup (M)
Sorbutuss Syrup (M)
Special Cough Formula Liquid
Synophylate-GG (M)
Synophylate-GG Syrup (M)
Synophylate-GG Tablets (M)
Tedral Expectorant Tablets (M)
Theo-Guaia Liquid (M)
Theo-Guaia Capsules (M)
Trind (M)
Uproco Capsules (M)
Verequad Suspension (M)
Verequad Tablets (M)
Vicks Cough Syrup (M)

HYDROCHLOROTHIAZIDE

Aldactazide (M)
Aldoril-15 Tablets (M)
Aldoril-25 Tablets (M)
Apresazide (M)
Apresoline-Esidrix (M)
Butaserpazide Tablets (M)
Butizide Tablets (M)
Diuchlor H
Diupres Tablets (M)
Esidrix
Esimil Tablets (M)
Hydrid

Hydro-Aquil
HydroDIURIL
Hydropres Tablets (M)
Hydroserp Tablets (M)
Hydrotensin Tablets (M)
Hydrotensin-Plus (M)
Hydrozide-Z-50
Hyperetic
Inderide (M)
Mallopress Tablets (M)
Naquival Tablets (M)
Neo-Codema

Novohydrazide
Oretic
Oreticyl Tablets (M)
Oreticyl-25 Tablets (M)
Oreticyl-Forte Tablets (M)
Reserpazide Tablets (M)
Ser-Ap-Es Tablets (M)
Serpasil-Esidrix Tablets (M)
Singoserp-Esidrix Tablets (M)
Thiuretic
Unipres Tablets (M)
Urozide
Zide

HYOSCYAMINE

Almezyme (M)
Anaspa 3
Anaspaz PB (M)
Bar-Cy-A-Tab (M)
Bar-Cy-Amine (M)
Bar-Don (M)
Barbella (M)
Barbeloid (M)
Barbidonna-CR (M)
Belbutal (M)
Belkaloids (M)
Bellafoline (M)
Brobella-PB (M)
Buren (M)
Cystospaz
Cytospa 3 (M)
Cytospa 3-SR (M)
De Tal (M)
Donnacin (M)
Donnagel (M)
Donnamine (M)
Donnatal #2 (M)

Donnatal (M)
Donnatal Extentabs
Donnazyme (M)
Eldonal (M)
Elixiril (M)
Ergobel (M)
Floramine
Gylanphen
Haponal (M)
Hyatal (M)
Hybephen (M)
Hyonal (M)
Hyonatol (M)
Hytrona (M)
Kinesed (M)
Koryza (M)
Levamine (M)
Levsin
Levsin (M)
Maso-Donna (M)
Neoquess (M)
Nevrotase (M)

Nilspasm (M)
Omnibel (M)
Peece (M)
Renalgin (M)
Restophen
Sedajen (M)
Sedamine (M)
Sedapar (M)
Sedatromine (M)
Sedralex (M)
Seds (M)
Spabelin (M)
Spasaid (M)
Spasdel (M)
Spasloids (M)
Spasmolin (M)
Spasquid (M)
Spastolate (M)
Ultabs (M)
Uriseptin (M)
Urogesic (M)
Zemarine (M)

INSULIN

Actrapid
Globin Insulin
Insulatard
Lentard
Lente Iletin II
Lente Insulin
Mixtard

Monotard
NPH
NPH Iletin II
PZI
Protamine Zinc & Iletin II
Regular Iletin II
Regular Insulin

Semilente
Semilente Iletin
Semitard
Ultralente
Ultralente Iletin
Ultratard
Velosulin

PHENDIMETRAZINE

Adphen
Anorex
B.O.F.
Bacarate
Bontril PDM
Delcozine
Di-Ap-Trol
Elephemet
Ex-Obese
Limit
Limitite

Melfiat
Minus
Obalan
Obe-Nil TR
Obestrol
Obeval
Obezine
P.S.P.R.X. 1, 2 & 3
Phendiet
Phenzine
Plegine

Prelu-2
Reducto
Slim-Tabs
Span-RD
Statobex
Symetra
Trimstat
Trimtabs
Weightrol

PHENIRAMINE

Citra Capsules (M)
Dri-Hist No. 2 Meta Caps (M)
Fiogesic Tablets (M)
Inhistor
Poly-Histine D Capsules (M)
Poly-Histine-D Elixir (M)
Robitussin-AC (M)

Symptrol Syrup (M)
Triaminic (M)
Triaminic Juvulets (M)
Triaminic Oral Infant Drops (M)
Triaminic Syrup (M)
Triaminicin (M)
Triaminicin Tablets (M)

Triaminicol (M)
Tussagesic (M)
Tussaminic (M)
Ursinus (M)
Ursinus Inlay Tablets (M)

PHENOBARBITAL

Aminophylline-Phenobarbital
  Tablets (M)
Aminophylline-Phenobarbital
  Suppositories (M)
Anaspaz-PB Liquid (M)
Anaspaz-PB Tablets (M)
Antrocol Capsules (M)

Antrocol Tablets (M)
Asminyl Tablets (M)
Banthine w/Phenobarbital
  Tablets (M)
Bar-Tropin Tablets (M)

Barbidonna #2 Tablets (M)
Barbidonna Elixir (M)
Barbidonna G.R. Capsules (M)
Barbidonna Tablets (M)
Bardase Filmseal (M)

ADDITIONAL BRAND NAMES

PHENOBARBITAL continued

Belap Elixir (M)
Belap Tablets (M)
Belbarb #2 Tablets (M)
Belbarb Tablets (M)
Belladenal Elixir (M)
Belladenal Spacetabs (M)
Belladenal Tablets (M)
Bellergal Tablets (M)
Bellkatal Tablets (M)
Bentyl 20 Tabs
  w/Phenobarbital (M)
Bentyl Phenobarbital Capsules
  (M)
Bentyl Phenobarbital Syrup (M)
Bronkolixir (M)
Bronkotabs (M)
Bronkotabs Hafs (M)
Cantil w/Phenobarbital Tablets
  (M)
Cantil-PHB Liquid (M)
Chardonna Tablets (M)
Cyclo-Bell Tablets (M)
Dactil Phenobarbital Capsules
  (M)
Dainite-KI Tablets (M)
Daricon PB Tablets (M)
Donna-Lix Elixir (M)
Donnatal #2 Tablets (M)
Donnatal Capsules (M)
Donnatal Elixir (M)
Donnatal Extentabs (M)
Donnatal Plus Elixir (M)
Donnatal Plus Tablets (M)
Donnatal Tablets (M)
Duovent Tablets (M)
Eskabarb
Gardenal
Gastrolic Tablets (M)

HASP Elixir (M)
HASP LA Capsules (M)
HASP Ovalets (M)
Hybephen Elixir (M)
Hybephen LA Capsules (M)
Hybephen Tablets (M)
Hytrona Tablets (M)
Iso-Asminyl Tablets (M)
Isuprel Compound (M)
Kinesed Tablets (M)
Levsin PB Drops (M)
Levsin w/Phenobarbital Elixir
  (M)
Levsin w/Phenobarbital
  Tablets (M)
Luasmin Capsules (M)
Luftodil Tablets (M)
Lufyllin-EPG Elixir (M)
Lufyllin-EPG Tablets (M)
Matropinal Elixir (M)
Matropinal Forte Tablets (M)
Matropinal Tablets (M)
Mesopin PB Tablets
Mudrane GG Elixir (M)
Mudrane GG Tablets (M)
Mudrane Tablets (M)
Neospect Tablets (M)
Nova-Pheno
Oxoids Tablets
Pamine PB Drops (M)
Pamine PB Elixir (M)
Pamine PB Tablets
  Half-strength (M)

Pathilon w/Phenobarbital
  Sequels (M)
Pathilon w/Phenobarbital
  Tablets (M)
Phyldrox Tablets (M)
Pro-Banthine w/Phenobarbital
  Tablets (M)
Probital Tablets
Pyrdonnal Spansules (M)
Quadrinal Suspension (M)
Qudrinal Tablets (M)
Robinul-PH Forte Tablets (M)
Robinul-PH Tablets (M)
SK-Phenobarbital
Sedadrops
Solfoton
Spasdel Capsules (M)
Spasticol PB Tablets (M)
Spasticol S.A. Tablets (M)
Tedral Elixir (M)
Tedral Expectorant Tablets (M)
Tedral S.A. Tablets (M)
Tedral Suspension (M)
Thalfed Tablets (M)
Theotabs Tablets (M)
Tral w/Phenobarbital Filmtabs
  (M)
Tral w/Phenobarbital
  Gradumet (M)
Valpin-PB Elixir (M)
Valpin-PB Tablets (M)
Verequad Suspension (M)
Verequad Tablets (M)

PHENYLBUTAZONE

Algoverine
Azolid
Butagesic
Butazolidin

Intrabutazone
Malgesic
Nadozone
Neo-Zoline

Novobutazone
Phenbutazone

PHENYLEPHRINE

4-Way Nasal Spray (M)
4-Way Tablets (M)
Alconefrin
Alka-Seltzer Plus Tablets (M)
Anamine T.D. Capsules (M)
Bromepaph Syrup (M)
Callergy Capsules
Cenagesic Tablets (M)
Children's Allerest Tablets (M)
Chlor-Histine Elixir (M)
Chlor-Trimeton (M)
Citra Capsules (M)
Clistin D Tablets (M)
Clistin-D
Co-Tylenol (M)
Codalex Syrup (M)
Colrex Capsules (M)

Colrex Decongestant (M)
Conar Expectorant (M)
Contac (M)
Coricidin Demilets (M)
Coricidin Mist
Coryzaid Capsules (M)
Cosea-D Capsules (M)
Covanamine Liquid (M)
Covangesic Tablets (M)
Dallergy Syrup (M)
Dehist Caps (M)
Demazin (M)
Demazin Repetabs (M)
Demazin Syrup (M)
Dimetapp Syrup (M)
Dri-Hist No. Meta-Caps (M)
Drinus Graduals (M)
Drize M Capsules (M)

Duadacin Capsules (M)
Duo-Medihaler (M)
Duphrene Tablets (M)
Emagrin Forte Tablets (M)
Extendryl (M)
Extendryl Syrup (M)
Extendryl Tablets (M)
Fendol Tablets (M)
Fernhist Tablets (M)
Ginospan Tablets (M)
Guaiahist Tablets (M)
Hista-Vadrin Tablets (M)
Histabid Duracaps (M)
Histalet Forte Tablets (M)
Histalet Syrup (M)
Histaspan-D Capsules (M)
Histaspan-Plus (M)
Histatapp Elixir (M)

PHENYLEPHRINE continued

Historal No. 2 Tablets (M)
Isophrin
Koryza Tablets (M)
Marhist Capsules (M)
Naldecon (M)
Naldecon Pediatric Drops (M)
Naldecon Pediatric Syrup (M)
Naldecon Syrup (M)
Naldecon Tablets (M)
Napril Plateau Capsules (M)
Narine Cyrocaps (M)
Narspan Capsules (M)
Nasahist Capsules (M)
Neo-Mist
Neo-Synephrine
NeoSynethrin Compound
  Tablets (M)
Neotep Granucaps (M)

Novahistine Fortis Capsules
  (M)
Novahistine LP Tablets (M)
Novahistine Melet Tablets (M)
Palohist Capsules (M)
Palohist Mild Capsules (M)
Phenate Tablets (M)
Prefrin
Pyma Timed Capsules (M)
Pyracort-D
Rhinall
Rhinex Tablets (M)
Rolabromophen Decongestant
  Elixir (M)
Rolahist Elixir
Rynatan Tablets (M)
Rynatan Pediatric Suspension
  (M)

Rynatapp Elixir (M)
Salphenyl Capsules (M)
Salphenyl Liquid (M)
Singlet Tablets (M)
Sinoran Timed Capsules (M)
Super Anahist
Synasal
T.P.I. Tablets (M)
Taltapp Elixir (M)
Tapp Elixir (M)
U.R.I. Capsules (M)
Vacon
Veltar Elixir (M)

PHENYLPROPANOLAMINE

4-Way Nasal Spray (M)
Allerest (M)
Allerest Time Capsules
Alumadrine Tablets (M)
Asbron Elixir (M)
Asbron Inlay-Tablets
Axon Capsules (M)
Blu-Hist Capsules (M)
Caldecon (M)
Children's Allerest Liquid (M)
Cinsospan Tablets
Citra Capsules
Coffee-Break
Colrex Decongestant
Conex DA Tablets
Conhist Capsules (M)
Contac (M)
Control
Coricidin "D" Decongestant
  Tablets (M)
Cornex Plus Tablets (M)
Coryban-D Capsules (M)
Coryztime Capsules (M)
Covanamine Liquid
D-Sinus Capsules
Dal-Sinus Capsules
Dietac
Dimetapp (M)
Dimetapp Elixir (M)
Dimetapp Extentabs (M)
Dri-Hist Meta-Kaps (M)
Dri-Hist No. 2 Meta-Capsules
  (M)
Drinus Syrup
Eldatapp Tablets

Endecon Tablets
Fiogesic Tablets (M)
Formula 44-D
Histabid Duracaps
Histalet Forte Tablets
Histapp Elixir (M)
Histatapp Tablets
Hycomine Syrup
Koryza Tablets
Kronohist Kronocaps
MSC Triaminic Tablets (M)
Naldecon (M)
Naldecon Pediatric Drops
Naldecon Pediatric Syrup
Naldecon Syrup
Naldecon Tablet
Napril Plateau Capsules
Nasahist Capsules
Nolamine Tablets
Novahistine Elixir
Obestat
Ornacol (M)
Ornacol Capsules
Ornade (M)
Ornex (M)
Ornex Capsules
Partuss T.D. Tablets (M)
Phenate Tablets (M)
Phenylin Capsules
Poly-Histine D Capsules
Poly-Histine-D Elixir (M)
Pro-Dax 21
Propadrine
Rhindecon
Rhinex Ty-Med (M)

Rhinidrin Tablets (M)
Rhinocaps Capsules
Robitussin-CF Liquid
Rolabromophen Decongestant
  Elixir (M)
Rynatapp Elixir (M)
Salelo-D Capsules
Sinarest (M)
Sine-Aid (M)
Sine-Off (M)
Sinubid (M)
Sinulin Tablets
Sinutab (M)
Sinutab Tablets (M)
Sinutab-II
Symtrol Capsules (M)
Symtrol Syrup (M)
T.P.I. Tablets (M)
Taltapp Duradisk Tablets
Taltapp Elixir (M)
Tapp Elixir (M)
Triaminic Juvulets
Triaminic Oral Infant Drops (M)
Triaminic Syrup (M)
Triaminic Tablets
Triaminicin (M)
Triaminicin Chewable Tablets
Triaminicol (M)
Tuss-Ornade (M)
Tussagesic (M)
Tussaminic (M)
U.R.I. Capsules
Ursinus (M)
Veltap Elixir (M)
Vernata Granucaps (M)

PSEUDOEPHEDRINE

Actifed (M)
Actifed Syrup (M)
Actifed Tablets (M)
Afrinol
Anamine Syrup (M)

Brexin Capsules (M)
Bronchobid Tablets (M)
Cenafed
Chlor-Trimeton Decongestant
  Tablets (M)
Chlorafed Syrup (M)

Co-Tylenol Liquid (M)
Co-Tylenol Tablets (M)
Codimal Tablets (M)
Codimal-L.A. Cenules (M)
Cosanyl Cough Syrup (M)
Cosanyl DM-Cough Syrup (M)

ADDITIONAL BRAND NAMES

PSEUDOEPHEDRINE continued

Cotrol-D Tablets (M)
D-Feda
Deconamine Capsules (M)
Deconamine Elixir (M)
Deconamine Tablets (M)
Dimacol (M)
Disophrol (M)
Disophrol Chronotabs (M)
Disphrol Tablets (M)
Drixoral (M)
Drixoral Tablets (M)
Eltor
Emprazil (M)
Emprazil Tablets (M)
Emprazil-C Tablets (M)
Fedahist Syrup (M)
Fedahist Tablets (M)
Fedrazil (M)

Hista-Clopane Tablets (M)
Histamic Tablets (M)
Historal Capsules (M)
Isoclor (M)
Isoclor Liquid (M)
Isoclor Tablets (M)
Isoclor Timesule (M)
Naldegesic Tablets (M)
Neobid
Novafed (M)
Novafed A Liquid (M)
Novahistine DMX Liquid (M)
Phenergan Compound (M)
Phenergan Compound Tablets (M)
Phenergan-D Tablets (M)
Poly-Histine-DX (M)
Poly-Histine-DX Elixir (M)
Pseudo-Hist Liquid (M)

Pseudofrin
Redahist Gyrocaps (M)
Ro-Fedrin
Robidrine
Rondec C Drops (M)
Rondec S Syrup (M)
Rondec T Tablets (M)
Sherafed Syrup
Sherafed Tablets
Suda-Prol Syrup
Suda-Prol Tablets (M)
Sudafed
Sudahist Tablets (M)
Sudolin Tablets (M)
Sudrin
Triphed Tablets (M)
Tussend Expectorant (M)
Tussend Liquid (M)
Tussend Tablets (M)

RESERPINE

Alkarau
Bonapene
Broserpine
Butiserpazide-50 Prestabs (M)
Buytizide-25 Prestabs (M)
Demi-Regroton (M)
Diupres-250 Tablets (M)
Diupres-500 Tablets (M)
Diutensin-R Tablets (M)
Dralserp Tablets (M)
Enduronyl Tablets (M)
Enduronyl-Forte Tablets (M)
Harmonyl-D (M)
Hydroserp 25 mg Tablets (M)
Hydroserp 50 mg Tablets (M)
Hydrotensin-50 Tablets (M)
Mallopress Tablets (M)

Metatensin (M)
Naquival Tablets (M)
Oreticyl-25 Tablets (M)
Oreticyl-50 Tablets (M)
Oreticyl-Forte Tablets (M)
Rau-Sed
Rauraine
Rautrax N Tablets (M)
Rautrax Tablets (M)
Rauzide (M)
Regroton (M)
Renese-R Tablets (M)
Reserpazide-25 Tablets (M)
Reserpazide-50 Tablets (M)
Reserpoid
Ruhexatal w/Reserpine Tablets (M)
SK-Reserpine

Salutensin Tablets (M)
Sandril
Ser-Ap-Es (M)
Serpalan
Serpanray
Serpasil
Serpasil-Apresoline Tablets (M)
Serpasil-Esidrix # 1 Tablets (M)
Serpasil-Esidrix #2 Tablets (M)
Serpate
Singoserp-Eisdrix #1 Tablets (M)
Singoserp-Esidrix #2 Tablets (M)
T-Serp
Unipres Tablets (M)

SCOPOLAMINE (HYOSCINE)

Allerspan
Almezyme (M)
Aluscop
Bar-Cy-A-Tab (M)
Bar-Cy-Amine (M)
Bar-Don (M)
Barbella (M)
Barbeloid (M)
Barbidonna-CR (M)
Belbutal (M)
Belkaloids (M)
Bobid
Brobella-PB (M)
Buren (M)
Cenahist
Chlorpel
Conalsyn
Dallergy
Donnacin (M)
Donnagel (M)
Donnamine (M)
Donnatal #2 (M)
Donnatal (M)

Donnatal Extentabs
Donnazyme (M)
Drinus
Drize
Eldonal (M)
Eulcin
Extendryl
Haponal (M)
Histaspan-D
Historal
Hyatal (M)
Hybephen (M)
Hydrochol-Plus
Hyonal (M)
Hyonatol (M)
Hytrona (M)
Kinesed (M)
Kleer
Kleer-Tuss
Koryza (M)
Levamine (M)
MSC Triaminic
Maso-Donna (M)

Methnite
Narine
Narspan
Nilspasm (M)
Omnibel (M)
Pamine
Pamine PB
Paraspan
Renalgin (M)
Sanhist
Scoline
Scoline-Amobarbital
Scotnord
Sedamine (M)
Sedapar (M)
Sedralex (M)
Seds (M)
Sinaprel
Sinodec
Sinoran
Sinunil
Spabelin (M)
Spasdel (M)

SCOPOLAMINE (HYOSCINE) continued

Spasloids (M)
Spasmid
Spasmolin (M)
Spasquid (M)

Spastolate (M)
Symptrol
Trisohist
Uriseptin (M)

Urogesic (M)
Vonodonnal (M)
Zemarine (M)

TETRACYCLINE

Achromycin
Achromycin V
Achrostatin V (M)
Bicycline
Bio-Tetra
Bristacycline
Cefacycline
Centet
Comycin (M)
Cyclopar
Desamycin
Fed-Mycin
G-Mycin
Kesso-Tetra
Lemtrex
Maytrex-BID
Medicycline

Muracine
Mysteclin F (M)
Neo-Tetrine
Nor-Tet
Novotetra
Paltet
Panmycin
Piracaps
Q'Dtet
Retet
Retet-S
Ro-Cycline
Robitet
SK-Tetracycline
Sarocyclin
Scotrex
Sumycin

T-125
T-250
T-Caps
Tet-Cy
Tetet
Tetra-Co
Tetrachel
Tetracyn
Tetracyrine
Tetralean
Tetram
Tetramax
Tetrastatin (M)
Tetrex
Trexin

THEOPHYLLINE

Accurbron
Aerolate
Amesec Enseals (M)
Amesec Pulvules (M)
Aminophylline and Amytal
    Pulvules (M)
Aminophylline-Phenobarbital
    Tablets (M)
Aminophylline-Phenobarbital
    Suppositories (M)
Amodrine Tablets (M)
Asbron Elixir (M)
Asbron G Elixir (M)
Asbron G Inlay-Tabs (M)
Asbron Inlay-Tabs (M)
Asma Syrup (M)
Asminyl Tablets (M)
Asthmophylline
Bronchobid Duracaps (M)
Broncholate Capsules (M)
Broncholate Elixir (M)
Brondecon Elixir (M)
Brondecon Tablets (M)
Brondilate Tablets (M)
Bronkodyl
Bronkolixir (M)
Bronkotabs (M)
Bronkotabs Hafs (M)
Choledyl
Co-Xan Elixir (M)
Dilor G Liquid (M)
Dilor G Tablets (M)
Duovent Tablets (M)
Elixicon
Elixophyllin

Emfaseem Capsules (M)
Emfaseem Liquid (M)
G-Bron Elixir
Iso-Asminyl Tablets (M)
Isuprel Compound Elixir
Klophyllin Tablets
Lixaminol AT Liquid (M)
Luasmin Capsules (M)
Luftodil Tablets (M)
Lufyllin-EPG Elixir (M)
Lufyllin-EPG Tablets (M)
Lufyllin-GG Elixir (M)
Lufyllin-GG Tablets (M)
Marax DF Syrup (M)
Marax Syrup (M)
Marax Tablets (M)
Mudrane GG Elixir (M)
Mudrane GG Tablets (M)
Mudrane GG-2 Tablets (M)
Mudrane Tablets (M)
Mudrane-2 Tablets (M)
Neospect Tablets (M)
Neothylline-G Elixir (M)
Neothylline-G Tablets (M)
Numa-Dura-Tabs (M)
Orthoxine & Aminophylline
    Capsules (M)
Phenylin Capsulets (M)
Phyldrox Tablets (M)
Physpan
Quadrinal Suspension (M)
Quadrinal Tablets (M)
Quibron Capsules (M)
Quibron Elixir (M)

Quibron Plus Capsules (M)
Quibron Plus Elixir (M)
Slo-Phyllin GG (M)
Slo-Phyllin-GG Syrup (M)
Slophyllin
Somophyllin-T
Sudolin Tablets (M)
Synophylate-GG (M)
Synophylate-GG Syrup (M)
Tedfern Tablets (M)
Tedral Anti-H Tablets (M)
Tedral Elixir (M)
Tedral Expectorant Tablets (M)
Tedral S.A. Tablets (M)
Tedral Suspension (M)
Tedral Tablets (M)
Tedral-25 Tablets (M)
Thalfed Tablets (M)
Theo-Dur
Theo-Guaia Capsules (M)
Theo-Guaia Liquid (M)
Theo-Nar 100 Tablets (M)
Theo-Organidin Elixir (M)
Theobid
Theoclear
Theolair
Theophyl
Theospan
Theotabs Tablets (M)
Verequad Suspension (M)
Verequad Tablets (M)

Additional Drug Interactions

The following lists of drugs and their interactions with other drugs are continuations of lists found in the alphabetized drug charts beginning on page 18. These lists are alphabetized by generic name, shown in large capital letters. Only those lists too long for the drug charts are included in this section. For complete information about any generic drug, see the alphabetized charts.

GENERIC NAME OR DRUG CLASS	COMBINED EFFECT	GENERIC NAME OR DRUG CLASS	COMBINED EFFECT

ACETOHEXAMIDE

Isoniazid	Decreased acetohexamide effect.	Probenecid	Increased acetohexamide effect.
MAO inhibitors	Increased acetohexamide effect.	Pyrazinamide	Decreased acetohexamide effect.
Oxyphenbutazone	Increased acetohexamide effect.	Sulfa drugs	Increased acetohexamide effect.
Phenylbutazone	Increased acetohexamide effect.	Sulfaphenazole	Increased acetohexamide effect.
Phenyramidol	Increased acetohexamide effect.	Thyroid hormones	Decreased acetohexamide effect.

ALLOPURINOL

Metolazone	Decreased allopurinol effect.	Probenecid	Increased allopurinol effect.

AMOBARBITAL

MAO inhibitors	Increased amobarbital effect.	Sedatives	Dangerous sedation. Avoid.
Mind-altering drugs	Dangerous sedation. Avoid.	Sleep inducers	Dangerous sedation. Avoid.
Narcotics	Dangerous sedation. Avoid.	Tranquilizers	Dangerous sedation. Avoid.
Pain relievers	Dangerous sedation. Avoid.	Valproic acid	Increased amobarbital effect.

ANISINDIONE

Carbamazepine	Decreased anisindione effect.	Cimetidine	Increased anisindione effect.
Chloral hydrate	Unpredictable increased or decreased anticoagulant effect.	Clofibrate	Unpredictable increased or decreased anisindione effect.
Chloramphenicol	Increased anisindione effect.	Contraceptives (oral)	Unpredictable increased or decreased anisindione effect.
Chlorpromazine	Decreased anisindione effect.		
Cholestyramine	Unpredictable increased or decreased anisindione effect.	Cortisone drugs	Unpredictable increased or decreased anisindione effect.

GENERIC NAME OR DRUG CLASS	COMBINED EFFECT	GENERIC NAME OR DRUG CLASS	COMBINED EFFECT

ANISINDIONE continued

GENERIC NAME OR DRUG CLASS	COMBINED EFFECT	GENERIC NAME OR DRUG CLASS	COMBINED EFFECT
Digitalis preparations	Decreased anisindione effect.	Nalidixic acid	Increased anisindione effect.
Disulfiram	Increased anisindione effect.	Nortriptyline	Increased anisindione effect.
Estrogens	Decreased anisindione effect.	Oxyphenbutazone	Increased anisindione effect.
Ethacrynic acid	Increased anisindione effect.	Para-aminosalicylic acid (PAS)	Increased anisindione effect.
Ethchlorvynol	Decreased anisindione effect.	Phenelzine	Increased anisindione effect.
Furosemide	Decreased anisindione effect.	Phenylbutazone	Unpredictable increased or decreased anisindione effect.
Glucagon	Increased anisindione effect.	Phenylpropanolamine	Decreased anticoagulant effect.
Glutethimide	Decreased anisindione effect.	Phenyramidol	Increased anisindione effect.
Griseofulvin	Decreased anisindione effect.	Probenecid	Increased anisindione effect.
Guanethidine	Increased anisindione effect.	Propoxyphene	Increased anisindione effect.
Haloperidol	Decreased anisindione effect.	Propylthiouracil	Increased anisindione effect.
Hydroxyzine	Increased anisindione effect.	Quinidine	Increased anisindione effect.
Indomethacin	Increased anisindione effect.	Rauwolfia alkaloids	Unpredictable increased or decreased anisindione effect.
Insulin	Increased insulin effect.		
Isocarboxazid	Increased anisindione effect.	Salicylates (including aspirin)	Increased anisindione effect.
Isoniazid	Increased anisindione effect.	Sulfa drugs	Increased anisindione effect.
Mefenamic acid	Increased anisindione effect.	Sulfinpyrazone	Increased anisindione effect.
Meprobamate	Decreased anisindione effect.	Tetracyclines	Increased anisindione effect.
Mercaptopurine	Increased anisindione effect.	Thyroid hormones	Increased anisindione effect.
Methyldopa	Increased anisindione effect.	Trimethoprim	Increased anisindione effect.
Methylphenidate	Increased anisindione effect.	Vitamin C (large doses)	Decreased anisindione effect.
Metronidazole	Increased anisindione effect.	Vitamin E (large doses)	Increased anisindione effect.

ASPIRIN

GENERIC NAME OR DRUG CLASS	COMBINED EFFECT	GENERIC NAME OR DRUG CLASS	COMBINED EFFECT
Probenecid	Decreased probenecid effect.	Spironolactone	Decreased spironolactone effect.
Propranolol	Decreased aspirin effect.	Sulfinpyrazone	Decreased sulfinpyrazone effect.
Rauwolfia alkaloids	Decreased aspirin effect.	Vitamin C (large doses)	Possible aspirin toxicity.
Salicylates (other)	Likely aspirin toxicity.		

ADDITIONAL DRUG INTERACTIONS

GENERIC NAME OR DRUG CLASS	COMBINED EFFECT	GENERIC NAME OR DRUG CLASS	COMBINED EFFECT

BETAMETHASONE

Ephedrine	Decreased betamethasone effect.	Insulin	Decreased insulin effect.
Estrogens	Increased betamethasone effect.	Isoniazid	Decreased isoniazid effect.
Ethacrynic acid	Potassium depletion.	Oxyphenbutazone	Possible ulcers.
Furosemide	Potassium depletion.	Phenylbutazone	Possible ulcers.
Glutethimide	Decreased betamethasone effect.	Rifampin	Decreased betamethasone effect.
Indomethacin	Increased betamethasone effect.	Sympathomimetics	Possible glaucoma.

BUTABARBITAL

MAO inhibitors	Increased butabarbital effect.	Sedatives	Dangerous sedation. Avoid.
Mind-altering drugs	Dangerous sedation. Avoid.	Sleep inducers	Dangerous sedation. Avoid.
Narcotics	Dangerous sedation. Avoid.	Tranquilizers	Dangerous sedation. Avoid.
Pain relievers	Dangerous sedation. Avoid.	Valproic acid	Increased butabarbital effect.

CALCIUM CARBONATE

Quinidine	Increased quinidine effect.	Tetracyclines	Decreased tetracycline effect.
Salicylates	Increased salicylate effect.	Vitamins A and C	Decreased vitamin effect.
Sulfa drugs	Decreased sulfa effect.		

CHLORPROPAMIDE

Isoniazid	Decreased chlorpropamide effect.	Pyrazinamide	Decreased chlorpropamide effect.
MAO inhibitors	Increased chlorpropamide effect.	Sulfa drugs	Increased chlorpropamide effect.
Oxyphenbutazone	Increased chlorpropamide effect.	Sulfaphenazole	Increased chlorpropamide effect.
Phenylbutazone	Increased chlorpropamide effect.	Thyroid hormones	Decreased chlorpropamide effect.
Phenyramidol	Increased chlorpropamide effect.		
Probenecid	Increased chlorpropamide effect.		

CHLORPROTHIXENE

Narcotics	Increased chlorprothixene effect. Excessive sedation.	Sleep inducers	Increased chlorprothixene effect. Excessive sedation.
Sedatives	Increased chlorprothixene effect. Excessive sedation.	Tranquilizers	Increased chlorprothixene effect. Excessive sedation.

ADDITIONAL DRUG INTERACTIONS

GENERIC NAME OR DRUG CLASS	COMBINED EFFECT	GENERIC NAME OR DRUG CLASS	COMBINED EFFECT

CIMETIDINE

Digitalis preparations	Increased digitalis effect.	Quinidine	Increased quinidine effect.
Penicillins	Increased penicillin effect.	Theophylline	Increased theophylline effect.
Propranolol	May increase propranolol effect.		

CONTRACEPTIVES (ORAL)

Phenothiazines	Increased phenothiazine effect.	Tetracyclines	Decreased contraceptive effect.
Rifampin	Decreased contraceptive effect.		

CORTISONE

Ephedrine	Decreased cortisone effect.	Insulin	Decreased insulin effect.
Estrogens	Increased cortisone effect.	Isoniazid	Decreased isoniazid effect.
Ethacrynic acid	Potassium depletion.	Oxyphenbutazone	Possible ulcers.
Furosemide	Potassium depletion.	Phenylbutazone	Possible ulcers.
Glutethimide	Decreased cortisone effect.	Rifampin	Decreased cortisone effect.
Indomethacin	Increased cortisone effect.	Sympathomimetics	Possible glaucoma.

DESERPIDINE

Narcotics	Increased narcotic effect.	Sedatives	Increased sedative effect.
Phenothiazines	Increased effect of deserpidine. Excessive sedation.	Sleep inducers	Increased sleep-inducer effect.
Quinidine	Irregular heartbeat.	Tranquilizers	Increased tranquilizer effect.

DEXAMETHASONE

Diuretics (thiazide)	Potassium depletion.	Insulin	Decreased insulin effect.
Ephedrine	Decreased dexamethasone effect.	Isoniazid	Decreased isoniazid effect.
Estrogens	Increased dexamethasone effect.	Oxyphenbutazone	Possible ulcers.
Ethacrynic acid	Potassium depletion.	Phenylbutazone	Possible ulcers.
Furosemide	Potassium depletion.	Rifampin	Decreased dexamethasone effect.
Glutethimide	Decreased dexamethasone effect.	Sympathomimetics	Possible glaucoma.
Indomethacin	Increased dexamethasone effect.		

ADDITIONAL DRUG INTERACTIONS

GENERIC NAME OR DRUG CLASS	COMBINED EFFECT	GENERIC NAME OR DRUG CLASS	COMBINED EFFECT

DICUMAROL

GENERIC NAME OR DRUG CLASS	COMBINED EFFECT	GENERIC NAME OR DRUG CLASS	COMBINED EFFECT
Chloral hydrate	Unpredictable increased or decreased anticoagulant effect.	Mefenamic acid	Increased dicumarol effect.
Chloramphenicol	Increased dicumarol effect.	Meprobamate	Decreased dicumarol effect.
Chlorpromazine	Decreased dicumarol effect.	Mercaptopurine	Increased dicumarol effect.
Cholestyramine	Unpredictable increased or decreased dicumarol effect.	Methyldopa	Increased dicumarol effect.
Cimetidine	Increased dicumarol effect.	Methylphenidate	Increased dicumarol effect.
Clofibrate	Unpredictable increased or decreased dicumarol effect.	Metronidazole	Increased dicumarol effect.
Contraceptives (oral)	Unpredictable increased or decreased dicumarol effect.	Nalidixic acid	Increased dicumarol effect.
Cortisone drugs	Unpredictable increased or decreased dicumarol effect.	Nortriptyline	Increased dicumarol effect.
Digitalis preparations	Decreased dicumarol effect.	Oxyphenbutazone	Increased dicumarol effect.
Disulfiram	Increased dicumarol effect.	Para-aminosalicylic acid (PAS)	Increased dicumarol effect.
Estrogens	Decreased dicumarol effect.	Phenelzine	Increased dicumarol effect.
Ethacrynic acid	Increased dicumarol effect.	Phenylbutazone	Unpredictable increased or decreased dicumarol effect.
Ethchlorvynol	Decreased dicumarol effect.	Phenylpropanolamine	Decreased anticoagulant effect.
Furosemide	Decreased dicumarol effect.	Phenyramidol	Increased dicumarol effect.
Glucagon	Increased dicumarol effect.	Probenecid	Increased dicumarol effect.
Glutethimide	Decreased dicumarol effect.	Propoxyphene	Increased dicumarol effect.
Griseofulvin	Decreased dicumarol effect.	Propylthiouracil	Increased dicumarol effect.
Guanethidine	Increased dicumarol effect.	Quinidine	Increased dicumarol effect.
Haloperidol	Decreased dicumarol effect.	Rauwolfia alkaloids	Unpredictable increased or decreased dicumarol effect.
Hydroxyzine	Increased dicumarol effect.	Salicylates (including aspirin)	Increased dicumarol effect.
Indomethacin	Increased dicumarol effect.	Sulfinpyrazone	Increased dicumarol effect.
Insulin	Increased insulin effect.	Sulfa drugs	Increased dicumarol effect.
Isocarboxazid	Increased dicumarol effect.	Tetracyclines	Increased dicumarol effect.
Isoniazid	Increased dicumarol effect.	Thyroid hormones	Increased dicumarol effect.
		Trimethoprim	Increased dicumarol effect.

ADDITIONAL DRUG INTERACTIONS

GENERIC NAME OR DRUG CLASS	COMBINED EFFECT	GENERIC NAME OR DRUG CLASS	COMBINED EFFECT

DICUMAROL continued

Vitamin C (large doses)	Decreased dicumarol effect.	Vitamin E (large doses)	Increased dicumarol effect.

ETHOTOIN

Griseofulvin	Increased griseofulvin effect.	Phenothiazines	Increased ethotoin effect.
		Phenylbutazone	Increased ethotoin effect.
Isoniazid	Increased ethotoin effect.	Propranolol	Increased propranolol effect.
Methadone	Decreased methadone effect.	Quinidine	Increased quinidine effect.
Methotrexate	Increased methotrexate effect.		
		Sedatives	Increased sedative effect.
Methylphenidate	Increased ethotoin effect.	Sulfa drugs	Increased ethotoin effect.
Oxyphenbutazone	Increased ethotoin effect.	Theophylline	Reduced anticonvulsant effect.
Para-aminosalicylic acid (PAS)	Increased ethotoin effect.		

FLUPREDNISOLONE

Diuretics (thiazide)	Potassium depletion.	Indomethacin	Increased fluprednisolone effect.
Ephedrine	Decreased fluprednisolone effect.	Insulin	Decreased insulin effect.
Estrogens	Increased fluprednisolone effect.	Isoniazid	Decreased isoniazid effect.
Ethacrynic acid	Potassium depletion.	Oxyphenbutazone	Possible ulcers.
Furosemide	Potassium depletion.	Phenylbutazone	Possible ulcers.
Glutethimide	Decreased fluprednisolone effect.	Rifampin	Decreased fluprednisolone effect.
		Sympathomimetics	Possible glaucoma.

FUROSEMIDE

Probenecid	Decreased probenecid effect.	Sedatives	Increased furosemide effect.
Salicylates (including aspirin)	Dangerous salicylate retention.		

HEXOBARBITAL

MAO inhibitors	Increased hexobarbital effect.	Sedatives	Dangerous sedation. Avoid.
Mind-altering drugs	Dangerous sedation. Avoid	Sleep inducers	Dangerous sedation. Avoid.
Narcotics	Dangerous sedation. Avoid.	Tranquilizers	Dangerous sedation. Avoid.
Pain relievers	Dangerous sedation. Avoid.	Valproic acid	Increased hexobarbital effect.

ADDITIONAL DRUG INTERACTIONS

GENERIC NAME OR DRUG CLASS	COMBINED EFFECT	GENERIC NAME OR DRUG CLASS	COMBINED EFFECT

HYDROCORTISONE (CORTISOL)

Ephedrine	Decreased hydrocortisone effect.	Insulin	Decreased insulin effect.
Estrogens	Increased hydrocortisone effect.	Isoniazid	Decreased isoniazid effect.
Ethacrynic acid	Potassium depletion.	Oxyphenbutazone	Possible ulcers.
Furosemide	Potassium depletion.	Phenylbutazone	Possible ulcers.
Glutethimide	Decreased hydrocortisone effect.	Rifampin	Decreased hydrocortisone effect.
Indomethacin	Increased hydrocortisone effect.	Sympathomimetics	Possible glaucoma.

INSULIN

Tetracyclines	Increased insulin effect.	Thyroid hormones	Decreased insulin effect.

ISOCARBOXAZID

Methyldopa	Blood-pressure rise to life-threatening level.	Sedatives	Excess sedation.
		Sleep inducers	Excess sedation.
Narcotics	Sudden, severe blood-pressure rise.	Sympathomimetics	Blood-pressure rise to life-threatening level.
Rauwolfia alkaloids	Blood-pressure rise to life-threatening level.	Tranquilizers	Excess sedation.

MAGNESIUM CARBONATE

Sulfa drugs	Decreased sulfa effect.	Vitamins A and C	Decreased vitamin effect.
Tetracyclines	Decreased tetracycline effect.	Vitamin D	Too much calcium in blood.

MAGNESIUM HYDROXIDE

Sulfa drugs	Decreased sulfa effect.	Vitamins A and C	Decreased vitamin effect.
Tetracyclines	Decreased tetracycline effect.	Vitamin D	Too much calcium in blood.

MAGNESIUM TRISILICATE

Sulfa drugs	Decreased sulfa effect.	Vitamins A and C	Decreased vitamin effect.
Tetracyclines	Decreased tetracycline effect.	Vitamin D	Too much calcium in blood.

MEPHENYTOIN

Isoniazid	Increased mephenytoin effect.	Para-aminosalicylic acid (PAS)	Increased mephenytoin effect.
Methadone	Decreased methadone effect.	Phenothiazines	Increased mephenytoin effect.
Methotrexate	Increased methotrexate effect.	Phenylbutazone	Increased mephenytoin effect.
Methylphenidate	Increased mephenytoin effect.	Propranolol	Increased propranolol effect.
Oxyphenbutazone	Increased mephenytoin effect.	Quinidine	Increased quinidine effect.

ADDITIONAL DRUG INTERACTIONS

GENERIC NAME OR DRUG CLASS	COMBINED EFFECT	GENERIC NAME OR DRUG CLASS	COMBINED EFFECT

MEPHENYTOIN continued

GENERIC NAME OR DRUG CLASS	COMBINED EFFECT	GENERIC NAME OR DRUG CLASS	COMBINED EFFECT
Sedatives	Increased sedative effect.	Theophylline	Reduced anticonvulsant effect.
Sulfa drugs	Increased mephenytoin effect.		

MEPHOBARBITAL

GENERIC NAME OR DRUG CLASS	COMBINED EFFECT	GENERIC NAME OR DRUG CLASS	COMBINED EFFECT
MAO inhibitors	Increased mephobarbital effect.	Sedatives	Dangerous sedation. Avoid.
Mind-altering drugs	Dangerous sedation. Avoid.	Sleep inducers	Dangerous sedation. Avoid.
Narcotics	Dangerous sedation. Avoid.	Tranquilizers	Dangerous sedation. Avoid.
Pain relievers	Dangerous sedation. Avoid.	Valproic acid	Increased mephobarbital effect.

METHARBITAL

GENERIC NAME OR DRUG CLASS	COMBINED EFFECT	GENERIC NAME OR DRUG CLASS	COMBINED EFFECT
MAO inhibitors	Increased metharbital effect.	Sedatives	Dangerous sedation. Avoid.
Mind-altering drugs	Dangerous sedation. Avoid.	Sleep inducers	Dangerous sedation. Avoid.
Narcotics	Dangerous sedation. Avoid.	Tranquilizers	Dangerous sedation. Avoid.
Pain relievers	Dangerous sedation. Avoid.	Valproic acid	Increased metharbital effect.

METHYLPREDNISOLONE

GENERIC NAME OR DRUG CLASS	COMBINED EFFECT	GENERIC NAME OR DRUG CLASS	COMBINED EFFECT
Contraceptives (oral)	Increased methylprednisolone effect.	Glutethimide	Decreased methylprednisolone effect.
Digitalis preparations	Dangerous potassium depletion. Possible digitalis toxicity.	Indomethacin	Increased methylprednisolone effect.
Diuretics (thiazide)	Potassium depletion.	Insulin	Decreased insulin effect.
Ephedrine	Decreased methylprednisolone effect.	Isoniazid	Decreased isoniazid effect.
		Oxyphenbutazone	Possible ulcers.
		Phenylbutazone	Possible ulcers.
Estrogens	Increased methylprednisolone effect.	Rifampin	Decreased methylprednisolone effect.
Ethacrynic acid	Potassium depletion.		
Furosemide	Potassium depletion.	Sympathomimetics	Possible glaucoma.

PARAMETHASONE

GENERIC NAME OR DRUG CLASS	COMBINED EFFECT	GENERIC NAME OR DRUG CLASS	COMBINED EFFECT
Diuretics (thiazide)	Potassium depletion.	Glutethimide	Decreased paramethasone effect.
Ephedrine	Decreased paramethasone effect.	Indomethacin	Increased paramethasone effect.
Estrogens	Increased paramethasone effect.	Insulin	Decreased insulin effect.
		Isoniazid	Decreased isoniazid effect.
Ethacrynic acid	Potassium depletion.		
Furosemide	Potassium depletion.	Oxyphenbutazone	Possible ulcers.

ADDITIONAL DRUG INTERACTIONS

GENERIC NAME OR DRUG CLASS	COMBINED EFFECT	GENERIC NAME OR DRUG CLASS	COMBINED EFFECT

PARAMETHASONE continued

Phenylbutazone	Possible ulcers.	Sympathomimetics	Possible glaucoma.
Rifampin	Decreased paramethasone effect.		

PARGYLINE

Methyldopa	Blood-pressure rise to life-threatening level.	Sedatives	Excess sedation.
		Sleep inducers	Excess sedation.
Narcotics	Sudden, severe blood-pressure rise.	Sympathomimetics	Blood-pressure rise to life-threatening level.
Rauwolfia alkaloids	Blood-pressure rise to life-threatening level.	Tranquilizers	Excess sedation.

PENTOBARBITAL

MAO inhibitors	Increased pentobarbital effect.	Sedatives	Dangerous sedation. Avoid.
Mind-altering drugs	Dangerous sedation. Avoid.	Sleep inducers	Dangerous sedation. Avoid.
Narcotics	Dangerous sedation. Avoid.	Tranquilizers	Dangerous sedation. Avoid.
Pain relievers	Dangerous sedation. Avoid.	Valproic acid	Increased pentobarbital effect.

PHENELZINE

Methyldopa	Blood-pressure rise to life-threatening level.	Sedatives	Excess sedation.
		Sleep inducers	Excess sedation.
Narcotics	Sudden, severe blood-pressure rise.	Sympathomimetics	Blood-pressure rise to life-threatening level.
Rauwolfia alkaloids	Blood-pressure rise to life-threatening level.	Tranquilizers	Excess sedation.

PHENOBARBITAL

MAO inhibitors	Increased phenobarbital effect.	Sedatives	Dangerous sedation. Avoid.
Mind-altering drugs	Dangerous sedation. Avoid.	Sleep inducers	Dangerous sedation. Avoid.
Narcotics	Dangerous sedation. Avoid.	Tranquilizers	Dangerous sedation. Avoid.
Pain relievers	Dangerous sedation. Avoid.	Valproic acid	Increased phenobarbital effect.

PHENPROCOUMON

Benzodiazepines	Unpredictable increased or decreased anticoagulant effect.	Chlorpromazine	Decreased phenprocoumon effect.
Carbamazepine	Decreased phenprocoumon effect.	Cholestyramine	Unpredictable increased or decreased phenprocoumon effect.
Chloral hydrate	Unpredictable increased or decreased anticoagulant effect.	Cimetidine	Increased phenprocoumon effect.
Chloramphenicol	Increased phenprocoumon effect.	Clofibrate	Unpredictable increased or decreased phenprocoumon effect.

GENERIC NAME OR DRUG CLASS	COMBINED EFFECT	GENERIC NAME OR DRUG CLASS	COMBINED EFFECT

PHENPROCOUMON continued

GENERIC NAME OR DRUG CLASS	COMBINED EFFECT	GENERIC NAME OR DRUG CLASS	COMBINED EFFECT
Contraceptives (oral)	Unpredictable increased or decreased phenprocoumon effect.	Nalidixic acid	Increased phenprocoumon effect.
Cortisone drugs	Unpredictable increased or decreased phenprocoumon effect.	Nortriptyline	Increased phenprocoumon effect.
		Oxyphenbutazone	Increased phenprocoumon effect.
Digitalis preparations	Decreased phenprocoumon effect.	Para-aminosalicylic acid (PAS)	Increased phenprocoumon effect.
Disulfiram	Increased phenprocoumon effect.	Phenelzine	Increased phenprocoumon effect.
Estrogens	Decreased phenprocoumon effect.	Phenylbutazone	Unpredictable increased or decreased phenprocoumon effect.
Ethacrynic acid	Increased phenprocoumon effect.	Phenylpropanolamine	Decreased anticoagulant effect.
Ethchlorvynol	Decreased phenprocoumon effect.	Phenyramidol	Increased phenprocoumon effect.
Furosemide	Decreased phenprocoumon effect.	Probenecid	Increased phenprocoumon effect.
Glucagon	Increased phenprocoumon effect.	Propoxyphene	Increased phenprocoumon effect.
Glutethimide	Decreased phenprocoumon effect.	Propylthiouracil	Increased phenprocoumon effect.
Griseofulvin	Decreased phenprocoumon effect.	Quinidine	Increased phenprocoumon effect.
Guanethidine	Increased phenprocoumon effect.	Rauwolfia alkaloids	Unpredictable increased or decreased phenprocoumon effect.
Haloperidol	Decreased phenprocoumon effect.	Salicylates (including aspirin)	Increased phenprocoumon effect.
Hydroxyzine	Increased phenprocoumon effect.		
Indomethacin	Increased phenprocoumon effect.	Sulfa drugs	Increased phenprocoumon effect.
Insulin	Increased insulin effect.	Sulfinpyrazone	Increased phenprocoumon effect.
Isocarboxazid	Increased phenprocoumon effect.	Tetracyclines	Increased phenprocoumon effect.
Isoniazid	Increased phenprocoumon effect.	Thyroid hormones	Increased phenprocoumon effect.
Mefenamic acid	Increased phenprocoumon effect.	Trimethoprim	Increased phenprocoumon effect.
Meprobamate	Decreased phenprocoumon effect.	Vitamin C (large doses)	Decreased phenprocoumon effect.
Mercaptopurine	Increased phenprocoumon effect.	Vitamin E (large doses)	Increased phenprocoumon effect.
Methyldopa	Increased phenprocoumon effect.		
Methylphenidate	Increased phenprocoumon effect.		
Metronidazole	Increased phenprocoumon effect.		

ADDITIONAL DRUG INTERACTIONS

GENERIC NAME OR DRUG CLASS	COMBINED EFFECT	GENERIC NAME OR DRUG CLASS	COMBINED EFFECT

PHENYTOIN

Griseofulvin	Increased griseofulvin effect.	Phenothiazines	Increased phenytoin effect.
Isoniazid	Increased phenytoin effect.	Phenylbutazone	Increased phenytoin effect.
Methadone	Decreased methadone effect.	Propranolol	Increased propranolol effect.
Methotrexate	Increased methotrexate effect.	Quinidine	Increased quinidine effect.
Methylphenidate	Increased phenytoin effect.	Sedatives	Increased sedative effect.
Oxyphenbutazone	Increased phenytoin effect.	Sulfa drugs	Increased phenytoin effect.
Para-aminosalicylic acid (PAS)	Increased phenytoin effect.	Theophylline	Reduced anticonvulsant effect.

PREDNISOLONE

Ephedrine	Decreased prednisolone effect.	Insulin	Decreased insulin effect.
Estrogens	Increased prednisolone effect.	Isoniazid	Decreased isoniazid effect.
Ethacrynic acid	Potassium depletion.	Oxyphenbutazone	Possible ulcers.
Furosemide	Potassium depletion.	Phenylbutazone	Possible ulcers.
Glutethimide	Decreased prednisolone effect.	Rifampin	Decreased prednisolone effect.
Indomethacin	Increased prednisolone effect.	Sympathomimetics	Possible glaucoma.

PREDNISONE

Ephedrine	Decreased prednisone effect.	Insulin	Decreased insulin effect.
Estrogens	Increased prednisone effect.	Isoniazid	Decreased isoniazid effect.
Ethacrynic acid	Potassium depletion.	Oxyphenbutazone	Possible ulcers.
Furosemide	Potassium depletion.	Phenylbutazone	Possible ulcers.
Glutethimide	Decreased prednisone effect.	Rifampin	Decreased prednisone effect.
Indomethacin	Increased prednisone effect.	Sympathomimetics	Possible glaucoma.

PRIMIDONE

Narcotics	Increased narcotic effect.	Sedatives	Increased sedative effect.
Oxyphenbutazone	Decreased oxyphenbutazone effect.	Sleep inducers	Increased effect of sleep inducer.
Phenylbutazone	Decreased phenylbutazone effect.	Tranquilizers	Increased tranquilizer effect.

PROBENECID

Salicylates	Decreased probenecid effect.	Sulfa drugs	Slows elimination. May cause harmful accumulation of sulfa.

ADDITIONAL DRUG INTERACTIONS

GENERIC NAME OR DRUG CLASS	COMBINED EFFECT	GENERIC NAME OR DRUG CLASS	COMBINED EFFECT

RAUWOLFIA SERPENTINA

Phenothiazines	Increased effect of rauwolfia serpentina. Excessive sedation.	Sleep inducers	Increased sleep-inducer effect.
Quinidine	Irregular heartbeat.	Tranquilizers	Increased tranquilizer effect.
Sedatives	Increased sedative effect.		

RESERPINE

Phenothiazines	Increased effect of reserpine. Excessive sedation.	Sleep inducers	Increased effect of sleep inducer.
Quinidine	Irregular heartbeat.	Tranquilizers	Increased tranquilizer effect.
Sedatives	Increased sedative effect.		

SECOBARBITAL

MAO inhibitors	Increased secobarbital effect.	Sedatives	Dangerous sedation. Avoid.
Mind-altering drugs	Dangerous sedation. Avoid.	Sleep inducers	Dangerous sedation. Avoid.
Narcotics	Dangerous sedation. Avoid.	Tranquilizers	Dangerous sedation. Avoid.
Pain relievers	Dangerous sedation. Avoid.	Valproic acid	Increased secobarbital effect.

TALBUTAL (BUTALBITAL)

MAO inhibitors	Increased talbutal (butalbital) effect.	Sedatives	Dangerous sedation. Avoid.
Mind-altering drugs	Dangerous sedation. Avoid.	Sleep inducers	Dangerous sedation. Avoid.
Narcotics	Dangerous sedation. Avoid.	Tranquilizers	Dangerous sedation. Avoid.
Pain relievers	Dangerous sedation. Avoid.	Valproic acid	Increased talbutal (butalbital) effect.

THIOTHIXENE

Sedatives	Increased thiothixene effect. Excessive sedation.	Tranquilizers	Increased thiothixene effect. Excessive sedation.
Sleep inducers	Increased thiothixene effect. Excessive sedation.		

TOLAZAMIDE

Isoniazid	Decreased tolazamide effect.	Phenyramidol	Increased tolazamide effect.
MAO inhibitors	Increased tolazamide effect.	Probenecid	Increased tolazamide effect.
Oxyphenbutazone	Increased tolazamide effect.	Pyrazinamide	Decreased tolazamide effect.
Phenylbutazone	Increased tolazamide effect.	Sulfaphenazole	Increased tolazamide effect.

ADDITIONAL DRUG INTERACTIONS

GENERIC NAME OR DRUG CLASS	COMBINED EFFECT	GENERIC NAME OR DRUG CLASS	COMBINED EFFECT

TOLAZAMIDE continued

GENERIC NAME OR DRUG CLASS	COMBINED EFFECT	GENERIC NAME OR DRUG CLASS	COMBINED EFFECT
Sulfa drugs	Increased tolazamide effect.	Thyroid hormones	Decreased tolazamide effect.

TOLBUTAMIDE

GENERIC NAME OR DRUG CLASS	COMBINED EFFECT	GENERIC NAME OR DRUG CLASS	COMBINED EFFECT
Isoniazid	Decreased tolbutamide effect.	Pyrazinamide	Decreased tolbutamide effect.
MAO inhibitors	Increased tolbutamide effect.	Sulfa drugs	Increased tolbutamide effect.
Oxyphenbutazone	Increased tolbutamide effect.	Sulfaphenazole	Increased tolbutamide effect.
Phenylbutazone	Increased tolbutamide effect.	Thyroid hormones	Decreased tolbutamide effect.
Phenyramidol	Increased tolbutamide effect.		
Probenecid	Increased tolbutamide effect.		

TRANYLCYPROMINE

GENERIC NAME OR DRUG CLASS	COMBINED EFFECT	GENERIC NAME OR DRUG CLASS	COMBINED EFFECT
Methyldopa	Blood-pressure rise to life-threatening level.	Sedatives	Excess sedation.
		Sleep inducers	Excess sedation.
Narcotics	Sudden, severe blood-pressure rise.	Sympathomimetics	Blood-pressure rise to life-threatening level.
Rauwolfia alkaloids	Blood-pressure rise to life-threatening level.	Tranquilizers	Excess sedation.

TRIAMCINOLONE

GENERIC NAME OR DRUG CLASS	COMBINED EFFECT	GENERIC NAME OR DRUG CLASS	COMBINED EFFECT
Ephedrine	Decreased triamcinolone effect.	Insulin	Decreased insulin effect.
Estrogens	Increased triamcinolone effect.	Isoniazid	Decreased isoniazid effect.
Ethacrynic acid	Potassium depletion.	Oxyphenbutazone	Possible ulcers.
Furosemide	Potassium depletion.	Phenylbutazone	Possible ulcers.
Glutethimide	Decreased triamcinolone effect.	Rifampin	Decreased triamcinolone effect.
Indomethacin	Increased triamcinolone effect.	Sympathomimetics	Possible glaucoma.

WARFARIN POTASSIUM

GENERIC NAME OR DRUG CLASS	COMBINED EFFECT	GENERIC NAME OR DRUG CLASS	COMBINED EFFECT
Chloral hydrate	Unpredictable increased or decreased anticoagulant effect.	Clofibrate	Unpredictable increased or decreased warfarin potassium effect.
Chloramphenicol	Increased warfarin potassium effect.	Contraceptives (oral)	Unpredictable increased or decreased warfarin potassium effect.
Chlorpromazine	Decreased warfarin potassium effect.	Cortisone drugs	Unpredictable increased or decreased warfarin potassium effect.
Cholestyramine	Unpredictable increased or decreased warfarin potassium effect.	Digitalis preparations	Decreased warfarin potassium effect.
Cimetidine	Increased warfarin potassium effect.		

ADDITIONAL DRUG INTERACTIONS

GENERIC NAME OR DRUG CLASS	COMBINED EFFECT	GENERIC NAME OR DRUG CLASS	COMBINED EFFECT

WARFARIN POTASSIUM continued

GENERIC NAME OR DRUG CLASS	COMBINED EFFECT	GENERIC NAME OR DRUG CLASS	COMBINED EFFECT
Disulfiram	Increased warfarin potassium effect.	Nortriptyline	Increased warfarin potassium effect.
Estrogens	Decreased warfarin potassium effect.	Oxyphenbutazone	Increased warfarin potassium effect.
Ethacrynic acid	Increased warfarin potassium effect.	Para-aminosalicylic acid (PAS)	Increased warfarin potassium effect.
Ethchlorvynol	Decreased warfarin potassium effect.	Phenelzine	Increased warfarin potassium effect.
Furosemide	Decreased warfarin potassium effect.	Phenylbutazone	Unpredictable increased or decreased warfarin potassium effect.
Glucagon	Increased warfarin potassium effect.	Phenylpropanolamine	Decreased anticoagulant effect.
Glutethimide	Decreased warfarin potassium effect.	Phenyramidol	Increased warfarin potassium effect.
Griseofulvin	Decreased warfarin potassium effect.	Probenecid	Increased warfarin potassium effect.
Guanethidine	Increased warfarin potassium effect.	Propoxyphene	Increased warfarin potassium effect.
Haloperidol	Decreased warfarin potassium effect.	Propylthiouracil	Increased warfarin potassium effect.
Hydroxyzine	Increased warfarin potassium effect.	Quinidine	Increased warfarin potassium effect.
Indomethacin	Increased warfarin potassium effect.	Rauwolfia alkaloids	Unpredictable increased or decreased warfarin potassium effect.
Insulin	Increased insulin effect.		
Isocarboxazid	Increased warfarin potassium effect.	Salicylates (including aspirin)	Increased warfarin potassium effect.
Isoniazid	Increased warfarin potassium effect.	Sulfa drugs	Increased warfarin potassium effect.
Mefenamic acid	Increased warfarin potassium effect.	Sulfinpyrazone	Increased warfarin potassium effect.
Meprobamate	Decreased warfarin potassium effect.	Tetracyclines	Increased warfarin potassium effect.
Mercaptopurine	Increased warfarin potassium effect.	Thyroid hormones	Increased warfarin potassium effect.
Methyldopa	Increased warfarin potassium effect.	Trimethoprim	Increased warfarin potassium effect.
Methylphenidate	Increased warfarin potassium effect.	Vitamin C (large doses)	Decreased warfarin potassium effect.
Metronizadole	Increased warfarin potassium effect.	Vitamin E (large doses)	Increased warfarin potassium effect.
Nalidixic acid	Increased warfarin potassium effect.		

WARFARIN SODIUM

GENERIC NAME OR DRUG CLASS	COMBINED EFFECT	GENERIC NAME OR DRUG CLASS	COMBINED EFFECT
Chloral hydrate	Unpredictable increased or decreased anticoagulant effect.	Cholestyramine	Unpredictable increased or decreased warfarin sodium effect.
Chloramphenicol	Increased warfarin sodium effect.	Cimetidine	Increased warfarin sodium effect.
Chlorpromazine	Decreased warfarin sodium effect.	Clofibrate	Unpredictable increased or decreased warfarin sodium effect.

ADDITIONAL DRUG INTERACTIONS

GENERIC NAME OR DRUG CLASS	COMBINED EFFECT	GENERIC NAME OR DRUG CLASS	COMBINED EFFECT

WARFARIN SODIUM continued

GENERIC NAME OR DRUG CLASS	COMBINED EFFECT	GENERIC NAME OR DRUG CLASS	COMBINED EFFECT
Contraceptives (oral)	Unpredictable increased or decreased warfarin sodium effect.	Metronidazole	Increased warfarin sodium effect.
Cortisone drugs	Unpredictable increased or decreased warfarin sodium effect.	Nalidixic acid	Increased warfarin sodium effect.
Digitalis preparations	Decrease warfarin sodium effect.	Nortriptyline	Increased warfarin sodium effect.
Disulfiram	Increased warfarin sodium effect.	Oxyphenbutazone	Increased warfarin sodium effect.
Estrogens	Decreased warfarin sodium effect.	Para-aminosalicylic acid (PAS)	Increased warfarin sodium effect.
Ethacrynic acid	Increased warfarin sodium effect.	Phenelzine	Increased warfarin sodium effect.
Ethchlorvynol	Decreased warfarin sodium effect.	Phenylbutazone	Unpredictable increased or decreased warfarin sodium effect.
Furosemide	Decreased warfarin sodium effect.	Phenylpropanolamine	Decreased anticoagulant effect.
Glucagon	Increased warfarin sodium effect.	Phenyramidol	Increased warfarin sodium effect.
Glutethimide	Decreased warfarin sodium effect.	Probenecid	Increased warfarin sodium effect.
Griseofulvin	Decreased warfarin sodium effect.	Propoxyphene	Increased warfarin sodium effect.
Guanethidine	Increased warfarin sodium effect.	Propylthiouracil	Increased warfarin sodium effect.
Haloperidol	Decreased warfarin sodium effect.	Quinidine	Increased warfarin sodium effect.
Hydroxyzine	Increased warfarin sodium effect.	Rauwolfia alkaloids	Unpredictable increased or decreased warfarin sodium effect.
Indomethacin	Increased warfarin sodium effect.	Salicylates (including aspirin)	Increased warfarin sodium effect.
Insulin	Increased insulin effect.	Sulfa drugs	Increased warfarin sodium effect.
Isocarboxazid	Increased warfarin sodium effect.	Sulfinpyrazone	Increased warfarin sodium effect.
Isoniazid	Increased warfarin sodium effect.	Tetracyclines	Increased warfarin sodium effect.
Mefenamic acid	Increased warfarin sodium effect.	Thyroid hormones	Increased warfarin sodium effect.
Meprobamate	Decreased warfarin sodium effect.	Trimethoprim	Increased warfarin sodium effect.
Mercaptopurine	Increased warfarin sodium effect.	Vitamin C (large doses)	Decrease warfarin sodium effect.
Methyldopa	Increased warfarin sodium effect.	Vitamin E (large doses)	Increased warfarin sodium effect.
Methylphenidate	Increased warfarin sodium effect.		

Glossary

The following medical terms are found in the drug charts.

A

Acute—Having a short and relatively severe course.

Addiction—Psychological or physiological dependence upon a drug.

Addison's Disease—Changes in the body caused by a deficiency of hormones manufactured by the adrenal gland. Usually fatal if untreated.

Adrenal Cortex—Center of the adrenal gland.

Adrenal Gland—Gland next to the kidney that produces cortisone and epinephrine (adrenalin).

Alkylating Agent—Chemical used to treat malignant diseases.

Allergy—Excessive sensitivity to a substance.

Amebiasis—Infection with amoeba, one-celled organisms. Causes diarrhea, fever and abdominal cramps.

Amphetamine—Drug that stimulates the brain and central nervous system, increases blood pressure, reduces nasal congestion and is habit-forming.

Analgesic—Agent that reduces pain without reducing consciousness.

Anaphylaxis—Severe allergic response to a substance. Symptoms are wheezing, itching, hives, nasal congestion, intense burning of hands and feet, collapse, loss of consciousness and cardiac arrest. Symptoms appear within a few seconds or minutes after exposure. Anaphylaxis is a severe medical emergency. Without appropriate treatment, it can cause death. Instructions for home treatment for anaphylaxis are on page 888.

Anemia—Not enough healthy red-blood cells in the bloodstream or too little hemoglobin in the red-blood cells. Anemia is caused by imbalance of blood loss and blood production.

Anemia, Hemolytic—Anemia caused by a shortened life span of red-blood cells. The body can't manufacture new cells fast enough to replace old cells.

Anemia, Iron-Deficiency—Anemia caused when iron necessary to manufacture red-blood cells is not available.

Anemia, Pernicious—Anemia caused by a vitamin B-12 deficiency. Symptoms include weakness, fatigue, numbness and tingling of the hands or feet, and degeneration of the central nervous system.

Anemia, Sickle-Cell—Anemia caused by defective hemoglobin that deprives red-blood cells of oxygen, making them sickle-shaped.

Anesthetic—Drug that eliminates the sensation of pain.

Angina (Angina Pectoris)—Chest pain with a sensation of suffocation and impending death. Caused by a temporary reduction in the amount of oxygen to the heart muscle through diseased coronary arteries.

Antacid—Chemical that neutralizes acid, usually in the stomach.

Antibiotic—Chemical that inhibits the growth of or kills germs.

Anticholinergic—Drug that chemically inhibits nerve impulses through the parasympathetic nervous system.

Anticoagulant—Drug that inhibits blood clotting.

Antiemetic—Drug that prevents or stops nausea and vomiting.

Antihypertensive—Medication to reduce blood pressure.

Appendicitis—Inflammation or infection of the appendix. Symptoms include loss of appetite, nausea, low-grade fever and tenderness in the lower right of the abdomen.

Artery—Blood vessel carrying blood away from the heart.

Asthma—Recurrent attacks of breathing difficulty due to spasms and contractions of the bronchial tubes.

B

Bacteria—Microscopic organism. Some bacteria contribute to health; others (germs) cause disease.

GLOSSARY

Basal Area of Brain—Part of the brain that regulates muscle control and tone.

Blood Count—Laboratory studies to count white-blood cells, red-blood cells, platelets and other elements of the blood.

Blood Pressure, Diastolic—Pressure (usually recorded in millimeters of mercury) in the large arteries of the body when the heart muscle is relaxed and filling for the next contraction.

Blood Pressure, Systolic—Pressure (usually recorded in millimeters of mercury) in the large arteries of the body at the instant the heart muscle contracts.

Blood Sugar (Blood Glucose)—Necessary element in the blood to sustain life.

C

Cataract—Loss of transparency in the lens of the eye.

Cell—Unit of protoplasm, the essential living matter of all plants and animals.

Cephalosporin—Antibiotic that kills many bacterial germs that penicillin and sulfa drugs can't destroy.

Cholinergic (also Parasympathomimetic)—Chemical that facilitates passage of nerve impulses through the parasympathetic nervous system.

Cirrhosis—Disease that scars and destroys liver tissue.

Cold Urticaria—Hives that appear in areas of the body exposed to the cold.

Colitis, Ulcerative—Chronic, recurring ulcers of the colon for unknown reasons.

Collagen—Support tissue of skin, tendon, bone, cartilage and connective tissue.

Colostomy—Surgical opening from the colon, the large intestine, to the outside of the body.

Congestive—Excess accumulation of blood. In congestive heart failure, congestion occurs in the lungs, liver, kidney and other parts to cause shortness of breath, swelling of the ankles and feet, rapid heartbeat and other symptoms.

Constriction—Tightness or pressure.

Contraceptive—Something that prevents pregnancy.

Convulsions—Violent, uncontrollable contractions of the voluntary muscles.

Corticosteroid (Adrenocorticosteroid)—Steroid hormones produced by the body's adrenal cortex or their synthetic equivalents.

Cystitis—Inflammation of the urinary bladder.

D

Delirium—Temporary mental disturbance characterized by hallucinations, agitation and incoherence.

Diabetes—Metabolic disorder in which the body can't use carbohydrates efficiently. This leads to a dangerously high level of glucose (a carbohydrate) in the blood.

Dialysis—Procedure to filter waste products from the bloodstream of patients with kidney failure.

Dilation—Enlarged.

Disulfiram Reaction—Disulfiram (Antabuse) is a drug to treat alcoholism. When alcohol in the bloodstream interacts with disulfiram, it causes a flushed face, severe headache, chest pains, shortness of breath, nausea, vomiting, sweating and weakness. Severe reactions may cause death.

A disulfiram reaction is the interaction of any drug with alcohol or another drug to produce these symptoms. See emergency first aid instructions, page 886.

Duodenum—The first 12 inches of the small intestine.

E

Eczema—Disorder of the skin with redness, itching, blisters, weeping and abnormal pigmentation.

Electrolyte—Substance that can transmit electrical impulses when dissolved in body fluids.

Embolism—Sudden blockage of an artery by a clot or foreign material in the blood.

Emphysema—Disease in which the lung's air sacs lose elasticity, and air accumulates in the lungs.

Endometriosis—Condition in which uterus tissue is found outside the uterus. Can cause pain, abnormal menstruation and infertility.

Enzyme—Protein chemical that can accelerate a chemical reaction in the body

Epilepsy—Episodes of brain disturbance that cause convulsions and loss of consciousness

Esophagitis—Inflammation of the lower part of the esophagus, the tube connecting the throat and the stomach.

Estrogens—Female sex hormones that stimulate female characteristics and prepare the uterus for fertilization.

Eustachian Tube—Small passage from the middle ear to the sinuses and nasal passages.

Extremity—Arm, leg, hand or foot.

F

Fecal Impaction—Condition in which feces become firmly wedged in the rectum.

Fibrocystic Breast Disease—Overgrowth of fibrous tissue in the breast, producing non-malignant cysts.

Fibroid Tumors—Non-malignant tumors of the muscular layer of the uterus.

Flu (Influenza)—A virus infection of the respiratory tract that lasts three to ten days. Symptoms include headache, fever, runny nose, cough, tiredness and muscle aches.

Folliculitis—Inflammation of a follicle.

G

G6PD—Deficiency of glucose 6-phosphate, necessary for glucose metabolism.

Gastritis—Inflammation of the stomach.

Gastrointestinal—Stomach and intestinal tract.

Gland—Cells that manufacture and excrete materials not required for their own metabolic needs.

Glaucoma—Eye disease in which increased pressure inside the eye damages the optic nerve, causes pain and changes vision.

Glucagon—Injectable drug that immediately elevates blood sugar by mobilizing glycogen from the liver.

H

Hangover Effect—The same feelings as a "hangover" after too much alcohol consumption. Symptoms include headache, irritability and nausea.

Hemochromatosis—Disorder of iron metabolism in which excessive iron is deposited in and damages body tissues, particularly liver and pancreas.

Hemoglobin—Pigment that carries oxygen in red-blood cells.

Hemorrhage—Heavy bleeding.

Hemosidcrosis—Increase of iron deposits in body tissues without tissue damage.

Hepatitis—Inflammation of liver cells, usually accompanied by jaundice.

Hiatal Hernia—Section of stomach that protrudes into the chest cavity.

Histamine—Chemical in body tissues that dilates the smallest blood vessels, constricts the smooth muscle surrounding the bronchial tubes and stimulates stomach secretions.

History—Past medical events in a patient's life.

Hives—Elevated patches on the skin that are redder or paler than surrounding skin and often itch severely.

Hormone—Chemical substance produced in the body to regulate other body functions.

Hypertension—High blood pressure.

Hypocalcemia—Abnormally low level of calcium in the blood.

Hypoglycemia—Low blood sugar (blood glucose). A critically low blood-sugar level will interfere with normal brain function and can damage the brain permanently.

I

Ichthyosis—Skin disorder with dryness, scaling and roughness.

Ileitis—Inflammation of the ileum, the last section of the small intestine.

Ileostomy—Surgical opening from the ileum, the end of the small intestine, to the outside of the body.

Impotence—Male's inability to achieve or sustain erection of the penis for sexual intercourse.

Insomnia—Sleeplessness.

Interaction—Change in the body's response to one drug when another is taken. Interaction may increase effect of one or both drugs, decrease the effect of one or both drugs or cause toxicity.

J

Jaundice—Symptoms of liver damage, bile obstruction or red-blood-cell destruction. Includes yellowed whites of the eyes, yellow skin, dark urine and light stool.

K

Keratosis—Growth that is an accumulation of cells from the outer skin layers.

Kidney Stones—Small, solid stones made from calcium, cholesterol, cysteine and other body chemicals.

GLOSSARY

L

Lupus—Serious disorder of connective tissue that primarily affects women. Varies in severity with skin eruptions, joint inflammation, low white-blood cell count and damage to internal organs, especially the kidney.

Lymph Glands—Glands in the lymph vessels throughout the body that trap foreign and infectious matter and protect the bloodstream from infection.

M

Manic-Depressive Illness—Psychosis with alternating cycles of excessive enthusiasm and depression.

Mast Cell—Connective-tissue cell.

Menopause—The end of menstruation in the female, often accompanied by irritability, hot flushes, changes in the skin and bones and vaginal dryness.

Metabolism—Process of using nutrients and energy to build and break down wastes.

Migraine—Periodic headaches caused by constriction of arteries to the skull. Symptoms include severe pain, vision disturbances, nausea, vomiting and light sensitivity.

Mind-Altering Drugs—Any drug that decreases alertness, perception, concentration, contact with reality or muscular coordination.

Myasthenia Gravis—Disease of the muscles characterized by fatigue and progressive paralysis. It is usually confined to muscles of the face, lips, tongue and neck.

N

Narcotic—Drug, usually addictive, that produces stupor.

O

Osteoporosis—Softening of bones caused by a loss of chemicals usually found in bone.

Ovary—Female sexual gland where eggs mature and ripen for fertilization.

P

Palpitations—Rapid heartbeat noticeable to the patient.

Pancreatitis—Serious inflammation or infection of the pancreas that causes upper abdominal pain.

Parkinson's Disease—Disease of the central nervous system. Characteristics are a fixed, emotionless expression of the face, tremor, slower muscle movements, weakness, changed gait and a peculiar posture.

Pellagra—Disease caused by a deficiency of the water-soluble vitamin, thiamine (vitamin B-1). Symptoms include brain disturbance, diarrhea and skin inflammation.

Penicillin—Chemical substance (antibiotic) originally discovered as a product of mold, which can kill some bacterial germs.

Phlegm—Thick mucus secreted by glands in the respiratory tract.

Pinworms—Common intestinal parasite that causes rectal itching and irritation.

Pituitary Gland—Gland at the base of the brain that secretes hormones to stimulate growth and other glands to produce hormones.

Platelet—Disc-shaped element of the blood, smaller than red- or white-blood cells, necessary for blood clotting.

Polyp—Growth on a mucous membrane.

Porphyria—Inherited metabolic disorder characterized by changes in the nervous system and kidney.

Post-partum—Following delivery of a baby.

Potassium—Important chemical found in body cells.

Potassium Foods—Foods high in potassium content, including dried apricots and peaches, lentils, raisins, citrus and whole-grain cereals.

Prostate—Gland in the male that surrounds the neck of the bladder and the urethra.

Prothrombin—Blood substance essential in clotting.

Prothrombin Time—Laboratory study used to follow prothrombin activity and keep coagulation safe.

Psoriasis—Chronic, inherited skin disease. Symptoms are lesions with silvery scales on the edges.

Psychosis—Mental disorder characterized by deranged personality, loss of contact with reality and possible delusions, hallucinations or illusions.

Purine Foods—Foods that are metabolized into uric acid. Foods high in purines include anchovies, liver, brains, sweetbreads, sardines, kidney, oysters, gravy and meat extracts.

R

RDA—Recommended daily allowance of a vitamin or mineral.

Rebound Effect—Return of a condition, often with increased severity, once the prescribed drug is withdrawn.

Renal—Pertaining to the kidney.

Retina—Innermost covering of the eyeball on which the image is formed.

Reye's Syndrome—Rare, sometimes fatal, disease of children that causes brain and liver damage.

Rickets—Bone disease caused by vitamin-D deficiency. Bones become bent and distorted during infancy or childhood.

S

Sedative—Drug that reduces excitement or anxiety.

Seizure—Brain disorder causing changes of consciousness or convulsions.

Sinusitis—Inflammation or infection of the sinus cavities in the skull.

Streptococcus—Bacteria that causes infections in the throat, respiratory system and skin. Improperly treated, can lead to disease in the heart, joints and kidneys.

Stroke—Sudden, severe attack. Usually sudden paralysis from injury to the brain or spinal cord caused by a blood clot or hemorrhage in the brain.

Stupor—Near unconsciousness.

Sublingual—Under the tongue. Some drugs are absorbed almost as quickly this way as by injection.

T

Tardive Dyskinesia—Involuntary movements of the jaw, lips and tongue caused by an unpredictable drug reaction.

Thrombophlebitis—Inflammation of a vein caused by a blood clot in the vein.

Thyroid—Gland in the neck that manufactures and secretes several hormones.

Tic-douloureaux—Painful condition caused by inflammation of a nerve in the face.

Toxicity—Poisonous reaction to a drug that impairs body functions or damages cells.

Tranquilizer—Drug that calms a person without clouding consciousness.

Tremor—Involuntary trembling.

Trichomoniasis—Infestation of the vagina by *trichomonas,* an infectious organism. The infection causes itching, vaginal discharge and irritation.

Triglyceride—Fatty chemical manufactured from carbohydrates for storage in fat cells.

Tyramine—Normal chemical component of the body that helps sustain blood pressure. Can rise to fatal levels in combination with some drugs.

Tyramine is found in many foods:

Beverages—Alcoholic beverages, especially Chianti or robust red wines, vermouth, ale, beer.

Breads—Homemade bread with a lot of yeast and breads or crackers containing cheese.

Fats—Sour cream.

Fruits—Bananas, red plums, avocados, figs, raisins.

Meats and meat substitutes—Aged game, liver, canned meats, salami, sausage, cheese, salted dried fish, pickled herring.

Vegetables—Italian broad beans, green-bean pods, eggplant.

Miscellaneous—Yeast concentrates or extracts, marmite, soup cubes, commercial gravy, soy sauce, any protein food that has been stored improperly or is spoiled.

U

Ulcer, Peptic—Open sore on the mucous membrane of the esophagus, stomach or duodenum caused by stomach acid.

Urethra—Hollow tube through which urine (and semen in men) is discharged.

Urethritis—Inflammation or infection of the urethra.

Uterus—Also called *womb.* A hollow muscular organ in the female in which the embryo develops into a fetus.

V

Vascular—Pertaining to blood vessels.

Virus—Infectious organism that reproduces in the cells of the infected host.

Y

Yeast—A single-cell organism that can cause infections of the mouth, vagina, skin and parts of the gastrointestinal system.

Guide to Index

Alphabetical entries in the index include three categories—generic names, brand names and drug-class names.

1. Generic names appear in capital letters, followed by their chart page number:

   ASPIRIN, 56.

2. Brand names appear in *italic,* followed by their generic ingredient and chart page number.

   Bayer—See ASPIRIN, 56.

   The letter M in parentheses (M) following a brand name indicates the brand is a mixture of two or more generic drugs. These generic ingredients are listed in capital letters following the brand name:

   Cefinal (M)—See
   ASPIRIN, 56
   CAFFEINE, 100

   Some brand names followed by (M) list additional generic ingredients not included in this book because of space limitations. These are designated by (NL), which means "not listed."

   Fedrazil (M)—See
   CHLORCYCLIZINE (NL)
   PSEUDOEPHEDRINE, 674

3. Drug-class names appear in regular type, capital and lower-case letters. All generic drug names in this book that fall into a drug class are listed after the class name.

   Analgesics
   ACETAMINOPHEN, 18
   ASPIRIN, 56
   CARBAMAZEPINE, 106
   PHENACETIN, 582

A

AL-R—See
CHLORPHENIRAMINE, 142

A-M-T (M)—See
ALUMINUM HYDROXIDE, 32
MAGNESIUM TRISILICATE, 424

APAP—See ACETAMINOPHEN, 18

A-P-A-P Tablets—See
ACETAMINOPHEN, 18

A.P.C. (M)—See
ASPIRIN, 56
CAFFEINE, 100
PHENACETIN, 582

A.P.C. with Codeine (M)—See
ASPIRIN, 56
CAFFEINE, 100
CODEINE, 176
PHENACETIN, 582

A.P.C. with Codeine Phosphate Tablets (M)—See
ASPIRIN, 56
CAFFEINE, 100
CODEINE, 176
PHENACETIN, 582

A.P.C —Demerol (M)—See
ASPIRIN, 56
CAFFEINE, 100
MEPERIDINE, 438
PHENACETIN, 582

A.S.A. & Codeine Compound (M)—See
ASPIRIN, 56
CODEINE, 176

A.S.A. Compound (M)—See
ASPIRIN, 56
CAFFEINE, 100

Accurbron—See
THEOPHYLLINE, 748

Acet-Am (M)—See
ACETAMINOPHEN, 18
EPHEDRINE, 274

Aceta with Codeine Tablets (M)—See
ACETAMINOPHEN, 18
CODEINE, 176

Acetaco Tablets (M)—See
ACETAMINOPHEN, 18
CODEINE, 176

ACETAMINOPHEN, 18

Acetaminophen Elixir—See
ACETAMINOPHEN, 18

Acetaminophen Suppositories—See
ACETAMINOPHEN, 18

Acetaminophen with Codeine (M)—See
ACETAMINOPHEN, 18
CODEINE, 176

ACETAZOLAMIDE, 20

ACETOHEXAMIDE, 22

Acetophen (M)—See
ASPIRIN, 56
CAFFEINE, 100
PHENACETIN, 582

ACETOPHENAZINE, 24

Achromycin—See
TETRACYCLINE, 746

Achrostatin V (M)—See
NYSTATIN, 532
TETRACYCLINE, 746

Acon—See VITAMIN A, 804

Actidil—See TRIPROLIDINE, 800

Actidil (M)—See
PSEUDOEPHEDRINE, 674
TRIPROLIDINE, 800

Actifed-C Expectorant (M)—See
CODEINE, 176
PSEUDOEPHEDRINE, 674
TRIPROLIDINE, 800

Actol Expectorant (M)—See
GUAIFENESIN, 346
NOSCAPINE (NL)

Actrapid—See INSULIN, 382

Acutuss Expectorant with Codeine (M)—See
CHLORPHENIRAMINE, 142
CODEINE, 176
GUAIFENESIN, 346
PHENYLEPHRINE, 606

Adapin—See DOXEPIN, 266
Adatuss Cough Syrup (M)—See
  CODEINE, 176
  GUAIFENESIN, 346
Adenex—See VITAMIN C
  (ASCORBIC ACID), 808
Adipex-D—See PHENTERMINE,
  602
Adphen—See
  PHENDIMETRAZINE, 586
Adrenalin—See EPINEPHRINE,
  276
ADRENOCORTICOIDS
  (TOPICAL), 26
Adroyd—See
  OXYMETHOLONE, 550
Adsorbocarpine—See
  PILOCARPINE, 614
Aero Caine Aerosol—See
  ANESTHETICS (TOPICAL), 52
Aero Caine-5 Aerosol—See
  ANESTHETICS (TOPICAL), 52
Aerolate—See
  THEOPHYLLINE, 748
Aerolone—See
  ISOPROTERENOL, 394
Aerophylline—See
  DYPHYLLINE, 272
Afaxin—See VITAMIN A, 804
Afko-Lube—See DOCUSATE
  SODIUM, 264
Afrin—See OXYMETAZOLINE,
  548
Afrinol—See
  PSEUDOEPHEDRINE, 674
A-hydroCort—See
  HYDROCORTISONE
  (CORTISOL), 364
Airet—See DYPHYLLINE, 272
Ak-Zol—See
  ACETAZOLAMIDE, 20
Akineton See BIPERIDINE, 84
Aladrine Tablets (M)—See
  EPHEDRINE, 274
  SECOBARBITAL, 704
Alaxin—See POLOXAMER 188,
  618
Alconefrin—See
  PHENYLEPHRINE, 606
Aldactazide (M)—See
  HYDROCHLOROTHIAZIDE,
  360
  SPIRONOLACTONE, 720
Aldactone—See
  SPIRONOLACTONE, 720
Aldoclor (M)—See
  CHLOROTHIAZIDE, 138
  METHYLDOPA, 478
Aldomet—See METHYLDOPA,
  478
Aldoril (M)—See
  HYDROCHLOROTHIAZIDE,
  360
  METHYLDOPA, 478
Alermine—See
  CHLORPHENIRAMINE, 142
Algodex—See
  PROPOXYPHENE, 668
Algoverine—See
  PHENYLBUTAZONE, 604
Alka-2—See CALCIUM
  CARBONATE, 102
Alka-Citrate Compound—See
  SODIUM BICARBONATE, 712
Alka-Seltzer Antacid—See
  SODIUM BICARBONATE, 712

Alka-Seltzer Effervescent
  Tablets (M)—See
  ASPIRIN, 56
  SODIUM BICARBONATE, 712
Alka-Seltzer Plus Tablets
  (M)—See
  ASPIRIN, 56
  CHLORPHENIRAMINE, 142
  PHENYLEPHRINE, 606
Alkarau—See RESERPINE, 698
Alkets—See
  CALCIUM CARBONATE, 102
  MAGNESIUM CARBONATE,
  416
Aller-chlor—See
  CHLORPHENIRAMINE, 142
Allerbid Tymcaps—See
  CHLORPHENIRAMINE, 142
Allerest (M)—See
  CHLORPHENIRAMINE, 606
  PHENYLPROPANOLAMINE,
  608
Allerform Tablets—See
  CHLORPHENIRAMINE, 142
Allergesic Tablets (M)—See
  CHLORPHENIRAMINE, 142
  PHENYLPROPANOLAMINE,
  608
Allernade—See
  ISOPROPAMIDE, 392
Allerspan—See SCOPOLAMINE
  (HYOSCINE), 702
Allertoc—See PYRILAMINE, 682
ALLOPURINOL, 28
Allylgesic (M)—See
  ASPIRIN, 56
  ENZYMES (NL)
Almezyme (M)—See
  ATROPINE, 60
  HYOSCYAMINE, 374
  SCOPOLAMINE
  (HYOSCINE), 702
Almocarpine—See
  PILOCARPINE, 614
Alophen See
  PHENOLPHTHALEIN, 596
Alpen—See AMPICILLIN, 50
Alpha Hedisol—See VITAMIN
  B-12 (CYANOCOBALAMIN),
  806
Alphadrol—See
  FLUPREDNISOLONE, 334
Alphalin—See VITAMIN A, 804
Alphamin—See VITAMIN B-12
  (CYANOCOBALAMIN), 806
Alphamul—See CASTOR OIL,
  120
ALPRAZOLAM, 30
Aludrox (M)—See
  ALUMINUM HYDROXIDE, 32
  MAGNESIUM HYDROXIDE,
  420
Alumadrine Tablets (M)—See
  CHLORPHENIRAMINE, 142
  PHENYLPROPANOLAMINE,
  608
Aluminum ASA Tablets
  Chewable (M)—See
  ASPIRIN, 56
  ALUMINUM HYDROXIDE, 32
ALUMINUM HYDROXIDE, 32
Alupent—See
  METAPROTERENOL, 448
Aluscop—See SCOPOLAMINE
  (HYOSCINE), 702
AMANTADINE, 34

Amaril D (M)—See
  CHLORPHENIRAMINE, 142
  PHENYLEPHRINE, 606
  PHENYLTOLOXAMINE, 610
AMBENONIUM, 36
Ambenyl Expectorant (M)—See
  CODEINE, 176
  BROMODIPHENHYDRAMINE,
  88
  DIPHENHYDRAMINE, 248
  GUAIFENESIN, 346
Ambodryl—See
  BROMODIPHENHYDRAMINE
  88
Amcill—See AMPICILLIN, 50
Amcort—See
  TRIAMCINOLONE, 776
Amen—See
  MEDROXYPROGESTERONE,
  434
Americaine—See
  ANESTHETICS (TOPICAL), 52
Amesec (M)—See
  EPHEDRINE, 274
  THEOPHYLLINE, 748
A-methaPred—See
  METHYLPREDNISOLONE,
  484
AMILORIDE, 38
Aminodur—See
  AMINOPHYLLINE, 40
Aminophyl—See
  AMINOPHYLLINE, 40
AMINOPHYLLINE, 40
Aminophylline and Amytal
  Pulvules (M)—See
  AMOBARBITAL, 44
  THEOPHYLLINE, 748
Aminophylline-Phenobarbital
  Suppositories (M)—See
  PHENOBARBITAL, 594
  THEOPHYLLINE, 748
Aminophylline-Phenobarbital
  Tablets (M)—See
  PHENOBARBITAL, 594
  THEOPHYLLINE, 748
Amitid—See AMITRIPTYLINE,
  42
Amitone—See CALCIUM
  CARBONATE, 102
Amitril—See AMITRIPTYLINE,
  42
AMITRIPTYLINE, 42
Amnestrogen—See
  ESTERIFIED ESTROGENS,
  298
Amnestrogen—See
  ESTROGEN, 302
AMOBARBITAL, 44
Amobel (M)—See
  AMOBARBITAL, 44
  BELLADONNA, 68
Amocine (M)—See
  AMOBARBITAL, 44
  ATROPINE, 60
Amodrine Tablets (M)—See
  EPHEDRINE, 274
  PHENOBARBITAL, 594
  THEOPHYLLINE, 748
AMOXICILLIN, 46
Amoxil—See AMOXICILLIN, 46
Amphaplex (M)—See
  AMPHETAMINE, 48
  DEXTROAMPHETAMINE, 218
AMPHETAMINE, 48

INDEX

Amphetamines—See
Central-nervous-
system stimulants
Amphicol—See
CHLORAMPHENICOL, 132
Amphylline—See
AMINOPHYLLINE, 40
AMPICILLIN, 50
Ampicin—See AMPICILLIN, 50
Amytal and Aspirin (M)—See
AMOBARBITAL, 44
ASPIRIN, 56
Amytal—See AMOBARBITAL,
44
Anabolin LA 100—See
NANDROLONE, 508
Anadrol-50—See
OXYMETHOLONE, 550
Analgesics
ACETAMINOPHEN, 18
ASPIRIN, 56
CARBAMAZEPINE, 106
PHENACETIN, 582
Analgesics (urinary)
PHENAZOPYRIDINE, 584
Anamine Syrup (M)—See
CHLORPHENIRAMINE, 142
PSEUDOEPHEDRINE, 674
*Anamine T.D. Capsules
(M)—See*
CHLORPHENIRAMINE, 142
PHENYLEPHRINE, 606
Anapap Tablets—See
ACETAMINOPHEN, 18
Anaphen (M)—See
ACETAMINOPHEN, 18
ASPIRIN, 56
CAFFEINE, 100
CODEINE, 176
Anapolon 50—See
OXYMETHOLONE, 550
Anaprox—See NAPROXEN, 510
Anaspaz—See HYOSCYAMINE,
374
Anaspaz PB (M)—See
HYOSCYAMINE, 374
PHENOBARBITAL, 594
Anatuss Syrup—See
CHLORPHENIRAMINE, 142
Anavar—See OXANDROLONE,
540
Anbesol—See ANESTHETICS
(TOPICAL), 52
Androgens (male sex hormone)
ETHYLESTRENOL, 318
FLUOXYMESTERONE, 330
METHANDROSTENOLONE,
456
METHYLTESTOSTERONE,
486
NANDROLONE, 508
OXANDROLONE, 540
OXYMETHOLONE, 550
STANOZOLOL, 722
TESTOSTERONE, 744
Android—See
METHYLTESTOSTERONE,
486
Androlone—See
NANDROLONE, 508
Anestacon Solution—See
ANESTHETICS (TOPICAL), 52
ANESTHETICS (TOPICAL), 52

*Anexsia with Codeine Tablets
(M)—See*
ASPIRIN, 56
CAFFEINE, 100
CODEINE, 176
Anhydron—See
CYCLOTHIAZIDE, 198
ANISINDIONE, 54
Anocobin—See VITAMIN B-12
(CYANOCOBALAMIN), 806
Anorex—See
PHENDIMETRAZINE, 586
Anoryol (M)—See
CONTRACEPTIVES (ORAL),
182
Anspor—See CEPHRADINE,
128
Antabuse—See DISULFIRAM,
258
Antacids
ALUMINUM HYDROXIDE, 32
CALCIUM CARBONATE, 102
MAGNESIUM CARBONATE,
416
MAGNESIUM HYDROXIDE,
420
MAGNESIUM TRISILICATE,
424
SODIUM BICARBONATE, 712
SODIUM CARBONATE, 714
Antagonate—See
CHLORPHENIRAMINE, 142
Anti-Tuss (M)—See
DEXTROMETHORPHAN, 220
GUAIFENESIN, 346
Antiacne drugs (topical)
BENZOYL PEROXIDE, 72
TRETINOIN, 774
Antianginal drugs
DILTIAZEM, 242
NIFEDIPINE, 516
VERAPAMIL, 802
Antianginal drugs (nitrate)
ERYTHRITYL
TETRANITRATE, 284
ISOSORBIDE DINITRATE, 396
NITROGLYCERIN
(GLYCERYL TRINITRATE),
520
PENTAERYTHRITOL
TETRANITRATE, 574
Antiarrhythmics
DILTIAZEM, 242
DISOPYRAMIDE, 256
NIFEDIPINE, 516
PROCAINAMIDE, 656
QUINIDINE, 690
VERAPAMIL, 802
Antiasthmatics
BECLOMETHASONE, 66
CROMOLYN, 186
Antibiopto—See
CHLORAMPHENICOL, 132
Antibiotics (antifungal)
GRISEOFULVIN, 344
Antibiotics
CHLORAMPHENICOL, 132
Antibiotics (cephalosporin)
CEFACLOR, 122
CEFADROXIL, 124
CEPHALEXIN, 126
CEPHRADINE, 128

Antibiotics (erythromycin)
ERYTHROMYCIN, 286
ERYTHROMYCIN
ESTOLATE, 288
ERYTHROMYCIN
ETHYLSUCCINATE, 290
ERYTHROMYCIN
GLUCEPTATE, 292
ERYTHROMYCIN
LACTOBIONATE, 294
ERYTHROMYCIN
STEARATE, 296
Antibiotics (lincomycin)
CLINDAMYCIN, 164
LINCOMYCIN, 406
Antibiotics (penicillin)
AMOXICILLIN, 46
AMPICILLIN, 50
BACAMPICILLIN, 64
CARBENICILLIN, 108
CLOXACILLIN, 174
CYCLACILLIN, 188
DICLOXACILLIN, 226
HETACILLIN, 354
METHICILLIN, 466
NAFCILLIN, 502
OXACILLIN, 538
PENICILLIN G, 570
PENICILLIN V, 572
TICARCILLIN, 762
Antibiotics (rifamycin)
RIFAMPIN, 700
Antibiotics (tetracycline)
DEMECLOCYCLINE, 208
DOXYCYCLINE, 268
METHACYCLINE, 450
MINOCYCLINE, 496
OXYTETRACYCLINE, 556
TETRACYCLINE, 746
Anticholinergics
ATROPINE, 60
BELLADONNA, 68
CLIDINIUM, 162
DICYCLOMINE, 230
HYOSCYAMINE, 374
ISOPROPAMIDE, 392
ORPHENADRINE, 536
PROPANTHELINE, 666
SCOPOLAMINE
(HYOSCINE), 702
TRIDIHEXETHYL, 782
Anticoagulants
ANISINDIONE, 54
DICUMAROL, 228
PHENPROCOUMON, 598
WARFARIN POTASSIUM, 816
WARFARIN SODIUM, 818
Anticonvulsants
CARBAMAZEPINE, 106
PHENOBARBITAL, 594
PRIMIDONE, 652
Anticonvulsants (hydantoin)
ETHOTOIN, 316
MEPHENYTOIN, 440
PHENYTOIN, 612
Anticonvulsants (succinimide)
ETHOSUXIMIDE, 314
METHSUXIMIDE, 472
PHENSUXIMIDE, 600
Antidepressants
ISOCARBOXAZID, 386
PARGYLINE, 566
PHENELZINE, 588
TRANYLCYPROMINE, 772

Antidepressants (tricyclic)
AMITRIPTYLINE, 42
DESIPRAMINE, 212
DOXEPIN, 266
IMIPRAMINE, 378
NORTRIPTYLINE, 528
PROTRIPTYLINE, 672
TRIMIPRAMINE, 796
Antidiabetics
INSULIN, 382
Antidiabetics (oral)
ACETOHEXAMIDE, 22
CHLORPROPAMIDE, 148
TOLAZAMIDE, 766
TOLBUTAMIDE, 768
Antidiarrheals
ALUMINUM HYDROXIDE, 32
DIPHENOXYLATE &
ATROPINE, 250
PAREGORIC, 564
POLYCARBOPHIL CALCIUM,
620
Antidotes (heavy-metal)
PENICILLAMINE, 568
Antidyskinetics
BENZTROPINE, 78
BIPERIDINE, 84
CYCRIMINE, 200
ETHOPROPAZINE, 312
PROCYCLIDINE, 660
TRIHEXYPHENIDYL, 788
Antiemetics
BUCLIZINE, 92
CHLORPROTHIXENE, 150
CYCLIZINE, 192
MECLIZINE, 430
THIOTHIXENE, 754
TRIMETHOBENZAMIDE, 792
Antiemetics (phenothiazine)
ACETOPHENAZINE, 24
BUTAPERAZINE, 96
CARPHENAZINE, 116
CHLORPROMAZINE, 146
FLUPHENAZINE, 332
MESORIDAZINE, 446
PERPHENAZINE, 580
PIPERACETAZINE, 616
PROCHLORPERAZINE, 658
PROMAZINE, 662
THIORIDAZINE, 752
TRIFLUOPERAZINE, 784
TRIFLUPROMAZINE, 786
Antiflatulents
SIMETHICONE, 710
Antifungals
NYSTATIN, 532
Antiglaucoma drugs
ACETAZOLAMIDE, 20
DICHLORPHENAMIDE, 224
EPINEPHRINE, 276
METHAZOLAMIDE, 462
PILOCARPINE, 614
Antigout drugs
ALLOPURINOL, 28
COLCHICINE, 178
Antigout drugs (uricosuric)
PROBENECID, 654
SULFINPYRAZONE, 730
Antihelminthics (antiworm
medication)
PYRVINIUM, 684
Antihistamines
AZATADINE, 62
BROMODIPHENHYDRAMINE,
88

Antihistamines—continued
BROMPHENIRAMINE, 90
BUCLIZINE, 92
CARBINOXAMINE, 112
CHLORPHENIRAMINE, 142
CLEMASTINE, 160
CYCLIZINE, 192
CYPROHEPTADINE, 202
DEXCHLORPHENIRAMINE,
216
DIMENHYDRINATE, 244
DIMETHINDENE, 246
DIPHENHYDRAMINE, 248
DIPHENYLPYRALINE, 252
DOXYLAMINE, 270
HYDROXYZINE, 372
MECLIZINE, 430
ORPHENADRINE, 536
PHENIRAMINE, 590
PHENYLTOLOXAMINE, 610
PROMETHAZINE, 664
PYRILAMINE, 682
TRIMEPRAZINE, 790
TRIPELENNAMINE, 798
TRIPROLIDINE, 800
Antihyperlipidemics
CHOLESTYRAMINE, 156
CLOFIBRATE, 166
NIACIN (NICOTINIC ACID),
514
Antihypertensives
BENDROFLUMETHIAZIDE, 70
BENZTHIAZIDE, 76
CAPTOPRIL, 104
CHLOROTHIAZIDE, 138
CHLORTHALIDONE, 152
CYCLOTHIAZIDE, 198
DESERPIDINE, 210
FUROSEMIDE, 340
GUANETHIDINE, 348
HYDRALAZINE, 358
HYDROCHLOROTHIAZIDE,
360
HYDROFLUMETHIAZIDE, 366
METHYCLOTHIAZIDE, 474
METHYLDOPA, 478
METOLAZONE, 490
POLYTHIAZIDE, 622
PRAZOSIN, 646
QUINETHAZONE, 688
RAUWOLFIA SERPENTINA,
696
RESERPINE, 698
SPIRONOLACTONE, 720
TRIAMTERENE, 778
TRICHLORMETHIAZIDE, 780
Antiinfectives (urinary)
METHENAMINE, 464
Antiinflammatory drugs
(salicylate)
ASPIRIN, 56
Antiinflammatory drugs
(non-steroid)
FENOPROFEN, 322
IBUPROFEN, 376
INDOMETHACIN, 380
MECLOFENAMATE, 432
MEFENAMIC ACID, 436
NAPROXEN, 510
OXYPHENBUTAZONE, 554
PHENYLBUTAZONE, 604
SULINDAC, 734
TOLMETIN, 770
Antimetabolites
METHOTREXATE, 470

Antimicrobials
NALIDIXIC ACID, 506
NITROFURANTOIN, 518
TRIMETHOPRIM, 794
Antiparkinsonism drugs
AMANTADINE, 34
BENZTROPINE, 78
BIPERIDINE, 84
CARBIDOPA & LEVODOPA,
110
CYCRIMINE, 200
ETHOPROPAZINE, 312
LEVODOPA, 402
ORPHENADRINE, 536
PROCYCLIDINE, 660
TRIHEXYPHENIDYL, 788
Antiprotozoal drugs
CHLOROQUINE, 136
HYDROXYCHLOROQUINE,
370
METRONIDAZOLE, 494
QUININE, 692
Antipruritics
CHOLESTYRAMINE, 156
Antipsoriatics
METHOTREXATE, 470
Antirheumatic drugs
CHLOROQUINE, 136
HYDROXYCHLOROQUINE,
370
PENICILLAMINE, 568
Antispasmodics
ATROPINE, 60
BELLADONNA, 68
CLIDINIUM, 162
DICYCLOMINE, 230
HYOSCYAMINE, 374
ISOPROPAMIDE, 392
SCOPOLAMINE
(HYOSCINE), 702
TRIDIHEXETHYL, 782
PROPANTHELINE, 666
Antituberculars
PARA-AMINOSALICYLIC
ACID (PAS), 560
Antituberculars (antimicrobial)
ISONIAZID, 390
Antivert—See MECLIZINE, 430
Antivirals
AMANTADINE, 34
Antrocol (M)—See
ATROPINE, 60
PHENOBARBITAL, 594
Anturan—See
SULFINPYRAZONE, 730
Anturane—See
SULFINPYRAZONE, 730
Anuphen Suppositories—See
ACETAMINOPHEN, 18
Apamide Tablets—See
ACETAMINOPHEN, 18
Aparkane—See
TRIHEXYPHENIDYL, 788
Apo-Oxazepam—See
OXAZEPAM, 542
A-poxide—See
CHLORDIAZEPOXIDE, 134
Appetite suppressants
PHENDIMETRAZINE, 586
BENZPHETAMINE, 74
CHLORPHENTERMINE, 144
CLORTERMINE, 172
DIETHYLPROPION, 232
FENFLUORAMINE, 320
MAZINDOL, 428

INDEX

Appetite
  suppressants—continued
  PHENMETRAZINE, 593
  PHENTERMINE, 602
Apresazide (M)—See
  HYDRALAZINE, 358
  HYDROCHLOROTHIAZIDE,
  360
Apresoline—See
  HYDRALAZINE, 358
Apresoline-Esidrix (M)—See
  HYDRALAZINE, 358
  HYDROCHLOROTHIAZIDE,
  360
AquaMEPHYTON—See
  VITAMIN K, 814
Aquachloral—See CHLORAL
  HYDRATE, 130
Aquasol A—See VITAMIN A, 804
Aquasol E—See VITAMIN E, 812
Aquastat—See BENZTHIAZIDE,
  76
Aquatag—See BENZTHIAZIDE,
  76
Aquatensen—See
  METHYCLOTHIAZIDE, 474
Aralen—See CHLOROQUINE,
  136
Arco-Lase (M)—See
  ATROPINE, 60
  ENZYMES (NL)
Arcoban—See
  MEPROBAMATE, 444
Aristocort—See
  ADRENOCORTICOIDS
  (TOPICAL), 26
Aristocort—See
  TRIAMCINOLONE, 776
Aristospan—See
  TRIAMCINOLONE, 776
Arlidin Forte—See NYLIDRIN,
  530
Arlidin—See NYLIDRIN, 530
Artane—See
  TRIHEXYPHENIDYL, 788
Arthralgen (M)—See
  ACETAMINOPHEN, 18
  CODEINE, 176
Asbron Elixir (M)—See
  GUAIFENESIN, 346
  PHENYLPROPANOLAMINE,
  608
  THEOPHYLLINE, 748
Ascodeen-30 Tablets (M)—See
  ASPIRIN, 56
  CODEINE, 176
Ascorbajen—See VITAMIN C
  (ASCORBIC ACID), 808
ASCORBIC ACID, 808
Ascorbicap—See VITAMIN C
  (ASCORBIC ACID), 808
Ascoril—See VITAMIN C
  (ASCORBIC ACID), 808
Ascriptin Tablets (M)—See
  ALUMINUM HYDROXIDE, 32
  ASPIRIN, 56
Ascriptin with Codeine
  (M)—See
  ALUMINUM HYDROXIDE, 32
  ASPIRIN, 56
  CODEINE, 76
Asma Syrup (M)—See
  GUAIFENESIN, 346
  THEOPHYLLINE, 748

Asminyl Tablets (M)—See
  EPHEDRINE, 274
  PHENOBARBITAL, 594
  THEOPHYLLINE, 748
Asmolin—See EPINEPHRINE,
  276
Asphac-G Tablets (M)—See
  ASPIRIN, 56
  CAFFEINE, 100
  PHENACETIN, 582
ASPIRIN, 56
Aspirin Compound with
  Codeine (M)—See
  ASPIRIN, 56
  CAFFEINE, 100
  CODEINE, 176
  PHENACTEIN, 582
Aspirin Suppositories—See
  ASPIRIN, 56
Aspirjen Jr.—See ASPIRIN, 56
Asthma Haler—See
  EPINEPHRINE, 276
Asthma Nefrin—See
  EPINEPHRINE, 276
Asthmophylline—See
  THEOPHYLLINE, 748
Atarax—See HYDROXYZINE,
  372
ATENOLOL, 58
Athrombin-K—See WARFARIN
  POTASSIUM, 816
Ativan—See LORAZEPAM, 414
Atrobarb (M)—See
  ATROPINE, 60
  PHENOBARBITAL, 594
Atrocap (M)—See
  ATROPINE, 60
  BELLADONNA, 68
  HYOSCYAMINE, 374
  HYOSCINE, 702
Atromal (M)—See
  ATROPINE, 60
  PHENOBARBITAL, 594
Atromid-S—See CLOFIBRATE,
  166
ATROPINE, 60
Atropine Bufopto—See
  ATROPINE, 60
Atropisol—See ATROPINE, 60
Atrosed (M)—See
  ATROPINE, 60
  BELLADONNA, 68
Aventyl—See NORTRIPTYLINE,
  528
Axon Capsules (M)—See
  ACETAMINOPHEN, 18
  CODEINE, 176
  PHENYLPROPANOLAMINE,
  608
Axotal (M)—See
  ACETAMINOPHEN, 18
  CODEINE, 176
Azapen—See METHICILLIN,
  466
AZATADINE, 62
Azo-100—See
  PHENAZOPYRIDINE. 584
Azo-Gantanol (M)—See
  PHENAZOPYRIDINE, 584
  SULFAMETHOXAZOLE, 726
Azo-Gantrisin (M)—See
  PHENAZOPYRIDINE, 584
  SULFISOXAZOLE, 732
Azo-Mandelamine (M)—See
  METHENAMINE, 464
  PHENAZOPYRIDINE, 584

Azo-Soxazole (M)—See
  PHENAZOPYRIDINE, 584
  SULFISOXAZOLE, 732
Azo-Standard—See
  PHENAZOPYRIDINE, 584
Azodine—See
  PHENAZOPYRIDINE, 584
Azolid—See
  PHENYLBUTAZONE, 604
Azotrex—See
  PHENAZOPYRIDINE, 584
Azulfidine—See
  SULFASALAZINE, 728

B

B & O Supprettes—See
  BELLADONNA, 68
B-Sed (M)—See
  BELLADONNA, 68
  PHENOBARBITAL, 594
B.O.F.—See
  PHENDIMETRAZINE, 586
BACAMPICILLIN, 64
Bacarate—See
  PHENDIMETRAZINE, 586
Bactocill—See OXACILLIN, 538
Bactopen—See CLOXACILLIN,
  174
Bactrim (M)—See
  SULFAMETHOXAZOLE, 726
  TRIMETHOPRIM, 794
Balminil DM (M)—See
  DEXTROMETHORPHAN, 220
  GUAIFENESIN, 346
Bamate—See MEPROBAMATE,
  444
Bamo 400—See
  MEPROBAMATE, 444
Ban-Drow 2—See CAFFEINE,
  100
Bancap with Codeine Capsules
  (M)—See
  ACETAMINOPHEN, 18
  ASPIRIN, 56
  CODEINE, 176
Banesin Forte Tablets (M)—See
  ACETAMINOPHEN, 18
  CODEINE, 176
Banlin—See PROPANTHELINE,
  666
Banthine with Phenobarbital
  Tablets (M)—See
  METHANTHLINE (NL)
  PHENOBARBITAL, 594
Barazole—See
  SULFISOXAZOLE, 732
Barbase Filmseal (M)—See
  BELLADONNA, 68
  PHENOBARBITAL, 594
Barbella (M)—See
  ATROPINE, 60
  HYOSCYAMINE, 374
  SCOPOLAMINE
  (HYOSCINE), 702
Barbeloid (M)—See
  ATROPINE, 60
  HYOSCYAMINE, 374
  SCOPOLAMINE
  (HYOSCINE), 702
Barbidonna (M)—See
  BELLADONNA, 68
  PHENOBARBITAL, 594

Barbidonna-CR (M)—See
ATROPINE, 60
HYOSCYAMINE, 374
SCOPOLAMINE
(HYOSCINE), 702
Bar-Cy-A-Tab (M)—See
ATROPINE, 60
HYOSCYAMINE, 374
SCOPOLAMINE, 702
Bar-Cy-Amine (M)—See
ATROPINE, 60
HYOSCYAMINE, 374
SCOPOLAMINE, 702
Bar-Don (M)—See
ATROPINE, 60
HYOSCYAMINE, 374
SCOPOLAMINE, 702
Bar-Tropin (M)—See
ATROPINE, 60
PHENOBARBITAL, 594
Bayer Aspirin—See ASPIRIN, 56
Baymethazine—See
PROMETHAZINE, 664
Bebatab (M)—See
BELLADONNA, 68
PHENOBARBITAL, 594
BECLOMETHASONE, 66
Beclovent Inhaler—See
BECLOMETHASONE, 66
Beconase—See
BETAMETHASONE, 80
Beesix—See PYRIDOXINE
(VITAMIN B-6), 680
Belap (M)—See
BELLADONNA, 68
PHENOBARBITAL, 594
Belatol (M)—See
BELLADONNA, 68
PHENOBARBITAL, 594
Belbarb (M)—See
BELLADONNA, 68
PHENOBARBITAL, 594
Bolbutal (M)—See
ATROPINE, 60
HYOSCYAMINE, 374
SCOPOLAMINE
(HYOSCINE), 702
Belkaloids (M)—See
ATROPINE, 60
HYOSCYAMINE, 374
SCOPOLAMINE
(HYOSCINE), 702
Bell/ans—See SODIUM
BICARBONATE, 712
Bellachai (M)—See
BELLADONNA, 68
CHARCOAL (NL)
PHENOBARBITAL, 594
Belladenal (M)—See
ATROPINE, 60
BELLADONNA, 68
PHENOBARBITAL, 594
BELLADONNA, 68
Bellafedrol (M)—See
BELLADONNA, 68
CHLORPHENIRAMINE, 142
PHENYLEPHRINE, 606
PYRALAMINE (NL)
Bellafoline (M)—See
BELLADONNA, 68
HYOSCYAMINE, 374
Bellergal (M)—See
ATROPINE, 60
BELLADONNA, 68
ERGOTAMINE, 282

Bellkatal Tablets (M)—See
BELLADONNA, 68
PHENOBARBITAL, 594
Bello-phen (M)—See
BELLADONNA, 68
PHENOBARBITAL, 594
Belphen (M)—See
BELLADONNA, 68
PHENOBARBITAL, 594
Benacen—See PROBENECID,
654
*Benadryl with Ephedrine
Capsules (M)*—See
DIPHENHYDRAMINE, 248
EPHEDRINE, 274
Benadryl—See
DIPHENHYDRAMINE, 248
Benedectin (M)—See
DOXYLAMINE, 270
PYRIDOXINE, 680
Bendopa—See LEVODOPA, 402
BENDROFLUMETHIAZIDE, 70
Bendylate—See
DIPHENHYDRAMINE, 248
Benemid—See PROBENECID,
654
Benoxyl—See BENZOYL
PEROXIDE, 72
Bensylate—See
BENZTROPINE, 78
Bentyl Phenobarbital (M)—See
DICYCLOMINE, 230
PHENOBARBITAL, 594
Bentyl—See DICYCLOMINE,
230
Bentylol—See DICYCLOMINE,
230
Benuryl—See PROBENECID,
654
Benylin Cough Syrup—See
DIPHENHYDRAMINE, 248
Benylin DM (M)—See
DEXTROMETHORPHAN, 220
DIPHENHYDRAMINE, 248
Benzac—See BENZOYL
PEROXIDE, 72
Benzagel—See BENZOYL
PEROXIDE, 72
Benzedrine—See
AMPHETAMINE, 48
Benzocaine Topical—See
ANESTHETICS (TOPICAL), 52
Benzocol Ointment—See
ANESTHETICS (TOPICAL), 52
Benzodiazepines—See
Tranquilizers
BENZOYL PEROXIDE, 72
BENZPHETAMINE, 74
BENZTHIAZIDE, 76
BENZTROPINE, 78
Bestorone—See ESTRONE, 304
Beta-adrenergic blockers
NADOLOL, 500
ATENOLOL, 58
METOPROLOL, 492
PROPRANOLOL, 670
TIMOLOL, 764
Betalin 12 Crystalline—See
VITAMIN B-12
(CYANOCOBALAMIN), 806
Betalin S—See THIAMINE
(VITAMIN B-1), 750
BETAMETHASONE, 80
Betapen-VK—See PENICILLIN
V, 572

Betaxin—See THIAMINE
(VITAMIN B-1), 750
BETHANECHOL, 82
Betnelan—See
BETAMETHASONE, 80
Betnesol—See
BETAMETHASONE, 80
Bewon—See THIAMINE
(VITAMIN B-1), 750
Bexophene Capsules (M)—See
ASPIRIN, 56
CAFFEINE, 100
Bicillin—See PENICILLIN G,
570
Bio-Tetra—See
TETRACYCLINE, 746
Biosone—See
HYDROCORTISONE
(CORTISOL), 364
Bioxatphen (M)—See
ATROPINE, 60
BISMUTH (NL)
PHENOBARBITAL, 594
BIPERIDINE, 84
Biphetamine (M)—See
AMPHETAMINE, 48
DEXTROAMPHETAMINE, 218
Biquin Durules—See
QUINIDINE, 690
BISACODYL, 86
Bisco-Lax—See BISACODYL,
86
Disodol Powder—See SODIUM
BICARBONATE, 712
Black Draught—See SENNA,
706
Blocadren—See TIMOLOL, 764
Blu-Hist Capsules (M)—See
ATROPINE, 60
CHLORPHENIRAMINE, 142
PHENYLPROPANOLAMINE,
608
Bobid—See SCOPOLAMINE
(HYOSCINE), 702
Bonapene—See RESERPINE,
698
Bonine—See MECLIZINE, 430
Bontril PDM—See
PHENDIMETRAZINE, 586
Brethine—See TERBUTALINE,
740
Brevicon (M)—See
CONTRACEPTIVES (ORAL),
182
Brexin Capsules (M)—See
GUAIFENESIN, 346
PSEUDOEPHEDRINE, 674
Briabell (M)—See
ATROPINE, 60
SCOPOLAMINE, 702
Briaspaz (M)—See
ATROPINE, 60
HYOSCYAMINE, 374
PHENOBARBITAL, 594
SCOPOLAMINE, 702
Bricanyl—See TERBUTALINE,
740
Brioschi—See SODIUM
BICARBONATE, 712
Bristacycline—See
TETRACYCLINE, 746
Bristamycin—See
ERYTHROMYCIN
STEARATE, 296

Brobella (M)—See
ATROPINE, 60
HYOSCYAMINE, 374
SCOPOLAMINE
(HYOSCINE), 702
Brocon Tablets (M)—See
BROMPHENIRAMINE, 90
PHENYLEPHRINE, 606
PHENYLPROPANOLAMINE,
608
Bromepaph (M)—See
BROMPHENIRAMINE, 90
PHENYLEPHRINE, 606
Bromo Seltzer (M)—See
ACETAMINOPHEN, 18
SODIUM BICARBONATE, 712
BROMODIPHENHYDRAMINE,
88
Bromphen—See
BROMPHENIRAMINE, 90
BROMPHENIRAMINE, 90
Brompheniramine Tablets—See
BROMPHENIRAMINE, 90
Bronchobid Duracaps (M)—See
PSEUDOEPHEDRINE, 674
THEOPHYLLINE, 748
Bronchodilators (xanthine)
OXTRIPHYLLINE, 544
AMINOPHYLLINE, 40
DYPHYLLINE, 272
THEOPHYLLINE, 748
Bronchodilators
ISOPROTERENOL, 394
METAPROTERENOL, 448
Broncholate (M)—See
BUTABARBITAL, 94
EPHEDRINE, 274
GUAIFENESIN, 346
THEOPHYLLINE, 748
Brondecon—See
GUAIFENESIN, 346
THEOPHYLLINE, 748
Brondilate Tablets (M)—See
BUTABARBITAL, 94
EPHEDRINE, 274
ISOPROTERENOL, 394
THEOPHYLLINE, 748
Bronitin—See EPINEPHRINE,
276
Bronkaid (M)—See
EPHEDRINE, 274
GUAIFENESIN, 346
THEOPHYLLINE, 748
Bronkaid Mist—See
EPINEPHRINE, 276
Bronkodyl—See
THEOPHYLLINE, 748
Bronkolixir (M)—See
EPHEDRINE, 274
GUAIFENESIN, 346
PHENOBARBITAL, 594
THEOPHYLLINE, 748
Bronkometer—See
ISOETHARINE, 388
Bronkosol (M)—See
AQUEOUS GLYCERIN (NL)
ISOETHARINE, 388
Bronkotabs (M)—See
EPHEDRINE, 274
GUAIFENESIN, 346
PHENOBARBITAL, 594
THEOPHYLLINE, 748
Broserpine—See RESERPINE,
698

Brown Mixture (M)—See
GLYCYRRHISA (NL)
PAREGORIC, 564
Bucladin-S—See BUCLIZINE,
92
BUCLIZINE, 92
Buff-A Tablets (M)—See
ASPIRIN, 56
BUTALBITAL, 736
CAFFEINE, 100
Buff-A-Comp (M)—See
ASPIRIN, 56
BUTALBITAL, 736
CAFFEINE, 100
CODEINE, 176
Buffadyne Tablets (M)—See
ASPIRIN, 56
CAFFEINE, 100
Buffered ASA Tablets (M)—See
ASPIRIN, 56
SODIUM BICARBONATE, 712
Buren (M)—See
ATROPINE, 60
HYOSCYAMINE, 374
SCOPOLAMINE
(HYOSCINE), 702
Burntame Aerosol—See
ANESTHETICS (TOPICAL), 52
Butabar Elixir—See
BELLADONNA, 68
BUTABARBITAL, 94
Butabell HMB (M)—See
BUTABARBITAL, 94
HOMATROPIDE METHYL
BROMIDE (NL)
Butagesic—See
PHENYLBUTAZONE, 604
BUTALBITAL, 736
BUTAPERAZINE, 96
Butaserpazide (M)—See
BUTABARBITAL, 94
HYDROCHLOROTHIAZIDE,
360
Butazolidin—See
PHENYLBUTAZONE, 604
Butesin Picrate Ointment—See
ANESTHETICS (TOPICAL), 52
Butibel (M)—See
ATROPINE, 60
BELLADONNA, 68
BUTABARBITAL, 94
Butibel-Zyme (M)—See
ATROPINE, 60
BELLADONNA, 68
BUTABARBITAL, 94
ENZYMES (NL)
Buticaps—See
BUTABARBITAL, 94
Butigetic (M)—See
BUTABARTIBAL, 94
CAFFEINE, 100
Butiserpazide (M)—See
BUTABARBITAL, 94
RESERPINE, 698
Butisol—See
BUTABARBITAL, 94
Butizide (M)—See
BUTABARBITAL, 94
HYDROCHLOROTHIAZIDE,
360
BUTORPHANOL, 98
Butyn Sulfate Solution—See
ANESTHETICS (TOPICAL), 52

C

C-Ject—See VITAMIN C
(ASCORBIC ACID), 808
C-Tran—See
CHLORDIAZEPOXIDE, 134
Cafacetin (M)—See
ACETAMINOPHEN, 18
CAFFEINE, 100
GELSEMIUM (trace)
Cafecon—See CAFFEINE, 100
Cafergot (M)—See
CAFFEINE, 100
ERGOTAMINE, 282
Cafergot-PB (M)—See
CAFFEINE, 100
ERGOTAMINE, 282
PHENOBARBITAL, 594
Cafermine (M)—See
CAFFEINE, 100
ERGOTAMINE, 282
Cafetrate—See CAFFEINE, 100
CAFFEINE, 100
Caine Spray—See
ANESTHETICS (TOPICAL), 52
Cal-Vi-Nol Ointment—See
ANESTHETICS (TOPICAL), 52
Calan—See VERAPAMIL, 802
Calcidrine (M)—See
CODEINE, 176
EPHEDRINE, 274
Calciferol—See VITAMIN D, 810
Calcifidiol—See VITAMIN D,
810
Calciphen Tablets (M)—See
ASPIRIN, 56
PHENOBARBITAL, 594
Calcitriol—See VITAMIN D, 810
CALCIUM CARBONATE, 102
Calcium-channel blockers
DILTIAZEM, 242
NIFEDIPINE, 516
VERAPAMIL, 802
Caldecon (M)—See
PHENYLPROPANOLAMINE,
608
VITAMIN C, 808
Calderol—See VITAMIN D, 810
Callergy Capsules—See
PHENYLEPHRINE, 606
Cama Inlay Tablets (M)—See
ALUMINUM HYDROXIDE, 32
ASPIRIN, 56
MAGNESIUM HYDROXIDE,
420
Camalox (M)—See
ALUMINUM HYDROXIDE, 32
CALCIUM CARBONATE, 102
MAGNESIUM HYDROXIDE,
420
Campain—See
ACETAMINOPHEN, 18
*Cantil with Phenobarbital
(M)*—See
MEPENZOLATE (NL)
PHENOBARBITAL, 594
Capade—See ISOPROPAMIDE,
392
Capital Tablets—See
ACETAMINOPHEN, 18
Capital with Codeine (M)—See
ACETAMINOPHEN, 18
CODEINE, 176
Capoten—See CAPTOPRIL, 104

CAPTOPRIL, 104
CARBAMAZEPINE, 106
CARBENICILLIN, 108
CARBIDOPA & LEVODOPA, 110
CARBINOXAMINE, 112
Carbolith—See LITHIUM, 412
Carbonic anhydrase
  inhibitors—See Diuretics
Carbrital (M)—See
  CARBROMAL (NL)
  PENTOBARBITAL, 578
Cardilate—See ERYTHRITYL
  TETRANITRATE, 284
Cardioquin—See QUINIDINE,
  690
Cardizem—See DILTIAZEM,
  242
CARISOPRODOL, 114
CARPHENAZINE, 116
Cartrax (M)—See
  HYDROXYZINE, 372
  PENTAETHYTHRITOL
  TETRANITRATE, 574
Cas-Evac—See CASCARA, 118
Casa-Fru—See SENNA, 706
CASCARA, 118
Cascara Sagrada—See
  CASCARA, 118
CASTOR OIL, 120
Causalin Tablets (M)—See
  ASPIRIN, 56
  MAGNESIUM SALICYLATE
  (NL)
Ce-Vi-Sol—See VITAMIN C
  (ASCORBIC ACID), 808
Ceclor—See CEFACLOR, 122
Cecon—See VITAMIN C
  (ASCORBIC ACID), 808
CEFACLOR, 122
CEFADROXIL, 124
Cefinal (M)—See
  ASPIRIN, 56
  CAFFEINE, 100
Cel-U-Sec—See
  BETAMETHASONE, 80
Celbenin—See METHICILLIN,
  466
Celestone—See
  ADRENOCORTICOIDS
  (TOPICAL), 26
Celestone—See
  BETAMETHASONE, 80
Cellothyl—See
  METHYLCELLULOSE, 476
Celontin—See
  METHSUXIMIDE, 472
Celostoject—See
  BETAMETHASONE, 80
Cenafed—See
  PSEUDOEPHEDRINE, 674
Cenagesic (M)—See
  CAFFEINE, 100
  PHENYLEPHRINE, 606
Cenahist—See SCOPOLAMINE
  (HYOSCINE), 702
Cenalax—See BISACODYL, 86
Cenocort Forte—See
  TRIAMCINOLONE, 776
Cenolate—See VITAMIN C
  (ASCORBIC ACID), 808
Central-nervous-system
  stimulants (amphetamine)
  AMPHETAMINE, 48
  DEXTROAMPHETAMINE, 218
  METHAMPHETAMINE, 454

Centrax—See PRAZEPAM, 644
Cephalac—See LACTULOSE,
  400
CEPHALEXIN, 126
CEPHRADINE, 128
Ceporex—See CEPHALEXIN,
  126
Cerebel (M)—See
  ATROPINE, 60
  HYOSCINE, 702
  HYOSCYAMINE, 374
  PHENOBARBITAL, 594
Cerebid—See PAPAVERINE,
  558
Cerespan—See PAPAVERINE,
  558
Ceri-Bid—See VITAMIN C
  (ASCORBIC ACID), 808
*Cerose Compound
  Capsules*—See
  CHLORPHENIRAMINE, 142
Cetacaine Liquid—See
  ANESTHETICS (TOPICAL), 52
Cetamide—See
  SULFAMETHOXAZOLE, 726
Cetazol—See
  ACETAZOLAMIDE, 20
Cetro Cirose Liquid (M)—See
  CODEINE, 176
  GUAIFENESIN, 346
Cevalin—See VITAMIN C
  (ASCORBIC ACID), 808
Cevita—See VITAMIN C
  (ASCORBIC ACID), 808
Chardonna (M)—See
  ATROPINE, 60
  BELLADONNA, 68
  PHENOBARBITAL, 594
Chelating agents
  PENICILLAMINE, 568
Chembicarb—See SODIUM
  BICARBONATE, 712
Chemgel—See ALUMINUM
  HYDROXIDE, 32
Chemovag—See
  SULFISOXAZOLE, 732
Cheracol (M)—See
  CODEINE, 176
  GUAIFENESIN, 346
Cheracol D (M)—See
  DEXTROMETHORPHAN, 220
  GUAIFENESIN, 346
Chew-E—See VITAMIN E, 812
Chiggerex Ointment—See
  ANESTHETICS (TOPICAL), 52
Children's Allerest (M)—See
  CHLORPHENIRAMINE, 142
  PHENYLEPHRINE, 606
  PHENYLPROPANOLAMINE,
  608
Chlor-Histine Elixir (M)—See
  CHLORPHENIRAMINE, 142
  PHENYLEPHRINE, 606
Chlor-Promanyl—See
  CHLORPROMAZINE, 146
Chlor-Span—See
  CHLORPHENIRAMINE, 142
*Chlor-Trimeton Decongestant
  (M)*—See
  CHLORPHENIRAMINE, 142
  PSEUDOEPHEDRINE, 674
*Chlor-Trimeton Expectorant
  with Codeine (M)*—See
  CHLORPHENIRAMINE, 142
  CODEINE, 176

Chlor-Trimeton—See
  CHLORPHENIRAMINE, 142
Chlorafed Liquid (M)—See
  CHLORPHENIRAMINE, 142
  PSEUDOEPHEDRINE, 674
CHLORAL HYDRATE, 130
Chloramate Unicelles—See
  CHLORPHENIRAMINE, 142
Chloramate—See
  CHLORPHENIRAMINE, 142
Chloramead—See
  CHLORPROMAZINE, 146
CHLORDIAZEPOXIDE, 134
CHLORAMPHENICOL, 132
Chlordiazachel—See
  CHLORDIAZEPOXIDE, 134
Chlormine—See
  CHLORPHENIRAMINE, 142
Chloromide—See
  CHLORPROPAMIDE, 148
Chloromycetin—See
  CHLORAMPHENICOL, 132
Chloronase—See
  CHLORPROPAMIDE, 148
Chlorophen—See
  CHLORPHENTERMINE, 144
Chloroptic—See
  CHLORAMPHENICOL, 132
CHLOROQUINE, 136
CHLOROTHIAZIDE, 138
CHLOROTRIANISENE, 140
Chlorpel—See SCOPOLAMINE
  (HYOSCINE), 702
CHLORPHENIRAMINE, 142
*Chlorpheniramine
  Maleate*—See
  CHLORPHENIRAMINE, 142
CHLORPHENTERMINE, 144
Chlorprom—See
  CHLORPROMAZINE, 146
CHLORPROMAZINE, 146
CHLORPROPAMIDE, 148
CHLORPROTHIXENE, 150
Chlortab—See
  CHLORPHENIRAMINE, 142
CHLORTHALIDONE, 152
CHLORZOXAZONE, 154
Cholan-DH—See
  DEHYDROCHOLIC ACID, 206
Cholan-HMB (M)—See
  BROMIDE (NL)
  DEHYDROCHOLIC ACID, 206
  HOMATROPINE (NL)
  METHYL (NL)
  PHENOBARBITAL, 594
Choledyl—See
  OXTRIPHYLLINE, 544
CHOLESTYRAMINE, 156
Cholinergics
  AMBENONIUM, 36
  BETHANECHOL, 82
  NEOSTIGMINE, 512
  PYRIDOSTIGMINE, 678
Chooz—See CALCIUM
  CARBONATE, 102
Chronulac—See LACTULOSE,
  400
CIMETIDINE, 158
Cin-Quin—See QUINIDINE, 690
Cino-40—See
  TRIAMCINOLONE, 776

INDEX

Cinsospan Tablets—See
PHENYLPROPANOLAMINE,
608
Ciramine T.R.—See
CHLORPHENIRAMINE, 142
Ciramine—See
CHLORPHENIRAMINE, 142
Circanol—See ERGOLOID
MESYLATES, 278
Circlidrin—See NYLIDRIN, 530
Ciriforte Capsules—See
CHLORPHENIRAMINE, 142
Cirin (M)—See
ASPIRIN, 56
VITAMIN C, 808
Citra (M)—See
PHENIRAMINE, 590
PHENYLEPHRINE, 606
PHENYLPROPANOLAMINE,
608
Citrate of Magnesia—See
MAGNESIUM CITRATE, 416
Citrated Caffeine Tablets—See
CAFFEINE, 100
Citro-Nesia—See MAGNESIUM
CITRATE, 416
Citroma—See MAGNESIUM
CITRATE, 416
Claripex—See CLOFIBRATE,
166
Clear By Design—See
BENZOYL PEROXIDE, 72
Clearasil BP (M)—See
BENZOYL PEROXIDE, 72
VANISHING BASE (NL)
CLEMASTINE, 160
Cleocin—See CLINDAMYCIN,
164
CLIDINIUM, 162
Clinazine—See
TRIFLUOPERAZINE, 784
CLINDAMYCIN, 164
Clinestone—See ESTROGEN,
302
Clinoril—See SULINDAC, 734
Clistin—See CARBINOXAMINE,
112
CLOFIBRATE, 166
Clomid—See CLOMIPHENE,
168
CLOMIPHENE, 168
CLORAZEPATE, 170
CLORTERMINE, 172
CLOXACILLIN, 174
Cloxapen—See CLOXACILLIN,
174
Clysodrast—See BISACODYL,
86
Co-Tylenol (M)—See
ACETAMINOPHEN, 18
CHLORPHENIRAMINE, 142
PHENYLEPHRINE, 606
PSEUDOEPHEDRINE, 674
Co-Xan (M)—See
CODEINE, 176
EPHEDRINE, 274
GUAIFENESIN, 346
THEOPHYLLINE, 748
Coastaldyne Tablets (M)—See
ACETAMINOPHEN, 18
CODEINE, 176
Coastalgesic (M)—See
ACETAMINOPHEN, 18
CAFFEINE, 100
CODEINE, 176

Coco-Quinine—See QUININE,
692
Codalan (M)—See
ASPIRIN, 56
CAFFEINE, 100
CODEINE, 176
Codalex (M)—See
CODEINE, 176
PHENYLEPHRINE, 606
Codap Tablets (M)—See
ACETAMINOPHEN, 18
CODEINE, 176
Codasa (M)—See
ASPIRIN, 56
CODEINE, 176
CODEINE, 176
Codeine Sulfate Tablets—See
CODEINE, 176
Codimal PH (M)—See
CODEINE, 176
PSEUDOEPHEDRINE, 674
CHLORPHENIRAMINE, 142
Codimal-L.A. Cenules (M)—See
CHLORPHENIRAMINE, 142
PSEUDOEPHEDRINE, 674
Coditrate Syrup (M)—See
CODEINE, 176
GUAIFENESIN, 346
Codone—See
HYDROCODONE, 362
Codylax—See BISACODYL, 86
Coffee-Break—See
PHENYLPROPANOLAMINE,
608
Cogentin—See BENZTROPINE,
78
ColBENEMID (M)—See
COLCHICINE, 178
PROBENECID, 654
Colace—See DOCUSATE
SODIUM, 264
Colax—See DOCUSATE
SODIUM, 264
COLCHICINE, 178
*Coldene Cough Formula
(Children)*—See
CHLORPHENIRAMINE, 142
Colidrate—See CHLORAL
HYDRATE, 130
Colisone—See PREDNISONE,
650
Cologel—See
METHYLCELLULOSE, 476
Colonil—See DIPHENOXYLATE
& ATROPINE, 250
Colrex (M)—See
ACETAMINOPHEN, 18
CAFFEINE, 100
CHLORPHENIRAMINE, 142
PHENYLEPHRINE, 606
*Colrex Compound Capsules
(M)*—See
CODEINE, 176
CHLORPHENIRAMINE, 142
PHENYLEPHRINE, 142
*Colrex Compound Elixir
(M)*—See
CHLORPHENIRAMINE, 142
CODEINE, 176
PHENYLEPHRINE, 606
*Colrex Decongestant Tablets
(M)*—See
CHLORPHENIRAMINE, 142
PHENYLEPHRINE, 606

Colrex—continued
PHENYLPROPANOLAMINE,
608
Combid (M)—See
ISOPROPAMIDE, 392
PROCHLORPERAZINE, 658
Comfolax—See DOCUSATE
SODIUM, 264
Compazine—See
PROCHLORPERAZINE, 658
Compocillin VK—See
PENICILLIN V, 572
Comtrex (M)—See
ACETAMINOPHEN, 18
CHLORPHENIRAMINE, 142
DEXTROMETHORPHAN, 220
PSEUDOEPHEDRINE, 674
Conalsyn—See
SCOPOLAMINE
(HYOSCINE), 702
Conar Expectorant (M)—See
GUAIFENESIN, 346
PHENYLEPHRINE, 606
*Conex with Codeine Liquid
(M)*—See
CHLORPHENIRAMINE, 142
CODEINE, 176
PHENYLPROPANOLAMINE,
608
Conhist (M)—See
ATROPINE, 60
CHLORPHENIRAMINE, 142
PHENYLPROPANOLAMINE,
608
CONJUGATED ESTROGENS,
180
Contac (M)—See
PHENYLEPHRINE, 606
PHENYLPROPANOLAMINE,
608
CONTRACEPTIVES (ORAL),
182
Contratuss (M)—See
CHLORPHENIRAMINE, 142
DEXTROMETHORPHAN, 220
Control—See
PHENYLPROPANOLAMINE,
608
Convangesic (M)—See
PHENYLPROPANOLAMINE,
608
Copavin (M)—See
CODEINE, 176
PAPAVERINE, 558
Cope (M)—See
ALUMINUM HYDROXIDE, 32
ASPIRIN, 56
CAFFEINE, 100
MAGNESIUM HYDROXIDE,
420
Cophene (M)—See
CHLORPHENIRAMINE, 142
PHENYLEPHRINE, 606
PHENYLPROPANOLAMINE,
608
Copin (M)—See
ATROPINE, 60
PHENOBARBITAL, 594
Coprobate—See
MEPROBAMATE, 444
Coralsone (M)—See
ALUMINUM HYDROXIDE, 32
ASPIRIN, 56
VITAMIN C, 808

Corax—See
   CHLORDIAZEPOXIDE, 134
Cordran—See
   ADRENOCORTICOIDS
   (TOPICAL), 26
Corgard—See NADOLOL, 500
Coricidin "D" (M)—See
   ASPIRIN, 56
   CHLORPHENIRAMINE, 142
   PHENYLPROPANOLAMINE,
   608
Coricidin Demilets (M)—See
   CHLORPHENIRAMINE, 142
   PHENYLEPHRINE, 606
Coricidin Mist—See
   PHENYLEPHRINE, 606
Coricidin Tablets—See
   CHLORPHENIRAMINE, 142
Coriforte (M)—See
   ASPIRIN, 56
   CAFFEINE, 100
   CHLORPHENIRAMINE, 142
   PHENACETIN, 582
   VITAMIN C, 808
Corilin Infant Liquid—See
   CHLORPHENIRAMINE, 142
Cornex Plus Tablets (M)—See
   PHENYLPROPANOLAMINE,
   608
Coronex—See ISOSORBIDE
   DINITRATE, 396
Corophyllin—See
   AMINOPHYLLINE, 40
Correctol—See
   PHENOLPHTHALEIN, 596
Cort-Dome—See
   ADRENOCORTICOIDS
   (TOPICAL), 26
Cortalone—See
   PREDNISOLONE, 648
Cortan—See PREDNISONE, 650
Cortef—See
   ADRENOCORTICOIDS
   (TOPICAL), 26
Cortef Fluid—See
   HYDROCORTISONE
   (CORTISOL), 364
Cortenema—See
   HYDROCORTISONE
   (CORTISOL), 364
Cortifoam—See
   HYDROCORTISONE
   (CORTISOL), 364
CORTISOL, 364
CORTISONE, 184
Cortisone drugs (adrenal
   corticosteroid)
   BECLOMETHASONE, 66
   BETAMETHASONE, 80
   CORTISONE, 184
   DEXAMETHASONE, 214
   FLUPREDNISOLONE, 334
   HYDROCORTISONE
   (CORTISOL), 364
   METHYLPREDNISOLONE,
   484
   PARAMETHASONE, 562
   PREDNISOLONE, 648
   PREDNISONE, 650
   TRIAMCINOLONE, 776
Cortone—See CORTISONE, 184
Cortril—See
   ADRENOCORTICOIDS
   (TOPICAL), 26

Corutol DH—See
   HYDROCODONE, 362
Coryban D (M)—See
   CAFFEINE, 100
   CHLORPHENIRAMINE, 142
   PHENYLPROPANOLAMINE,
   608
Coryza Brengle Capsules
   (M)—See
   CHLORPHENIRAMINE, 142
   EPHEDRINE, 274
   PHENYLPROPANOLAMINE,
   608
Coryzaid (M)—See
   CAFFEINE, 100
   CHLORPHENIRAMINE, 142
   PHENYLEPHRINE, 606
Coryztime (M)—See
   BELLADONNA, 68
   PHENYLPROPANOLAMINE,
   608
Cosanyl (M)—See
   DEXTROMETHORPHAN, 220
   PSEUDOEPHEDRINE, 674
Cosea—See
   CHLORPHENIRAMINE, 142
Cosea-D Capsules (M)—See
   CHLORPHENIRAMINE, 142
   PHENYLEPHRINE, 606
Cotrol-D Tablets (M)—See
   CHLORPHENIRAMINE, 142
   PSEUDOEPHEDRINE, 674
Cotussis (M)—See
   TERPIN HYDRATE, 742
   CODEINE, 176
Cough suppressants
   DEXTROMETHORPHAN, 220
Cough/cold preparations
   GUAIFENESIN, 346
Coumadin—See WARFARIN
   SODIUM, 818
Covanamine (M)—See
   CHLORPHENIRAMINE, 142
   PHENYLEPHRINE, 606
   PHENYLPROPANOLAMINE,
   608
Covangesic (M)—See
   ACETAMINOPHEN, 18
   CHLORPHENIRAMINE, 142
   PHENYLEPHRINE, 606
Creamalin (M)—See
   ALUMINUM HYDROXIDE, 32
   MAGNESIUM HYDROXIDE,
   420
CROMOLYN, 186
Crystapen—See PENICILLIN G,
   570
Crysticillin—See PENICILLIN
   G, 570
Crystodigin—See DIGITOXIN,
   238
Cuprimine—See
   PENICILLAMINE, 568
CYANOCOBALAMIN, 806
Cyantin—See
   NITROFURANTOIN, 518
CYCLACILLIN, 188
Cyclaine Solution—See
   ANESTHETICS (TOPICAL), 52
CYCLANDELATE, 190
Cyclapen-W—See
   CYCLACILLIN, 188
CYCLIZINE, 192

Cyclo-Bell Tablets (M)—See
   BUTABARBITAL, 94
   PHENOBARBITAL, 594
CYCLOBENZAPRINE, 194
Cyclobec—See DICYCLOMINE,
   230
Cyclopar—See
   TETRACYCLINE, 746
CYCLOPHOSPHAMIDE, 196
Cyclospasmol—See
   CYCLANDELATE, 190
CYCLOTHIAZIDE, 198
CYCRIMINE, 200
Cyprodine—See
   CYPROHEPTADINE, 202
CYPROHEPTADINE, 202
Cyraso-400—See
   CYCLANDELATE, 190
Cystospaz—See
   HYOSCYAMINE, 374
Cytolen—See THYROXINE
   (T-4, LEVOTHYROXINE), 760
Cytomel—See LIOTHYRONINE,
   408
Cytospaz-(M) Capsules—See
   BUTABARBITAL, 94
   HYOSCYAMINE, 374
Cytoxan—See
   CYCLOPHOSPHAMIDE, 196

D

D-Feda—See
   PSEUDOEPHEDRINE, 674
D-Sinus Capsules (M)—See
   ACETAMINOPHEN, 18
   PHENYLPROPANOLAMINE,
   608
D-Tran—See DIAZEPAM, 222
D.E.P.—75—See
   DIETHYLPROPION, 232
DES—See
   DIETHYLSTILBESTROL, 234
DM Plus Cough Syrup (M)—See
   CHLORPHENIRAMINE, 142
   DEXTROMETHORPHAN, 220
Dactil Phenobarbital Capsules
   (M)—See
   BELLADONNA, 68
   PHENOBARBITAL, 594
Dainite (M)—See
   EPHEDRINE, 274
   PHENOBARBITAL, 594
Dal-Sinus Capsules—See
   PHENYLPROPANOLAMINE,
   608
Dalacin C—See CLINDAMYCIN,
   164
Dalalon L.A.—See
   DEXAMETHASONE, 214
Dallergy (M)—See
   ATROPINE, 60
   CHLORPHENIRAMINE, 142
   PHENYLEPHRINE, 606
   SCOPOLAMINE
   (HYOSCINE), 702
Dalmane—See FLURAZEPAM,
   336
Daltose—See VITAMIN E, 812
Danabol—See
   METHANDROSTENOLONE,
   456
DANTHRON, 204
Dantoin—See PHENYTOIN, 612

Dapa Tablets—See
ACETAMINOPHEN, 18
Dapase Tablets (M)—See
ACETAMINOPHEN, 18
CODEINE, 176
Daranide—See
DICHLORPHENAMIDE, 224
Darbid—See ISOPROPAMIDE, 392
Daricon PB Tablets (M)—See
OXYPHENCYCLAMINE (NL)
PHENOBARBITAL 594
Darvocet-N (M)—See
ACETAMINOPHEN, 18
PROPOXYPHENE, 668
Darvon Compound (M)—See
ASPIRIN, 56
CAFFEINE, 100
PROPOXYPHENE, 668
Darvon—See
PROPOXYPHENE, 668
Dasicon Capsules (M)—See
ASPIRIN, 56
CAFFEINE, 100
Datril Elixir—See
ACETAMINOPHEN, 18
Datril Tablets—See
ACETAMINOPHEN, 18
Datril—See ACETAMINOPHEN, 18
De Tal (M)—See
ATROPINE, 60
HYOSCYAMINE, 374
HYOSCINE, 702
PHENOBARBITAL, 594
Deapril-ST—See ERGOLOID
MESYLATES, 278
Deca-Durabolin—See
NANDROLONE, 508
Decadron L.A.—See
DEXAMETHASONE, 214
Decadron Respihaler—See
DEXAMETHASONE, 214
Decadron with Xylocaine (M)—See
ADRENOCORTICOIDS
(TOPICAL), 26
DEXAMETHASONE, 214
Decadron—See
ADRENOCORTICOIDS
(TOPICAL), 26
Decadron—See
DEXAMETHASONE, 214
Decagesic (M)—See
ASPIRIN, 56
DEXAMETHASONE, 214
Decapryn—See DOXYLAMINE, 270
Decaspray—See
ADRENOCORTICOIDS
(TOPICAL), 26
Decholin—See
DEHYDROCHOLIC ACID, 206
Declobese (M)—See
AMPHETAMINE, 48
DEXTROAMPHETAMINE, 218
Declomycin—See
DEMECLOCYCLINE, 208
Declostatin (M)—See
DEMECLOCYCLINE, 208
NYSTATIN, 532
Decobel (M)—See
BELLADONNA, 68
CHLORPHENIRAMINE, 142

Decobel—continued
PHENYLPROPANOLAMINE, 608
Deconamine Capsules (M)—See
CHLORPHENIRAMINE, 142
PSEUDOEPHEDRINE, 674
Deficol—See BISACODYL, 86
Dehist (M)—See
CHLORPHENIRAMINE, 142
PHENYLEPHRINE, 606
DEHYDROCHOLIC ACID, 206
Delatestryl—See
TESTOSTERONE, 744
Delaxin—See
METHOCARBAMOL, 468
Delcid (M)—See
ALUMINUM HYDROXIDE, 32
MAGNESIUM HYDROXIDE, 420
Delcozine—See
PHENDIMETRAZINE, 586
Delestrogen—See ESTRADIOL, 300
Delestrogen—See ESTROGEN, 302
Delta-Cortef—See
PREDNISOLONE, 648
Deltalin—See VITAMIN D, 810
Deltasone—See PREDNISONE, 650
Demazin (M)—See
CHLORPHENIRAMINE, 142
PHENYLEPHRINE, 606
DEMECLOCYCLINE, 208
Demer-Idine—See
MEPERIDINE, 438
Demerol—See MEPERIDINE, 438
Demi-Regroton (M)—See
CHLORTHALIDONE, 152
RESERPINE, 698
Demo-Cincol—See
DEXTROMETHORPHAN, 220
Demulen (M)—See
CONTRACEPTIVES (ORAL), 182
Denta-Fl—See SODIUM
FLUORIDE, 716
Depen—See PENICILLAMINE, 568
Depletite—See
DIETHYLPROPION, 232
Depo-Medrol—See
METHYLPREDNISOLONE, 484
Depo-Pred—See
METHYLPREDNISOLONE, 484
Depo-Provera—See
MEDROXYPROGESTONE, 434
Depo-Testosterone—See
TESTOSTERONE, 744
Deprol (M)—See
BENACTYCINE (NL)
MEPROBAMATE, 444
Depronal-SA—See
PROPOXYPHENE, 668
*Derma-Medicone
Ointment*—See
ANESTHETICS (TOPICAL), 52
Dermo-Gen Dressing—See
ANESTHETICS (TOPICAL), 52
Dermodex—See BENZOYL
PEROXIDE, 72

DESERPIDINE, 210
DESIPRAMINE, 212
Desoxyn—See
METHAMPHETAMINE, 454
Desquam-X—See BENZOYL
PEROXIDE, 72
DEXAMETHASONE, 214
Dexampex—See
DEXTROAMPHETAMINE, 218
Dexamyl—See AMOBARBITAL, 44
Dexasone—See
DEXAMETHASONE, 214
DEXCHLORPHENIRAMINE, 216
Dexedrine—See
DEXTROAMPHETAMINE, 218
Dexone—See
DEXAMETHASONE, 214
Dextro-Tussin (M)—See
CHLORPHENIRAMINE, 142
DEXTROMETHORPHAN, 220
DEXTROAMPHETAMINE, 218
*Dextromal Cough Syrup
(M)*—See
CHLORPHENIRAMINE, 142
DEXTROMETHORPHAN, 220
DEXTROMETHORPHAN, 220
Di-Ap-Trol—See
PHENDIMETRAZINE, 586
Di-Azo—See
PHENAZOPYRIDINE, 584
Di-Gel (M)—See
ALUMINUM HYDROXIDE, 32
MAGNESIUM CARBONATE, 416
MAGNESIUM HYDROXIDE, 420
SIMETHICONE, 710
Di-Phen—See PHENYTOIN, 612
Diabinese—See
CHLORPROPAMIDE, 148
Diacin—See NIACIN
(NICOTINIC ACID), 514
Diafen—See
DIPHENYLPYRALINE, 252
Dialog (M)—See
ACETAMINOPHEN, 18
CODEINE, 176
Dialose—See DOCUSATE
SODIUM, 264
Diamox—See
ACETAZOLAMIDE, 20
Dianabol—See
METHANDROSTENOLONE, 456
DIAZEPAM, 222
Diban (M)—See
ATROPINE, 60
PAREGORIC, 564
Dibucaine Ointment—See
ANESTHETICS (TOPICAL), 52
Dicarbosil—See CALCIUM
CARBONATE, 102
DICHLORPHENAMIDE, 224
DICLOXACILLIN, 226
Dicodid—See HYDROCODONE, 362
DICUMAROL, 228
DICYCLOMINE, 230
Didrex—See BENZPHETAMINE, 74
Dietac—See
PHENYLPROPANOLAMINE, 608

Dietec—See
  DIETHYLPROPION, 232
DIETHYLPROPION, 232
DIETHYLSTILBESTROL, 234
Digifortis—See DIGITALIS, 236
DIGITALIS, 236
Digitalis preparations
  DIGITALIS, 236
  DIGITOXIN, 238
  DIGOXIN, 240
  GITALIN, 342
DIGITOXIN, 238
DIGOXIN, 240
Dihydrotachysterol—See
  VITAMIN D, 810
Dilabron—See ISOETHARINE,
  388
Dilantin—See PHENYTOIN, 612
Dilatrate-SR—See
  ISOSORBIDE DINITRATE, 396
Dilaudid Cough Syrup (M)—See
  GUAIFENESIN, 346
  HYDROMORPHONE, 368
Dilaudid—See
  HYDROMORPHONE, 368
Dilin—See DYPHYLLINE, 272
Dilor (M)—See
  DYPHYLLINE, 272
  GUAIFENESIN, 346
  THEOPHYLLINE, 748
DILTIAZEM, 242
Dimacol (M)—See
  DEXTROMETHORPHAN, 220
  GUAIFENESIN, 346
  PSEUDOEPHEDRINE, 674
Dimelor—See
  ACETOHEXAMIDE, 22
DIMENHYDRINATE, 244
Dimentabs See
  DIMENHYDRINATE, 244
Dimetane Expectorant (M)—See
  GUAIFENESIN, 346
  PHENYLEPHRINE, 606
*Dimetane Expectorant-DC
  (M)*—See
  CODEINE, 176
  GUAIFENESIN, 346
  PHENYLEPHRINE, 606
Dimetane—See
  BROMPHENIRAMINE, 90
Dimetapp (M)—See
  BROMPHENIRAMINE, 90
  PHENYLPROPANOLAMINE,
  608
DIMETHINDENE, 246
*Dioctyl Sodium
  Sulfosuccinate*—See
  DOCUSATE SODIUM, 264
Diothane Ointment—See
  ANESTHETICS (TOPICAL), 52
Dipav—See PAPAVERINE, 558
DIPHENHYDRAMINE, 248
DIPHENOXYLATE &
  ATROPINE, 250
Diphenylan—See PHENYTOIN,
  612
Diphenylhydantoin—See
  PHENYTOIN, 612
DIPHENYLPYRALINE, 252
DIPYRIDAMOLE, 254
Disipal—See ORPHENADRINE,
  536
Disophrol (M)—See
  PSEUDOEPHEDRINE, 674
  BROMPHENIRAMINE, 90

DISOPYRAMIDE, 256
Dispatabs—See VITAMIN A, 804
DISULFIRAM, 258
Diucardin—See
  HYDROFLUMETHIAZIDE, 366
Diuchlor H—See
  HYDROCHLOROTHIAZIDE,
  360
Diulo—See METOLAZONE, 490
Diupres (M)—See
  HYDROCHLOROTHIAZIDE,
  360
  RESERPINE, 698
Diuretics
  AMILORIDE, 38
  FUROSEMIDE, 340
  SPIRONOLACTONE, 720
  TRIAMTERENE, 778
Diuretics (carbonic anhydrase
  inhibitor, sulfonamide)
  ACETAZOLAMIDE, 20
  DICHLORPHENAMIDE, 224
  METHAZOLAMIDE. 462
Diuretics (thiazide)
  BENDROFLUMETHIAZIDE, 70
  BENZTHIAZIDE, 76
  CHLOROTHIAZIDE, 138
  CHLORTHALIDONE, 152
  CYCLOTHIAZIDE, 198
  HYDROCHLOROTHIAZIDE,
  360
  HYDROFLUMETHIAZIDE, 366
  METHYCLOTHIAZIDE, 474
  METOLAZONE, 490
  POLYTHIAZIDE, 622
  QUINETHAZONE, 688
  TRICHLORMETHIAZIDE, 780
Diuril—See CHLOROTHIAZIDE,
  138
Diutensin-R Tablets (M)—See
  CRYPTENAMINE (NL)
  METHYCLOTHIAZIDE, 474
DOCUSATE CALCIUM, 260
DOCUSATE POTASSIUM, 262
DOCUSATE SODIUM, 264
Dolanex Elixir—See
  ACETAMINOPHEN, 18
Dolene (M)—See
  ACETAMINOPHEN, 18
  ASPIRIN, 56
  CODEINE, 176
  PROPOXYPHENE, 668
Dolophine—See METHADONE,
  452
Dolor (M)—See
  ACETAMINOPHEN, 18
  ASPIRIN, 56
  CAFFEINE, 100
  CODEINE, 176
Donabarb (M)—See
  BELLADONNA, 68
  PHENOBARBITAL, 594
Donna-Lix Elixir (M)—See
  BELLADONNA, 68
  PHENOBARBITAL, 594
Donnacin (M)—See
  ATROPINE, 60
  HYOSCYAMINE, 374
  SCOPOLAMINE
  (HYOSCINE), 702
Donnafed Jr. (M)—See
  BELLADONNA, 68
  EPHEDRINE, 274

Donnagel (M)—See
  ATROPINE, 60
  HYOSCYAMINE, 374
  SCOPOLAMINE
  (HYOSCINE), 702
Donnagel-PG (M)—See
  ATROPINE, 60
  HYOSCYAMINE, 374
  PAREGORIC, 564
  SCOPOLAMINE
  (HYOSCINE), 702
Donnamine (M)—See
  ATROPINE, 60
  HYOSCYAMINE, 374
  SCOPOLAMINE
  (HYOSCINE), 702
Donnatal (M)—See
  ATROPINE, 60
  BELLADONNA, 68
  HYOSCYAMINE, 374
  SCOPOLAMINE
  (HYOSCINE), 702
  PHENOBARBITAL, 594
Donnazyme (M)—See
  ATROPINE, 60
  BELLADONNA, 68
  ENZYMES (NL)
  HYOSCYAMINE, 374
  SCOPOLAMINE
  (HYOSCINE), 702
Dopamet—See METHYLDOPA,
  478
Dopar—See LEVODOPA, 402
Dorbane—See DANTHRON, 204
Dormarex—See PYRILAMINE,
  682
Dormethan—See
  DEXTROMETHORPHAN, 220
Dowmycin—See
  ERYTHROMYCIN, 286
DOXEPIN, 266
Doxidan (M)—See
  DOCUSATE SODIUM, 264
  DANTHRON, 204
Doxy-Lemmon—See
  DOXYCYCLINE, 268
Doxy-Tabs—See
  DOXYCYCLINE, 268
Doxychel—See
  DOXYCYCLINE, 268
DOXYCYCLINE, 268
DOXYLAMINE, 270
*Dr. Caldwell's Senna
  Laxative*—See SENNA, 706
Dralserp (M)—See
  HYDRALAZINE, 358
  RESERPINE, 698
Dralzine—See HYDRALAZINE,
  358
Dramaban—See
  DIMENHYDRINATE, 244
Dramamine—See
  DIMENHYDRINATE, 244
Dri-Hist (M)—See
  PHENIRAMINE, 590
  PHENYLPROPANOLAMINE,
  608
Drinus (M)—See
  ATROPINE, 60
  CHLORPHENIRAMINE, 142
  PHENYLEPHRINE, 606
  PHENYLPROPANOLAMINE,
  608
  SCOPOLAMINE
  (HYOSCINE), 702

INDEX

Drisdol—See VITAMIN D, 810
Dristan Cough Formula (M)—See
DEXTROMETHORPHAN, 220
GUAIFENESIN, 346
Drixoral (M)—See
BROMPHENIRAMINE, 90
PSEUDOEPHEDRINE, 674
Drize M Capsules (M)—See
CHLORPHENIRAMINE, 142
PHENYLEPHRINE, 606
SCOPOLAMINE
(HYOSCINE), 702
Dry and Clean—See BENZOYL
PEROXIDE, 72
Duad Koff Balls (M)—See
DEXTROMETHORPHAN, 220
PHENYLPROPANOLAMINE, 608
Duadacin (M)—See
ACETAMINOPHEN, 18
CAFFEINE, 100
CHLORPHENIRAMINE, 142
PHENYLEPHRINE, 606
Ducon (M)—See
ALUMINUM HYDROXIDE, 32
CALCIUM CARBONATE, 102
MAGNESIUM HYDROXIDE, 420
Dufalone—See DICUMAROL, 228
Dularin (M)—See
ACETAMINOPHEN, 18
CAFFEINE, 100
CODEINE, 176
Dulcolax—See BISACODYL, 86
Duo-Medihaler (M)—See
ISOPROTERENOL, 394
PHENYLEPHRINE, 606
Duotrate—See
PENTAERYTHRITOL
TETRANITRATE, 574
Duovent (M)—See
EPHEDRINE, 274
GUAIFENESIN, 346
PHENOBARBITAL, 594
THEOPHYLLINE, 748
Duphrene Tablets (M)—See
CHLORPHENIRAMINE, 142
PHENYLEPHRINE, 606
Durabolin—See
NANDROLONE, 508
Duracillin—See PENICILLIN G, 570
Duragesic Tablets (M)—See
ASPIRIN, 56
MAGNESIUM HYDROXIDE, 420
Duralone—See
METHYLPREDNISOLONE, 484
Duraquin—See QUINIDINE, 690
Duration—See
OXYMETAZOLINE, 548
Duretic—See
METHYCLOTHIAZIDE, 474
Duricef—See CEFADROXIL, 124
Duvoid—See BETHANECHOL, 82
Dyazide (M)—See
HYDROCLOROTHIAZIDE, 360
TRIAMTERENE, 778
Dycill—See DICLOXACILLIN, 226

Dyclone Solution—See
ANESTHETICS (TOPICAL), 52
Dylate—See PAPAVERINE, 558
Dymelor—See
ACETOHEXAMIDE, 22
Dynapen—See
DICLOXACILLIN, 226
Dynosal Tablets (M)—See
ACETAMINOPHEN, 18
ASPIRIN, 56
CAFFEINE, 100
CODEINE, 176
DYPHYLLINE, 272
Dyrenium—See
TRIAMTERENE, 778
Dysne-Inhal—See
EPINEPHRINE, 276
Dyspas—See DICYCLOMINE, 230

E

E-Biotic—See
ERYTHROMYCIN, 286
E-Mycin E—See
ERYTHROMYCIN
ETHYLSUCCINATE, 290
E-Pam—See DIAZEPAM, 222
E.E.S.—See ERYTHROMYCIN
ETHYLSUCCINATE, 290
Econochlor—See
CHLORAMPHENICOL, 132
Ecotrin—See ASPIRIN, 56
Ectasule—See EPHEDRINE, 274
Efed—See EPHEDRINE, 274
Effersyllium—See PSYLLIUM, 676
Elavil—See AMITRIPTYLINE, 42
Eldadryl—See
DIPHENHYDRAMINE, 248
Eldafed (M)—See
PSEUDOEPHEDRINE, 674
TRIPROLIDINE, 800
Eldatapp Tablets (M)—See
BROMPHENIRAMINE, 90
PHENYLPROPANOLAMINE, 608
Elder 65 Compound (M)—See
ASPIRIN, 56
CAFFEINE, 100
Eldodram—See
DIMENHYDRINATE, 244
Eldonal (M)—See
ATROPINE, 60
HYOSCYAMINE, 374
SCOPOLAMINE
(HYOSCINE), 702
Elephemet—See
PHENDIMETRAZINE, 586
Elixicon—See THEOPHYLLINE, 748
Elixiral (M)—See
ATROPINE, 60
HYOSCYAMINE, 374
PHENOBARBITAL, 594
Elixophyllin—See
THEOPHYLLINE, 748
Elthroxin—See THYROXINE
(T-4, LEVOTHYROXINE), 760
Eltor—See
PSEUDOEPHEDRINE, 674
Emagrin (M)—See
ASPIRIN, 56
CAFFEINE, 100
PHENYLEPHRINE, 606

Emfaseem Capsules (M)—See
GUAIFENESIN, 346
THEOPHYLLINE, 748
Empirin Compound (M)—See
ASPIRIN, 56
CAFFEINE, 100
PHENACETIN, 582
Empirin Compound with Codeine (M)—See
ASPIRIN, 56
CAFFEINE, 100
CODEINE, 176
PHENACETIN, 582
Empirin with Codeine (M)—See
ASPIRIN, 56
CODEINE, 176
Empracet with Codeine (M)—See
ACETAMINOPHEN, 18
CODEINE, 176
Emprazil (M)—See
ASPIRIN, 56
CAFFEINE, 100
PHENACETIN, 582
PSEUDOEPHEDRINE, 674
Emprazil-C Tablets (M)—See
ASPIRIN, 56
CAFFEINE, 100
CODEINE, 176
PSEUDOEPHEDRINE, 674
Emulsoil—See CASTOR OIL, 120
Enarax (M)—See
HYDROXYZINE, 372
OXYPHENCYCLAMINE (NL)
Endecon Tablets (M)—See
ACETAMINOPHEN, 18
PHENYLPROPANOLAMINE, 608
Endep—See AMITRIPTYLINE, 42
Endotussin-NN (M)—See
DEXTROMETHORPHAN, 220
PYRALAMINE, 682
Enduron—See
METHYCLOTHIAZIDE, 474
Enduronyl Tablets (M)—See
METHYCLOTHIAZIDE, 474
RESERPINE, 698
Eno—See SODIUM
BICARBONATE, 712
Enovid (M)—See
CONTRACEPTIVES (ORAL), 182
Entrophen—See ASPIRIN, 56
Ephed-Organidin (M)—See
EPHEDRINE, 274
IODINATED GLYCEROL (NL)
EPHEDRINE, 274
Ephedrine and Amytal Pulvules (M)—See
AMOBARBITAL, 44
EPHEDRINE, 274
Ephedrine and Nembutal-25 Capsules (M)—See
EPHEDRINE, 274
PENTOBARBITAL, 578
Ephedrine and Seconal Pulvules (M)—See
EPHEDRINE, 274
SECOBARBITAL, 704
Ephedrol with Codeine Liquid (M)—See
CODEINE, 176
EPHEDRINE, 274

Epi-Clear—See BENZOYL
  PEROXIDE, 72
Epifrin—See EPINEPHRINE, 276
EPINEPHRINE, 276
Epitrate—See EPINEPHRINE,
  276
Eppy—See EPINEPHRINE, 276
Epragen—See EPHEDRINE, 274
Eprolin—See VITAMIN E, 812
Epsom Salts—See
  MAGNESIUM SULFATE, 422
Equagesic (M)—See
  ASPIRIN, 56
  MEPROBAMATE, 444
Equanil—See MEPROBAMATE,
  444
Ergobel (M)—See
  ERGOTAMINE, 282
  HYOSCYAMINE, 374
  PHENOBARBITAL, 594
ERGOLOID MESYLATES, 278
Ergomar—See ERGOTAMINE,
  282
ERGONOVINE, 280
Ergostat—See ERGOTAMINE,
  282
Ergot preparations
  ERGOLOID MESYLATES, 278
  ERGOTAMINE, 282
Ergot preparations (uterine
  stimulant)
  ERGONOVINE, 280
  METHYLERGONOVINE, 480
ERGOTAMINE, 282
Ergotrate—See ERGONOVINE,
  280
Ery-Tab—See
  ERYTHROMYCIN, 286
Ery-derm—See
  ERYTHROMYCIN, 286
EryPed—See ERYTHROMYCIN
  ETHYLSUCCINATE, 290
Eryc—See ERYTHROMYCIN,
  286
Erypar—See ERYTHROMYCIN
  STEARATE, 296
ERYTHRITYL TETRANITRATE,
  284
Erythrocin—See
  ERYTHROMYCIN
  LACTOBIONATE, 294
Erythromid—See
  ERYTHROMYCIN, 286
ERYTHROMYCIN, 286
ERYTHROMYCIN ESTOLATE,
  288
ERYTHROMYCIN
  ETHYLSUCCINATE, 290
ERYTHROMYCIN
  GLUCEPTATE, 292
ERYTHROMYCIN
  LACTOBIONATE, 294
ERYTHROMYCIN STEARATE,
  296
Esgic (M)—See
  ACETAMINOPHEN, 18
  CAFFEINE, 100
  CODEINE, 176
Esidrix—See
  HYDROCHLOROTHIAZIDE,
  360
Esimil (M)—See
  GUANETHIDINE, 348
  HYDROCHLOROTHIAZIDE,
  360

Eskabarb—See
  PHENOBARBITAL, 594
Eskalith—See LITHIUM, 412
Eskatrol (M)—See
  DEXTROAMPHETAMINE, 218
  PROCHLORPERAZINE, 658
Espotabs—See
  PHENOLPHTHALEIN, 596
ESTERIFIED ESTROGENS, 298
Estinyl—See ESTROGEN, 302
Estinyl—See ETHINYL
  ESTRADIOL, 310
Estomed—See ESTROGEN, 302
ESTRADIOL, 300
Estrace—See ESTRADIOL, 300
Estrace—See ESTROGEN, 302
ESTROGEN, 302
Estrogens—See Female sex
  hormones (estrogens)
ESTRONE, 304
ESTROPIPATE, 306
Estrovis—See ESTROGEN, 302
Estrovis—See QUINESTROL,
  686
ETHCHLORVYNOL, 308
ETHINYL ESTRADIOL, 310
Ethril—See ERYTHROMYCIN
  STEARATE, 296
ETHOPROPAZINE, 312
ETHOSUXIMIDE, 314
ETHOTOIN, 316
ETHYLESTRENOL, 318
Etrafon (M)—See
  PERPHENAZINE, 580
  AMITRIPTYLINE, 42
Eulcin—See SCOPOLAMINE
  (HYOSCINE), 702
Euthroid (M)—See
  LIOTRIX, 410
  THYROXINE (T-4,
  LEVOTHYROXINE), 760
Eutonyl—See PARGYLINE, 566
Evac-U-Gen—See
  PHENOLPHTHALEIN, 596
Evac-U-Lax—See
  PHENOLPHTHALEIN, 596
Evex—See ESTERIFIED
  ESTROGENS, 298
Evex—See ESTROGEN, 302
Ex-Lax—See
  PHENOLPHTHALEIN, 596
Ex-Obese—See
  PHENDIMETRAZINE, 586
Excedrin (M)—See
  ACETAMINOPHEN, 18
  ASPIRIN, 56
  CAFFEINE, 100
Exdol—See ACETAMINOPHEN,
  18
Exna—See BENZTHIAZIDE, 76
Expectorants
  TERPIN HYDRATE, 742
Expectrosed Syrup—See
  CHLORPHENIRAMINE, 142
Extendryl (M)—See
  CHLORPHENIRAMINE, 142
  GUAIFENESIN, 346
  PHENYLEPHRINE, 606
  SCOPOLAMINE
  (HYOSCINE), 702

F

*FL-Tussex Cough Syrup
  (M)*—See
  CODEINE, 176
  PHENYLPROPANOLAMINE,
  608
Fastin—See PHENTERMINE,
  602
Febrogesic Capsules—See
  ACETAMINOPHEN, 18
Febrogesic Tablets—See
  ACETAMINOPHEN, 18
Feco-T—See FERROUS
  FUMARATE, 324
Fedahist Tablets (M)—See
  CHLORPHENIRAMINE, 142
  PSEUDOEPHEDRINE, 674
Fedrazil (M)—See
  CHLORCYCLIZINE (NL)
  PSEUDOEPHEDRINE, 674
Feen-A-Mint—See
  PHENOLPHTHALEIN, 596
Fellozine—See
  PROMETHAZINE, 664
Female hormones
  CONTRACEPTIVES (ORAL),
  182
Female sex hormones (estrogen)
  CHLOROTRIANISENE, 140
  CONJUGATED ESTROGENS,
  180
  DIETHYLSTILBESTROL, 234
  ESTERIFIED ESTROGENS,
  298
  ESTRADIOL, 300
  ESTROGEN, 302
  ESTRONE, 304
  ESTROPIPATE, 306
  ETHINYL ESTRADIOL, 310
  QUINESTROL, 686
Female sex hormones
  (progestin)
  MEDROXYPROGESTONE,
  434
  NORETHINDRONE, 522
  NORETHINDRONE
  ACETATE, 525
  NORGESTREL, 526
Feminone—See ESTROGEN,
  302
Feminone—See ETHINYL
  ESTRADIOL, 310
Femiron—See FERROUS
  FUMARATE, 324
Femogen—See ESTROGEN,
  302
Fendol Tablets (M)—See
  ACETAMINOPHEN, 18
  CAFFEINE, 100
  PHENYLEPHRINE, 606
FENFLURAMINE, 320
FENOPROFEN, 322
Fenylhist—See
  DIPHENHYDRAMINE, 248
Feosol—See FERROUS
  SULFATE, 328
Feostat—See FERROUS
  FUMARATE, 324
Fer-In-Sol—See FERROUS
  SULFATE, 328
Fergon—See FERROUS
  GLUCONATE, 326
Ferndex—See
  DEXTROAMPHETAMINE, 218

Fernhist Tablets (M)—See
CHLORPHENIRAMINE, 142
PHENYLEPHRINE, 606
Fernisolone-P—See
PREDNISOLONE, 648
Fernisone—See
HYDROCORTISONE
(CORTISOL), 364
Fero-Gradumet—See
FERROUS SULFATE, 328
Fero-folic-500 (M)—See
FERROUS SULFATE, 328
FOLIC ACID (VITAMIN B-9),
338
Ferralet Plus—See FERROUS
GLUCONATE, 326
Ferralet—See FERROUS
GLUCONATE, 326
Ferralyn—See FERROUS
SULFATE, 328
Ferrofume—See FERROUS
FUMARATE, 324
Ferro-sequels (M)—
FERROUS FUMERATE, 324
DOCUSATE SODIUM, 264
Ferrous-G—See FERROUS
GLUCONATE, 326
FERROUS FUMARATE, 324
FERROUS GLUCONATE, 326
FERROUS SULFATE, 328
Fersamal—See FERROUS
FUMARATE, 324
Fesofor—See FERROUS
SULFATE, 328
Fever reducers
ACETAMINOPHEN, 18
ASPIRIN, 56
PHENACETIN, 582
Fiogesic Tablets (M)—See
PHENIRAMINE, 590
PHENYLPROPANOLAMINE,
608
Fiorinal (M)—See
CAFFEINE, 100
PHENACETIN, 582
TALBUTAL (BUTALBITAL),
736
Fiorinal with Codeine (M)—See
CAFFEINE, 100
PHENACETIN, 582
TALBUTAL (BUTALBITAL),
736
CODEINE, 176
Fitacol (M)—See
ATROPINE, 60
CHLORPHENIRAMINE, 142
PHENYLPROPANOLAMINE,
608
Fizrin—See SODIUM
BICARBONATE, 712
Flagyl—See METRONIDAZOLE,
494
Fletcher's Castoria—See
SENNA, 706
Flexeril—See
CYCLOBENZAPRINE, 194
Flexoject—See
ORPHENADRINE, 536
Flexon—See ORPHENADRINE,
536
Flo-Tab—See SODIUM
FLUORIDE, 716
Floramine—See
HYOSCYAMINE, 374

Fluorident—See SODIUM
FLUORIDE, 716
Fluoritab—See SODIUM
FLUORIDE, 716
Fluorodex—See SODIUM
FLUORIDE, 716
FLUOXYMESTERONE, 330
FLUPHENAZINE, 332
FLUPREDNISOLONE, 334
Flura—See SODIUM
FLUORIDE, 716
FLURAZEPAM, 336
Foille Liquid—See
ANESTHETICS (TOPICAL), 52
Foille Ointment—See
ANESTHETICS (TOPICAL), 52
FOLIC ACID (VITAMIN B-9), 338
Folvite—See FOLIC ACID
(VITAMIN B-9), 338
Forbaxin—See
METHOCARBAMOL, 468
Forhistal—See
DIMETHINDENE, 246
Formatrix—See ESTROGEN,
302
Formula 44-D (M)—See
DEXTROMETHORPHAN, 220
GUAIFENESIN, 346
PHENYLPROPANOLAMINE,
608
Formulex—See DICYCLOMINE,
230
Fostex BPO—See BENZOYL
PEROXIDE, 72
4-Way Nasal Spray (M)—See
PHENYLEPHRINE, 606
PHENYLPROPANOLAMINE,
608
4-Way Tablets (M)—See
PHENYLEPHRINE, 606
PHENYLPROPANOLAMINE,
608
Fulvicin P/B—See
GRISEOFULVIN, 344
Fulvicin U/F—See
GRISEOFULVIN, 344
Fumasorb—See FERROUS
FUMARATE, 324
Fumerin—See FERROUS
FUMARATE, 324
Furadantin—See
NITROFURANTOIN, 518
Furalan—See
NITROFURANTOIN, 518
Furaloid—See
NITROFURANTOIN, 518
Furantoin—See
NITROFURANTOIN, 518
FUROSEMIDE, 340
Furoside—See FUROSEMIDE,
340

G

G-1 Tablets—See
ACETAMINOPHEN, 18
G-2 (M)—See
ACETAMINOPHEN, 18
CODEINE, 176
G-Bron Elixir—See
THEOPHYLLINE, 748
G-Sox—See SULFISOXAZOLE,
732
G.B.S. (M)—See
ATROPINE, 60
DEHYDROCHOLIC ACID, 206

Ganphen—See
PROMETHAZINE, 664
Gantanol—See
SULFAMETHOXAZOLE, 726
Gantrisin—See
SULFAMETHOXAZOLE, 726
Gantrisin—See
SULFISOXAZOLE, 732
Gardenal—See
PHENOBARBITAL, 594
Gas-X—See SIMETHICONE,
710
Gastrolic (M)—See
BELLADONNA, 68
PHENOBARBITAL, 594
Gaviscon (M)—See
ALUMINUM HYDROXIDE, 32
MAGNESIUM TRISILICATE,
424
Gaysal (M)—See
ACETAMINOPHEN, 18
CODEINE, 176
Gelcomul—See BELLADONNA,
68
Gelusil (M)—See
MAGNESIUM HYDROXIDE,
420
MAGNESIUM TRISILICATE,
424
SIMETHICONE, 710
Gemonil—See METHARBITAL,
460
Geocillin—See
CARBENICILLIN, 108
Geopen—See CARBENICILLIN,
108
Geritol Tablets (M)—See
FERROUS SULFATE, 328
NIACINAMIDE (NL)
OTHER VITAMINS (NL)
PYRIDOXINE (VITAMIN B-6),
680
Ginospan Tablets (M)—See
CHLORPHENIRAMINE, 142
PHENYLEPHRINE, 606
Gitaligin—See GITALIN, 342
GITALIN, 342
Glaucon—See EPINEPHRINE,
276
Globin Insulin—See INSULIN,
382
GLYCERYL TRINITRATE, 520
Glycotuss (M)—See
DEXTROMETHORPHAN, 220
GUAIFENESIN, 346
Glysennid—See SENNOSIDES
A & B, 708
Glytuss—See GUAIFENESIN,
346
Gonad stimulants
CLOMIPHENE, 168
Gravol—See
DIMENHYDRINATE, 244
Grifulvin V—See
GRISEOFULVIN, 344
Gris-PEF—See
GRISEOFULVIN, 344
Grisactin—See
GRISEOFULVIN, 344
GRISEOFULVIN, 344
Grisovin-FP—See
GRISEOFULVIN, 344
grisOwen—See
GRISEOFULVIN, 344
GUAIFENESIN, 346

Guaiahist (M)—See
  CHLORPHENIRAMINE, 142
  GUAIFENESIN, 346
  PHENYLEPHRINE, 606
Guaiamine Capsules (M)—See
  ACETAMINOPHEN, 18
  CHLORPHENIRAMINE, 142
GUANETHIDINE, 348
Guistrey Fortis Tablets (M)—See
  CHLORPHENIRAMINE, 142
  PHENYLEPHRINE, 606
Gustalac—See CALCIUM
  CARBONATE, 102
Gylanphen—See
  HYOSCYAMINE, 374
Gynergen—See ERGOTAMINE,
  282

H
HASP (M)—See
  ATROPINE, 60
  PHENOBARBITAL, 594
HALAZEPAM, 350
Haldol—See HALOPERIDOL,
  352
Haldrone—See
  PARAMETHASONE, 562
HALOPERIDOL, 352
Halotestin—See
  FLUOXYMESTERONE, 330
Haponal (M)—See
  ATROPINE, 60
  HYOSCYAMINE, 374
  SCOPOLAMINE
  (HYOSCINE), 702
Harmonyl—See DESERPIDINE,
  210
Harmonyl-D—See
  RESERPINE, 698
Harratrate (M)—See
  ATROPINE, 60
  PHENOBARBITAL, 594
Hasacode Tablets (M)—See
  ACETAMINOPHEN, 18
  CODEINE, 176
Hepahydrin—See
  DEHYDROCHOLIC ACID, 206
HETACILLIN, 354
Hexa-Betalin—See
  PYRIDOXINE (VITAMIN B-6),
  680
Hexacrest—See PYRIDOXINE
  (VITAMIN B-6), 680
Hexadrol—See
  DEXAMETHASONE, 214
Hexathricin Aerospra—See
  ANESTHETICS (TOPICAL), 52
Hexavibex—See PYRIDOXINE
  (VITAMIN B-6), 680
HEXOBARBITAL, 356
Hi-Temp Tablets—See
  ACETAMINOPHEN, 18
Hiprex—See METHENAMINE,
  464
Hispril—See
  DIPHENYLPYRALINE, 252
Hista-Clopane (M)—See
  CHLORPHENIRAMINE, 142
  PSEUDOEPHEDRINE, 674
Hista-Derfule (M)—See
  ATROPINE, 60
  CHLORPHENIRAMINE, 142
  PAREGORIC, 564
  PHENACETIN, 582

Hista-Vadrin (M)—See
  CHLORPHENIRAMINE, 142
  PHENYLEPHRINE, 606
Histabid (M)—See
  CHLORPHENIRAMINE, 142
  PHENYLEPHRINE, 606
  PHENYLPROPANOLAMINE,
  608
Histadyl Compound (M)—See
  CAFFEINE, 100
  CHLORPHENIRAMINE, 142
  EPHEDRINE, 274
Histadyl and ASA Compound
  (M)—See
  ASPIRIN, 56
  CAFFEINE, 100
  CHLORPHENIRAMINE, 142
  EPHEDRINE, 274
Histalet (M)—See
  CHLORPHENIRAMINE, 142
  PHENYLEPHRINE, 606
  PHENYLPROPANOLAMINE,
  608
Histalon—See
  CHLORPHENIRAMINE, 142
Histamic Tablets (M)—See
  CHLORPHENIRAMINE, 142
  PSEUDOEPHEDRINE, 674
Histamine H-2 antagonists
  CIMETIDINE, 158
  RANITIDINE, 694
Histapp Elixir (M)—See
  PHENYLEPHRINE, 606
  PHENYLPROPANOLAMINE,
  608
Histaspan—See
  CHLORPHENIRAMINE, 142
Histaspan-D (M)—See
  PHENYLEPHRINE, 606
  SCOPOLAMINE
  (HYOSCINE), 702
Histaspan-Plus (M)—See
  CHLORPHENIRAMINE, 142
  PHENYLEPHRINE, 606
Histatapp Elixir (M)—See
  BROMPHENIRAMINE, 90
  PHENYLEPHRINE, 606
Histatapp Tablets (M)—See
  BROMPHENIRAMINE, 90
  PHENYLPROPANOLAMINE,
  608
Histex—See
  CHLORPHENIRAMINE, 142
Historal (M)—See
  CHLORPHENIRAMINE, 142
  PHENYLEPHRINE, 606
  PSEUDOEPHEDRINE, 674
  SCOPOLAMINE
  (HYOSCINE), 702
Hormonin—See ESTROGEN,
  302
Hurricaine—See ANESTHETICS
  (TOPICAL), 52
Hyatal (M)—See
  ATROPINE, 60
  HYOSCYAMINE, 374
  SCOPOLAMINE
  (HYOSCINE), 702
Hybephen (M)—See
  ATROPINE, 60
  HYOSCYAMINE, 374
  SCOPOLAMINE
  (HYOSCINE), 702

Hycodan (M)—See
  HYDROCODONE, 362
  HOMATROPINE
  METHYLBROMIDE (Atropine
  actions), 60
Hycoff Cold Caps (M)—See
  BELLADONNA, 68
  CHLORPHENIRAMINE, 142
Hycomine (M)—See
  CHLORPHENIRAMINE, 142
  PHENYLPROPANOLAMINE,
  608
Hycotuss Expectorant (M)—See
  CODEINE, 176
  GUAIFENESIN, 346
Hydeltra-TBA—See
  PREDNISOLONE, 648
Hydeltrasol—See
  PREDNISOLONE, 648
Hydergine—See ERGOLOID
  MESYLATES, 278
HYDRALAZINE, 358
Hydralazide (M)—See
  HYDRALAZINE, 358
  HYDROCHLOROTHIAZIDE,
  360
Hydrex—See BENZTHIAZIDE
  76
Hydrid—See
  HYDROCHLOROTHIAZIDE,
  360
Hydro-Aquil—See
  HYDROCHLOROTHIAZIDE,
  360
HydroDIURIL—See
  HYDROCHLOROTHIAZIDE,
  360
HYDROCHLOROTHIAZIDE, 360
Hydrocil—See PSYLLIUM, 676
HYDROCODONE, 362
HYDROCORTISONE
  (CORTISOL), 364
Hydrocortone—See
  ADRENOCORTICOIDS
  (TOPICAL), 26
Hydrocortone—See
  HYDROCORTISONE
  (CORTISOL), 364
HYDROFLUMETHIAZIDE, 366
Hydrolose—See
  METHYLCELLULOSE, 476
HYDROMORPHONE, 368
Hydromox—See
  QUINETHAZONE, 688
Hydropres Tablets (M)—See
  HYDROCHLOROTHIAZIDE,
  360
  RESERPINE, 698
Hydroserp (M)—See
  HYDROCHLOROTHIAZIDE,
  360
  RESERPINE, 698
Hydrotensin (M)—See
  HYDROCHLOROTHIAZIDE,
  360
  RESERPINE, 698
HYDROXYCHLOROQUINE, 370
HYDROXYZINE, 372
Hydrozide-Z-50—See
  HYDROCHLOROTHIAZIDE,
  360

INDEX

Hygroton—See
CHLORTHALIDONE, 152
Hykaterol—See VITAMIN D, 810
Hynaldyne (M)—See
BELLADONNA, 68
PHENOBARBITAL, 594
Hyobid—See PAPAVERINE, 558
Hyonal (M)—See
ATROPINE, 60
HYOSCYAMINE, 374
SCOPOLAMINE
(HYOSCINE), 702
Hyonatol (M)—See
ATROPINE, 60
HYOSCYAMINE, 374
SCOPOLAMINE
(HYOSCINE), 702
HYOSCINE, 702
HYOSCYAMINE, 374
Hyperetic—See
HYDROCHLOROTHIAZIDE,
360
Hypnotics
CHLORAL HYDRATE, 130
METHAQUALONE, 458
Hypnotics (barbiturate)
AMOBARBITAL, 44
BUTABARBITAL, 94
HEXOBARBITAL, 356
MEPHOBARBITAL, 442
METHARBITAL, 460
PENTOBARBITAL, 578
PHENOBARBITAL, 594
SECOBARBITAL, 704
TALBUTAL (BUTALBITAL),
736
Hytinic—See
IRON-POLYSACCHARIDE,
384
Hytrona (M)—See
ATROPINE, 60
HYOSCYAMINE, 374
PHENOBARBITAL, 594
SCOPOLAMINE
(HYOSCINE), 702
Hytuss—See GUAIFENESIN,
346

I

ICN 65 Compound (M)—See
ASPIRIN, 56
CAFFEINE, 100
INH—See ISONIAZID, 390
Iberet—See FERROUS
SULFATE, 328
Iberet-Folic-500 (M)—See
FERROUS SULFATE, 328
FOLIC ACID (VITAMIN B-9),
338
IBUPROFEN, 376
Ilosone—See ERYTHROMYCIN
ESTOLATE, 288
Ilotycin—See ERYTHROMYCIN
GLUCEPTATE, 292
Imavate—See IMIPRAMINE, 378
IMIPRAMINE, 378
Immunosuppressives
CYCLOPHOSPHAMIDE, 196
Inderal—See PROPRANOLOL,
670

Inderide (M)—See
HYDROCHLOROTHIAZIDE,
360
PROPRANOLOL, 670
Indocid—See INDOMETHACIN,
380
Indocin SR—See
INDOMETHACIN, 380
Indocin—See INDOMETHACIN,
380
INDOMETHACIN, 380
Inhistor—See PHENIRAMINE,
590
Insomnal—See
DIPHENHYDRAMINE, 248
Insulatard—See INSULIN, 382
INSULIN, 382
Intal—See CROMOLYN, 186
Intrabutazone—See
PHENYLBUTAZONE, 604
Ionamin—See PHENTERMINE,
602
Iprenol—See
ISOPROTERENOL, 394
Ircon—See FERROUS
FUMARATE, 324
IRON-POLYSACCHARIDE, 384
Iron supplements—See Mineral
supplements (iron)
Ismelin—See GUANETHIDINE,
348
Ismelin-Esidrix (M)—See
GUANETHIDINE, 348
HYDROCHLOROTHIAZIDE,
360
Iso-Asminyl Tablets (M)—See
EPHEDRINE, 274
PHENOBARBITAL, 594
THEOPHYLLINE, 748
Iso-Bid—See ISOSORBIDE
DINITRATE, 396
Isobec—See AMOBARBITAL,
44
ISOCARBOXAZID, 386
Isoclor (M)—See
CHLORPHENIRAMINE, 142
CODEINE, 176
PSEUDOEPHEDRINE, 674
ISOETHARINE, 388
Isogard—See ISOSORBIDE
DINITRATE, 396
ISONIAZID, 390
Isophrin—See
PHENYLEPHRINE, 606
ISOPROPAMIDE, 392
ISOPROTERENOL, 394
Isoptin—See VERAPAMIL, 802
Isopto Atropine—See
ATROPINE, 60
Isopto Carpine—See
PILOCARPINE, 614
Isordil—See ISOSORBIDE
DINITRATE, 396
ISOSORBIDE DINITRATE, 396
Isotraine Cream—See
ANESTHETICS (TOPICAL), 52
ISOXSUPRINE, 398
Isptrate—See ISOSORBIDE
DINITRATE, 396
Isuprel Compound (M)—See
PHENOBARBITAL, 594
POTASSIUM IODIDE (NL)
THEOPHYLLINE, 748
Isuprel—See
ISOPROTERENOL, 394

J

Janimine—See IMIPRAMINE,
378

K

K-10—See POTASSIUM
GLUCONATE, 642
K-Lor—See POTASSIUM
CHLORIDE, 636
K-Lyte—See POTASSIUM
BICARBONATE & CITRIC
ACID, 626
K-Lyte/Cl—See POTASSIUM
BICARBONATE, POTASSIUM
CHLORIDE & CITRIC ACID,
632
K-Phen—See PROMETHAZINE,
664
KEFF—See POTASSIUM
BICARBONATE, POTASSIUM
CARBONATE & POTASSIUM
CHLORIDE, 628
KLOR-10%—See POTASSIUM
CHLORIDE, 636
KLOR-CON—See POTASSIUM
CHLORIDE, 636
Kalmedic—See ATROPINE, 60
Kalmn—See MEPROBAMATE,
444
Kamabel (M)—See
ATROPINE, 60
HYOSCYAMINE, 374
KAOLIN (NL)
PECTIN (NL)
Kaochlor-Eff—See POTASSIUM
BICARBONATE, POTASSIUM
CHLORIDE & POTASSIUM
CITRATE, 634
Kaon—See POTASSIUM
GLUCONATE, 642
Kaon-Cl—See POTASSIUM
CHLORIDE, 636
Kaoparin (M)—See
KAOLIN (NL)
PAREGORIC, 564
PECTIN (NL)
Kappadione—See VITAMIN K,
814
Karidium—See SODIUM
FLUORIDE, 716
Kasof—See DOCUSATE
POTASSIUM, 262
Kato—See POTASSIUM
CHLORIDE, 636
Kavrin—See PAPAVERINE, 558
Kay-Ciel—See POTASSIUM
CHLORIDE, 636
Kaybovite—See VITAMIN B-12
(CYANOCOBALAMIN), 806
Kaytrate—See
PENTAERYTHRITOL
TETRANITRATE, 574
Keflex—See CEPHALEXIN, 126
Kemadrin—See
PROCYCLIDINE, 660
Kenacort—See
TRIAMCINOLONE, 776
Kenalog—See
ADRENOCORTICOIDS
(TOPICAL), 26
Kenalog—See
TRIAMCINOLONE, 776

Kengesin (M)—See
ASPIRIN, 56
CAFFEINE, 100
Kesso-mycin—See
ERYTHROMYCIN, 286
Kestrin—See ESTRONE, 304
Kinesed (M)—See
ATROPINE, 60
BELLADONNA, 68
HYOSCYAMINE, 374
PHENOBARBITAL, 594
SCOPOLAMINE
(HYOSCINE), 702
Kirkaffeine Tablets—See
CAFFEINE, 100
Kistanil—See PROMETHAZINE,
664
Kleer—See SCOPOLAMINE
(HYOSCINE), 702
Kleer-Tuss—See
SCOPOLAMINE
(HYOSCINE), 702
Klophyllin Tablets—See
THEOPHYLLINE, 748
Klorvess—See POTASSIUM
BICARBONATE &
POTASSIUM CHLORIDE, 630
Klotrix—See POTASSIUM
CHLORIDE, 636
Koachlor—See POTASSIUM
CHLORIDE, 636
Kolantyl (M)—See
ALUMINUM HYDROXIDE, 32
MAGNESIUM HYDROXIDE,
420
Kolyum—See POTASSIUM
CHLORIDE & POTASSIUM
GLUCONATE, 638
Konakion—See VITAMIN K, 814
Konsyl—See PSYLLIUM, 676
Korostatin—See NYSTATIN,
532
Koryza (M)—See
ATROPINE, 60
CHLORPHENIRAMINE, 142
HYOSCYAMINE, 374
PHENYLEPHRINE, 606
PHENYLPROPANOLAMINE,
608
SCOPOLAMINE
(HYOSCINE), 702
Kronohist (M)—See
CHLORPHENIRAMINE, 142
PHENYLPROPANOLAMINE,
608

L

L-T-S—See THYROXINE (T-4,
LEVOTHYROXINE), 760
L.A. Formula—See PSYLLIUM,
676
Lan-Dol—See MEPROBAMATE,
444
LACTULOSE, 400
Lanatuss Expectorant (M)—See
CHLORPHENIRAMINE, 142
GUAIFENESIN, 346
PHENYLPROPANOLAMINE,
608
Laniazid C.P.—See ISONIAZID,
390
Lanorinal (M)—See
ASPIRIN, 56
CAFFEINE, 100

Lanothal (M)—See
BELLADONNA, 68
PHENOLPHTHALEIN, 596
Lanoxin—See DIGOXIN, 240
Largactil—See
CHLORPROMAZINE, 146
Larodopa—See LEVODOPA,
402
Larotid—See AMOXICILLIN, 46
Lasix—See FUROSEMIDE, 340
Laud-Iron—See FERROUS
FUMARATE, 324
Laxatives
MAGNESIUM HYDROXIDE,
420
MAGNESIUM TRISILICATE,
424
Laxatives (bulk-forming)
MALT SOUP EXTRACT, 426
METHYLCELLULOSE, 476
POLYCARBOPHIL CALCIUM,
620
PSYLLIUM, 676
Laxatives (emollient)
DOCUSATE CALCIUM, 260
DOCUSATE POTASSIUM, 262
DOCUSATE SODIUM, 264
POLOXAMER 188, 618
Laxatives (hyperosmotic)
MAGNESIUM CITRATE, 416
LACTULOSE, 400
MAGNESIUM HYDROXIDE,
420
MAGNESIUM SULFATE, 422
MAGNESIUM TRISILICATE,
424
SODIUM PHOSPHATE, 718
Laxatives (stimulant)
BISACODYL, 86
CASCARA, 118
CASTOR OIL, 120
DANTHRON, 204
DEHYDROCHOLIC ACID, 206
PHENOLPHTHALEIN, 596
SENNA, 706
SENNOSIDES A & B, 708
Ledercillin VK—See
PENICILLIN V, 572
Lemidyne with Codeine
(M)—See
ASPIRIN, 56
CAFFEINE, 100
CODEINE, 176
Lentard—See INSULIN, 382
Lente Iletin II—See INSULIN,
382
Lente Insulin—See INSULIN,
382
Letter—See THYROXINE (T-4,
LEVOTHYROXINE), 760
Levamine (M)—See
ATROPINE, 60
BUTABARBITAL, 94
HYOSCYAMINE, 374
SCOPOLAMINE
(HYOSCINE), 702
Levo-Dromoran—See
LEVORPHANOL, 404
LEVODOPA, 402
Levoid—See THYROXINE (T-4,
LEVOTHYROXINE), 760
Levopa—See LEVODOPA, 402
LEVORPHANOL, 404
Levothroid—See THYROXINE
(T-4, LEVOTHYROXINE), 760

LEVOTHYROXINE, 760
Levsin—See
HYOSCYAMINE, 374
Levsin with Phenobarbital
(M)—See
HYOSCYAMINE, 374
PHENOBARBITAL, 594
Levsin—See HYOSCYAMINE
374
Librax (M)—See
CHLORDIAZEPOXIDE, 134
CLIDINIUM, 162
Libritabs—See
CHLORDIAZEPOXIDE, 134
Librium—See
CHLORDIAZEPOXIDE, 134
Lida-Mantle Cream—See
ANESTHETICS (TOPICAL) 52
Lidex—See
ADRENOCORTICOIDS
(TOPICAL), 26
Lidocaine Ointment—See
ANESTHETICS (TOPICAL), 52
Limit—See
PHENDIMETRAZINE, 586
Limitite—See
PHENDIMETRAZINE, 586
Lincocin—See LINCOMYCIN,
406
LINCOMYCIN, 406
LIOTHYRONINE, 408
LIOTRIX, 410
Lipo Gantrisin—See
SULFISOXAZOLE, 732
Liprinal—See CLOFIBRATE,
166
Liquamar—See
PHENPROCOUMON, 598
Liqui-Cee—See VITAMIN C
(ASCORBIC ACID), 808
Liquid-Pred—See
PREDNISONE, 650
Liquiprin Drops—See
ACETAMINOPHEN, 18
Liquiprin—See
ACETAMINOPHEN, 18
Liquix-C Capsules (M)—See
ACETAMINOPHEN, 18
CODEINE, 176
Lithane—See LITHIUM, 412
LITHIUM, 412
Lithizine—See LITHIUM, 412
Lithobid—See LITHIUM, 412
Lithonate—See LITHIUM, 412
Lithotabs—See LITHIUM, 412
Lixaminol (M)—See
AMINOPHYLLINE, 40
DEXTROMETHORPHAN, 220
THEOPHYLLINE, 748
Lo-Ovral (M)—See
CONTRACEPTIVES (ORAL),
182
Lo-Tussin Syrup (M)—See
CHLORPHENIRAMINE, 142
CODEINE, 176
GUAIFENESIN, 346
PHENYLEPHRINE, 606
Locorten—See
ADRENOCORTICOIDS
(TOPICAL), 26
Loestrin (M)—See
CONTRACEPTIVES (ORAL),
182

INDEX

Lomotil—See
DIPHENOXYLATE &
ATROPINE, 250
Lopressor—See
METOPROLOL, 492
Lopurin—See ALLOPURINOL,
28
LORAZEPAM, 414
Lotusate—See TALBUTAL
(BUTALBITAL), 736
Luasmin (M)—See
EPHEDRINE, 274
PHENOBARBITAL, 594
THEOPHYLLINE, 748
Luftodil (M)—See
GUAIFENESIN, 346
PHENOBARBITAL, 594
THEOPHYLLINE, 748
Lufyllin (M)—See
DYPHYLLINE, 272
EPHEDRINE, 274
GUAIFENESIN, 346
PHENOBARBITAL, 594
THEOPHYLLINE, 748
Luride—See SODIUM
FLUORIDE, 716
Lyteca Elixir—See
ACETAMINOPHEN, 18
Lyteca Tablets—See
ACETAMINOPHEN, 18

M

M-Mycin—See
ERYTHROMYCIN, 286
MAO inhibitors (monamine
oxidase inhibitor)
PHENELZINE, 588
ISOCARBOXAZID, 386
PARGYLINE, 566
TRANYLCYPROMINE, 772
MSC Triaminic (M)—See
PHENYLPROPANOLAMINE,
608
SCOPOLAMINE
(HYOSCINE), 702
Maalox (M)—See
ALUMINUM HYDROXIDE, 32
MAGNESIUM HYDROXIDE,
420
Macrodantin—See
NITROFURANTOIN, 518
Magnased (M)—See
ATROPINE, 60
MAGNESIUM TRISILICATE,
424
MAGNESIUM HYDROXIDE,
420
Magnatril (M)—See
ALUMINUM HYDROXIDE, 32
MAGNESIUM HYDROXIDE,
420
MAGNESIUM TRISILICATE,
424
MAGNESIUM CARBONATE, 416
MAGNESIUM CITRATE, 418
MAGNESIUM HYROXIDE, 420
MAGNESIUM SULFATE, 422
MAGNESIUM TRISILICATE, 424
Magnox—See
ATROPINE, 60
MAGNESIUM HYDROXIDE,
420

Malgesic—See
PHENYLBUTAZONE, 604
Mallenzyme (M)—See
BELLADONNA, 68
PLUS ENZYMES (NL)
Mallopress Tablets (M)—See
HYDROCHLOROTHIAZIDE,
360
RESERPINE, 698
Malotuss—See
GUAIFENESIN, 346
MALT SOUP EXTRACT, 426
Maltsupex—See MALT SOUP
EXTRACT, 426
Mandelamine—See
METHENAMINE, 464
Mandelets—See
METHENAMINE, 464
Mandrax—See
METHAQUALONE, 458
Maniron—See FERROUS
FUMARATE, 324
Marax (M)—See
EPHEDRINE, 274
HYDROXYZINE, 372
Marbaxin-750—See
METHOCARBAMOL, 468
Marblen—See MAGNESIUM
CARBONATE, 416
Marcumar—See
PHENPROCOUMON, 598
Marezine—See CYCLIZINE, 192
Marflex—See ORPHENADRINE,
536
Marhist Capsules (M)—See
CHLORPHENIRAMINE, 142
PHENYLEPHRINE, 606
Marine—See
DIMENHYDRINATE, 244
Marplan—See
ISOCARBOXAZID, 386
Maso-Donna (M)—See
ATROPINE, 60
HYOSCYAMINE, 374
SCOPOLAMINE
(HYOSCINE), 702
Matropinal—See
PHENOBARBITAL, 594
Maxamag (M)—See
ALUMINUM HYDROXIDE, 32
MAGNESIUM HYDROXIDE,
420
Maxibolin—See
ETHYLESTRENOL, 318
Maxigesic Capsules (M)—See
CODEINE, 176
ACETAMINOPHEN, 18
PROMETHAZINE, 664
MAZINDOL, 428
Mazinor—See MAZINDOL, 428
Measurin Timed-release
Tablets—See ASPIRIN, 56
Mebaral—See
MEPHOBARBITAL, 442
MECLIZINE, 430
MECLOFENAMATE, 432
Meclomen—See
MECLOFENAMATE, 432
Medache (M)—See
ACETAMINOPHEN, 18
CAFFEINE, 100
Medi-Spas (M)—See
BELLADONNA, 68
HYOSCYAMINE, 374
PHENOBARBITAL, 594
ATROPINE, 60

Medi-Tran—See
MEPROBAMATE, 444
Medicone Dressing—See
ANESTHETICS (TOPICAL), 52
Medicycline—See
TETRACYCLINE, 746
Medihaler-Epi—See
EPINEPHRINE, 276
Medihaler-Ergotamine—See
ERGOTAMINE, 282
Medihaler-Iso—See
ISOPROTERENOL, 394
Medilium—See
CHLORDIAZEPOXIDE, 134
Medimet-250—See
METHYLDOPA, 478
Medralone—See
METHYLPREDNISOLONE,
484
Medrol Enpak—See
METHYLPREDNISOLONE,
484
Medrol—See
ADRENOCORTICOIDS
(TOPICAL), 26
Medrol—See
METHYLPREDNISOLONE,
484
Medrone-80—See
METHYLPREDNISOLONE,
484
MEDROXYPROGESTERONE,
434
MEFENAMIC ACID, 436
Megacillin—See PENICILLIN G,
570
Megascorb—See VITAMIN C
(ASCORBIC ACID), 808
Melfiat—See
PHENDIMETRAZINE, 586
Melitoxin—See DICUMAROL,
228
Mellaril—See THIORIDAZINE,
752
Menadiol—See VITAMIN K, 814
Menadione—See VITAMIN K,
814
Menest—See ESTROGEN, 302
Menospasm—See
DICYCLOMINE, 230
Menotrol—See ESTROGEN, 302
Menrium—See ESTROGEN, 302
Mep-E—See MEPROBAMATE,
444
Mepergan Fortis (M)—See
MEPERIDINE, 438
PROMETHAZINE, 664
MEPERIDINE, 438
MEPHENYTOIN, 440
MEPHOBARBITAL, 442
Mephyton—See VITAMIN K, 814
Mepred-40—See
METHYLPREDNISOLONE,
484
MEPROBAMATE, 444
Meprocon—See
MEPROBAMATE, 444
Meprospan—See
MEPROBAMATE, 444
Meprotabs—See
MEPROBAMATE, 444
Mequelon—See
METHAQUALONE, 458
Mequin—See
METHAQUALONE, 458

Meribam—See
MEPROBAMATE, 444
Mesantoin—See
MEPHENYTOIN, 440
Mesopin PB Tablets—See
PHENOBARBITAL, 594
MESORIDAZINE, 446
Mestinon—See
PYRIDOSTIGMINE, 678
Metalone-TBA—See
PREDNISOLONE, 648
Metamucil—See PSYLLIUM,
676
Metandren—See
METHYLTESTOSTERONE,
486
Metaprel—See
METAPROTERENOL, 448
METAPROTERENOL, 448
Metatensin (M)—See
RESERPINE, 698
TRICHLORMETHIAZIDE, 780
METHACYCLINE, 450
METHADONE, 452
Methadorm—See
METHAQUALONE, 458
Methahydrin—See
TRICHLORMETHIAZIDE, 780
Methampex—See
METHAMPHETAMINE, 454
METHAMPHETAMINE, 454
METHANDROSTENOLONE, 456
METHAQUALONE, 458
METHARBITAL, 460
METHAZOLAMIDE, 462
METHENAMINE, 464
Methergine—See
METHYLERGONOVINE, 480
METHICILLIN, 466
Methidate—See
METHYLPHENIDATE, 482
Methnite—See SCOPOLAMINE
(HYOSCINE), 702
Metho-500—See
METHOCARBAMOL, 468
METHOCARBAMOL, 468
Methoin—See MEPHENYTOIN,
440
METHOTREXATE, 470
METHSUXIMIDE, 472
METHYCLOTHIAZIDE, 474
METHYLCELLULOSE, 476
METHYLDOPA, 478
METHYLERGONOVINE, 480
Methylone—See
METHYLPREDNISOLONE,
484
METHYLPHENIDATE, 482
METHYLPREDNISOLONE, 484
METHYLTESTOSTERONE, 486
METHYSERGIDE, 488
Meticortelone—See
PREDNISOLONE, 648
Meticorten—See PREDNISONE,
650
METOLAZONE, 490
METOPROLOL, 492
Metrogesic (M)—See
ASPIRIN, 56
ACETAMINOPHEN, 18
CODEINE, 176
METRONIDAZOLE, 494
Metryl—See METRONIDAZOLE,
494

Mexate—See
METHOTREXATE, 470
microNEFRIN—See
EPINEPHRINE, 276
Micronor (M)—See
CONTRACEPTIVES (ORAL),
182
Midamor—See AMILORIDE, 38
Migraine (M)—See
ERGOTAMINE, 282
ACETAMINOPHEN, 18
Migrastat (M)—See
ERGOTAMINE, 282
ASPIRIN, 56
CAFFEINE, 100
Milk of Magnesia—See
MAGNESIUM HYDROXIDE,
420
Milocarpine—See
PILOCARPINE, 614
Milontin—See PHENSUXIMIDE,
600
Milpath (M)—See
TRIDIHEXETHYL, 782
MEPROBAMATE, 444
Milprem—See ESTROGEN, 302
Miltown—See MEPROBAMATE,
444
Min-Ovral (M)—See
CONTRACEPTIVES (ORAL),
182
Mineral supplements (iron)
FERROUS FUMARATE, 324
FERROUS GLUCONATE, 326
FERROUS SULFATE, 328
IRON-POLYSACCHARIDE,
384
Mineral supplements (fluoride)
SODIUM FLUORIDE, 716
Mineral supplements
(potassium)

POTASSIUM ACETATE,
POTASSIUM BICARBONATE
& POTASSIUM CITRATE, 624

POTASSIUM BICARBONATE
& CITRIC ACID, 626

POTASSIUM BICARBONATE,
POTASSIUM CARBONATE &
POTASSIUM CHLORIDE, 628

POTASSIUM BICARBONATE
& POTASSIUM CHLORIDE,
630

POTASSIUM BICARBONATE,
POTASSIUM CHLORIDE &
CITRIC ACID, 632

POTASSIUM BICARBONATE,
POTASSIUM CHLORIDE &
POTASSIUM CITRATE, 634

POTASSIUM CHLORIDE, 636

POTASSIUM CHLORIDE &
POTASSIUM GLUCONATE,
638

POTASSIUM CITRATE &
POTASSIUM GLUCONATE,
640

POTASSIUM GLUCONATE,
642
Mini-Lix—See
AMINOPHYLLINE, 40

Minipress—See PRAZOSIN, 646
Minizide (M)—See
PRAZOSIN, 646
POLYTHIAZIDE, 622
MINOCYCLINE, 496
Minocin—See MINOCYCLINE,
496
Minotal (M)—See
ACETAMINOPHEN, 18
CODEINE, 176
Minus—See
PHENDIMETRAZINE, 586
Miradon—See ANISINDIONE, 54
Mitrolan—See
POLYCARBOPHIL CALCIUM,
620
Mixtard—See INSULIN, 382
Mobenol—See TOLBUTAMIDE,
768
Mobidin Tablets—See
ASPIRIN, 56
Modacon (M)—See
CONTRACEPTIVES (ORAL),
182
Modane Bulk—See PSYLLIUM,
676
Modane—See DANTHRON, 204
Modecate—See
FLUPHENAZINE, 332
Modicon (M)—See
CONTRACEPTIVES (ORAL),
182
Moditen—See FLUPHENAZINE,
332
Mol-Iron—See FERROUS
SULFATE, 328
Monotard—See INSULIN, 382
MORPHINE, 498
Morusan Ointment—See
ANESTHETICS (TOPICAL), 52
Motion Cure—See MECLIZINE,
430
Motrin—See IBUPROFEN, 376
Mucilose—See PSYLLIUM, 676
Mucotin (M)—See
ALUMINUM HYDROXIDE, 32
MAGNESIUM HYDROXIDE,
420
Mudrane GG Elixir (M)—See
EPHEDRINE, 274
GUAIFENESIN, 346
PHENOBARBITAL, 594
THEOPHYLLINE, 748
Murcil—See
CHLORDIAZEPOXIDE, 134
Muscle relaxants (skeletal)
CARISOPRODOL, 114
CHLORZOXAZONE, 154
CYCLOBENZAPRINE, 194
METHOCARBAMOL, 468
ORPHENADRINE, 536
Mychel—See
CHLORAMPHENICOL, 132
Mycolog (M)—See
ADRENOCORTICOIDS,
(TOPICAL), 26
GRAMACIDIN (NL)
NEOMYCIN (NL)
NYSTATIN, 532
TRIAMCINOLONE, 776
Mycostatin—See NYSTATIN,
532

Mylanta (M)—See
ALUMINUM HYDROXIDE, 32
MAGNESIUM HYDROXIDE,
420
Mylicon—See SIMETHICONE,
710
Myobid—See PAPAVERINE, 558
Myolin—See ORPHENADRINE,
536
Myotonachol—See
BETHANECHOL, 82
Mysoline—See PRIMIDONE,
652
Mytelase—See AMBENONIUM,
36

N

N-Caps—See NIACIN
(NICOTINIC ACID), 514
NPH Iletin II—See INSULIN, 382
NPH—See INSULIN, 382
NADOLOL, 500
Nadostine—See NYSTATIN,
532
Nadozone—See
PHENYLBUTAZONE, 604
NAFCILLIN, 502
Nafcil—See NAFCILLIN, 502
Nafeen—See SODIUM
FLUORIDE, 716
Nafrine—See
OXYMETAZOLINE, 548
NALBUPHINE, 504
Naldecol (M)—See
PHENYLTOLOXAMINE, 610
PHENYLEPHRINE, 606
PHENYLPROPANOLAMINE,
608
PHENYLTOLOXAMINE, 610
Naldegesic Tablets (M)—See
ACETAMINOPHEN, 18
PSEUDOEPHEDRINE, 674
Naldetuss Syrup (M)—See
CHLORPHENIRAMINE, 142
ACETAMINOPHEN, 18
DEXTROMETHORPHAN, 220
PHENYLPROPANOLAMINE,
608
PHENYLTOLOXAMINE, 610
Nalfon—See FENOPROFEN,
322
NALIDIXIC ACID, 506
NANDROLONE, 508
NAPAP Capsules—See
ACETAMINOPHEN, 18
Napril (M)—See
CHLORPHENIRAMINE, 142
PHENYLEPHRINE, 606
PHENYLPROPANOLAMINE,
608
Naprosyn—See NAPROXEN,
510
NAPROXEN, 510
Naptrate—See
PENTAERYTHRITOL
TETRANITRATE, 574
Naqua—See
TRICHLORMETHIAZIDE, 780
Naquival Tablets (M)—See
HYDROCHLOROTHIAZIDE,
360
RESERPINE, 698

Narcotics
BUTORPHANOL, 98
CODEINE, 176
HYDROCODONE, 362
HYDROMORPHONE, 368
LEVORPHANOL, 404
MEPERIDINE, 438
METHADONE, 452
MORPHINE, 498
NALBUPHINE, 504
OPIUM, 534
OXYCODONE, 546
OXYMORPHONE, 552
PAREGORIC, 564
PENTAZOCINE, 576
PROPOXYPHENE, 668
Nardil—See PHENELZINE, 588
Narine Gyrocaps (M)—See
CHLORPHENIRAMINE, 142
PHENYLEPHRINE, 606
Narine—See SCOPOLAMINE
(HYOSCINE), 702
Narspan (M)—See
CHLORPHENIRAMINE, 142
PHENYLEPHRINE, 606
SCOPOLAMINE
(HYOSCINE), 702
Nasahist (M)—See
CHLORPHENIRAMINE, 142
PHENYLEPHRINE, 606
PHENYLPROPANOLAMINE,
608
Naturetin—See
BENDROFLUMETHIAZIDE, 70
Navane—See THIOTHIXENE,
754
Nebs—See ACETAMINOPHEN,
18
NegGram—See NALIDIXIC
ACID, 506
Nemasol—See
PARA-AMINOSALICYLIC
ACID (PAS), 560
Nembutal—See
PENTOBARBITAL, 578
Neo-Betalin—See VITAMIN
B-12 (CYANOCOBALAMIN),
806
Neo-Calme—See DIAZEPAM,
222
Neo-Codema—See
HYDROCHLOROTHIAZIDE,
360
Neo-Codenyl-M Syrup (M)—See
GUAIFENESIN, 346
CODEINE, 176
SODIUM CITRATE (NL)
Neo-Cortef (M)—See
ADRENOCORTICOIDS,
(TOPICAL), 26
NEOMYCIN, (TOPICAL) (NL)
Neo-Decadron (M)—See
ADRENOCORTICOIDS,
(TOPICAL), 26
NEOMYCIN, (TOPICAL) (NL)
Neo-Dibetic—See
TOLBUTAMIDE, 768
Neo-Mist—See
PHENYLEPHRINE, 606
Neo-Renal—See FUROSEMIDE,
340
Neo-Rubex—See VITAMIN
B-12 (CYANOCOBALAMIN),
806

Neo-Synephrine—See
PHENYLEPHRINE, 606
Neo-Tetrine—See
TETRACYCLINE, 746
Neo-Tran—See
MEPROBAMATE, 444
Neo-Tric—See
METRONIDAZOLE, 494
Neo-Zoline—See
PHENYLBUTAZONE, 604
Neobid—See
PSEUDOEPHEDRINE, 674
Neocholan—See
DEHYDROCHOLIC ACID, 206
Neocyten—See
ORPHENADRINE, 536
Neogel with sulfa (M)—See
ATROPINE, 60
Neoloid—See CASTOR OIL, 120
Neopap Supprettes—See
ACETAMINOPHEN, 18
Neoquess (M)—See
ATROPINE, 60
BUTABARBITAL, 94
HYOSCINE, 702
PHENOBARBITAL, 594
Neospect (M)—See
GUAIFENESIN, 346
PHENOBARBITAL, 594
THEOPHYLLINE, 748
NEOSTIGMINE, 512
Neotep Granucaps (M)—See
CHLORPHENIRAMINE, 142
PHENYLEPHRINE, 606
Neothylline—See
DYPHYLLINE, 272
Neothylline-G Tablets (M)—See
GUAIFENESIN, 346
THEOPHYLLINE, 748
Neptazane—See
METHAZOLAMIDE, 462
Nevrotose (M)—See
HYOSCYAMINE, 374
PHENOBARBITAL, 594
CAMPHOR (NL)
Niac—See NIACIN (NICOTINIC
ACID), 514
NIACIN (NICOTINIC ACID), 514
Niacin—See NIACIN
(NICOTINIC ACID), 514
Nicalex—See NIACIN
(NICOTINIC ACID), 514
Nico-400—See NIACIN
(NICOTINIC ACID), 514
Nico-Span—See NIACIN
(NICOTINIC ACID), 514
Nicobid—See NIACIN
(NICOTINIC ACID), 514
Nicocap—See NIACIN
(NICOTINIC ACID), 514
Nicolar—See NIACIN
(NICOTINIC ACID), 514
NICOTINIC ACID, 514
Nicotinex—See NIACIN
(NICOTINIC ACID), 514
Nicotym—See NIACIN
(NICOTINIC ACID), 514
NIFEDIPINE, 516
Niferex—See
IRON-POLYSACCHARIDE,
384
Nilcol (M)—See
CHLORPHENIRAMINE, 142
DEXTROMETHORPHAN, 220
GUAIFENESIN, 346

Nilcol—continued
PHENYLPROPANOLAMINE, 608
Nilspasm (M)—See
ATROPINE, 60
BELLADONNA, 68
HYOSCYAMINE, 374
SCOPOLAMINE
(HYOSCINE), 702
Nilstat—See NYSTATIN, 532
Nitrates—See Antianginal drugs
Nitrex—See
NITROFURANTOIN, 518
Nitro-Bid—See
NITROGLYCERIN
(GLYCERYL TRINITRATE), 520
Nitrodan—See
NITROFURANTOIN, 518
Nitrodisc—See
NITROGLYCERIN
(GLYCERYL TRINITRATE), 520
Nitro-Dur—See
NITROGLYCERIN
(GLYCERYL TRINITRATE), 520
NITROFURANTOIN, 518
NITROGLYCERIN (GLYCERYL
TRINITRATE), 520
Nitroglyn—See
NITROGLYCERIN
(GLYCERYL TRINITRATE), 520
Nitrol—See NITROGLYCERIN
(GLYCERYL TRINITRATE), 520
Nitrong—See NITROGLYCERIN
(GLYCERYL TRINITRATE), 520
Nitrospan—See
NITROGLYCERIN
(GLYCERYL TRINITRATE), 520
Nitrostabilin—See
NITROGLYCERIN
(GLYCERYL TRINITRATE), 520
Nitrostat—See
NITROGLYCERIN
(GLYCERYL TRINITRATE), 520
Nobesine-75—See
DIETHYLPROPION, 232
Noctec—See CHLORAL
HYDRATE, 130
Nodaca Timed-release
Capsules—See CAFFEINE, 100
Nodoz Tablets—See
CAFFEINE, 100
Nodoz—See CAFFEINE, 100
Nolamine (M)—See
CHLORPHENIRAMINE, 142
PHENYLPROPANOLAMINE, 608
Nor-Pred-TBA—See
PREDNISOLONE, 648
Nor-Q.D. (M)—See
CONTRACEPTIVES (ORAL), 182
Nor-tet—See TETRACYCLINE, 746
Nordryl—See
DIPHENHYDRAMINE, 248

NORETHINDRONE ACETATE, 524
NORETHINDRONE, 522
Norflex—See ORPHENADRINE, 536
NORGESTREL, 526
Norgesic (M)—See
ASPIRIN, 56
CAFFEINE, 100
ORPHENADRINE, 536
Norinyl—See
CONTRACEPTIVES (ORAL), 182
Norisodrine Aerotrol—See
ISOPROTERENOL, 394
Norlestrin (M)—See
CONTRACEPTIVES (ORAL), 182
Norlutate—See
NORETHINDRONE
ACETATE, 525
Norlutin—See
NORETHINDRONE, 522
Noroxine—See THYROXINE
(T-4, LEVOTHYROXINE), 760
Norpace—See
DISOPYRAMIDE, 256
Norpanth—See
PROPANTHELINE, 666
Norpramin—See
DESIPRAMINE, 212
NORTRIPTYLINE, 528
Norzine—See PROMAZINE, 662
Nova-Carpine—See
PILOCARPINE, 614
Nova-Phase—See ASPIRIN, 56
Nova-Pheno—See
PHENOBARBITAL, 594
Nova-Rectal—See
PENTOBARBITAL, 578
Novafed (M)—See
CHLORPHENIRAMINE, 142
PSEUDOEPHEDRINE, 674
Novahistine DH (M)—See
CHLORPHENIRAMINE, 142
CODEINE, 176
Novahistine DMX (M)—See
DEXTROMETHORPHAN, 220
GUAIFENESIN, 346
PSEUDOEPHEDRINE, 674
Novahistine Elixir (M)—See
CHLORPHENIRAMINE, 142
PHENYLPROPANOLAMINE, 608
Novahistine Expectorant
(M)—See
CHLORPHENIRAMINE, 142
CODEINE, 176
Novahistine Fortis (M)—See
CHLORPHENIRAMINE, 142
PHENYLEPHRINE, 606
Novahistine LP Tablets
(M)—See
CHLORPHENIRAMINE, 142
PHENYLEPHRINE, 606
Novahistine Melet (M)—See
CHLORPHENIRAMINE, 142
PHENYLEPHRINE, 606
Novamoxin—See
AMOXICILLIN, 46
Novapen V—See PENICILLIN V, 572
Novasen—See ASPIRIN, 56
Novo-Mepro—See
MEPROBAMATE, 444

Novobutamide—See
TOLBUTAMIDE, 768
Novobutazone—See
PHENYLBUTAZONE, 604
Novocloxin—See
CLOXACILLIN, 174
Novocolchine—See
COLCHICINE, 178
Novodimenate—See
DIMENHYDRINATE, 244
Novodipam—See DIAZEPAM, 222
Novoferrosulfa—See FERROUS
SULFATE, 328
Novoflupam—See
FLURAZEPAM, 336
Novoflurazine—See
TRIFLUOPERAZINE, 784
Novofolacid—See FOLIC ACID
(VITAMIN B-9), 338
Novohydrazide—See
HYDROCHLOROTHIAZIDE, 360
Novomedopa—See
METHYLDOPA, 478
Novoniacin—See NIACIN
(NICOTINIC ACID), 514
Novonidazol—See
METRONIDAZOLE, 494
Novopheniram—See
CHLORPHENIRAMINE, 142
Novopoxide—See
CHLORDIAZEPOXIDE, 134
Novopropanthil—See
PROPANTHELINE, 666
Novoproproxyn—See
PROPOXYPHENE, 668
Novoridazine—See
THIORIDAZINE, 752
Novorythro—See
ERYTHROMYCIN, 286
Novosemide—See
FUROSEMIDE, 340
Novosoxazole—See
SULFISOXAZOLE, 732
Novotetra—See
TETRACYCLINE, 746
Novothalidone—See
CHLORTHALIDONE, 152
Nu-Dispoz—See
DIETHYLPROPION, 232
Nu-Iron—See
IRON-POLYSACCHARIDE, 384
Nubain—See NALBUPHINE, 504
Nulac—See BISACODYL, 86
Numa-Dura-Tablets (M)—See
BUTABARBITAL, 94
EPHEDRINE, 274
THEOPHYLLINE, 748
Numorphan—See
OXYMORPHONE, 552
Nupercainal Cream—See
ANESTHETICS (TOPICAL), 52
Nupercainal Ointment—See
ANESTHETICS (TOPICAL), 52
Nupercainal Spray—See
ANESTHETICS (TOPICAL), 52
Nydrazid—See ISONIAZID, 390
NYLIDRIN, 530
Nyquil (M)—See
ACETAMINOPHEN, 18
DEXTROMETHORPHAN, 220
EPHEDRINE, 274

NYSTATIN, 532
Nytol—See
DIPHENHYDRAMINE, 248

O

O-V statin—See NYSTATIN, 532
Obalan—See
PHENDIMETRAZINE, 586
Obe-Nil TR—See
PHENDIMETRAZINE, 586
Obephen—See PHENTERMINE,
602
Obermine—See
PHENTERMINE, 602
Obestat—See
PHENYLPROPANOLAMINE,
608
Obestrin-30—See
PHENTERMINE, 602
Obestrol—See
PHENDIMETRAZINE, 586
Obetrol (M)—See
DEXTROAMPHETAMINE, 218
AMPHETAMINE, 48
Obeval—See
PHENDIMETRAZINE, 586
Obezine—See
PHENDIMETRAZINE, 586
Obotan—See
DEXTROAMPHETAMINE, 218
Octapav—See PAPAVERINE,
558
Ocusert—See PILOCARPINE,
614
Oestrilin—See ESTROGEN, 302
Ogen—See ESTROPIPATE, 306
Omni-Tuss Suspension
(M)—See
CHLORPHENIRAMINE, 142
CODEINE, 176
EPHEDRINE, 274
PHENYLTOLOXAMINE, 610
Omnibel (M)—See
HYOSCYAMINE, 374
SCOPOLAMINE
(HYOSCINE), 702
Omnipen—See AMPICILLIN, 50
Onset—See ISOSORBIDE
DINITRATE, 396
Ophthochlor—See
CHLORAMPHENICOL, 132
OPIUM, 534
Opium Tincture—See
PAREGORIC, 564
Opticrom—See CROMOLYN,
186
Optimine—See AZATADINE, 62
Ora-Testryl—See
FLUOXYMESTERONE, 330
Oradrate—See CHLORAL
HYDRATE, 130
Oramide—See TOLBUTAMIDE,
768
Oraminic (M)—See
ATROPINE, 60
CHLORPHENIRAMINE, 142
Orasone—See PREDNISONE,
650
Oratestin—See
FLUOXYMESTERONE, 330
Oratrol—See
DICHLORPHENAMIDE, 224

Oretic—See
HYDROCHLOROTHIAZIDE,
360
Oreticyl Tablets (M)—See
HYDROCHLOROTHIAZIDE,
360
RESERPINE, 698
Oreton Methyl—See
METHYLTESTOSTERONE,
486
Oreton—See TESTOSTERONE,
744
Orinase—See TOLBUTAMIDE,
768
Ornacol (M)—See
DEXTROMETHORPHAN, 220
PHENYLPROPANOLAMINE,
608
Ornade (M)—See
ISOPROPAMIDE, 392
PHENYLPROPANOLAMINE,
608
Ornex (M)—See
ACETAMINOPHEN, 18
PHENYLPROPANOLAMINE,
608
ORPHENADRINE, 536
Ortho-Novum (M)—See
CONTRACEPTIVES (ORAL),
182
Orthoxine & Aminophylline
Capsules (M)—See
THEOPHYLLINE, 748
Ossonate-Plus (M)—See
ACETAMINOPHEN, 18
CODEINE, 176
Ostoforte—See VITAMIN D, 810
Otrivin—See
OXYMETAZOLINE, 548
Ovcon (M)—See
CONTRACEPTIVES (ORAL),
182
ETHINYL ESTRADIOL, 310
Ovol—See SIMETHICONE, 710
Ovral (M)--See
CONTRACEPTIVES (ORAL),
182
Ovrette (M)—See
CONTRACEPTIVES (ORAL),
182
Ovulen (M)—See
CONTRACEPTIVES (ORAL),
182
Ox-Pam—See OXAZEPAM, 542
OXACILLIN, 538
Oxalid—See
OXYPHENBUTAZONE, 554
OXANDROLONE, 540
OXAZEPAM, 542
Oxlopar—See
OXYTETRACYCLINE, 556
Oxoids Tablets—See
PHENOBARBITAL, 594
OXTRIPHYLLINE, 544
Oxy-10—See BENZOYL
PEROXIDE, 72
Oxy-Kesso-Tetra—See
OXYTETRACYCLINE, 556
Oxybutazone—See
OXYPHENBUTAZONE, 554
OXYCODONE, 546
Oxydess II—See
DEXTROAMPHETAMINE, 218
OXYMETAZOLINE, 548
OXYMETHOLONE, 550

OXYMORPHONE, 552
OXYPHENBUTAZONE, 554
OXYTETRACYCLINE, 556

P

P & A (M)—See
ATROPINE, 60
PHENOBARBITAL, 594
P-200—See PAPAVERINE, 558
P-A-C Compound with Codeine
(M)—See
ASPIRIN, 56
CAFFEINE, 100
CODEINE, 176
P.A.C. Compound (M)—See
ASPIRIN, 56
CAFFEINE, 100
PHENACETIN, 582
PAMA (M)—See
ATROPINE, 60
METHAMPHETAMINE, 454
PYRILAMINE, 682
PAS, 560
P.A.S. Acid—See
PARA-AMINOSALICYLIC
ACID (PAS), 560
P.A.S.—See
PARA-AMINOSALICYLIC
ACID (PAS), 560
P-A-V—See PAPAVERINE, 558
PBZ—See TRIPELENNAMINE,
798
PBZ-Lontabs—See
TRIPELENNAMINE, 798
PBZ-SR—See
TRIPELENNAMINE, 798
P.E.T.N.—See
PENTAERYTHRITOL
TETRANITRATE, 574
PMB-200—See ESTROGEN,
302
PMB-400—See ESTROGEN,
302
P.R. Syrup—See
CHLORPHENIRAMINE, 142
P.S.P.R.X.—See
PHENDIMETRAZINE, 586
P.V. Carpine—See
PILOCARPINE, 614
PZI—See INSULIN, 382
Pabirin Buffered (M)—See
ALUMINUM HYDROXIDE, 32
ASPIRIN, 56
Pagitane—See CYCRIMINE, 200
Palafer—See FERROUS
FUMARATE, 324
Palbar No. 2 (M)—See
ATROPINE, 60
HYOSCYAMINE, 374
PHENOBARBITAL, 594
SCOPOLAMINE,
(HYOSCINE), 702
Palohist (M)—See
CHLORPHENIRAMINE, 142
PHENYLEPHRINE, 606
Pamelor—See
NORTRIPTYLINE, 528
Pamine PB (M)—See
PHENOBARBITAL, 594
SCOPOLAMINE
(HYOSCINE), 702
Pamine—See SCOPOLAMINE
(HYOSCINE), 702
Pan-B-1—See THIAMINE
(VITAMIN B-1), 750

INDEX

Panectyl—See TRIMEPRAZINE, 790
Panmycin—See TETRACYCLINE, 746
Panoxyl—See BENZOYL PEROXIDE, 72
Panthocal A & D—See ANESTHETICS (TOPICAL), 52
Pantopon—See OPIUM, 534
Panwarfin—See WARFARIN SODIUM, 818
PAPAVERINE, 558
PARA-AMINOSALICYLIC ACID (PAS), 560
Paracort—See PREDNISONE, 650
Paraflex—See CHLORZOXAZONE, 154
Parafon Forte (M)—See ACETAMINOPHEN, 18 CHLORZOXAZONE, 154
PARAMETHASONE, 562
Parasal—See PARA-AMINOSALICYLIC ACID (PAS), 560
Paraspan—See SCOPOLAMINE (HYOSCINE), 702
PAREGORIC, 564
Parepectolin (M)—See KAOLIN (NL) PAREGORIC, 564 PECTIN (NL)
Purest—See METHAQUALONE, 458
Pargesic 65—See PROPOXYPHENE, 668
Pargesic Compound 65 (M)—See ASPIRIN, 56 CAFFEINE, 100
PARGYLINE, 566
Parmine—See PHENTERMINE, 602
Purnate—See TRANYLCYPROMINE, 772
Parsidol—See ETHOPROPAZINE, 312
Parsitan—See ETHOPROPAZINE, 312
Partuss Tablets (M)—See ACETAMINOPHEN, 18 CHLORPHENIRAMINE, 142 PHENYLPROPANOLAMINE, 608
Pasna—See PARA-AMINOSALICYLIC ACID (PAS), 560
Pathibamate (M)—See MEPROBAMATE, 444 TRIDIHEXETHYL, 782
Pathilon with Phenobarbital (M)—See PHENOBARBITAL, 594 TRIDIHEXETHYL, 782
Pathilon—See TRIDIHEXETHYL, 782
Pathocil—See DICLOXACILLIN, 226
Pavabid—See PAPAVERINE, 558
Pavacap—See PAPAVERINE, 558
Pavadon Elixir (M)—See ACETAMINOPHEN, 18 CODEINE, 176

Pavadon—See PAPAVERINE, 558
Pavakey—See PAPAVERINE, 558
Pavased—See PAPAVERINE, 558
Pavasule—See PAPAVERINE, 558
Pavatest—See PAPAVERINE, 558
Pavatran—See PAPAVERINE, 558
Paverolan—See PAPAVERINE, 558
Pax 400—See MEPROBAMATE, 444
Paxipam—See HALAZEPAM, 350
Pediacof Cough Syrup (M)—See CHLORPHENIRAMINE, 142 CODEINE, 176 PHENYLEPHRINE, 606 POTASSIUM IODIDE (NL)
Pediaflor—See SODIUM FLUORIDE, 716
Pediamycin—See ERYTHROMYCIN ETHYLSUCCINATE, 290
Peece (M)—See ATROPINE, 60 HYOSCYAMINE, 374 PHENOBARBITAL, 594
Peganone—See ETHOTOIN, 316
Pen-Vee K—See PENICILLIN V, 572
Penamox—See AMOXICILLIN, 46
Penapar VK—See PENICILLIN V, 572
Penbritin—See AMPICILLIN, 50
PENICILLAMINE, 568
PENICILLIN G, 570
PENICILLIN V, 572
Penioral—See PENICILLIN G, 570
PENTAERYTHRITOL TETRANITRATE, 574
Pentazine—See PROMETHAZINE, 664 TRIFLUOPERAZINE, 784
PENTAZOCINE, 576
Pentestan—See PENTAERYTHRITOL TETRANITRATE, 574
Pentids—See PENICILLIN G, 570
PENTOBARBITAL, 578
Pentogen—See PENTOBARBITAL, 578
Pentraspan—See PENTAERYTHRITOL TETRANITRATE, 574
Pentritol—See PENTAERYTHRITOL TETRANITRATE, 574
Pepsogel—See ALUMINUM HYDROXIDE, 32
Pepto-Bismol—See CALCIUM CARBONATE, 102
Percocet (M)—See ACETAMINOPHEN, 18 CODEINE, 176
Percodan (M)—See ASPIRIN, 56

Percodan—continued CAFFEINE, 100 OXYCODONE, 546 PHENACETIN, 582
Percogesic (M)—See ACETAMINOPHEN, 18 PHENYLTOLOXAMINE, 610
Peri-Colase (M)—See DOCUSATE SODIUM, 264 CASANTHROL (NL)
Periactin—See CYPROHEPTADINE, 202
Peritrate—See PENTAERYTHRITOL TETRANITRATE, 574
Permapen—See PENICILLIN G, 570
Permitil—See FLUPHENAZINE, 332
PERPHENAZINE, 580
Persa-Gel—See BENZOYL PEROXIDE, 72
Persadox—See BENZOYL PEROXIDE, 72
Persantine—See DIPYRIDAMOLE, 254
Persistin Tablets (M)—See ASPIRIN, 56 SALICYLSALICYLIC ACID (NL)
Pertofrane—See DESIPRAMINE, 212
Pethadol—See MEPERIDINE, 438
Pevadil—See NYLIDRIN, 530
Pfi-Lithium—See LITHIUM, 412
Pfizer-E—See ERYTHROMYCIN STEARATE, 296
Pfizerpen G—See PENICILLIN G, 570
Pfizerpen VK—PENCILLIN V, 572
Phebe (M)—See BELLADONNA, 68 PHENOBARBITAL, 594
Phen-Azo—See PHENAZOPYRIDINE, 584
Phen-o-bel (M)—See BELLADONNA, 68 PHENOBARBITAL, 594
PHENACETIN, 582
Phenacol-DM Syrup (M)—See CHLORPHENIRAMINE, 142 DEXTROMETHORPHAN, 220
Phenaphen with Codeine (M)—See ACETAMINOPHEN, 18 CODEINE, 176
Phenaphen—See ACETAMINOPHEN, 18
Phenate Tablets (M)—See CHLORPHENIRAMINE, 142 PHENYLEPHRINE, 606 PHENYLPROPANOLAMINE, 608
PHENAZOPYRIDINE, 584
Phenazine—See PERPHENAZINE, 580
Phenazodine—See PHENAZOPYRIDINE, 584
Phenbutazone—See PHENYLBUTAZONE, 604
Phendex Tablets—See ACETAMINOPHEN, 18 PHENDIMETRAZINE, 586

INDEX 875

INDEX

Phendiet—See
  PHENDIMETRAZINE, 586
PHENELZINE, 588
Phenergan Compound (M)—See
  PSEUDOEPHEDRINE, 674
  PROMETHAZINE, 664
Phenergan Expectorant with
  Codeine (M)—See
  CODEINE, 176
  PROMETHAZINE, 664
Phenergan—See
  PROMETHAZINE, 664
Phenerhist—See
  PROMETHAZINE, 664
Phenetron—See
  CHLORPHENIRAMINE, 142
PHENIRAMINE, 590
PHENOLPHTHALEIN, 596
PHENMETRAZINE, 593
PHENOBARBITAL, 594
Phenobarbital and Belladonna
  (M)—See
  BELLADONNA, 68
  PHENOBARBITAL, 594
Phenodyne Tablets (M)—See
  ASPIRIN, 56
  CAFFEINE, 100
Phenodyne with Codeine
  Capsules (M)—See
  ASPIRIN, 56
  CAFFEINE, 100
  CODEINE, 176
Phenolax—See
  PHENOLPHTHALEIN, 596
Phenothiazines—See
  Tranquilizers or Antiemetics
PHENPROCOUMON, 598
Phensal Tablets (M)—See
  ASPIRIN, 56
  CAFFEINE, 100
PHENSUXIMIDE, 600
PHENTERMINE, 602
Phentrol—See PHENTERMINE,
  602
PHENYLBUTAZONE, 604
PHENYLEPHRINE, 606
Phenylin (M)—See
  PHENYLPROPANOLAMINE,
  608
  THEOPHYLLINE, 748
PHENYLPROPANOLAMINE,
  608
PHENYLTOLOXAMINE, 610
PHENYTOIN, 612
Phenzine—See
  PHENDIMETRAZINE, 586
Pheryl-E—See VITAMIN E, 812
Phospho-Soda—See SODIUM
  PHOSPHATE, 718
Phrenilin (M)—See
  ACETAMINOPHEN, 18
  CAFFEINE, 100
  CODEINE, 176
Phyldrox Tablets (M)—See
  EPHEDRINE, 274
  PHENOBARBITAL, 594
  THEOPHYLLINE, 748
Physpan—See
  THEOPHYLLINE, 748
Phytonadione—See VITAMIN K,
  814
Pil-Digis—See DIGITALIS, 236
PILOCARPINE, 614

Pilocar—See PILOCARPINE,
  614
Pilocel—See PILOCARPINE,
  614
Pilomiotin—See PILOCARPINE,
  614
PIPERACETAZINE, 616
Piperazine Estrone
  Sulfate—See ESTROPIPATE,
  306
Placidyl—See
  ETHCHLORVYNOL, 308
Plaquenil—See
  HYDROXYCHLOROQUINE,
  370
Plegine—See
  PHENDIMETRAZINE, 586
Plexonal (M)—See
  DIHYDROERGOTAMINE (NL)
  PHENOBARBITAL, 594
  SCOPOLAMINE
  (HYOSCINE), 702
  TALBUTAL (BUTALBITAL),
  736
Plova—See PSYLLIUM, 676
Polaramine Expectorant
  (M)—See
  CHLORPHENIRAMINE, 142
  DEXCHLORPHENIRAMINE,
  216
  GUAIFENESIN, 346
  PSEUDOEPHEDRINE, 674
Polaramine—See
  DEXCHLORPHENIRAMINE,
  216
POLOXAMER 188, 618
Poly-Histine (M)—See
  PHENIRAMINE, 590
  PHENYLPROPANOLAMINE,
  608
Poly-Histine Expectorant with
  Codeine (M)—See
  BROMPHENIRAMINE, 90
  CODEINE, 176
Poly-Histine-DX (M)—See
  PSEUDOEPHEDRINE, 674
  BROMPHENIRAMINE, 90
POLYCARBOPHIL CALCIUM,
  620
Polycillin—See AMPICILLIN, 50
Polymox—See AMOXICILLIN,
  46
POLYTHIAZIDE, 622
Pomalin—See PAREGORIC, 564
Pondimin—See
  FENFLURAMINE, 320
Ponstan—See MEFENAMIC
  ACID, 436
Ponstel—See MEFENAMIC
  ACID, 436
Pontocaine Cream—See
  ANESTHETICS (TOPICAL), 52
Pontocaine Ointment—See
  ANESTHETICS (TOPICAL), 52
Porox 7—See BENZOYL
  PEROXIDE, 72
POTASSIUM ACETATE,
  POTASSIUM BICARBONATE
  & POTASSIUM CITRATE, 624
POTASSIUM BICARBONATE &
  CITRIC ACID, 626
POTASSIUM BICARBONATE &
  POTASSIUM CHLORIDE, 630

POTASSIUM BICARBONATE,
  POTASSIUM CARBONATE &
  POTASSIUM CHLORIDE, 628
POTASSIUM BICARBONATE,
  POTASSIUM CHLORIDE &
  CITRIC ACID, 632
POTASSIUM BICARBONATE,
  POTASSIUM CHLORIDE &
  POTASSIUM CITRATE, 634
POTASSIUM CHLORIDE &
  POTASSIUM GLUCONATE,
  638
POTASSIUM CHLORIDE, 636
POTASSIUM CITRATE &
  POTASSIUM GLUCONATE,
  640
Potassium chloride solution
  USP—See POTASSIUM
  CHLORIDE, 636
POTASSIUM GLUCONATE, 642
POTASSIUM CITRATE, 624
Potassium supplements—See
  Mineral supplements
  (potassium)
Potassium Triplex—See
  POTASSIUM ACETATE,
  POTASSIUM BICARBONATE
  & POTASSIUM CITRATE, 624
POTASSIUM CHLORIDE, 628
Povan—See PYRVINIUM, 684
Poxy Compound-65 (M)—See
  ASPIRIN, 56
  CAFFEINE, 100
PRAZEPAM, 644
PRAZOSIN, 646
Pre-sate—See
  CHLORPHENTERMINE, 144
Pred Cor-TBA—See
  PREDNISOLONE, 648
PREDNISOLONE, 648
PREDNISONE, 650
Prefrin—See PHENYLEPHRINE,
  606
Prelu-2—See
  PHENDIMETRAZINE, 586
Preludin—See
  PHENMETRAZINE, 593
Premarin—See CONJUGATED
  ESTROGENS, 180
Presalin Tablets (M)—See
  ACETAMINOPHEN, 18
  ASPIRIN, 56
  CODEINE, 176
Presamine—See IMIPRAMINE,
  378
Primatene Mist—See
  EPINEPHRINE, 276
PRIMIDONE, 652
Principen—See AMPICILLIN, 50
Pro-65—See PROPOXYPHENE,
  668
Pro-Banthine with
  Phenobarbital Tablets
  (M)—See
  PHENOBARBITAL, 594
  PROPANTHELINE, 666
Pro-Banthine—See
  PROPANTHELINE, 666
PROBENECID, 654
Pro-Dax—See
  PHENYLPROPANOLAMINE,
  608
Pro-Dep—See
  METHYLPREDNISOLONE,
  484

Probalan—See PROBENECID, 654

Probital Tablets—See PHENOBARBITAL, 594

PROCAINAMIDE, 656

Procamide—See PROCAINAMIDE, 656

Procan SR—See PROCAINAMIDE, 656

Procan—See PROCAINAMIDE, 656

Procapan—See PROCAINAMIDE, 656

Procardia—See NIFEDIPINE, 516

PROCHLORPERAZINE, 658

PROCYCLIDINE, 660

Procytox—See CYCLOPHOSPHAMIDE, 196

Prodolor (M)—See ACETAMINOPHEN, 18 CAFFEINE, 100 CODEINE, 176

Progesic Compound-65 (M)—See ASPIRIN, 56 CAFFEINE, 100 PHENACETIN, 582 PROPOXYPHENE, 668

Progestins—See Female sex hormones

Prokotazine—See CARPHENAZINE, 116

Prolixin—See FLUPHENAZINE, 332

Proloid—See THYROGLOBULIN, 756

Promanyl—See PROMAZINE 662

Promapar—See CHLORPROMAZINE, 146

PROMAZINE, 662

PROMETHAZINE, 664

Promethazine HCl Expectorant with Codeine (M)—See CODEINE, 176 PROMETHAZINE, 664

Promosol—See CHLORPROMAZINE, 146

Pronestyl—See PROCAINAMIDE, 656

Propadrine—See PHENYLPROPANOLAMINE, 608

PROPANTHELINE, 666

Propanthel—See PROPANTHELINE, 666 PROPOXYPHENE, 668

Propoxychel Compound (M)—See ASPIRIN, 56 CAFFEINE, 100

PROPRANOLOL, 670

Prorex—See PROMETHAZINE, 664

Prosedin—See PROMETHAZINE, 664

Prostaphlin—See OXACILLIN, 538

Prostigmin—See NEOSTIGMINE, 512

Protamine Zinc & Iletin II—See INSULIN, 382

Proternol—See ISOPROTERENOL, 394

Protophylline—See DYPHYLLINE, 272

Protoprim—See TRIMETHOPRIM, 794

PROTRIPTYLINE, 672

Prov-U-Sep—See METHENAMINE, 464

Proval Drops—See ACETAMINOPHEN, 18

Proval Elixir—See ACETAMINOPHEN, 18

Provel Tablets—See ACETAMINOPHEN, 18

Provera—See MEDROXYPROGESTONE, 434

Provigan—See PROMETHAZINE, 664

Proxagesic—See PROPOXYPHENE, 668

Proxene—See PROPOXYPHENE, 668

Prulet—See PHENOLPHTHALEIN, 596

Prunicodeine (M)—See TERPIN HYDRATE, 742 CODEINE, 176

Prydon—See ATROPINE, 60

Pseudo-Hist Liquid (M)—See CHLORPHENIRAMINE, 142 PSEUDOEPHEDRINE, 674

PSEUDOEPHEDRINE, 674

Pseudofrin See PSEUDOEPHEDRINE, 674

PSYLLIUM, 676

Psyquil—See TRIFLUPROMAZINE, 786

Purge—See CASTOR OIL, 120

Purinol—See ALLOPURINOL, 28

Purodigin—See DIGITOXIN, 238

Pyma Timed Capsules (M)—See CHLORPHENIRAMINE, 142 PHENYLEPHRINE, 606

Pyopen—See CARBENICILLIN, 108

Pyracort-D—See PHENYLEPHRINE, 606

Pyrdonnal Spansules (M)—See ATROPINE, 60 BELLADONNA, 68 PHENOBARBITAL, 594

Pyribenazmine with Ephedrine Tablets (M)—See EPHEDRINE, 274 TRIPELENNAMINE, 798

Pyribenzamine—See TRIPELENNAMINE, 798

Pyridiate—See PHENAZOPYRIDINE, 584

Pyridium Plus (M)—See BUTABARBITAL, 94 HYOSCINE, 702 PHENAZOPYRIDINE, 584

Pyridium—See PHENAZOPYRIDINE, 584

PYRIDOSTIGMINE, 678

PYRIDOXINE (VITAMIN B-6), 680

PYRILAMINE, 682

Pyrodine—See PHENAZOPYRIDINE, 584 PYRIDOXINE (VITAMIN B-6), 680

Pyrroxate (M)—See CAFFEINE, 100 CHLORPHENIRAMINE, 142

Pyrroxate with Codeine Capsules (M)—See CAFFEINE, 100 CODEINE, 176 CHLORPHENIRAMINE, 142

PYRVINIUM, 684

Q

Quaalude—See METHAQUALONE, 458

Quadrinal (M)—See EPHEDRINE, 274 PHENOBARBITAL, 594 THEOPHYLLINE, 748

Quarzan—See CLIDINIUM, 162

Quelidrine (M)—See EPHEDRINE, 274 CHLORPHENIRAMINE, 142

Queltuss (M)—See CHLORPHENIRAMINE, 142 DEXTROMETHORPHAN, 220 GUAIFENESIN, 346

Questran—See CHOLESTYRAMINE, 156

Quibron (M)—See GUAIFENESIN, 346 THEOPHYLLINE, 748

Quide—See PIPERACETAZINE, 616

Quietal—See MEPROBAMATE, 444

Quinaglute Dura-Tabs—See QUINIDINE, 690

Quinamm (M)—See AMINOPHYLLINE, 40 QUININE, 692

Quinate—See QUINIDINE, 690

Quine—See QUININE, 692

QUINESTROL, 686

QUINETHAZONE, 688

QUININE, 692

QUINIDINE, 690

Quinidex Extentabs—See QUINIDINE, 690

Quinobarb (M)—See QUINIDINE, 690

Quinora—See QUINIDINE, 690

Quless—See PENTOBARBITAL, 578

Quotane Lotion—See ANESTHETICS (TOPICAL), 52

Quotane Ointment—See ANESTHETICS (TOPICAL), 52

R

RP-Mycin—See ERYTHROMYCIN, 286

Radiostol Forte—See VITAMIN D, 810

Radiostol—See VITAMIN D, 810

Ralabromophen Decongestant Elixir—See BROMPHENIRAMINE, 90

RANITIDINE, 694

Ratio—See CALCIUM CARBONATE, 102

Rau-Sed—See RESERPINE, 698

Raudixin—See RAUWOLFIA SERPENTINA, 696

Raulfia—See RAUWOLFIA SERPENTINA, 696

Raunormine—See DESERPIDINE, 210

Raupoid—See RAUWOLFIA SERPENTINA, 696

Rauraine—See RESERPINE, 698

Rauserpa—See RAUWOLFIA SERPENTINA, 696

Rautrax N Tablets (M)—See BENDROFLUMETHIAZIDE, 70 RESERPINE, 698

Rautrax Tablets (M)—See FLUMETHIAZIDE (NL) RESERPINE, 698

Rauwolfia alkaloids—See Tranquilizers

RAUWOLFIA SERPENTINA, 696

Rauzide (M)—See BENDROFLUMETHIAZIDE, 70 RESERPINE, 698

Re-Orphena—See ORPHENADRINE, 536

Rectacort (Topical) (M)—See BELLADONNA, 68 BISMUTH (NL) EPHEDRINE, 274 HYDROCORTISONE, 364

Rectal Medicone—See ANESTHETICS (TOPICAL), 52

Rectoid—See HYDROCORTISONE (CORTISOL), 364

Redahist Gyrocaps (M)—See CHLORPHENIRAMINE, 142 PSEUDOEPHEDRINE, 674

Redi-Dent—See SODIUM FLUORIDE, 716

Redisol—See VITAMIN B-12 (CYANOCOBALAMIN), 806

Redoxon—See VITAMIN C (ASCORBIC ACID), 808

Reducto—See PHENDIMETRAZINE, 586

Regibon—See DIETHYLPROPION, 232

Regonol—See PYRIDOSTIGMINE, 678

Regroton (M)—See CHLORTHALIDONE, 152 RESERPINE, 698

Regular Iletin II—See INSULIN, 382

Regular Insulin—See INSULIN, 382

Rela—See CARISOPRODOL, 114

Relaxil—See CHLORDIAZEPOXIDE, 134

Relium—See CHLORDIAZEPOXIDE, 134

Remsed—See PROMETHAZINE, 664

Renalgin (M)—See ATROPINE, 60 HYOSCYAMINE, 374 METHENAMINE, 464 SCOPOLAMINE (HYOSCINE), 702

Renese—See POLYTHIAZIDE, 622

Renese-R Tablets (M)—See POLYTHIAZIDE, 622 RESERPINE, 698

Renoquid—See SULFACYTINE, 724

Repoise—See BUTAPERAZINE, 96

Reposans—See CHLORDIAZEPOXIDE, 134

Repro Compound 65 (M)—See CAFFEINE, 100 ASPIRIN, 56 PHENACETIN, 582 PROPOXYPHENE, 668 RESERPINE, 698

Reserpazide Tablets (M)—See HYDROCHLOROTHIAZIDE, 360 RESERPINE, 698

Reserpoid—See RESERPINE, 698

Restophen—See HYOSCYAMINE, 374

Restoril—See TEMAZEPAM, 738

Retet—See TETRACYCLINE, 746

Retin-A—See TRETINOIN, 774

Rhinall—See PHENYLEPHRINE, 606

Rhindecon—See PHENYLPROPANOLAMINE, 608

Rhinex (M)—See CHLORPHENIRAMINE, 142 PHENYLEPHRINE, 606

Rhinex Ty-Med (M)—See CHLORPHENIRAMINE, 142 PHENYLPROPANOLAMINE, 608

Rhinidrin Tablets (M)—See CHLORPHENIRAMINE, 142 PHENYLPROPANOLAMINE, 608

Rhinocaps Capsules (M)—See ACETAMINOPHEN, 18 ASPIRIN, 56 PHENYLPROPANOLAMINE, 608

Rhinspec Tablets (M)—See ACETAMINOPHEN, 18 GUAIFENESIN, 346 PHENYLEPHRINE, 606

Rifadin—See RIFAMPIN, 700

RIFAMPIN, 700

Rifamate (M)—See ISONIAZID, 390 RIFAMPIN, 700

Rifomycin—See RIFAMPIN, 700

Rimactane—See RIFAMPIN, 700

Ritalin—See METHYLPHENIDATE, 482

Rival—See DIAZEPAM, 222

Ro Trim (M)—See AMPHETAMINE, 48 ATROPINE, 60 PHENOBARBITAL, 594

Ro-Diet—See DIETHYLPROPION, 232

Ro-Fedrin—See PSEUDOEPHEDRINE, 674

Ro-Hist—See TRIPELENNAMINE, 798

Ro-Papan—See PAPAVERINE, 558

Ro-Thyronine—See LIOTHYRONINE, 408

Ro-Thyroxine—See THYROXINE (T-4, LEVOTHYROXINE), 760

Robalate—See ALUMINUM HYDROXIDE, 32

Robamate—See MEPROBAMATE, 444

Robamol—See METHOCARBAMOL, 468

Robamox—See AMOXICILLIN, 46

Robaxin—See METHOCARBAMOL, 468

Robaxisal—See METHOCARBAMOL, 468

Robicillin VK—See PENICILLIN V, 572

Robidone—See HYDROCODONE. 362

Robidrine—See PSEUDOEPHEDRINE, 674

Robigesic—See ACETAMINOPHEN, 18

Robimycin—See ERYTHROMYCIN, 286

Robinul-PH Forte (M)—See GLYCOPYRROLATE (NL) PHENOBARBITAL, 594

Robitet—See TETRACYCLINE, 746

Robitussin A-C (M)—See CODEINE, 176 GUAIFENESIN, 346 PHENIRAMINE, 590

Robitussin-CF (M)—See DEXTROMETHORPHAN, 220 GUAIFENESIN, 346 PHENYLPROPANOLAMINE, 608

Robitussin-DM (M)—See DEXTROMETHORPHAN, 220 GUAIFENESIN, 346

Rocaltrol—See VITAMIN D, 810

Rofact—See RIFAMPIN, 700

Rolabromophen Decongestant Elixir (M)—See PHENYLEPHRINE, 606 PHENYLPROPANOLAMINE, 608

Rolahist—See PHENYLEPHRINE, 606

Rolaids (M)—See ALUMINUM HYDROXIDE, 32 SODIUM CARBONATE, 714

Rolazine—See HYDRALAZINE, 358

Rolidrin—See NYLIDRIN, 530

Romilar (M)—See DEXTROMETHORPHAN, 220 PHENYLPROPANOLAMINE, 608

Rondec (M)—See CARBINOXAMINE (NL) PSEUDOEPHEDRINE, 674

Rondomycin—See METHACYCLINE, 450

Ronuvex—See ACETAMINOPHEN, 18

Ropanth—See PROPANTHELINE, 666

Rosoxol—See SULFISOXAZOLE, 732

Rotitussin-DAC (M)—See
CODEINE, 176
GUAIFENESIN, 346
PSEUDOEPHEDRINE, 674
Rouqualone-300—See
METHAQUALONE, 458
Rubramin—See VITAMIN B-12
(CYANOCOBALAMIN), 806
Rubramin-PC—See VITAMIN
B-12 (CYANOCOBALAMIN),
806
Rufen—See IBUPROFEN, 376
Ruhexatal with Reserpine
Tablets (M)—See
MANNITOL HEXANITRATE
(NL)
RESERPINE, 698
Rynacrom—See CROMOLYN,
186
Rynatan Pediatric Suspension
(M)—See
CHLORPHENIRAMINE, 142
PHENYLEPHRINE, 606
Rynatan Tablets (M)—See
CHLORPHENIRAMINE, 142
PHENYLEPHRINE, 606
Rynatapp Elixir (M)—See
BROMPHENIRAMINE, 90
PHENYLEPHRINE, 606
PHENYLPROPANOLAMINE,
608
Rynatuss (M)—See
CHLORPHENIRAMINE, 142
EPHEDRINE, 274
PHENYLEPHRINE, 606
Rythmodan—See
DISOPYRAMIDE, 256

S

S-A-C Tablets (M)—See
ACETAMINOPHEN, 18
CAFFEINE, 100
CODEINE, 176
SAS-500—See
SULFASALAZINE, 728
SK-65 Compound (M)—See
ASPIRIN, 56
CAFFEINE, 100
PHENACETIN, 582
PROPOXYPHENE, 668
SK-65—See PROPOXYPHENE,
668
SK-APAP—See
ACETAMINOPHEN, 18
SK-APAP with Codeine Tablets
(M)—See
ACETAMINOPHEN, 18
CODEINE, 176
SK-Amitriptyline—See
AMITRIPTYLINE, 42
SK-Ampicillin—See
AMPICILLIN, 50
SK-Bamate—See
MEPROBAMATE, 444
SK-Chloral Hydrate—See
CHLORAL HYDRATE, 130
SK-Chlorothiazide—See
CHLOROTHIAZIDE, 138
SK-Dexamethasone—See
DEXAMETHASONE, 214
SK-Diphenhydramine—See
DIPHENHYDRAMINE, 248
SK-Diphenoxylate—See
DIPHENOXYLATE &
ATROPINE, 250

SK-Erythromycin—See
ERYTHROMYCIN
STEARATE, 296
SK-Furosemide—See
FUROSEMIDE, 340
SK-Lygen—See
CHLORDIAZEPOXIDE, 134
SK-Niacin—See NIACIN
(NICOTINIC ACID), 514
SK-Phenobarbital—See
PHENOBARBITAL, 594
SK-Pramine—See IMIPRAMINE,
378
SK-Prednisone—See
PREDNISONE, 650
SK-Probenecid—See
PROBENECID, 654
SK-Propantheline—See
PROPANTHELINE, 666
SK-Reserpine—See
RESERPINE, 698
SK-Soxazole—See
SULFISOXAZOLE, 732
SK-Tetracycline—See
TETRACYCLINE, 746
SK-Tolbutamide—See
TOLBUTAMIDE, 768
SMZ-TMP (M)—See
SULFAMETHOXAZOLE, 726
TRIMETHOPRIM, 794
S-P-T—See THYROID, 758
Sal Hepatica—See SODIUM
PHOSPHATE, 718
Sal-Adult—See ASPIRIN, 56
Sal-Infant—See ASPIRIN, 56
Salatin Capsules (M)—See
ACETAMINOPHEN, 18
ASPIRIN, 56
CAFFEINE, 100
Salatin with Codeine Tablets
(M)—See
ACETAMINOPHEN, 18
ASPIRIN, 56
CAFFEINE, 100
CODEINE, 176
Salazopyrin—See
SULFASALAZINE, 728
Saleto Tablets (M)—See
ACETAMINOPHEN, 18
ASPIRIN, 56
CAFFEINE, 100
CODEINE, 176
Saleto-D Capsules (M)—See
ACETAMINOPHEN, 18
CAFFEINE, 100
PHENYLPROPANOLAMINE,
608
Salimeph Forte (M)—See
ACETAMINOPHEN, 18
ASPIRIN, 56
CODEINE, 176
Salocol Tablets (M)—See
ASPIRIN, 56
CAFFEINE, 100
Salphenyl (M)—See
ACETAMINOPHEN, 18
CHLORPHENIRAMINE, 142
PHENYLEPHRINE, 606
Salsprin Tablets (M)—See
ALUMINUM ACETATE (NL)
ASPIRIN, 56
Saluron—See
HYDROFLUMETHIAZIDE, 366
Salutensin (M)—See
HYDROFLUMETHIAZIDE, 366
RESERPINE, 698

Sandoptal—See TALBUTAL
(BUTALBITAL), 736
Sandril—See RESERPINE, 698
Sanhist—See SCOPOLAMINE
(HYOSCINE), 702
Sanorex—See MAZINDOL, 428
Sansert—See
METHYSERGIDE, 488
Sarodant—See
NITROFURANTOIN, 518
Satric—See METRONIDAZOLE,
494
Savacort 50 & 100—See
PREDNISOLONE, 648
Scolate Tablets—See
BUTABARBITAL, 94
Scoline—See SCOPOLAMINE
(HYOSCINE), 702
Scoline-Amobarbital—See
SCOPOLAMINE
(HYOSCINE), 702
SCOPOLAMINE (HYOSCINE),
702
Scotnord—See SCOPOLAMINE
(HYOSCINE), 702
SECOBARBITAL, 704
Secogen—See
SECOBARBITAL, 704
Seconal—See
SECOBARBITAL, 704
Sedadrops—See
PHENOBARBITAL, 594
Sedajen (M)—See
HYOSCYAMINE, 374
PHENOBARBITAL, 594
Sedalone—See
METHAQUALONE, 458
Sedamine (M)—See
ATROPINE, 60
HYOSCYAMINE, 374
SCOPOLAMINE
(HYOSCINE), 702
Sedapap (M)—See
ACETAMINOPHEN, 18
CODEINE, 176
Sedapar (M)—See
ATROPINE, 60
BELLADONNA, 68
HYOSCYAMINE, 374
SCOPOLAMINE
(HYOSCINE), 702
Sedatabs (M)—See
ATROPINE, 60
PHENOBARBITAL, 594
Sedatives
AMOBARBITAL, 44
BUTABARBITAL, 94
HEXOBARBITAL, 356
MEPHOBARBITAL, 442
METHARBITAL, 460
PENTOBARBITAL, 578
PHENOBARBITAL, 594
SECOBARBITAL, 704
TALBUTAL (BUTALBITAL),
736
Sedatromine (M)—See
ATROPINE, 60
BELLADONNA, 68
HYOSCYAMINE, 374
Sedatuss—See
DEXTROMETHORPHAN, 220
Sedralex (M)—See
ATROPINE, 60
HYOSCYAMINE, 374

Sedralex—continued
  SCOPOLAMINE
  (HYOSCINE), 702
Seds (M)—See
  ATROPINE, 60
  HYOSCYAMINE, 374
  SCOPOLAMINE
  (HYOSCINE), 702
Seidlitz Powder—See SODIUM
  BICARBONATE, 712
Semilente Iletin—See INSULIN,
  382
Semilente—See INSULIN, 382
Semitard—See INSULIN, 382
Senexon—See SENNA, 706
SENNA, 706
SENNOSIDES A & B, 708
Senokot with Psyllium (M)—See
  PSYLLIUM, 676
  SENNA, 706
Senokot—See SENNA, 706
Septra (M)—See
  SULFAMETHOXAZOLE, 726
  TRIMETHOPRIM, 794
Ser-Ap-Es (M)—See
  HYDRALAZINE, 358
  HYDROCHLOROTHIAZIDE,
  360
  RESERPINE, 698
Seral—See SECOBARBITAL,
  704
Serax—See OXAZEPAM, 542
Sereen—See
  CHLORDIAZEPOXIDE, 134
Serentil—See MESORIDAZINE,
  446
Serpalan—See RESERPINE,
  698
Serpanray—See RESERPINE,
  698
Serpasil—See RESERPINE, 698
Serpasil-Apresoline (M)—See
  HYDRALAZINE, 358
  RESERPINE, 698
*Serpasil-Esidrix #2 Tablets
  (M)*—See
  RESERPINE, 698
  HYDROCHLOROTHIAZIDE,
  360
Serpate—See RESERPINE, 698
Sertan—See PRIMIDONE, 652
Sherafed Syrup—See
  PSEUDOEPHEDRINE, 674
Siblin—See PSYLLIUM, 676
Sidonna Tablets—See
  BUTABARBITAL, 94
Silain—See SIMETHICONE, 710
Silain-Gel (M)—See
  MAGNESIUM CARBONATE,
  416
  MAGNESIUM HYDROXIDE,
  420
*Silence is Golden Cough
  Syrup*—See
  DEXTROMETHORPHAN, 220
Silexin Cough Syrup (M)—See
  DEXTROMETHORPHAN, 220
  GUAIFENESIN, 346
SIMETHICONE, 710
Simplene—See EPINEPHRINE,
  276
Sinaprel—See SCOPOLAMINE
  (HYOSCINE), 702

Sinarest (M)—See
  ACETAMINOPHEN, 18
  CAFFEINE, 100
  CHLORPHENIRAMINE, 142
  PHENYLPROPANOLAMINE,
  608
*Sinate-M 1/2 Strength
  Tablets*—See
  BUTABARBITAL, 94
Sinate-M Tablets—See
  BUTABARBITAL, 94
Sine-Aid (M)—See
  ACETAMINOPHEN, 18
  PHENYLPROPANOLAMINE,
  608
Sine-Off (M)—See
  ACETAMINOPHEN, 18
  PHENYLPROPANOLAMINE,
  608
Sinemet—See CARBIDOPA &
  LEVODOPA, 110
Sinequan—See DOXEPIN, 266
Sinex—See
  PHENYLEPHRINE, 606
Singlet Tablets (M)—See
  CHLORPHENIRAMINE, 142
  PHENYLEPHRINE, 606
*Singoserp-Esidrix Tablets
  (M)*—See
  RESERPINE, 698
  HYDROCHLOROTHIAZIDE,
  360
Sinodec—See SCOPOLAMINE
  (HYOSCINE), 702
Sinoran (M)—See
  CHLORPHENIRAMINE, 142
  PHENYLEPHRINE, 606
  SCOPOLAMINE
  (HYOSCINE), 702
Sinubid (M)—See
  PHENACETIN, 582
  PHENYLPROPANOLAMINE,
  608
  PHENYLTOLOXAMINE, 610
Sinulin Tablets (M)—See
  CHLORPHENIRAMINE, 142
  PHENYLPROPANOLAMINE,
  608
  SCOPOLAMINE
  (HYOSCINE), 702
Sinutab (M)—See
  ACETAMINOPHEN, 18
  PHENYLPROPANOLAMINE,
  608
  PHENYLTOLOXAMINE, 610
642—See PROPOXYPHENE,
  668
Sleep inducers (hypnotic)
  ETHCHLORVYNOL, 308
Slim-Tabs—See
  PHENDIMETRAZINE, 586
Slo-Fedrin—See EPHEDRINE,
  274
Slo-Phyllin (M)—See
  GUAIFENESIN, 346
  THEOPHYLLINE, 748
Slow-Fe—See FERROUS
  SULFATE, 328
Slow-K—See POTASSIUM
  CHLORIDE, 636
Soda Mint—See SODIUM
  BICARBONATE, 712
SODIUM BICARBONATE, 712
SODIUM CARBONATE, 714
SODIUM FLUORIDE

SODIUM PHOSPHATE, 718
Sof-Cil—See PSYLLIUM, 676
Solarcaine—See
  ANESTHETICS (TOPICAL), 52
Solazine—See
  TRIFLUOPERAZINE, 784
Solfoton—See
  PHENOBARBITAL, 594
Solium—See
  CHLORDIAZEPOXIDE, 134
Solu-Cortef—See
  HYDROCORTISONE
  (CORTISOL), 364
Soma Compound (M)—See
  CARISOPRODOL, 114
  PHENACETIN, 582
*Soma Compound with Codeine
  (M)*—See
  CARISOPRODOL, 114
  CODEINE, 176
  PHENACETIN, 582
Soma—See CARISOPRODOL,
  114
Sombulex—See
  HEXOBARBITAL, 356
Sominex—See
  DIPHENHYDRAMINE, 248
Somnicaps—See PYRILAMINE,
  682
Somophyllin—See
  AMINOPHYLLINE, 40
Somophyllin-T—See
  THEOPHYLLINE, 748
Sopor—See METHAQUALONE,
  458
Soprodol—See
  CARISOPRODOL, 114
Sorate—See ISOSORBIDE
  DINITRATE, 396
Sorbase Cough Syrup (M)—See
  DEXTROMETHORPHAN, 220
  GUAIFENESIN, 346
*Sorbase II Cough Syrup
  (M)*—See
  CODEINE, 176
  DEXTROMETHORPHAN, 220
  GUAIFENESIN, 346
Sorbide—See ISOSORBIDE
  DINITRATE, 396
Sorbitrate—See ISOSORBIDE
  DINITRATE, 396
Sorbutuss Syrup (M)—See
  DEXTROMETHORPHAN, 220
  GUAIFENESIN, 346
Sosol—See SULFISOXAZOLE,
  732
Soxa—See SULFISOXAZOLE,
  732
Spabelin (M)—See
  ATROPINE, 60
  BELLADONNA, 68
  HYOSCYAMINE, 374
  SCOPOLAMINE
  (HYOSCINE), 702
Span-Niacin—See NIACIN
  (NICOTINIC ACID), 514
Span-RD—See
  PHENDIMETRAZINE, 586
Spancap No. 1—See
  DEXTROAMPHETAMINE, 218
Sparine—See PROMAZINE, 662
Spasaid (M)—See
  ATROPINE, 60
  HYOSCYAMINE, 374

Spasdel (M)—See
  ATROPINE, 60
  HYOSCYAMINE, 374
  SCOPOLAMINE
  (HYOSCINE), 702
  PHENOBARBITAL, 594
Spasidon (M)—See
  ATROPINE, 60
  BELLADONNA, 68
Spasloids (M)—See
  ATROPINE, 60
  HYOSCYAMINE, 374
  SCOPOLAMINE
  (HYOSCINE), 702
Spasmate—See ATROPINE, 60
Spasmid—See SCOPOLAMINE
  (HYOSCINE), 702
Spasmoban—See
  DICYCLOMINE, 230
Spasmolin (M)—See
  ATROPINE, 60
  HYOSCYAMINE, 374
  SCOPOLAMINE
  (HYOSCINE), 702
Spasnil (M)—See
  ATROPINE, 60
  BELLADONNA, 68
  HYOSCYAMINE, 374
Spasquid (M)—See
  ATROPINE, 60
  HYOSCYAMINE, 374
  SCOPOLAMINE
  (HYOSCINE), 702
Spasticol (M)—See
  ATROPINE, 60
  PHENOBARBITAL, 594
Spastolate (M)—See
  ATROPINE, 60
  HYOSCYAMINE, 374
  SCOPOLAMINE
  (HYOSCINE), 702
Spastosed (M)—See
  ATROPINE, 60
  PHENOBARBITAL, 594
Special Cough Formula
  Liquid—See GUAIFENESIN,
  346
Spectrobid—See
  BACAMPICILLIN, 64
Spinaxin—See
  METHOCARBAMOL, 468
SPIRONOLACTONE, 720
St. Joseph Aspirin—See
  ASPIRIN, 56
St. Joseph Cough Syrup—See
  DEXTROMETHORPHAN, 220
St. Joseph Decongestant for
  Children—See
  OXYMETAZOLINE, 548
Stadol—See BUTORPHANOL,
  98
Stannitol (M)—See
  ATROPINE, 60
  SCOPOLAMINE
  (HYOSCINE), 702
STANOZOLOL, 722
Staphcillin—See METHICILLIN,
  466
Statobex—See
  PHENDIMETRAZINE, 586
Stay-Flo—See SODIUM
  FLUORIDE, 716
Stelazine—See
  TRIFLUOPERAZINE, 784

Stemetil—See
  PROCHLORPERAZINE, 658
Sterane—See PREDNISOLONE,
  648
Sterapred—See PREDNISONE,
  650
Sterazolidin (M)—See
  ALUMINUM HYDROXIDE, 32
  MAGNESIUM TRISILICATE,
  424
  PREDNISONE, 650
  PHENYLBUTAZONE, 604
Stero-Darvon (M)—See
  ASPIRIN, 56
  PROPOXYPHENE, 668
StieVAA—See TRETINOIN, 774
Stilbestrol—See
  DIETHYLSTILBESTROL, 234
Stilphostrol—See
  DIETHYLSTILBESTROL, 234
  ESTROGEN, 302
Stimulants (xanthine)
  CAFFEINE, 100
Strascogesic Tablets (M)—See
  ACETAMINOPHEN, 18
  CODEINE, 176
Stress-Pam—See DIAZEPAM,
  222
Studaflor—See SODIUM
  FLUORIDE, 716
Sub-Quin—See
  PROCAINAMIDE, 656
Suda-Prol Syrup—See
  PSEUDOEPHEDRINE, 674
Sudafed—See
  PSEUDOEPHEDRINE, 674
Sudahist Tablets (M)—See
  CHLORPHENIRAMINE, 142
  PSEUDOEPHEDRINE, 674
Sudolin Tablets (M)—See
  PSEUDOEPHEDRINE, 674
  THEOPHYLLINE, 748
Sudrin—See
  PSEUDOEPHEDRINE, 674
Sulfa drugs (sulfonamide)
  SULFACYTINE, 724
  SULFAMETHOXAZOLE, 726
  SULFASALAZINE, 728
  SULFISOXAZOLE, 732
SULFACYTINE, 724
Sulfagen—See
  SULFISOXAZOLE, 732
SULFAMETHOXAZOLE, 726
SULFASALAZINE, 728
SULFINPYRAZONE, 730
SULFISOXAZOLE, 732
Sulfizin—See
  SULFISOXAZOLE, 732
Sulfizole—See
  SULFISOXAZOLE, 732
Sulfonurea drugs
  ACETOHEXAMIDE, 22
  CHLORPROPAMIDE, 148
  TOLAZAMIDE, 766
  TOLBUTAMIDE, 768
SULINDAC, 734
Sumox—See AMOXICILLIN, 46
Sumycin—See
  TETRACYCLINE, 746
Supac (M)—See
  ACETAMINOPHEN, 18
  ASPIRIN, 56
  CAFFEINE, 100
  CODEINE, 176
Supen—See AMPICILLIN, 50

Super Anahist—See
  PHENYLEPHRINE, 606
Surfacaine Cream—See
  ANESTHETICS (TOPICAL), 52
Surfacaine Ointment—See
  ANESTHETICS (TOPICAL), 52
Surfak—See DOCUSATE
  CALCIUM, 260
Surmontil—See
  TRIMIPRAMINE, 796
Sus-phrine—See
  EPINEPHRINE, 276
Susadrin—See
  NITROGLYCERIN
  (GLYCERYL TRINITRATE),
  520
Sust-A—See VITAMIN A, 804
Sustaverine—See
  PAPAVERINE, 558
Swiss Kriss—See SENNA, 706
Sylapar Tablets (M)—See
  ACETAMINOPHEN, 18
  CODEINE, 176
Syllact—See PSYLLIUM, 676
Symetra—See
  PHENDIMETRAZINE, 586
Symmetrel—See AMANTADINE,
  34
Sympathomimetics
  (bronchodilator)
  ISOETHARINE, 388
Sympathomimetics
  EPHEDRINE, 274
  EPINEPHRINE, 276
  ISOPROTERENOL, 394
  METAPROTERENOL, 448
  METHYLPHENIDATE, 482
  OXYMETAZOLINE, 548
  PHENYLEPHRINE, 606
  PHENYLPROPANOLAMINE,
  608
  PSEUDOEPHEDRINE, 674
  TERBUTALINE, 740
Symptom 3—See
  BROMPHENIRAMINE, 90
Symptrol (M)—See
  PHENIRAMINE, 590
  PHENYLPROPANOLAMINE,
  608
  SCOPOLAMINE
  (HYOSCINE), 702
Synalar—See
  ADRENOCORTICOIDS
  (TOPICAL), 26
Synalgos (M)—See
  ASPIRIN, 56
  CAFFEINE, 100
  PHENACETIN, 582
  PROMETHAZINE, 664
Synasal—See
  PHENYLEPHRINE, 606
Synkayvite—See VITAMIN K,
  814
Synophylate-GG (M)—See
  GUAIFENESIN, 346
  THEOPHYLLINE, 748
Synthroid—See THYROXINE
  (T-4, LEVOTHYROXINE), 760
Syraprim—See
  TRIMETHOPRIM, 794
Sytobex—See VITAMIN B-12
  (CYANOCOBALAMIN), 806

T

T-4, 760
T-Serp—See RESERPINE, 698
T.P.I. (M)—See
  ACETAMINOPHEN, 18
  CHLORPHENIRAMINE, 142
  PHENYLEPHRINE, 606
  PHENYLPROPANOLAMINE, 608
Tace—See
  CHLOROTRIANISENE, 140
Tagamet—See CIMETIDINE, 158
TALBUTAL (BUTALBITAL), 736
Taltapp (M)—See
  BROMPHENIRAMINE, 90
  PHENYLPROPANOLAMINE, 608
  PHENYLEPHRINE, 606
Taltapp Elixir—See
  BROMPHENIRAMINE, 90
Talwin Compound
  Caplets—See ASPIRIN, 56
Talwin—See PENTAZOCINE, 576
Tandearil—See
  OXYPHENBUTAZONE, 554
Tapar Elixir—See
  ACETAMINOPHEN, 18
Tapar Tablets—See
  ACETAMINOPHEN, 18
Tapar—See ACETAMINOPHEN, 18
Tapp Elixir (M)—See
  BROMPHENIRAMINE, 90
  PHENYLEPHRINE, 606
  PHENYLPROPANOLAMINE, 608
Taractan—See
  CHLORPROTHIXENE, 150
Tarasan—See
  CHLORPROTHIXENE, 150
Tavist—See CLEMASTINE, 160
Tedfern Tablets (M)—See
  EPHEDRINE, 274
  THEOPHYLLINE, 748
Tedral Anti-H Tablets (M)—See
  CHLORPHENIRAMINE, 142
  EPHEDRINE, 274
  THEOPHYLLINE, 748
Tedral Tablets (M)—See
  EPHEDRINE, 274
  THEOPHYLLINE, 748
  PHENOBARBITAL, 594
Teebacin—See
  PARA-AMINOSALICYLIC
  ACID (PAS), 560
Teen—See BENZOYL
  PEROXIDE, 72
Tega-Dyne Ointment—See
  ANESTHETICS (TOPICAL), 52
Tega-Flex—See
  ORPHENADRINE, 536
Tega-Span—See NIACIN
  (NICOTINIC ACID), 514
Tegamide—See
  TRIMETHOBENZAMIDE, 792
Tegopen—See CLOXACILLIN, 174
Tegretol—See
  CARBAMAZEPINE, 106
Teldrin Spansules—See
  CHLORPHENIRAMINE, 142
Temaril—See TRIMEPRAZINE, 790

TEMAZEPAM, 738
Temlo Syrup—See
  ACETAMINOPHEN, 18
Temlo Tablets—See
  ACETAMINOPHEN, 18
Tempra Drops—See
  ACETAMINOPHEN, 18
Tempra Syrup—See
  ACETAMINOPHEN, 18
Tempra Tablets—See
  ACETAMINOPHEN, 18
Tempra—See
  ACETAMINOPHEN, 18
Tenax—See
  CHLORDIAZEPOXIDE, 134
Tenlap Elixir—See
  ACETAMINOPHEN, 18
Tenormin—See ATENOLOL, 58
Tenuate—See
  DIETHYLPROPION, 232
Tepanil—See
  DIETHYLPROPION, 232
TERBUTALINE, 740
Terfluzine—See
  TRIFLUOPERAZINE, 784
TERPIN HYDRATE, 742
Terpin Hydrate Elixir—See
  TERPIN HYDRATE, 742
Terpin Hydrate with Codeine
  (M)—See
  CODEINE, 176
  TERPIN HYDRATE, 742
Terramycin—See
  OXYTETRACYCLINE, 556
Terrastatin (M)—See
  NYSTATIN, 532
  TERRAMYCIN (NL)
Tertroxin—See
  LIOTHYRONINE, 408
TESTOSTERONE, 744
Testred—See
  METHYLTESTOSTERONE, 486
TETRACYCLINE, 746
Tetrachel—See
  TETRACYCLINE, 746
Tetracyn—See
  TETRACYCLINE, 746
Tetracyrine—See
  TETRACYCLINE, 746
Tetramine—See
  OXYTETRACYCLINE, 556
Tetrastatin (M)—See
  NYSTATIN, 532
  TETRACYCLINE, 746
Tetrex—See TETRACYCLINE, 746
Tex Six T.R.—See PYRIDOXINE
  (VITAMIN B-6), 680
Thalfed Tablets (M)—See
  EPHEDRINE, 274
  PHENOBARBITAL, 594
  THEOPHYLLINE, 748
Theelin—See ESTRONE, 304
Theo-Dur—See
  THEOPHYLLINE, 748
Theo-Guaia Capsules (M)—See
  GUAIFENESIN, 346
  THEOPHYLLINE, 748
Theo-Nar 100 Tablets (M)—See
  NOSCAPINE (NL)
  THEOPHYLLINE, 748
Theo-Organidin Elixir (M)—See
  IODINATED GLYCEROL (NL)
  THEOPHYLLINE, 748

Theobid—See THEOPHYLLINE, 748
Theoclear—See
  THEOPHYLLINE, 748
Theogen—See ESTRONE, 304
Theolair—See THEOPHYLLINE, 748
Theolixir—See
  THEOPHYLLINE, 748
THEOPHYLLINE, 748
Theophyl—See
  THEOPHYLLINE, 748
Theospan—See
  THEOPHYLLINE, 748
Theotabs Tablets (M)—See
  EPHEDRINE, 274
  PHENOBARBITAL, 594
  THEOPHYLLINE, 748
Theralax—See BISACODYL, 86
THIAMINE (VITAMIN B-1), 750
THIORIDAZINE, 752
Thioril—See THIORIDAZINE, 752
Thiosulfil-A (M)—See
  PHENAZOPYRIDINE, 584
  SULFAMETHIAZOLE (NL)
THIOTHIXENE, 754
Thioxanthines—See
  Tranquilizers
Thitrate—See ATROPINE, 60
Thiuretic—See
  HYDROCHLOROTHIAZIDE, 360
Thorazine—See
  CHLORPROMAZINE, 146
Thyrar—See THYROID, 758
Thyrocrine—See THYROID, 758
THYROGLOBULIN, 756
Thyroid hormones
  LIOTHYRONINE, 408
  LIOTRIX, 410
  THYROGLOBULIN, 756
  THYROID, 758
  THYROXINE (T-4, LEVOTHYROXINE), 760
THYROID, 758
Thyrolar (M)—See
  LIOTRIX, 410
  THYROXINE (T-4, LEVOTHYROXINE), 760
THYROXINE (T-4, LEVOTHYROXINE), 760
Ticar—See TICARCILLIN, 762
TICARCILLIN, 762
Tigan—See
  TRIMETHOBENZAMIDE, 792
TIMOLOL, 764
Tindal—See
  ACETOPHENAZINE, 24
Tirend—See CAFFEINE, 100
Titralac—See CALCIUM
  CARBONATE, 102
Tofranil—See IMIPRAMINE, 378
Tofranil-PM—See IMIPRAMINE, 378
Tolabromophen Decongestant
  Elixir—See
  BROMPHENIRAMINE, 90
TOLAZAMIDE, 766
TOLBUTAMIDE, 768
Tolbutone—See
  TOLBUTAMIDE, 768
Tolectin DS—See TOLMETIN, 770
Tolectin—See TOLMETIN, 770

Toleron—See FERROUS
  FUMARATE, 324
Tolfrinic—See FERROUS
  FUMARATE, 324
Tolifer—See FERROUS
  FUMARATE, 324
Tolinase—See TOLAZAMIDE,
  766
TOLMETIN, 770
Topex—See BENZOYL
  PEROXIDE, 72
Topicort—See
  ADRENOCORTICOIDS
  (TOPICAL), 26
Totacillin—See AMPICILLIN, 50
Tramacort—See
  TRIAMCINOLONE, 776
Tranquilizers
  HYDROXYZINE, 372
  LITHIUM, 412
  MEPROBAMATE, 444
Tranquilizers (antipsychotic)
  HALOPERIDOL, 352
Tranquilizers (benzodiazepine)
  ALPRAZOLAM, 30
  CHLORDIAZEPOXIDE, 134
  CLORAZEPATE, 170
  DIAZEPAM, 222
  FLURAZEPAM, 336
  HALAZEPAM, 350
  LORAZEPAM, 414
  OXAZEPAM, 542
  PRAZEPAM, 644
  TEMAZEPAM, 730
Tranquilizers (phenothiazine)
  ACETOPHENAZINE, 24
  BUTAPERAZINE, 96
  CARPHENAZINE, 116
  CHLORPROMAZINE, 146
  FLUPHENAZINE, 332
  MESORIDAZINE, 446
  PERPHENAZINE, 580
  PIPERACETAZINE, 618
  PROCHLORPERAZINE, 658
  PROMAZINE, 662
  PROMETHAZINE, 664
  THIORIDAZINE, 752
  TRIFLUOPERAZINE, 784
  TRIFLUPROMAZINE, 786
  TRIMEPRAZINE, 790
Tranquilizers (rauwolfia
  alkaloid)
  DESERPIDINE, 210
  RAUWOLFIA SERPENTINA,
  696
  RESERPINE, 698
Tranquilizers (thioxanthine)
  CHLORPROTHIXENE, 150
  THIOTHIXENE, 754
Transderm-Nitro—See
  NITROGLYCERIN
  (GLYCERYL TRINITRATE),
  520
Trantoin—See
  NITROFURANTOIN, 518
Tranxene—See
  CLORAZEPATE, 170
TRANYLCYPROMINE, 772
Travamine—See
  DIMENHYDRINATE, 244
Tremin—See
  TRIHEXYPHENIDYL, 788
TRETINOIN, 774
Tri-K—See POTASSIUM
  ACETATE POTASSIUM

Tri-K—continued
  BICARBONATE &
  POTASSIUM CITRATE, 624
Triacort—See
  TRIAMCINOLONE, 776
Triactin—See DICYCLOMINE,
  230
Triador—See
  METHAQUALONE, 458
Trialka—See CALCIUM
  CARBONATE, 102
TRIAMCINOLONE, 776
Triaminic (M)—See
  ASPIRIN, 56
  CAFFEINE, 100
  PHENIRAMINE, 590
  PHENYLPROPANOLAMINE,
  608
Triaminicin (M)—See
  ACETAMINOPHEN, 18
  CAFFEINE, 100
  CHLORPHENIRAMINE, 142
  PHENIRAMINE, 590
  PHENYLPROPANOLAMINE,
  608
Triaminicol (M)—See
  PHENIRAMINE, 590
  PHENYLPROPANOLAMINE,
  608
TRIAMTERENE, 778
TRICHLORMETHIAZIDE, 780
TRIDIHEXETHYL, 782
TRIFLUOPERAZINE, 784
TRIFLUPROMAZINE, 786
Triflurin—See
  TRIFLUOPERAZINE, 784
Trigesic Tablets (M)—See
  ACETAMINOPHEN, 18
  ASPIRIN, 56
  CAFFEINE, 100
  CODEINE, 176
TRIHEXYPHENIDYL, 788
Trikacide—See
  METRONIDAZOLE, 494
Trikates—See POTASSIUM
  ACETATE, POTASSIUM
  BICARBONATE &
  POTASSIUM CITRATE, 624
Trilafon—See PERPHENAZINE,
  580
Trilium—See
  CHLORDIAZEPOXIDE, 134
TRIMEPRAZINE, 790
TRIMETHOPRIM, 794
TRIMETHOBENZAMIDE, 792
TRIMIPRAMINE, 796
Trimox—See AMOXICILLIN, 46
Trimpex—See TRIMETHOPRIM,
  794
Trimstat—See
  PHENDIMETRAZINE, 586
Trimtabs—See
  PHENDIMETRAZINE, 586
Trind (M)—See
  ACETAMINOPHEN, 18
  DEXTROMETHORPHAN, 220
  GUAIFENESIN, 346
Tripazine—See
  TRIFLUOPERAZINE, 784
Triphed Tablets (M)—See
  PSEUDOEPHEDRINE, 674
  TRIPROLIDINE, 800
TRIPELENNAMINE, 798
TRIPROLIDINE, 800

Trisohist—See SCOPOLAMINE
  (HYOSCINE), 702
Triten—See DIMETHINDENE,
  246
Trocal—See
  DEXTROMETHORPHAN, 220
Tronolane—See ANESTHETICS
  (TOPICAL), 52
Tronothane—See
  ANESTHETICS (TOPICAL), 52
Tualone—See
  METHAQUALONE, 458
Tuinal (M)—See
  AMOBARBITAL, 44
  SECOBARBITAL, 704
Tumol—See
  METHOCARBAMOL, 468
Tums—See CALCIUM
  CARBONATE, 102
Turbinaire Decadron—See
  DEXAMETHASONE, 214
Tusquelin Syrup—See
  CHLORPHENIRAMINE, 142
Tuss-Ornade (M)—See
  CHLORPHENIRAMINE, 142
  PHENYLPROPANOLAMINE,
  608
Tussagesic (M)—See
  DEXTROMETHORPHAN, 220
  PHENIRAMINE, 590
  PHENYLPROPANOLAMINE,
  608
Tussaminic (M)—See
  DEXTROMETHORPHAN, 220
  PHENIRAMINE, 590
  PHENYLPROPANOLAMINE,
  608
Tussar SF Cough Syrup
  (M)—See
  CHLORPHENIRAMINE, 142
  CODEINE, 176
Tussend Expectorant (M)—See
  CODEINE, 176
  PSEUDOEPHEDRINE, 674
Tussi-Organidin (M)—See
  CHLORPHENIRAMINE, 142
  CODEINE, 176
Tussionex (M)—See
  CODEINE, 176
  PHENYLTOLOXAMINE, 610
Twin-K—See POTASSIUM
  CITRATE & POTASSIUM
  GLUCONATE, 640
2/G-DM Liquid (M)—See
  DEXTROMETHORPHAN, 220
  GUAIFENESIN, 346
Tylenol Chewable Tablets—See
  ACETAMINOPHEN, 18
Tylenol Drops—See
  ACETAMINOPHEN, 18
Tylenol Elixir—See
  ACETAMINOPHEN, 18
Tylenol Extra Strength
  Capsules—See
  ACETAMINOPHEN, 18
Tylenol Tablets—See
  ACETAMINOPHEN, 18
Tylenol with Codeine Tablets
  (M)—See
  ACETAMINOPHEN, 18
  CODEINE, 176
Tylenol—See
  ACETAMINOPHEN, 18

INDEX

U

U-Tract—See BELLADONNA, 68
U.R.I. Capsules (M)—See
CHLORPHENIRAMINE, 142
PHENYLEPHRINE, 606
PHENYLPROPANOLAMINE,
608
Ultabs (M)—See
BELLADONNA, 68
HYOSCYAMINE, 374
Ultracef—See CEFADROXIL,
124
Ultralente Iletin—See INSULIN,
382
Ultralente—See INSULIN, 382
Ultramycin—See
MINOCYCLINE, 496
Ultratard—See INSULIN, 382
Unipen—See NAFCILLIN, 502
Unipres Tablets (M)—See
HYDROCHLOROTHIAZIDE,
360
RESERPINE, 698
Uniserp—See HYDRALAZINE,
358
Unisom Nighttime Sleep
Aid—See DOXYLAMINE, 270
Unitral—See ATROPINE, 60
Univol—See MAGNESIUM
HYDROXIDE, 420
Unproco Capsules (M)—See
DEXTROMETHORPHAN, 220
GUAIFENESIN, 346
Urecholine—See
BETHANECHOL, 82
Urex—See METHENAMINE, 464
Uridon—See
CHLORTHALIDONE, 152
Urilief—See BELLADONNA, 68
Urised (M)—See
BELLADONNA, 68
METHENAMINE, 464
Uriseptin (M)—See
ATROPINE, 60
HYOSCYAMINE, 374
SCOPOLAMINE
(HYOSCINE), 702
Urisoxin—See
SULFISOXAZOLE, 732
Uritol—See FUROSEMIDE, 340
Uro-phosphate (M)—See
METHENAMINE, 464
SODIUM PHOSPHATE (NL)

Urobiotic (M)—See
OXYTETRACYCLINE, 556
PHENAZOPYRIDINE, 584
Urogesic (M)—See
ATROPINE, 60
HYOSCYAMINE, 374
SCOPOLAMINE
(HYOSCINE), 702
Urolocaine Liquid—See
ANESTHETICS (TOPICAL), 52
Uroquid-Acid (M)—See
METHENAMINE, 464
SODIUM ACID PHOSPHATE
(NL)
Urotoin—See
NITROFURANTOIN, 518
Urozide—See
HYDROCHLOROTHIAZIDE,
360
Ursinus (M)—See
PHENIRAMINE, 590
PHENYLPROPANOLAMINE,
608
Uticillin VK See PENICILLIN V,
572
Utimox—See AMOXICILLIN, 46

V

V-Cillin See PENICILLIN V, 572
V-Lax—See PSYLLIUM, 676
Vacon—See PHENYLEPHRINE,
606
Valadol Liquid—See
ACETAMINOPHEN, 18
Valadol Tablets—See
ACETAMINOPHEN, 18
Valadol—See
ACETAMINOPHEN, 18
Valdrene—See
DIPHENHYDRAMINE, 248
Valisone—See
ADRENOCORTICOIDS
(TOPICAL), 26
Valium—See DIAZEPAM, 222
Valpin-PB Elixir (M)—See
ANISOTROPINE (NL)
PHENOBARBITAL, 594
Vancerace—See
BETAMETHASONE, 80
Vanceril Inhaler—See
BECLOMETHASONE, 66

Vapo-Iso—See
ISOPROTERENOL, 394
Vaponefrin—See
EPINEPHRINE, 276
Vasoconstrictors
CAFFEINE, 100
ERGOTAMINE, 282
Vasoconstrictors (antiserotonin)
METHYSERGIDE, 488
Vasodilan—See ISOXSUPRINE,
398
Vasodilators
CYCLANDELATE, 190
ISOXSUPRINE, 398
NIACIN (NICOTINIC ACID)
514
NITROGLYCERIN
(GLYCERYL TRINITRATE),
520
NYLIDRIN, 530
PAPAVERINE, 558
Vasoglyn—See
NITROGLYCERIN
(GLYCERYL TRINITRATE),
520
Vasoprine—See ISOXSUPRINE,
398
Vasospan—See PAPAVERINE,
558
Vasotherm—See NIACIN
(NICOTINIC ACID), 514
Veetids—See PENICILLIN V,
572
Velosef—See CEPHRADINE,
128
Velosulin—See INSULIN, 382
Veltap Elixir (M)—See
BROMPHENIRAMINE, 90
PHENYLEPHRINE, 606
PHENYLPROPANOLAMINE,
608
VERAPAMIL, 802
Verequad (M)—See
EPHEDRINE, 274
GUAIFENESIN, 346
PHENOBARBITAL, 594
THEOPHYLLINE, 748
Vernate Granucaps (M)—See
ATROPINE, 60
CHLORPHENIRAMINE, 142
PHENYLPROPANOLAMINE,
608

Versapen—See HETACILLIN, 354
Vesprin—See TRIFLUPROMAZINE, 786
Vibra-Tabs—See DOXYCYCLINE, 268
Vibramycin—See DOXYCYCLINE, 268
Vicks Cough Syrup (M)—See DEXTROMETHORPHAN, 220 GUAIFENESIN, 346
Vimicon—See CYPROHEPTADINE, 202
Vioform—See ADRENOCORTICOIDS, (TOPICAL), 26 IODOCHLORHYDROXYQUIN, (TOPICAL), (NL)
Viscerol—See DICYCLOMINE, 230
Vistaril—See HYDROXYZINE, 372
Vistrax (M)—See HYDROXYZINE, 372 OXYPHENCYCLAMINE (NL)
Vitalone—See METHAQUALONE, 458
VITAMIN A, 804
VITAMIN B-1, 750
VITAMIN B-12 (CYANOCOBALAMIN), 806
VITAMIN B-6, 680
VITAMIN B-9, 338
VITAMIN C (ASCORBIC ACID), 808
VITAMIN D, 810
VITAMIN E, 812
VITAMIN K, 814
Vitamin supplements
  FOLIC ACID (VITAMIN B-9), 338
  NIACIN (NICOTINIC ACID), 514
  PYRIDOXINE (VITAMIN B-6), 680
  THIAMINE (VITAMIN B-1), 750
  VITAMIN A, 804
  VITAMIN B-12 (CYANOCOBALAMIN), 806
  VITAMIN C (ASCORBIC ACID), 808
  VITAMIN D, 810
  VITAMIN E, 812
  VITAMIN K, 814

Vitron C—See FERROUS FUMARATE, 324
Vivactil—See PROTRIPTYLINE, 672
Vivarin—See Caffeine, 100
Vivol—See DIAZEPAM, 222
Voranil—See CLORTERMINE, 172

W

WARFARIN POTASSIUM, 816
WARFARIN SODIUM, 818
Warfilone—See WARFARIN SODIUM, 818
Warnerin—See WARFARIN SODIUM, 818
Wehvert—See MECLIZINE, 430
Weightrol—See PHENDIMETRAZINE, 586
Wesmatic Capsules (M)—See CHLORPHENIRAMINE, 142 EPHEDRINE, 274 PHENOBARBITAL, 594
Wigraine (M)—See BELLADONNA, 68 CAFFEINE, 100 ERGOTAMINE, 282 PHENACETIN, 582
Wilpowr—See PHENTERMINE, 602
Win-Gel (M)—See ALUMINUM HYDROXIDE, 32 MAGNESIUM HYDROXIDE, 420
Winpred—See PREDNISONE, 650
Winstrol—See STANOZOLOL, 722
Woltac (M)—See ATROPINE, 60 BELLADONNA, 68 HYOSCYAMINE, 374 PHENIRAMINE, 590 PHENYLPROPANOLAMINE, 608 SCOPOLAMINE (HYOSCINE), 702
Wyamycin E—See ERYTHROMYCIN ETHYLSUCCINATE, 290

Wyamycin S—See ERYTHROMYCIN STEARATE, 296
Wyanoids Suppositories (M)—See BELLADONNA, 68 EPHEDRINE, 274
Wycillin—See PENICILLIN G, 570
Wygesic Tablets (M)—See ACETAMINOPHEN, 18 CODEINE, 176
Wymox—See AMOXICILLIN, 46

X

X-Otag—See ORPHENADRINE, 536
X-Prep—See SENNA, 706
Xanax—See ALPRAZOLAM, 30
Xerac BP—See BENZOYL PEROXIDE, 72
Xylocaine Ointment—See ANESTHETICS (TOPICAL), 52

Z

Zactirin Compound-100 Tablets (M)—See ASPIRIN, 56 CAFFEINE, 100
Zantac—See RANITIDINE, 694
Zarontin—See ETHOSUXIMIDE, 314
Zaroxolyn—See METOLAZONE, 490
Zemarine (M)—See ATROPINE, 60 HYOSCYAMINE, 374 SCOPOLAMINE (HYOSCINE), 702
Zetran—See CHLORDIAZEPOXIDE, 134
ZiPan—See PROMETHAZINE, 664
Zide—See HYDROCHLOROTHIAZIDE, 360
Zyloprim—See ALLOPURINOL, 28
Zynol—See SULFINPYRAZONE, 730

Emergency Guide for Overdose Victims

This section lists *basic* steps in recognizing and treating immediate effects of drug overdose.

Study the information before you need it. If possible, take a course in first aid and learn external cardiac massage and mouth-to-mouth breathing techniques, called *cardiopulmonary resuscitation* (CPR). A detailed reference is *How to Save a Life Using CPR* by Lindsay R. Curtis, M.D., published by HPBooks.

For quick reference, list emergency telephone numbers in the spaces provided on page 888 for fire department paramedics, ambulance, poison-control center and your doctor. These numbers, except for doctor, are usually listed on the inside cover of your telephone directory.

If Victim is Unconscious, Not Breathing:

1. Yell for help. Don't leave victim.
2. Begin mouth-to-mouth breathing immediately.
3. If there is no heartbeat, give external cardiac massage.
4. Have someone call O (operator) or 911 (emergency) for an ambulance or medical help.
5. Don't stop CPR until help arrives.
6. Don't try to make victim vomit.
7. If vomiting occurs, save vomit to take to emergency room for analysis.
8. Take medicine or empty bottles with you to emergency room.

If Victim is Unconscious and Breathing:

1. Dial 0 (operator) or 911 (emergency) for an ambulance or medical help.
2. If you can't get help immediately, take victim to the nearest emergency room.
3. Don't try to make victim vomit.
4. If vomiting occurs, save vomit to take to emergency room for analysis.
5. Watch victim carefully on the way to the emergency room. If heart or breathing stops, use cardiac massage and mouth-to-mouth breathing (CPR).
6. Take medicine or empty bottles with you to emergency room

If Victim is Drowsy:

1. Dial 0 (operator) or 911 (emergency) for an ambulance or medical help.
2. If you can't get help immediately, take victim to the nearest emergency room.
3. Don't try to make victim vomit.
4. If vomiting occurs, save vomit to take to emergency room for analysis.
5. Watch victim carefully on the way to the emergency room. If heart or breathing stops, use cardiac massage and mouth-to-mouth breathing (CPR).
6. Take medicine or empty bottles with you to emergency room.

If Victim is Alert:

1. Dial 0 (operator) or 911 (emergency) for an ambulance or emergency medical help.
2. Call poison-control center or doctor for specific instructions.
3. If you can't get instructions, make victim swallow as much water as possible to dilute drug in the stomach. Don't use milk or other beverages.
4. If you are instructed to make victim vomit, use syrup of ipecac according to instructions from your doctor, poison-control center or ipecac label.
5. If you have no ipecac, induce vomiting by pushing your finger far back in victim's throat.
6. Save vomit for analysis.
7. If you can't get paramedic help quickly, take victim to nearest emergency room.
8. Take medicine or empty bottles with you to emergency room.

If Victim has No Symptoms but You Suspect Overdose:

1. Call poison-control center.
2. Describe the suspect drug with as much information as you can quickly gather. The center will give emergency instructions.
3. Or call victim's doctor or your doctor for instructions.
4. If you have no telephone, take victim to the nearest emergency room.
5. Take medicine or empty bottles with you to emergency room.

Emergency Guide for Anaphylaxis Victims

The following are *basic* steps in recognizing and treating immediate effects of severe allergic reaction, which is called *anaphylaxis*.

Some people may be highly sensitive to certain drugs. An anaphylactic reaction to a drug can be life-threatening! Persons suffering these allergic symptoms should receive immediate emergency treatment!

Study the information before you need it. If possible, take a course in first aid and learn external cardiac massage and mouth-to-mouth breathing techniques, called *cardiopulmonary resuscitation* (CPR).

Symptoms of Anaphylaxis:

- Itching
- Rash
- Hives
- Runny nose
- Wheezing
- Paleness
- Cold sweats
- Low blood pressure
- Coma
- Cardiac arrest

If Victim is Unconscious, *Not* Breathing:

1. Yell for help. Don't leave victim.
2. Begin mouth-to-mouth breathing immediately.
3. If there is no heartbeat, give external cardiac massage.
4. Have someone call O (operator) or 911 (emergency) for an ambulance or medical help.
5. Don't stop cardiopulmonary resuscitation (CPR) until help arrives.
6. Take medicine or empty bottles with you to the emergency room.

If Victim is Unconscious *and* Breathing:

1. Dial O (operator) or 911 (emergency) for an ambulance or emergency medical help.
2. If you can't get help immediately, take patient to nearest emergency room.
3. Take medicine or empty bottles with you to emergency room for analysis.

Emergency Telephone Numbers

Fire Department (Paramedic)

Ambulance

Doctor

Poison-Control Center